EQUINE INFECTIOUS DISEASES

Second Edition

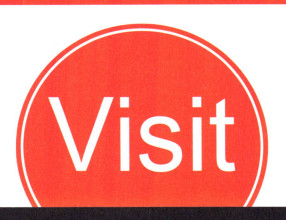
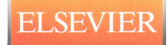

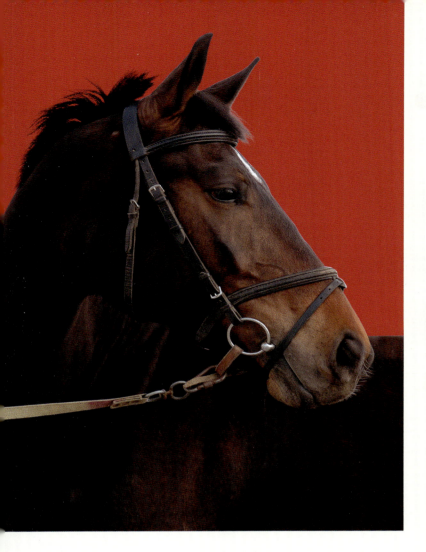

EQUINE INFECTIOUS DISEASES

Second Edition

Debra C. Sellon, DVM, PhD, DACVIM
Professor
Equine Medicine
Department of Veterinary Clinical Sciences
Associate Dean, Graduate School
College of Veterinary Medicine
Washington State University
Pullman, Washington

Maureen T. Long, DVM, PhD, DACVIM
Associate Professor
Large Animal Medicine
College of Veterinary Medicine
University of Florida
Gainesville, Florida

With 574 illustrations

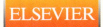

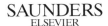

3251 Riverport Lane
St. Louis, Missouri 63043

Equine Infectious Diseases   ISBN: 978-1-4557-0891-8

Notices

Knowledge and best practice in this field are constantly changing. As new research and experience broaden our understanding, changes in research methods, professional practices, or medical treatment may become necessary.

Practitioners and researchers must always rely on their own experience and knowledge in evaluating and using any information, methods, compounds, or experiments described herein. In using such information or methods they should be mindful of their own safety and the safety of others, including parties for whom they have a professional responsibility.

With respect to any drug or pharmaceutical products identified, readers are advised to check the most current information provided (i) on procedures featured or (ii) by the manufacturer of each product to be administered, to verify the recommended dose or formula, the method and duration of administration, and contraindications. It is the responsibility of practitioners, relying on their own experience and knowledge of their patients, to make diagnoses, to determine dosages and the best treatment for each individual patient, and to take all appropriate safety precautions.

To the fullest extent of the law, neither the Publisher nor the authors, contributors, or editors, assume any liability for any injury and/or damage to persons or property as a matter of products liability, negligence or otherwise, or from any use or operation of any methods, products, instructions, or ideas contained in the material herein.

Library of Congress Cataloging-in-Publication Data

Equine infectious diseases (Sellon)
    Equine infectious diseases / [edited by] Debra C. Sellon, Maureen T. Long. – Second edition.
       p. cm.
    Includes bibliographical references and index.
    ISBN 978-1-4557-0891-8 (hbk. : alk. paper) 1. Horses–Diseases. 2. Horses–Infections.
I. Sellon, Debra C., editor of compilation.   II. Long, Maureen T., editor of compilation.   III. Title.
    [DNLM: 1. Horse Diseases. 2. Bacterial Infections–veterinary. 3. Infection–veterinary.
4. Virus Diseases–veterinary. SF 951]
    SF951.E557 2013
    636.1089–dc23
                                                                              2013028894

Vice President and Publisher: Linda Duncan
Content Strategy Director: Penny Rudolph
Content Manager: Shelly Stringer
Publishing Services Manager: Catherine Jackson
Senior Project Manager: Rachel E. McMullen
Design Direction: Brian Salisbury

Printed in China

Last digit is the print number: 9 8 7 6 5 4 3 2 1

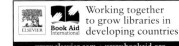
Working together to grow libraries in developing countries

www.elsevier.com • www.bookaid.org

This book is dedicated to our mothers and sister, Leah Etheleen Clabough, Lenore Genevieve Long, and Christine Marie Long, who brought great beauty to our lives and will always inspire us to love our families, value our intellect, and have the courage to achieve academic excellence.

Contributors

Udeni B.R. Balasuriya, BVSc, MS, PhD
Professor of Virology
Veterinary Science
Maxwell H. Gluck Equine Research Center
University of Kentucky
Lexington, Kentucky
Equine Viral Arteritis

Joy L. Barbet, DVM, MRCVS, DACVD
Courtesy Faculty
Department of Small Animal Clinical Sciences
University of Florida
College of Veterinary Medicine
Gainesville, Florida
Ectoparasites of Horses

Susan E. Barnett, DVM
Resident in Equine Medicine
Veterinary Clinical Sciences
Washington State University
College of Veterinary Medicine
Pullman, Washington
Candidiasis

Melissa Ann Bourgeois, DVM, PhD, DACVIM
(Virology)
Associate Service Fellow
Influenza Division
Molecular Virology and Vaccines Branch
Centers for Disease Control and Prevention
Atlanta, Georgia
Laboratory Diagnosis of Viral Infections

Brandy A. Burgess, DVM, MSc, DACVIM
Infection Control Officer
Clinical Sciences
James L. Voss Veterinary Teaching Hospital
Colorado State University
Fort Collins, Colorado
Biosecurity and Control of Infectious Disease Outbreaks

Barbara A. Byrne, DVM, PhD
Associate Professor of Clinical Microbiology
Pathology, Microbiology, and Immunology
University of California, Davis
Davis, California
Laboratory Diagnosis of Bacterial Infections
Laboratory Diagnosis of Fungal Infections

Julia A. Conway, DVM, DACVP
Clinical Assistant Professor
Infectious Diseases and Pathology
University of Florida
College of Veterinary Medicine
Gainesville, Florida
Skin Infections

Elizabeth G. Davis, DVM, PhD, DACVIM
Associate Professor
Clinical Sciences
Kansas State University
Manhattan, Kansas
Respiratory Infections

Jennifer L. Davis, DVM, PhD, DACVIM (LA),
DACVCP
Assistant Professor of Equine Medicine
Department of Clinical Sciences
North Carolina State University
Raleigh, North Carolina
Antimicrobial Therapy
Antimicrobial Drug Formulary

Gretchen Henry Delcambre, DVM
Graduate Assistant
Infectious Diseases & Pathology
University of Florida
Gainesville, Florida
Flavivirus Encephalitides

Thomas J. Divers, DVM, ACVECC, DACVIM
Professor of Medicine
Clinical Sciences
Cornell University
Ithaca, New York
Lyme Disease
Miscellaneous Parasitic Diseases

Paulo C. Duarte, DVM, MPVM, PhD
Scientist
Secretariat of International Affairs
Brazilian Agricultural Research Corporation (Embrapa)
Brasilia, DF, Brazil
Epidemiology of Equine Infectious Disease

Maria Julia Bevilaqua Felippe, DVM, MS, PhD,
DACVIM
Associate Professor of Medicine
Clinical Sciences
Cornell University
College of Veterinary Medicine
Ithaca, New York
Immunotherapy

David E. Freeman, MVB, PhD, DACVS
Large Animal Clinical Sciences
College of Veterinary Medicine
University of Florida
Gainesville, Florida
Respiratory Infections

Connie J. Gebhart, PhD
Professor
Department of Veterinary and Biomedical Sciences
College of Veterinary Medicine
University of Minnesota
St. Paul, Minnesota
Lawsonia intracellularis

Liberty M. Getman, DVM, DACVS
Surgeon
Tennessee Equine Hospital
Thompson's Station, Tennessee
Infections of Muscle, Joint, and Bone

Pamela E. Ginn, DVM, DACVP
Associate Dean for Students and Instruction
College of Veterinary Medicine
University of Florida
Gainesville, Florida
Skin Infections

Ellis C. Greiner, PhD
Professor Emeritus
Department of Infectious Diseases and Pathology
University of Florida
College of Veterinary Medicine
Gainesville, Florida
Laboratory Diagnosis of Parasitic Diseases

Amy M. Grooters, DVM, DACVIM
Professor
Companion Animal Medicine
Veterinary Clinical Sciences
Louisiana State University
Baton Rouge, Louisiana
Pythiosis and Zygomycosis

Jorge A. Hernandez, DVM, MPVM, PhD
Professor
College of Veterinary Medicine
University of Florida
Gainesville, Florida
Salmonellosis

Ashley E. Hill, DVM, MPVM, PhD
Assistant Professor, Epidemiology
Department of Clinical Sciences
College of Veterinary Medicine & Biomedical Sciences
Colorado State University
Fort Collins, Colorado
Epidemiology of Equine Infectious Disease

Kenneth William Hinchcliff, BVSc, MS, PhD, DACVIM
Dean and Professor
Faculty of Veterinary Science
University of Melbourne
Melbourne, Victoria, Australia
Miscellaneous Viral Diseases

Melissa T. Hines, DVM, PhD, DACVIM
Professor
Large Animal Clinical Sciences
University of Tennessee
Knoxville, Tennessee
Rhodococcus equi
Leptospirosis

Anthony N.B. Kettle, BVSc, BSc, MSc, MBA, MRCVS, MACVSc
Head of Department
Veterinary Department
Dubai Racing Club
Dubai, United Arab Emirates
Glanders and Farcy

Donald P. Knowles, DVM, PhD, DACVP
Professor
Veterinary Microbiology and Pathology
Washington State University
Pullman, Washington
Research Leader, Animal Disease Research Unit (ADRU)
Agricultural Research Service, USDA-PWA
Pullman, Washington
Piroplasmosis

Michaela Kristula, DVM, MS
Associate Professor of Medicine
Clinical Studies
University of Pennsylvania
Philadelphia, Pennsylvania
Contagious Equine Metritis

Gabriele A. Landolt, DVM, MS, PhD, DACVIM
Associate Professor
Equine Medicine
Department of Clinical Sciences
Colorado State University
Fort Collins, Colorado
Equine Influenza Infection

Katharina L. Lohmann, MedVet, PhD, DACVIM
Associate Professor
Large Animal Clinical Sciences
Western College of Veterinary Medicine
University of Saskatchewan
Saskatoon, Saskatchewan, Canada
Systemic Inflammatory Response Syndrome

Maureen T. Long, DVM, PhD, DACVIM
Associate Professor
Large Animal Medicine
College of Veterinary Medicine
University of Florida
Gainesville, Florida
Central Nervous System Infections
African Horse Sickness
Equine Alphaviruses
Flavivirus Encephalitides
Borna Disease
Salmonellosis
Coccidiomycosis
Immunoprophylaxis
Infectious Disease Rule-Outs for Medical Problems
Laboratory Testing for Infectious Diseases
Diagnostic Test Kits

D. Paul Lunn, BVSc, MS, PhD, MRCVS, DACVIM
Dean
College of Veterinary Medicine
North Carolina State University
Raleigh, North Carolina
Equine Influenza Infection

Robert J. MacKay, BVSc (Dist), PhD
Professor
Large Animal Clinical Sciences
University of Florida
Gainesville, Florida
Tetanus
Sporotrichosis

K. Gary Magdesian, DVM, DACVIM, DACVECC,
  DACVCP
Professor and Henry Endowed Chair in Emergency Medicine
  and Critical Care
Veterinary Medicine: Medicine & Epidemiology
University of California, Davis
Davis, California
Viral Diarrhea

Martha Mallicote, DVM, DACVIM
Staff Veterinarian
Large Animal Clinical Sciences
College of Veterinary Medicine University of Florida
Gainesville, Florida
Gastrointestinal and Peritoneal Infections

Celia M. Marr, BVMS, MVM, PhD, DEIM, DECEIM,
  MRCVS
Specialist, Internal Medicine
Rossdale and Partners
Newmarket, Suffolk, United Kingdom
Cardiovascular Infections

Rosanna Marsella, DVM, DACVD
Small Animal Clinical Sciences
College of Veterinary Medicine
University of Florida
Gainesville, Florida
Dermatophilosis
Dermatophytosis

Brian J. McCluskey, DVM, MS, PhD, DACVPM
Chief Epidemiologist
USDA
APHIS Veterinary Services
Fort Collins, Colorado
Vesicular Stomatitis

Robert H. Mealey, DVM, PhD, DACVIM
Associate Professor
Department of Veterinary Microbiology and Pathology
Washington State University
Pullman, Washington
Equine Infectious Anemia

Deborah Middleton, BVSc, MVSc, PhD
CSIRO
Australian Animal Health Laboratory
Geelong, Victoria, Australia
Miscellaneous Viral Respiratory Diseases

Linda D. Mittel, MSPH, DVM
Cornell University
College of Veterinary Medicine
Ithaca, New York
Miscellaneous Parasitic Diseases

Paul S. Morley, DVM, PhD, DACVIM
Professor
Department of Clinical Sciences
College of Veterinary Medicine and Biomedical Sciences
Director of Infection Control
James L. Voss Veterinary Teaching Hospital
Colorado State University
Fort Collins, Colorado
Professor
Department of Epidemiology
Colorado School of Public Health
Fort Collins, Colorado
Epidemiology of Equine Infectious Diseases

Sally Anne L. Ness, DVM
Internal Medicine Resident
Cornell University
College of Veterinary Medicine
Equine and Farm Animal Hospital
Ithaca, New York
Miscellaneous Parasitic Diseases

Martin K. Nielsen, DVM, PhD, DEPVC
Assistant Professor
Maxwell H. Gluck Equine Research Center
Department of Veterinary Science
University of Kentucky
Lexington, Kentucky
Nematodes

Lisa K. Pearson, DVM, MS
Resident
Large Animal Theriogenology
Veterinary Clinical Sciences
Washington State University
Pullman, Washington
Reproductive Tract Infections

Caryn E. Plummer, DVM, DACVO
Assistant Professor
Comparative Ophthalmology
Gainesville, Florida
Ocular Infections

Nicola Pusterla, Dr Med Vet, Dr Med Vet Habil, FVH, DACVID
Associate Professor
Medicine and Epidemiology
School of Veterinary Medicine
University of California, Davis
Davis, California
Lawsonia intracellularis
Anaplasma phagocytophilum Infection
Neorickettsia risticii
Immunoprophylaxis

Craig R. Reinemeyer, DVM, PhD
President
East Tennessee Clinical Research Inc.
Knoxville, Tennessee
Nematodes

Chris Sanchez, DVM, PhD, DACVIM
Associate Professor
Department of Large Animal Clinical Sciences
College of Veterinary Medicine
University of Florida
Gainesville, Florida
Gastrointestinal and Peritoneal Infections
Neonatal Sepsis

C.J. (Kate) Savage, BVSc (Hons), MS, PhD, DACVIM
Specialist in Equine Internal Medicine
South Eastern Equine Hospital
Narre Warren, Victoria, Australia
Miscellaneous Viral Respiratory Diseases

Kelly P. Sears, DVM
Resident in Equine Internal Medicine
Veterinary Clinical Sciences
Washington State University
Pullman, Washington
Papillomavirus Infections

Kathy K. Seino, DVM, MS, PhD
Assistant Professor
Equine Medicine
Pullman, Washington
Central Nervous System Infections

Debra C. Sellon, DVM, PhD, DACVIM
Professor of Equine Medicine
Department of Veterinary Clinical Sciences
Associate Dean, Graduate School
College of Veterinary Medicine
Washington State University
Pullman, Washington
Papillomavirus Infections
Brucellosis
Systemic Clostridial Infections
Miscellaneous Bacterial Infections
Aspergillosis
Miscellaneous Fungal Diseases
Infectious Disease Rule-Outs for Medical Problems

Josh Slater, BVM&S, PhD, DECEIM, MRCVS
Professor of Equine Clinical Studies
Clinical Sciences and Services
Royal Veterinary College
Hatfield, Herts, United Kingdom
Equine Herpesviruses

Sharon J. Spier, DVM, PhD, DACVIM
Professor
Department of Medicine and Epidemiology
University of California, Davis
Davis, California
Miscellaneous Bacterial Infections

Ahmed Tibary, DMV, MS, DSc, PhD, DACT
Professor
Veterinary Clinical Sciences
Washington State University
Pullman, Washington
Reproductive Tract Infections

Peter J. Timoney, MVB, MS, PhD, FRCVS
Gluck Equine Research Center
Department of Veterinary Science
University of Kentucky
Lexington, Kentucky
Infectious Diseases and International Movement of Horses

Hugh G.G. Townsend, BSc, DVM, MSc
Professor
Large Animal Clinical Sciences
Western College of Veterinary Medicine
Senior Research Scientist and Program Manager
Vaccine and Infectious Disease Organization/International Vaccine Center
University of Saskatchewan
Saskatoon, Saskatchewan
Equine Influenza Infection

Josie L. Traub-Dargatz, DVM, MS
Professor
Equine Medicine
Clinical Sciences
Colorado State University
Fort Collins, Colorado
Biosecurity and Control of Infectious Disease Outbreaks

Karl van Laaren, BVSc
Veterinarian
Borrowdale Park Veterinary Hospital
Harare, Zimbabwe
Miscellaneous Parasitic Diseases

Heather Stockdale Walden, MS, PhD
Research Assistant Professor
Infectious Diseases and Pathology
College of Veterinary Medicine
University of Florida
Gainesville, Florida
Cestodes
Miscellaneous Parasitic Diseases

Andrew Stephen Waller, PhD, BSc
Head of Bacteriology
Department of Bacteriology
Animal Health Trust
Newmarket, Suffolk, United Kingdom
Streptococcal Infections

J. Scott Weese, DVM, DVSc, DACVIM
Professor
Pathobiology
Chief of Infection Control
Ontario Veterinary College
Health Sciences Centre
University of Guelph
Guelph, Ontario, Canada
Staphylococcal Infections
Enteric Clostridial Infections

Mary Beth Whitcomb, DVM
University of California, Davis
Davis, California
Miscellaneous Bacterial Infections

Pamela A. Wilkins, DVM, PhD, DACVIM (LAIM), DACVECC
Professor of Equine Medicine and Emergency and Critical Care
Veterinary Clinical Medicine
College of Veterinary Medicine
University of Illinois
Champaign-Urbana, Illinois
Rabies
Botulism

W. David Wilson
Professor
Large Animal Medicine
Department of Medicine and Epidemiology (VME)
School of Veterinary Medicine
University of California, Davis
Davis, California
Immunoprophylaxis

L. Nicki Wise, DVM, MS, DACVIM
Veterinary Microbiology & Pathology
Washington State University
Pullman, Washington
Piroplasmosis

Sharon Witonsky, DVM, PhD, DACVIM
Associate Professor
Large Animal Clinical Sciences
Virginia Maryland Regional College of Veterinary Medicine
Virginia Tech
Blacksburg, Virginia
Equine Protozoal Myeloencephalitis

Dana N. Zimmel, DVM, DACVIM, DABVP
Clinical Associate Professor and Chief of Staff
Department of Large Animal Clinical Sciences
University of Florida
Gainesville, Florida
Urinary Tract Infections

Preface

Because of the excellent contributions of our authors and publisher, the first edition of *Equine Infectious Diseases* was a critical success. Our goal for the second edition is to continue to provide "anyone interested in equine health with a single source summary" of worldwide equine infectious diseases that meets the achievement of the first book. We hope we achieved this overall goal by redefining the goals of several chapters, relying on many of the same equine and infectious disease scholars of the first edition, and turning over the authorship in about 15% to 20% of the new edition to offer fresh perspectives through new expertise.

In the 6 years since publication of the first book, equine infectious diseases continue to dominate equine clinical medicine, while researchers in the equine sciences have contributed new knowledge to our understanding of many devastating infectious conditions that plague the industry. In the face of these losses and gains, world markets underwent seismic shifts that have definitely changed the equine industry and created new challenges because of limited resources for controlling and studying old and new pathogens.

Modern science is defining the way in which we process clinical information; pursue diagnostic testing, treatment, and prevention of diseases; and investigate host-pathogen interactions of infectious diseases. Some of the seminal changes that are reflected in this book include enhanced chapters on biosecurity and international movement of horses to give practitioners and young clinicians an understanding of the complexities of the industry and more web-based information regarding diagnostic testing. With the increased availability of rapid molecular and antigen-based test kits, our authors have provided much evidence-based discussion on the merits of these tests, and we have provided an appendix of the tests now available with information on diagnostic laboratory availability as of April 2013. Methods of treatment have been updated for all viral, bacterial, and fungal diseases, and sections on prevention of infectious diseases have been updated. An important trend has been for more equine-specific information on pathogenesis, in part as a result of the publication of the equine genome. Many of the previous discussions have included rodent models for many diseases, but wherever possible our authors and we as editors have tried to minimize this information in lieu of the more recent work made possible only by pioneers in equine molecular medicine.

Many new diseases are being discovered as we publish this book, and many old diseases are recurring worldwide, and several subjects in this book will require updating even as it comes off the press. We have tried to capture as much information on the recent outbreaks of equine viral arteritis, equine infectious anemia, contagious equine metritis, and equine herpesvirus 1. Our thoughtful authors included biocontainment and updated their chapters again even during review. For example, we have current information on control of contagious equine metritis in the United States with recommended protocols, the formation of which was ongoing as the book was written.

We hope to provide a tool that serves students, practitioners, and post-DVM trainees as they develop their own expertise in diagnostic medicine. World recession and monetary restrictions in education demand that we all become responsible seekers of information and use evidence-based methods to help our clients maintain healthy livestock and minimize risk to our precious industry.

Finally, we provide a nod once again to Dr. Craig Green, author of *Infectious Diseases of the Dog and Cat*, who was our inspiration for this book. At the end of our second edition, we acknowledge his initial foresight and his perseverance through four editions, each one as fresh and knowledgeable as the one before it.

Acknowledgments

First, we are grateful for the exceptional competence and talent of the Elsevier professionals who worked with us on this edition. Penny Rudolph, our Publisher for two editions, has become a friend and is vigorously committed to broadening and creating excellent veterinary textbooks. Shelley Stringer, our Content Manager, is always there for us, keeping us on track, running her team smoothly whether there was an author/editor scarcity or a last minute blizzard, and filling in the gaps as things came up long on deadlines. Her patience, understanding, kindness, and professionalism will always be valued. Rachel McMullen, our Project Manager, tirelessly pushed the page proofs through and helped us keep this book on track even though I am sure it was like herding cats. Rachel's attention to detail and eye for layout has maintained and even improved on the exceptional quality of the first edition.

To all authors of the first and second edition, thank you for the amazing material you provided. The very favorable reviews that were received for the first edition of this book were the direct result of strong collaborative efforts between specialists in equine medicine, surgery, reproduction, critical care, and infectious diseases. To our new authors, we are grateful for your willingness to contribute to this effort, sometimes at the last minute. Your contributions allowed us to keep material fresh and increase the global context of the information provided.

We are grateful to the members of the ACVIM-LA list serve for providing great ideas for the new edition. In addition, many practitioners and reviewers of the first edition made excellent suggestions, such as using more international expertise. Finally, we would like to acknowledge members of our University staff, especially Sally Beachboard for assistance in editing.

Debra C. Sellon
Maureen T. Long

Contents

Section 1: Clinical Problems   1

1. Respiratory Infections   1
   *Elizabeth G. Davis, David E. Freeman, Joanne Hardy**
2. Cardiovascular Infections   21
   Celia M. Marr
3. Gastrointestinal and Peritoneal Infections   42
   Martha Mallicote and Chris Sanchez
4. Central Nervous System Infections   47
   Kathy K. Seino and Maureen T. Long
5. Infections of Muscle, Joint, and Bone   60
   Liberty M. Getman, W. Wesley Sutter,
   *and Alicia L. Bertone**
6. Neonatal Sepsis   70
   Chris Sanchez
7. Skin Infections   78
   *Julia A. Conway, Pamela E. Ginn, and Dawn Logas**
8. Reproductive Tract Infections   84
   *Ahmed Tibary, Lisa K. Pearson, and Cheryl L. Fite**
9. Urinary Tract Infections   106
   Dana N. Zimmel
10. Ocular Infections   109
    Caryn E. Plummer, Carmen M.H. Colitz,
    *and Vanessa Kuonen**
11. Systemic Inflammatory Response Syndrome   119
    *Katharina L. Lohmann and Michelle H. Barton**

Section 2: Viral Diseases   132

12. Laboratory Diagnosis of Viral Infections   132
    *Melissa Ann Bourgeois and J. Lindsay Oaks**
13. Equine Influenza Infection   141
    Grabriele A. Landolt, Hugh G.G. Townsend,
    and D. Paul Lunn
14. Equine Herpesviruses   151
    Josh Slater
15. Equine Viral Arteritis   169
    *Udeni B.R. Balasuriya and N. James MacLachlan**
16. African Horse Sickness   181
    *Maureen T. Long and Alan J. Guthrie**
17. Adeno, Hendra, and Equine Rhinitis Viral Respiratory
    Diseases   189
    C.J. (Kate) Savage, Deborah Middleton,
    *and Michael J. Studdert **
18. Viral Diarrhea   198
    K. Gary Magdesian, Roberta M. Dwyer,
    *and Marta Gonzalez Arguedas**

19. Rabies   203
    *Pamela A. Wilkins and Fabio Del Piero**
20. Equine Alphaviruses   210
    *Maureen T. Long and E. Paul J. Gibbs**
21. Flavivirus Encephalitides   217
    Gretchen Henry Delcambre and Maureen T. Long
22. Borna Disease   226
    Maureen T. Long, Juergen A. Richt, Arthur Grabner,**
    Sibylle Herzog, Wolfgang Garten,* and Christiane Herden**
23. Equine Infectious Anemia   232
    Robert H. Mealey
24. Vesicular Stomatitis   239
    Brian J. McCluskey
25. Papillomavirus Infections   244
    Kelly P. Sears and Debra. C. Sellon
26. Miscellaneous Viral Diseases   251
    Kenneth William Hinchcliff

Section 3: Bacterial and Rickettsial Diseases   257

27. Laboratory Diagnosis of Bacterial Infections   257
    Barbara A. Byrne
28. Streptococcal Infections   265
    *Andrew Stephen Waller, Debra C. Sellon,**
    Corinne R. Sweeney, Peter J. Timoney,**
    J. Richard Newton, and Melissa T. Hines**
29. Staphylococcal Infections   278
    J. Scott Weese
30. Dermatophilosis   283
    Rosanna Marsella
31. *Rhodococcus equi*   287
    Melissa T. Hines
32. Leptospirosis   302
    Melissa T. Hines
33. Lyme Disease   311
    Thomas J. Divers
34. *Lawsonia intracellularis*   316
    *Nicola Pusterla, Connie J. Gebhart, Jean-Pierre Lavoie,**
    *and Richard Drolet**
35. Salmonellosis   321
    Jorge A. Hernandez, Maureen T. Long,
    Josie L. Traub-Dargatz, and Thomas E. Besser**
36. Glanders   333
    *Anthony N.B. Kettle and Paul L. Nicoletti**
37. Brucellosis   337
    *Debra C. Sellon and Paul L. Nicoletti**

*The authors acknowledge and appreciate the original contributions of these authors, whose work has been incorporated into this chapter.

38. Contagious Equine Metritis 339
Michaela Kristula

39. *Anaplasma phagocytophilum* Infection 344
*Nicola Pusterla and John E. Madigan**

40. *Neorickettsia risticii* 347
*Nicola Pusterla and John E. Madigan**

41. Enteric Clostridial Infections 352
J. Scott Weese

42. Systemic Clostridial Infections 359
*Debra C. Sellon and Simon F. Peek**

43. Botulism 364
Pamela A. Wilkins

44. Tetanus 368
Robert J. MacKay

45. Miscellaneous Bacterial Infections 373
*Debra C. Sellon, Sharon J. Spier, Mary Beth Whitcomb,
Marta Gonzalez Arguedas,* Maureen T. Long,*
J. Lindsay Oaks,* and Melissa T. Hines**

Section 4: Fungal Diseases 393

46. Laboratory Diagnosis of Fungal Diseases 393
Barbara A. Byrne

47. Coccidioidomycosis 399
Maureen T. Long, Demosthenes Pappagianis,
and Jill Higgins**

48. Sporotrichosis 406
Robert J. MacKay

49. Candidiasis 408
*Susan E. Barnett and Natalie Ann Carrillo**

50. Dermatophytosis 411
Rosanna Marsella

51. Pythiosis and Zygomycosis 415
Amy M. Grooters

52. Aspergillosis 421
*Debra C. Sellon and Catherine Kohn**

53. Miscellaneous Fungal Diseases 433
*Debra C. Sellon, Maureen T. Long, and Catherine Kohn**

Section 5: Parasitic Diseases 449

54. Laboratory Diagnosis of Parasitic Diseases 449
Ellis C. Greiner

55. Equine Protozoal Myeloencephalitis 456
Sharon Witonsky, Debra C. Sellon, and J.P. Dubey**

56. Piroplasmosis 467
*L. Nicki Wise, Donald P. Knowles, and
Chantal M. Rothschild**

57. Nematodes 475
*Martin K. Nielsen, Craig R. Reinemeyer,
and Debra C. Sellon**

58. Cestodes 490
Heather Stockdale Walden, Merijo Eileen Jordan,
and Joseph A. DiPietro**

59. Ectoparasites of Horses 495
Joy L. Barbet

60. Miscellaneous Parasitic Diseases 505
*Heather Stockdale Walden, Sally Anne L. Ness,
Linda D. Mittel, Thomas J. Divers, Karl van Laaren,
and Debra C. Sellon**

**Section 6: Prevention and Control
of Infectious Diseases 515**

61. Epidemiology of Equine Infectious Disease 515
Paulo C. Duarte, Ashley E. Hill, Paul S. Morley

62. Biosecurity and Control of Infectious
Disease Outbreaks 530
Brandy A. Burgess and Josie L. Traub-Dargatz

63. Infectious Diseases and International Movement
of Horses 544
Peter J. Timoney

64. Immunoprophylaxis 551
W. David Wilson, Nicola Pusterla, and Debra C. Long

65. Antimicrobial Therapy 571
*Jennifer L. Davis and Mark G. Papich**

66. Immunotherapy 584
Maria Julia Bevilaqua Felippe

Appendices 598

Appendix A: Infectious Disease Rule-Outs
for Medical Problems 598
Maureen T. Long and Debra C. Sellon

Appendix B: Laboratories Molecular Testing for Infectious
Diseases 604
Maureen T. Long

Appendix C: Diagnostic Test Kits 614
Maureen T. Long

Appendix D: Antimicrobial Drug Formulary 615
*Jennifer L. Davis and Mark G. Papich**

CHAPTER

1

Respiratory Infections

Elizabeth G. Davis, David E. Freeman, Joanne Hardy*

Equine Respiratory Tract

Normal Respiratory Flora

Bacterial flora plays an important role in host health in a variety of tissues and organ systems such as the skin, gastrointestinal tract, and urogenital system, as well as the respiratory system.[1] The upper airway of healthy horses contains many bacteria, including a variety of aerobic and anaerobic species. This flora competes with pathogenic species that, when present in large numbers, can colonize the epithelial surface. Normal equine respiratory flora include *Streptococcus* spp., *Pasteurella* spp., *Escherichia coli*, and *Actinomyces* spp. Anaerobes predominate in the normal equine oral cavity with a population consisting of several bacterial genera, including *Bacteroides fragilis*, *Fusobacterium* spp., *Eubacterium* spp., *Clostridium* spp., *Veillonella* spp., and *Megasphaera* spp.[2] Commonly, horses suffering from infectious lower airway disease are contaminated with one of these bacteria, consistent with the concept that contamination of the lower respiratory tract originates from the upper airways. Aspiration is not an uncommon mechanism for contamination to occur, evidenced by the fact that head elevation and long distance transport contribute to lower airway contamination and accumulation of mucus.[3-5] Contamination of the lower airway is a common occurrence in apparently healthy horses, and many horses will have positive bacterial cultures when examined by tracheobronchial aspirate.

Pulmonary Defense Mechanisms

Endogenous pulmonary defense involves components of nonspecific and specific clearance mechanisms. Components of nonspecific clearance include anatomic barriers, mucosal lining, mucous secretions, and the mucociliary escalator. These nonspecific mechanisms are distinguished from specific immune effector molecules because they lack antigenic specificity and memory.

An effective mediator of nonspecific clearance of debris and pathogens from the respiratory tract is the mucociliary escalator. The mucociliary escalator is comprised of a double layer of mucus that extends from the pharynx to the respiratory bronchioles. This mucous layer is propelled in an upward fashion by the ciliated respiratory epithelium. The mucus is produced by goblet cells that line the walls of the upper respiratory tract. The mucous gel adsorbs soluble host defense molecules that include defensins, lysozyme, and immunoglobulin A (IgA), thereby providing a valuable layer of innate immune protection. Inhaled particles and debris are propelled in a proximal direction by a constant wave of upward movement by the cilia and mucus from the level of the bronchioles up to the bronchi and trachea by the ciliary action. The mucociliary system can become damaged by smoke inhalation and direct viral destruction.[6,7]

Retrograde movement of material can occur from mucus that has adhered to material from the nasal cavity to the pharynx. This "dirty" mucus is subsequently swallowed and removed through digestive mechanisms in the gastrointestinal tract. Particles that are less than 5 μm in size may bypass the mucociliary escalator and reach the alveoli, with clearance occurring via phagocytosis by alveolar macrophages. Leukocytes that include macrophages will migrate with the mucous escalator to the pharynx. Respiratory mucus provides a valuable physical barrier for removal of pathogens and debris but also contains several antimicrobial molecules, including defensins and surfactant proteins (SPs) such as the collectins SP-A and SP-D.[8]

Influenza and herpes viruses replicate within and destroy ciliated epithelium, which then requires approximately 21 days for regeneration. In addition, environment may play a role in clearance mechanisms because high ammonia concentrations, such as those associated with a high degree of urinary and fecal waste, will result in depressed ciliary motility.[9-11] Dehydration may also contribute to reduced pulmonary clearance because effective ciliary movement will be depressed with reduced fluidity of the mucous layer.

The major mediators of specific pulmonary clearance mechanisms are within the bronchial-associated lymphoid tissue (BALT). Bronchial-associated lymphoid tissue exists within the submucosa of the segmental bronchi and terminal bronchioles. As with other lymphoid organs, BALT is an area where antigen-specific responses stimulate cell-mediated and humoral immune defense. B lymphocytes within BALT can switch to all classes of antibodies, yet the predominant antibody produced in the upper respiratory tract is IgA; IgG is secreted in greater quantities in the lower airways[12] (Fig. 1-1). The advantage of upper respiratory secretion of IgA is the blockage of adherence of pathogens to the upper respiratory tract epithelium, a process referred to as *immune exclusion*. Memory is conferred by this arm of the immune system and thereby results in long-term protection from infectious disease.

The goal of immunization against pathogens is to produce high concentrations of antigen-specific responses that will confer resistance at the site of infectious challenge. A disadvantage of many intramuscular vaccines is that high levels of IgG are induced in circulation, with minimal levels of IgA produced at the mucosal surface. The intent of intranasally delivered vaccines is to induce local IgA production. The IgG production becomes essential when pathogens gain entrance to the lower airways. This antibody isotype is critical for opsonization and removal of bacteria and foreign material. Effective opsonization will result in effective phagocytosis and removal from the lower airways and pulmonary parenchyma. Some pathogens such as herpesviruses are capable of surviving and replicating within BALT, resulting in necrosis of lymphoid nodules. This contributes to a postviral state of immunocompromise in which the patient is susceptible to infection with secondary, often bacterial, pathogens.

Below the level of the mucociliary escalator and the BALT, cellular responses are critical for immune protection of the

*The authors acknowledge and appreciate the original contributions of these authors, whose work has been incorporated into this chapter.

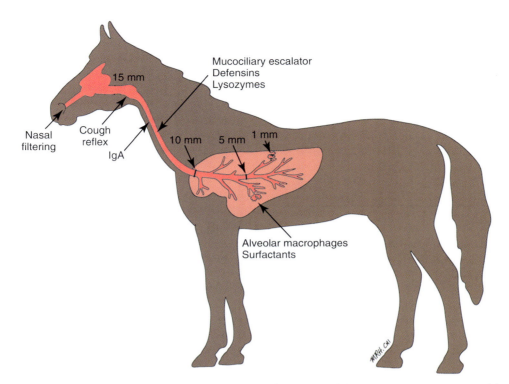

Figure 1-1 Diagram of the equine respiratory tract demonstrating the relationship of the upper and lower respiratory components and the immunologic factors that play a role in maintaining host health. *IgA*, Immunoglobulin A. *(Courtesy Mal Hoover, College of Veterinary Medicine, Kansas State University.)*

equine host. The first phagocyte of importance is the alveolar macrophage located in the terminal bronchioles and alveoli. The alveolar macrophage provides a bridge between innate and adaptive immune responses. Although these cells can nonspecifically ingest foreign material, they also serve as important antigen-presenting cells for T lymphocytes and the development of adaptive immunity. Particles that are inhaled and reach the alveolar spaces are removed by local alveolar macrophages. Once they contain foreign material, these cells may be coughed up and swallowed or they may move from the alveolar space and enter general circulation, resulting in clearance by the lymphatic system. The function of these cells depends on host health status; long distance transport or viral infection will destroy these cells.[13]

Another important cell in the pulmonary system of horses is the pulmonary intravascular macrophage (PIM). These cells are important for removal of particulate matter such as bacteria or toxins from general circulation. Mammalian species that contain PIMs include horses, pigs, ruminants, and cats. Species that do not have PIMs utilize hepatic Kupffer's cells and splenic macrophages for similar purposes. Of note, PIMs are critical for removal of bacteria or endotoxin on the first pass through the lungs, yet contribute to the systemic inflammatory response that is induced following pathogen challenge.[14,15] Disadvantages of PIMs include the resultant inflammatory reactions that follow their activation.[14] For example, phagocytosis of endotoxin is associated with pronounced inflammatory mediator release, microthrombus formation, neutrophilic influx, vasoconstriction, pulmonary edema, and endothelial damage that may lead to other systemic disorders. Species variation in sensitivity to endotoxin relates to the presence of PIMs, and intensified sensitivity to endotoxin is related to the number of PIMs in the pulmonary vasculature.

Epithelial protection of the respiratory tract is provided not only by the mucosal lining and leukocytes within the submucosa but also by mechanisms of the innate immune system.

Host defense peptides play an important role in innate immune protection in the pulmonary system of many species.[16] Cathelicidin peptides have been identified in pulmonary equine neutrophils collected from heaves-affected individuals.[17] This class of defense peptide plays a role in pathogen clearance, having broad-spectrum activity against bacterial pathogens.[18] Other similar peptides are expressed in epithelial cells, as well as within leukocyte subsets.[19,20]

Anatomic and Physiologic Considerations

The horse is an obligate nasal airway breather, which means that even under strenuous exercise, no air is obtained through the oral cavity or oropharynx. This consideration impacts the pathogenesis of equine infectious disease in two ways. First, an initial upper airway contamination may lead to lower airway challenge by bacteria that originated from the oral cavity and oropharynx. Risk factors include prolonged changes in head placement that occur with long distance transport, fatigue of the pharynx secondary to intense physical exertion, or changes in the local immunity of the nasopharynx subsequent to viral infection. Additionally, any physiologic change in the upper airway results in an immediate decrease in the exercise capacity of the horse. Thus any inflammatory condition, even as "innocuous" as lymphoid hyperplasia, will have a profound impact on performance and health of the lower respiratory tract.

The equine airway has a monopodial branching pattern, meaning that each branch gives rise to daughter branches. The respiratory tree is lined by mucous membrane and supported by lamina propria with cartilage and smooth muscle, depending on site. Ciliated cells and goblet cells (which produce mucus) line the bronchioles. The secretory cells change to Clara cells in the bronchioles. The alveoli are lined by a single layer of epithelial cells consisting of type I and type II pneumocytes. These cells are supported by a thin interstitium and a small amount of smooth muscle at each opening.

Clinical Findings Associated with Infectious Respiratory Disease

In general, proper diagnosis of infectious respiratory disease depends on information gleaned from the history and physical examination, identification of abnormalities (problem list), and development of a diagnostic plan. Age, signalment, and recent exposure to new arrivals may indicate viral respiratory disease. Long distance travel before onset of respiratory signs indicates a horse is at high risk for pleuropneumonia. *Rhodococcus equi* infection occurs primarily in foals between 3 and 5 months of age.

Clinical signs of infectious respiratory disease may initially be nonspecific, including fever, depression, and possible anorexia. Signs referable to the respiratory system may include nasal discharge, cough, and tachypnea. Either upper or lower respiratory disease can cause these clinical signs. Respiratory stridor (usually upper respiratory tract disease) and respiratory distress (upper or lower respiratory tract disease) may also be present. Other nonspecific signs include epistaxis and cyanosis. With either acute viral infection or chronic lower airway disease, exercise intolerance is a consistent clinical finding. Weight loss may occur with chronic respiratory infection.

Physical examination should be thorough and include examination of all body systems. Normal respiratory rate of foals is between 20 and 40 breaths/minute; in adults, a normal respiratory rate is between 12 and 24 breaths/minute. Breathing should be slow and deliberate with no nostril flare. Auscultation of horses can be difficult due to the normally slow rate and character of breathing. Depth of breathing can be increased by performing a rebreathing examination with a plastic bag placed over the nares of the horse. Normal horses generally do not cough when asked to take a deep breath with rebreathing. Normal horses do not cough when the trachea is palpated. Concomitant percussion during auscultation may indicate a fluid line.

Diagnostic Approach to Infectious Respiratory Disease

Endoscopy may be used to confirm the presence of upper airway disease and to perform diagnostic tests such as transtracheal aspirate (TTA) or bronchoalveolar lavage (BAL). Diagnosis of rhinitis, pharyngeal lymphoid hyperplasia, guttural pouch diseases, and retropharyngeal lymphadenopathy (presumably from *Streptococcus equi* subsp. *equi* infection; Fig. 1-2) may be facilitated by endoscopic examination. Radiographs of the sinuses are essential for identification of fluid or masses within sinuses, guttural pouches, and thorax. Diagnostic quality thoracic radiography is difficult with most field equipment. Lower airway radiography is important for determining the type of pattern present but is not specific for identification of any particular etiologic agents. Thoracic ultrasound is easily performed in the field and, although nonspecific for etiology, is particularly useful to detect lower airway disease, including consolidation of the peripheral lung lobes and identification of pulmonary fluid. Optimal image quality will be obtained with a 3.5-MHz curvilinear probe; however, a 5.0-MHz linear probe (used for most rectal ultrasound examinations) will typically provide general diagnostic information (e.g., presence of pleural fluid, pulmonary consolidation, measurement of peripheral abscess).

Ancillary diagnostic testing is critical for correct etiologic identification of potentially contagious pathogens. Nasopharyngeal or nasal passage swabs are particularly useful for diagnosis of viral respiratory tract disease. Polyester-tipped swabs are

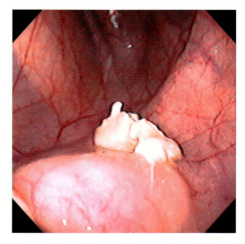

Figure 1-2 Endoscopic view of the medial compartment of the guttural pouch in a horse suffering from *Streptococcus equi* subsp. *equi* infection. Exudate may become inspissated if not completely cleared with recovery from infection.

recommended because viruses may adhere to cotton fibers, decreasing the likelihood of isolating virus or viral deoxyribonucleic acid (DNA) from the sample. Swabs should be placed in sterile viral transport medium and kept on ice until analysis. Maintaining moisture with physiologic saline is an alternative for very short-term transport. Swabs for viral isolation need to be only a standard length (6 inches); the only requirement is contact with the nasal mucosa. Viral swabs may be analyzed in three ways: viral culture, polymerase chain reaction (PCR), and antigen enzyme-linked immunosorbent assay (ELISA). Virus isolation and paired serum titers can be obtained to confirm the diagnosis of specific viral infections. Clinical signs of disease, local population, history, and vaccination status will influence the likelihood of viral infection.

Diagnosis of equine influenza (see Chapter 13) is based on virus isolation, virus antigen detection, and paired serum testing. An ELISA test is commercially available for the detection of influenza virus particles in nasal secretions (Directigen FLU-A, BD Diagnostic Systems, Franklin Lakes, NJ). This potential stall-side test was not designed for equine use but has been validated for use in this species.[21]

Diagnosis of infection with equine herpesvirus type 1 (EHV-1) and EHV-4 depends somewhat on disease manifestation (see Chapter 14). For example, diagnosis of infectious respiratory disease is based on real-time quantitative PCR (RT-qPCR) or virus isolation of nasal swab samples, PCR or virus isolation of buffy coat samples, or detection of increasing serum antibody titers to the virus. EHV-1 RT-qPCR or virus isolation from a buffy coat smear, nasal swab, or postmortem tissues may provide valuable diagnostic information. DNA testing through PCR will provide the clinician with evidence of the specific strain of EHV-1 associated with clinical disease. A definitive association has been established with DNA open reading frame (ORF30) mutation and the potential development of equine herpesvirus myeloencephalopathy (EHM); appropriate biosecurity precautions therefore should be employed when dealing with any suspected case of EHM. Cerebrospinal fluid (CSF) analysis should be performed in horses suspected of having EHM; cytologic findings are typically characterized by xanthochromia and albuminocytologic dissociation. Antibody titer analysis of CSF is of limited value for diagnosis of EHM because significant disruption of the blood-brain barrier has frequently occurred in affected horses.

Diagnosis of EHV-2 is most effectively performed using PCR analysis; however, not all diagnostic laboratories routinely perform PCR for this pathogen. Alternate diagnostic methods such as culture may be challenging because virus isolation does not provide consistently positive results. Paired serologic titers may provide suggestive information for establishing a diagnosis of upper respiratory disease in horses.[22]

Definitive diagnosis of equine viral arteritis (EVA) infection is made on the basis of virus isolation from nasopharyngeal, vaginal, or semen samples (see Chapter 15). Polymerase chain reaction testing has improved sensitivity and specificity for detection of the virus in these samples. Acute and convalescent serum titers may provide additional information to facilitate confirmation of the diagnosis in suspect cases. Gross examination of fetuses postmortem typically reveals edema, pleural effusion, and petechiation on mucosal surfaces or on the inner ear.

Equine rhinoviruses are a cause of upper respiratory tract infection in horses (see Chapter 17). They can be more challenging to diagnose than other viral respiratory tract infections because seroprevalence can be high.[23] Of 28 cases in which the virus was isolated from infected horses, only 6 showed serologic evidence of viral exposure.[24] Therefore, when equine rhinitis B virus (ERBV) infection is a diagnostic differential, virus isolation is the preferred diagnostic test. Although another rhinovirus, ERBV2, has been investigated as a possible etiologic agent of equine viral respiratory tract disease, its role remains unconfirmed.[25]

Culture of nasopharyngeal swabs or wash samples are useful for diagnosis of *S. equi* subsp. *equi* (strangles; subsequently referred to as *S. equi*) infection in horses (see Chapter 28). Detection of *S. equi* DNA using the PCR test is also confirmatory for a respiratory infection secondary to *S. equi* infection. Infection in carrier horses may be challenging to identify without endoscopic evaluation that includes examination of the guttural pouches. Culture and PCR of samples obtained from the guttural pouch of these horses are recommended. If both tests are negative, the horse is unlikely to be an *S. equi* carrier. Polymerase chain reaction testing for *S. equi* is more sensitive than standard microbiologic culture techniques.[26]

Serology for diagnosis of equine respiratory viruses must be performed on paired sera obtained at least 2 to 4 weeks apart. An individual serum titer is nondiagnostic and a waste of laboratory time and owner resources. Whenever possible, paired sera testing should be pursued and can be extremely useful if the index case is no longer shedding virus and for assessment of herd exposure. For herd testing, testing of a minimum of 10% of the herd or group is necessary.

Communication with the appropriate diagnostic laboratory regarding differential diagnoses under consideration is recommended. Not all laboratories perform all types of diagnostic tests.

Fluid analysis of the trachea and lungs is often helpful in the diagnosis of lower airway disease. Transtracheal wash technique is discussed in more detail later in this chapter. Bronchoalveolar lavage is essential for analysis of the alveolar spaces; however, this technique provides regional sampling at best. Samples of both types may be submitted for cytologic evaluation, viral detection, and bacterial and fungal culture.

Upper Respiratory Tract Infections

Diseases of the Upper Respiratory Tract

Rhinitis and Sinusitis

Nasal airways can be infected with a variety of viral, bacterial, fungal, and parasitic agents with resultant sinusitis and/or rhinitis. In this chapter, rhinitis in the horse is defined as infection of the nasal passage independent of the sinus. Infection may include the nasal concha but does not involve the conchal sinuses unless caused by viral agents. Specific viral agents include equine influenza virus, EHV-1 and EHV-4, equine rhinoviruses, and equine adenovirus.[23,25,27-32] Bacterial rhinitis is not common and usually occurs secondary to trauma or foreign body. *Mycoplasma* spp. have been isolated at postmortem examination from horses with rhinitis.[7,24,32,33] A variety of mycotic agents such as *Aspergillus* spp. (see Chapter 52), *Conidiobolus* spp. (usually *C. coronatus*) (see Chapter 51), and *Cryptococcus neoformans* (see Chapter 53) may cause rhinitis in horses.[34-37] The most common cause of parasitic rhinitis is myiasis caused by *Habronema, Draschia*, and the Russian gadfly, *Rhinoestrus purpureus*.[38] Enzootic lymphangitis or glanders caused by *Burkholderia mallei* causes a specific granuloma within the sinus cavity[39-45] (see Chapter 36).

Horses with sinusitis most commonly have unilateral disease unless the infection is viral or there is extensive involvement of the nasal septa. Most horses present with respiratory stridor and nasal discharge with diminished airflow.[27,29,31,32] Therapy is usually aimed at surgical debridement, debulking of nasal granuloma, and local therapy for the specific agent.[31,46-48] Orally administered itraconazole has been described for treatment of recurrent nasal mycoses.[31,47] Although successful in this case, the pharmacokinetics of this agent are variable. Fluconazole may be a viable alternative.

Sinonasal disease is very common in the horse. The horse has six pairs of sinuses, including the conchal sinuses, that exchange air with the nasal airway. The frontal sinuses may be affected with granulomatous masses (usually fungal or parasitic) or empyema (bacterial). The most common bacterial isolates are *Streptococcus* spp. with *S. equi* subsp. *zooepidemicus* and *S. equi* subsp. *equi* as the most common isolates. *Staphylococcus* spp. are the next most frequent isolates.[49-52] Mixed bacterial infections are not uncommon. *Cryptococcus neoformans* and *Coccidioides immitis* also may cause granuloma formation within the paranasal sinuses (see Chapter 47).[34-37]

In a study of 277 horses with sinusitis, 24% of the horses had primary sinusitis with no history of predisposing trauma or dental infection.[52] Dental disease of the third to sixth maxillary cheek teeth was the most common predisposing factor for secondary sinusitis (22% of horses) followed by sinus cysts, neoplasia, progressive ethmoidal hematoma, trauma, mycotic infection, sinonasal polyps, and nasal epidermal inclusion cysts. Primary infection of a rostral maxillary cheek root infection was identified in only 4% of cases, although computed tomography (CT) evaluation was not used for diagnosis of many of these cases. Nasal discharge (most commonly unilateral but occasionally bilateral) and facial swelling were the most common clinical signs. These findings were supported by a more recent report that compared diagnostic modalities: sinoscopy, radiography, and scintigraphy.[53] Discharge can be mucopurulent to serosanguineous fluid with a foul smell. Clinical signs frequently persisted over several weeks (without other progressive systemic clinical signs). Other signs of frontal and maxillary sinus involvement included lacrimal discharge and exophthalmia. Headshaking syndrome is an uncommon clinical manifestation of fungal sinusitis in horses.[54]

Diagnostic techniques that may facilitate identification and characterization of sinusitis in horses include endoscopy, radiography, CT, and magnetic resonance imaging (MRI).[55-57] Endoscopy can detect changes in airway structure (84% of cases) and rule out ethmoidal hematoma.[51,52] Sinoscopy can also be performed through a space created in the skull by trephination in the standing horse.[29,34,51,52]

Radiography is essential for identification of fluid and masses within sinuses (Fig. 1-3). If there is no fluid, this modality is valuable for detection of tooth root abscess.[50,52,55,56-60] Usually the first molar is involved. Computed tomography and MRI are

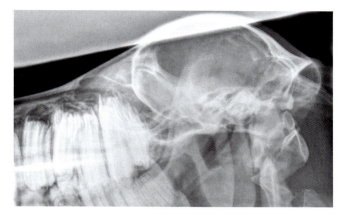

Figure 1-3 Lateral skull radiograph that demonstrates a soft tissue opacity and fluid lines in the region of the frontal sinus, consistent with a chronic sinusitis and accumulation of exudate.

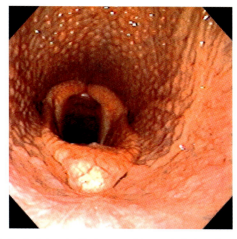

Figure 1-4 Grade 3 lymphoid pharyngeal hyperplasia in a 2-year-old Thoroughbred colt (see Box 1-1).

exceptionally valuable for detection of tooth root involvement and bony changes, which often involve the maxillary bone and facial crest.

Appropriate and effective treatment of sinusitis requires that underlying or predisposing conditions be accurately identified and treated, that debris be flushed from the sinus, and that associated infectious agents are properly identified. When fluid is present within a sinus, medical treatment with antibiotics alone is unlikely to be successful. Trephination and flushing or surgical debridement and drainage through a sinus flap are indicated.[31,47,48,51,61-64] Establishment of ventral drainage of the affected sinuses may be required. Local flushing is likely to be the most important component of therapy, although systemic antimicrobial therapy may be indicated for any horse with signs of osteomyelitis. Prognosis is guarded for complete resolution of clinical signs, especially when apical dental disease is present. Frequently, tooth removal is indicated. Recurrence is most common with ethmoidal hematoma and neoplasia.[52]

Lymphoid Pharyngeal Hyperplasia

Lymphoid pharyngeal hyperplasia is a common condition involving the upper respiratory tract of 2- and 3-year-old racehorses (Fig. 1-4 and Box 1-1). Most mild cases respond favorably to reduced athletic activity combined with systemic and topical antiinflammatory therapy. Dexamethasone can be administered at a dose of 0.02 to 0.05 mg/kg orally daily for 1 week, followed by one-half of the original dose given orally for 1 week, then the same dose administered orally every other day for an additional week. A throat spray composed of nitrofurazone, dexamethasone, and dimethyl sulfoxide is reported to be beneficial when administered topically.[61] Systemic immune modulation is reported to be effective for treatment of horses with lower airway inflammation and may also have some benefit in horses suffering from upper airway inflammation.[61,65,66] Occasionally, chronic disease occurs; reports have suggested that these horses may respond favorably to cautery of the dorsal roof of the pharynx.[67]

Organisms associated with a more prolonged course of pharyngeal hyperplasia include *S. equi* subsp. *equi*, equine influenza, EHV-1, EHV-2, and EHV-4. The condition is thought to result from chronic inflammation of the localized lymphoid tissues, particularly since these structures have a diffuse distribution within the mucosa in this species. Although some investigators have cultured the oropharynx of affected horses, no consistent etiologic agent has been identified. Normal inhabitants of the equine upper respiratory tract, such as *S. equi* subsp.

Box 1-1 Grading Scheme for Lymphoid Pharyngeal Hyperplasia

Grade 1: Small number of white follicles scattered over dorsal pharyngeal wall. The follicles are small and inactive. This appearance is normal in horses of all ages.

Grade 2: Many small, inactive white follicles over dorsal and lateral walls of pharynx to level of guttural pouches. Numerous follicles are larger, pink, edematous, and interspersed throughout.

Grade 3: Many large, pink follicles and some shrunken white follicles distributed over dorsal and lateral walls of pharynx. In some individuals the follicles extend onto the dorsal surface of the soft palate and into the dorsal pharyngeal diverticula.

Grade 4: More numerous pink and edematous follicles packed close together, covering entire pharynx, dorsal surface of soft palate, and epiglottis and lining guttural pouches. Large accumulations appear as polyps.

Modified from Raker CW: The nasopharynx. In Mansmann RA, McAllister ES, editors: *Equine medicine and surgery,* Santa Barbara, CA, 1982, American Veterinary Publications.

---

zooepidemicus, *Bordetella bronchiseptica,* and *Moraxella,* have been isolated; however, the direct association with the condition has not been determined. A grading system has been established for this condition; those horses with more severe inflammation have greater numbers of bacterial organisms isolated from their upper respiratory tract.[68]

Arytenoid Chondritis

Arytenoid chondritis is a progressive inflammatory condition of the arytenoid cartilages in adult horses, originating as an infectious condition. Most commonly, upper airway dysfunction is reflected in poor athletic performance and respiratory stridor. Diagnosis is based on upper airway endoscopy (Fig. 1-5). One manifestation of chondritis is the development of granulomas on the axial surface of the arytenoid cartilages. Clinical management of affected patients involves medical or surgical therapy. Although broad-spectrum antibiotic therapy has been attempted in many cases, it is rarely curative. Also important in the management of some of these cases is placement of a tracheostomy tube. Several techniques are described for placement of a permanent tracheostomy.[6]

Viral Diseases

Equine influenza virus is classified as an orthomyxovirus with a single-stranded, segmented ribonucleic acid (RNA) genome[69]

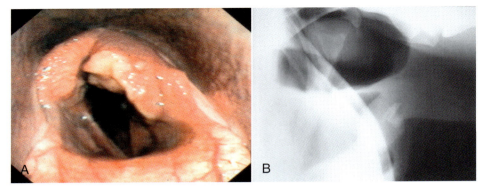

Figure 1-5 Arytenoid chondritis as viewed in an affected horse. **A,** Upper airway endoscopy showing severe inflammation and purulent exudate of the affected arytenoid cartilage. **B,** Chronic inflammation in a horse suffering from arytenoid chondritis resulted in mineralization of affected cartilaginous structures.

(see Chapter 13). Influenza viruses are classified on the basis of surface and internal protein antigens into three types: A, B, and C; only type A influenza is reported to infect horses. Major viral antigens include neuraminidase (NA) and hemagglutinin (HA). Two type A viral subtypes are known to cause disease in horses: H7N7 and H3N8.[69] The strain H7N7 was initially isolated in 1956 in Prague and designated A/equine/Prague/56. This H7N7 variant, termed *equine-1 influenza*, has not been isolated since 1980 and is believed to have disappeared from the equine population.[68] The H3N8 equine influenza virus, called *equine-2*, is a strain that was initially isolated in Miami in 1963 and designated A/equine/Miami/63.[70-72] Antigenic drift has subsequently resulted in many subtypes of variant equine-2 among horses, including A/equine/Fontainebleau/79, A/equine/Kentucky/81, A/equine/Saskatoon/90, and A/equine/Newmarket 2/93. Although antigenic drift has been observed for many years, antigenic shift, a larger scale change in the antigenic nature of the equine influenza viruses, has not been documented to date.

Equine herpesviruses (see Chapter 14) are classified among the alpha (EHV-1, EHV-3, and EHV-4) and gamma (EHV-2 and EHV-5) herpesviruses. Those viruses associated with respiratory disease of the greatest significance in the horses are EHV-1 and EHV-4. These alpha-herpesviruses are responsible for sporadic respiratory disease, abortion, and myeloencephalopathy. Equine herpesvirus-4 is less likely than EHV-1 to be associated with disease other than respiratory infection. Fatal neonatal sepsis has been reported in association with EHV-4 infection, but EHV-1 is more commonly involved in this form of disease.[73,74] Because EHV is neurotropic, latency is possible and generally associated with the trigeminal (cranial nerve [CN] V) ganglion or lymphocytes.[75] During times of severe stress or immune suppression, disease transmission is possible when latent virus is reactivated. In a stressful situation such as hospitalization, viral shedding with EHV-1 is not necessarily more likely to occur.

Equine herpesvirus-2, often referred to as *cytomegalovirus*, is a slow-replicating virus that typically results in self-limiting viral respiratory disease in young horses.[68] Many investigators question the role of this virus as a primary etiologic agent of fulminant respiratory disease in horses. The virus has been recovered from both normal horses and young horses with clinical signs of respiratory tract disease.[76-79] Studies of seroprevalence and virus isolation reveal that young foals are commonly exposed to the virus. The virus could also be isolated from fluid collected by TTA of young horses with clinical respiratory tract disease, whereas it was rare to isolate the virus from tracheal fluid of clinically normal foals. Experimental inoculation of foals with EHV-2 results in chronic pharyngitis.[80] This organism may

be a pathogen of concern in predisposing foals to bacterial pathogens such as *Rhodococcus equi*.[76]

Although most commonly recognized for its association with the equine reproductive tract, EVA causes a mild to moderate respiratory disease (see Chapter 15). The virus is maintained in equine populations in carrier stallions because testosterone is required for persistence and maintenance of the virus in vivo. Carrier stallions maintain the virus within the ampulla and vas deferens. Variations in the severity of clinical signs result from strain differences in virulence, pathogen dose, and host immune function. Incubation requires several days to 2 weeks, with a more rapid course of disease after venereal transmission. Most infections are self-limiting, although edema may be severe and respiratory distress evident. Abortion typically occurs within a month of exposure and disease development. Abortion may occur, although other clinical signs of EVA have not been observed. Neonatal foals infected with the virus demonstrate respiratory difficulty and rarely recover from viral infection.[81-83]

Equine rhinoviruses have been divided into two serogroups: equine rhinitis virus A and B (ERAV and ERBV; see Chapter 17). Equine rhinitis virus A is grouped in the *Aphthovirus* genus based on genotype and similarity with other members of this genus such as foot and mouth virus, as well as the characteristic viremia and persistent shedding that occurs following infection with the virus.[22,30] Equine rhinitis B virus is the sole member of the genus *Erbovirus*. A third serotype has been identified and proposed to be called *ERBV2*, classified among the Erboviruses as well; currently, this virus is referred to as P13/75 and is classified within the family *Picornaviridae*.[25]

Strangles

Clinical disease in horses associated with *S. equi* subsp. *equi* infection (strangles) is most common in horses younger than 5 years of age but very uncommon in young foals (<3 months of age) born to mares previously exposed to the organism (see Chapter 28). Natural infection results from direct contact with an infected or carrier individual that may have overt clinical disease or has maintained the organism within the upper airway, most frequently the guttural pouch.[63] Transmission may also occur via fomites such as contaminated clothing or cleaning instruments. Infection with *S. equi* primarily occurs through oral and nasal routes. Incubation from time of infection to manifestation of clinical signs varies from a few days to a few weeks and is influenced by pathogen virulence, dose of inoculum, and host immunity at the time of challenge. Some of the earliest clinical signs include fever, depression, and reduced appetite. Nasal discharge may initially be serous but with disease progression will become mucopurulent. Lymph node enlargement and abscess maturation generally require approximately 7 days to occur. Early in the course of infection, affected lymph nodes are sensitive to palpation and firm in nature. As rupture becomes eminent, a soft center develops and a serous crust on the surface may be observed. Submandibular and retropharyngeal nodes are most commonly affected; edema may be severe, resulting in dysphagia and respiratory stridor. After rupture of abscess(es), swelling will diminish rapidly. Severe obstruction may necessitate that a tracheostomy be performed. Most common hematologic abnormalities in horses infected with *S. equi* include leukocytosis caused by neutrophilia, hyperfibrinogenemia, and anemia of chronic disease. Definitive diagnosis is based on aerobic culture of nasal secretions, preferably obtained from the abscessed lymph nodes, the guttural pouch, or a nasopharyngeal wash (see Chapter 28).

Therapy of Upper Respiratory Viral Infections

Specific recommendations for treatment of *S. equi* and acute viral respiratory tract disease of horses are discussed in detail in the relevant chapters of this text. Because of the severity of epithelial surface damage and the potential for secondary bacterial infection, all virally affected horses should be rested from race training during the course of disease and recovery. A significant cough may persist for weeks after onset of clinical signs of viral respiratory disease. A standard rule of thumb is to implement a week of rest from strenuous exercise for each day the horse demonstrates a fever. Recovery of the respiratory epithelium should be complete before reintroduction of strenuous exercise. During periods of high fever, depression, anorexia, and myalgia, nonsteroidal antiinflammatory therapy is recommended. If significant nasal discharge and fever are persistent, additional testing is warranted to rule out secondary infection.

Lower Respiratory Tract Infections

Etiology and Epidemiology

Bacterial Pneumonia

Under normal conditions the equine lung contains only small numbers of potential bacterial or fungal pathogens; when present they are considered transient contaminants. These bacteria are typically cleared by the normal defense mechanisms that have been previously discussed. However, when the normal defense mechanisms are overwhelmed or pulmonary immune defense is impaired, proliferation of such contaminants may become pathogenic to the host. The most common source for contamination of the lower airways is aspiration of microorganisms from the upper respiratory tract. Gram-positive pathogens include *S. equi* subsp. *zooepidemicus*, *Staphylococcal aureus*, and *S. pneumoniae*. Gram-negative pathogens affecting the lower airways of horses include *Pasteurella*, *Actinobacillus* spp., *Escherichia coli*, *Klebsiella pneumoniae*, and *Bordetella bronchiseptica*. Anaerobic organisms that may infect the lower airways of horses include *Bacteroides fragilis*, *Peptostreptococcus anaerobius*, and *Fusobacterium* spp.

Miscellaneous Causes of Pneumonia

Infectious disease involving the lower respiratory tract is most commonly associated with bacterial infection, although fungal[35-37,84,85] and viral[75,84-87] pathogens are also potential invaders of the lower respiratory tract. Septic thrombophlebitis is considered a risk factor for metastatic spread of septic foci.[88] The presence of anaerobic organisms have been suggested to warrant a more guarded prognosis when cultured from horses suffering from pleuropneumonia.[89] Polymicrobial infection may

result from synergy among pathogens, particularly aerobic organisms that can exist as facultative anaerobes or those that are purely anaerobic organisms, which favor survival of the organism that would otherwise not survive.

The best-described pathogen of the lower airways involves the gamma-herpesvirus pathogen EHV-5, which is an important component for the development of multinodular pulmonary fibrosis (MNPF), or interstitial pneumonia of adult horses.[90]

Pulmonary Abscess

Pulmonary abscess formation most commonly occurs in weanling age foals in association with *Rhodococcus equi* infection (see Chapter 31). *Streptococcus equi* subsp. *zooepidemicus* is the organism most commonly cultured from the lungs of horses with generalized pneumonia and rarely results in abscess formation. Complications from *S. equi* infection include metastatic spread to various organs, including possible pulmonary abscess formation. Aspiration is another cause of focal pulmonary infection and abscessation. Aspiration pneumonia is a potential complication of esophageal obstruction or dysphagia in horses. Neonatal foals may suffer from dysphagia in association with hypoxic ischemic encephalopathy or nutritional muscular dystrophy, whereas adult horses may develop aspiration pneumonia after complete esophageal obstruction.

Pathogenesis

Bronchopneumonia occurs after colonization of the lower respiratory tract with bacteria. This colonization may occur after damage from viral infection or after an episode of impaired pulmonary clearance, as might occur after strenuous exercise or long distance transport. Bacterial contamination of the lower airways may also lead to concurrent or subsequent pleuropneumonia or pulmonary abscess formation.

Primary viral respiratory tract infection predisposes adult horses to bacterial infection because of disruption of the surface epithelium and loss of the mucociliary elevator and surfactant production by type II alveolar epithelial cells. Pulmonary inflammation leads to increased capillary permeability and pulmonary exudate, which is conducive to the survival and replication of contaminating pathogens, particularly those that survive under conditions of low oxygen tension (anaerobes).

Elite performance horses may be predisposed to lower airway infection because alveolar macrophages are reduced in efficacy after strenuous exercise.[13] In addition, challenge is enhanced because horses in training are at greater risk for aspiration of pathogens and particulate matter. Horses used for performance activities often travel long distances, and persistent head elevation, as might occur in a trailered horse, reduces pulmonary clearance mechanisms within 6 to 12 hours.[3] Although many strategies have been utilized to enhance protection in such individuals, neither antibiotic therapy nor intermittent lowering of the head appears to dramatically reduce the incidence of pulmonary infection.[89] Transportation for a distance greater than 500 miles within the preceding 2 weeks is an important risk factor for the development of pleuropneumonia in horses. Although uncommon, horses that have suffered from severe gastrointestinal disease or those with pulmonary infection that remains unresponsive to antibiotic therapy may be suffering from pulmonary mycotic colonization.[37] Diagnostic testing should be implemented to rule out fungal organisms as primary or secondary invaders.

Clinical Findings

Clinical findings in horses with pulmonary disease most commonly include depression, fever, and reduced food intake.

Coughing is most frequently observed during physical exertion or with advanced disease. With disease progression, horses may show respiratory distress, as well as marked weight loss. Purulent nasal discharge with a fetid odor, evidence of thoracic pain, and epistaxis may occur in association with rupture of a pulmonary abscess. A sequelae to severe disease may be laminitis; therefore abnormal gait or intermittent recumbency may accompany evidence of pulmonary infection.

Diagnosis

Although clinical evidence may suggest pulmonary infection as the primary problem in equine patients, a thorough evaluation is warranted to ensure that all problems and diagnoses are appropriately managed. Physical examination should include careful auscultation to evaluate the patient for pulmonary air movement. In the event that respiratory distress is observed, further manipulation for auscultation should not be performed. However, if pulmonary sounds are difficult to detect, a rebreathing bag may be applied to enhance the ability to detect air movement. When diminished pulmonary sounds are present, an ultrasound examination should be performed to determine if pleural fluid or pulmonary consolidation exists.

Hematologic findings that are consistent with bacterial infection include a neutrophilic leukocytosis with a left shift, toxic changes in neutrophils, hyperglobulinemia, and hyperfibrinogenemia. Mild to moderate anemia may exist in association with chronic disease.

Thoracic radiographs are useful to determine the extent and severity of pulmonary disease; ultrasonographic examination will only be helpful for detection of peripheral parenchymal conditions or those associated with pleural effusions.

Sterile TTA samples should be obtained from the respiratory tract for culture and antimicrobial susceptibility testing. Although endoscopy is a useful diagnostic test for horses with pulmonary disease, this is rarely the preferred method for collection of sterile samples for culture and sensitivity analysis. If *Pseudomonas* spp. are cultured from samples obtained by endoscopic TTA, results should be interpreted with caution because this organism is rarely a pathogen of the equine pulmonary system.

Therapy

Treatment of horses with historical, clinical, and hematologic evidence of pulmonary bacterial infection should include broad-spectrum antimicrobial therapy (pending sensitivity testing of isolates and implementation of more targeted antimicrobial therapy) and excellent supportive care. Although bacterial culture results are not available immediately upon diagnosis of pulmonary infection, cytologic evaluation of pulmonary aspirates should give the clinician some indication of the type (Gram stain) and population (single versus multiple classes of pathogens) of pathogens in the patient. β-Lactam antibiotics combined with aminoglycosides provide good coverage for a variety of pathogens that may infect the lower airways of horses. Caution should be used in individuals that are debilitated or dehydrated.[75] Because of nephrotoxicity, aminoglycosides are contraindicated for use in patients at risk for renal impairment.

The prognosis for recovery from bacterial pneumonia is generally considered favorable for horses that have been managed appropriately in a timely fashion. Horses with severe disease that have not recovered or incompletely respond to antimicrobial therapy may subsequently develop pleuropneumonia, which may worsen the prognosis for complete recovery and return to previous level of athletic function, particularly for elite athletes.

Pneumonias

Pleuropneumonia

Etiology and Epidemiology

Pleuropneumonia is a condition in which infection associated with bronchopneumonia has spread to involve the pleura and the pleural space.[91] This disorder most commonly occurs in performance horses, frequently after long distance transport.[68,75,92] Although apparently spontaneous cases of pleuropneumonia may occur in some horses, most affected horses have experienced one or more predisposing risk factors such as long distance transport, recent viral or bacterial respiratory tract disease, or a recent episode of general anesthesia.[89,93,94]

Most cases of equine pleuropneumonia result from bacterial infection, but reports also demonstrate that *Mycoplasma* spp.,[33] viral agents, and mycotic agents[37] may be isolated or the disease may occur as a complication of septic thrombophlebitis.[88] Rarely, pulmonary hydatidosis may be a cause of equine pleuropneumonia[95] (see Chapter 60). Bacterial pleuropneumonia can be associated with a single pathogen but more commonly results from a mixed infection that may include aerobic and anaerobic organisms.[89,94,96,97] The single most important factor for the development of transport-associated pleuropneumonia is head position during long distance transport.[89,92,98-100] The most compelling evidence to demonstrate this claim is the observation that horses transported long distances without restraint of head position do not develop changes in lower airway cytologic findings. In contrast, horses without any other stress had an estimated 75% increased likelihood of developing lower airway accumulation of bacteria and inflammatory debris after a minimum of 24 hours of head restraint.[3,89,91,94] High intensity exercise in combination with long distance transport further contributes to development of lower airway inflammation and impaired immune clearance mechanisms.[13]

Striving to prevent equine pleuropneumonia is important because the prognosis for return to previous level of athletic function may be guarded to poor in severe cases.[89,94] Complications associated with pleuropneumonia, such as laminitis and chronic abscess formation, may negatively influence the future athletic performance of affected individuals.[89]

Clinical Findings

Horses suffering from pleuropneumonia may demonstrate a variety of clinical signs, but disease should be suspected in horses with an appropriate history and in those that demonstrate evidence of lethargy, pyrexia, cough (may be a quiet cough due to pleural pain), nasal discharge (bilateral, may be bloody), shallow breathing pattern, increased laryngeal excursions, or painful, stilted gait. During the acute stages of the disease, horses are likely to have signs referable to pleurodynia. Pain may be demonstrated by pawing, reluctance to move, abducted elbows, stiff gait, guarded breathing pattern, or shallow respiration. Ballottement or percussion of the thorax typically reveals reduced air resonance and may elicit a painful grunt. Differential diagnoses for such cases include exertional rhabdomyolysis, laminitis, and colic.

Thoracic auscultation usually reveals abnormal pulmonary sounds. When pleural effusion is present, the most common finding is attenuation of audible bronchovesicular sounds over the ventral lung fields. In the dorsal lung fields, normal pulmonary sounds may be heard; more commonly, however, increased bronchovesicular sounds are heard, accompanied by crackles or wheezes. Before significant pleural fluid accumulation, abnormal pulmonary sounds may be heard diffusely.[101,102] With chronicity, friction rubs are common, reflecting fibrin accumulation along the parietal and visceral pleural surfaces.

Tachycardia and tachypnea are common findings in horses with pleuropneumonia. Jugular pulsation and severe respiratory distress may occur. Nasal discharge is often present and can vary from serous to mucopurulent to mucohemorrhagic in character. A fetid odor associated with nasal discharge, breath, or pleural fluid should increase the clinicians' suspicion of anaerobic infection. Mucous membrane color may be dark red to injected, depending on whether the horse is experiencing significant toxemia or ventilatory compromise (Fig. 1-6). Horses with subacute to chronic pleuropneumonia will often demonstrate weight loss, which may be dramatic.

Diagnosis

History and physical examination findings are often highly suggestive of pleuropneumonia. Definitive diagnosis is made on the basis of identification of septic fluid within the pleural space. Ultrasonographic examination (3.5- to 5.0-MHz transducer) will reveal evidence of pleural effusion.[68,75,103,104] Ultrasonographic examination is a superior diagnostic test when compared with radiography for the confirmation of a diagnosis of pleuropneumonia because of the presence of fluid accumulation within the thoracic cavity (Fig. 1-7). Ultrasonography may also reveal evidence of pleural irregularities or changes within the pulmonary parenchyma such as atelectasis, abscess

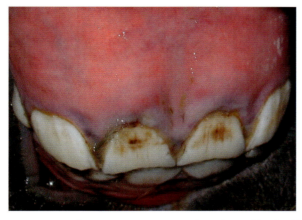

Figure 1-6 Equine pleuropneumonia in a yearling Thoroughbred gelding. Mucous membrane color is dark pink with severe injection of mucosal vessels and a prominent toxic line visible surrounding the incisors.

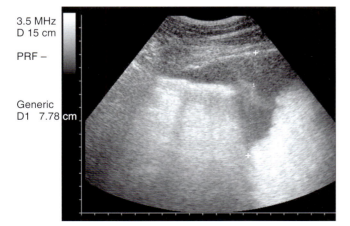

Figure 1-7 Thoracic ultrasound using a 3.5-MHz transducer showing significant pleural effusion and pulmonary consolidation in a horse with pleuropneumonia.

formation, consolidation, and pulmonary hepatization.[104] Comet tail artifacts on pleural surfaces denote foci of inflammation or fibrosis on the visceral pleura.[75] The ultrasonographic character of pleural fluid in horses with pleuropneumonia may range from anechoic to hyperechoic, depending on the relative cellularity and fibrin accumulation.[104] Evidence of bright gas echoes within the pleural fluid is indicative of anaerobic colonization within the pleural fluid. Other considerations for gas accumulation within the pleural space include previous thoracocentesis or severe parenchymal disease resulting in a bronchopleural fistula, with communication between the pleural space and conducting airways. Fibrin accumulation can be detected with ultrasound examination, commonly visualized by strands or loculated cavitations. Familiarity with pleural ultrasonographic examination is important because in some cases the pericardiodiaphragmatic ligament may be confused with fibrin accumulation.[104]

Thoracocentesis is required to determine specific characteristics of pleural fluid such as leukocyte cell count and differential and total protein concentration. Fine-needle aspiration of parenchymal lesions may be indicated in horses with suspected pulmonary abscess formation. Samples of pleural fluid, pulmonary abscess aspirates, and percutaneous transtracheal wash samples should be submitted for bacterial culture (aerobic and anaerobic) with antimicrobial susceptibility testing and cytologic analysis. Because pleuropneumonia in most horses begins as severe bronchopneumonia, culture of tracheal secretions is particularly important for identification of primary bacterial pathogens (Fig. 1-8).[75,91,93,101] Early in the course of disease, pleural fluid may be inflammatory but sterile, and an etiologic diagnosis would be missed if only pleural fluid samples were cultured. If, however, the pleural sepsis results from a penetrating thoracic wound, then transtracheal wash analysis is not indicated and the primary etiologic agents are best identified by culture and sensitivity testing of pleural fluid samples.[105]

Cytologic examination of pleural fluid is important diagnostically and may influence prognosis. Pleural fluid obtained from healthy individuals will be characterized as an ultrafiltrate of plasma and is appropriately classified as a transudate. It is transparent, straw colored, and nonfetid. The total nucleated cell count should be <10,000 cells/μL, and the protein concentration should be <2.5 g/dL. Differential analysis of normal pleural fluid reveals the majority of cells to be neutrophils, with few monocytes and mesothelial cells. Additional analysis may include measurement of glucose, lactate, and pH. Pleural fluid samples from horses with bacterial pleuropneumonia are commonly acidic with low glucose and increased lactate concentrations.[106,107] Pleural fluid glucose concentration is reported to be a reliable indicator of sepsis when concentrations are less than 2.22 mmol/L.[108]

Pneumothorax is a potential complication of pleuropneumonia with a reported incidence of up to 43%.[109] Clinical evidence of pneumothorax may include depression, dyspnea, tachypnea, loss of auscultable pulmonary sounds in the dorsal thorax, anxiety, and cough. Radiography and ultrasonography are useful diagnostic tests that aid in the confirmation of pneumothorax. When pneumothorax occurs as a complication to pleuropneumonia, it is commonly unilateral.[109] In general, horses with pneumothorax secondary to pleuropneumonia have a more guarded prognosis for recovery and survival as compared to horses with uncomplicated pleuropneumonia.[109]

Pleuropneumonia with secondary hemorrhagic pulmonary infarction has been described in Thoroughbred racehorses shortly after a bout of strenuous exercise.[110] Affected horses showed evidence of acute respiratory distress with serosanguineous nasal discharge shortly after strenuous exercise. Thoracic radiography and ultrasound revealed evidence of pulmonary consolidation and pleural effusion in affected individuals; in

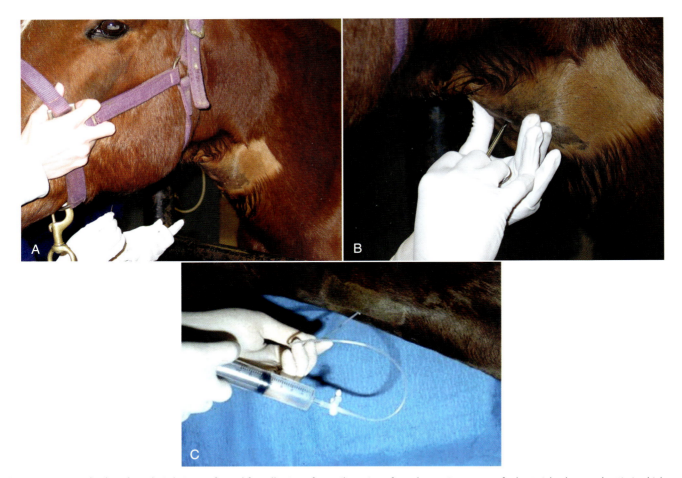

Figure 1-8 Transtracheal wash analysis being performed for collection of a sterile aspirate from the respiratory tract for bacterial culture and antimicrobial sensitivity testing. Sterile preparation **(A)** is followed by local instillation of anesthetic and a small stab incision **(B)** and placement of a trochar into the tracheal lumen to allow for sterile aspiration of tracheal secretions **(C).**

contrast to many cases of pleuropneumonia, thoracocentesis revealed serosanguineous to hemorrhagic effusion. Although an underlying bacterial etiology was demonstrated in most affected horses, conventional management with antibiotic and anti-inflammatory therapy was unsuccessful in resolving most cases. Therefore, although various manifestations of pleuropneumonia may occur, those individuals with a history and clinical evidence of pulmonary infarction should receive a more guarded prognosis.[110]

An uncommon but serious manifestation of pulmonary disease in horses is the development of pulmonary thrombo-embolism (PTE). A recent report described a severe form of this disease in a series of six seriously ill equine patients.[111] Pulmonary thromboembolism should be included as a differential consideration among equine patients that suffer from severe clinical disease, such as infectious gastrointestinal disease or neoplasia, and subsequently develop marked tachypnea. An important risk factor is the development of extrapulmonary vascular thrombosis, notably jugular vein thrombophlebitis in horses. In humans that suffer from PTE, peripheral venous thrombi are the source of pulmonary thrombi and a similar pathogenesis is suspected in horses. Therapeutic management of high risk individuals may include aspirin (12-18 mg/kg body weight orally [PO] every 24-48 hours [q24-48h]); additional therapy may include administration of low molecular weight heparin (dalteparin, 50 IU/kg body weight subcutaneous [SC] q24h), although this therapy may prove cost-prohibitive in

some equine clinical settings. Clinical manifestation of PTE in equine patients is a serious complicating factor to systemic disease, but with supportive care and attention to avoidance of bacterial colonization of the devitalized region of lung with broad-spectrum antimicrobial therapy, the prognosis may remain fair to favorable.

Therapy

The primary goals of therapy in horses with pleuropneumonia include resolution of sepsis, clearance of effusion from the pleural space, and provision of excellent nursing care to avoid or manage the onset of complicating factors associated with the primary disease.

Antimicrobial therapy should provide broad-spectrum coverage for a wide variety of bacterial pathogens, including gram-positive and gram-negative aerobic and anaerobic organisms.[102] Combination therapy with β-lactam (e.g., penicillin at 22,000 IU/kg intravenous [IV] every 6 hours [q6h]) and aminoglycoside (e.g., gentamicin at 6.6 mg/kg IV q24h) antibiotics are the mainstay of antimicrobial therapy in horses suffering from pleuropneumonia. Metronidazole (15-25 mg/kg q6-8h PO) is added to the treatment regimen if anaerobic infection is suspected. Identification of all bacterial species present is an important component of clinical diagnosis because the presence of obligate anaerobic organisms will influence patient prognosis.[89,94] Anaerobic organisms frequently isolated from horses with pleuropneumonia include *Bacteroides* spp.,

Peptostreptococcus spp., *Clostridium* spp., and *Fusobacterium* spp. Although most of these anaerobic pathogens are sensitive to penicillin, some strains of *Bacteroides* are resistant to β-lactam therapy as the result of elaboration of β-lactamase enzymes that inactivate this class of antimicrobial. Metronidazole is a nitroimidazole antibiotic that is metabolized to its active form in the reducing environment produced exclusively by anaerobic organisms and is highly efficacious against this class of bacteria.[112]

Supportive care for horses with pleuropneumonia frequently includes IV fluid therapy, particularly during the acute stages of disease when affected horses are depressed, anorectic, and dehydrated. Dehydration results from reduced voluntary fluid intake, as well as a redistribution of fluid to the pleural space. Intravenous fluid therapy aids in control of pyrexia and maintaining secretions that can easily be removed by the mucociliary escalator, rather than remaining inspissated within the pleural cavity. Nonsteroidal antiinflammatory therapy is indicated in the euhydrated patient to aid in management of pain, endotoxemia, and pyrexia associated with infection.[113]

Drainage of the pleural cavity is required in patients with moderate to severe pleural fluid accumulation. Without appropriate removal, development of severe respiratory distress may ensue. If large volumes of pleural fluid exist within the pleural space, antibiotic therapy alone will be unsuccessful at pathogen clearance.

Insertion of a teat cannula or female urinary (canine) catheter may be effective for removal of small amounts of fluid. In horses with accumulation of a large volume of fluid within the pleural space, indwelling thoracic tubes are indicated to maintain constant fluid removal. A one-way valve system is required on the end of such a tube to avoid the introduction of free air into the pleural space or iatrogenic pneumothorax will occur.

Placement of the thoracic tube should be determined after ultrasonographic identification of the dependent region of greatest fluid accumulation. Tube position should reflect the ventral-most site of fluid accumulation. After the site has been selected and aseptically prepared, local anesthetic is generously infused from the skin surface to the pleural surface just cranial to the rib of interest. A stab incision large enough to allow for placement of the thoracic tube (24-32 French) is made using a #10 surgical blade. The tube is inserted into the incision site, and firm pressure is continued until a "pop" is felt, indicating the pleural space has been entered. Most horses will tolerate this procedure adequately with proper local anesthesia; however, in fractious animals, sedation may be required, recalling that most patients are in critical condition and heavy sedation may compromise their clinical stability. The thoracic tube should be introduced into the thoracic cavity to a depth of 7 to 9 cm, ensuring that the trochar needle remains in place, just penetrating the parietal pleura. The trochar needle is removed to check for fluid accumulation. A pair of Kelly forceps should be available as the potential exists for air aspiration and subsequent pneumothorax as fluid is evacuated from the pleural space. After the initial fluid drainage is complete, the tube is sutured into place with a one-way stop valve on the end (e.g., Heimlich valve). In some horses in which the mediastinum remains incomplete, particularly in the early stages of disease, evacuation of one hemithorax will be successful in removal of fluid from the contralateral hemithorax (Fig. 1-9). Thoracic drainage tubes are left in place until significant fluid accumulation ceases, which may be days to weeks, depending on the severity of disease. With chronic disease, fibrin accumulation will result in a complete mediastinum, which may necessitate bilateral thoracic drainage. In some horses, pleural lavage is indicated to aid in removal of inspissated material. Surgical intervention is indicated in horses that do not recover after thoracic drainage through an indwelling tube.[114] A thoracotomy may be

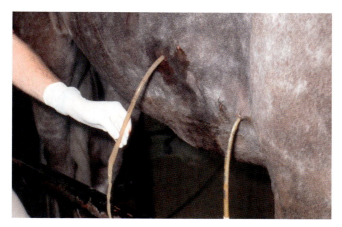

Figure 1-9 Indwelling thoracic tubes have been placed into the pleural space of an equine patient suffering from pleuropneumonia.

performed between rib spaces or may necessitate removal of a portion of rib. Surgical drainage is typically reserved for patients that have not fully recovered from pleural disease, yet are clinically stable. Description of the entire surgical procedure is beyond the scope of this discussion but is recommended to be performed over the area of chronic septic accumulation (identified by ultrasonographic examination). In some horses, a surgical entry site needs to be reopened because of rapid closure, or bilateral procedures are required for horses with severe involvement of both hemithoraces.

Supportive care is focused on prevention of secondary complications that may include pulmonary abscess formation, bronchopleural fistula, pneumothorax, cranial mediastinal abscess, restrictive pericarditis, laminitis, colic, antibiotic-associated colitis, and jugular vein thrombosis.[93,115]

The prognosis for horses with pleuropneumonia depends on the inciting pathogen(s) and the duration of disease before seeking veterinary assistance. As noted, infarctive pleuropneumonia is associated with a more guarded prognosis.

Interstitial Pneumonia

Interstitial pneumonia is a pulmonary disorder that may affect horses of various age groups. Adult horses with interstitial pneumonia have a more guarded prognosis for recovery and survival[75] when compared to foals and weanlings. Horses less than 1 year of age that are provided with appropriate therapy and supportive care tend to have a favorable prognosis for complete recovery.[116]

Etiology

Some cases of interstitial pneumonia result from a primary toxic or infectious insult, but, at the time of presentation, determination of the exact etiology can be challenging.[116-119] Toxic pulmonary disease has been associated with ingestion of Crofton weed, pyrrolizidine alkaloids (*Crotalaria, Trichodesma,* and *Senecio*), perilla ketones, silicosis, and prolonged oxygen therapy. Hepatic metabolites of pyrrolizidine alkaloids cause cellular damage and death in the pulmonary endothelium.[118,120] Inhaled irritants or toxins may contribute to direct pulmonary damage such as occurs after inhalation of smoke or agrichemicals.[121-123] Silicosis is a highly specific chronic granulomatous pneumonia of horses and should be considered in horses with compatible clinical signs that originate from the Carmel Valley in California.[75]

The most recent evidence for an infectious etiology associated with interstitial disease in horses is EHV-5–associated

MNPF. Supportive evidence for the association was recently described by investigators who characterized findings of 24 adult horses that suffered from progressive nodular fibrotic lung disease associated with EHV-5.[90] Herpes viral DNA was identified in 79.2% of affected individuals compared with 8.7% of the control animals.[90] Similarly, a case series of five horses suffering from respiratory distress with clinical evidence of interstitial disease were confirmed to have EHV-5 in pulmonary tissue or secretions supporting previous findings of the association of this disorder and viral infection.[124] An additional report of two horses confirmed similar clinical manifestation of disease, radiographic and histopathologic evidence of multinodular granulomatous disease, and the presence of EHV-5.[125] The exact association of viral involvement remains speculative in some circumstances—in a prospective investigation of mares and foals in central Kentucky, up to 88% of the foals were positive for the virus in peripheral blood, yet they remained clinically healthy.[126] Although EHV-5 has been isolated from the upper respiratory tract in horses with respiratory disease, similar to a related gamma-herpesvirus EHV-2, clinical disease associated with EHV-5 has been suggested to result in lymphadenopathy, immune suppression, depression, and primary respiratory tract disease. Adult onset of severe respiratory disease characterized by multinodular granulomatous pulmonary lesions should be strongly suspected to be associated with EHV-5 infection.

The initial infectious or toxic agent causes alveolar damage resulting in cell death and increased permeability at the level of the alveoli. Pulmonary congestion, interstitial edema, erythrocyte extravasation, and alveolar edema occur during the exudative phase of the disease. Subsequently, alveolar infiltrates with inflammatory leukocytes and fibrin and increased permeability lead to fluid accumulation, impairing normal gas exchange mechanisms, hyaline membrane formation, and clinical respiratory distress. Acutely affected patients typically demonstrate respiratory distress, injected mucous membranes, and impaired pulmonary function. Subacute to chronic disease results in alveolar regeneration with alveolar type II pneumocyte proliferation to replace damaged type I pneumocytes. Fibroplasia leads to cellular proliferation and septae thickening, fibrous development, and ultimately to reduced pulmonary compliance.

Clinical Findings

Horses presenting with interstitial pneumonia are typically in severe respiratory distress with labored breathing, dark mucous membranes, poor pulse quality, and tachycardia. Some patients are mistakenly considered to have an obstructive disease like heaves, yet interstitial pneumonia is characterized by a restrictive, rapid, and shallow breathing pattern. Additional clinical features of disease include hypoxemia, a stress or inflammatory leukogram, hyperfibrinogenemia, and hypoxemia that may be severe. More chronic disease may be observed in mildly affected individuals with exercise intolerance and chronic cough.

Diagnosis

Definitive diagnosis of interstitial pneumonia in horses is based on histopathologic evaluation of a pulmonary biopsy (Fig. 1-10). Examination for EHV-5 viral DNA can be performed on a tissue sample or BAL fluid. Thoracic radiographs can be helpful in establishing a preliminary diagnosis of interstitial pneumonia. Two patterns of interstitial disease have been described in horses with interstitial pneumonia: as discrete or diffuse nodules suggestive of neoplasia or mycotic disease or as a diffuse increase in radiographic interstitial pattern (Fig. 1-11). Serum titers may indicate recent exposure or infection with viral respiratory disease. Histopathologic evaluation of lung biopsies or specimens obtained at postmortem will confirm

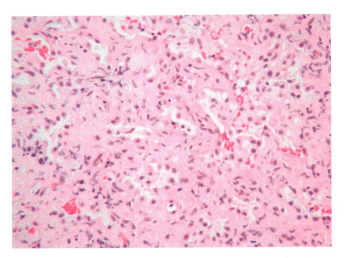

Figure 1-10 Histopathology from a middle-aged horse diagnosed with interstitial pneumonia. Fibrosis and inflammation have resulted in a loss of the normal parenchymal architecture; note the loss of alveolar spaces for adequate gas exchange to occur.

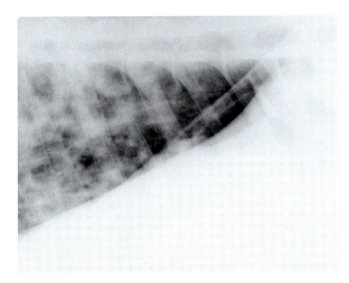

Figure 1-11 Adult interstitial pneumonia in an equine patient. Thoracic radiographs obtained at the time of presentation demonstrate a heavy bronchointerstitial pattern.

the diagnosis of interstitial pneumonia. If silicosis remains a differential, diagnosis is based on x-ray diffraction techniques on lung tissue preparations.[75]

Therapy

The prognosis for adult horses with interstitial pneumonia remains guarded. In horses that present with mild to moderate disease, treatment should be aimed at improving oxygenation. Intranasal insufflation of oxygen is warranted for patients that are severely hypoxemic. Antiinflammatory therapy should initially include systemic corticosteroids (dexamethasone 0.05-0.1 mg/kg IV daily), with transition to aerosolized corticosteroids (beclomethasone 1500 μg intranasally 2 or 3 times daily [BID or TID])[127] as clinical improvement is observed. Corticosteroid therapy should be continued until clinical resolution is observed or no further improvement is noted with therapy. Prolonged corticosteroid therapy of several weeks to months should be anticipated because of the severity of lower airway inflammation associated with this condition. Bronchodilator therapy is indicated when severe bronchoconstriction exists. β_2-adrenergic receptor agonists are the drugs of choice for immediate bronchodilation and subsequent improvement of air movement to the lower airways (albuterol 360-720 mcg/kg q3-12h)[128,129] Enteral bronchodilator therapy with clenbuterol 0.8-3.0 μg/kg PO q12h (Ventipulmin, Boehringer Ingelheim, Canada) can provide additional support in cases with marked bronchoconstriction. Following initial stabilization, an additional therapeutic option is the use of a combined parasympatholytic agent (ipratropium 360-470 total q6-12h)[130] with a β_2-adrenergic receptor agonist (albuterol [Combivent, Boehringer Ingelheim, Canada]) to improve oxygen delivery to the lower airways with the added advantage of having an increased half-life when compared with β_2-adrenergic agonist therapy alone.

In addition to supportive care and antiinflammatory therapy, specific antiviral therapy may be selected for cases of EHV-5–associated MNPF, typically in combination with antiinflammatory therapy. Although pharmacokinetic evaluation has been determined for valacyclovir with a protocol that includes 27 mg/kg PO every 8 hours for 48 hours followed by 20 mg/kg every 12 hours thereafter additional reports have demonstrated evidence of clinical benefit when doses as high as 40 mg/kg PO every 8 hours have been administered to patients suffering from EMPF[131-133a] Duration of therapy should be based on clinical response to treatment. In some circumstances, this therapeutic protocol may be cost-prohibitive or only possible for a limited time. Investigations are ongoing with regard to optimizing antiviral therapeutic protocols for horses that suffer from herpesviral infection, but supportive evidence is provided by the use of such agents in human patients who are at risk for serious cytomegalovirus infection postorgan transplantation.[134,135]

Prognosis

The prognosis for return to function is guarded for adult horses and favorable for foals that are managed appropriately. Supportive and antiinflammatory therapy may improve clinical status, but high-level athletic activity may be impaired.

Parasitic Pneumonia

Etiology

Parasitic pneumonia is a condition that may affect foals or adult horses. Parasites associated with this condition include *Parascaris equorum* larvae or the adults of *Dictyocaulus arnfieldi* (see Chapter 57). Clinically affected horses have obvious evidence of respiratory disease that includes exercise intolerance and coughing that may be accompanied by nasal discharge, fever, and depression, particularly when secondary bacterial infection has occurred. *Parascaris equorum* infection is most common in foals and weanlings, particularly those raised on breeding farms where the parasite resides in the environment and soil. *Dictyocaulus arnfieldi* infection may occur in horses of any age, but this parasite requires a donkey as a primary host to complete its life cycle.

Clinical Findings

Chronic coughing, mucoid to mucopurulent nasal discharge, respiratory distress, and poor overall body condition provide nonspecific evidence of parasitic disease in foals. Poor body condition, abnormal pulmonary sounds represented by increased bronchovesicular sounds, crackles, and wheezes are common findings on thoracic auscultation of horses with parasitic pneumonia. Poor body condition is a common finding because of intestinal involvement of parasitic infection. Colic may be a component of the history or may result following therapeutic anthelminthic treatment in severely affected individuals. Frequently, the history also includes a poor response to appropriate antimicrobial therapy for suspected bronchopneumonia.

Diagnosis

Hematologic evaluation commonly reveals an inflammatory leukogram consisting of mature neutrophilia, hyperfibrinogenemia, and hyperglobulinemia. In some instances, particularly early in the course of disease, hematologic evaluation may reveal few abnormalities. Hepatic parasitic migration (*P. equorum*) may result in mild to moderate hepatic enzyme elevation.[136] Thoracic radiography is a useful diagnostic test in affected individuals. A moderate to severe bronchointerstitial pattern is a common finding, whereas granuloma or abscess formation may be detected by radiographs with advanced disease. Thoracic ultrasonographic examination will allow the clinician to detect the presence of pleural fluid or peripheral pulmonary consolidation.

Cytologic examination of a sterile tracheobronchial aspirate will often reveal abundant eosinophils (5%-50% [normal: <2%]), neutrophilic inflammation may exist concurrently, particularly when secondary bacterial infection is present. Microorganisms are apparent with significant bacterial infection; culture is recommended to determine the presence of bacterial infection and to determine the antimicrobial sensitivity pattern for pathogens of concern. Fecal flotation is indicated to determine the presence of parasite ova being shed from the host. *Dictyocaulus arnfieldi* requires a donkey or mule host for life cycle completion; therefore parasite eggs will only infrequently be detected in adult horses with lungworm infection. It is difficult to diagnose *P. equorum* infection on fecal floatation because tissue migration occurs during the prepatent period. Therefore, diagnosis is based on clinical signs, lack of evidence of bacterial infection and tracheal wash cytology indicating eosinophilic pneumonitis. Response to therapy is supportive of the diagnosis, although antibiotic therapy may be required in combination with anthelminthic therapy.

Therapy

Severely hypoxemic patients may require oxygen insufflation. Severe pulmonary inflammation is induced by eosinophilic infiltrates necessitating bronchodilator and potentially aerosolized corticosteroid therapy (see previous recommendations on aerosol therapy). Oral anthelminthics used to treat *P. equorum* infection include an initial low dose of fenbendazole (5 mg/kg). Careful monitoring for approximately 24 hours is recommended to observe the foal for evidence of deterioration or gastrointestinal distress. Laxative therapy may be required if gastrointestinal ascarid impaction is suspected to occur. After the foal has received an initial low dose of fenbendazole without complication, the dose can be increased (10 mg/kg PO daily) and repeated daily for 5 days. This therapy will be effective in killing adult and migrating larvae. Because this is a farm problem, other individuals of similar age on the same property should be managed appropriately, even if clinical evidence of disease is not apparent. Other anthelminthics that have been used include pyrantel pamoate (6.6 mg/kg) and ivermectin (200 μg/kg). *Dictyocaulus arnfieldi* infection can be successfully treated with oral doses of ivermectin (200 μg/kg), moxidectin (adults horses only, 400 μg/kg), thiabendazole (44 mg/kg/day twice), or levamisole (10 mg/kg).

Benzimidazole anthelminthic agents inhibit microtubule formation, which impairs the parasites ability to move and ingest food. Energy metabolism is also impaired due to the inhibition of fumarate reductase.[4] Although many benzimidazoles are efficacious against intestinal larvae, they are not uniformly effective at killing migrating parasite larvae; however, at higher doses fenbendazole is safe and effective at killing intestinal and tissue larvae. Anecdotal and personal observations have suggested this anthelminthic to be highly effective, particularly in cases where ivermectin resistance is suspected.

Pyrantel pamoate is an acetylcholine agonist that results in parasite paralysis.[137] At the recommended dose, this agent is effective at killing intestinal larvae but not migrating larvae.[4,136] Avermectins are effective due to their ability to bind glutamate-gated chloride channels and this class is effective against both *P. equorum* and *D. arnfieldi* adults and migrating larvae. Ivermectin has a reported efficacy of 76.9% for removal of intestinal *P. equorum* and 100% effective for removal of pneumonic larvae.[4,46] Overall, ivermectin and moxidectin have similar efficacy as effective anthelminthics in horses for many gastrointestinal parasites other than *Anoplocephala perfoliata*.[138] Based on these reports regarding anthelminthic efficacy, recommendations include combining therapeutic agents to maintain maximal efficacy. Initial treatment with fenbendazole (10 mg/kg PO daily for 5 days) followed in 14 days with an avermectin product at the appropriate dose should clear the individual of both intestinal and pneumonic parasites.

Prognosis

Foals or adult horses with primary parasitic pneumonia and secondary bacterial infection will require concurrent antibiotic and anthelminthic therapy. The prognosis is excellent for recovery from parasitic pneumonitis. It is important to emphasize the need for complete deworming, including donkeys and mules because they harbor the adult *Dictyocaulus* parasites that serve as a source for parasite contamination to horses in the immediate environment.

Guttural Pouch

David E. Freeman and Joanne Hardy

Guttural pouches are paired extensions of the eustachian tubes that connect the pharynx to the middle ear.[139] They are found in perissodactyls such as equids, tapirs, some species of rhinoceros (except the white rhinoceros), some bats, a South American forest mouse, and hyraxes.[140-142]

Anatomy

The guttural pouches are separated from each other on the midline by the rectus capitis ventralis and the longus capitis muscles and the median septum.[139] Each pouch is in close contact rostrally with the basisphenoid bone; ventrally with the retropharyngeal lymph nodes, pharynx, and esophagus; caudally with the atlanto-occipital joint; laterally with the digastricus muscle and the parotid and mandibular salivary glands; and dorsally with the petrous part of the temporal bone, tympanic bulla, and auditory meatus. Each guttural pouch is divided ventrally into a medial and a lateral compartment by the stylohyoid bone, and it communicates with the pharynx through the pharyngeal orifice of the eustachian tube. The pharyngeal orifice is a funnel-shaped opening in the dorsolateral aspect of the pharynx that forms an oblique slit, rostral and ventral to the dorsal pharyngeal recess. The small end of the funnel opens into the guttural pouch. The medial lamina of each opening is composed of fibrocartilage directed in a rostroventral-to-caudodorsal direction. The capacity of guttural pouches in adult horses is 472 ± 12.4 mL, and the lateral compartment is approximately one third of the capacity of the medial compartment.[143]

Pathogenesis

Clinical signs of important guttural pouch diseases are referable to injury of specific nerves and arteries in the guttural pouch and acoustic system. The internal carotid artery (ICA), cranial cervical ganglion, cervical sympathetic trunk, and the vagus, glossopharyngeal, hypoglossal, and spinal accessory nerves are all contained in a fold of mucous membrane along the caudal wall of the medial compartment[139] (Fig. 1-12). The cranial laryngeal nerve and the pharyngeal branch of the vagus nerve lie beneath the mucosa on the floor of the medial compartment. The external carotid artery (ECA) lies along the wall of the

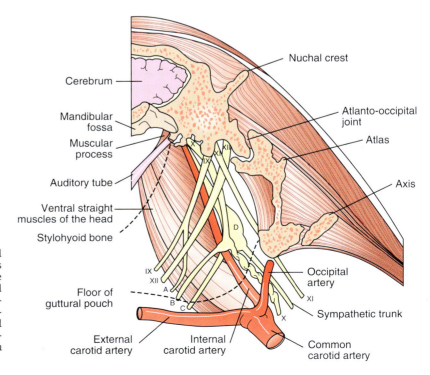

Figure 1-12 Interior of medial compartment of left guttural pouch viewed from lateral aspect in sagittal section of a horse's head. The section is cut through the styloid process of the petrous temporal bone on a line that divides the guttural pouch into medial and lateral compartments. *IX*, Glossopharyngeal nerve; *X*, vagus nerve; *XI*, accessory nerve; *XII*, hypoglossal nerve; *A*, pharyngeal branch of glossopharyngeal nerve; *B*, pharyngeal branch of vagus nerve; *C*, cranial laryngeal nerve; *D*, cranial cervical ganglion. *(Redrawn from Freeman DE, Donawick WJ: J Am Vet Med Assoc 176:236, 1980.)*

Cerebrum
Nuchal crest
Mandibular fossa
Atlanto-occipital joint
Muscular process
Atlas
Auditory tube
Axis
Ventral straight muscles of the head
Stylohyoid bone
Floor of guttural pouch
Occipital artery
External carotid artery
Internal carotid artery
Sympathetic trunk
Common carotid artery

lateral compartment and gives off the caudal auricular artery and superficial temporal artery, and it continues as the maxillary artery (MA) along the roof of the guttural pouch. The facial nerve (CN VII) passes for a short distance over the caudodorsal aspect of the lateral compartment after it emerges from the stylomastoid foramen. The vestibulocochlear nerve (CN VIII) enters the internal acoustic meatus caudal to the facial nerve and divides into vestibular and cochlear branches that innervate components of the middle ear. CN VIII does not enter the guttural pouch but can become involved in guttural pouch diseases that affect the middle ear (e.g., temporohyoid osteoarthropathy). The mandibular nerve, a branch of the trigeminal nerve (CN V), emerges from the foramen lacerum, passes close to the muscular process of the petrous part of the temporal bone, and continues rostrally along the roof of the lateral compartment of the guttural pouch.

The guttural pouch is lined with pseudostratified ciliated epithelium containing goblet cells[139] in both adults and foals.[144] The guttural pouch mucosa has the ability to clear foreign substances, but this ability varies among different regions of the epithelium.[144] In a study on the distribution of various immunoglobulin (Ig) isotypes and subisotypes in the guttural pouch mucosa of healthy horses, IgGa was found in the guttural pouch mucosa, mucosal lymph nodules, and submucosal lymph nodules.[145] IgM was scattered in the mucosal lymph nodules and in the germinal centers of the submucosal lymph nodules. The Ig previously referred to as subisotype IgGc (IgG5)[146] was recognized only in the submucosal lymph nodules, and IgA was detected in glandular epithelial cells and the surface layer of the mucosal epithelium.

Possible functions of the guttural pouches include pressure equilibration across the tympanic membrane, contribution to air warming, a resonating chamber for vocalization, and a flotation device.[147] A more recently proposed role is brain cooling, based on measurement of lower arterial temperatures in the cerebral side of the ICA compared with the cardiac side.[148,149] As shown by cadaver studies, opening of the pharyngeal orifice of the guttural pouch involves the levator and tensor veli palatini muscles and the pterygopharyngeus and palatopharyngeus muscles. Passive opening of the auditory tube involves a reduced tone in the stylopharyngeus and pterygopharyngeus muscles, accompanied by increased inspiratory pressure.[150] Although guttural pouch filling was previously reported to occur on expiration, the latter study demonstrated that filling occurs on inspiration.[150]

Clinical Examination

External palpation, endoscopy, and radiography are used to examine the guttural pouches. Enlargement caused by empyema (purulent material in the pouches), but particularly by tympany (air engorgement), can be palpated externally. Guttural pouch endoscopy provides the most information regarding guttural pouch disease. Nonspecific evidence of guttural pouch disease, such as collapse of the pharynx and blood or pus draining from the pharyngeal orifice, can be found on endoscopic examination of the pharynx. However, blood or pus from other respiratory sources may be aspirated into the guttural pouch opening and appear to drain from it, so that direct endoscopic examination of the pouches must be performed (Fig. 1-13). With the horse mildly sedated, the biopsy instrument is passed through the biopsy channel of the endoscope and used to guide the endoscope into the guttural pouch. The endoscope is placed so that the biopsy forceps is as close as possible to the lateral wall of the pharynx until successful insertion into the guttural pouch is achieved. Both pouches can be entered in this manner with the endoscope in the same nostril. Alternatively, the pharyngeal opening can be levered

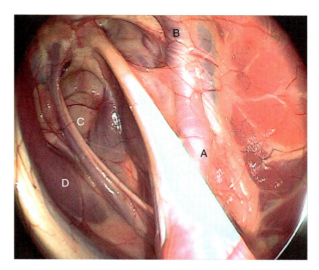

Figure 1-13 Normal endoscopic anatomy of left guttural pouch. The narrow, pale structure that runs from dorsal to ventral is the stylohyoid bone that divides the caudoventral part into lateral (to right) and medial (to left) compartments. Sources of hemorrhage from guttural pouch: *A,* external carotid artery; *B,* maxillary artery; *C,* internal carotid artery; *D,* ventral straight muscles. *(From Freeman DE, Hardy J: Guttural pouch. In Auer JA, Stick JA, editors: Equine surgery, ed 3, St Louis, 2006, Elsevier, p 592.)*

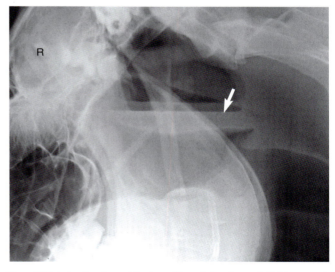

Figure 1-14 Lateral radiographic view of horse's head reveals fluid accumulation in guttural pouches *(arrow)* caused by bilateral guttural pouch empyema.

open with a Chamber's catheter to allow the endoscope to enter the pouches.

Lateral radiographic projections of the guttural pouches can demonstrate fluid lines, fractures and exostoses of the stylohyoid bone, radiopaque foreign bodies, and space-occupying masses[151] (Fig. 1-14). Air distention, as in tympany, can increase dimensions of the affected guttural pouch, sometimes beyond the second cervical vertebra. A dorsoventral or ventrodorsal projection is best used to image the stylohyoid bones and temporohyoid articulation. Computed tomography can provide an alternate imaging modality,[152-155] especially for imaging of the stylohyoid bone, inner ear, and petrous temporal bone in cases of temporohyoid osteoarthropathy.[155] Ultrasonography can be used to demonstrate soft tissue lesions in the guttural pouches

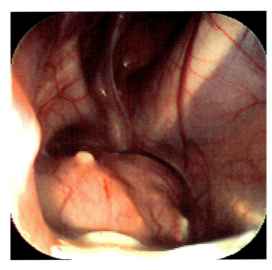

Figure 1-15 Endoscopic view of interior of right guttural pouch of horse with enlargement and drainage from retropharyngeal lymph node on floor of medial compartment. Note purulent material on floor of the medial compartment. *(From Freeman DE, Hardy J: Guttural pouch. In Auer JA, Stick JA, editors: Equine surgery, ed 3, St Louis, 2006, Elsevier, p 594.)*

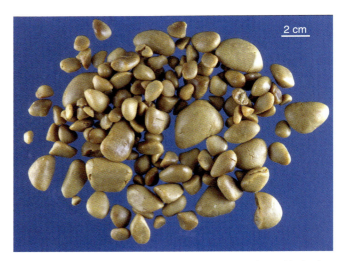

Figure 1-16 Guttural pouch chondroids removed through modified White-house approach. *(From Freeman DE, Hardy J: Guttural pouch. In Auer JA, Stick JA, editors: Equine surgery, ed 3, St Louis, 2006, Elsevier, p 594.)*

such as tumors[156] or muscle damage and associated submucosal hemorrhage.[157]

A percutaneous centesis technique through Viborg's triangle has been described for guttural pouch lavage and collection of samples for cytologic and microbiologic examinations.[158] The normal cytologic pattern is less than 5% neutrophils, a large proportion of ciliated columnar epithelial cells, a few nonciliated cuboidal epithelial cells, and less than 1% monocytes, lymphocytes, and eosinophils. The proportion of neutrophils is important, with less than 5% considered normal and greater than 25% considered abnormal. A high correlation exists between high cytologic score and presence of pathogenic bacteria such as *S. equi* subsp. *equi*.[159,160] The cytologic gradings and neutrophil concentrations of guttural pouch washings are increased in horses whose heads are restrained for more than 12 hours such as during long distance transport. Washings from these horses are more likely to contain bacteria and yield potentially pathogenic bacteria.[161]

Empyema

Empyema of the guttural pouches is defined as the presence of purulent material (Fig. 1-15) or chondroids within one or both guttural pouches. Chondroids consist of inspissated purulent material in the form of numerous individual balls of varying shapes and sizes (Fig. 1-16). Empyema can affect horses of any age but is more common in young animals.

Etiology

Causes of empyema are numerous and include upper respiratory tract infections (especially those caused by *Streptococcus*), abscessation and rupture of retropharyngeal lymph nodes into the guttural pouch, infusion of irritant drugs, fracture of the stylohyoid bone, congenital or acquired stenosis of the pharyngeal orifice, and pharyngeal perforation by a nasogastric tube.[149,150,163] Persistence of guttural pouch infection in unsuspected long-term carriers could be responsible for recurrent outbreaks of strangles.[164]

Clinical Findings

Clinical signs of guttural pouch empyema include intermittent nasal discharge, swelling of adjacent lymph nodes, parotid swelling and pain, extended head carriage, excessive respiratory noise, and difficulties in swallowing and breathing. In rare cases, guttural pouch empyema can cause pharyngeal and laryngeal paresis.[165] In one study of 91 horses with guttural pouch empyema, 21% had chondroids, and the horses with chondroids were more likely to have retropharyngeal and pharyngeal swelling than those without this complication.[166] The number of chondroids present is variable, ranging from one to many, and both guttural pouches can be affected. Duration of infection does not appear to correlate with development of chondroids.

Diagnosis

Purulent discharge can be seen at the pharyngeal orifice of the affected side on endoscopic examination, with pharyngeal collapse in some horses. Fluid accompanied by masses seen within the guttural pouch on standing lateral radiographs suggests chondroids.[167] Fluid aspirates or saline washings can be obtained from the guttural pouch for culture and sensitivity testing; however, results should be interpreted with caution because microorganisms can be retrieved from the normal guttural pouch and upper respiratory tract. Horses that are carriers of or infected with *S. equi* subsp. *equi* in the guttural pouches can be identified by culture and PCR tests with repeated swabs[168] (see Chapter 28).

Medical Therapy

Daily irrigation with physiologic saline solution is usually effective in acute cases. An indwelling catheter, devised from polyethylene 240 tubing with heat-formed coils at one end, can be used for this purpose. Alternatively, a commercially available guttural pouch catheter (Cook Veterinary Projects, Bloomington, IN; Mila International, Florence, KY) or one made from a polypropylene canine urinary catheter can be used. Coiled catheters can be straightened to facilitate insertion by inserting a coaxial wire or by passage through a larger, curved catheter. The coiled end of the catheter is placed under endoscopic guidance within the pouch, and the free end is secured by a suture to the alar fold. A Foley catheter can also be used, but it should be advanced until the end is completely in the pouch because distention of the balloon within the pharyngeal opening could cause pressure necrosis. In larger horses, standard Foley catheters are not long enough to reach the guttural pouch. Delivery of large volumes of fluid under pressure through large-bore tubes can provide effective lavage, but this is not recommended because of the risk of rupturing the lining of the guttural pouch and forcing the infection into inaccessible tissue planes.[169,170] Alternatively, the pouch can be flushed through the biopsy channel of the endoscope, which has the advantage of delivery of the flush solution to areas coated with purulent material. After 7 to 10 days, irrigation should be interrupted briefly to assess the response, with the awareness that this treatment can cause some inflammation.

In horses that are severely dyspneic because of guttural pouch distention, a tracheotomy should be performed. If the response to medical treatment is poor or if the purulent material becomes inspissated or forms chondroids, surgical drainage of the guttural pouch should be considered (see later discussion). Chondroids can also be removed by maceration, followed by saline lavage or extraction by endoscopically guided grabbing forceps, a basket snare, or a memory-helical polyp retrieval basket (Cook, Bloomington, IN).[168] Another technique involves repeated section of each mass by a diathermic snare (Olympus Optical, Irving, TX) or a wire loop, with removal by suction, lavage, or extraction by basket-type endoscopic forceps (Gomco Equipment, Chemetron Medical Products, Buffalo, NY).[171] In one study, 44% of horses with chondroids were treated successfully by these noninvasive methods,[153] although these methods can be tedious and slow. If empyema is the result of occlusion of guttural pouch openings by adhesions, this occlusion may be relieved by blunt division through a surgical approach to the guttural pouch interior.[168] Chronic empyema of the guttural pouches that does not respond to medical therapy because of poor drainage through the pharyngeal ostia can be successfully treated by using a laser to establish a permanent pharyngeal fistula into the guttural pouch.[172]

If only one guttural pouch is affected, the medial septum can be fenestrated by laser to allow removal of chondroids and pus through the healthy guttural pouch.[173] Response to medical treatment is usually satisfactory, and surgery is rarely indicated. Neurologic signs usually resolve once the infection is brought under control by medical or surgical treatment.

Surgical Therapy

Surgery of the guttural pouch through any approach should be a last resort because of risks of iatrogenic nerve damage. Identification of the guttural pouch lining and underlying nerves is difficult, especially in horses in which there is no distention, and can be facilitated by a lighted endoscope inserted into the medial compartment. A fixed structure, such as the stylohyoid bone, should be used as a guide for deep dissection. The mucosa should not be incised with sharp instruments, and retractors should be applied with care to avoid nerve damage. Because all approaches enter the pouch cavity in the same approximate area, none provides less risk of nerve damage than the others. Several approaches can be used to open the guttural pouch for removal of pus, mycotic plaques, and foreign bodies and to establish drainage. These include hyovertebrotomy, approach through Viborg's triangle (tendon of sternocephalicus muscle, linguofacial vein, vertical ramus of mandible), Whitehouse approach, modified Whitehouse approach, and a modified Garm's technique.[174] Advantages of both Whitehouse approaches are direct access to the roof of the guttural pouch, digital access to the lateral compartment, excellent ventral drainage, and simultaneous access through the septum to both pouches. Although both approaches involve deep dissection, they do not appear to have a higher rate of complications than other approaches. The modified Whitehouse approach is also suitable as a standing procedure for removal of chondroids.[169]

Open incisions in the guttural pouch are cleaned daily, and the guttural pouch cavity should be flushed daily with a nonirritating solution. Open incisions close spontaneously within

14 days, and the infection should also resolve within this time. Postoperative antibiotics can be given.

Guttural Pouch Mycosis

Etiology

Guttural pouch mycosis is usually unilateral, but rarely it may affect both pouches. There is no apparent age, gender, breed, or geographic predisposition to this disease. The cause of guttural pouch mycosis is unknown, although *Aspergillus* spp. can frequently be identified in the lesion. *Aspergillus fumigatus* is the most common isolate and can be identified more readily in direct examination of biopsies than by culture.[175] The typical lesion of guttural pouch mycosis is a diphtheritic membrane of variable size, composed of necrotic tissue, cell debris, a variety of bacteria, and fungal mycelia.[162] Aneurysm formation does not appear to precede or follow arterial invasion consistently and therefore is not essential to the pathogenesis of arterial rupture.

Clinical Findings

The most common clinical sign of guttural pouch mycosis is moderate to severe epistaxis, which is caused by fungal erosion of the ICA in most cases[176-179] (Fig. 1-17) and of the ECA and MA in approximately one third of cases[180,181] (Fig. 1-18). However, any branch of the ECA, such as the caudal auricular artery, can be affected. Several bouts of hemorrhage usually precede a fatal episode. Mucus and dark blood continue to drain from the nostril on the affected side for days after acute hemorrhage ceases.

Dysphagia is the second most common clinical sign and is caused by damage to the pharyngeal branches of the vagus and glossopharyngeal nerves.[171] Aspiration pneumonia may develop in severe or protracted cases. Abnormal respiratory noise can arise from pharyngeal paresis or from laryngeal hemiplegia, which results from recurrent laryngeal nerve damage.[171] Horner's syndrome may develop from damage to the cranial cervical ganglion and postganglionic sympathetic fibers. The classic signs associated with this denervation are ptosis, miosis, and enophthalmos; patchy sweating; and congestion of the nasal mucosa. The reason equine sweat glands increase their activity when

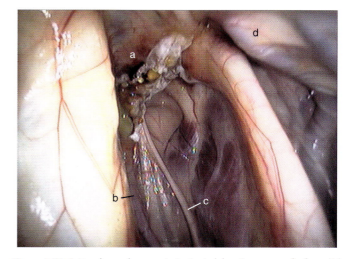

Figure 1-17 Guttural pouch mycosis in typical location on roof of medial compartment (left guttural pouch), overlying internal carotid artery. *a,* Lesion; *b,* internal carotid artery; *c,* mucosal reflection that contains glossopharyngeal and hypoglossal nerves; *d,* maxillary artery lateral to stylohyoid bone. This small lesion did not cause epistaxis but did cause dysphagia that necessitated euthanasia. *(From Freeman DE, Hardy J: Guttural pouch. In Auer JA, Stick JA, editors: Equine surgery, ed 3, St Louis, 2006, Elsevier, p 596.)*

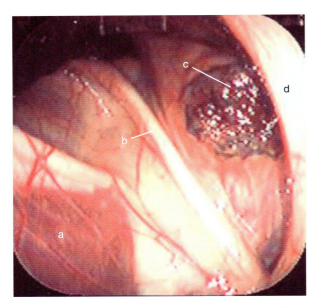

Figure 1-18 Roof of left guttural pouch as viewed through retroflexion of endoscope. *a,* Insertion of ventral straight muscles of head; *b,* cartilaginous flap of eustachian tube; *c,* mycotic lesion on left maxillary artery; *d,* dorsal edge of stylohyoid bone. This approach provides an excellent view of these structures when the rostral end of the guttural pouch is obscured with hemorrhage. *(From Freeman DE, Hardy J: Guttural pouch. In Auer JA, Stick JA, editors: Equine surgery, ed 3, St Louis, 2006, Elsevier, p 596.)*

denervated is unclear.[182] Equine sweat gland myoepithelium is predominantly under α_2-adrenergic control, with additional α-adrenergic input from receptors. However, sweating after neurectomy may be caused by increased peripheral vasodilation, which increases blood flow and skin temperature. Ptosis is caused by a decreased tone of the superior tarsus muscle, and it is assessed by observing eyelash angles from a frontal view. Pupillary response to decreased sympathetic tone in horses is variable, and the maximal difference in pupil size is usually slight. Enophthalmos, which is the result of decreased smooth muscle retrobulbar tone and unopposed activity of the striated retractor bulbi muscle, is rarely obvious and usually evident as a slight protrusion of the nictitating membrane.[182]

Less common signs of guttural pouch mycosis are parotid pain, nasal discharge, abnormal head posture, head shyness, sweating and shivering, corneal ulcers, colic, blindness, locomotion disturbances, facial nerve paralysis, paralysis of the tongue, and septic arthritis of the atlanto-occipital joint.[176,177,183-186]

Diagnosis

Diagnosis of guttural pouch mycosis should be based on history and clinical signs, with endoscopy of the guttural pouch providing definitive confirmation. On endoscopic examination of a horse with epistaxis, blood can be seen draining from the pharyngeal orifice. In horses with dysphagia the roof of the pharynx can be collapsed, the soft palate can be displaced, and the nasopharynx may contain food material. The typical lesion appears as a white, tan, and black diphtheritic membrane on the roof of the affected guttural pouch, and its size can vary but bears no relationship to the severity of clinical signs. Part of the diphtheritic membrane can coat the stylohyoid bone and the bone can be thickened, but clinical signs usually do not develop from this change. Fistulas may form into the opposite guttural pouch and pharynx.[179] The presence of serum antibodies to *Aspergillus fumigatus* detected by ELISA cannot distinguish between horses with guttural pouch mycosis and healthy horses.[187]

Medical Therapy

The response to topical treatment is generally slow and inconsistent. Daily direct lavage through the endoscope can macerate the diphtheritic membrane, and the biopsy forceps or cytology brush of the endoscope can be used to detach it, provided any eroded artery was occluded beforehand. Topical povidone-iodine or thiabendazole, with or without dimethyl sulfoxide, has been used with mixed results.[179,180,183,188,189] Nystatin, natamycin, and miconazole have little activity against *Aspergillus,*[171] but amphotericin B is effective against this organism, although its use in the horse is limited by its toxicity.[190] Topical antifungal medication can be effectively delivered to the lesion on the roof of the guttural pouch by transendoscopic infusion of a liquid or by insufflating a powder through a Neilson catheter using an enema syringe.[191]

Successful treatment of dysphagia from guttural pouch mycosis has been reported with a combination of oral itraconazole (5 mg/kg) and topical enilconazole (60 mL of 33.3 mg/mL solution per daily flush) in one horse[188] and with topical enilconazole alone in another.[192] Itraconazole 3 mg/kg twice a day in the feed can be effective against *Aspergillus* and other fungi in the nasal passage of horses, but treatment may be required for up to 4 or 5 months.[193] Bioavailability of another triazole antifungal agent, fluconazole, can be sufficiently high after oral and IV administration in horses to suggest a potential value in treatment of fungal infections.[194] The response to any treatment method that is measured solely by disappearance of the mycotic lesion should be interpreted with caution because spontaneous regression of the lesion over a variable time course is typical. Horses with blood loss should be treated with polyionic fluids and, if necessary, with blood transfusions, and horses with dysphagia should be fed by nasogastric tube or by esophagostomy and should receive nonsteroidal antiinflammatory drugs (NSAIDs) to reduce neuritis.

Surgical Therapy

The diphtheritic membrane can be detached by gentle swabbing and lavage through a modified Whitehouse approach. This treatment does not eliminate the risk of hemorrhage completely, it does not affect progression of neurologic signs, and it does carry the risk of iatrogenic nerve damage and hemorrhage. In horses with epistaxis the affected artery should be identified by endoscopy and surgically occluded. Anecdotal but widely accepted evidence indicates that occlusion of the affected artery hastens spontaneous resolution of the mycotic lesion and thereby renders medical therapy unnecessary.[195] However, this is unproved and at least one report would appear to refute this claim.[196]

Fatal hemorrhage from guttural pouch mycosis can be prevented by occluding the involved artery or arteries as soon as the diagnosis is made. The vessel to be occluded is determined by endoscopy. If accurate identification is impossible because landmarks are obscured by blood and diphtheritic membrane, all arteries in the pouch should be occluded.[181] Arteriography may be used to identify the affected vessel and to identify unusual anatomy. It is not required in all methods or in all cases; however, it does allow more precise and selective occlusion.[197]

In horses with guttural pouch mycosis, fatal or severe hemorrhage has followed ligation of the affected ICA and could be attributed to occlusion of the wrong vessel or to retrograde flow from the cerebral arterial circle (circle of Willis).[176,178,198,199] Ligation of the ipsilateral common carotid artery (CCA) in a horse bleeding from the ICA would increase flow in the affected artery and would be contraindicated.[200] However, the same procedure may provide some immediate benefit in horses bleeding from the ECA and its branches, although any such benefit could be temporary. Ligation of the affected ICA would decrease flow but not pressure, so bleeding could persist or recur.[201] However, if access to definitive occlusion procedures is not immediate during a severe bleeding crisis, induction of general anesthesia to quiet the horse and ligation of the affected ICA could be attempted as temporary measures.

Success with ICA ligation can be attributed to thrombosis extending distal to the ligature to occlude the arterial wall defect at some time after surgery.[176,178] To prevent backflow, an additional ligature has been placed distal to the mycotic infection[199]; however, this is difficult because the artery must be ligated deep within the guttural pouch, where it and adjacent critical nerves are difficult to see and likely to be obscured by the diphtheritic membrane. The site for ligation of the ICA is immediately distal to its origin, outside the guttural pouch, using a similar but more ventral approach than for a hyovertebrotomy. The ICA is identified on the cardiac side of the occipital artery and deep to that vessel. In some horses, both arteries arise as a single trunk. If necessary, both ICAs can be ligated simultaneously without any apparent risk.[178,198]

The ECA can be ligated distal to the origin of the linguofacial trunk through an incision similar to that used for the ICA ligation but after extensive rostral dissection.[180] However, this procedure is generally unsuccessful because the ECA and MA have numerous collateral channels that allow retrograde flow to the affected segment.[139,181] Although ligation of the major palatine artery could prevent retrograde flow, a combination of this procedure with ligation of the ECA and ICA can cause ischemic optic neuropathy and permanent blindness.[202]

The balloon catheter technique is preferable to ligation because it allows immediate intravascular occlusion of the artery and prevents retrograde flow from the cerebral arterial circle.[179,203] Risk of retrograde flow through an arterial defect is not diminished immediately by ligation alone because this does not decrease blood pressure in the distal segment of artery.[202] Complications associated with balloon catheter occlusion are rare[162,182] and usually arise from inappropriate placement. Failure to prevent fatal hemorrhage in one case was caused by inadvertent catheterization and occlusion of an aberrant branch from the ICA, which left the affected segment of artery open to retrograde blood flow.[204] To prevent this mishap, approximately 6 cm of the ICA should be exposed to locate any aberrant branch. Such a branch should be ligated so that the catheter can be maintained in the ICA.[202] The catheter rarely penetrates the defect in the artery, and if it does, it can be withdrawn and redirected. Incisional infection can be resolved by removal of the catheter.

Balloon occlusion of the MA combined with ligation or balloon occlusion of the ECA is more effective than ligation of the ECA only. In addition, blindness associated with ECA ligation (resulting in loss of flow to ophthalmic branch of MA) does not occur when the ECA and MA are occluded.[139,181,202,205] However, the owner should still be warned of the risk of blindness.

A detachable, self-sealing latex balloon can be used to occlude the ICA successfully,[206] without the need for catheter removal, as required in some patients treated with the nondetachable balloons. Combined with angiography, the detachable system can also be used to occlude aberrant vessels that originate at a distance from the origin of the ICA.[207]

A transarterial coil embolization technique can selectively occlude the arterial segments involved in a mycotic lesion in horses with guttural pouch mycosis.[208-211] The coil embolization technique combines angiographic studies to image the affected vessels and identify any unusual vessels and sites of bleeding, followed by a selective embolization of the affected vessels. Compared with the balloon catheter technique, transarterial coil embolization allows visualization of affected vessels throughout the procedure because it is performed under fluoroscopic guidance.[208] This is critical because aberrant vasculature has been described in horses with guttural pouch mycosis, and failure to identify and occlude such aberrant branches may result in fatal hemorrhage.[204,212] Coil embolization is less invasive than the original balloon catheter procedures, requires shorter anesthesia and shorter hospitalization, and can be performed during active bleeding. The surgical approach for all arteries in the guttural pouch is the CCA exposed through a single incision. Nitinol plugs have been used to occlude affected arteries in horses with guttural pouch mycosis[213] and offer advantages over transarterial coils. The disadvantages of both coils and plugs are the need for fluoroscopy (and the specialized equipment and expertise involved), positioning of the horse's head for fluoroscopy, and apparel and equipment for radiation shielding.

Prognosis

Approximately 50% of horses with hemorrhage from guttural pouch mycosis die from this complication,[177] but this risk can be eliminated or greatly reduced by appropriate occlusion procedures. These procedures must be performed as soon as possible after the first bout of hemorrhage to prevent subsequent bouts that could complicate anesthesia. Although the mycotic lesion disappears with time, neurologic signs can persist. Laryngeal hemiplegia is usually permanent, but recovery has been reported.[176] Some horses with dysphagia do eventually recover, but 6 to 18 months may be required and recovery may be incomplete.[176,177] Horses can recover from Horner's syndrome and facial nerve paralysis.

Temporohyoid Osteoarthropathy

Etiology

Temporohyoid osteoarthropathy (THO) is a progressive disease of the middle ear and temporohyoid joint that can affect the stylohyoid bone, the cartilaginous tympanohyoid, and the squamous portion of the temporal bone. Horses of a wide age range and of any breed or either gender can be affected. The most likely cause is an inner or a middle ear infection of hematogenous origin that spreads to the bones listed, causing them to thicken and the temporohyoid joint to fuse.[214] Other possible causes range from extension of otitis media/externa or guttural pouch infection to a nonseptic osteoarthritis.[214-218] Although guttural pouch mycosis can involve the same bony structures and temporohyoid articulation,[177] clinical signs of THO are uncommon with this disease. Recent histopathologic and CT evidence of bilateral age-related worsening of degenerative changes in the temporohyoid joint of normal horses suggests a degenerative rather than infectious cause for THO.[219]

Once the temporohyoid joint fuses and the associated bones thicken, forces generated by movement of the tongue and larynx during swallowing, vocalizing, combined head and neck movements, oral or dental examinations, and teeth floating may induce fractures of the petrous part of the temporal bone, resulting in facial nerve (CN VII) and vestibulocochlear nerve (CN VIII) dysfunction.[214-218,220] Severe new bone production and inflammation can damage the glossopharyngeal and vagus nerves where they leave the medulla caudal to the vestibulocochlear nerve.[139,221] After fracture of the petrous temporal bone, middle or inner ear infection could extend around the brainstem and involve additional cranial nerves and hindbrain structures.

Clinical Findings and Diagnosis

Early clinical signs include head tossing, ear rubbing, refusing to take the bit, refusing to position the head properly when saddled, resistance to digital pressure around the base of the ears or on the basihyoid bone, and other nonspecific behavior changes. The onset of signs can be acute and referable to facial

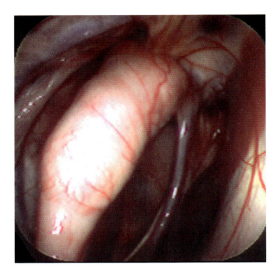

Figure 1-19 Thickened stylohyoid bone with involvement of temporohyoid articulation in horse with clinical signs of damage to vestibulocochlear and facial nerves. *(From Freeman DE, Hardy J: Guttural pouch. In Auer JA, Stick JA, editors: Equine surgery, ed 3, St Louis, 2006, Elsevier, p 599.)*

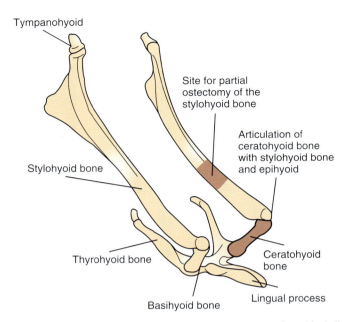

Figure 1-20 Hyoid apparatus, showing sites for ostectomy procedures *(shaded)* for horses with temporohyoid osteoarthropathy. *(From Freeman DE, Hardy J: Guttural pouch. In Auer JA, Stick JA, editors: Equine surgery, ed 3, St Louis, 2006, Elsevier, p 599.)*

and vestibulocochlear nerve deficits, including asymmetric ataxia, head tilt with the poll to the affected side, and spontaneous nystagmus with the slow component to the affected side.[214] These signs can be revealed or exacerbated by blindfolding. Signs of facial nerve damage, including paresis or paralysis of the ear on the affected side, deviation of the upper lip away from the affected side, decreased tear production, and inability to close the eyes, are evident in most cases. Decreased tear production and inability to close the eyes may cause corneal ulcers, keratoconjunctivitis sicca, and exposure keratitis.[220,221] Dysphagia is rare but can result from damage to the glossopharyngeal and vagus nerves.[214]

Radiographs of the skull may demonstrate proliferation and osteitis of the affected bones; however, endoscopy of the guttural pouch is in most cases a more sensitive method for detection of stylohyoid bone and temporohyoid joint involvement and thus for making the diagnosis[221] (Fig. 1-19). Computed tomography or MRI can precisely demonstrate bony and soft tissue changes in the middle and inner ear.[155] Computed tomography can demonstrate bilateral changes in the relevant bones in horses that have signs of unilateral disease, with more pronounced changes on the affected side.[222]

Therapy

Broad-spectrum antibiotics for infection, NSAIDs to relieve pain and inflammation, and dimethyl sulfoxide to relieve inflammation are typically used for medical treatment of THO.[193,223] Unilateral partial ostectomy of the stylohyoid bone has been used to create a pseudoarthrosis between the cut ends of the bone, which decreases the forces on the ankylosed temporohyoid and thereby prevents skull fractures[223] (Fig. 1-20). In this procedure, approximately 2 to 3 cm of the midbody of the stylohyoid bone is removed. Although this procedure appears to have merit as a prophylactic measure against more severe bone damage and associated neurologic consequences, it may cause transient dysphagia or injury to the hypoglossal nerve. When performed as a bilateral procedure, it causes permanent problems with prehension.[223]

An additional complication of partial ostectomy is regrowth of the stylohyoid bone approximately 6 months after surgical resection, with recurrence of clinical signs. Because of this complication, a ceratohyoidectomy has been recommended as a

safer, easier, and more permanent surgical alternative.[221] Although the prognosis is good according to one report,[224] neurologic signs may persist,[225] especially if treatment is delayed. In general, the prognosis for stylohyoid arthropathy depends on the severity of clinical signs. Some degree of facial and vestibulocochlear nerve paresis can persist.[147] In a recent report, 89% of horses that had a ceratohyoidectomy and 87% of those that had a partial stylohyoid ostectomy improved substantially over the first 6 months after surgery, with continued improvement for the remainder of the first year.[226] Corneal ulcers are difficult to treat because there is an underlying problem with lid closure and tear production. A temporary tarsorrhaphy may help manage the ocular complications until facial nerve function returns.

Suggested Readings

Guttural Pouch

Alexander K, Baird JD, Dobson H, et al: What is your diagnosis? J Am Vet Med Assoc 220:297, 2002.

Bayly WM, Robertson JT: Epistaxis caused by foreign body penetration of a guttural pouch. J Am Vet Med Assoc 180:1232, 1982.

Bentz BG, Dowd AL, Freeman DE: Treatment of guttural pouch empyema with acetylcysteine irrigation. Equine Pract 18:33, 1996.

Blazyczek I, Hamann H, Deegen E, et al: Retrospective analysis of 50 cases of guttural pouch tympany in foals. Vet Rec 154:261, 2004.

Blazyczek I, Hamann H, Ohnesorge B, et al: Guttural pouch tympany in German warmblood foals: influence of sex, inbreeding and blood proportions of founding breeds as well as estimation of heritability. Berl Munch Tierarztl Wochenschr 116:346, 2003.

Blazyczek I, Hamann H, Ohnesorge B, et al: Population genetic analysis of the heritability of guttural pouch tympany in Arabian purebred foals. Dtsch Tierarztl Wochenschr 110:417, 2003.

Blazyczek I, Hamann H, Ohnesorge B, et al: Inheritance of guttural pouch tympany in the Arabian horse. J Hered 95:195, 2004.

Darien BJ, Watrous BJ, Huber MJ, et al: What is your diagnosis? J Am Vet Med Assoc 198:1799, 1991.

Fintl C, Dixon PM: A review of five cases of parotid melanoma in the horse. Equine Vet Educ 13:17–24, 2001.

Greene HJ, O'Connor JP: Hemangioma of the guttural pouch of a 16-year-old Thoroughbred mare: clinical and pathological findings. Vet Rec 118:445, 1986.

Hance SR, Robertson JT, Bukowiecki CF: Cystic structures in the guttural pouch (auditory tube diverticulum) of two horses. J Am Vet Med Assoc 200:1981, 1992.

Harvey SC: Antiseptics and disinfectants; fungicides; ectoparasiticides. In Gilman A, Goodman LS, Rall TW, et al, editors: Goodman and Gilman's the pharmacological basis of therapeutics, New York, 1985, Macmillan.

May KA, Howard RD: Exercise intolerance secondary to parotid melanomas in a mare. Equine Vet Educ 13:195–197, 2001.

McConnico RS, Blas-Machado U, Cooper VL, et al: Bilateral squamous cell carcinoma of the guttural pouches and the left middle ear in a horse. Equine Vet Educ 13:175–178, 2001.

McCue PM, Freeman DE, Donawick WJ: Guttural pouch tympany: 15 cases (1977-1986). J Am Vet Med Assoc 194:1761, 1989.

Merriam JG: Guttural pouch fibroma in a mare. J Am Vet Med Assoc 161:487, 1972.

Milne DW, Fessler JR: Tympanitis of the guttural pouch in a foal. J Am Vet Med Assoc 161:61, 1972.

Moulton JE, editor: Tumors in domestic animals, Los Angeles, 1978, University of California Press.

Raker CW: The nasopharynx. In Mannsmann RA, McAllister ES, editors: Equine medicine and surgery, ed 3, Santa Barbara, CA, 1982, American Veterinary Publications.

Sullins KE: Endoscopic application of cutting current for upper respiratory surgery in the standing horse. Proc Am Assoc Equine Pract 36:439, 1990.

Tate LP, Blikslager AT, Little ED: Transendoscopic laser treatment of guttural pouch tympanites in eight foals. Vet Surg 24:367, 1995.

Tetens J, Tulleners EP, Ross MW, et al: Transendoscopic contact neodymium:yttrium aluminum garnet laser treatment of tympany of the auditory tube diverticulum in two foals. J Am Vet Med Assoc 204:1927, 1994.

Trigo RJ, Nickels FA: Squamous cell carcinoma of a horse's guttural pouch. Mod Vet Pract 62:456, 1981.

The complete reference list is available online at www.expert-consult.com.

CHAPTER

2

Cardiovascular Infections

Celia M. Marr

All components of the cardiovascular system, from cardiac tissues to blood vessels, are susceptible to infection. Fortunately, these conditions are relatively uncommon in the horse, but they can be devastating when they occur. Viral or bacterial infection can also act as a trigger for immune-mediated disorders such as pericarditis and myocarditis. Fever is a common clinical feature of cardiovascular infections, and localizing signs will vary, depending on the site of infection. In general, successful treatment relies on appropriate antimicrobial therapy. In many cases, however, systemic inflammatory response syndrome (SIRS) is a prominent feature (see Chapter 11), and supportive therapy is important and challenging in these severely compromised individuals.

Infective Endocarditis

Etiology and Pathogenesis

Infective endocarditis (IE) is an uncommon but frequently fatal disorder in horses. Endocardial lesions have been reported in association with a wide range of microorganisms. *Borrelia burgdorferi*,[1] *Shigella equirulis*,[2] *Actinobacillus equuli* subsp. *equlli*,[3-6] *Pasteurella caballi*,[7] *Pasteurella/Actinobacillus* spp.,[8,9] *Pseudomonas* spp.,[10,11] *Escherichia coli*,[8,12] *Corynebacterium* spp.,[8] *Bacillus* spp.,[8] *Serratia marcescens*,[13] *Erysipelothrix rhusiopathiae*,[14] coagulase-positive *Staphylococcus* spp.,[15] α-hemolytic[8] and β-hemolytic[16] *Streptococcus* spp., *Streptococcus equi* subsp. *equi*,[17] and *Klebsiella* spp.[18] are reported as causes of IE in horses, with no one organism emerging as distinctly more prevalent than the others. Fungal IE has been attributed to *Aspergillus* species in a horse with disseminated aspergillosis affecting the lungs, intestine, and peritoneal cavity, as well as the mitral valve and left ventricular wall.[19] In another report, *Candida* species affected the aortic valve and right atrial wall in an 11-year-old Thoroughbred.[10]

In many cases of IE the causative microorganisms cannot be determined. Analysis of 34 cases published between 1980 and 2002 together with a further 6 cases seen at the author's clinic has demonstrated that neither blood nor postmortem cultures allowed identification of a causative organism in 7 of 32 horses (22%; CI 7.6%-36.2%) in which culture was attempted.[8,10,20,21] *Pasteurella/Actinobacillus* spp. (six cases, 18.8%; 95% confidence intervals [CI] 5.2%-32.3%) and *Pseudomonas* spp. (three cases, 9.4%; CI 0%-19.5%) occur more than once in this series, whereas the other organisms were each identified in one case only. *Rhodococcus equi* was isolated from synovial and bony material removed surgically from a foal with septic osteoarthritis and mural IE, but blood culture from that foal yielded *E. coli*.[12] A blood culture from a 14-year-old mixed-breed gelding with aortic IE in the author's clinic also yielded *R. equi*. That horse had no apparent immunosuppression or other reason to have become infected with *R. equi* and recovered after 6 weeks of treatment with trimethoprim-sulfonamide and rifampin. Although not a typical skin commensal, *R. equi* may have been a contaminant introduced during the blood collection.

A combination of endothelial damage and bacteremia are prerequisites for the development of IE.[22,23] Preexisting heart disease is present in 42% to 98% of human IE patients, and 4% to 13% have congenital defects such as ventricular septal defect (VSD), with preexisting valvular regurgitation in most of the remaining patients.[24] Endothelial damage caused by the effects of high-velocity jets and turbulence leads to deposition of complexes of platelets and fibrin, which in turn are susceptible to colonization by bacteria or fungi during bacteremia or fungemia.[22,23] In horses the structures on the left side of the heart are most likely to be affected by IE, with the mitral valve affected slightly more often than the aortic valve, despite that preexisting valvular lesions are most likely to be present on the aortic valve[25] (Table 2-1). Mural endocarditis occurs less often in horses, possibly because an association between IE and VSD, which is an important predisposing factor in human IE, has not been identified in the horse, although this is a fairly common congenital abnormality in certain breeds, such as the Standardbred, Arabian,[26] and Welsh Mountain pony,[27] and tricuspid endocarditis has been reported in one horse with VSD.[28]

Table 2-1 Location of Lesions in 40 Cases of Infective Endocarditis*

Location	Number Affected	Prevalence (%)	Lower Confidence Limit (%)	Upper Confidence Limit (%)
Cases with Single Site Involvement				
Mitral valve only	11	27.5	13.7	41.3
Aortic valve only	9	22.5	9.6	35.4
Tricuspid valve only	5	12.5	2.3	22.7
Pulmonic valve only	1	2.5	0	7.3
Mural: left atrium	11	27.5	0	7.3
Cases with Single or Multisite Involvement				
Mitral valve	21	52.5	37.0	68.0
Aortic valve	15	37.5	22.5	52.5
Tricuspid valve	8	20.0	7.6	32.4
Pulmonic valve	2	5.0	0	11.8
Mural sites	4	10.0	0.7	19.3
"Left heart" structures	26	65.0	50.2	79.8
"Right heart" structures	7	17.5	5.7	29.3
Both sides of heart	5	12.5	2.3	22.7

*With 34 cases from references 4-17, 19, 20, 32, 34, and 35, plus 6 cases from the author's clinic.

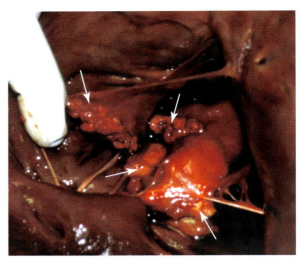

Figure 2-1 Pathologic specimen from 8-year-old Thoroughbred stallion with infective endocarditis. Ventricular surfaces of tricuspid valve are normal, but vegetations *(arrows)* are visible protruding from the atrial aspect, at the line of closure. *(Courtesy P. Ramzan, Rossdale and Partners, Newmarket, Suffolk, United Kingdom.)*

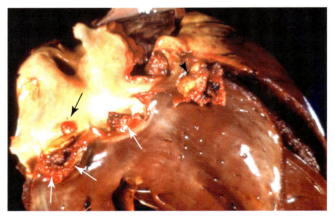

Figure 2-2 Pathologic specimen from 4-year-old Thoroughbred colt with infective endocarditis. Vegetations are attached to both the ventricular *(white arrows)* and the aortic *(black arrowhead)* aspects of the aortic valve. An additional small vegetation is attached to the intimal surface of the aorta *(black arrow)*. The tear in the left coronary cusp was created postmortem.

The portal of entry of the causative microorganism is often not apparent. In humans, potential routes include dental infection and procedures, surgery, endoscopy, intravenous (IV) catheters, drug abuse, and infection of the skin, lungs, bowel, and urinary tract.[24] No strongly established association exists between bacteremia and dental procedures in horses, but IE has occurred after dental procedures, associated with *Fusobacterium necrophorum* in one case[29] and a mixed growth of *Klebsiella* spp., gram-positive cocci and gram-positive rods in another.[18] A 13-year-old mixed-breed mare at the author's clinic had concurrent temporohyoid osteoarthropathy and guttural pouch empyema from which β-hemolytic *Streptococcus* spp. were isolated, although blood culture was negative. Septic jugular thrombophlebitis is considered a risk factor for tricuspid IE in horses. Two of eight reported cases of tricuspid IE[8] had recent jugular thrombophlebitis; a third case had an inactive thrombosis related to treatment for an unrelated condition 1 year earlier.[5] Permanent IV devices, such as transvenous pacing devices, are rarely used in horses but can predispose to IE.[30] IE has also been reported in foals with sepsis, umbilical infection,[8] and osteoarthritis,[12] but in most adult cases the route of infection remains unclear.

Once a critical mass of bacteria has been deposited on an area of damaged endothelium, vegetations consisting of platelets, fibrin, microorganisms, exopolysaccharides, inflammatory cells, and associated necrotic debris begin to develop.[31] Mitral and tricuspid vegetations typically occur on the atrial surface of the valve (Fig. 2-1), whereas aortic vegetations are more likely to develop on the ventricular surface. However, vegetations may occur on any endocardial surface, including the valve leaflets, ventricular or atrial endocardium, and the intimal surface of the great vessels[31] (Figs. 2-2 to 2-4). Vegetations usually form at the line of valve closure.[23] "Kissing lesions" develop by spreading between adjacent cusps[23,31] (Fig. 2-5). IE can extend to involve adjacent structures, such as the chordae tendineae[8,13,32] and papillary muscles,[31] or can form myocardial abscesses through metastatic infection or direct extension.[9,33,34] Infected areas may perforate, leading to defects in the septum or aorta[34] or septic pericarditis.[31] Valve cusps[35] and chordae

tendineae[8,13,32] can rupture (see Fig. 2-5), causing catastrophic regurgitation. Valve obstruction can arise due to distortion of the valve orifice or the presence of vegetative masses[36] (Fig. 2-6).

The hemodynamic consequences of IE involve the combined effects of regurgitation and SIRS. Severe mitral regurgitation results in pulmonary hypertension and pulmonary congestion and may lead to right-sided heart failure.[37] In acute cases, there may be clinical and radiographic signs of pulmonary edema. Horses that survive the initial episode of acute mitral IE may develop signs of congestive heart failure (CHF), and the resultant chronic pulmonary hypertension can lead to pulmonary artery rupture.[16] In general, aortic IE appears to be better tolerated in horses than in humans, in whom severe hemodynamic collapse occurs more often with aortic IE or myocarditis than with mitral IE.[23] Nevertheless, in equine aortic IE, signs consistent with low cardiac output, left-sided heart

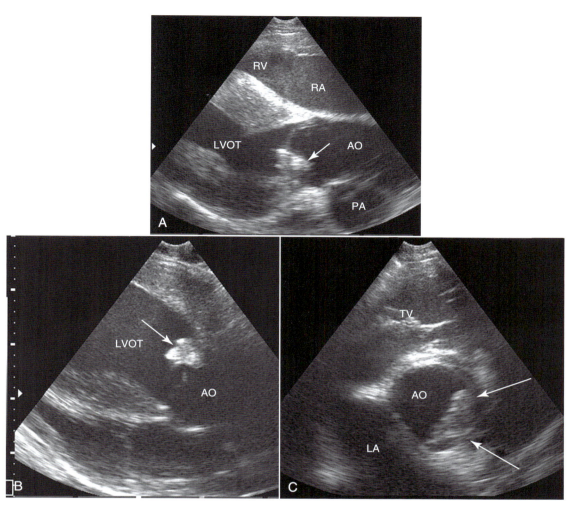

Figure 2-3 Right **(A)** and left **(B)** long-axis echocardiograms of the left ventricular outflow tract *(LVOT)* and right short-axis **(C)** echocardiogram of the ascending aorta *(AO)* from a 5-year-old Thoroughbred mare with infective endocarditis diagnosed 6 days earlier. Large, heterogenous vegetations *(arrows)* are attached to upper and lower aspects of the aortic valve and to the intimal surface of the aorta. *LA,* Left atrium; *PA,* pulmonary artery; *RA,* right atrium; *RV,* right ventricle; *TV,* tricuspid valve. *(Courtesy H Dillon, Troytown Equine Hospital, Kildare, Ireland.)*

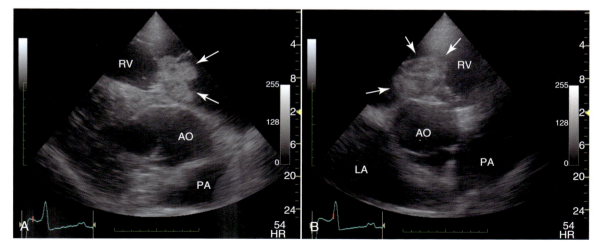

Figure 2-4 Right long- **(A)** and short-axis **(B)** echocardiograms of the tricuspid valve and left ventricular outflow tract from a cross-breed gelding with infective endocarditis. There are large, slightly heterogenous vegetations on the tricuspid valve. *AO,* Aorta; *LA,* left atrium; *PA,* pulmonary artery; *RA,* right atrium; *RV,* right ventricle.

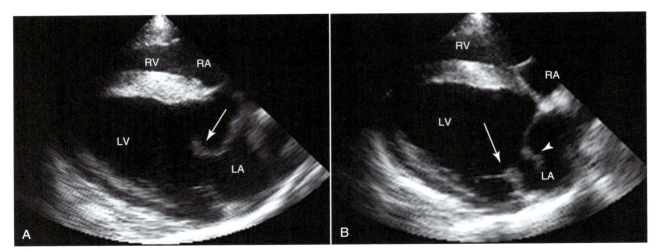

Figure 2-5 Right long-axis echocardiograms from 8-year-old polo pony gelding with infective endocarditis diagnosed 2 days earlier. Vegetations *(arrows)* are visible on adjacent aspects of the septal and nonseptal cusps of the mitral valve, and rupture of a chorda tendinea is allowing a portion of the septal cusp *(arrowhead)* to prolapse into the left atrium *(LA)*. *RA,* Right atrium; *RV,* right ventricle; *LV,* left ventricle.

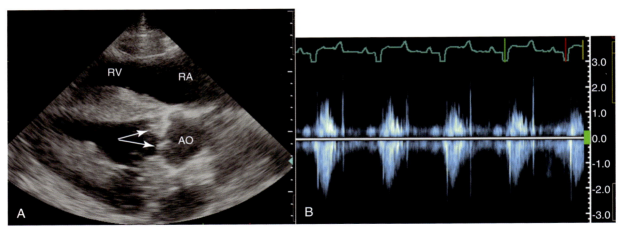

Figure 2-6 A, Right long-axis echocardiogram from a yearling Welsh Mountain pony filly with infective endocarditis. Vegetations *(arrows)* are visible on the ventricular aspect of the aortic valve. **B,** Continuous-wave Doppler echocardiography demonstrates that the velocity of blood flow through the aortic valve is very rapid, confirming that the vegetations are obstructing blood flow. *AO,* Aorta; *RA,* right atrium; *RV,* right ventricle.

failure, and CHF are reported.[21,34] Concurrent myocarditis or myocardial abscesses compromise myocardial function further, and dysrhythmias are common (Fig. 2-7). Clearly, the more extensive the left-sided valvular pathology, the more severe are the hemodynamic consequences. Regurgitation caused by tricuspid IE is likely to have less direct hemodynamic impact,[8] although systemic venous and hepatic congestion can be expected.[11]

Regardless of the site of the vegetation, bacteremia is likely to induce SIRS and, consequently, distributive shock. The self-amplifying cascade of inflammatory mediators that is triggered in SIRS dysregulates hemodynamic control mechanisms. The pathogenesis of SIRS is described in Chapter 11. In brief, widespread vasodilation produces vascular blood pooling, decreased venous return, and decreased cardiac output.[38] This is exacerbated by a direct myocardial suppression, and when these changes are superimposed on mitral or aortic insufficiency, the situation worsens synergistically.[39]

Once IE is established, in addition to valvular pathology, local infection, bacteremia, and related hemodynamic consequences, embolic complications and immunologic events contribute to disease progression.[39,40] Myocarditis results from microabscesses, coronary vasculitis, immune complex deposition, and injury from microbial toxin production.[33] Myocardial infarcts,[9,10,32] coronary artery thrombosis,[7,9] and pulmonary artery thrombosis[2,7] may further compromise cardiac function. Embolic pneumonia occurs secondary to tricuspid IE.[5,11] Testicular, adrenal, and pancreatic infarcts have been described in a horse with aortic IE and a history of testicular torsion.[21] Renal infarcts are found in two thirds of humans who succumb to IE and were present in 8 of 28 horses (28.6%; CI 11.8%-45.3%) at postmortem examination.[6,8,10,21] All of the equine cases of renal infarct involved IE in the left side of the heart; however, renal infarcts are occasionally associated with right-sided IE in humans, in whom the presumed source of emboli is thrombosed pulmonary vessels resulting from embolic pneumonia.[33]

Immunologically mediated glomerulonephritis, prerenal azotemia, and disseminated intravascular coagulation (DIC) are also potential sequelae to IE.[5,11,33] The compromised individual with IE is at increased risk of developing acute tubular nephrosis in association with use of antimicrobials such as the aminoglycosides.[33] Lameness and synovial effusion are common.

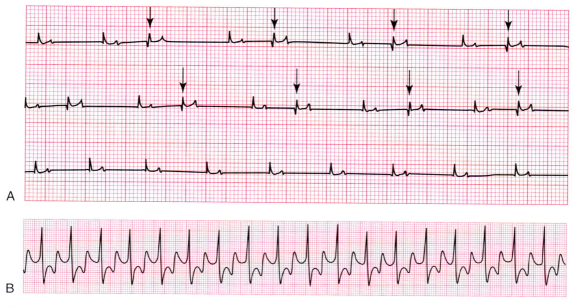

Figure 2-7 A, Electrocardiogram (ECG) from 13-year-old mixed-breed mare with aortic infective endocarditis (IE) and concurrent myocarditis diagnosed 12 weeks earlier showing numerous isolated ventricular premature depolarizations. The mare's clinical status had improved considerably since this initial diagnosis, but she continued to have episodes of distress and weakness that were attributed to a paroxysmal ventricular dysrhythmia (modified base-apex lead; see also Fig. 2-8). **B,** ECG from 5-year-old Thoroughbred mare with aortic IE diagnosed 6 days earlier showing an episode of monomorphic ventricular tachycardia that resolved after treatment with magnesium sulfate and lidocaine. One week later, 24-hour ambulatory ECG revealed normal sinus rhythm (base-apex lead; see also Fig. 2-3).

Multifocal synovial distention is generally immunologic in origin[7,13,16,20]; however, septic embolism can lead to synovial sepsis, particularly in the digital sheath.[5,15] Various forms of neuropathology occur in approximately 30% of humans with IE, about half of whom have associated clinical signs and a high mortality rate.[41] These complications are relatively rare in horses, but their prevalence may be underreported (3 of 28 reported cases, 10.7%; CI 0%-22.25%) because of the lack of large, high-quality case series. Meningeal infarcts were described in two horses with IE, one of which had neurologic signs.[8] An additional horse with mitral and aortic IE developed unilateral blindness, optic neuritis, uveitis with endophthalmitis, and multifocal suppurative meningoencephalitis in association with *Actinobacillus equuli* infection.[6]

Clinical Findings

IE appears to be a disease of younger adults,[4-20,32,34,35] but there is no apparent breed predisposition.[42] In the case series described previously the ratio of males to females is 1.85:1, which is similar to that described in humans.[26] However, a retrospective case-control study comparing nine cases of IE to other horses in which IE was included on the differential list based on clinical findings did not show any gender predisposition.[42] Fever is the most common presenting sign in horses with IE (Table 2-2). Cardiac murmurs are likely to be present in all animals with left-sided involvement but may be absent in horses with tricuspid IE.[5,8,15] In the sole reported equine case of pulmonic IE, no murmur was detected.[5,8,15] Therefore it is important to remember that absence of a cardiac murmur does not exclude a diagnosis of IE.[43] Murmurs are most likely to be absent in IE caused by a virulent microorganism that induces rapid, severe disease,[33] and interestingly, two equine reports of tricuspid IE that lacked murmurs include horses that died shortly after the onset of signs.[5,8] When present, the murmur of tricuspid regurgitation has its point of maximal intensity (PMI) over the right fourth

Table 2-2 Major Clinical Findings in 35 Cases of Infective Endocarditis*

Clinical Sign	Number Affected	Prevalence (%)	Lower Confidence Limit (%)	Upper Confidence Limit (%)
Fever and depression†	30	88.2	77.4	99.1
Cardiac murmur‡	28	87.5	76.0	99.0
Cardiac dysrhythmia	11	31.4	16.0	46.8
Ventral edema	5	14.3	2.7	25.9
Lameness	9	25.7	11.2	40.2
Joint and/or tendon sheath distention	11	31.4	16.0	46.8
Weight loss	13	37.1	21.1	53.2
Respiratory signs	7	20.0	6.7	33.3

*With 29 cases from references 4-17, 19, 20, 32, 34, and 35, plus 6 from the author's clinic.

†Not reported = 1.

‡Not reported = 3.

intercostal space and is usually holosystolic. Mitral regurgitant murmurs are also holosystolic, with their PMI over the left fifth intercostal space. Aortic regurgitant murmurs are holodiastolic, with their PMI over the left fourth intercostal space, high in the axilla. With aortic obstruction, there is a coarse crescendo-decrescendo murmur in the same location. Mitral IE and aortic IE are usually associated with very loud murmurs that radiate over a wide area. Aortic IE murmurs, as with the murmur caused by severe degenerative aortic valve disease, typically have a squeaking or buzzing quality. A mitral regurgitant murmur with a honking quality should raise the suspicion of rupture of one or more chordae tendineae.

Additional signs of cardiovascular compromise that are not specific for IE include tachycardia, weak pulses, congested or pale mucous membranes, and petechiation. Affected horses are usually depressed, lethargic, anorexic, and weak.

Cardiac dysrhythmias occur in approximately one third of horses with IE (see Table 2-2). Ventricular dysrhythmias may include isolated ventricular premature depolarizations or monomorphic or polymorphic ventricular tachycardias (see Fig. 2-7). Episodic collapse or distress can be associated with dysrhythmic episodes in both acute and chronic stages. Although no statistical association has been documented, horses with aortic IE appear to be most likely to develop ventricular dysrhythmias. In humans, these are the patients most likely to develop coronary thrombosis and myocardial microabscess.[33] Supraventricular premature depolarizations[8,12,16] and atrial fibrillation[12] may occur, particularly in horses with mitral or left-sided atrial mural IE. Signs consistent with CHF, including ventral edema, pleural and peritoneal effusion, and venous congestion, may be detected on presentation or develop as disease progresses.

Lameness is a frequent presenting complaint for horses with IE (see Table 2-2). This is often shifting in nature and may be associated with distention of one or more synovial structures.[8,13,16,20,42] IE should be considered as a potential source of hematogenous synovial sepsis.[5,15] Right-sided IE generally presents with clinical and radiographic signs relating to embolic pneumonia in humans.[43] Other clinical signs reported in horses with IE include weight loss, ataxia or other neurologic abnormalities,[42] blindness,[6] laminitis,[8] guttural pouch empyema, sinusitis,[29] umbilical infection,[32] and physitis.[12]

Diagnosis

Hematologic and blood biochemical abnormalities are not specific for IE but include leukocytosis, hyperfibrinogenemia, anemia, and less often, thrombocytopenia.[4-20,32,34,35] A case-control study comparing horses with IE with a group that presented with similar signs confirmed that hyperfibrinogenemia, leukocytosis, hypoalbuminemia, and hyperglobulinemia, but not anemia, were associated with a diagnosis of IE.[44] C-reactive protein (CRP), an acute-phase protein that increases in response to infection and inflammation, is considered particularly useful in the diagnosis of IE in humans and is used to monitor therapy.[45] Increased serum amyloid A concentrations can also be expected and may serve as a suitable alternative in horses.[5] Increases in serum concentrations of creatinine and blood urea nitrogen warrant a guarded prognosis because they may indicate renal infarct.[8,21] Measurement of cardiac troponin I[46,47] and the cardiac isoenzyme of creatine kinase (CK-MB) can be useful in identifying myocardial lesions. The half-life of cardiac troponin I is extremely short,[48] thus it is helpful in identifying acute myocardial damage, but concentrations are likely to rapidly fall and it may not be increased in the presence of chronic disease. Cardiac dysrhythmias should be characterized; ambulatory electrocardiographic (ECG) monitoring may be useful in detecting paroxysmal dysrhythmias that are not evident on a short rhythm strip.

The Duke diagnostic criteria for IE in humans, based on laboratory and echocardiographic findings, were developed to categorize patients as definite, possible, or rejected IE cases. Major criteria are (1) persistently positive blood cultures (the specific number of cultures required is defined by the specific organism in question) and (2) echocardiographic evidence of endocardial involvement. Minor criteria include (1) fever, (2) predisposition (e.g., preexisting heart condition), (3) vascular phenomenon (e.g., renal infarcts), (4) immunologic events (e.g., glomerulonephritis, positive rheumatoid factor), (5) positive blood cultures that fall short of the definitions of persistent bacteremia, and (6) suspicious but not definitive echocardiograms. Cases are rejected when (1) a firm alternative diagnosis is made, (2) the clinical signs resolve with antimicrobial therapy in 4 days or less, or (3) pathologic evidence is lacking at surgery or autopsy.[49] The Duke criteria are primarily a tool to allow comparison of patient groups in clinical research[33] but serve to emphasize the importance of blood culture and echocardiography in the diagnosis of IE. Echocardiography achieves improved sensitivity and equivalent specificity when these criteria are compared with older classification systems based on clinical and laboratory findings alone.[50-52] Similarly, in horses the majority of premortem diagnoses of IE are based on echocardiographic findings combined with laboratory findings.[6-9,11-13,15-17,20,34]

Blood culture is extremely important in the diagnostic evaluation of horses with IE because it may allow identification of a specific microorganism that will help define therapy. In IE, there is continuous bacteremia, therefore timing culture with fever spikes has no advantage. Furthermore, because of continuous bacteremia, positive results from only one of several blood cultures should be regarded with caution.[53] The optimal number of cultures is not known,[33] but recent guidelines for best practice in human IE recommend obtaining three samples at intervals greater than 6 hours before commencing antimicrobial therapy in patients with a chronic or subacute presentation. In patients with severe sepsis or septic shock at the time of presentation, two samples at different times within 1 hour before commencing antimicrobial therapy are recommended.[53] Meticulous aseptic technique is required when taking samples to avoid contamination with skin commensals, and sampling from intravascular catheters should be avoided.[53] Once a microbiologic diagnosis has been made, routine repeat blood cultures are not necessary, but blood cultures should be repeated if a patient is still febrile after 7 days of antimicrobial treatment.[53] Where possible, in addition to conventional disk diffusion antimicrobial sensitivity testing, the minimum inhibitory concentration (MIC) of candidate drugs should be evaluated for the specific organisms to aid therapeutic decision making.[53]

Prior antimicrobial therapy limits the likelihood of positive cultures.[22,50,54-56] Negative blood culture can occur with fastidious or slow-growing organisms, and these include *Streptococcus* spp., *Haemophilus* spp., *Actinobacillus* spp., *Brucella* and fungi, or intracellular organisms.[53,57] Additional reasons for negative blood culture include extended course of illness and mural endocarditis.[45] Microorganisms were identified in 13 of 20 horses (68.4%; CI 47.5%-89.3%) when one to four cultures were submitted (median of two). In these cases, samples were obtained before antimicrobial therapy was initiated in these horses at the secondary care stage of treatment, although most horses had received antimicrobial medication before admission to the secondary care. Passage of the blood sample through a device designed to remove antimicrobials before inoculation of blood onto culture media may enhance bacterial recovery rates. Cultures should be incubated for a minimum of 4 days before they are classified as negative because prior antimicrobial therapy may delay the growth of microorganisms.[22]

Because blood culture-negative endocarditis occurs in a similar proportion of human patients,[60] several nonculture methods, including genetic and serologic techniques, have been introduced and led to the recognition of a wide spectrum of causal organisms in blood culture-negative IE in humans.[58,59] Serologic analysis is used to identify some microorganisms; *Mycoplasma* spp. and *Brucella* spp. should potentially be considered in equine patients.[53,60] In many human cases, tissue from excised valves is available for testing, but in its absence, bacterial DNA extraction from blood is performed.[60]

Echocardiography has a pivotal role in the diagnosis of IE and should be performed as soon as possible after the suspicion of IE arises.[36,53,57] For humans, transthoracic echocardiography is fairly specific, but in the horse, it is not very sensitive[36] and cases can be missed particularly early in the disease process. In humans, the sensitivity is improved by performing transesophageal echocardiography.[36,53,61] Currently, equipment and expertise for transesophageal imaging in horses is limited in its availability and the procedure requires general anesthesia.[62] Even with a combination of transthoracic and transesophageal imaging, a negative echocardiogram is observed in approximately 15% of human cases, with nonoscillating and atypically located lesions particularly difficult to detect.[36] Because conventional transthoracic echocardiography in horses requires transducers of relatively low frequency, it is even more likely that equine IE may go undetected in some cases. Guidelines for the diagnosis of IE in humans state that in suspicious cases with normal echocardiographic findings early in the clinical course, the examination should be repeated before the condition can be ruled out.[36]

The presence of an oscillating soft tissue mass attached to the valve cusps, endocardial surfaces of the cardiac chambers, or the intimal surface of the great vessels represents definitive evidence of a vegetation (see Figs. 2-3 to 2-5). Many disease processes can cause thickening of the valve cusps, and it can be difficult to distinguish vegetations from other forms of nodular pathology. Recognition of oscillatory movement of a mass independent of movement of the valve confirms that it is a vegetation, but not all vegetations oscillate and it is the nonoscillating masses that are the most difficult to identify.[36] Abscesses typically have a zone of reduced echogenicity and may perforate to form pseudoaneurysms.[36] Destructions of adjacent structures may be identified, such as ruptured chordae tendineae, which cause portions of the valve (flail cusp) or chordae to prolapse into the atrium[33] (see Fig. 2-5).

Echocardiography is not 100% specific for the diagnosis of IE.[36] Differentiating severe degenerative valvular disease from IE can be difficult. When severe nodular changes are detected in younger animals at low risk of severe degenerative valvular disease, particularly if the nodules are located on the low-pressure aspect of the valve (ventricular surface for aortic valve, atrial surfaces for mitral and tricuspid valves) and are accompanied by clinical and laboratory evidence of infection, a diagnosis of probable IE should be considered, with appropriate treatment instituted (at least until this diagnosis can be rejected after reaching an alternative diagnosis). In the early stages of the disease, vegetations tend to be fairly homogenous (see Figs. 2-3 to 2-5), and as they become more organized, they become more echogenic and heterogenous.

Doppler echocardiography allows identification of regurgitation and permits semiquantitation of its degree,[63] which is usually moderate to severe with IE (Fig. 2-8). Jet dimensions provide only a subjective impression of the degree of regurgitation, and these measurements are not very repeatable. Limitations are created by several factors; suboptimal image angulation leads to underestimation of jet size, particularly in the mitral valve, where regurgitant jets are often running at right angles to the image plane, and variation of the image plane is difficult because of anatomic constraints.[64] Additional Doppler echocardiographic findings indicative of severe regurgitation include proximal flow convergence and velocity characteristics. Proximal flow convergence is recognized where nonturbulent, retrograde flow can be seen to speed up as it is approaching the regurgitant orifice, represented by bands of color on the proximal aspect of the regurgitating valve (see Fig. 2-8). The velocity of flow across a regurgitant orifice or other intracardiac shunt is determined by the pressure difference between the two chambers in question.[64] With severe aortic regurgitation, flow

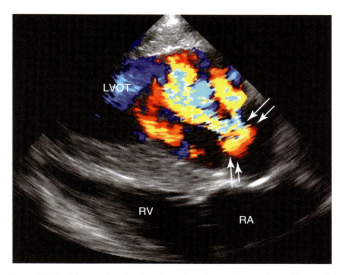

Figure 2-8 Left long-axis color-flow Doppler echocardiogram from 13-year-old mixed-breed mare with aortic infective endocarditis (IE) and concurrent myocarditis of 12 weeks' duration. Two large (yellow and turquoise) jets of aortic regurgitation occupy most of the left ventricular outflow tract (*LVOT*), and proximal flow convergence is present (between *arrows*). *RV*, Right ventricle; *RA*, right atrium. (See also Fig. 2-7.)

early in diastole will have high velocity, but as left ventricular pressures rapidly increase as a result of entry of the additional regurgitant volume, there will be a rapid deceleration of the regurgitant jet. In the presence of normal left atrial pressures that would be expected with mild mitral regurgitation, regurgitant flow between the left ventricle and left atrium is fast (usually >5 ms^{-1}), whereas with severe regurgitation, the jet velocities are lower. However, accurate flow velocities also depend greatly on the operator, machine, and angle, and these velocities should be interpreted with extreme caution because they have not been validated as indices of severity of regurgitation in the horse. A useful rule of thumb is that if Doppler echocardiographic findings suggest that there is severe regurgitation, this is probably true. However, if Doppler echocardiography fails to demonstrate severe regurgitation in a horse in which clinical findings suggest otherwise, the clinician should remember that the Doppler echocardiographic findings may be misleading. Forward flow velocities will increase in the presence of valve obstruction (see Fig. 2-6).

Two-dimensional and M-mode echocardiography are also useful in assessing the hemodynamic impact of valvular regurgitation.[37,65] In long-standing degenerative valve disease, the most accurate assessment of severity is gained by measurement of the diameter of the left ventricle, and these M-mode measurements correlate with heart failure score better than Doppler echocardiographic indices. Because equine IE usually presents as an acute severe condition, cardiac remodeling will not have occurred, and often the ventricular dimensions are normal despite the presence of severe regurgitation. Nonetheless, the ventricle may be hyperkinetic with exaggerated movement of the septum and the free wall caused by volume overload (Fig. 2-9). Fractional shortening* may be increased provided that myocardial function is maintained, but it may be decreased if there is concurrent myocardial failure. With reduced cardiac output, the diameter of the aortic root may be decreased and the movement of the aortic root depressed on M-mode

---

*Fractional shortening = (LVIDd − LVIDs) ÷ LVIDd where LVIDd = left ventricular internal dimension in diastole and LVIDs = left ventricular internal dimension in systole.

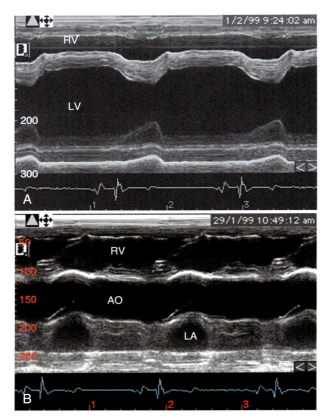

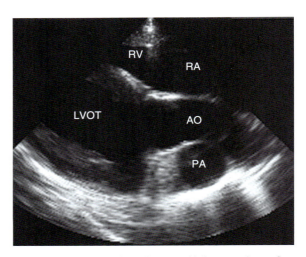

Figure 2-10 Right long-axis echocardiogram of left ventricular outflow tract (*LVOT*) from 8-year-old polo pony gelding with infective endocarditis (IE) diagnosed 2 days previously. The pulmonary artery (*PA*) is dilated, and in this view, it can be compared directly with the aorta (*AO*). Note that measurements of the PA are made from this view and the right inflow-outflow view. *RA,* Right atrium; *RV,* right ventricle. (See also Figs. 2-5 and 2-9.)

Figure 2-9 M-mode echocardiograms from 8-year-old polo pony gelding with infective endocarditis (IE) diagnosed 2 days earlier. **A,** Ventricular image demonstrates that although there is no ventricular enlargement, the septal movement is exaggerated because the left ventricle is hyperkinetic. **B,** Left ventricular outflow image demonstrates flattening of the aortic root secondary to decreased cardiac output. *AO,* Aorta; *LA,* left atrium; *LV,* Left ventricle; *RV,* right ventricle. (See also Figs. 2-5 and 2-10.)

echocardiography (see Fig. 2-9). Dilation of the pulmonary artery is a sensitive indicator of pulmonary hypertension[37]; it can be identified by comparing the diameter of the pulmonary artery in a long-axis image of the right ventricular outflow tract with the diameter of the aorta in a long-axis image of the left ventricular outflow tract[66] (Fig. 2-10). In long-standing cases, signs of ventricular remodeling can be expected. As it enlarges, the left ventricle will typically take on a rounded or globoid shape at the apex, and M-mode measurements of the ventricular dimensions and septal-mitral E-point separation will increase.[37,65]

Therapy

The first goal of therapy is sterilization of the vegetations.[45,67] Successful treatment of IE requires bactericidal therapy over a prolonged period. It is extremely important to attempt to isolate the organism and determine antimicrobial sensitivity patterns and specific information on MIC if possible.[45,53] In the absence of specific culture results, broad-spectrum antimicrobial therapy should be instituted. Penicillin and gentamicin are the most common choices,* but previous reports have also described using ampicillin,[9,18] trimethoprim-sulfonamide,[4,8] metronidazole,[19] oxytetracycline,[7] ceftoxamine,[12] and rifampicin,[15] with no antimicrobial regimen emerging as superior to

the others. Bactericidal drugs are preferable to bacteriostatic drugs in this life-threatening bacteremia.[45,53,57,68] Based on the literature, *Pasteurella* spp. and *Actinobacillus* spp. represent about 20% of equine cases with *Pseudomonas* spp. isolated from about 10% of cases. Consequently, penicillin with an aminoglycoside[67] or a fluoroquinolone, such as enrofloxacin,[69] can be predicted to have an appropriate spectrum of activity. Serum bactericidal titers can be used to monitor therapeutic efficacy.

Other microbial ancillary testing can be used. Serial dilutions of the patient's serum, collected at the end of dosing, can be tested for their ability to inhibit growth of the bacteria previously isolated from the patient. Serum bactericidal titers of 1:16 or higher have been associated with successful outcomes in human IE.[67]

Studies relating specifically to the pharmacokinetics and pharmacodynamics of common antimicrobials used in equine IE are lacking. Drug efficacy may be compromised by poor penetration of the vegetation, high bacterial numbers, and slow growth of deep-seated organisms.[67] The diffusion of antimicrobials within vegetations varies; ceftriaxone and penicillin generate a concentration gradient with decreasing levels toward the center, whereas others, such as fluoroquinolones, permeate the vegetation homogenously,[69] which, at least theoretically, should confer a therapeutic advantage. Rifampin has excellent tissue penetration and should be effective against gram-positive organisms but should not be used in isolation because of concerns over the development of resistance. Rifampin also has the potential to induce drug interactions with phenylbutazone and digoxin.[68] Successful treatment of fungal IE has not been described in horses, although successful treatment of systemic candidiasis in foals with IV amphotericin B and oral fluconazole has been reported.[70] In humans, amphotericin B,[45] possibly combined with rifampin,[71] is used to treat IE caused by candidiasis. Fluconazole is less successful but avoids the nephrotoxic effects of amphotericin.[45]

In human patients, treatments for at least 4 and typically 6 or more weeks is recommended.[36,53] The echocardiographic appearance of vegetations alters over time, becoming denser and more echogenic, but this does not necessarily provide any information on the sterility of the lesion (Fig. 2-11). Repeat blood cultures do not differentiate between complete and

*References 5, 8, 12, 13, 15, 17, 19, 28.

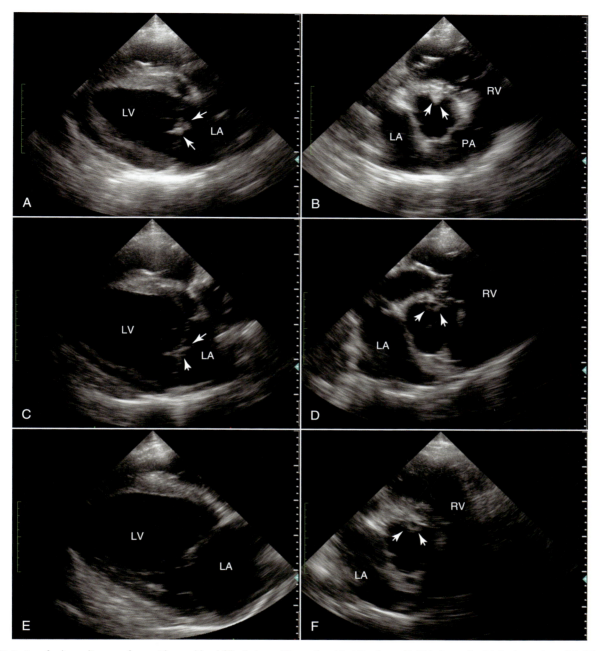

Figure 2-11 Series of echocardiograms from a Thoroughbred filly that was 15 months old at the time of initial diagnosis of infective endocarditis (IE). At initial diagnosis, vegetations are visible on both cusps of the mitral valve (*arrows* in **A**) and on the right and noncoronary cusps of the aortic valve (*arrows* in **B**). Two months later, these are much smaller (*arrows* in **C** and **D**). Fourteen months after diagnosis, the mitral valve has nodular thickening (*arrows* in **D**), and this long-axis echocardiogram **(E)** shows that there is rounding of the apex of the left ventricle *(LV)* and subjectively the left atrium *(LA)* is also larger. Note the imaging depth is the same in all images (30 cm); some but not all of the increase in size is due to the filly's growth. **F,** The nodules are still visible on the aortic valve cusps, but these have become much smaller and denser than at the time of initial diagnosis. *PA,* Pulmonary artery; *RV,* right ventricle.

incomplete healing because vegetations may contain deep-seated organisms.[31] On the other hand, repeat cultures may be useful in identifying treatment failure.[67] In horses, antimicrobial therapy should be continued until the white blood cell count, serum fibrinogen, and serum amyloid A concentrations have returned to normal. This may involve many weeks of treatment. After treatment is discontinued, these laboratory parameters, as well as clinical signs (e.g., rectal temperature), should be evaluated frequently to ensure early detection of any relapse.

Embolic events are difficult to predict but large, highly mobile vegetations, particularly those located on the mitral

valve, are the main risk factors.[57] Experimental studies have shown that aspirin may reduce embolism.[72,73] Treatment with aspirin did not reduce the risk of embolism but did increase risk of bleeding in a randomized controlled study.[74,75] Current recommendations are that there is no indication for the initiation of antithrombotic drugs, thrombolytic drugs, anticoagulants, or antiplatelet therapy during the active phase of IE.[57]

Specific measures to combat SIRS are important in the early stages of therapy (see Chapter 11). All serum and plasma products containing antibodies to the lipopolysaccharide molecule, polymyxin B, pentoxifylline, and flunixin meglumine, low-molecular-weight heparin, and aspirin are potentially useful in SIRS cases in general.[38] However, as noted previously, heparin and aspirin should be used with caution in IE, and renal function must be monitored carefully when polymyxin B and non-steroidal antiinflammatory drugs (NSAIDs) are used in patients that may have preexisting renal pathology or have volume compromise, as is often the case with IE.

Provision of cardiovascular support presents a particular problem in horses with IE. In conditions involving SIRS, high volumes of IV crystalloid and colloid fluids together with inotropic agents are advocated.[38] With severe regurgitation, however, increased preload and consequently increased stroke volume are likely to result in an increased regurgitant fraction, therefore it is difficult to improve cardiac output with volume replacement.[39] In left-sided heart failure from other causes, vasodilators are used to support forward flow and cardiac output. The decrease in systemic vascular resistance (SVR) induced by SIRS may temporarily have a similar beneficial action in maintaining forward flow, and forward flow may decrease as SVR is restored when treating SIRS.[39] Drugs such as dopamine should be used cautiously because their beneficial effects in producing vasodilation of the renal, mesenteric, coronary, and intracerebral vasculature are present only with low doses (1-3 μg/kg/min), whereas dopamine stimulates α-adrenoreceptors at higher doses, causing vasoconstriction. Similarly, because of its α-adrenoreceptor activity, norepinephrine is likely to be counterproductive in IE. The inotropic effects of dopamine and dobutamine mediated through β_1-adrenoreceptors are unlikely to be beneficial in many horses with IE. These drugs increase forward stroke volume by decreasing end-systolic volume; in acute mitral IE with normal left ventricular function, however, the afterload reduction created by the regurgitant pathway already allows for ejection to the point of minimum end-systolic volume.[39]

The arteriovenous dilator sodium nitroprusside along with diuretics is used to stabilize humans with left-sided IE, provided the arterial pressure is adequate for organ perfusion. Angiotensin-converting enzyme (ACE) inhibitors such as enalapril have a similar effect, but the oral bioavailability is extremely low.[76] If arteriovenous dilation fails, the arterial dilator hydralazine is a therapeutic consideration[39] and based on the pharmacokinetics of hydralazine established in the horse, a dose of 0.5 mg/kg IV is recommended.[77] Sodium nitroprusside, hydralazine, and alternative ACE inhibitors have yet to be critically evaluated in equine patients with acute heart failure. Monitoring of arterial pressure is mandatory if these agents are employed.[78] Furosemide is indicated if pulmonary edema is present and should be administered intravenously in the critically ill patient (1 mg/kg IV three times a day [TID]). The oral bioavailability is poor,[79] and the clinical response with oral administration is often inadequate.

Prognosis

The prognosis for equine IE is extremely guarded. Thirty-two of 40 horses (fatality rate 80%; CI 67.6%-92.4%) died or were euthanized (7 died, 19 euthanized, 6 not specified).[4-20,32,34,35] Even if the vegetation can be sterilized with antimicrobial therapy, unfortunately the structural damage to the heart valves is often so severe that CHF ensues. Clinical and laboratory signs of renal insufficiency and rupture of chordae tendineae have a poor prognosis.[32,33,37] Examination of the associations between survival and age, gender, affected cardiac sites, presence of dysrhythmias, and clinical and laboratory findings has shown that horses with IE of the mitral valve, either alone or in combination with other sites, have an increased risk of not surviving (proportion of cases affecting mitral valve in nonsurvivors, 62.5%; in survivors, 12.5%; p = 0.0174; odds ratio 12.09;

CI 1.27-106.9). No other factor was significantly associated with survival. This demonstrates that horses with mitral vegetations are less likely to survive, although clearly with such a small study group, the magnitude of the increased risk is difficult to quantify.

Inflammatory Valvulitis

Inflammatory valvulitis is an uncommon cause of valvular regurgitation in horses, occurring much less frequently than degenerative valvular disease.[80] Its pathologic features have not been documented rigorously, and detailed clinical descriptions are lacking. Early work on equine valvular pathology demonstrated inflammatory cell infiltrates in valvular lesions, and it was proposed at that time that this might represent a parallel condition to human rheumatic heart disease, but this hypothesis has not been explored critically. The pathogenesis of rheumatic heart disease involves an exaggerated immune response to streptococcal epitopes in a susceptible host and probably involves molecular mimicry between epitopes on the pathogen and host tissues. Structural similarities between streptococcal M protein and myosin (α-helical, coiled molecules) are proposed; valvular tissue does not contain myosin, and the involvement of the valve results from the presence of laminin, which has a similar molecular structure to myosin and M protein.[81]

Inflammatory valvulitis is difficult to diagnose with certainty but should be considered in horses with valvular regurgitation and echocardiographically visible valve thickening. The main differential diagnoses are degenerative valvular disease, congenital valvular dysplasia, and IE. In particular, inflammatory valvulitis should be suspected in individuals with concurrent mild ventricular dysfunction when the regurgitation improves or resolves after a period of rest, with or without corticosteroid therapy, because the other forms of valvular disease are unlikely to respond in this way. In offering a prognosis for horses presenting with cardiac murmurs of valvular regurgitation, it is important for the clinician to recognize that valvular regurgitation may occasionally be reversible if caused by inflammatory valvulitis. Further studies are needed to define this condition and its pathogenesis, management, and prognosis.

Myocarditis

Etiology and Pathogenesis

Infection with bacteria, viruses,[82] and fungi[80,83] can cause myocardial inflammation. Clinical signs consistent with myocarditis may also occur as sequelae to viral or bacterial respiratory infection.[80] Frequently, viruses are anecdotally stated to be involved in generalized cardiomyopathy or in horses presenting with dysrhythmias in which focal myocardial disease is suspected. Viruses, including equine arteritis virus,[84] morbillivirus,[85] and African horse sickness virus,[86] have been demonstrated within cardiac myocytes. The "cardiac form" is one of the various important presentations of African horse sickness (see Chapter 16). However, these viral infections are not as common and widespread as exposure to the equine herpesviruses and equine influenza virus. Necrosis of cardiac myocytes has been demonstrated in equine fetuses infected with equid herpesvirus 1.[87] Three of 23 ponies experimentally infected with equine influenza virus had transient increases in cardiac troponin I, confirming that this virus can induce myocardial injury.[88] Nevertheless, detailed and robust of reports of clinically significant cardiac disease are currently lacking.

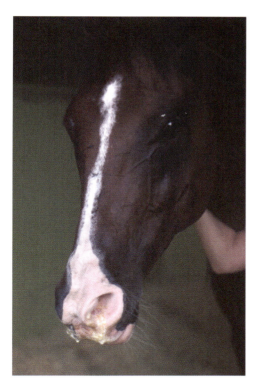

Figure 2-12 Frothy nasal discharge consistent with pulmonary edema in 11-year-old Arabian mare with acute myocarditis.

Clinical Findings

Horses with myocarditis can present with signs of varying severity depending on the extent of the pathology. With focal myocarditis, horses may display fairly mild signs (e.g., impaired performance) evident only on maximal exercise, whereas horses with generalized myocarditis will present with signs of acute heart failure (Fig. 2-12). In more severe cases, respiratory distress, weakness, ataxia, collapse, weak pulses, tachycardia, dysrhythmias, cardiac murmurs, and pulmonary and ventral edema occur.

Diagnosis

All forms of cardiac dysrhythmias can occur with both generalized and focal myocarditis. Ambulatory ECG monitoring is useful in identifying intermittent dysrhythmias and assessing response to therapy. Radiotelemetric techniques are invaluable for identification of exercise-induced dysrhythmias. Ventricular dilation and abnormal wall movement are the echocardiographic hallmarks of severe myocardial dysfunction. The ventricles may be subjectively enlarged with a globoid appearance at the apex (Fig. 2-13). Global myocardial dysfunction leads to reduction in movement of the ventricular walls (Fig. 2-14) and reduction in the fractional shortening. Focal myocardial disease may produce regional wall movement abnormalities, but often the echocardiogram is unremarkable. With ventricular dilation the septal-mitral E-point separation increases (Fig. 2-14, *B*), and reduced cardiac output leads to flattening of the aortic root on M-mode echocardiography, prolongation of the preejection period, and decreases in the left ventricular ejection periods.

Cardiac troponin I is considered the most specific biochemical marker of myocardial disease,[46,47] and increases in the serum concentration of CK-MB or lactate dehydrogenase (LDH) also suggest myocardial injury.[80] Marked increases in cardiac troponin I should prompt further investigations; however, minor increases are often encountered in biochemical profiles performed at the in-house laboratory at the author's clinic, and these horses rarely have any other evidence of myocardial disease when investigated with echocardiography or exercising and 24-hour ambulatory ECG monitoring. Evaluation of seven horses with myocardial pathology presenting to the author's clinic suggests that cardiac troponin I is not more sensitive than CK-MB for detection of myocardial disease in horses. Cardiac troponin I is rapidly eliminated,[48] and increases in CK-MB, but not in cardiac troponin I, were found in horses that had myocardial disease of more than 2 weeks' duration.* Further work is required to determine the sensitivity and specificity of biochemical markers of myocardial injury.

Therapy

Treatment of myocarditis has not been well defined. If a bacterial origin is suspected, broad-spectrum antimicrobials are indicated. With other forms of myocardial pathology, corticosteroids are often prescribed. Dobutamine (1-5 µg/kg/min) may improve cardiac output.[78] Furosemide may relieve pulmonary congestion, and digoxin has potentially beneficial positive inotropic effects and negative chronotropic effects. Digoxin can be associated with ventricular dysrhythmias, and phenytoin is recommended for treatment of digoxin-induced dysrhythmias.[89] In the horse, supraventricular premature depolarizations are often prevented from reaching the ventricles by the action of the vagus nerve on the atrioventricular (AV) node, such that the ventricular rate remains fairly stable in their presence, rendering specific antidysrhythmic therapy unnecessary. Digoxin may be used concurrently to suppress conduction at the AV node if necessary. Ventricular dysrhythmias are much more likely to require antidysrhythmic therapy. Accepted guidelines suggest that antidysrhythmics should be considered when the heart rate is rapid (>100 beats/min), the dysrhythmia is polymorphic, and R-on-T phenomenon is present. In all cases, the most important factor in the consideration of usage of antidysrhythmic drugs should be the presence or absence of signs of low cardiac output (e.g., weakness, cold extremities, pallor, hypotension, azotemia). Lidocaine and quinidine gluconate are the most common first choices for emergency treatment of unstable ventricular tachycardia. Magnesium sulfate is inexpensive and readily available and can be efficacious alone or in combination with other antidysrhythmic agents.[90] Phenytoin may be effective in cases refractory to therapy with other antidysrhythmics[91] (Table 2-3).

Prognosis

The prognosis for myocarditis is variable. Horses with suspected focal myocarditis, manifested by cardiac dysrhythmias and poor performance, will usually have a good prognosis for life. Athletic performance may be limited, however, and rider safety is an issue if persistent, exercise-induced dysrhythmias are present. The prognosis for horses with generalized myocardial disease is poor.

Pericarditis

Etiology and Pathogenesis

Similar to other animals and humans, pericarditis in the horse can be effusive, noneffusive, or constrictive. Effusive pericarditis is most often fibrinous and neutrophilic in nature.[92-96] Much less often, nonfibrinous, eosinophilic, and histocytic effusions have

---

*Unpublished data courtesy J. Sento and C. Marr.

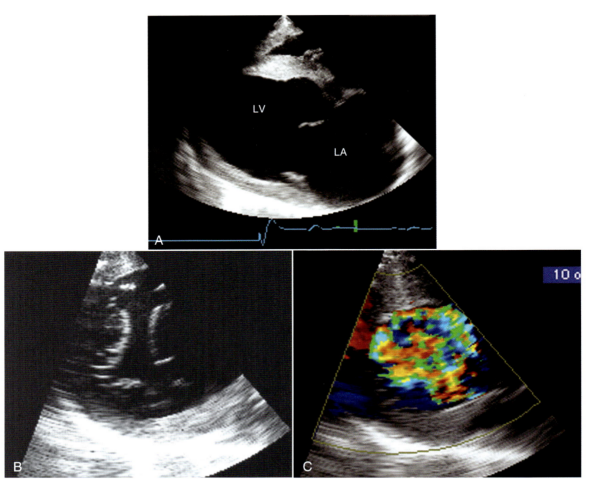

Figure 2-13 Right long-axis echocardiogram of ventricles and atria **(A)** and left short-axis echocardiograms at level of mitral valve **(B)** and just above the mitral valve **(C)** from 7-year-old Thoroughbred gelding with myocarditis of unknown etiology. There is marked dilation of the left ventricle *(LV)* and left atrium *(LA)*. The mitral valve annulus is incompetent secondary to ventricular dilation in **B**, and severe mitral regurgitation (green/yellow/turquoise) is evident on the color-flow Doppler image **(C)**.

been described.[93] Constrictive pericarditis occurs when fibrin matures to fibrous tissue or when pericardial or myocardial injury results in fibrosis.[97] Noneffusive pericarditis is not well described in horses but should be considered in individuals presenting with signs consistent with pericardial disease in which no effusion is identified.[95] Pericarditis can be accompanied by myocarditis, and if so, it is termed *myopericarditis*.[98]

In terms of etiology, pericarditis appears to be of two major types: (1) idiopathic, immune-mediated, and/or related to viral infection and (2) septic pericarditis of bacterial origin. Rarely, pericarditis is due to trauma arising from external thoracic injury,[99] penetrating foreign bodies entering through the gastrointestinal (GI) tract,[100] and iatrogenic penetration during bone marrow aspiration.[101] Until recently, the vast majority of reported cases were classified as idiopathic.[102] In humans, idiopathic pericarditis can be viral in origin and is attributed to direct cytopathic effects, infiltration of tissues in which virus is evidenced by cytotoxic lymphocytes, and immune-mediated processes. Similar mechanisms likely occur in the horse. Horses with pericarditis often have a recent or current history of respiratory disease,[92,94,95] and rising titers to equine herpesvirus type 1 (EHV-1) have been observed on paired serology in 2 of 18 cases in one study.[95] Nevertheless, the evidence for a viral etiology in equine pericarditis, whether directly or through immune-mediated mechanisms, remains scant. Idiopathic pericarditis has also been observed as a sequela to pleuritis and peritonitis,[92,94,95]

and occasionally there is evidence of concurrent immune-mediated disorders such as vasculitis and hemolytic anemia.[95]

Pericarditis has been associated with *Mycoplasma felis* infection,[103] but bacterial infection is the other major cause of fibrinoeffusive and constrictive pericarditis. *Escherichia coli*, *Enterococcus faecalis*, *Streptococcus equi* subsp. *zooepidemicus*,[96] *Streptococcus bovis*,[81] *Corynebacterium pseudotuberculosis*,[104] and *Clostridium perfringens*[105] have been reported in individual cases.

Actinobacillus spp. are the most commonly reported isolates from pericardial fluid of horses with bacterial pericarditis. In an epidemic of equine pericarditis that occurred in association with early and late fetal losses in Kentucky (mare reproductive loss syndrome [MRLS]), bacteria were isolated from 13 of 32 pericarditis cases, with *Actinobacillus* spp. most commonly identified (11 of 13 horses).[96] In other reports, *Actinobacillus* spp. were found in three of four[103] and one of four[92] horses in other reports unrelated to MRLS. *Streptococcus* spp., *Pasteurella multocida*, *Staphylococcus aureus*, *Pseudomonas* spp., *Acinetobacter*, and *Enterococcus faecalis* were isolated in some of the MRLS cases,[96,98] and β-hemolytic *Streptococcus* spp. were isolated in 1 of 6[94] and 2 of 18 non-MRLS related cases of equine pericarditis.[95]

The MRLS outbreak was an occasion in which multiple horses were affected by pericarditis. Exposure to Eastern tent caterpillars was the greatest risk factor for the development of pericarditis, and the temporal distribution of cases was

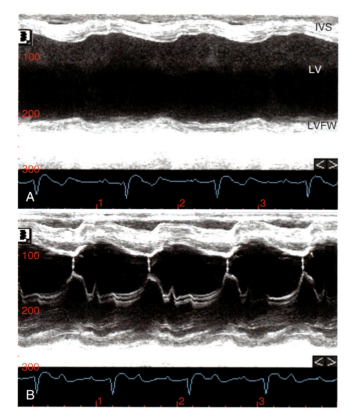

Figure 2-14 M-mode echocardiograms at level of ventricles **(A)** and mitral valve **(B)** from 11-year-old Arabian mare with acute myocarditis. Movement of interventricular septum *(IVS)* and left ventricular free wall *(LVFW)* is greatly reduced, and there is increase in the septal-mitral E-point separation (*arrows* in **B**). *LV,* Left ventricle. (See also Fig. 2-12.)

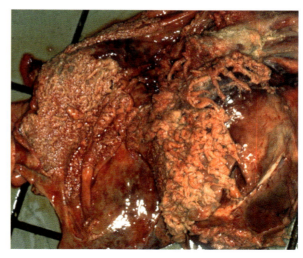

Figure 2-15 Pathologic specimen from 14-year-old Thoroughbred gelding with septic fibrinoeffusive pericarditis of about 3 weeks' duration. Both the pericardial (*left* of image) and the epicardial (*right* of image) surface is covered with villonodular deposits of fibrin.

Table 2-3 Agents Used in the Emergency Treatment of Tachydysrhythmia in Horses

Drug	Indications	Dose
Amiodarone	Ventricular tachycardia, atrial fibrillation	5 mg/kg/hr for 1 hr, then 0.83 mg/kg/hr for 23 hr
Bretylium tosylate	Ventricular fibrillation	3-5 mg/kg IV, can repeat up to 10 mg/kg
Digoxin	Supraventricular tachycardia	0.0022 mg/kg IV 0.011 mg/kg PO, q12h
Diltiazem	Supraventricular tachycardia	0.125 mg/kg IV over 2 min, repeated every 12 min
Lidocaine	Ventricular tachycardia	0.25-0.5 mg/kg IV bolus, can repeat in 5-10 min Loading bolus of 1.3 mg/kg IV over 5 min, followed by CRI at 0.05 mg/kg/min
Magnesium sulfate	Ventricular tachycardia	2.2-4.4 mg/kg IV boluses, q5min intervals up to 12 times
Phenytoin sodium	Ventricular and supraventricular tachycardia	7.5-8.8 mg/kg IV single bolus Loading dose 20 mg/kg PO, followed by 10-15 mg/kg PO q12h
Procainamide	Ventricular and supraventricular tachycardia	1 mg/kg/min IV to 20 mg/kg
Propranolol	Ventricular and supraventricular tachycardia	0.03-2 mg/kg IV 25-35 mg/kg PO, q12h
Quinidine gluconate	Ventricular and supraventricular tachycardia	2.2 mg/kg q10min until 8-10 mg/kg total
Verapamil	Supraventricular tachycardia	0.025-0.05 mg/kg IV q30min to 0.2 mg/kg

IV, Intravenously, intravenous; *PO,* orally; *CRI,* continuous rate infusion; *q5min,* every 5 minutes; *q12h,* every 12 hours.

consistent with a point-source epidemic. The *Actinobacillus* spp. isolates recovered from pericardial fluid samples of MRLS horses were identical to those found in the oral cavity and alimentary tracts of healthy horses.[106] Isolation of fastidious species from pericardial fluid can be difficult, but using an insect cell culture growth medium, additional species (*Propionibacterium acnes, Staphylococcus equorum, Streptococcus,* and *Pseudomonas rhodesiae*) were found in some of the MRLS cases, but none of these species were specifically linked to catepillars.[107] A toxin produced by Eastern tent caterpillars may have compromised immune defenses or alternatively, some unidentified mechanism may have led to a breakdown of GI mucosal barriers, facilitating opportunistic infection in these horses.[96] There is evidence that when ingested in large quantities, the barbed setae on the caterpillar exoskeleton may migrate through tissues carrying bacteria and/or toxins.[108] *Actinobacillus* spp. are commensal bacteria of mucosal surfaces that appear to be pericardiotrophic in the horse.

The hemodynamic effects of effusive pericarditis depend on the volume of fluid within the pericardial sac and its rate of accumulation. Fibrin tends to accumulate in a villonodular arrangement on both inner surfaces of the pericardial sac (Fig. 2-15). Fluid and fibrin restrict diastolic filling of the heart and have the most impact on the low-pressure right side of the heart. With larger amounts of fluid and fibrin, all cardiac chambers may be reduced in volume. Venous return is compromised, and diastolic myocardial perfusion and contractility are decreased, resulting in decreased stroke volume and cardiac output.[97] With constrictive pericarditis, the initial phase of diastolic filling is unimpeded, but when a critical diastolic volume

is reached, filling ceases rapidly as the limit of the noncompliant pericardium is reached. Ventricular preload is decreased, leading to decreased stroke volume.[109] In both situations, there is a compensatory tachycardia to maintain cardiac output, and signs of right-sided failure predominate.

Clinical Findings

No specific breed predispositions for pericarditis have been identified. Younger horses may be at increased risk, although in the sole case-control study that has examined this risk factor, the study design may have biased this result.[110] Intact males were overrepresented and geldings underrepresented compared with the general hospital population in another study.[95] Common presenting complaints include fever, anorexia, and lethargy. Specific cardiovascular signs include tachycardia, weak peripheral arterial pulses, muffled heart sounds, cardiac murmurs, and pericardial friction rubs, which are usually biphasic or triphasic sounds that coincide with the heart rate and that may not become apparent until the pericardial effusion is removed. Pericarditis cannot be excluded in the absence of these signs, and horses often present with signs relating to concurrent respiratory disease. Right-sided heart failure is manifested by ventral edema, venous distention, and pleural and peritoneal effusions evident on ultrasonography.[92,94,97,109]

Diagnosis

Echocardiography

Echocardiography is the most important tool for diagnosis of pericarditis. Pericardial fluid creates an anechoic space between the parietal pericardium and the epicardial surface of the heart, and a subjective assessment of its volume can be made. Fibrin typically appears as tags of tissue that are slightly more echogenic than the myocardium (Fig. 2-16). Echocardiographic findings suggestive of cardiac tamponade include right atrial collapse, right ventricular early-diastolic collapse, overall decreases in chamber size, reduced fractional shortening, and decreased opening and slowing of the closure of the anterior leaflet of the mitral valve.[76]

The main alternative differential diagnoses for fluid within the pericardial sac are hemopericardium and neoplastic effusion; neither is typically associated with the accumulation of large amounts of fibrin. In hemopericardium the fluid is usually slightly echogenic, and diagnostic ultrasonography may reveal the source of hemorrhage such as fractured ribs or a ruptured sinus of Valsalva aneurysm. Therefore these structures should be examined carefully when fluid is detected within the pericardium. With neoplastic effusion, masses within the pericardial sac or heart may be visible, and cytologic characterization of the pericardial fluid may be diagnostic.

In constrictive pericarditis, pericardial thickening may or may not be evident (Fig. 2-17). Characteristically, there is abrupt cessation of ventricular filling during early diastole, diastolic flattening of the left ventricular free-wall (see Fig. 2-17), and abnormal increases in tricuspid flow with abnormal decreases in mitral flow during inspiration.[97,109]

Electrocardiography, Thoracic Radiography, and Cardiac Catheterization

The most common ECG findings in horses with pericarditis are decreased QRS amplitude and electrical alternans (variations in amplitude).[92,93] Decreased QRS amplitude is caused by fluid dampening and short circuiting of the electrical signal (Fig. 2-18). This QRS decrease is not specific to pericarditis and can also be seen in horses with obesity, chronic respiratory disease, diaphragmatic hernia, and thoracic masses.[97]

Thoracic radiography adds little to the information obtained with echocardiography. Enlargement of the cardiac silhouette

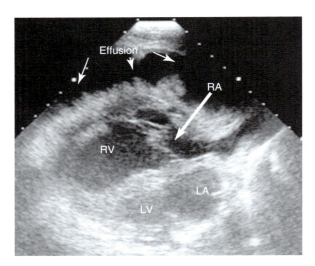

Figure 2-16 Right long-axis echocardiogram from 2-week-old Thoroughbred colt with septic fibrinoeffusive pericarditis. Right atrium *(RA)* is collapsed from cardiac tamponade, and left cardiac chambers are small. *RV,* Right ventricle; *LV,* left ventricle; *LA,* left atrium. (See also Fig. 2-19.) *(Courtesy Dr. Jan Bright, College of Veterinary Medicine and Biomedical Sciences, Colorado State University.)*

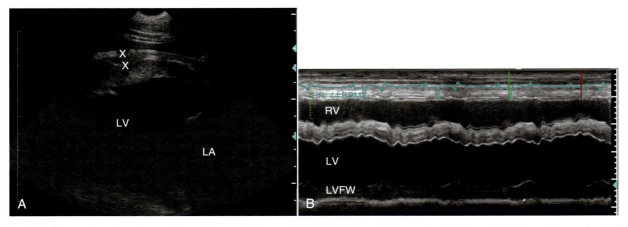

Figure 2-17 A, Left long-axis echocardiogram from a 2-year-old Thoroughbred colt with constrictive pericarditis. The colt had been diagnosed with fibrinous pericarditis 5 months previously, associated with high titers to both equine herpesvirus type 1 (EHV-1) and type 4 (EHV-4), and this was treated with pericardial lavage, antimicrobials, and dexamethasone. Although there was an initial clinical improvement and reduction in the fibrinous deposits, the pericardium is now thickened (between X). **B,** M-mode echocardiogram of the ventricles shows diastolic flattening of the left ventricular free wall *(LVFW)*, suggesting the presence of pericardial constriction. *LA,* Left atrium; *LV,* left ventricle; *RV,* right ventricle.

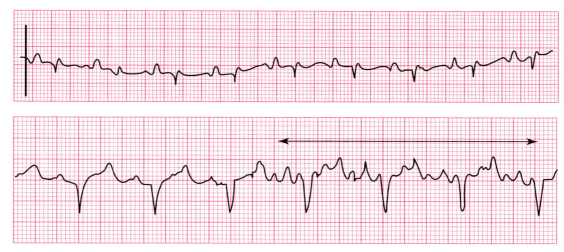

Figure 2-18 Electrocardiograms (ECGs) from 18-month-old Standardbred filly with fibrinoeffusive idiopathic pericarditis. *Upper panel,* Small complexes that increase in size during pericardial drainage (*lower panel,* which has induced artifact resulting from muscle tremors [under *double arrow*]). Vertical bar indicates 1 mV; paper speed 25 ms⁻¹.

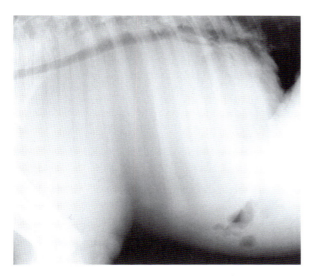

Figure 2-19 Lateral thoracic radiograph from a 2-week-old Thoroughbred colt with septic fibrinoeffusive pericarditis. The cardiac silhouette is increased in size, with marked tracheal elevation. (See also Fig. 2-16.) *(Courtesy Dr. Jan Bright, College of Veterinary Medicine and Biomedical Sciences, Colorado State University.)*

may be present (Fig. 2-19), but in many cases, pleural effusion obscures the heart.[93,109]

Cardiac catheterization provides the definitive diagnosis of constrictive pericarditis. There is equalization of the right atrial and right ventricular pressures, and a dip-and-plateau configuration of the right ventricular pressure curve reflects the abrupt termination of diastolic filling when the limit of compliance of the pericardium is reached.[109]

Laboratory Investigations

Leukocytosis, neutrophilia, and hyperfibrinogenemia are common but nonspecific findings in pericarditis. Paired serology for influenza, equine herpesvirus, and equine viral arteritis may be useful. Renal function should be assessed because prerenal azotemia is often present.

Box 2-1 lists guidelines for collection of pericardial fluid. Pericardial fluid should contain less than 1500×10^6/L total

---

Box 2-1 Technique for Pericardiocentesis

1. Location for pericardiocentesis
   - Left 4 to 6 intercostal spaces, approximately 6 cm ventral to point of shoulder.
   - Selection of site is facilitated by echocardiography.
2. Sedation for pericardiocentesis
   - May not be necessary depending on the horse's clinical status.
   - If necessary, use with caution; these drugs may exacerbate cardiovascular compromise.
3. Monitoring for pericardiocentesis
   - Monitor the cardiac rhythm for ventricular dysrhythmias.
   - Have appropriate doses of procainamide, quinidine, or lidocaine at hand (see Table 2-3).
   - If ventricular dysrhythmia occurs, the needle should be retracted immediately.
   - If ventricular dysrhythmia persists, antidysrhythmic drugs are necessary (see Table 2-3).
4. Preparation of site
   - Clip and surgical scrub.
   - Infiltration of lidocaine in skin, subcutaneous layers, and intercostal muscles.
5. Selection of catheter and drain
   - For small sample collection: over-the-needle intravenous catheters (14 g, 15 cm) or blunt-ended teat cannulae.
   - For lavage: chest drains (16-24 French).
6. Insertion of catheter and drain
   - Stab incision.
   - Insert catheter and drain carefully using the minimum force while observing the ECG continuously.
   - Withdraw trocar promptly once pericardial sac has been penetrated.
   - Be prepared to seal the catheter with an artery forceps or similar instrument if air enters.
7. Maintenance of drain
   - Secure drain using purse-string suture.
   - After lavage, flush with a small volume of heparinized saline.
   - Seal drain with a clamp or sterile syringe.
   - Clean drain entry site twice daily.
   - Cover with gauze, tape, and bandage material to keep the site clean.

---

nucleated cells and have a protein content less than 2.5 g/dL.[111] Samples of pericardial fluid should be submitted for bacteriologic culture, and culture of mycoplasmal species may also be useful. Ideally, culture should be performed before antimicrobial therapy is instituted. The diagnosis of septic pericarditis is based on the identification of increased numbers of degenerative neutrophils, with or without cytologic evidence of bacteria. Idiopathic or immune-mediated pericarditis is characterized by the presence of increased numbers of well-preserved neutrophils. Monitoring glucose concentrations in the pericardial effusion may be helpful as an immediate assessment of sepsis. Glucose concentrations of less than 2.2 mmol/L (40 mg/dL) suggest sepsis, and concentrations greater than 3.3 mmol/L (60 mg/dL) probably indicate a sterile effusion.[103]

Therapy

Broad-spectrum antimicrobial therapy is indicated for horses with documented sepsis and while awaiting pericardial fluid cytology.[67] Antimicrobials are also often used prophylactically in horses with suspected nonseptic immune-mediated pericarditis.[95] Antimicrobial therapy is ideally based on pericardial fluid culture results, but these are often negative. Given the high prevalence of infection with *Actinobacillus* and *Streptococcus* spp., appropriate empiric choices include penicillin and an aminoglycoside or cephalosporins. Experimental studies in dogs suggest that these drugs should penetrate the pericardium effectively.[67] Sodium penicillin G (10×10^6 units in a 420-kg mare),[95,112] gentamicin (no dose reported),[94,97] or cefquinome (1.35 g in an adult Hanoverian gelding)[113] can be instilled at the end of drainage as adjunctive antimicrobial therapy.

Pericardial drainage and possibly lavage should be considered for horses with moderate to severe pericardial effusion.[95,112] Echocardiographic signs of cardiac tamponade, particularly marked right atrial collapse (see Fig. 2-16), should prompt emergency pericardiocentesis to restore cardiac function (see Box 2-1). During the procedure, ECG monitoring can identify ventricular dysrhythmias and facilitate prompt treatment (see Fig. 2-18). After drainage, 1 to 2 L of 0.9% saline may be infused and left in place for 30 to 60 minutes before removal. Another liter of saline solution is then inserted and left in place until the next drainage-lavage cycle. Drainage-lavage may be repeated twice daily until the volume of fluid removed at the beginning of a drainage session is less than the amount infused at the end of the preceding session.[97]

The fibrinolytic effect of tissue plasminogen activator (tPA) has been shown to be beneficial in fibrinous pericarditis to promote breakdown of fibrinous material and promote effective drainage in human patients.[114,115] In horses, tPA has been used in both septic pleuropneumonia[116] and in fibrinous pericarditis.[98] In the latter case, a 2-year-old Thoroughbred colt, 50 mg of tissue plasminogen activator in 300 mL normal saline were instilled into the pericardial space and the pericardial drain was closed for 24 hours. The authors reported that the following day, 4 L of serosanguineous pericardial fluid was removed and the colt went on to make a full recovery.[98]

Corticosteroids have been advocated for treatment of idiopathic or immune-mediated pericarditis.[93,95] Decision making in these cases is complicated by the concern of possible active viral infection, but the majority of affected horses apparently are not viremic. Supportive therapy includes NSAIDs, and if the patient has prerenal azotemia, the cautious use of IV fluids is warranted. In these horses, it is helpful to monitor central venous pressure so that fluid therapy can be closely titrated. The administration of furosemide is contraindicated as it reduces preload and tends to exacerbate azotemia.

Prognosis

The prognosis for idiopathic or immune-mediated pericarditis appears to be very favorable.[75,77] Similarly, there are several reports of successful treatment of septic pericarditis using drainage or drainage-lavage techniques.[94,97,105] Constrictive pericarditis warrants a poor prognosis. A partial pericardiectomy technique has been reported but was ultimately unsuccessful because the pericardial fibrosis returned.[109] Chronic pericarditis has been associated with chronic lameness resulting from hypertrophic osteopathy in one horse.[117]

Jugular Thrombophlebitis

Etiology and Pathogenesis

Jugular thrombophlebitis is defined as vein thrombosis accompanied by mural inflammation and is a common complication of IV catheterization.[118] Rarely, it can occur as a result of direct extension of infection from a traumatic oral lesion.[119] The prevalence of jugular thrombosis in horses being treated for a variety of GI diseases has ranged from 6% to 22%. Combining data from these studies suggests that the prevalence in this patient group is approximately 18% (CI 13.0%-22.8%).[120-122] A similar proportion (15%) of neonatal foals receiving parenteral nutrition developed catheter-related problems.[123] Many proven and putative positive risk factors exist for thrombophlebitis. Use of home-produced fluid solutions, fever, diarrhea, and duration of IV treatment increase risk.[118] Foals and horses with colic or diarrhea are more likely to have bacteria isolated from catheters after removal.[124] Horses with GI disease are at risk of developing coagulopathies, which contributes to the propensity to develop jugular thrombophlebitis during treatment, and endotoxemia, salmonellosis, hypoproteinemia, and large intestinal disease increased the odds of catheter-associated thrombophlebitis by approximately 18, 68, 5, and 4 times, respectively, in one study.[125] Other indicators that GI disease was a significant underlying contributor in that study were that, of the horses admitted to the medicine section, those receiving antidiarrheal or antiulcer medications were at increased risk.[125] Another study examining risk factors associated with subclinical venous catheter-related diseases showed that horses with fever were at increased risk while the administration of NSAIDs reduced the risk.[126] Nevertheless, putative but unproven risk factors for thrombophlebitis include administration of drugs that irritate the vascular endothelium (e.g., oxytetracycline and phenylbutazone), rapid IV fluid infusion rates, and standing with the head down for prolonged periods. These latter two factors may predispose to thrombophlebitis because they promote turbulent blood flow.[127]

Studies investigating catheter types and materials have lacked statistical power, but both catheter material and design are likely to be important. Flexible polyurethane over-the-wire catheters are assumed to have less risk than the more rigid polyurethane over-the-needle catheters, and Teflon or polytetrafluoroethylene catheters are likely to carry the greatest risk.[127] Jugular thrombophlebitis may be septic or nonseptic. Microorganisms most often isolated from the tips of IV catheters are coagulase-negative *Staphylococcus* spp., *Corynebacterium* spp., *Enterobacter* spp., and *Streptococcus* spp.[124]

Clinical Findings

Swelling or palpable thickening of the jugular vein is characteristic of thrombophlebitis. There may be variable degrees of perivenous swelling. Heat, pain, fever, and discharge from the site of venipuncture suggest sepsis. Acute-onset, severe thrombophlebitis may result in obstruction to venous drainage of the head, and swelling may occur in the supraorbital area, muzzle, and cheek on the affected side. Bilateral thrombosis may be associated with swelling of the tongue and airway obstruction. Chronic thrombophlebitis can lead to distention of the facial veins and discharging abscesses.

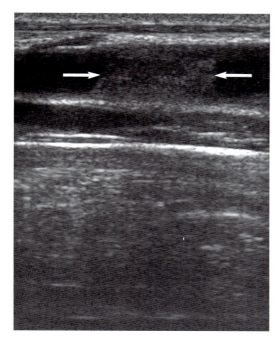

Figure 2-20 Longitudinal ultrasonogram of jugular vein from 3-year-old Thoroughbred colt that developed jugular thrombosis after surgery to correct colon torsion. A small, homogenous, nonseptic thrombus is visible *(arrows)*.

Diagnosis

Diagnostic Ultrasonography

Diagnostic ultrasonography is useful to characterize the nature and extent of thrombophlebitis. Nonseptic thrombi are usually uniformly echogenic and fairly small (Fig. 2-20). Septic thrombophlebitis has a heterogenous appearance, and in the early stages, there may be numerous anechoic areas representing areas of fluid accumulation or necrosis (Fig. 2-21, *A*) and hyperechoic areas with reverberation artifacts representing gas formation (Fig. 2-21, *B*). The thrombus will often have an onion-layer appearance on transverse images (Fig. 2-21, *C*). This layering is also evident on longitudinal images, reflecting the layers of platelets and fibrin that are deposited on the thrombus (Fig. 2-21, *D*). Variable degrees of thickening of the vessel wall are apparent. Perivenous swelling can readily be distinguished from thrombophlebitis, and perivascular edema typically has a honeycomb appearance. As thrombophlebitis resolves, the thrombus usually becomes more echogenic because of fibrosis and eventually contracts into irregular shapes as it shrinks away from the vessel wall (Fig. 2-22). Generally, it is possible to assess patency of the vein and visualize flow with conventional B-mode images; however, color-flow Doppler imaging may depict this more elegantly (see Fig. 2-22). Because jugular flow is sluggish and acute thrombi can be hypoechoic, in early thrombosis the blood may be more echogenic than the thrombus (see Fig. 2-21).

Laboratory Investigations

As in IE and pericarditis, leukocytosis, neutrophilia, and hyperfibrinogenemia are common but nonspecific findings in septic thrombophlebitis. If DIC is suspected, platelet count, prothrombin time, activated partial thromboplastin time, fibrinolytic degradation products, and antithrombin III should be measured. Abnormality in four of five of these coagulation variables is considered indicative of DIC. The tips of catheters removed from an affected vein should be sterilely inserted into thioglycolate broth for bacterial culture. Blood cultures, swabs of discharging tracts at the catheter insertion site, and aspirates of fluid pockets obtained in a sterile manner may also be submitted for bacterial culture and antimicrobial sensitivity testing.

Therapy

Intravenous catheters should be removed at the first sign of potential problems. If possible, further IV therapy should be avoided. If continued IV therapy is needed and unilateral jugular thrombosis is present, it is prudent to place a catheter at an alternative site, such as the lateral thoracic or cephalic vein rather than the opposite jugular vein. Penicillin with an aminoglycoside, enrofloxacin, and cephalosporins are appropriate choices for antimicrobial therapy while awaiting results of microbiologic sensitivity testing. The presence of gas echoes may indicate anaerobic infection, and in these cases, metronidazole therapy should be considered. Generally, parenteral administration of antimicrobials is preferred in the acute stages of thrombophlebitis. Some horses with chronic septic thrombophlebitis require several weeks of antimicrobial therapy and oral administration of enrofloxacin, with or without metronidazole, or a combination of trimethoprim-sulfonamide and rifampin may be more practical. Horses with head swelling should be tied with the head elevated, ideally with the option of resting the head on straw bales or another suitable support. Oral aspirin (18 mg/kg every other day) and topical treatments, such as hot packing and application of gels containing dimethyl sulfoxide or hydroxyethyl salicylate, may be helpful. Jugular vein thrombectomy can be effective in horses with chronic septic jugular thrombophlebitis that has failed to resolve with antimicrobial therapy and in which an abscess cavity has developed together with complete occlusion of the vein. The procedure is performed with standing sedation, and two or three incisions are made to open the abscess cavity, which is subsequently lavaged on a daily basis and allowed to heal by secondary intention.[128] Reconstructive surgery using saphenous vein grafts[129] or synthetic vessel prostheses[130] have been effective in horses with permanent thrombophlebitic occlusion. Experimental studies comparing different types of grafts have demonstrated that polytetrafluoroethylene and autografts of saphenous veins show most promise with respect to host acceptance, presence of endothelium, and subsequent vessel patency.[131]

Prognosis

Jugular thrombophlebitis resolves uneventfully in most affected horses but can occasionally prolong treatment and delay hospital discharge for patients with primary GI disorders. Septic jugular thrombosis can be associated with a variety of serious complications (including IE),[8] temporary or permanent damage to the sympathetic and recurrent laryngeal nerves, and upper airway edema that affects the horse's athletic performance. In most individuals, even with complete loss of the jugular vein, collateral circulation will develop to allow adequate venous drainage of the head. Thrombophlebitis did not affect subsequent athletic performances in nonracing horses and had only a slight impact on racehorses in that 84% returned to racing after treatment for this condition, and those that did performed as well as previously.[132]

Prevention

Thrombophlebitis can be minimized with (1) early identification and appropriate treatment of the coagulation disturbances associated with GI disease and SIRS (see Chapter 11); (2) careful selection, insertion, and use of IV catheters; (3) avoidance of homemade IV fluid solutions; (4) appropriate

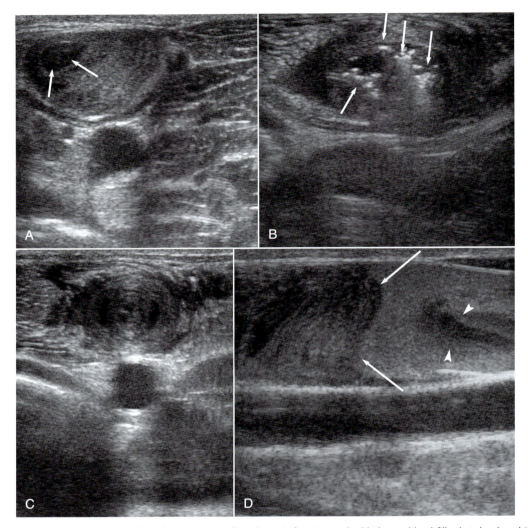

Figure 2-21 Transverse (**A** to **C**) and longitudinal (**D**) ultrasonograms of jugular vein from 5-month-old Thoroughbred filly that developed jugular thrombosis associated with colitis. An anechoic pocket (*arrows* in **A**) and echogenic gas echoes (*arrows* in **B**) are visible within a thrombus, confirming sepsis. The thrombus has an "onion ring" appearance in the transverse image (**C**), and in the longitudinal image (**D**) the blood that is stationary proximal to the thrombus (*arrows*) is swirling and creating movement patterns within the vein (*arrowheads*) and the layered structure of the thrombus is evident.

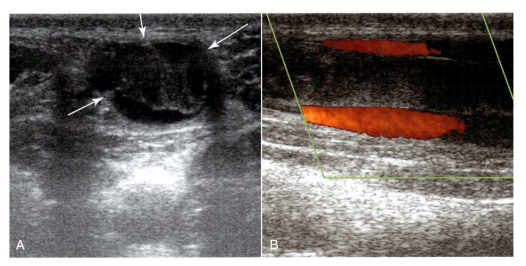

Figure 2-22 Transverse (**A**) and longitudinal (**B**) ultrasonograms of jugular vein from 5-year-old Warmbred gelding that developed jugular thrombosis after severe colitis. Eight days after the onset of signs, as the thrombus begins to resolve, it contracts to an irregular shape with attachments to the vessel wall (*arrows*). Power Doppler imaging confirms that the vein is patent.

dilution of irritant drugs; and (5) avoidance of needlesticks in veins that are or recently have been catheterized. Catheters should be flushed frequently with heparinized saline (1 IU/mL) when not in continuous use, and Teflon over-the-needle catheters should be left in place for no more than 72 hours. Polyurethane over-the-needle catheters can be maintained for up to 5 days. Fluid lines should be changed every 24 hours in high-risk patients. It may be helpful to cover the catheter with bandage material in foals or horses that are frequently recumbent, although this is not done routinely in adult horses in most veterinary hospitals.[127]

Caudal Vena Cava Thrombosis Syndrome

Caudal vena cava thrombosis syndrome is recognized in cattle. Hepatic abscesses arise in association with rumenitis and can lead to septic thrombosis of the vena cava and ultimately embolic pneumonia. In horses, liver abscesses are uncommon but have been associated with septic caudal vena cava thrombosis.[133] There is one report of a horse developing embolic pneumonia related to hepatic thrombosis, caudal vena cava thrombosis, and pulmonary thromboembolism.[134] The relevant portion of the caudal vena cava and the hilar portion of the liver are difficult to image with ultrasonography, but this condition should be considered a possibility when embolic pneumonia is identified.

Arterial Thrombosis, Arteritis, and Aortitis

Horses with aortoiliac thrombosis are typically adults presenting for evaluation of hindlimb lameness, difficulty in breeding, or acute pain. Affected horses have cold extremities and reduced arterial pulses in the affected limbs. The condition can be diagnosed with ultrasonography or nuclear scintigraphy (Fig. 2-23). The etiology is unknown. Rational medical therapy includes the administration of antithrombotics such as aspirin; however, the outcome has often been disappointing. Intraluminal thrombectomy using a graft thrombectomy device[135] and an ultrasound-guided balloon thrombectomy procedure[136] have been described. With the former procedure, 11 of 17 cases (65%) returned to exercise, with 9 (53%) performing at their previous level,[137] thus surgical intervention appears to offer promising results.

Arterial thrombosis associated with sepsis is rare but has been documented in association with neonatal sepsis affecting the aortoiliac quadrification ("saddle thrombus")[138,139] in the digital,[140,141] metacarpal, and metatarsal arteries[141]; in the pulmonary artery[142]; and in the major vessels of the metatarsal and metacarpal regions in older animals with enterocolitis.[141] In an additional case of brachial artery thrombosis in a foal with an atrial septal defect, it was suggested that the condition may have arisen following embolism from an atrial thrombus.[143] In sepsis and endotoxemia, abnormalities of hemostasis and fibrinolytic pathways may lead to arterial thrombosis. Thrombocytopenia and deficiencies in antithrombin III, caused by either excessive consumption or loss through the GI tract in protein-losing enteropathy, have been observed in affected patients.[141,143] Activation of procoagulants by endotoxin, dehydration, hypoxia, and acidosis may also contribute to the pathogenesis.[141] Clinical examination reveals that the affected limbs are cold, and there may be partial or complete sloughing of the hoof. Arterial thrombosis can be documented using two-dimensional and Doppler ultrasonography,[142] nuclear scintigraphy,[139,144] thermography,[145] and contrast angiography.[143] Attempts to remove the thrombus by surgical embolectomy[144] and the use of tPA[139] and urokinase[140] have not yet produced successful results.

Cranial mesenteric arteritis is associated with migrating strongyle species and even has been documented in foals as young as 3 months.[146] As it migrates through the mesenteric arteries, *Strongylus vulgaris* induces thrombosis, inflammation, and intimal and adventitial fibrosis, and the accumulation of collagen leads to decreased arterial elasticity.[147] Affected animals present with recurrent or persistent colic, and a firm mass can sometimes be palpated at the mesenteric root. The condition is no longer common, presumably as a result of the widespread use of anthelmintics that are effective in reducing the burden of *S. vulgaris*. The diagnosis can be confirmed with transrectal ultrasonography[148]; typically a complex solid mass is visualized, representing fibrous tissue surrounding the mesenteric blood vessels (Fig. 2-24). Appropriate anthelmintic regimens should minimize the risk of cranial mesenteric arteritis (see Chapter 57).

Aortitis and aortic root abscess are rare conditions described in a horse with concurrent aortic valve IE[149] and also reported as isolated conditions in a horse presenting with clinical signs similar to those of IE: fever, hindlimb swelling, lethargy, tachycardia, and a systolic murmur. The diagnosis was confirmed with echocardiography; blood culture yielded *Streptococcus* spp. Treatment with penicillin G and gentamicin was unsuccessful in this latter case.[150]

Cardiac Complications in Systemic Inflammatory Response Syndrome and Sepsis

Cardiac Dysrhythmias

Dysrhythmias occurring secondary to other systemic diseases, particularly GI diseases accompanied by SIRS,[151,152] are encountered more frequently in horses than rhythm disturbances associated with primary myocardial pathology. In a group of 67 horses with duodenitis or proximal jejunitis, 6 (9%; CI 2.1%-15.8%) had dysrhythmias,[151] and ambulatory electrocardiograms (ECGs) obtained from 50 horses within 3 days of exploratory celiotomy demonstrated that 11 horses (22%; CI 10.5%-33.5%) developed isolated supraventricular premature depolarizations,[120] and 8 horses (16%; CI 5.8%-26.2%) developed isolated ventricular premature depolarizations, including 4 (8%; CI 0.5%-15.5%) with idioventricular rhythms or paroxysmal monomorphic ventricular tachycardia. These dysrhythmias are often self-limiting, requiring no specific treatment,[153,154] and often the dysrhythmia is not recognized on physical examination. Occasionally, more clinically significant dysrhythmias are encountered in critical care patients, and concurrent clinical signs of reduced cardiac output and marked tachycardia are recognized. Such dysrhythmias can occur with other systemic diseases[152] and conditions associated with SIRS, such as IE and metritis (see Fig. 2-7).

In these horses, arrhythmogenesis is likely related to multiple confounding factors, including the direct effects of endotoxin on the myocardium, autonomic imbalance resulting from GI distention, and metabolic, electrolyte, or acid-base imbalances.[151] Overall electrolyte balance is more important than isolated disturbances, although the electrolytes usually associated with dysrhythmias are potassium, calcium, and magnesium.[120] With potassium, hyperkalemia leads to decreased P-wave amplitude and increased T-wave amplitude. Hypokalemia is associated with ventricular dysrhythmias in humans[155] and horses[154] and has been implicated in the development of atrial fibrillation in horses.[156] Calcium principally affects the ST segment, and both hypocalcemia and hypercalcemia are associated with fatal ventricular dysrhythmias.[156] Magnesium is an

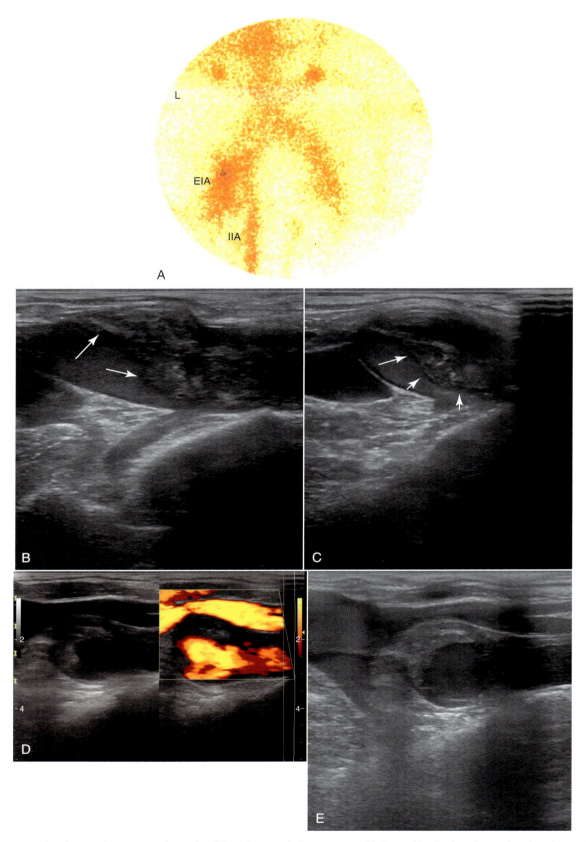

Figure 2-23 **A,** Vascular phase nuclear scintigraphic study of the pelvic vessels from a 3-year-old Thoroughbred colt with aortoiliac thrombosis, obtained by placing the gamma camera dorsal to the pelvis, demonstrates reduction in blood flow within the right internal iliac artery *(IIA)*. *L,* Left; *EIA,* external iliac artery. **B** and **C,** At the time of diagnosis, ultrasonograms positioned along the long- and short-axis of the right internal iliac artery demonstrate that there is a heterogeneous thrombus *(arrows)* occupying a large portion of the lumen. **D,** Eight weeks later, following treatment with fenbendazole, phenylbutazone, and aspirin, the thrombus is smaller and power Doppler demonstrates blood flow within the vessel. **E,** At 14 weeks, 6 weeks after the discontinuation of aspirin and introduction of a progressive incremental exercise program, the thrombus has reduced in size considerably and occupies less than one third of the vessel lumen. The colt returned to racing with no further recurrence of clinical signs. *(Courtesy W. Schofield, Troytown Equine Hospital, Kildare, Ireland.)*

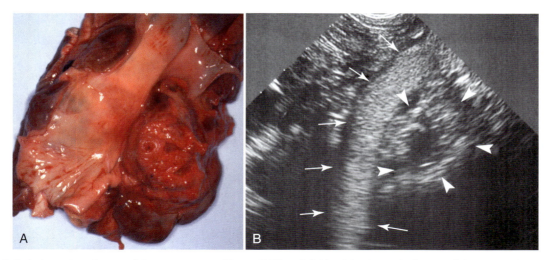

Figure 2-24 **A,** Pathologic specimen from aged Connemara mare with pyrrolizidine alkaloid toxicity. A mass in the area of the mesenteric root was detected as an incidental finding. **B,** Transrectal abdominal ultrasonogram shows thick-walled blood vessels surrounded by fibrous tissue in longitudinal *(arrows)* and transverse *(arrowheads)* planes resulting from mesenteric arteritis.

important cofactor in the sodium-potassium adenosine triphosphatase (ATPase) pump that regulates action potentials; hypomagnesemia is associated with ventricular dysrhythmias.[155]

In addition to electrolyte imbalances at the intracellular or extracellular level, metabolic and acid-base disturbances and alterations of the autonomic nervous system play a role in the genesis of dysrhythmias.[120] Addressing underlying and contributory factors is the main therapeutic goal. Strong evidence to support decisions on which specific antidysrhythmic agent to use in equine patients is lacking, and the decision to institute specific antidysrhythmic therapy is generally based on an assessment of whether it is likely that the dysrhythmia will destabilize to a life-threatening state. Guidelines for treatment of tachydysrhythmia are provided earlier in the section on myocarditis (see Table 2-3).

Cardiac Involvement in Multiple Organ Dysfunction

The distributive shock that occurs with endotoxemia and SIRS is principally caused by dysregulation of systemic vascular function and is accompanied by microthrombosis. However, a direct myocardial depressant mechanism may also come into play. Compared with measurement of cardiac output by thermodilution or lithium dilution techniques, echocardiography is not a particularly useful tool for critical care monitoring. Horses and foals with endotoxemia or sepsis can have echocardiographic signs of global cardiac dysfunction (Fig. 2-25) such as reduced fractional shortening, spontaneous contrast, and poor ventricular wall movement. Hypovolemic patients may have reduced cardiac chamber size, and in septic patients, mild pericardial effusions are fairly common. Thus, in addition to primary myocardial or pericardial diseases, endotoxemia and sepsis should be considered as major differential diagnoses when these echocardiographic findings are observed.

Mild fibrinous pericarditis, right atrial and ventricular enlargement, myocardial depression, and ventricular tachycardia have been observed in streptococcal toxic shock with multiple organ dysfunction in a horse.[157] Treatment of streptococcal shock consists of supportive care and symptomatic therapy. Maintaining adequate tissue perfusion with IV crystalloid and colloidal fluids and pressor agents is critical. Antimicrobial therapy is important and should be guided by the results of blood culture and antimicrobial sensitivity tests. In humans, fluoroquinolones are not recommended because these agents

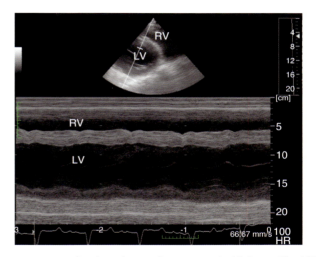

Figure 2-25 M-mode echocardiogram from a 4-month-old Thoroughbred filly with moderately severe pneumonia. The movement of the septum and left ventricular wall is reduced, suggesting myocardial dysfunction secondary to sepsis. In addition to antimicrobial therapy, the filly was treated with an infusion of dobutamine, titrated to blood pressure and digoxin, and the ventricular movement was restored over the subsequent 3 days. *LV*, Left ventricle; *RV*, right ventricle.

have a poor spectrum of activity against streptococci. Interestingly, in the single reported equine case, clinical deterioration was noted when initial treatment with ceftiofur, penicillin, and metronidazole was changed to enrofloxacin, although the microorganism that was identified on blood culture, *Streptococcus mitis*, was sensitive in vitro to enrofloxacin. Streptococcal toxic shock was previously associated specifically with *Streptococcus pyogenes* infection in humans, but it is now recognized in association with a wide range of *Streptococcus* spp. in both humans[158] and dogs.[159] In the last 20 years, this condition has been increasingly diagnosed in humans,[158] and streptococcal toxic shock may become more important in horses in the future.[157]

The complete reference list is available online at www.expert-consult.com.

Gastrointestinal and Peritoneal Infections

3

Martha Mallicote and Chris Sanchez

The pathophysiologic mechanisms of the primary etiologic agents responsible for infectious diseases of the gastrointestinal (GI) tract are covered in depth individually elsewhere in this text. Thus the primary goals of this chapter are to present the normal microflora throughout the GI tract and to briefly discuss an approach to the diagnosis and management of the primary clinical syndromes associated with these infectious processes.

Oral Cavity

Normal Flora

Most work describing the normal flora of bacteria in the equine pharynx relates to upper respiratory tract infection and lower respiratory tract infection attributed to aspiration. But, relatively few studies have examined the normal flora of the oral cavity in horses. Several aerobic and facultative anaerobic organisms have been isolated from various locations throughout the pharynx, most notably *Streptococcus equi* subsp. *zooepidemicus*.[1-3] Commonly isolated anaerobes included those from the genera *Bacteroides*, *Eubacterium*, *Fusobacterium*, *Clostridium*, *Veillonella*, *Peptostreptococcus*, and *Megasphera*.[3]

Infectious Disorders

Unlike in small animals, infectious diseases of the oral cavity are relatively rare in horses. Primary problems with a possible infectious etiology include periodontitis and tooth root abscesses, pharyngitis, and dysphagia. Anaerobic organisms are frequently associated with tooth root abscesses.[4] Other infectious problems with potential impact on the oral cavity include *Actinobacillus lignieresii*, the organism associated with wooden tongue[5,6]; various fungal organisms such as *Candida* spp., which can cause thrush in foals; viral diseases such as vesicular stomatitis[7]; infectious causes of dysphagia such as *Clostridium botulinum* (botulism)[8,9]; and equine protozoal myeloencephalitis.

Esophagus and Stomach

Normal Flora

The esophagus and stomach are not sterile environments, and the stomach harbors a relatively diverse microbial population. In one study, 2.78×10^9 total (2.00×10^8 viable) bacteria per gram of ingesta were recovered from the fundic region of normal ponies, with 1.92×10^9 total (1.0×10^7 viable) bacteria per gram of ingesta recovered from the pyloric region.[10] In both regions, gram-positive organisms (rods and cocci) predominated, and very few cellulolytic (100 to 300/g) bacteria were isolated.[10] Both the total anaerobic bacterial population and the lactobacilli concentration appeared to increase in a linear fashion in live horses after a meal.[11] Colonization of and attachment to the gastric squamous mucosa by several indigenous *Lactobacillus* spp. have also been documented.[12] Similar bacteria have been identified within different regions of the gastric mucosa using fluorescent in-situ hybridization,[13,14] although the microbial population can vary by individual.[13]

Infectious Disorders

Infectious diseases of the esophagus mainly occur secondary to perforation, thus involving a mixed population of aerobic and anaerobic bacteria. In the equine stomach, although polymerase chain reaction (PCR) fragments unique to gastric-dwelling *Helicobacter* spp. have been identified in horses, an association between *H. pylori* and ulceration has not been established in adult horses or foals.[15,16] More recent studies have failed to identify *Helicobacter* spp. in equine gastric mucosa using fluorescent in-situ hybridization,[13] including those with antral pathology.[14] One case of emphysematous gastritis due to *Clostridium perfringens* has been reported.[17]

Small Intestine

Normal Flora

Few studies have evaluated normal equine small intestinal microbial populations. Total bacterial counts and proportion of gram-positive bacteria recovered from the ileum were similar to that seen in the stomach,[10] but viable bacteria numbered 3.6×10^7. In a study analyzing only anaerobic bacteria, increasing numbers of both culturable and proteolytic bacteria were identified in the duodenum, jejunum, and ileum.[18] Proteolytic bacteria composed a high proportion of the total bacteria in all regions but accounted for almost all in the duodenum. Numbers of bacteria identified from the GI lumen outnumbered those recovered from the mucosa in all segments.[18]

Infectious Disorders Causing Diarrhea in Foals

Most infectious causes of diarrhea in foals, unlike those causes in adult horses, affect the small intestine either alone or in combination with the large colon.

Bacterial Disorders

Foals diagnosed with systemic sepsis (see Chapter 6) commonly develop diarrhea in association with their primary disease, with reported incidence between 16% and 42%.[19-23] As such, although *Escherichia coli* is the most common causative organism associated with sepsis, it is not typically recognized as a primary cause of enteritis and/or enterocolitis in foals. One report demonstrated an increased probability of diarrhea in foals with *Actinobacillus* sepsis when compared to those foals from which other organisms were isolated.[19] Further, up to 50% of foals presenting with diarrhea have a positive blood culture at admission, supporting the usefulness of this diagnostic test for foals less than 30 days of age.[24,25]

Another common bacterial cause of enterocolitis in foals is *Salmonella enteritidis* (see Chapter 35). In addition to diarrhea, affected foals typically display clinical signs of sepsis. Diagnosis is confirmed via aerobic culture of blood and/or feces. Treatment is supportive and should always include directed systemic antimicrobial therapy.

Clostridial organisms can act as primary pathogens in foals (see Chapter 41), and these agents can cause disease in individual animals or present as outbreaks in affected farms. *Clostridium perfringens* typically affects foals younger than 10 days of age. *Clostridium perfringens* serotypes A and C are most commonly implicated, with serotype C resulting in more severe disease, hemorrhagic diarrhea, and higher mortality than that seen with serotype A.[26,27] Serotype A is commonly isolated from the feces of normal foals, but the organism in general is more commonly isolated from foals with diarrhea.[28,29] A diagnosis is typically based on the presence of compatible clinical signs and culture of the organism from feces, preferably with genotyping of the obtained isolate. Observation of large, gram-positive rods or spores on a fecal Gram stain should raise the index of suspicion.[26] *Clostridium difficile* has also been implicated as a cause of diarrhea in foals. Disease severity can vary from mild to hemorrhagic diarrhea. As with *C. perfringens*, *C. difficile* can be isolated from asymptomatic foals, thus toxin detection in feces is useful for confirmation of a diagnosis.[30,31] Commercial immunoassays are available for the detection of toxins A and B in feces, as well as the enterotoxin of *C. perfringens*.[32] Treatment is supportive with the addition of directed antimicrobial therapy, typically with metronidazole. In some geographic locations, documented metronidazole resistance in *C. difficile* isolates has prompted therapy with vancomycin in select cases.[33] Infection with *Lawsonia intracellularis* has been described in older foals.[34-37] Infection with this obligate intracellular pathogen results in a proliferative enteropathy and should be suspected in any weanling age foal with severe hypoproteinemia. Clinical signs include weight loss, ill thrift, depression, colic, peripheral edema, and variable fecal consistency, ranging from soft normal to watery diarrhea. Protein loss can be severe. Diagnosis is based on clinical signs in combination with results of fecal PCR and serum antibody testing. Treatment includes supportive care, predominantly with colloid replacement, and directed antimicrobial therapy. Common specific recommendations include chloramphenicol and oxytetracycline followed by doxycycline, erythromycin, or clarithromycin.[38-40] Duration of treatment is dictated by clinical status and improvement of clinicopathologic findings; a minimum of 3 weeks of treatment is typically indicated.

Viral Disorders

The most commonly encountered viral pathogen causing diarrhea in foals is rotavirus. Typically, rotavirus is thought to affect foals between 5 and 35 days of age,[41] although recent data suggest the mean age of affected foals can be as high as 81 days.[24] Older foals appear to be less severely affected.[42] The most common and obvious clinical sign is diarrhea, and fecal consistency can vary greatly. Other signs relate to disease severity, including depression, anorexia, dehydration, and other similar findings. The virus causes blunting of the small intestinal microvilli, resulting in malabsorption and maldigestion. Diagnosis can be confirmed with fecal electron microscopy, which

has a significant lag time, or commercial immunoassays, also performed on feces. Treatment is principally supportive. Emphasis must be placed on biosecurity protocols to prevent spread of new outbreaks. Because this is a nonenveloped virus, typical antiviral disinfectant compounds, such as quaternary ammonium mixtures, are ineffective against rotavirus. The virus is extremely contagious, with morbidity often approaching 100% in farm outbreaks. Prognosis is very good to excellent with supportive care, and mortality is typically very low in uncomplicated cases. Other viral disorders occur much less frequently and include coronavirus[43-45] and adenovirus.[46,47]

Protozoal Disorders

Cryptosporidium spp. are the most common protozoal cause of diarrhea in foals.[28,45,48] These organisms are generally regarded as less significant than the major bacterial and viral diseases discussed previously.

Small Intestinal Disease in Adult Horses

Etiology and Pathophysiology

Proven infectious disorders of the small intestine in horses are rare. Horses do not appear predisposed to small intestinal bacterial overgrowth, which is common in dogs and human beings. One disorder that has a suspected, but to this point unsubstantiated, infectious origin is duodenitis/proximal jejunitis (DPJ), a syndrome of small intestinal inflammation primarily characterized by copious quantities of gastric reflux. This syndrome has also been termed *anterior enteritis* or *proximal enteritis*. In most cases, an underlying etiology cannot be determined. In some cases, *Salmonella* spp. or *Clostridium* spp. can be isolated from culture of gastric reflux. Salmonella has not been consistently identified in a majority of cases, and many horses with documented infections by these organisms do not develop DPJ. Recently, toxigenic strains of *C. difficile* were isolated from the reflux of 10 of 10 horses with DPJ and 1 of 16 control horses with other causes of nasogastric reflux.[49] Further investigation of this organism is clearly warranted. Another suspected infectious cause is *Fusarium* spp.[50] In one epidemiologic report, affected horses were fed significantly more concentrate and were more likely to have grazed pasture than unaffected controls.[51] Regardless of the initiating cause, inflammatory-mediated alterations in secretion and motility contribute to a functional obstruction and a vicious cycle of events. Intestinal inflammation can result in alterations in normal sensory-motor function, mucosal function, ion transport, and transepithelial permeability. The blanket term *duodenitis/proximal jejunitis* may actually encompass a wide spectrum of inflammatory small intestinal disorders resulting in a similar clinical syndrome.

Clinical Signs and Laboratory Findings

The most characteristic clinical findings in horses with DPJ include moderate to severe pain that often improves after gastric decompression, large volumes of gastric reflux, clinical signs of endotoxemia, and small intestinal distention evident on rectal palpation and ultrasonographic examination.

Abnormal clinicopathologic findings can include hemoconcentration, neutropenia, acidemia, prerenal azotemia, hyponatremia, hypochloremia, hypokalemia, and increased hepatic enzymes.[52] Typically, peritoneal tap findings include a mild to moderate increase in total nucleated cell count (TNCC), which can be elevated to 20,000/μL with a moderate to marked increase in total solids (up to 5 g/dL). However, the nucleated cell count has been reported to vary widely in some cases. These findings are often a useful method of differentiation from horses with strangulating small intestinal disease, which tend to have higher numbers of red blood cells, as well as increased TNCC;

however, peritoneal tap findings should be used in conjunction with other parameters.[53]

Therapy

Treatment consists primarily of supportive care, with an emphasis on fluid therapy and gastric decompression. Particular care should be taken to provide maintenance fluid requirements while also replacing the volume lost through gastric reflux. Therapy should also include nonsteroidal antiinflammatory therapy for analgesic as well as antiinflammatory purposes, as long as renal function remains normal, and directed therapy to combat endotoxemia. When cases either deteriorate or do not improve with medical therapy, surgical exploration can be considered.[54] Surgical exploration can offer manual decompression of the small intestine and rule out any physical obstruction, although surgical treatment did not improve patient outcome in one report.[55] In protracted cases or in horses with hypertriglyceridemia, supplemental parenteral nutritional support should be considered. Prokinetic therapy with either erythromycin lactobionate, metoclopramide, bethanechol, or lidocaine can also be considered[56-58]; one should note that these therapies may be less effective in the inflamed intestine.[59]

With prompt medical therapy, horses with DPJ generally carry a good prognosis. Factors associated with a decreased risk of survival include increased peritoneal fluid protein concentration and increased anion gap,[60] as well as failure to respond to prokinetic therapy within 24 hours.[56] Potential complications include laminitis, thrombophlebitis, peritonitis, adhesions, pharyngitis and/or esophagitis, and cardiac dysrhythmias.[61]

Large Intestine

Normal Flora

Much more is known about the resident microflora in the equine large intestine relative to the more orad portions of the GI tract. The cecum and large colon have a large capacity and the capability for extensive fermentation by bacteria and protozoa. Total protozoal concentrations in the large colon appear to increase in horses fed a diet high in forage, relative to a diet high in concentrate.[62] In the same study, the colon had concentrations of both total and cellulolytic fungi more than 10 times greater than those found in the cecum.[62] Increasing the grain component of a diet appears to have a greater impact in the colon, relative to the cecum; total bacterial concentration increased and cellulolytic bacterial concentration decreased in horses fed a primarily concentrate diet.[63] Cecal microflora remained predominantly cellulolytic regardless of diet.[64] At least two species of anaerobic phycomycetes capable of digesting plant cellulose and hemicellulose have been isolated from the equine cecum,[65] and *Ruminococcus flavefaciens* has recently been identified as the predominant cellulolytic cecal bacterial species.[66] At least two types of spirochetes have been documented in the equine cecum.[67] Bacteriophages have been documented infecting spirochetes from the equine cecum,[67] and bacteriophage-like particles have been demonstrated in various regions of the large intestine by electron microscopy.[68]

Acute Diarrhea in Adult Horses

Etiology

The most common infectious agents associated with colitis in adult horses include *Salmonella* spp. (see Chapter 35), *Neorickettsia* (formerly *Ehrlichia*) *risticii* (equine monocytic ehrlichiosis, Potomac horse fever [PHF]; see Chapter 40), *C. difficile* (see Chapter 42), and *C. perfringens* (see Chapter 42). *Aeromonas* spp. are often isolated from horses with diarrhea, but true

causality as an etiologic agent in acute diarrhea has not been determined. Parasites are not typically associated with acute diarrhea in adult horses, with the exception of larval cyathostomiasis in Europe, the northern part of the United States, and Canada. The most common cause of outbreaks of colitis in horses is salmonellosis. Outbreaks of PHF and clostridial colitis are rare, although the latter may occur as a clustering of cases of foals or hospitalized horses.

Diagnostic Approach

In evaluation of horses with acute diarrhea, laboratory evaluation should include complete blood count (CBC) with fibrinogen and a biochemical profile. If available, venous blood gas analysis is desirable. Additional tests aimed at identification of an etiologic agent can be performed both on blood and feces. The potential for co-infections should be considered when determining an appropriate diagnostic plan.

Diagnostic Tests on Whole Blood or Serum

Neorickettsia risticii

Although an enzyme-linked immunosorbent assay (ELISA) has been described for the diagnosis of *N. risticii*, most laboratories use an immunofluorescent assay (IFA) or PCR.[69] Infected horses develop high titers (>640) within days, often before clinical signs are apparent. Paired serum samples (acute and convalescent) should be collected within 5 to 7 days rather than the conventional interval of 2 to 4 weeks because infected horses rapidly develop high titers. Several laboratories interpret a single serum titer of ≥80 at the onset of signs as consistent with PHF once horses develop diarrhea. However, given the variation in the immune response of individual horses and the variation in clinical signs wherein some horses do not develop diarrhea, paired serum must be utilized even if the first sample was negative. Vaccination for PHF results in positive titers that usually disappear by 6 to 9 months, and previous subclinical exposure has prolonged waxing and waning titers for over a year. Polymerase chain reaction detects the presence of antigen and has excellent sensitivity without the potential for interference from vaccination,[70,71] and both feces and blood should be tested since the organism may not be present in both fluids concurrently.[69,70] This testing can be performed on postmortem tissues even if formalin-fixed.[69]

Diagnostic Tests on Feces

Aerobic Culture

The main organism of interest is *Salmonella enterica*. Enrichment culture is required, and antiserum assays are required for identification to serogroup. Most accredited laboratories identify to serogroup, and the National Veterinary Services Laboratory (Ames, IA) will identify all isolates to serotype. Multiple cultures are preferable, and recovery of pathogens can be difficult when feces are very watery. Culture of a rectal mucosal biopsy sample may improve the recovery rate.[72] Polymerase chain reaction has been reported as a more sensitive method of detecting salmonella in feces relative to culture.[73-76] In a horse with clinical signs, detection using a validated real-time assay PCR recently had a specificity as high as 98%.[77]

Anaerobic Culture

Anaerobic culture of fecal samples is primarily used to identify the presence of *Clostridium* spp. Strict anaerobic handling of the feces is critical to successful culture, especially for *C. difficile*.[78] Recovery of *C. difficile* organisms is dramatically reduced after storage for 72 hours in aerobic conditions at 4° C.[78]

Because clostridia can be cultured from the feces of some normal horses, direct detection of specific clostridial toxins from feces enhances diagnostic specificity. Toxins are detected by bioassay for the *C. perfringens* pathogens and by cytoxic bioassay or ELISA for *C. difficile*. *Clostridium difficile* toxins are more stable in aerobic conditions than the organisms themselves.[78] Commercial assays (ELISA) are available for *C. difficile* toxins A and B, as well as the enterotoxin of *C. perfringens*.[32] For *C. perfringens*, PCR analysis of isolates cultured from feces is the preferred method for detection of toxin and confirmation of a diagnosis of clinically relevant disease. Many diagnostic laboratories will perform toxin testing, and some will provide packages including both culture and toxin analysis.

Feces should be examined by sedimentation for sand and microscopically for increased fecal leukocytes. A Gram stain may be useful as an initial screen for *Clostridial* organisms (long gram-positive rods). Cyathostome larvae are best detected by direct examination of feces.

Therapy

The primary goal of therapy for adult horses with diarrhea is restoration and maintenance of fluid, electrolyte, and acid-base balance. Specific pathogen-directed antimicrobial therapy may be indicated, depending on the etiologic agent identified, but generalized, prophylactic antimicrobial administration is not recommended for most adult horses with diarrhea. For many horses with acute diarrhea, initial intravenous (IV) fluid replacement is required as the result of tremendous volume losses. Typically, mild to moderate acidemia is corrected by restoration of plasma volume with a balanced polyionic replacement fluid. Acidifying solutions (such as 0.9% sodium chloride) are not recommended but may be used if another fluid option is unavailable. In cases of severe dehydration, initial therapy with hypertonic saline or synthetic colloid (such as hydroxyethyl starch) can be used to restore circulatory volume, but these must be followed by administration of isotonic fluids.

Other goals of therapy include reducing inflammation, pain control, and limiting the effects of endotoxemia. Drugs commonly used for these purposes include nonsteroidal antiinflammatory drugs (NSAIDs), such as flunixin meglumine which has analgesic and antiinflammatory properties.[79] As with other NSAIDs, one must take care to avoid use of this agent in horses with renal compromise, moderate to severe dehydration, NSAID toxicity, or right dorsal colitis. Adjunctive therapy with polymyxin B sulfate[80-82] and/or pentoxifylline[79,83-85] is suggested to combat the effects of endotoxemia.

Chronic Diarrhea in Adult Horses

Etiology

Chronic diarrhea is usually defined as diarrhea persisting for more than 4 weeks.[86] Fecal consistency can vary widely. Although many specific diseases can result in chronic diarrhea, the actual inciting cause at the time of presentation is usually elusive. Occasionally, problems of a non-GI nature, such as hepatic disease or abdominal abscessation, result in diarrhea. More common infectious causes of chronic diarrhea include chronic salmonellosis and parasitism with large and/or small strongyles. Recently, the spirochete *Brachyspira pilosicoli* was implicated in a herd outbreak of chronic diarrhea in weanling age horses.[87] Noninfectious inflammatory causes include inflammatory bowel diseases (granulomatous enteritis or colitis, lymphocytic-plasmacytic enterocolitis, and eosinophilic enterocolitis), neoplasia (most commonly lymphosarcoma), sand enteropathy, and right dorsal colitis. Noninflammatory causes encompass a range of problems with the common theme of disruption of the large colonic intestinal flora or mucosal function. This may or may not be related to a dietary disruption, and many of these horses have few other clinical signs. Regardless of the inciting cause, horses with chronic diarrhea remain very difficult to treat and afford a guarded prognosis for long-lasting return to normal fecal consistency.

Diagnostic Approach

Laboratory evaluation for the individual horse with chronic diarrhea typically includes CBC with fibrinogen, serum biochemical profile, venous blood gas analysis, rectal examination, abdominal ultrasound, and analysis of peritoneal fluid. Results of all the aforementioned diagnostic procedures are commonly normal, and further recommended analyses include a comprehensive fecal examination, gastro-duodenoscopy with biopsy, and rectal biopsy.

Comprehensive fecal analysis should include assessment for parasites (grossly and by fecal flotation/McMasters quantification), aerobic culture for *Salmonella* (5 samples at a minimum 12-hour interval, as for acute diarrhea), sand sedimentation, unstained wet mount for protozoa and parasites, new methylene blue stain for fecal leukocytes, and Gram stain to evaluate the gram-positive:gram-negative bacteria ratio.

Gastro-duodenoscopy allows both visual inspection of the stomach and proximal duodenum and the collection of biopsy specimens for histopathology. Rectal biopsy is a simple, relatively noninvasive procedure.[88] Samples should be submitted for both culture *(Salmonella)* and histopathology. The main diagnoses obtained with use of histopathology are the inflammatory bowel diseases.

Therapy

If a specific diagnosis is achieved, directed therapy should be initiated according to the etiologic agent. In all cases, free-choice access to fresh water is critical to maintenance of hydration. Many horses will consume balanced, isotonic electrolyte-spiked water, if such a solution is offered. Alternatively, access to a salt or mineral block can serve as a substitute source of electrolyte replacement. Typical feeding recommendations include good quality grass hay with limited legume hay and concentrate intake. Dietary changes alone are unlikely to effect a cure but may provide improvement.

Nonspecific therapy for horses with chronic diarrhea can include transfaunation and iodochlorhydroxyquin. Exact recommendations for the transfaunation procedure are sparse in the veterinary literature, as are reported benefits. Typically, cecal liquor is obtained either from an animal recently euthanized for non-GI reasons or from an animal implanted with a cecal cannula. Once appropriate transfaunate is obtained, one must also decide whether to pretreat the recipient. Frequently, recipients are pretreated with acid-suppressing agents to enhance viability of transplanted bacteria and protozoa as they pass through the gastric environment. The efficacy of such treatment has not been validated to date in the horse, although the potential value of transfaunation was recently highlighted during a herd outbreak potentially related to the spirochete *Brachyspira pilosicoli*.[89]

Iodochlorhydroxyquin, an 8-hydroxyquinolone derivative, has long been recommended for the treatment of chronic diarrhea, although this therapy was initially proposed for the treatment of trichomoniasis.[90] Although the described disease entity likely involved disruption of the normal intestinal flora rather than an infectious cause, some horses responded favorably to therapy. The response to treatment with iodochlorhydroxyquin is highly variable, from no change to worsening of the diarrhea. Often, therapy will result in more normal fecal consistency, but unfortunately many will revert to diarrhea within a few days of drug withdrawal.[89]

Prognosis

Regardless of the inciting cause, the prognosis for complete recovery is guarded when the duration of diarrhea exceeds

1 month; the prognosis worsens as the course of disease progresses.

Peritoneal Infections

Peritonitis refers to inflammation of the mesothelial lining of the peritoneal cavity and is typically caused by mechanical, chemical, or infectious insult to the parietal peritoneum. In addition to classification based on the causative insult, further classification can include onset (acute or chronic), distribution (localized or diffuse), origin (primary or secondary), and infectious component (septic or aseptic). Acute, diffuse, septic peritonitis secondary to GI disease is the most common manifestation.[91]

Etiology and Clinical Findings

Most cases of peritonitis occur secondary to a GI event such as perforation of the GI tract, intestinal ischemia, DPJ, colitis, neoplasia, verminous arteritis, intestinal mural abscess, or other causes.[92-94] Iatrogenic causes include rectal tear, enterocentesis, castration, and abdominal surgery. Other causes include traumatic events (including uterine or vaginal perforation during foaling or breeding), mesenteric abscess (including those associated with *Streptococcus equi* subsp. *equi*), cholelithiasis, and others. Causes specific to the young foal include rupture of the urinary bladder or urachus, omphalitis and/or omphalophlebitis, sepsis, and *Rhodococcus equi* abscessation.

Organisms associated with GI rupture include a mixed population of gram-positive and gram-negative aerobic and anaerobic organisms, typically with no clear predominance. Enterobacteriaceae, *Streptococcus* spp., and *Staphylococcus* spp. have been most commonly isolated from septic peritoneal fluid samples.[93,95,96] Common anaerobes include *Bacteroides*, *Clostridium*, and *Bacillus* spp. In foals, peritonitis is more commonly associated with *Streptococcus* and *R. equi* infections. Several case series involving peritonitis associated with *Actinobacillus equuli* have been reported.[97-99] Initial reports of *A. equuli* peritonitis originated solely in Australia, but individual cases have been reported from the United Kingdom and United States.[100,101]

Clinical signs of peritonitis in horses are variable but include fever, depression and abdominal pain. Individuals may present with diarrhea or weight loss.[92,94] Based on severity and localization, signs can also include those of endotoxemia and shock. In horses with *A. equuli* peritonitis, clinical signs commonly include depression, inappetence, lethargy, and mild to moderate abdominal pain acutely or weight loss in a chronic form.[98,99] Postpartum mares with peritonitis secondary to a uterine perforation typically present with fever and depression, with or without abdominal pain.[102]

Horses with acute peritonitis are more likely to present with subclinical disseminated intravascular coagulation (DIC), as indicated by increased plasma and peritoneal D-dimer concentrations and prolonged clotting times, relative to those with other causes of acute colic.[111,112]

Diagnosis

Definitive diagnosis is based on an increased TNCC in peritoneal fluid (generally >10,000 cells/μL) with an increased total solids or protein that is often >5.0 mg/dL. Cytologic examination of the fluid is imperative to identify toxic changes and degenerating neutrophils and detect any intracellular or extracellular bacteria or plant materials. If GI contents or plant material are evident, one should take care to differentiate between GI rupture and enterocentesis. Aerobic and anaerobic

bacterial culture of peritoneal fluid should be performed in all suspected cases, but this procedure has a low sensitivity, with only 9.5% to 41% of samples yielding positive growth.[92,93,95,96] Total cell count in peritoneal fluid may be increased following enterocentesis, abdominal surgery, or open castration.[103-107] It is important to differentiate between peritonitis secondary to gastrointestinal rupture or leakage and iatrogenic enterocentesis. If fluid samples show abnormalities in TNCC and cytology, peritonitis is most likely present; enterocentesis can result in an elevated TNCC in abdominal fluid within 4 hours.[106] If a differentiation between peritonitis and enterocentesis cannot be clearly made, a sample should be taken from an alternate location, preferably with ultrasound guidance. In postfoaling mares, the percentage of neutrophils in the peritoneal fluid may be increased for up to 7 days, but the total protein and TNCC should remain within normal limits.[108,109] Other parameters, if available, can aid in the diagnosis. Ultrasonographic findings of abundant hypoechoic or variably echogenic peritoneal fluid is supportive of a septic process. A decrease in peritoneal fluid pH (<7.3) or glucose (<30 mg/dL) or an increase in the peritoneal lactate concentration can indicate aseptic peritonitis.[107,110]

Therapy

Treatment of horses with peritonitis should begin with identification and correction of the underlying problem, if possible. If a GI source is suspected, an exploratory celiotomy is likely indicated. Supportive care is also critical to the treatment protocol. This should include correction of fluid deficits, acid-base and electrolyte imbalances, and colloid oncotic pressure. Antiinflammatory and antiendotoxic therapy are also clearly of benefit. Additional analgesic and prokinetic drugs should be provided if necessary.

Antimicrobial therapy is critical to the management of septic peritonitis. Broad-spectrum coverage should be instituted pending results of peritoneal fluid culture and sensitivity. If positive results with sensitivity testing are obtained, therapy can be adjusted accordingly. A typical initial regimen includes penicillin, gentamicin, and metronidazole to cover gram-positive, gram-negative, and anaerobic spectrums, respectively (see Appendix D for dosages). Metronidazole should be included if anaerobic involvement is suspected because of the known resistance of multiple *Bacteroides* spp. to penicillins. Enrofloxacin can replace gentamicin in the treatment regimen because the lipophilic nature of this compound can provide increased penetration to the peritoneum. Neonatal foals with peritonitis should receive a similar regimen to that suggested for adults, although amikacin is frequently substituted for gentamicin due to increased sensitivity of commonly isolated organisms.[111] A combination of azithromycin or clarithromycin plus rifampin provides reasonable coverage for older foals or weanlings, as *Streptococcus* or *R. equi* are commonly associated with disease in that population if a primary GI lesion is not suspected.[111] Although *A. equuli* is typically sensitive to either penicillin or trimethoprim-sulfonamide combinations, initial broad-spectrum coverage with penicillin and gentamicin is suggested pending culture results as the result of microbial resistance of some isolates.[99]

Abdominal drainage and lavage can help remove excess fluid, foreign materials, fibrin, and bacterial products from horses with peritonitis, and postoperative lavage has been shown to decrease the incidence of experimentally-induced abdominal adhesions.[112] Open surgical exploration provides the most effective and thorough examination of all peritoneal surfaces and is recommended if GI perforation or ischemia is suspected or in any other case in which correction of a primary lesion is indicated. A ventral abdominal drain can either be placed at the time of surgery or in the standing horse with sedation and local anesthesia. Techniques have been described in detail elsewhere.[111,113] Medical and surgical treatment of postpartum peritonitis had similar outcomes in 49 recently described cases; but the severity of injury that can safely be treated medically is unknown.[102]

Peritoneal lavage is typically performed with 10 to 20 L of a balanced isotonic electrolyte solution (such as lactated Ringer's solution or Normosol-R) twice a day for 3 to 5 days, until the lavage solution becomes clear or the catheter loses its patency because of fibrin deposition or omentum. Hypertonic solutions should be avoided because they can result in fluid shifts into the peritoneum. The addition of povidone-iodine to a balanced solution is contraindicated since concentrations as low as 3% can induce peritoneal inflammation.[114] Other agents, such as antibiotics or heparin, have also been suggested as components of the lavage solution, but data demonstrating their benefit are not currently available. Active (or closed suction) abdominal drains have also been advocated, with similar benefits and potential complications to other methods.[113] Lavage with a plain isotonic solution did not alter the pharmacokinetics of gentamicin administered systemically.[115] Thus alteration of antimicrobial dosing does not appear necessary if lavage with plain solutions is part of the therapeutic regimen.

Prognosis

The prognosis is grave for peritonitis associated with GI rupture. Reported survival rates for horses with peritonitis vary but can be as high as 84%.[93,94,96] Some of the variability in reported survival percentages can be related to inclusion criteria, mainly whether horses with GI rupture were included. Septic peritonitis following abdominal surgery is reportedly associated with high mortality (56%).[93] Peritonitis associated with *A. equuli* carries a very favorable prognosis, and all horses in these reports responded to medical therapy if attempted.[97-99]

The complete reference list is available online at www.expertconsult.com.

CHAPTER

4

Central Nervous System Infections

Kathy K. Seino and Maureen T. Long

Infections of the central nervous system (CNS) of horses, although uncommon, are some of the most devastating and frequently fatal diseases in horses. Diseases such as equine protozoal myeloencephalitis (EPM) and West Nile virus encephalomyelitis (WNE), recent outbreaks of equine herpesvirus myeloencephalopathy (EHM), and resurgence of clusters of horses affected by eastern equine encephalomyelitis (EEE) have a significant economic impact on the equine industry and have stimulated investigations into preventive, diagnostic, and therapeutic alternatives for CNS infections in horses.

Viral, bacterial, rickettsial, protozoal, parasitic, and fungal pathogens may cause CNS infections in horses (Table 4-1). In small animals and humans, the causes of meningoencephalitis, in order of decreasing frequency, are viral, bacterial, protozoal, rickettsial, parasitic, and fungal, whereas in the horse the most frequently diagnosed CNS infections are probably of viral and protozoal origin.[1,2] In an Australian study, 30 of 450 horses with neurologic disease had an infectious or inflammatory disease, and 11 of these 30 had meningitis.[3] This study did not reflect the emergence of West Nile virus (WNV) in the United States in 1999 or account for CNS diseases that are present in North America such as EEE or EPM.

Regardless of the type of etiologic agent involved, CNS infections require an accurate and rapid diagnosis and implementation of an appropriate course of treatment by the attending clinician. CNS infection should be suspected in horses with abnormal mentation, seizures, blindness, multiple cranial nerve abnormalities, and general proprioceptive deficits. Infections involving primarily the spinal cord may manifest as limb weakness, incoordination, and stiffness, with or without associated cerebral dysfunction. The reader is referred to chapters on individual diseases for detailed description and discussion of EPM (see Chapter 55), WNV (see Chapter 21), alphavirus encephalitides (see Chapter 20), rabies (see Chapter 19), equine herpesvirus myelopathy (see Chapter 14), *Streptococcus equi* subsp. *equi* (see Chapter 28), and *Anaplasma phagocytophilum* (see Chapter 39). This chapter provides an overview of CNS infection, pathogenesis, diagnosis, and treatment, with discussion of miscellaneous CNS infections not covered elsewhere in this text.

CNS infection and resultant inflammation is defined by the specific area of the nervous system affected. Inflammation of the brain, meninges, spinal cord, and peripheral nerves is termed encephalitis, meningitis, myelitis, and neuritis, respectively. Rhombencephalitis and cerebellitis refer to localized inflammation of the brainstem and cerebellum, respectively.[4,5] Frequently, more than one tissue or anatomic site may be affected. Meningoencephalitis is inflammation of the meninges and brain, and meningoencephalomyelitis is inflammation of the meninges, brain, and spinal cord. Inflammation of the brain and spinal cord, without meningeal involvement, is termed *myeloencephalitis.*

Infection of the CNS can also result in focal suppuration of the brain parenchyma or spinal cord and formation of abscesses. Localized areas of infection between the outermost meningeal layer (dura mater) and the skull and vertebral column are termed *epidural abscesses.* Inflammation between the outer two layers of the meninges (dura mater and arachnoid) is termed *subdural empyema.*[1]

Table 4-1 Equine Central Nervous System Pathogens

Pathogen	Select References
Viral	
West Nile virus	15, 20, 22, 67, 153-157
Western equine encephalomyelitis virus	159-167
Eastern equine encephalomyelitis virus	160, 165, 167, 169-177
Venezuelan equine encephalomyelitis virus	181, 182
St. Louis virus	184
Murray Valley virus	187-189
Louping ill virus	191-195
California group/snowshoe hare virus	197-202
Main Drain virus	208
Semliki Forest virus	209
Japanese encephalitis virus	210
Hendra virus	211
Nipah virus	211
Powassan virus	214
Aujeszky's disease virus	218
Equine herpesvirus type 1	47, 48, 219-225
Equine infectious anemia virus	226, 227
Rhabdovirus (rabies)	230
Kunjin virus	189, 232
Borna virus	233
Parasitic	
Setaria	158
Habronema	168
Hypoderma (lineatum, bovis, diana)	178-180
Parastrongylus spp.	183
Strongylus vulgaris	168, 185, 186
Halicephalobus gingivalis	127-129, 134, 135, 139, 141-147, 151, 152, 190
Draschia megastoma	196
Trypanosoma evansi	203-207
Bacterial	
Escherichia coli	9, 91
Actinobacillus equuli	91, 114
Streptococcus (equi, zooepidemicus, suis)	7, 27, 91, 99, 212, 213
Salmonella	91, 92, 122
Pasteurella caballi	11, 215-217
Pseudomonas aeruginosa	7
Enterococcus	8
Actinomyces	228, 229
Rhodococcus equi*	25, 114-116, 120, 123, 231
Brucella abortus*	123
Mycobacterium bovis*	11, 234-236
Staphylococcus spp.*	107
Actinobacillus lignieresii*	113
Klebsiella pneumoniae, type 1	97
Listeria monocytogenes	38, 93
Protozoal	
Balamuthia mandrillaris	149
Sarcocystis neurona	18, 62, 237-241
Fungal	
Cryptococcus neoformans	101-103
Aspergillus niger, A. fumigatus*	104
Rickettsial	
Anaplasma phagocytophilum	242

* Denotes vertebral body osteomyelitis.

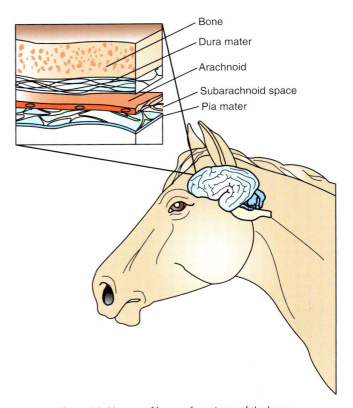

Figure 4-1 Diagram of layers of meninges of the horse.

(Labels: Bone; Dura mater; Arachnoid; Subarachnoid space; Pia mater)

Neuroanatomy and Disease

Brain and Meninges

Inside the protective barrier of the skull, the brain is surrounded by three layers of meninges: the outermost dura mater, or pachymeninges, and the leptomeninges, consisting of the inner arachnoid membrane and pia mater (Fig. 4-1).[1] The pia mater is adherent to the external surface of the brain and spinal cord, forming cuffs around penetrating vessels and merging with the ependymal lining of the fourth ventricle. Cerebrospinal fluid (CSF) occupies the subarachnoid space between the pia mater and arachnoid. Acute bacterial infections within the subarachnoid space typically begin with the leptomeninges of the brain and spinal cord and spread inward through the foramina of the fourth ventricle. Infections between the dura mater and arachnoid (subdural empyema) can spread over the entire cerebral hemisphere. The dura mater adheres to the periosteum of the skull and limits the spread of epidural abscesses (between the dura and skull), except where it invaginates into the cranial cavity to form four rigid septa: the falx cerebri, falx cerebelli, tentorium cerebelli, and diaphragma selli.[1]

The brain rests within the anterior, middle, and posterior cranial fossae, which are associated with the paranasal sinuses.[6-10] The anterior fossa forms the roof of the frontal and ethmoidal sinuses. The sella turcica is located between the left and right middle fossa and forms the roof of the sphenoid sinuses. Infection in these paranasal sinuses can spread through the respective fossa centrally to the brain, resulting in epidural abscesses and subdural empyema. In the horse, these infections can be either bacterial or fungal.[6-10] Middle ear infections (otitis media) within the petrous temporal bone may extend into the middle fossa to involve the temporal lobe of the brain or into the posterior fossa to involve the cerebellum or brainstem.[1,11]

Neuroanatomic localization of brain disease in the horse has been well described.[12-14] Briefly, infectious neurologic disease in the horse either is diffuse (e.g., viral or protozoal) or can have a single neuroanatomic signal (e.g., brain abscess). Neuroanatomic localization should be defined in terms of the five major regions of the CNS (and the cranial nerves): disease of the cerebrum, basal nuclei, rostral brainstem, caudal brainstem, and cerebellum.[14]

Seizure activity and moderate to severe obtundation are the most common signs of cerebral disease in the horse. Although the cortex controls conscious proprioception, this is difficult to localize to the cerebrum in the horse and in the absence of other clinical signs. Blindness occurs secondary to lesions in the visual cortex. Cortical blindness presents as decreased normal reactions to visual cues, with normal pupillary light reflexes. A full ophthalmic examination is paramount to assessing cortical blindness. The most common clinical sign of focal disease of the basal nuclei is the inability to chew and form coordinated eating movements with the tongue, teeth, and oropharynx.[12-14] However, diffuse disease in this area involves the caudate nucleus, globus pallidus, putamen, and substantia nigra and should result in loss of coordination of movement. Extension to the reticular formation may result in abnormalities of the wake/sleep cycle.[15]

Clinical signs referable to lesions of the rostral brainstem can be differentiated on the basis of signs of abnormalities of cranial nerve (CN) II through CN IV. Vision, pupillary responses, and eyeball placement can be affected by disease in these areas. Postganglionic Horner's syndrome (ipsilateral ptosis, miosis, enophthalmos, and localized ipsilateral sweating) can occur if lesions are rostral to the foramen lacerum involving the sympathetic fibers as they course to the sphincter pupillae muscle (see Chapter 10).[12-14]

The hypothalamus, reticular formation, and pituitary gland are included within the diencephalon and mesencephalon of the brainstem. Hypothalamic and pituitary disease generally result in endocrine dyscrasia. The reticular formation is very important for arousal and coordination of motor function. Lesions associated with the caudal brainstem can be identified based on clinical signs indicating abnormalities of CN V through XII.

Cranial Nerves

All the cranial nerves exit through the meninges at the base of the brain and are susceptible to injury in horses with meningitis because of direct spread of infection or increased intracranial pressure. The clinical signs of multiple versus single cranial nerve abnormalities are important for ruling out specific etiologies.[12-14] For example, a weak horse with primary dysphagia and slow pupillary light responses has evidence of a multifocal or diffuse disease process such as botulism. Unilateral masseter atrophy consistent with CN V paralysis is a common finding in horses with clinical disease caused by *Sarcocystis neurona* infection.

Spinal Cord

The spinal cord has a central core of gray matter surrounded by the ascending and descending nerve tracts of the white matter. Intramedullary lesions (within the spinal cord) produce neuronal injury at one or more spinal cord segments and then expand laterally to involve motor and sensory nerve tracts. Clinical signs are observed caudal to the site of the spinal cord lesion because of damage to descending motor tracts.[12-14] Although clinical signs of spinal cord disease are most often bilateral in horses, severity is frequently asymmetric; a close examination will reveal that most intramedullary lesions, unless extremely focal, will have some degree of abnormality associated with the contralateral limb. On the other hand, extramedullary lesions, or lesions of the peripheral nerves, will involve a single limb. Peripheral or extramedullary lesions can produce signs of nerve root irritation. When a lesion is compressive on the spinal cord, from outward to inward, there is a stepwise loss of proprioception, then weakness. After onset of weakness, further compression results in loss of sensation, followed by loss of deep pain. A typical presentation for a horse with cervical vertebral myelopathy is a young, strong 2-year-old racehorse

with spontaneous loss of balance.[16,17] Diffuse spinal cord disease is often observed in viral infections such as arbovirus infection, neurologic equine herpesvirus syndrome, rabies, and verminous infection, whereas multifocal, asymmetric disease is observed in horses with EPM.[18,19] West Nile virus can be highly variable, with either diffuse spinal signs or highly asymmetric clinical signs.[15,20-22]

Spread of infectious agents can be limited by neuroanatomic boundaries. The anatomic arrangements of the spinal meningeal layers (pia mater, arachnoid, and dura mater) are the same as described for the brain, and a plane of infection is possible between the arachnoid and dura. The spinal dura and periosteum diverge at the foramen magnum. At the level of the seventh cervical vertebra (C7), they are separated by a fat-filled epidural space that cannot prevent longitudinal spread of infection, and thus infection may extend over many segments.[1] In the horse the spinal cord ends as the cauda equina as the cord tapers into the conus medullaris, with distally coursing spinal nerve roots. Unlike in other species, the meninges end caudally between the second and third sacral vertebrae (S2 and S3) in the horse.[12,16] The cauda equina is a site associated with CNS inflammatory diseases and occasional peripheral neuritis.[23]

Vascularization

The blood supply to the CNS includes an extensive network of intercranial arterial and venous vessels fed by two sources, the basilar and internal carotid arteries, with multiple communications to the external circulatory vessels via the circle of Willis to ensure collateral circulation of the brain. The horse is distinct from other species because the internal carotid artery does not receive any blood from the maxillary artery. The details are beyond the scope of this review; however, some salient features are worth mentioning. The ophthalmic artery is a branch of the internal carotid artery, which is a branch of the main intercranial artery, the basilar artery. Therefore CNS infection could result in septic emboli to the ophthalmic artery and consequent retinal lesions and loss of some visual fields. The middle cerebral artery has the greatest blood flow volume and is considered the area of greatest risk for septic embolization and mycotic aneurysms in the brain.[3] Brain infection most likely arises from infections with *Aspergillosis* and mucoraceous fungi in lungs, uterus, and intestine[24] (see Chapters 52 and 53). In descending order of frequency, the internal carotid artery, external carotid artery, and maxillary arteries are the most common equine vessels to be affected with mycotic aneurysm and extracranial (guttural pouch) infection[1] (see Chapter 1).

Despite an extensive network of collateral circulation, three areas of the brain are supplied by only one or two vessels. Highly vulnerable to ischemic injury and abscess formation, these areas include (1) the middle and posterior cerebral arteries at the junction of the parietal, occipital, and temporal lobes; (2) the medial surface of the hemispheres of the cerebellum; and (3) cerebral white matter. No valves are present in the venous supply to the CNS, and the direction of flow may change with hemodynamic changes caused by pressure changes in the CSF and conditions such as cerebral edema. The anterior spinal cord is supplied by the cervical and intercostal arteries from the descending aorta and generally has a higher likelihood of infection than other parts of the spinal cord.[1,3] Data that support this have not been evaluated in the horse, although osteomyelitis of the cervical and thoracic spinal column may occur in foals.[25,26]

Blood-Brain Barrier and Cerebrospinal Fluid

The capillary system of the CNS is unique in that it consists of endothelial cells with tight junctions and no fenestrations, creating an effective blood-brain barrier (BBB).[1] The BBB is the primary protective barrier of the CNS and acts as a filter preventing access of large proteins, immunoglobulins, antigens, pathogens, and some antimicrobial agents (e.g., gentamicin, amphotericin B) to the brain.[1] Injury to the BBB by ischemic insult (e.g., septic emboli), vasculitis induced by inflammation, or increased levels of tumor necrosis factor alpha (TNF-α) can disrupt this protective barrier and predispose to CNS infection. Disruption of the BBB permits the entry of radiodense agents into the CNS for early visualization of abscesses on contrast magnetic resonance imaging (MRI) and computed tomography (CT) studies.[7,27] The blood supply to the pituitary gland, choroid plexus, and brainstem does not have tight junctions, and these areas are considered to exist outside the BBB.

Cerebrospinal fluid is an ultrafiltrate of plasma produced by active secretion from the choroid plexus in the lateral, third, and fourth ventricles and by diffusion across the meninges.[1,28-30] CSF protects and sustains the CNS.[31,32] It circulates outward through the ventricular foramina into the subarachnoid space and is reabsorbed over 3 to 4 hours through cells of the arachnoid villi along the superior sagittal sinuses. Blockage of the villi from inflammation, blood in the subarachnoid space, or occlusion of the superior sagittal or lateral sinuses prevents the reabsorption of CSF, and communicating hydrocephalus develops. Obstructive hydrocephalus results from blockage of CSF circulation at the ventricles caused by inflammation or compression of the ventricles, as might occur with abscess or hemorrhage. Unlike communicating hydrocephalus, redistribution of increased quantities of CSF and cerebral edema into the subarachnoid space is not possible in obstructive hydrocephalus, and there is increased likelihood of brain herniation and death.[1,32] In the horse, this event has been described primarily for neonates.[33,34]

Pathogenesis

Entry of Pathogens

Most neurotropic viruses gain initial entry to the body through the bite of an infected mosquito or insect (e.g., arboviruses), the bite of an infected mammal (e.g., rabies), the respiratory tract (e.g., herpesvirus), or the gastrointestinal (GI) tract. Dendritic cells or phagocytes at the site of initial infection transport virus to local lymph nodes where it undergoes primary replication with subsequent viremia. Initial infection with bacterial or fungal organisms most often occurs through the respiratory, GI, reproductive, and urinary tracts.[2] Septic emboli from vegetative endocarditis are another potential source of bacteria or fungi for hematogenous spread to the CNS. Regardless of the initial route of infection, the majority of CNS pathogens probably enter the nervous system of the host by a hematogenous route.[1,2,5]

The exact mechanism by which pathogens cross the BBB and enter the CNS is uncertain for most viruses and bacteria, but several mechanisms have been proposed. Bacterial infections of the CNS frequently involve the meninges. A breakdown in the BBB caused by ischemia of meningeal vessels secondary to emboli and inflammation may provide a route of access to the brain parenchyma with subsequent abscessation.[35-37] The initial systemic immune response to viral infection in the periphery results in release of cytokines, which stimulate increased expression of adhesion molecules on CNS endothelial cells and increased surveillance of the CNS by activated T cells.[5] Some viruses enter the CNS using these cells as a "Trojan horse." Other viruses use endothelial adhesion molecules to gain entry or induce release of TNF-α, with subsequent increased BBB permeability.[5] Intracellular pathogens, such as *Listeria*

monocytogenes and rickettsial species, gain entry into the CNS by penetrating endothelial cells of the BBB or by traveling within phagocytes.[38]

Other than hematogenous spread, pathogens may access the CNS by direct invasion (trauma or iatrogenic introduction), spread from contiguous structures (e.g., paranasal sinuses, otitis media), or retrograde entry along nerve roots.[2,5,35,39] Despite the frequency of infections involving the equine head (e.g., sinusitis, tooth root abscesses, guttural pouch empyema), the number of CNS infections resulting from direct spread to the CNS appears to be low in horses.[39] An excellent general review has been recently published regarding the entry of toxins and viruses into the CNS utilizing axonal transport.[40] Rabies virus gains entry to the CNS by retrograde axonal transport along peripheral nerves. Herpesvirus is thought to infect the peripheral trigeminal nerve during latent phases.[2] The potential for entry to the brain through the free nerve endings of the olfactory nerve in the nasal cavity has been proposed for rabies virus and arboviruses.[41] Recent work with WNV has demonstrated that the virus can be transported axonally and is likely important in the pathogenesis of flaccid paralysis.[42]

Immune Response of Central Nervous System

The response of the CNS to infection plays an important role in the pathogenesis of disease. In bacterial CNS infections, CSF concentrations of complement and immunoglobulin G (IgG) are low compared with concentrations in the peripheral circulation.[35] Complement and specific antibody are important for opsonization of bacteria, and a diminution of this function may be a critical factor in the pathogenesis of bacterial infections in the CNS. The presence of bacterial cell wall components in the CSF elicits the release of cytokines (e.g., interleukin-6 [IL-6], TNF-α, macrophage inflammatory protein [MIP-1a, -1b, -2]), which stimulate the entry of neutrophils, increased BBB permeability, and vasculitis; CNS edema; and inflammation of tissues surrounding the meninges.

The peak inflammatory response is observed 72 hours after the start of infection.[35] Degenerating leukocytes release toxins that stimulate vasospasm, local ischemia, and further tissue edema. Inflammation of the arachnoid villi where CSF is absorbed could result in communicating hydrocephalus; inflammation of the ependymal lining and ventricles where CSF is circulated may result in obstructive hydrocephalus. Initially, there is redistribution of increased CSF and cerebral edema into the subarachnoid space with communicating hydrocephalus, but with severe edema and obstructive hydrocephalus, this redistribution is not possible. Within the confining structures of the skull, the increase in intracranial pressure may result in pressure necrosis of the brain parenchyma or death due to herniation of the cerebellum through the foramen magnum.[36] Vasogenic edema of the CNS is now viewed as a potentially fatal consequence of bacterial infection, and treatment of human patients with both antimicrobial and antiinflammatory medications has dramatically decreased the mortality associated with CNS infection.[41]

When infection occurs, the CNS must mount a controlled adaptive immune response that minimizes damage to brain cells.[5] Initially there is an innate immune response, with production of interferon beta (IFN-β), chemokines, and proinflammatory cytokines. These mediators activate microglia to express interleukin-1 (IL-1), TNF-α, and chemokines that stimulate increased expression of endothelial adhesion molecules (e.g., vascular cell adhesion molecule [VCAM-1], intracellular adhesion molecule [ICAM]). By 3 to 4 days after infection, peripheral inflammatory cells that were activated in secondary lymphoid tissues enter the CNS. Unlike in the periphery, nonlytic clearance of viruses and infected cells occurs in the CNS to prevent secondary damage to surrounding neurons and tissues. Viruses that remain latent in neurons are controlled by continued secretion of antibody, IFN-β, and IFN-γ by long-term lymphocytes.

As with bacterial CNS infections, control or elimination of viral infection in the CNS, without inducing unacceptable damage to neural tissue, requires a delicate balance of the CNS immune response. Induction of apoptosis (cell death) of neurons by microglia and stimulation of migration of T cells into the CNS are possible contributing factors to the neurodegeneration observed in degenerative diseases such as Parkinson's disease and Alzheimer's disease.[43] Overexpression of C protein, important in the complement system, causes bystander neurodegeneration and oligodendrocyte damage.[44] There is growing recognition of the role matrix metalloproteinases (MMPs) play in the immunopathogenesis of CNS diseases. They are widely expressed in the CNS and are important for CNS development and normal function and repair (i.e., synaptic plasticity, angiogenesis, and myelin turnover). In response to inflammation, trauma, and infection, however, overexpression of MMPs have been implicated in the further deterioration of the CNS by inducing demyelination, cytotoxicity, disruption of the BBB, neuronal and axonal death, and oxidative stress. Increased expression of MMP-2 and -9 have been detected in the CNS of patients with human immunodeficiency virus (HIV-1).[45] In another study, MMP-9 and endogenous tissue inhibitor of MMP (TIMP) -1 were significantly higher in the serum and CSF of patients with meningitis.[46]

The immune response to equine herpesvirus type 1 (EHV-1) may be important in the pathogenesis of the neurologic form of this pathogen. Localization of EHV-1 in the CNS endothelium induces vasculitis. Subsequent CNS damage results from ischemia rather than direct neuronal insult; thus the disease is termed *myeloencephalopathy* rather than myeloencephalitis.[47] The exact pathogenesis of herpesvirus neurologic disease in horses remains unclear. The disease is sporadic and seems to be more common in horses with a previous history of exposure to this ubiquitous pathogen and in pregnant or lactating mares. Evidence of antigen-antibody complexes between EHV-1 antigen and EHV-4 antibody and decreased levels of complement activation have been observed in experimentally infected ponies.[48,49]

Other factors also play a role in the pathogenesis of viral infections. Nonsurvivors of Japanese encephalitis virus (JEV), a flavivirus infection, have increased levels of IL-6, INF-α, and IL-8. Viruses have developed strategies to facilitate evasion of the CNS immune response. For example, WNV may block the signaling pathway for IFN-α.[50]

Host genetic factors influencing the type and quality of the immune response may be a factor[51] and may explain why, with certain diseases, only a small percentage of those infected develop neurologic disease. In WNV infection, for example, less than 1% (1 out 150) of humans and less than 10% of horses develop WNE. Variation in expression of a brain chemokine receptor, CCR5, has been found to have either deleterious or protective effects in the progression of a number of infections in the CNS.[52] In particular, the CCR5Δ32 deletion promotes increased viral spread and mortality to WNV in humans homozygous for the mutation.[53] This has not been demonstrated in horses; mutations in the INF-inducible Oas1b gene, however, contribute to increased susceptibility in horses to WNV. The mutation in the Oas1b gene results in the truncation of the 2'5' oligoadenylate synthetase protein that normally mediates the activation of cellular ribonuclease (RNase) L that cleaves viral double-stranded ribonucleic acid (dsRNA).[54] Understanding host response to infection is also important in explaining improper or inadequate immune responses that allows the establishment of persistent infection. In human patients, certain

types of vaccination or viral infection result in a multifocal inflammatory demyelinating process or acute disseminated encephalomyelitis (ADEM).[55,56] An immune-mediated attack against antigen in brain myelin appears to be the cause of ADEM. The poliomyelitis-like acute flaccid paralysis observed in some people with WNE may be an example of ADEM.[55,56]

The old paradigm of the CNS as incapable of mounting an immune response to infection and being "immunologically privileged" has given way to our current recognition of the CNS as a specialized immune organ.[43] The innate and adaptive immune responses of the host play an important role in CNS infections. Increasing availability in the past several years of equine specific reagents has opened the door not only to better characterization of the immune response to CNS infections in horses beyond measuring antibody response, but also profiling cytokine expression, cell-mediated immunity, functional immune assays, identification of T cell epitopes, and characterizing innate immune responses.[57-60] The availability of more powerful molecular diagnostic tools and bioinformatics will also play a profound impact in the exponential learning curve in neuroimmunology. Gene expression profiling in the thalamus and cerebrum of horses experimentally infected with WNV demonstrated significant differences in gene expression of neurologic, immunologic, and apoptotic pathways based on virus exposure, survival, and location, providing not only insight into the immunopathogenesis of WNV in the CNS of the horse but also knowledge for viral encephalitis in general.[61] Increasing knowledge of the role of the CNS in immunity will ultimately lead to developing novel therapeutic and preventive strategies.

Cerebrospinal Fluid Characteristics

Collection Techniques

Cerebrospinal fluid may be obtained antemortem from two sites in horses: the atlanto-occipital (cerebellomedullary) space (Fig. 4-2) and the lumbosacral (LS) space (Fig. 4-3). The optimal site for sample collection is determined on the basis of the neuroanatomic localization of the suspected lesion and practical considerations regarding patient systemic health status and restraint options. In general, better diagnostic results are

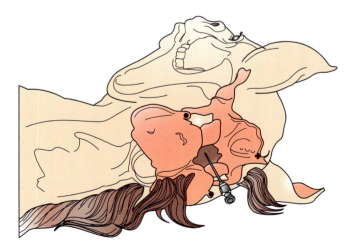

Figure 4-2 Atlanto-occipital (AO) cerebrospinal fluid collection from recumbent horse. Spinal needle in position with stylet removed. Palpable landmarks are the cranial borders of the atlas (•—•) and the external occipital protuberance (+) on the dorsal midline. *(Redrawn from Mayhew IG: Cornell Vet 65: 500-511, 1975.)*

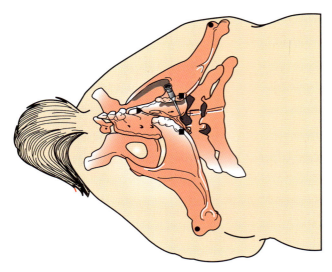

Figure 4-3 Lumbosacral (LS) cerebrospinal fluid collection from standing horse. Spinal needle in position with stylet removed. Palpable landmarks are the caudal borders of each tuber coxa (•—•), caudal edge of the spine of the sixth lumbar vertebra (L6) (+), cranial edge of the spine of the second sacral vertebra (S2) (▸), and cranial edge of each tuber sacrale (■—■). *(Redrawn from Mayhew IG: Cornell Vet 65:500-511, 1975.)*

achieved if CSF is obtained from the site closest to the suspected lesion. The atlanto-occipital (AO) space is sampled under general anesthesia and may be preferable in nervous horses, horses undergoing anesthesia for another reason, or in horses with conformation preventing successful LS taps (LS subluxation). Conversely, an LS tap performed standing under sedation may be advantageous in an animal in which recovery from general anesthesia is considered a risk because of the severity of neurologic disease.

Collection techniques for both AO and LS taps have been described in detail.[11,28,30] Briefly, atlanto-occipital CSF collection is performed with the horse under general anesthesia and lying in lateral recumbency. An area of the poll and neck (15-20 cm caudal to ears and 8-10 cm on either side of mane) is clipped and surgically prepped. The head is flexed so that the median axis of the head is at right angles to the median axis of the cervical vertebrae. A sterile 8.9-cm, 20-gauge spinal needle with stylet is inserted at the intersection of the cranial borders of the atlas and the external occipital protuberance along the dorsal midline. The needle should be parallel to the ground, perpendicular to the skin, and aimed toward the nose of the horse. The needle is gradually advanced until a "popping" sensation is felt with penetration of the AO membrane and cervical dura. The stylet is withdrawn, and the appearance of clear CSF at the hub indicates a successful procedure. If no CSF appears when the stylet is removed, the needle is rotated 90 degrees. If fluid is still not obtained, the stylet is replaced, and the needle is advanced carefully. The approximate depth of needle insertion for entry into the subarachnoid space is 5 to 8 cm. If the needle contacts bone at a depth of 2 to 5 cm, it should be withdrawn and repositioned appropriately. If blood appears at the hub of the needle when the stylet is removed and does not clear with CSF in 15 to 20 seconds, the stylet is replaced and the needle removed; a fresh needle is used for the next attempt. When CSF flows freely from the hub of the needle, the sample is collected by free flow or gentle aspiration into an appropriate tube. After the sample has been collected and the needle is withdrawn, the head of the horse is extended to a normal or slightly extended position to prevent leakage of CSF from the puncture site.[30]

Lumbosacral CSF collection in the horse is typically performed with the sedated horse standing as squarely as possible.[12,30] Landmarks for the LS site are the intersection of imaginary lines joining the caudal borders of the tuber coxae along the dorsal midline or at the highest point of the gluteal region of the horse. In addition to sedation, adequate restraint with a twitch and use of stocks are advisable. In response to penetration of the dura mater, sedated horses may show no reaction, or tail movement and slight flexion of the pelvic limbs, or violent kicking responses that can endanger the patient and the veterinarian. A 10×10-cm site is clipped and sterilely prepped. A 20-gauge, 15.2-cm spinal needle with stylet is inserted in a sterile manner and advanced carefully a few millimeters at a time. Care should be taken to keep the needle perpendicular to the dorsum and on midline. A "popping" sensation may be felt with penetration of the LS interarcuate ligament, dorsal dura mater, and arachnoid membrane. The stylet is removed to check for CSF at the hub. Gentle aspiration with a syringe may be necessary to initiate flow of spinal fluid. If no fluid is obtained, the needle (with the stylet replaced) is advanced to the floor of the vertebral canal and then withdrawn with slow rotation of the needle a millimeter at a time. A needle depth of 12 to 14 cm is usually required for successful CSF collection. Large-breed horses or obese horses may require longer needles. Queckenstedt's maneuver (bilateral occlusion of the jugular veins) may be performed by an assistant to increase intracranial and intraspinal pressure and facilitate CSF flow up the spinal needle. Rotation of the needle 90 degrees to remove occluding meningeal tissue and nerve roots from the needle point may also be helpful. Indirect aspiration with a syringe through an extension set connected to the spinal needle hub is recommended to minimize hemorrhage from excessive suction pressure and resultant occlusion of the needle with meninges. After adequate CSF is obtained, the stylet is replaced in the spinal needle, and the needle is removed. Collection of CSF from the LS space while the horse is in lateral recumbency (under general anesthesia or in a tetraplegic horse) is possible but is considered more difficult than in the standing horse. Attempts may be facilitated by elevating the upper pelvic limb so that the tuber coxae are perpendicular to the floor or by advancing the pelvic limbs cranially to flex the pelvis and LS joint.

Both AO and LS collection techniques are regarded as safe procedures in the horse. A common complication is blood contamination of the sample with puncture of meningeal or spinal cord vessels. Initial blood contamination of CSF frequently clears after a few milliliters during collection; however, even microscopic amounts of blood in the CSF sample may result in false-positive results in testing for EPM in horses.[62] In humans, cerebellar herniation through the foramen magnum and herniation of the temporal cortex under the tentorium cerebelli are considered potential complications of CSF collection, especially in patients with increased intracerebral pressure, severe meningitis, or brain abscesses with deteriorating condition.[1] This complication has not been reported as a frequent sequela to CSF collection in horses. Evidence of extradural hemorrhage or formation of fibrous adhesions between the LS ligament and dorsal LS dura mater have been observed in experimental subjects post mortem. Penetration of the AO joint is another potential complication. Cellulitis and septic abscesses secondary to CSF collection in horses are rare.

Techniques utilizing ultrasound-guided collection of CSF from the LS[63] and AO[64] sites and most recently from cervical centesis at C1-C2[65] have been described in the literature and may potentially gain increased use in equine practice. These techniques have the benefit of better visualization of the vertebral anatomy, which may be beneficial in the case of larger horses (i.e., Warmbloods, drafts, heavily conditioned horses), particularly at the LS site in which anatomic landmarks are not easily palpable. Use of ultrasound resulted in less repeated insertion of the spinal needle, less trauma, and less blood contamination of the CSF and acquisition of a better diagnostic sample. Additionally, the ultrasound-guided collection was quite useful in a lateral recumbent animal at the LS site in which positioning resulted in displacement of palpable pelvic and sacral bony structures and subsequent shift in midline positioning of the spinal needle. The ultrasound-guided cervical centesis technique was performed with the horses under heavy sedation, and this may be a more viable option in a neurologic patient in which recovery from general anesthesia may be a potential risk.[65]

Analysis

Analysis of the CSF may include measurement of CSF pressure and examination of sample cytology, total protein concentration, glucose concentration, biochemical alteration, turbidity, and color.[28,30] Cerebrospinal fluid pressure is measured by attachment of a manometer to the hub of the spinal needle before collection. Normal CSF pressure in the horse is approximately 300 mm H_2O (150 to 500 mm H_2O).[16,30,66] Increased opening pressure, when CSF is first obtained, may result from obstructive hydrocephalus. In addition to noninfectious congenital abnormalities, potential causes of obstruction include tumor, abscess, hemorrhage, and edema. An increased opening pressure that decreases by 20% to 50% after removal of 1 to 2 mL of CSF is indicative of an intracranial mass or spinal cord lesion cranial to the site of collection. Because CSF flows caudad from the ventricles of the brain and because jugular compression causes increased blood volume in the cranial cavity with subsequent increases in CSF pressure, failure of the CSF pressure to increase in the LS site with bilateral jugular vein compression may indicate a compressive thoracic or cervical lesion.

Appearance

Normal CSF is clear and colorless and does not clot. Xanthochromia (yellow discoloration) of the CSF after centrifugation is caused by preexisting trauma, vasculitis, increased protein concentration (150 mg/dL), direct bilirubin leakage from high serum concentration, or breakdown of the BBB.[16,30,66] Xanthochromia with increased protein concentration is typical of equine encephalomyelopathy caused by vascular inflammation and increased BBB permeability.[48,49]

Clots may result from increased fibrinogen caused by inflammation. A CSF sample may appear turbid if there is an increase in quantity of white blood cells (>200 WBCs/μL), red blood cells (>400 RBCs/μL), or epidural fat cells, or if significant numbers of bacterial, fungal, or amebic organisms are present.

Cellular Evaluation

Cell counts and cytologic evaluation performed within 30 minutes of CSF collection are diagnostic. In normal horses and foals, less than 10 WBCs/μL is expected in the CSF. Cells are predominantly small (70% to 90%) and large (10% to 30%) mononuclear cells.[30,66] An initial neutrophilic pleocytosis followed by mononuclear pleocytosis is characteristic of EEE infections. However, CSF from horses with Western equine encephalomyelitis (WEE) and WNE is characterized by predominantly lymphocytic cells.[67] The increase in CSF nucleated cell count with viral infections is typically less (100 to 1000 cells/μL) than with bacterial meningitis. Eosinophilic pleocytosis with xanthochromia and increased protein concentration may be observed in CSF from horses with parasitic meningitis.[13,68] Infrequently, horses with parasitic meningitis can have a neutrophilic pleocytosis. Fungal organisms may be observed in the CSF of horses with fungal meningitis.[13] Although CSF analysis is useful to confirm the presence of an inflammatory process, to determine antibody titers to specific pathogens, and to monitor for therapeutic response, culture of viral or bacterial pathogens from CSF of horses with infectious neurologic disease is often difficult. Identification of viral etiologic agents in CSF is rare.[4]

Protein

Normal protein concentration in equine CSF ranges from 20 to 124 mg/dL and is typically higher in CSF obtained from the LS site (93.0 ± 16.0 [65 to 124] mg/dL) than from the AO site (87.0 ± 17.0 [59 to 118] mg/dL).[13,66,69] Differences in CSF protein between AO and LS samples that are greater than 25 mg/dL may indicate a lesion closer to the site of origin of the sample with greater CSF protein. Cerebrospinal fluid IgG and albumin concentrations may be determined by electrophoresis and radial immunodiffusion. These values are compared with serum IgG and albumin concentrations. An increase in the albumin quotient ([Alb CSF]/[Alb serum] × 100) is considered indicative of an increase in BBB permeability, as may be seen with EHM. An increase in the IgG index ([IgG CSF]/[IgG serum] × [Alb serum]/[Alb CSF]) may reflect intrathecal IgG production caused by inflammatory disease (e.g., EPM, meningitis, tumors, equine motor neuron disease).[69] Additional CSF antibody coefficients routinely used in the diagnosis of human neuroinfections such as *Toxoplasma gondii* and *Trypanosoma brucei* were recently evaluated for the diagnosis of EPM. Antibody index (AI), Goldman-Witmer coefficient (C-value), IgG concentration, and anti-*S. neurona* titers were significantly higher in horses with EPM versus horses with cervical vertebral malformation (CVM), and results were not affected by red blood cell contamination of the CSF.[70]

Biochemical Parameters

Increases in CSF creatine kinase (CK) are an unreliable indicator of neurologic disease in the horse and may be falsely elevated by contamination of the sample with epidural fat or dura during collection.[71-74] Lactic acid concentrations in the CSF may increase with some CNS diseases (e.g., EEE), head trauma, and brain abscesses.[13,69]

Immunologic Testing and Molecular Diagnostics

Detection of specific antibodies or antigens within the CSF may be helpful for the diagnosis of some viral, fungal, or rickettsial diseases. Use of polymerase chain reaction (PCR) for the diagnosis of viral encephalitis has become an important and sensitive tool.[4] Details of testing for specific diseases are presented in appropriate chapters.

In the wake of the recent outbreaks of neuropathogenic EHV-1, rapid diagnosis has become crucial for the management of these outbreaks. Real-time PCR tests for EHV-1 (differentiating the neuropathogenic strain from the nonneuropathogenic strain) that can be performed in a matter of hours have been developed.[75] Rapid diagnosis is based on nasal and whole blood samples that are taken at the onset of clinical signs from febrile horses (increased rectal temperature >101.5° F [38.6° C]).[76,77] Laboratories frequently offer cost-effective viral pathogen panels where one can simultaneously test for EHV-1, EHV-4, equine influenza virus, equine viral arteritis virus, and *Streptococcus equi* subsp. *equi* to rule out potential common differentials for an outbreak of respiratory disease or fevers in groups of horses.

General Therapeutic Considerations

Antimicrobial Agents

Antimicrobial selection for treatment of horses with bacterial infections of the CNS is based on initial Gram stain, culture, and susceptibility results whenever possible.[78] Desirable antimicrobial traits include the ability to penetrate the CNS and predicted activity in the low-pH and high-protein environment of infected CSF.[37] Low-molecular-weight antimicrobial agents that are lipid soluble and have a degree of protein binding and ionization at physiologic pH are favored.[37,78] With inflammation, BBB permeability increases to allow penetration and accumulation of drugs that are normally actively transported out of the CNS (e.g., penicillin, cephalosporins).

To allow for maximum peak plasma concentrations, intravenous (IV) administration of antimicrobials is recommended initially. The rapid bactericidal killing needed for CNS infections in human patients requires drug concentrations that exceed the minimal bactericidal concentration by tenfold to twentyfold.[35] Expected duration of therapy varies, depending on the nature of the infection but generally is 10 to 14 days.[35,78]

Antimicrobial agents with poor CNS penetration across the intact BBB include penicillins, cephalothin, cefazolin, ceftiofur, tetracycline, and aminoglycosides.[11,37,78] Good penetration is observed with fluoroquinolones, third-generation cephalosporins (e.g., cefotaxime, ceftazidime, ceftizoxime, ceftriaxone), sulfonamides, trimethoprim, pyrimethamine, doxycycline, chloramphenicol, rifampin, metronidazole, and macrolides. Enrofloxacin obtains therapeutic concentrations in the CSF for many gram-negative pathogens (e.g., *Escherichia coli*, *Salmonella*, *Actinobacillus*, *Klebsiella*) but is ineffective for treatment of most streptococcal and anaerobic pathogens. Its association with arthropathies in foals limits its use for treatment of neonatal bacterial meningitis. Potentiated sulfonamides (e.g., trimethoprim-sulfa combinations) are attractive therapeutic agents for CNS infections because they have a broad spectrum of activity, are inexpensive, and are administered orally, but unfortunately, antimicrobial resistance is common. Additionally, potentiated sulfonamides have been associated with adverse drug reactions resulting in aseptic meningitis in people in a rare number of cases[79] and were also recently described in a case series to be associated with the onset of neurologic signs (hypermetric gaits, agitation, and erratic behavior) in five horses.[80]

Third-generation cephalosporins are considered the antimicrobial of choice in human patients with bacterial CNS infection because of their activity against gram-negative bacteria, but these agents may be cost-prohibitive for use in horses. Although ceftiofur sodium is similar to true third-generation cephalosporins, it does not effectively cross the intact BBB in horses.[78] Chloramphenicol is a bacteriostatic broad-spectrum antibiotic with activity against gram-positive, gram-negative, and anaerobic bacteria and is administered orally, but the associated human health risk (i.e., aplastic anemia) must be considered. Rifampin has activity against gram-positive and anaerobic bacteria and is distributed into the CSF, but it must be used in combination with other antimicrobials (e.g., erythromycin) because of the frequent development of bacterial resistance when used alone. Fluoroquinolones should not be used with rifampin because it is an inhibitor of RNA synthesis. Metronidazole is effective against anaerobic bacteria and is used in combination with third-generation cephalosporins for treatment of human patients with bacterial CNS infections.

Advances in the field of CNS drug delivery to enhance uptake and penetration of the BBB have been the focus of human CNS research. Potential novel systems include lipid-mediated transport, microspheres, nanoparticles, and endogenous receptor (i.e., insulin, glucose, transferase) -mediated transport systems. Development of synthetic drugs with better CNS penetration and antiinflammatory effects, such as minocycline, have also been studied. Minocycline is a second-generation, semisynthetic tetracycline with increased lipophilicity, less protein binding, and broader antimicrobial spectrum than other drugs in the tetracycline class. Minocycline has been shown to have good distribution in various body tissues, including the CSF and aqueous humor in a variety of species, including IV administration (2.2 mg/kg every 12 hours [q12h] with a long half-life) in horses[81] and oral administration (4 mg/kg q12h) in horses.[82] The minimum inhibitory concentration (MIC) of oral minocycline for equine pathogens was comparable to doxycycline and not better as in humans. No adverse effects, such as diarrhea or anorexia, from minocycline administration were reported in either of the equine studies. Cardiovascular collapse seen with other tetracycline antimicrobials given intravenously was not seen with IV administration of minocycline at 2.2 mg/kg.[81] Minocycline has also been shown in experimental murine infection models of JEV to have neuroprotective properties by reducing cytokines such as TNF-α, IL-1β, and MMPs that have been implicated in BBB damage. Intraperitoneal injection of minocycline at 24 hours in mice infected with JEV resulted in reduced BBB damage, significant decrease in MMP-9 activity in brain tissue homogenates, decreased expression of inducible nitric oxide, cyclooxygenase-2, vascular endothelial cell growth factor, chemokine receptors, and adhesion molecules in the brain.[83] Based on its bioavailability, spectrum, and potential neuroprotective effects, minocycline may be beneficial in the treatment of CNS infections in horses, including *Borrelia burgdorferi*.

Glucocorticoids, Osmotic Agents, and Diuretics

Increased intracranial pressure (ICP) caused by vasogenic edema or obstructive hydrocephalus is common in patients with bacterial CNS infections, and its control is critical for successful treatment of these patients.[37,78] The use of corticosteroids in patients with CNS infection is controversial because of their immunosuppressive effects; however, mortality was unaffected with corticosteroid administration to humans with brain abscesses.[84] Moreover, corticosteroids reverse the increased permeability of the BBB induced by inflammatory mediators (e.g., IL-6, TNF-α, prostaglandins, leukotrienes, IL-1). Administration of dexamethasone (0.25 to 0.75 mg/kg) to two horses successfully treated for intracranial abscesses was thought to be beneficial.[9]

Mannitol causes an osmotic shift of water into the vascular space, decreases blood viscosity, and increases cerebral blood flow and oxygen delivery.[9,78] The net result is vasoconstriction of the cerebral arterioles and a decrease in cerebral blood volume and ICP. A single dose of mannitol (0.15 to 2.5 g/kg IV) decreases ICP experimentally within 5 minutes, with peak effects at 10 to 40 minutes and lasting 90 to 120 minutes. Adequate hydration of the patient must be maintained.

Hypertonic saline (1232 mmol of sodium/L) as a continuous IV infusion of 1 mL/kg/hr for 6 hours and then 0.2 mL/kg/hr for 12 hours has been advocated to be beneficial in the treatment of brain swelling in traumatic brain injury of horses and has additional effects such as plasma volume expansion, antiinflammatory properties, and reduction of microvascular permeability.[85] Hypertonic saline is used to manage ICP in human patients with tuberculosis meningitis[86] and may potentially have improved effects to reduce cerebral edema compared with mannitol based on a rabbit bacterial meningitis model.[87]

The benefits of dimethyl sulfoxide (DMSO) for reduction of ICP are unclear, and most research has been performed in rodent models.[88] In one clinical trial, DMSO reduced ICP and improved clinical course of neurologic recovery. In another trial, continued therapy was necessary for maintenance of decreased ICP.[89] Objective studies regarding the efficacy of DMSO in horses for reducing ICP are lacking.[6,9]

Furosemide prolongs the effects of mannitol, but its effect as a sole agent for ICP reduction is inconsistent and delayed. Controlled ventilation to prevent hypercapnia and subsequent cerebral arteriolar vasodilation is advocated in human patients for the control of ICP.[1] Barbiturates reduce cerebral oxygen demand and are neuroprotective against brain injury.

Supportive Therapy

Properly trained nursing personnel and facilities equipped to handle horses with CNS dysfunction are essential because the size and behavioral abnormalities associated with severe neurologic disease in some horses may render provision of adequate care extremely demanding and dangerous.[90] Rapid progression of disease is common in horses, resulting in imbalance and recumbency and necessitating the use of padded stalls and protective head gear, removal of shoes, and placement of leg wraps. Adequate bedding, periodic turning of the patient from side to side, or the use of slings to prevent formation of decubital ulcers is essential in the care of recumbent horses. Control of hyperthermia with ice water, alcohol baths, and fans may be required. Supportive care with IV fluids, parenteral nutrition, and electrolytes is necessary in an inappetent animal.

Miscellaneous Bacterial Infections

Bacterial and Fungal Meningitis and Meningoencephalitis

Etiology

Bacterial meningitis most often occurs in septicemic foals, often caused by infection with *E. coli*, *Actinobacillus* spp., *Klebsiella* spp., *Streptococcus* spp., and *Staphylococcus* spp. *Listeria* has been isolated from affected immunosuppressed foals (see Chapter 45) and adult horses and is associated with a pyogranulomatous meningoencephalitis.[8,91-95] Bacterial meningitis occurs rarely in older horses and may be caused by a variety of organisms.[37,96-100]

Clinical Findings

Early clinical signs of bacterial CNS infection include fever, stiff neck, obtundation, malaise, lethargy, anorexia, and photophobia.[6,11,35,90,101] The stiff neck (meningismus) is caused by a reflex spasm of the neck muscles caused by traction on inflamed cervical nerve roots.

Extension of infection from the meninges into the brain parenchyma (meningoencephalitis) via blood supply through the Virchow-Robin spaces occurs rapidly and will manifest as multifocal or diffuse cortical disease. Forebrain disease is characterized by behavioral and mentation changes and may manifest as hyperexcitability, hyperesthesia, obtundation, and self-mutilation. Blindness, lack of menace, compulsive walking, circling, and anorexia may also be seen. Depressed consciousness, head tilt, loss of balance, ataxia, limb weakness, and cranial nerve deficits (e.g., facial paralysis, nystagmus, tongue paresis, pharyngeal paresis) indicate brainstem involvement. Cerebellar disorders are characterized by ataxia, intention tremor, and nystagmus. With increasing severity of disease, seizures and coma are likely.[11,90] Clinical signs in foals may be more subtle because meningitis in the foal may be secondary to generalized sepsis.[95] Presentation in foals can vary from the ambulatory foal with increased body temperature and mild hyperesthesia to the fully recumbent and comatose foal. Foals may present with fever of unknown origin and increased irritability. Seizures are likely in foals with meningitis. Foals may or may not have abnormalities of blood work that support clinical signs; CSF analysis is mandatory to confirm meningitis in the foal.

In horses, fungal encephalitis is associated with *Cryptococcus neoformans* infection (see Chapter 53) secondary to immunodeficiency and with extension from guttural pouch mycosis (see Chapter 1). Clinical signs are similar to those of bacterial meningitis. In the horse with guttural pouch involvement, signs associated with the primary disease may include epistaxis, dysphagia, laryngeal hemiplegia, facial paralysis, and mydriasis.[11,101-103] *Aspergillus niger* infection with mycotic vasculitis and right cerebral infarction was reported in one horse, associated with acute bacterial typhlocolitis[104] (see Chapter 52). The mare presented with a 10-day history of watery diarrhea, fever, increased heart rate, dehydration, dysphagia, and depression.

Diagnosis

As with any clinical problem, accurate diagnosis of CNS infection depends on obtaining a thorough history and a detailed physical examination of the patient. Neuroanatomic localization of the lesion in the CNS should be emphasized to facilitate development of an accurate list of differential diagnoses. Further diagnostic tests are chosen to support or eliminate specific differential diagnoses for that patient.

Bacterial meningitis should be suspected in a neonate with clinical signs and history of questionable immune status or concurrent septicemia.[95] A history of systemic infection, ethmoidal hematoma, otitis media, or guttural pouch empyema in adult horses with bacterial meningitis is common.[11,39] Diagnostic investigation to identify possible primary systemic infection is warranted in both adult horses and foals. Confirmation of a diagnosis of bacterial meningitis is usually obtained on the basis of clinical signs, CSF analysis, and imaging of the CNS.

Diagnostic evaluation is done to identify underlying systemic infection that may be associated with meningitis. This evaluation may include complete blood count (CBC), serum biochemical profile, urinalysis, thoracic or abdominal imaging, serology, and blood or urine culture, depending on the patient's clinical signs and presenting complaints. In foals, clinical signs may mirror metabolic encephalopathies associated with septicemia. The CBC and serum biochemistry panel are warranted to rule out hypoglycemia, hyponatremia, and hepatic dysfunction.

Analysis of CSF is often invaluable for diagnosis of bacterial meningitis. In human patients, opening CSF pressures of 180 to 600 mm H_2O are reported. Increased WBC count (100-10,000 cells/μL) with a predominantly neutrophilic profile and the presence of intracellular organisms are the hallmark of suppurative bacterial meningitis. A low WBC count with high numbers of bacteria is considered indicative of a poor prognosis. Decreased CSF glucose concentration, increased lactate concentration, and increased protein concentration are also observed in many patients.[35,36,66,69]

The utility of CT and MRI is increasing as aids in the diagnosis of diseases of equids (e.g., neoplasia, intracranial abscesses)[35,36] (Fig. 4-4). Recent retrospective studies have found CT to be a useful diagnostic tool for evaluation of horses presenting with abnormal mentation and cranial nerve signs.[105] In particular, CT is useful in the horse for early recognition of temporohyoid osteoarthropathy changes not evident on endoscopy or radiographs.[106] Standard radiographic imaging of the skull or vertebral bodies may facilitate identification of predisposing conditions such as fractures, vertebral body abscess, sinusitis, and otitis media. Electroencephalography (EEG) is a sensitive tool for the diagnosis of intracranial disease in horses.[10] Abnormal EEGs appear as high-voltage waves with discrete paroxysmal activity.

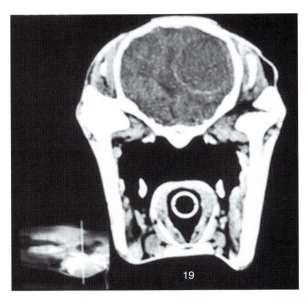

Figure 4-4 Computed tomographic image of foal that presented with circling and blindness. Large abscess with ring enhancement is visible in the foal's right hemisphere. This lesion was confirmed by surgical exploration and drainage. *(Courtesy Dr. Rodney Belgrave.)*

Differential diagnoses for bacterial meningitis in foals include metabolic encephalopathies associated with septicemia, Tyzzer's disease, idiopathic epilepsy, cerebellar abiotrophy, intracranial abscesses, neonatal maladjustment syndrome, hydrocephalus, hydranencephaly, and hypoxia.[11] In adult horses, differential diagnoses for bacterial meningitis include mycotic meningitis and encephalitis, viral encephalitides, neoplasia, rabies, migrating parasites, metabolic derangement, hepatoencephalopathy, intracranial abscesses, leukoencephalomalacia, endotoxemia, botulism, tetanus, brain trauma, and intoxication with organophosphate, strychnine, metaldehyde, lead, arsenic, mercury, or bracken fern.

Postmortem findings are diagnostic in most horses with bacterial meningitis. Grossly congested, swollen, opalescent meninges with petechiation are observed. Histopathologic lesions include infiltration of the tissues with neutrophils and lymphocytes, choroiditis, bacterial colonies around blood vessels, and meningeal hemorrhage. In foals, evidence of septicemia and concurrent infection of the joints, umbilical cord, respiratory system, and GI system may be observed.[11] Culture of lesions will identify specific etiologic agents.

Therapy

Treatment of bacterial meningitis emphasizes elimination of bacterial pathogens and limiting the severe and often fatal consequences of the immune response within the CNS. Third-generation cephalosporins and metronidazole remain antibiotics of choice in human medicine, administered in combination with nonsteroidal antiinflammatory drugs (NSAIDs). The use of antiinflammatory medications with bactericidal drugs has reduced the mortality in children with bacterial meningitis from 30% to less than 5%.[41,78,107] Antimicrobials that do not induce cell lysis (e.g., imipenem) rather than traditional β-lactam antimicrobials have been recommended to reduce the amount of inflammatory bacterial debris created.

Prognosis for survival of horses with meningoencephalitis is fair to poor. Early diagnosis is critical, but vague clinical signs in horses early in the disease process often prevent timely medical care.[90]

Prevention

Although chemoprophylaxis with antibiotics is a mainstay in the prevention of bacterial meningitis in humans,[35-37,108] vaccines against bacterial CNS pathogens are not available for horses. As stated previously, bacterial meningitis should be suspected in a neonate with clinical signs and history of questionable immune status or concurrent septicemia.[95]

Intracranial Abscesses

Etiology

Brain and spinal abscesses are rare in horses.[7,27] In adult horses, evidence indicates that CNS infections may occur secondary to extension of infections involving other structures in the head (e.g., sinuses, otitis media, traumatic injury, tooth root abscesses).[39] In a recent report of cerebral listeriosis in a 6-year-old Freiberger gelding after being fed hay silage, the route of entry to the CNS was unknown. It was proposed to be either (1) via damaged oral, nasal, or ocular mucosa and entry into the CNS through branches of the trigeminal nerve or (2) systemically via ingestion and invasion of the bacteria in the intestinal epithelial cells and dissemination to neighboring cells.[109] Similar to bacterial meningitis, intracranial and spinal abscesses in foals are associated with neonatal septicemia and questionable immune status and are likely to result from hematogenous spread. *Rhodococcus equi* was isolated from an intracranial abscess and concurrent occipital osteomyelitis in a 3-month-old colt. The colt had presented for respiratory distress and a mild left-sided head tilt. The intracranial abscess was suspected to have resulted from dissemination of the pulmonary infection. *Listeria monocytogenes* has been isolated from the CNS in septicemic neonatal foals[110,111] and in a 1-month Arabian foal with combined immunodeficiency.[112] *Streptococcus* spp., however, are common isolates from brain abscesses in both foals and adult horses. Other species isolated include *Klebsiella pneumonia*, *Actinobacillus equuli*, and *Pasteurella caballi*.[39] There is one report of iatrogenic spinal epidural abscess secondary to CSF aspiration.[113]

Clinical Findings

Horses with intracranial abscesses are often presented for evaluation of compulsive circling toward the side of the lesion, head pressing, focal neurologic deficits, seizures, mentation changes, papilledema, and ophthalmic tract deficits. Fever is often present. Impaired vision has been frequently reported with brain abscesses in horses. Unilateral cortical abscesses result in loss of vision in the contralateral eye because of the high percentage of optic nerve fibers (85%) that cross at the optic chiasm in the horse compared with other species.[6] Although pituitary abscess is considered rare in horses because of the lack of defined rete mirabile vessels, six abscesses involving the pituitary were observed in four of five horses with intracranial abscesses.[39]

Diagnosis

Previous history of a severe purulent infection, such as *Streptococcus equi* subsp. *equi* ("strangles") and other systemic bacterial infections (respiratory, GI, reproductive, urinary, cardiovascular), are frequently reported in horses with intracranial abscesses.[6,9,27,39] Primary infections of the head (sinusitis, periocular lesions, dental disease, submandibular lymphadenopathy) without concomitant systemic disease are also considered risk factors. In horses, antemortem diagnosis of intracranial abscess is primarily made on the basis of clinical signs, neuroanatomic localization of the lesion, CSF analysis, ancillary diagnostic testing, and imaging of the brain and spinal cord. Human patients with suspected intracranial abscesses are empirically treated with antibiotics before ancillary testing with CT, MRI, and skull radiographs. Involvement of the pituitary gland may result in hyponatremia caused by inappropriate antidiuretic hormone secretion.[1]

Cerebrospinal fluid changes in horses with intracranial abscessation may be minimal and nonspecific. Increased protein concentration, decreased glucose concentration, and a mononuclear pleocytosis may be observed in affected horses.* Culture of the lesion itself through CT-guided stereotactic aspiration is preferred over culture of CSF for identification of a causative organism. Culture of a pathogen from the CSF of human patients with brain abscesses is successful in only 11% to 17% of cases, whereas culture of aspirates from intracranial lesions is 95% successful in untreated patients and 70% to 82.6% successful in patients treated with antibiotics before sample collection. Collection of CSF is contraindicated in neurologically unstable patients because of the risk of brain herniation.

Computed tomography is considered superior to standard radiographs for anatomic visualization of brain abscesses. An intracranial abscess is seen as a hypodense area of avascular necrotic tissue and purulent discharge. With injection of iodinated contrast material, the hypodense area appears to be surrounded by an "enhancement ring," representing a region of hypercellularity and hypervascularity encapsulated by fibrous tissue (see Fig. 4-4). Surrounding the ring may be a hypodense area of brain edema.[9] Stereotactic CT-guided techniques are useful for direct aspiration of abscesses, with minimal damage to surrounding tissue.[84]

In humans, MRI is more sensitive and accurate than CT for the diagnosis of brain abscesses.[35,36,84] MRI is also more sensitive than CT for detection of cerebritis and cerebral edema, which frequently precede overt abscess formation.[84] With CT, small pathologic changes in the tissue are masked by "hardening artifacts," which are streaklike artifacts of low density caused by absorption of lower-energy photons in the x-ray beam by large radiodense structures. MR images are generated with T1-weighted, T2-weighted, proton density (PD)–weighted, and inversion recovery (IR)–weighted spin-echo sequences. Intracranial abscesses appear hypointense to isointense, with a hyperintense rim if there is capsule formation.[27] The contrast agent chelated gadolinium is excluded from the normal CNS. Its appearance in neural tissue after systemic injection indicates breakdown of the BBB.[7] The sensitivity of MRI has allowed clinicians to define four stages of intracranial abscess formation: early cerebritis (days 1-3), late cerebritis (days 4-9), early capsule formation (days 10-13), and late capsule formation (day 14 and onward). Initiation of treatment during the early stages of abscess formation before encapsulation of the lesion allows for better penetration of antibiotics and better prognosis for response to therapy.[84]

There are two reports of MRI for the diagnosis of intracranial abscesses in horses. In one horse, comparison of MRI and CT found that MRI demonstrated better spatial resolution and soft tissue contrast in delineating the surrounding tissue edema. MR findings of a chronic brain abscess in a 10-month-old filly correlated with the characteristics of a mature brain abscess and were confirmed by histopathologic changes.[7,27]

Differential diagnostic considerations for intracranial abscesses in horses include otitis media, central vestibular disease, cholesterol granuloma, neoplasia, rabies, tetanus, EPM, EHM, polyneuritis equi, meningoencephalitis (viral, bacterial, fungal, protozoal), subdural empyema, aberrant parasite migration, intracranial hemorrhage, brain trauma, cerebral infarction, and intracarotid injection.[11]

Intracranial abscesses are usually obvious lesions if the brain is evaluated grossly during a postmortem examination. They are usually focal lesions of encephalomalacia with surrounding dense, fibrous connective tissue and dense aggregates of microglia.

Therapy

Long-term antimicrobial therapy and surgical intervention are recommended for treatment of horses with intracranial abscesses. Surgical intervention with craniotomy has been described in three horses.[6,9,39] In all three cases, poor response and/or progression of neurologic signs despite systemic antimicrobial therapy prompted surgical intervention.[9]

Of the three horses with a reported successful outcome for treatment of brain abscesses, antimicrobial agents initially administered included crystalline penicillin or procaine penicillin intramuscularly (IM) with or without sulfa-trimethoprim.[6,9,39] Therapy was switched to procaine penicillin for 10 to 14 days, and then horses were discharged from the hospital with recommendations for treatment with sulfa-trimethoprim for 28 days. Cefazolin was infused into the craniotomy site in one affected horse.

Empiric therapy with antimicrobials is immediately instituted in all human patients with suspected intracranial abscesses.[84] Course of therapy is determined by whether the patient is a surgical candidate. Nonsurgical patients include those with stable neurologic condition, multiple abscesses, deep location of abscesses, abscesses in a sensitive area of the brain, concomitant meningitis or ependymitis, lesions less than 3 cm in size, and response to empiric antimicrobial therapy. Surgery is also contraindicated in patients with early cerebritis because of the risk of hemorrhage with aspiration. Surgery is considered in patients with rapidly deteriorating neurologic conditions (likely caused by increased intracranial pressure) or chronic encapsulated lesions that are nonresponsive to prolonged antimicrobial treatment. CT-guided stereotactic aspiration is the preferred technique; however, full-excision craniotomy may be necessary in rapidly deteriorating patients; patients with inaccessible lesions in the brainstem, thalamus, or basal ganglia; and lesions with gas abscesses. Fungal abscesses have a poor prognosis in the horse as they require direct infusion of antimicrobial drugs into the lesion because of the poor concentrations achieved by systemic administration of most drugs. Use of corticosteroids in patients with intracranial abscesses is controversial because it decreases antibiotic entry into the CNS and decreases collagen formation and glial response, but it may be indicated in rapidly deteriorating patients to reduce ICP.[84]

The veterinary literature suggests that the prognosis for horses with intracranial abscesses is poor. Of 13 affected horses, three horses were successfully treated, but one of the three succumbed to secondary laminitis.[8,9,15,30,31] Use of CT or MRI, long-term antimicrobial therapy, concomitant antiinflammatory therapy, and surgical intervention were common factors in the horses that survived.[30]

Spinal Abscessation and Vertebral Osteomyelitis

Etiology and Epidemiology

Spinal abscesses are rare in horses.[3,11] Most reported cases originate from a preexisting vertebral osteomyelitis (more likely in foals) or diskospondylitis.[11] Common etiologic agents found in vertebral infections in foals include *Salmonella* spp., *Actinobacillus equuli*, *Escherichia coli*, *Streptococcus* spp., *Rhodococcus equi*, and *Klebsiella* spp.[11,25,120-122] Less common agents isolated from horses include *Mycobacterium avium*, *Actinobacillus lignieresii*, *Aspergillus* spp., *Eikenella corrodens*, and *Brucella* spp.[11,113,121,123,124] These bone infections are likely the result of hematogenous spread of the pathogen from primary systemic infection sites

---

*References 6-9, 25, 27, 39, 107, 113-119.

(lung, heart, GI) or probably secondary to septicemia in neonates.

The unique vascular anatomy of the vertebrae contributes to the pathogenesis of infection. The decreased blood flow of the tortuous metaphyseal arteries as they approach the vertebral physis creates an ideal environment for the embolization of septic thrombi. Furthermore, the metaphyseal vessels communicate with the ventral vertebral plexus, which in turn drains into the post cava, the portal vein, and the pulmonary veins. The ventral vertebral plexus does not contain valves, and when blood flow reverses with an increase in abdominal or pleural pressure, regurgitated blood from infected sites in the body cavities showers the vertebrae and spinal cord with bacteria. As previously described, the posterior spinal cord blood supply is rarely involved in infections because it is supplied by an irregular portion of arterial plexuses, whereas the anterior spinal cord is supplied by the cervical and intercostal arteries from the descending aorta.[11]

Bone lesions may also develop from sequestra that have fragmented off fractured vertebrae. Injection of contaminated vaccines or drugs in the proximity of the spinal column is another potential route of infection. Septic arthritis of the AO joint resulting from extension of a mycotic guttural pouch lesion has also been reported.[11] Spinal epidural infection secondary to epidural anesthesia is not considered a likely potential complication in horses.[125] There is one report of iatrogenic spinal epidural abscess secondary to CSF aspiration.[113]

Clinical Findings

Clinical signs depend on the anatomic area involved and the extent of infection. Horses with cervical spinal abscesses may appear stiff, exhibit signs of neck pain, and be reluctant to eat from the ground. Additional signs may include pain, heat, swelling, and crepitus over the affected areas and associated signs of bacteremia (e.g., fever, depression, anorexia).[11,121,124] Neurologic deficits depend on the degree of spinal cord compression, the degree of inflammation, and the area of the lesion. Hindlimb lameness, ataxia, weakness, paresis, cauda equine syndrome, and urinary incontinence have been described in horses with epidural abscesses, pelvic osteomyelitis, and sacral diskospondylitis.[11,72,115,116] If infection is extensive and erodes through the dura mater, septic meningitis may develop. Extensive bone infection may also result in vertebral bone fracture and development of acute signs of spinal trauma.

Diagnosis

In horses, antemortem diagnosis of a spinal abscess is primarily made on the basis of clinical signs, neuroanatomic localization of the lesion, CSF analysis, ancillary diagnostic testing, and imaging of the spinal cord. Plain radiographs are considered the most diagnostic for spinal abscesses, with osteomyelitis manifesting as hyperlucency and increased bone density in the affected vertebrae (Fig. 4-5). Myelography may be used to define spinal cord compression further.[126] Nuclear scintigraphy (^{99m}Tc–methylene diphosphonate [MDP] and labeled leukocytes) may be beneficial when bone lesions are not well defined on plain-film radiography, as with extradural abscesses.[116] In foals, CT or MRI may be beneficial.

The CBC in affected horses is often consistent with a chronic inflammatory focus and may include hyperfibrinogenemia, neutrophilia, monocytosis, nonresponsive anemia, and left shift. In neonates with inadequate colostral immunoglobulin transfer, plasma globulin levels may or may not be increased. CSF evaluation may not be as beneficial because most spinal abscesses do not infiltrate through the dura and into the pachymeninges. Normal or mild increases in protein concentration may be seen.[11,121,124] Diagnostic testing to evaluate underlying primary infection is indicated.

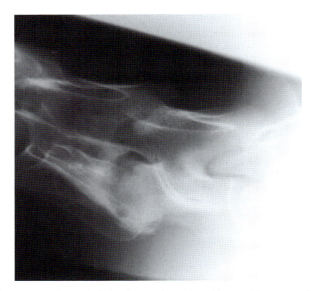

Figure 4-5 Radiograph of distal cervical vertebra of horse with osteomyelitis (diskospondylitis) at C6-C7. Initial films demonstrated a large, lytic lesion. The horse recovered after long-term antibiotic therapy with mild residual spinal deficits. *(Courtesy Dr. Steeve Giguere.)*

Therapy

As with intracranial abscesses, prolonged systemic antimicrobial therapy is indicated for the treatment of vertebral abscesses. Selection of a broad-spectrum antimicrobial is advocated but ideally should be based on results obtained from culture of the primary underlying systemic infection. Access to the vertebral lesion may be difficult because of the large epaxial muscles of the horse.[11] Surgical drainage and curettage of necrotic bone constituted successful therapy in one horse.[124] Use of NSAIDs may be beneficial to reduce inflammation and musculoskeletal pain. Use of a supportive fiberglass neck cast has been described to stabilize infected cervical vertebrae in smaller and compliant patients. Easier access to water and food by lifting the feed buckets may be beneficial for horses with neck pain.

As with intracranial abscesses, vertebral osteomyelitis and spinal cord abscesses are potentially life threatening, and prognosis is guarded.[11,121]

Miscellaneous Parasitic Infection

Maureen T. Long

Verminous encephalitis is rare in horses but does occur in the Midwest and Southeast United States and throughout the world. Specific causes to consider include *Strongylus vulgaris*, *Setaria* spp. filariae, *Halicephalobus gingivalis*, *Draschia megastoma*, *Hypoderma* spp., and *Parelaphostrongylus tenuis* (see Chapter 60). *Setaria* and *Strongylus* spp. can cause brain or spinal cord disease. Signs are ipsilateral and sudden, resulting from an infarctive process. *Halicephalobus* and *Hypoderma* usually are intracranial.

Halicephalobus gingivalis Encephalomyelitis

Halicephalobus gingivalis, previously known as *Micronema deletrix* and *Halicephalobus deletrix*, causes sporadic brain infection in horses, resulting from an aberrant infection. This parasite was identified and named in 1954.[127-129] Infection has been identified in humans as well.

Etiology and Epidemiology

Halicephalobus parasites are free-living nematodes of the order Rhabditida (family *Rhabditidae*) that normally reside in soil and humus.[129] In Florida, infection with *H. gingivalis* is anecdotally associated with a swampland environment, although stabled horses have developed the disease. Actual species characterization had been limited until recent molecular techniques were applied to analysis of this organism.[130] The nematode identified as *H. deletrix* is one of seven nematodes that belong to the *Halicephalobus* genus.

Recent genetic analysis demonstrates several different clades.[130] Isolates from clinical cases and from the environment are not aligned geographically, although there are differences among isolates from cases in Tennessee compared with California. Only one type of *Halicephalobus* is associated with mammalian infection; all other species have been obtained solely from environmental sampling. Recent case reports include locales such as Iceland,[131] the United Kingdom,[132] and Japan.[133]

The life cycle of *H. gingivalis* has not been completely determined; only females have been recovered from tissue sections.[127,128,134] Eggs and immature larvae are present in these infections, indicating an asexual reproductive cycle in tissues. Free-living male worms have been recovered from soil, indicating sexual reproduction does occur.

Pathogenesis

Disease in horses infected with *H. gingivalis* may affect the CNS; the renal, ocular, and reproductive tracts; and the skeletal system.[128,129,135-137] Little is known about the pathogenesis of this disease in horses. High numbers of organisms are observed in tissue sections. Regardless of infection site, the tissue burden of this organism is dense, and there is an extremely severe tissue reaction with suppurative inflammation and eosinophilic localization within tissue. Abscess and severe, fulminant pyogranulomatous disease is associated with infection.

Site of entry for the parasite is hypothesized to be through breaks in the skin or mucous membranes. Mammary, uterine, and renal infection has been reported independent of CNS infection.[136,138,139] In one horse with CNS infection, a large, oral granulomatous lesion was observed.[140] Breaks in urogenital mucosa may also provide an important pathway for invasion. Two stallions with renal infection, one with concurrent testicular involvement, have been described.[141] Vertical transmission may also occur in horses.[142] Localization to the kidney may occur through ascending infection, resulting in perirenal granulomas. These frequently coincide with CNS infection. Ocular and periocular infections have also been described in horses.[135,141]

Clinical Findings

Horses with CNS infection usually present with signs of fulminant encephalitis. Rarely, peripheral CNS infection has been described. Most horses have a rapid onset of progressive cerebral signs, with head pressing, coma, extensive loss of proprioception, recumbency, and death.[135,142-143b] Onset can be insidious initially, but with cerebral and hindbrain infestation, signs rapidly progress. One horse has been described with cauda equina clinical signs consisting of ataxia, flaccid tail, fecal impaction, and urinary incontinence.[144] Parasitic granulomas were associated only with spinal nerve roots of the cauda equina.

Diagnosis

There is no specific antemortem test for diagnosis of *H. gingivalis* in horses. The CBC is usually normal except for possibly an eosinophilia. Hypergammaglobulinemia has been inconsistently described in the literature. CSF total nucleated cell count and total protein concentration are usually markedly increased. CSF that contains eosinophils is highly suggestive of a parasitic infection. Very high numbers of nondegenerate and degenerate neutrophils have been observed cytologically in the CSF of affected horses.

CNS infection with *H. gingivalis* is usually confirmed by histopathology; however, renal involvement with perirenal granulomas is highly suspicious for *H. gingivalis*.* Histopathologic identification of the parasite in tissues is the most common way in which the organism is diagnosed. In tissue section the parasite has a smooth, thin cuticle with what is called a *plymyarian-meromyarian* musculature, and the nematode body ends in a tapered tail. The pendocoelom and rhabditiform esophagus is composed of a corpus, isthmus, and bulb. The parasite has an intestinal tract lined by single, nucleated cuboidal cells. The ovary and uterus can be visualized as a "flexed" structure.

Therapy

Reports are limited on treatment of *H. gingivalis* infection.[145,151,152] A 12-year-old gelding with a granuloma in the orbit was successfully treated with oral ivermectin (0.55 mg/kg every 14 days) and surgical debulking. There was no evidence of infection in any other organ system. Although ivermectin is likely active against systemic infection, it is unlikely that CNS levels obtained after oral therapy are high enough to treat intracerebral *H. gingivalis*. High-dose treatment with fenbendazole in addition to ivermectin is indicated for neurologic disease caused by *H. gingivalis*, although the prognosis for survival is exceedingly poor.

Prevention and Control

Because limited information is available regarding the epidemiology of *H. gingivalis* infection, no specific control measures can be recommended. Good pasture management and restriction of horses from marsh or swamp environments are indicated.

Zoonotic Potential

Zoonotic infection is reported in humans, although infection has never been reported from direct contact with an infected horse. Nonetheless, one of the most recent case reports in the literature describes prophylactic treatment of all people in contact with a horse with *H. gingivalis* osteomyelitis.[137]

The complete reference list is available online at www.expertconsult.com.

---

*References 127, 130, 134, 136, 139, 141, 143, and 145-150.

Infections of Muscle, Joint, and Bone

5

Liberty M. Getman, W. Wesley Sutter,* and Alicia L. Bertone*

Musculoskeletal infections are a common clinical problem encountered in equine practice. Infections in the adult horse are often associated with trauma or are iatrogenically induced via surgery or joint injections. Conversely, musculoskeletal infections in the foal are more likely to be of hematogenous origin. In both foals and adults, musculoskeletal infections are associated with significant morbidity and mortality. A rapid, accurate diagnosis and prompt initiation of appropriate therapy are important for a successful outcome.

Muscle Infections

Infectious myositis may be caused by bacteria, viruses, or parasites as either a primary or a secondary disease process. Primary infectious myositis occurs when inflammation is caused by active infection of muscle tissue with a pathogen. In secondary infectious myositis, muscle inflammation occurs as a response to current or past infection at other body sites, and viable pathogens are not usually present in the affected muscle tissue. Primary infectious myositis may result from direct inoculation of a pathogen (through the skin) or hematogenous localization to a single muscle or multiple muscle groups.

Primary Bacterial Myositis

Etiology

Bacterial infection occurring in association with trauma is the most common form of primary infectious myositis. *Streptococcus equi* subsp. *equi* (see Chapter 28), *Clostridium* spp. (see Chapter 42), and *Staphylococcus* spp. (see Chapter 29) are common bacterial isolates from these cases.[1] Mixed gram-negative and anaerobic bacterial muscle infection with abscessation can occur secondary to infection of deeper structures.[1,2] Many different bacterial agents can colonize muscle from a hematogenous route, including *S. equi* subsp. *equi* and *Clostridium* spp.[3-6] *Salmonella enterica* can cause localized myonecrosis and infection secondary to septicemia in both adult horses and foals[7] (see Chapter 35).

Clinical Findings

In general, clinical signs of primary bacterial myositis reflect whether the infection is generalized or localized. Presentation may vary, depending on the virulence of the organism and whether the infection is localized or if the horse has signs of systemic infection (i.e., toxemia). Clinical findings of localized infection include signs typical of impending or fully mature abscess formation such as increased rectal temperature; pain on palpation; hot, pitting edema; and localized swelling. Localized myositis may be insidious if deep muscular structures are involved. Mild to non–weight-bearing lameness can be the primary clinical sign. Horses with injection site abscesses caused by non–toxin-producing organisms can present with moderately painful swelling and no other clinical signs. Infections with organisms such as *S. equi* subsp. *equi*, *Corynebacterium pseudotuberculosis*, and *Staphylococcus aureus* can be accompanied by generalized edema, serum leakage, vasculitis, and cellulitis. Signs of systemic toxemia include red to injected mucous membranes, tachycardia, tachypnea, increased rectal temperature, poor peripheral pulses, and reluctance to move.

Diagnosis

A diagnosis of primary bacterial myositis can be quite obvious if the lesion is localized; however, if generalized myositis or localized myositis without external swelling is present, identification of infectious myositis can be problematic. A detailed history of recent injections, trauma, travel, and other systemic complaints should be closely considered. A complete blood count (CBC) may reveal an inflammatory leukogram (neutrophilia with or without a left shift) and hyperfibrinogenemia. If chronic or viral infection is present, these tests may be normal. Increased serum creatine kinase (CK) and aspartate transaminase (AST) activities indicate muscle inflammation or necrosis but are not specific for infectious myositis or an etiologic agent. Muscle enzymes may not be significantly elevated when localized or occult infection exists or in the acute stages of the disease.

For localized infection, ultrasound evaluation, radiography, and scintigraphy may assist in the diagnosis and treatment of infectious myositis. Even with an obvious abscess, ultrasound of the affected muscle can be useful for evaluating the extent of the lesion, directing therapy (by helping obtain samples for culture and sensitivity testing and identifying areas to lance), and assessing response to therapy. Radiographs of the affected area may be indicated if skeletal involvement is suspected. Nuclear scintigraphy has been suggested to aid in localization of deep abscesses in muscle, either by soft tissue phase imaging or by the use of radiolabeled autologous white blood cells.[8]

Diagnostic testing should include efforts to identify the causative agent. For localized infections, aspiration and culture of soft or fluid-filled swellings is recommended. Culture of samples obtained by deep swab of draining tracts is important. Both of these techniques should be performed aseptically. Culture of fine-needle aspirates from swollen, inflamed muscles may yield inciting organisms such as *S. aureus* and *C. pseudotuberculosis*. Muscle biopsy may be indicated in some cases to confirm the presence of myositis and obtain diagnostic culture results. Aerobic and anaerobic cultures should always be performed, and fungal cultures should be requested when indicated. Identification of parasites is usually accomplished with histopathology. Serology can aid diagnosis of *C. pseudotuberculosis* (see

*The authors acknowledge and appreciate the original contributions of these authors, whose work has been incorporated into this chapter.

Chapter 45). High *S. equi* subsp. *equi* titer may reflect recent exposure or active infection if vaccination has not been recent.

Therapy

Therapy for infectious myositis depends on the etiologic agent, presentation (generalized or localized), and other organ involvement. For localized infection without signs of toxemia, local drainage and lavage with an isotonic solution is essential and may be the only indicated treatment. When there is evidence of cellulitis, systemic infection, or toxemia, antimicrobial and antiinflammatory therapy is indicated. If an infectious etiology is suspected, therapy should be initiated prior to culture results with broad-spectrum and anaerobic coverage. With life-threatening infection, all medication available as such should be administered parenterally. Once obtained, antimicrobial therapy should reflect culture and sensitivity results.

Clostridial Myonecrosis

Clostridial myonecrosis is a rapidly progressing infection of muscle with *Clostridium* spp. that results in severe myonecrosis and systemic toxemia (see Chapter 42).

Primary Fungal Myositis

Etiology

Primary fungal myositis may occur after direct inoculation of the etiologic agent, as may occur with phycomycoses (see Chapter 51). Alternatively, hematogenous dissemination of systemic fungi may result in infectious myositis[9,10] (see Chapter 47).

Clinical Findings

Most fungal infections are usually localized and reflect a deeper invasion of the subcutis and underlying muscle, as seen in *Pythium* infections (see Chapter 51) and less commonly with *Aspergillus* infections (see Chapter 52), mycosis fungoides (see Chapter 53), and sporotrichosis infections (see Chapter 48). Coccidioidomycosis may be localized or may have concomitant widespread systemic disease with infection of the lung and liver (see Chapter 47).

Diagnosis and Therapy

Diagnosis of localized fungal myositis is similar to that described for diagnosis of bacterial myositis. Treatment of fungal myositis may include local therapy, surgical excision of lesions, and local or systemic administration of antifungal drugs.

Primary Parasitic Myositis

Etiology

The most common causes of parasitic myositis include *Sarcocystis* spp.,[1,11,12] *Trichinella* spp.,[13-15] and *Trypanosoma evansi*.[16] Aberrant parasitic migrations from various nematodes can occur. Rarely, hydatidosis has been associated with infectious myositis.[17]

Clinical Findings

With parasitic myositis, horses usually have generalized muscle infection (unless there is a localized area of aberrant parasite migration). Trichinellosis in the horse is often occult. Affected horses have variable clinical signs, ranging from mild generalized stiffness to signs of severe generalized pain with reluctance to move. Horses with chronic parasitic infections, such as sarcocystosis or trypanosomiasis, may present with weight loss or ill thrift and moderate to severe muscle wasting. Horses with hydatid disease usually have widespread systemic infection of internal organs leading to chronic wasting.

Diagnosis and Therapy

Diagnosis of parasitic myositis is usually accomplished by biopsy and histopathologic examination of the affected muscle. Treatment of specific parasitic infections is discussed elsewhere in this text. The most important health risk for humans associated with equine muscle infection is related to consumption of parasitized horse meat.[12,14,18-22] Outbreaks of human trichinellosis occur fairly regularly in the countries of the European Union. Horse meat is screened for infected muscle in slaughter plants; however, it is advisable that preparation of human meals with horse meat follow appropriate guidelines for inactivation of *Trichinella* larvae in equine muscle before consumption.

Secondary Infectious Myositis

Etiology

Streptococcal infections and several viruses may contribute to development of secondary myositis in which viable infectious agents are not present in the affected muscle tissue.[3-6] Lesions are usually generalized, affecting several muscle groups. The primary infectious agent triggers myositis as an inflammatory or an immune-mediated process. *Streptococcus equi* subsp. *equi* is associated with two types of myositis in horses: acute severe myositis, characterized by infarction of muscle, and chronic generalized muscle wasting. Both manifestations of streptococcal myositis are thought to be immune-mediated disorders and are discussed in more detail in Chapter 28. Myositis may occur concomitant with or as a sequela to acute viral infection. Viral myositis has been demonstrated or postulated to occur secondary to infection with equine herpesvirus (see Chapter 14), equine influenza virus (see Chapter 13), and African horse sickness (see Chapter 16).

Clinical Findings

Horses with myositis secondary to systemic infection present with generalized stiffness and lameness. Most affected horses demonstrate reluctance to move, and laminitis is the most common differential diagnosis. Muscles may or may not be painful on palpation. Horses with muscle infarction or necrosis may have areas of localized edema and pain. When widespread, these horses can have signs of circulatory failure accompanied by poor peripheral perfusion.[23,24]

Diagnosis and Therapy

Diagnosis of secondary myositis is accomplished by muscle biopsy to demonstrate histopathologic lesions of immune-mediated or inflammatory myositis. The approach to diagnosis of a specific underlying systemic infection depends on the type of infection that is suspected. Diagnosis of *S. equi* subsp. *equi* infection is discussed in Chapter 28. Diagnosis of equine influenza, equine herpesvirus, and African horse sickness is discussed in Chapters 13, 14, and 16, respectively.

Cellulitis

Etiology

Cellulitis is a diffuse infection of the subcutaneous tissue.[25,26] The disease is relatively common in horses, occurring either as a primary disease process with no obvious underlying cause or as a secondary infection after trauma, iatrogenic procedures, or systemic disease.[25] Primary cellulitis seems to be particularly common in Thoroughbred racehorses but can occur in any type of horse.[25,27] Causes of secondary cellulitis include infections that occur following surgery, joint injections, wounds, or blunt trauma. However, only about half of the reported cases of equine cellulitis occur secondary to a known event. The most common bacteria isolated are *Staphylococcus* and *Streptococcus* spp., but gram-negative bacteria and polymicrobial infections are also common.

Clinical Findings

Typically, horses with cellulitis have marked swelling and lameness of one limb (more commonly a hindlimb than a front limb). The lameness develops acutely and may precede the marked swelling that follows within a few hours. Owners often initially suspect that the horse has a fracture due to the severity of the lameness. By the time of the veterinarian's evaluation, most horses with cellulitis will be febrile (temperature >101.5° F [38.6° C]) and have marked swelling from the stifle or elbow to the foot. The swelling is usually hot, painful, and pitting when firm pressure is applied.

Diagnosis

On initial evaluation, other causes of the lameness, such as fractures or septic joints, should be ruled out. This can be done largely based on clinical examination findings, but sometimes adjunctive diagnostics, such as radiography, ultrasonography, and blood work values, can be helpful in establishing the diagnosis. Findings consistent with cellulitis include generalized painful pitting edema, increased rectal temperature, and marked thickening and increased echogenicity of subcutaneous tissues, with or without areas of fluid accumulation seen on ultrasonographic evaluation. Complete blood count often reveals leukocytosis or leukopenia with a left shift and hyperfibrinogenemia. Bacteria are commonly isolated from aspirates taken from subcutaneous fluid, therefore culture is recommended in all cases to direct antimicrobial therapy.

Therapy

Conventional treatment consists of broad-spectrum intravenous (IV) antimicrobial therapy that is ideally based on the results of bacterial culture and sensitivity testing.[28] Adjunctive therapy aimed at decreasing pain and inflammation generally includes nonsteroidal antiinflammatory drugs (NSAIDs), cold hosing the affected limb, and bandaging, with or without application of various topical preparations. Even with treatment, life-threatening complications, such as contralateral limb laminitis and skin necrosis and sloughing, may occur. Survival rates between 55% and 89% have been reported, with horses that are febrile on admission to referral hospitals or those that develop laminitis more likely to be euthanized.[25,27] Of horses that survive, the prognosis for return to full function is guarded; many horses continue to have an abnormal contour of the limb, and about one-third will experience lameness when resuming exercise or recurrence of infection.

Local antimicrobial delivery may be beneficial to attain higher levels of antimicrobials in the affected tissues. Intravenous regional limb perfusions may be performed daily during the acute phase of disease; the antimicrobial used is typically an aminoglycoside, but alternative choices may be indicated by results of bacterial culture and sensitivity testing. Other methods of local delivery, such as antimicrobial impregnated polymethyl methacrylate (PMMA) beads or collagen sponges, are used less commonly to treat primary cellulitis, but if wounds or surgical incisions are present in cases of secondary cellulitis, they can be placed in those areas to further increase antimicrobial concentrations.

The application of various topical preparations to the limb is aimed at reducing inflammation and edema and is largely chosen based on clinician preference. Many products contain a combination of NSAIDs, dimethyl sulfoxide (DMSO), corticosteroids, and antimicrobials. These preparations probably do have some therapeutic effect, but care should be taken to ensure that no overly harsh or irritating products are used because horses with cellulitis often have compromised skin with areas of cracks and full-thickness tears. As mentioned previously, the author prefers to apply topical diclofenac with or without a solution of 10% DMSO and 1% amikacin to the entire limb, avoiding any open wounds, incisions, or areas of full-thickness skin defects. Gloves should be worn when applying these substances to the limb.

Cellulitis in horses is markedly painful, and pain may not be adequately controlled with NSAIDs alone. In those horses, additional analgesic therapy is indicated to increase the horse's comfort as rapidly as possible and to prevent the development of contralateral limb laminitis. Opioids, α-2 agonists, local anesthetics, and ketamine can be used alone or in various combinations as single intramuscular (IM) or IV injections or as a continuous rate infusion (CRI).[29] In horses with hindlimb cellulitis, epidural administration of these agents should be considered.[29] This can be done as a single injection or more practically via an epidural catheter. Topical application of 1% diclofenac sodium (Surpass, Boehringer Ingelheim, Canada) to the affected area may also be helpful in decreasing the inflammation and associated pain in the limb. Continuous icing of the contralateral foot may be indicated in horses that remain markedly painful beyond ~24 hours after the initiation of treatment to help prevent the development of laminitis.

Physical therapy is extremely important in the treatment of horses with cellulitis. The edema and inflammation associated with acute cellulitis may persist even after infection has resolved, resulting in chronic lameness. Principles of therapy aimed at minimizing inflammation, edema accumulation, and swelling include compression and cryotherapy.[30] Compression is effective in stimulating tissue healing, minimizing edema, and increasing blood flow. Cryotherapy reduces the inflammatory response in the tissue, reduces the metabolic demand of the tissue, and provides a short-term analgesic effect. Compression can be provided by bandaging the limb or with the use of boots or other devices that provide intermittent pneumatic compression. Cryotherapy can be performed via a variety of ice boots or whirlpool systems. Minimally, hydrotherapy and hand walking (if the horse is comfortable enough to walk) two to three times daily helps decrease edema and improve circulation and comfort. After walking, the topical preparation of choice is applied to the leg and then a compressive full-limb bandage is applied.

New rehabilitation tools that have shown promise as adjunctive treatments are becoming more widely available. The Game Ready Equine system (CoolSystems, Inc., Concord, CA) has specific boots designed for equine use that provide both intermittent pneumatic compression and cryotherapy. This system has been used successfully by the author for treatment of horses with cellulitis. Typically, the system is applied to the limb 1 to 2 times daily for 20 to 30 minutes at a time. Cold saltwater spas provide cold, hypertonic water with aeration that combines the efficacy of cryotherapy with the osmotic action of salt water in order to decrease soft tissue inflammation and provide analgesia. Hyperbaric oxygen (HBO) chambers are becoming increasingly available for equine patients; they increase the oxygen content delivered to the tissues by having the horse breathe 100% oxygen within a pressurized hyperbaric chamber. Proposed therapeutic effects of HBO therapy that would be beneficial for treatment of cellulitis include hypoxia reversal, reduction in edema, modulation of nitric oxide production, acceleration of microbial oxidative killing, improvement of antibiotic exchange across membranes, and decreasing ischemia-reperfusion injury.[31] In humans, HBO therapy is an accepted treatment for conditions similar to equine cellulitis such as clostridial myositis, crush injuries, compartment syndrome, and necrotizing soft tissue infections.[32]

Synovial Infections

Septic arthritis and tenosynovitis are common clinical problems in horses with potentially devastating consequences. Mortality estimates vary between 15% and 50%.[33-37] In adult horses, these infections are most often caused by direct bacterial contamination of a synovial structure resulting from trauma or as a sequela to surgery or intrathecal injection. Hematogenous spread of infection is rare in adult horses but should not be overlooked as a differential diagnosis in the acutely lame horse. In foals, most synovial infections are of hematogenous origin. Failure of transfer of passive immunity, respiratory infection, and gastrointestinal infection should be considered as potential concurrent problems in foals diagnosed with septic synovial structures (see Chapter 6).

Etiology and Pathogenesis

Bacterial inoculation into a synovial structure causes a severe inflammatory response with the production of inflammatory mediators that damage the synovial lining and joint. A variety of bacteria may be isolated from synovial infections that are traumatic in origin. *Enterobacteriaceae* and anaerobes are most common. Horses that develop infection as a sequela to surgery or intrathecal injection are more likely to have staphylococcal infections.[33]

Historically, synovial infections in foals were postulated to originate from umbilical infections, but these infections may originate from other sources, including the respiratory and gastrointestinal tracts. Foals with poor acquisition of passive immunity are predisposed to developing septic arthritis.[38] The pathogens most frequently isolated from foals with neonatal sepsis are also the bacteria most often isolated from joints of foals with septic arthritis (see Chapter 6). Young foals (<3 weeks) are more likely to have infection of multiple joints, whereas older foals (>4 weeks) generally have only one affected joint.[39] The most common bacterial organisms isolated from septic arthritis in foals are *Enterobacteriaceae*, most notably *Escherichia coli*. Other gram-negative organisms, such as *Salmonella enterica*, are relatively common isolates. The most common gram-positive organisms isolated from foals with septic arthritis include *Staphylococcus*, *Streptococcus*, and *Rhodococcus equi*.[33]

Fungal infections of synovial structures are rare but should be considered, especially if a fungal organism is cultured from more than one site or more than one sample from the same site, or if the infection fails to respond to prompt and aggressive antimicrobial therapy. Fungal infection of synovial structures may originate either hematogenously or by direct inoculation.[40]

Clinical Findings

The hallmark clinical sign of synovial infection is severe lameness. The onset and severity of clinical signs depend on the mode of contamination, degree of contamination, virulence of the organism involved, amount of open drainage from the synovial structure, previous treatment with intraarticular corticosteroids, and any recent treatment with NSAIDs. Although clinical signs are evident within 24 hours of experimental inoculation of equine joints with bacteria,[41,42] the onset of clinical signs from noniatrogenic infection appears to be slower. In one study, joint infections on average became apparent on day 8 after surgery, with a range of 1 to 25 days.[34] It is questionable whether all affected joints were inoculated at surgery.

Anecdotally, postoperative joint infections can be separated into two groups: (1) those showing clinical signs within 3 to 5 days, presumably inoculated at surgery, and (2) those showing clinical signs 2 to 4 weeks after surgery, presumably resulting from extension of superficial infection. Incomplete removal of sutures and extension of infection through the suture tracts after removal appear to be major contributing factors to delayed infection.

The onset of clinical signs of synovial infection after trauma is variable, depending on whether there is open drainage present (horses with sealed synovial infections are more lame), the degree of inflammation present, the amount of pain associated with the inciting trauma (which may be indistinguishable from that caused by synovial infection), and delayed recognition by owners or trainers. The onset of lameness and clinical signs of synovial infection after intrathecal injections is also somewhat variable, depending on the factors just listed, as well as whether intrathecal corticosteroids were administered. Tulamo et al[42] showed that co-administration of corticosteroids with an infective dose of bacteria significantly delayed clinical signs and synovial fluid changes for up to 2 days. In two retrospective studies describing infection after intrathecal injection, the onset of clinical signs varied from 2.5 to 7 days.[33,37]

Synovial effusion, localized cellulitis, heat, and sensitivity to palpation are usually observed in horses with synovial infection. Experimental models of infection suggest that these signs may briefly precede clinical lameness.[41,42] Affected horses are usually febrile,[42] but the lack of an increased rectal temperature does not rule out joint sepsis, especially in adult horses or those treated with NSAIDs. Foals typically have higher increased rectal temperatures than adult horses. In one study, 45% of foals with septic arthritis had a body temperature of 102° F (38.9° C) or higher.[33]

Diagnosis

Synovial Fluid Analysis

Synovial fluid analysis is necessary for the definitive diagnosis of infection. Grossly, synovial fluid from an infected joint is serosanguineous and/or turbid (increased cellularity) with decreased viscosity resulting from decreased hyaluronic acid content. Samples from affected joints may contain visible fibrin and debris. The sample should be submitted for total and differential cell count, total protein measurement, and immediate culture. Most samples from infected synovial structures have a total white blood cell (WBC) count greater than 30,000 cells/μL (normal <1000/μL, predominantly mononuclear cells), a differential with 90% or more neutrophils, and a total protein concentration greater than 4.0 g/dL (normal <2.0 g/dL). Cytology with a Gram stain should be performed; positive findings indicate infectious arthritis and may guide initial antimicrobial therapy. A sample of synovial fluid should be cultured aerobically and anaerobically. The fluid should be cultured in a broth culture system designed for culturing body fluids[43] (see Chapter 27). Synovial biopsy and culture do not yield better results than culture of synovial fluid.[44]

Diagnostic Imaging

The primary goal of diagnostic imaging of synovial infections is to determine if the infection has extended into surrounding bone or resulted in cartilage damage. This information can be used as an adjunct to determine prognosis and modify treatment strategies if necessary. Radiographs should be obtained in most horses with synovial infections.

Septic osteitis or osteomyelitis may precede or follow septic arthritis. Septic epiphysitis and physitis must be ruled out in all foals with septic arthritis. Osteomyelitis and osteitis are less common with tendon sheath infections than with joint sepsis; however, the sesamoid bones may be affected.[45]

Articular bone destruction and joint collapse are not early findings in septic arthritis and indicate that the infection has been present for at least 2 to 3 weeks. Comparative views of the contralateral extremity may be necessary to recognize subtle changes. Although not necessary in most cases, advanced imaging techniques, such as computed tomography (CT) and magnetic resonance imaging (MRI), can provide additional information regarding the extent of lesions, especially in horses with septic physitis, and nuclear scintigraphy can be useful in identifying sources of infection in cases in which localizing clinical signs are not definitive (i.e., joints of the upper limbs and appendicular skeleton).

Therapy

Synovial infections in horses are a medical emergency. The three basic principles for treating bacterial infection of synovial structures are systemic antimicrobial therapy, local antimicrobial therapy, and lavage. Successful outcomes are associated with early diagnosis and aggressive treatment.[33,46-48] Negative prognostic indicators include the presence of large conglomerates of fibrin, osteochondral lesions, navicular bursa sepsis, and concurrent septic osteitis/osteomyelitis.[48-50]

Debridement and lavage can be accomplished using many different techniques. For horses with acute iatrogenic sepsis or many foals with septic joints, needle lavage of the joint using large (i.e., 16-14 gauge) needles can often be done standing with local analgesia and sedation in adults or under short-acting IV anesthetics in foals. This procedure may need to be repeated every 24 to 48 hours depending on the horse's clinical signs. Needle lavage is most likely to be effective only in acute cases because, as the duration of sepsis increases, so does the amount of fibrin within the joint, which necessitates a more aggressive approach to thoroughly clear the joint of all infected and necrotic debris. In these cases or in horses with sepsis secondary to lacerations or puncture wounds, debridement and lavage via an arthrotomy or using arthroscopy with the horse under general anesthesia is the preferred approach[33,48] (Fig. 5-1).

If there is a laceration, it should be thoroughly debrided and either closed primarily if the majority of contaminating material and fibrin can be removed, or left open to provide a portal for drainage. Other options for continued drainage include leaving the arthrotomy sites open or placing active or passive drains at the time of surgery. However, if thorough debridement of the joint is performed, open drainage is not necessary and all surgical incisions or traumatic wounds can be closed.

Arthroscopic debridement of septic or contaminated joints has several advantages, including the ability to see the joint surface, which increases the ability to recognize and remove debris and foreign material and to identify concurrent osteochondral damage.[47,49] With an arthroscopic approach, almost all areas of the joint can be accessed for debridement and lavage, and since all contaminated tissues and foreign material can be removed, the incisions can be closed. Arthroscopy is a minimally invasive surgical procedure associated with low postoperative morbidity. Finally, the information gained from performing arthroscopy can be used to estimate prognosis for survival and future athletic activity.[48,50] Arthroscopic treatment of septic joints has been associated with shorter hospital times, a shorter duration of IV antimicrobial drug administration, higher survival rates, and a greater percentage of horses returning to athletic activity when compared to studies that used conventional open surgical techniques.[47,49]

Broad-spectrum systemic antimicrobial therapy should be initiated immediately if a septic joint is suspected; however, it is important to obtain samples of synovial fluid for bacterial culture and antimicrobial sensitivity testing prior to initiating antimicrobial therapy.[33,35,48,51] In foals with septic joints or horses that show signs of systemic sepsis, it is useful to obtain a blood culture. The initial antimicrobial drugs will need to be chosen prior to obtaining culture and sensitivity results and should be based on the knowledge of common equine bacterial isolates. For horses with traumatically-induced synovial sepsis, the most common isolates are *Enterobacter* spp., *Staphylococcus* spp., *Streptococcus* spp., and *Pseudomonas* spp.; these are often present as mixed bacterial infections that may include anaerobic bacteria.[49,52] Septic arthritis in foals is often hematogenous in origin; common bacterial isolates include *Escherichia coli*, *Klebsiella* spp., *Actinobacillus equuli*, *Streptococcus* spp., *Salmonella* spp., and *Rhodococcus equi*.[50] A good initial choice for antimicrobial drug therapy is a penicillin or cephalosporin in combination with an aminoglycoside. This combination provides broad-spectrum coverage that will be effective for most of the common infecting microorganisms.

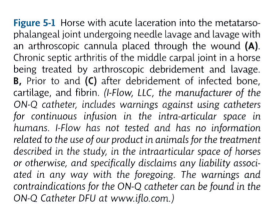
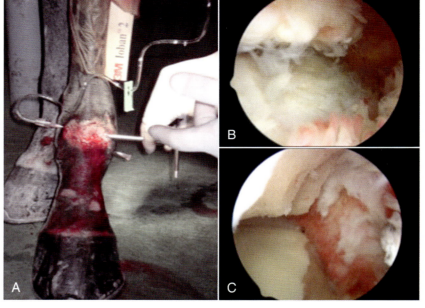

Figure 5-1 Horse with acute laceration into the metatarsophalangeal joint undergoing needle lavage and lavage with an arthroscopic cannula placed through the wound (**A**). Chronic septic arthritis of the middle carpal joint in a horse being treated by arthroscopic debridement and lavage. **B,** Prior to and (**C**) after debridement of infected bone, cartilage, and fibrin. (*I-Flow, LLC, the manufacturer of the ON-Q catheter, includes warnings against using catheters for continuous infusion in the intra-articular space in humans. I-Flow has not tested and has no information related to the use of our product in animals for the treatment described in the study, in the intraarticular space of horses or otherwise, and specifically disclaims any liability associated in any way with the foregoing. The warnings and contraindications for the ON-Q catheter can be found in the ON-Q Catheter DFU at www.iflo.com.*)

Techniques to improve local concentrations of antimicrobial drugs should also be performed, such as intraarticular administration (via injection or continuous infusion), IV regional limb perfusion, or placing antimicrobial impregnated material (e.g., Plaster of Paris or collagen sponges) into the joint. These local techniques increase the concentration of the antimicrobial within the synovial fluid, surrounding soft tissues, and bone compared with systemic therapy alone. Amikacin is the initial drug of the choice for local therapy because most common equine bacterial isolates that cause joint sepsis are sensitive to it and antimicrobial resistance to amikacin is less common than for gentamicin. The antimicrobial drug used should be modified as needed based on bacterial culture and sensitivity testing results. For sepsis that is completely contained within the joint, intraarticular therapy (either by injection or continuous infusion) (Fig. 5-2) is preferred because higher concentrations of the antimicrobial drug (≥100 times the minimal inhibitory concentration [MIC] of many organisms) are achieved in the synovial fluid compared to concentrations after performing IV regional limb perfusions (up to 50 times the MIC of many organisms). If the infection is more diffuse or extends further into the surrounding soft tissues and bones or if there is a large degree of periarticular cellulitis present, then IV regional limb perfusion should be performed. This can be done alone but is often combined with intraarticular treatments. To perform an IV regional limb perfusion, the horse is sedated, a tourniquet is applied above the affected area, and antimicrobials are injected into a vein below the tourniquet (Fig. 5-3). The author typically uses 2.5 g of amikacin diluted to 60 mL total volume with saline if the tourniquet is placed above the carpus or tarsus in adults, or diluted to 30 mL if the tourniquet is placed below these joints. In foals the systemic dose of amikacin can be divided between the regional limb perfusion and intraarticular injection. The tourniquet is typically left in place for approximately 20 minutes. This procedure is performed daily initially until improvement in clinical signs is noted. In general, either of these techniques (intraarticular injections or IV regional limb perfusions) will maintain concentrations of the chosen antimicrobial drug above the MIC for most organisms for 24 to 48 hours. Therefore local antimicrobial drug therapy should be repeated daily or every other day until the horse's clinical signs resolve.

Antiinflammatory therapy is also indicated for the treatment of joint sepsis, although some clinicians prefer to use systemic NSAIDs sparingly in these cases. In some authors' opinions, horses with septic joints should receive systemic antiinflammatory drugs at moderate doses to reduce the inflammation within the joint and decrease the damage caused to the joint and periarticular structures by the inflammatory response. Additionally, topical therapy with antiinflammatory substances (e.g.,

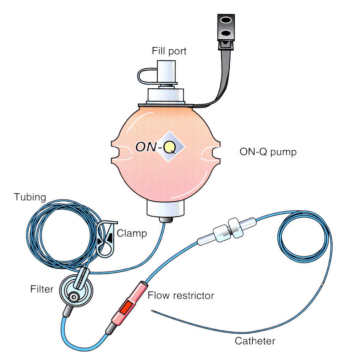

Figure 5-2 Example of constant-rate infusion system (ON-Q PainBuster) that can deliver antimicrobials and anesthetics to synovial structure. *(Courtesy I-Flow Corp., Lake Forest, CA. I-Flow, LLC, the manufacturer of the ON-Q catheter, includes warnings against using catheters for continuous infusion in the intra-articular space in humans. I-Flow has not tested and has no information related to the use of our product in animals for the treatment described in the study, in the intraarticular space of horses or otherwise, and specifically disclaims any liability associated in any way with the foregoing. The warnings and contraindications for the ON-Q catheter can be found in the ON-Q Catheter DFU at www.iflo.com.)*

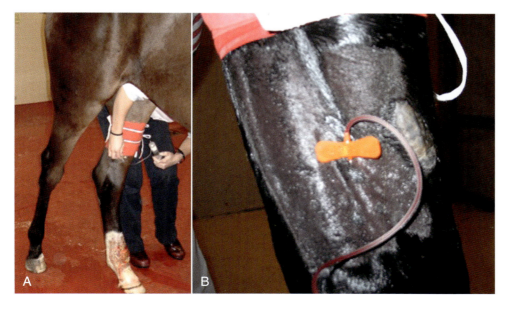

Figure 5-3 Intravenous regional limb perfusion performed in the saphenous vein of a hindlimb **(A)** and the cephalic vein in a forelimb **(B)**.

diclofenac or DMSO) can also be used to help prevent the development of capsulitis and periarticular fibrosis.

Bone Infection (Septic Osteomyelitis and Osteitis)

Etiology and Pathogenesis

Infection of bone can be caused by direct trauma, hematogenous spread, extension of a contiguous focus of infection, or inoculation at surgery. One key conceptual difference is that hematogenous infections spread from the "inside out," whereas most other causes of osteomyelitis spread from the "outside in." The pathogenesis after trauma to bone involves acute inflammation of bone, with vascular engorgement, edema, cellular infiltration, and abscess formation. The associated increase in intramedullary pressure spreads pathogens throughout the bone cortex, with intracortical extension facilitated by the haversian systems and Volkmann's canals. With continued extension, the periosteal space may become involved.[51]

In foals, hematogenous spread of infection into the bone is a common cause of osteomyelitis.[52] Typically, the metaphyses of long bones are affected. In young animals, blood flow is slow and turbulent in the venous sinuses of the metaphyses near the site of endochondral ossification. Bacteria can become lodged at these sites and readily establish infection. In the neonatal foal the metaphyseal blood supply communicates with the epiphyseal blood supply via the transphyseal vessels. The epiphyseal blood supply communicates with the blood supply of the joint synovium.[53-55] This provides a direct route for infection from the joint to spread to the bone, or vice versa. As the animal ages, the epiphyseal and metaphyseal blood supplies become independent. In foals the transphyseal vessels start to regress at 14 days of age and disappear almost completely by 45 days of age.[56] Generally, this protects the epiphysis from infection,[57] and septic arthritis and septic physitis/epiphysitis are less likely to coexist in older foals.

In adult horses, there is a paucity of information regarding the most likely etiologic agents of osteomyelitis. Retrospective studies suggest that most horses with traumatic osteomyelitis have mixed antimicrobial infections, with *Enterobacteriaceae*, β-hemolytic streptococci, and staphylococci being the most frequently isolated organisms.[33,49] Osteomyelitis after surgery is often caused by staphylococci, but mixed infections may also occur. In foals, *Enterobacteriaceae* are the most common organisms isolated from osteomyelitis. In older foals, *Rhodococcus equi* osteomyelitis should be considered as a differential diagnosis[58] (see Chapter 31). Mycotic or phycomycotic infections can be found in the bone in horses but are less common than bacterial infections (see Chapter 51).

Clinical Findings

The clinical signs of osteomyelitis are variable. Most horses with osteomyelitis of the limbs will present with moderate to marked lameness. Soft tissue swelling, heat, and sensitivity to palpation are almost always present and may be the only clinical signs of osteomyelitis involving the head. Exceptions are osteomyelitis involving bones heavily covered by muscle or hoof capsule. In these horses, lameness may be the only clinical sign. Laboratory findings are variable. Leukocytosis or hyperfibrinogenemia may be present but are certainly not diagnostic.

The most common sites of osteomyelitis in the foal are the distal tibial physes and the distal third metacarpal/tarsal physes.[59] Affected foals will generally present with marked lameness and palpable heat, pain, and swelling, which often can be distinguished from joint effusion if the joint is not involved. The swelling in affected foals may be soft and fluctuant, in contrast to swelling in affected adults, which usually is firm. This difference is caused by the relatively loosely attached periosteum and thin cortex in young animals, which allows suppuration and expansion.[57] In more proximal limb locations (e.g., proximal humerus, femur), swelling may not be obvious because of surrounding muscle mass.

The most common sites of osteomyelitis in the adult horse are the metacarpal and metatarsal bones and the phalanges.[60] In these areas, lameness is a common clinical finding, whereas in the head and axial skeleton, painful soft tissue swelling with or without draining tracts may be the only clinical sign.

Diagnosis

Diagnosis of osteomyelitis and osteitis is usually confirmed by radiography; however, radiographic changes may not be present in the early stages of the disease so the absence of radiographic abnormalities in these cases does not rule out osteomyelitis.

Radiographic changes require 30% to 50% bone density (mineralization) with at least 1 cm of affected area.[61] This may result in delayed recognition of lesions, especially early in the disease process. Radiographs of the contralateral limb can assist in detecting subtle changes, but it may take 10 to 14 days after injury or onset of clinical signs to see radiographic evidence of infection. Unfortunately, this can delay the diagnosis and therefore timely treatment of osteomyelitis. When present, lesions typically appear lytic, with varying degrees of sclerosis and periosteal new bone production (Fig. 5-4). Osseous sequestra are a relatively common feature of osteomyelitis in horses, especially in areas with minimal soft tissue covering. With periosteal damage or wound infection, the outer cortex of the bone is susceptible to ischemia and infection. If the bone becomes necrotic, it will separate from the parent bone, forming a sequestrum.

In human patients, advanced imaging techniques, such as nuclear scintigraphy, MRI, and CT, are often used to improve the accuracy of diagnosis of osteomyelitis. These modalities are widely accessible to private practitioners and are being increasingly used for diagnosis of osteomyelitis in horses.

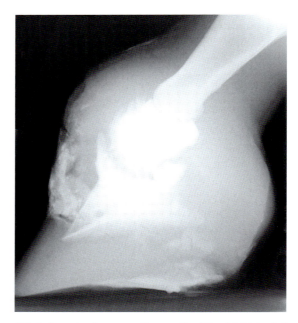

Figure 5-4 Radiograph of severe septic synovitis of the distal interphalangeal joint with osteomyelitis of the second and third phalanx demonstrating sclerosis, lysis, and periosteal new bone production.

A three-phase scintigraphic scan with methylene diphosphonate (MDP) can aid in the diagnosis of equine osteomyelitis. Increased uptake of the radiopharmaceutical in all three phases (flow, pool, bone) is supportive of osteomyelitis. However, the diagnosis may be complicated by recent trauma, surgery, or orthopedic implants. These coexisting conditions significantly decrease the specificity (as low as 38% in human patients) of results.[62] White blood cell scans can be performed in horses using hexamethylpropyleneamine oxime (HMPAO)–labeled WBCs.[17,63] The main advantage to this technique is an increase in specificity for detection of osteomyelitis. False-negative scans are possible with chronic or partially treated osteomyelitis. In the future, newer techniques (e.g., ciprofloxacin labeling) may provide more accurate and less technically demanding methods to detect osteomyelitis.

Computed tomography provides high spatial and contrast resolution of bone and its surrounding tissue and is best used for determining cortical changes associated with osteomyelitis and providing a three-dimensional image that can be used to guide surgical treatment or biopsy. In horses, complex joints such as the hock can be difficult to evaluate with plain radiography. Computed tomography is especially useful for localizing and characterizing these lesions.[64] The presence of metallic implants often precludes the use of CT because of beam-hardening artifact. Other limitations in the horse include the necessity for general anesthesia and gantry aperture limitations. In adult horses, CT is often limited to the distal extremities and head. Large horses may be difficult to image, except for lesions distal to the tarsus or carpus.

Magnetic resonance imaging is one of the most sensitive tools for diagnosis of osteomyelitis in human patients.[61] Magnetic resonance imaging can detect the differences between normal and abnormal bone from the differences in their density of water protons. Several clinically available imaging sequences and contrast agents can be used to increase the accuracy of detection. In the area of lesions, T1-weighted images will show low signal intensity (fluid is dark, fat is bright), and T2-weighted images will show increased signal intensity (fluid is bright, fat is dark). Magnetic resonance imaging can clearly define the extent of osteomyelitis lesions and provide information related to the chronicity of the infection. Images cannot be obtained from horses with ferrous implants. Nonferrous implants are routinely used in human patients and allow subsequent MRI. Magnetic resonance imaging shares some of the limitations of CT regarding aperture size and ability to image much of the adult equine skeleton. Ultrasound may be used to evaluate soft tissue swelling and is especially useful for detection of increased quantities of synovial fluid or abscesses in severely swollen or heavily muscled areas. Subperiosteal fluid or pus may be visible, which can support the clinical diagnosis of osteomyelitis. These fluid pockets can be aspirated for culture. Sequestra and foreign bodies may be detectable and aid in treatment planning or the decision for further diagnostic efforts. With experience, ultrasound can be used to detect early changes (not radiographically apparent) of osteomyelitis. A thin fluid layer immediately adjacent to the bone is usually detectable, and occasionally, periosteal lysis or proliferation may be observed.[65]

Biopsy, culture, and sensitivity are necessary to confirm septic osteomyelitis and to determine the best course of antimicrobial treatment. However, because many horses with osteomyelitis require surgical debridement, these diagnostic procedures are often done at treatment.

Therapy

The treatment of osteomyelitis can be involved and often requires intensive care best provided in a hospital environment. Many of these horses should be referred to veterinary hospitals where the appropriate diagnostic testing and necessary treatments are routinely performed.

Systemic antimicrobial treatment for osteomyelitis should be selected after consideration of the most likely pathogens. Whenever possible, the causative organism(s) should be identified and antimicrobial sensitivity patterns determined. Long-term antimicrobial therapy is often necessary, and adverse effects and economics should be considered. Initial empiric therapy in horses generally consists of broad-spectrum IV antimicrobials (e.g., combination of β-lactam and aminoglycoside antibiotic).

Oral antimicrobial options are limited but can be used effectively. Trimethoprim-sulfa (TMS) antimicrobials are often effective against β-hemolytic streptococcal infection; however, resistance is common, and the use of TMS alone is questionable for treatment of most horses with osteomyelitis. Chloramphenicol is effective against many organisms typically isolated from equine osteomyelitis lesions; however, human health concerns and controversy over its oral absorption in horses tend to limit its use by many clinicians. In the authors' opinions, chloramphenicol remains one of the few clinically effective oral antibiotics for osteomyelitis that can be safely used long term. Rifampin in combination with a macrolide or azalide antimicrobial drug is often used to treat *Rhodococcus equi* infections (see Chapter 31). Additionally, the authors have used rifampin in combination with TMS or enrofloxacin to treat osteomyelitis. In human patients, rifampin is considered one of the most effective antistaphylococcal agents and is useful in eradicating intraleukocytic bacteria and penetrating the bacterial glycocalyx. Rifampin should not be used alone because resistance will quickly develop.[57] As a general rule, antimicrobial administration should be continued for several weeks after the resolution of clinical signs.

Unfortunately, by the time most cases of osteomyelitis in the horse are diagnosed, they have advanced beyond the point when systemic antimicrobial therapy alone is effective. Surgical debridement is indicated when nonviable tissue is present. Nonviable tissue can provide a continuous nidus of infection, leading to persistence or recrudescence of infection. Debridement removes debris, eliminates dead space, restores soft tissue integrity, encourages vascular supply, and thus encourages complete healing and resolution of infection.[57] Large defects in the bone may require cancellous bone grafts to restore structural integrity and promote healing.

Local antimicrobial delivery techniques, such as IV regional limb perfusion and antimicrobial-impregnated substances, are indicated for treatment of horses with osteomyelitis (Boxes 5-1 and 5-2). Antimicrobial-impregnated beads made with PMMA may be especially useful for treatment of osteomyelitis because they can be implanted and left to deliver antimicrobials for an extended time. They can be prepared at surgery or stored for future use. Antimicrobial release from PMMA occurs in a bimodal manner. First, in a rapid phase, approximately 5% of the antimicrobial is released within the first 24 to 48 hours. A slow-release phase then provides bactericidal concentrations for the next few weeks to months.[66] Single agents or combinations of antimicrobials may be used. Several factors affect release of antimicrobials from PMMA beads, including heat stability and water solubility. Table 5-1 lists some common antimicrobials that effectively elute from PMMA. PMMA beads are nonabsorbable, and removal at a later date may be required. Tissue irritation often leads to some degree of fibrous tissue formation. In difficult osteomyelitis cases, the benefits of therapy with PMMA beads generally outweigh these disadvantages.

Plaster of Paris beads can also be used to deliver antimicrobials. Plaster of Paris beads have the advantage of being absorbable and have reported osteoinductive and osteoconductive properties. Disadvantages are that most of the antimicrobial is released

---

Box 5-1 Intravenous Regional Limb Perfusion

- Prepare appropriate dose of antimicrobial drug. A general rule is one-third of the systemic dose of the chosen antimicrobial diluted in saline to a final volume of 30 mL for lower limb perfusions or for foals or 60 mL for upper limb perfusions. The author typically uses 2.5 g of amikacin in adult horses, and the full systemic dose of amikacin in foals as an empiric choice.
- Appropriate anesthesia or sedation should be administered, depending on whether the procedure is performed in the anesthetized or standing horse. If the procedure is to be performed standing, the horse should be heavily sedated to prevent movement. The author routinely uses 5 mg of detomidine + 5 mg of butorphanol IV ± 10 mg of acepromazine IV in adult horses.
- Apply a tourniquet proximal to the region to be perfused. Tourniquets should be wide to be effective (i.e., Esmarch bandages, wide rubber tourniquets, or pneumatic tourniquets—NOT IV simplex tubing or Penrose drains).
- Insert small (i.e., 25 gauge) butterfly catheter into the appropriate blood vessel.
- Begin injection of the perfusate. The volume should be injected slowly over 5 to 10 minutes to avoid damage to small blood vessels. If the perfusion is performed standing, it is recommended to tape the extension set to the tourniquet to prevent movement of the horse and inadvertent removal of the catheter.
- During the injection, periodically aspirate with the syringe to confirm that the needle remains appropriately situated in the blood vessel.
- After completion of the regional perfusion, the catheter may be removed and a small pressure bandage placed over the vessel puncture site. Alternatively, the catheter may be left in place for the duration of the soaking time and the extension set secured to avoid backflow of blood.
- The tourniquet should be left in place for 20 to 25 minutes after completion of the injection.
  - Treatment of a wound, lavage of a joint, and other therapies may be performed while the regional perfusion is being performed; however, do not perform procedures that will cause the horse to move the limb because this will decrease the tourniquet's efficacy.
- After the procedure is completed, apply topical 1% diclofenac to the venipuncture site and bandage the area where the regional limb perfusion was performed, as well as the rest of the limb (if indicated). This will decrease the amount of cellulitis that develops at the venipuncture site and allow for continued use of the vessel.

Box 5-2 Antimicrobial-Impregnated Polymethylmethacrylate (PMMA) Beads

Items Needed
- Half-dose PMMA bone cement (Surgical Simplex P Radiopaque Bone Cement, Howmedica Osteonics, Mahwah, NJ). This package contains 20 g of sterile PMMA powder and 10 mL of sterile liquid that is 97.4% v/v methylmethacrylate.
- Mixing bowl (sterile) with spatula or mixing device
- Sterile gloves
- Sterile field (table cover or drape)
- Scissors (sterile)
- Antibiotics

Recommended Antibiotic Doses
- Cefazolin, 1 g
- Amikacin, 1 g
- Imipenem, 500 mg

Procedure
1. Using sterile technique, open packet with 20 g of sterile PMMA powder and empty into sterile bowl.
2. Add antimicrobials to dry powder. If antibiotics are in dry powder form, add them to the PMMA powder dry, without reconstitution.
3. Mix sterile PMMA powder and antimicrobials well.
4. Add 10 mL of liquid methylmethacrylate and mix until tacky and starting to set.
5. Immediately begin rolling portions of resultant mixture into small, cigar-shaped rods or small, round beads. After the mixture starts to set, only a brief time is available to change the shape of the beads. Therefore several people with sterile gloves may be required to prepare all beads within the available time.
6. Beads are ready to use within 10 to 15 minutes.
7. Remaining beads may be sealed in sterilization pouches and gas-sterilized for later use.

---

in the first 48 hours (80% with gentamicin), they are unlikely to maintain concentrations above MIC for longer than 2 weeks, and they require fabrication and gas sterilization in advance of implantation.[67] In the future, better carriers for antimicrobials will likely be available, providing better biocompatibility, longer release times, and enhancement of new bone production.

Foals with septic osteomyelitis involving the metaphysis, physis, and epiphysis are difficult to manage. The diagnosis is generally not evident until radiographic changes are apparent (Fig. 5-5). Typically, an area of soft tissue swelling with pus formation can be found at the affected site. This is usually adjacent to the affected side of the physis. The prognosis generally worsens after radiographic changes are evident. If elected, treatment should be aggressive. If osteomyelitis involves the physis and metaphysis, drainage should be established through the skin. Often, a curette can be used to open and debride the affected area of bone. Care should be taken to avoid excessive damage to the physis and surrounding bone when debriding. Implanted antibiotic-impregnated beads combined with regional perfusion techniques can be used for local antimicrobial therapy. Less frequently, osteomyelitis will involve the epiphysis. Infection of the adjacent joint is almost always present concurrently. Lesions may be debrided arthroscopically. However, every effort should be made to preserve the weight-bearing surface and structural integrity of the epiphysis. If peripheral, the lesion can be opened and debrided through the skin and joint capsule.

Infected orthopedic implants generally must be removed before infection can be resolved; however, in many cases this cannot be done for a period of time because of the instability that doing so would cause. In situations in which it is not practical to remove the implant(s), efforts must be made to minimize extension of the infection and further destruction of the implant bone interface. Surgery to remove any implants not providing stability, all possible glycocalyx (bacterial slime), dead bone, and any other foreign material is necessary for host defenses to fight infection effectively.[68]

Many factors affect the prognosis for horses with osteomyelitis. Unfortunately, the body of knowledge regarding osteomyelitis largely consists of retrospective studies with relatively small case numbers, and information often must be extrapolated from other species. Duration of osteomyelitis is one of the most important factors affecting prognosis. Delays in diagnosis and referral are major factors contributing to treatment failure.

Horses with significant radiographic evidence of osteomyelitis have a guarded to poor prognosis and require aggressive surgical intervention. Extensive joint or other synovial structure involvement also has a significant negative impact on prognosis. Osteomyelitis in these locations complicates surgical treatment, and necessary debridement may result in loss of cartilage and joint congruity. Only in select joints, such as the proximal interphalangeal joint, fetlock, carpus, or distal tarsal joints, can arthrodesis or facilitated ankylosis be considered an option. In these cases, immobilization combined with debridement, bone graft, and potentially limited implants can result in salvage of the animal. Conversely, osteomyelitis in areas of the head, metacarpals and tarsals, and coffin bone can often be treated

Table 5-1 Systemic Antibiotics Used to Treat Osteomyelitis and Septic Synovial Structures

Drug	Manufacturer	Systemic Dose	Other Uses
Amikacin	Amiglyde (Fort Dodge)	*Adult:* 15 mg/kg IV q24h	RP, IA, AIB
		Foal: 21-25 mg/kg IV q24h	
Ampicillin	Amp-equine (Pfizer)	20 mg/kg IV q6h	
Ceftriaxone	Rocephin (Roche Laboratories)	50 mg/kg IV q24h	RP, IA, AIB
Cefazolin	Ancef (GlaxoSmithKline)	10-20 mg/kg IV q6h	AIB
Ceftazidime	Fortaz (GlaxoSmithKline)	30-50 mg/kg IV q6-12h	RP, IA, AIB
Ceftiofur	Naxcel (Pharmacia & Upjohn)	2-8 mg/kg IV q6-24h	IA, AIB
Cefotaxime	Claforan (Aventis)	25 mg/kg IV q6h	
Chloramphenicol	Generic	50 mg/kg PO q6h	Human health risk
Doxycycline	Generic	10 mg/kg PO q12h	Variable oral absorption
Enrofloxacin	Baytril (Bayer Corp)	2.5-10 mg/kg IV q12-24h	Arthropathies (foals), tendon weakening or rupture
Erythromycin	Generic	20-30 mg/kg PO q8h	May cause hyperthermia and diarrhea
Fluconazole	Diflucan (Roerig)	5 mg/kg PO q24h	Susceptible fungal infections; AIB
Gentamicin	Gentocin (Schering-Plough)	6-7 mg/kg IV q24h	RP, IA, AIB
Imipenem-cilastatin	Primaxin (Merck)	10-20 mg/kg IV q6h	RP, IA, AIB
Metronidazole	Generic	15-25 mg/kg PO q6h	AIB
Oxytetracycline		8-10 mg/kg IV q12h	
Procaine penicillin G		22,000-40,000 IU/kg IM q12h	
Potassium penicillin G		10,000-40,000 IU/kg IV q4-6h	
Rifampin	Rifadin (Hoechst Marion Roussel)	5-10 mg/kg PO q12h	Do not use alone
Ticarcillin/clavulanate	Timentin (SmithKline Beecham)	50 mg/kg IV q6h	Antipseudomonal
Trimethoprim-sulfa	Generic	20-30 mg/kg PO q12h (based on sulfa portion)	
		15-24 mg/kg IV q8-12h	
Vancomycin	Vancocin (Eli Lilly)	6 mg/kg IV q8h	AIB; use slow infusion

IV, Intravenously; *q24h,* every 24 hours; *PO,* orally; *IM,* intramuscularly; *RP,* regional perfusion; *IA,* intraarticular; *AIB,* antibiotic-impregnated beads.

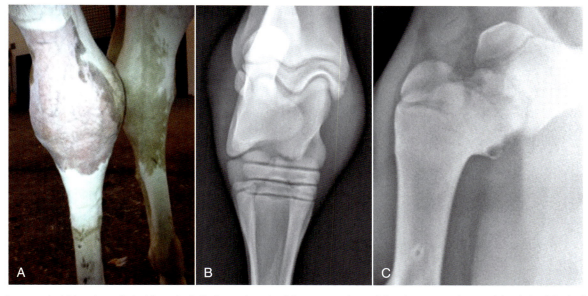

Figure 5-5 One-month-old Appaloosa foal with marked effusion and sepsis of the tarsocrural joint **(A)** with septic epiphysitis of distal tibia **(B)**. The foal also had septic synovitis and osteomyelitis of the scapulohumeral joint **(C).**

effectively with debridement and antimicrobial therapy. In general, if osteomyelitis is focal and surgically accessible, debridement may be curative, and often the joint infection will resolve after bone removal. The horse with diffuse, multifocal, or surgically inaccessible osteomyelitis, particularly with concurrent joint infection, has a poor or guarded prognosis.

Supportive Care for Horses with Severe Lameness from Infection

The management of pain in acute and chronic equine musculoskeletal infections can be difficult. The physiologic consequences of severe pain are beyond the scope of this chapter. However, in the adult horse, support-limb laminitis is a major concern in all horses in which the unaffected limb bears the majority of the weight. Nonsteroidal antiinflammatory drugs, primarily phenylbutazone, are indicated in almost all cases. Unfortunately, NSAIDs may be insufficient in controlling pain and promoting weight bearing on the injured limb. A simple method of providing additional analgesia is to use morphine (0.05-0.10 mg/kg IM every 6 hours [q6h]) with acepromazine (5-10 mg). Other options include regional nerve blocks, epidural anesthesia (hindlimb pain), lidocaine patches, and continuous-rate infusions of lidocaine, ketamine, morphine, or butorphanol (or combinations of these drugs). If an infusion pump or catheter is being used to deliver antimicrobials constantly and locally into the joint, mepivacaine or other local analgesic can be added if it is compatible.

Horses developing support-limb laminitis may exhibit a sudden increase in weight bearing on the injured limb or greater time spent in recumbency. Differentiating clinical improvement in the affected limb from the development of laminar pain in the support limb is critical. It is not unusual for pain from laminitis to supersede pain from severe infection. Careful monitoring of digital pulses and willingness to bear weight on the support limb is important. Providing adequate sole support, primarily in the heel region, appears to be beneficial for prevention and treatment of laminitis in some horses. This can be accomplished with soft bedding (ideally sand), foam pads taped to the bottom of the foot, or dental impression material molded to the sole. Systemic IV infusion of lidocaine (50 µg/kg/min) has some antiinflammatory properties that may be beneficial in management of pain associated with early support-limb

laminitis. Continuous cryotherapy (icing) of the feet has been shown to prevent the development of laminitis in experimental metabolic models, but it is unknown if icing will prevent laminitis induced by increased weight bearing.[69] However, it is the authors' opinion that cryotherapy is indicated for the contralateral limb in horses in extreme pain caused by orthopedic infection.

Pain management to encourage weight bearing on the injured limb is important in foals. Increased loading of the support limb can create varus angular limb deformities and pain from physitis, whereas decreased weight bearing on the injured limb can result in limb contracture. These complications can occur within 1 to 2 weeks in foals and can become the limiting factor in recovery if the infection resolves. Support of the infected limb with bandages or splints may be necessary to encourage loading.

The complete reference list is available online at www. expertconsult.com.

Neonatal Sepsis

Chris Sanchez

Sepsis represents a major disease process of clinical and economic importance worldwide. Sepsis has been implicated as the major cause of morbidity and mortality in the equine neonate.[1,2] Because the body's response to microbial invasion of the bloodstream involves a systemic inflammatory response, foals can deteriorate rapidly despite aggressive treatment.

Pathophysiology and Associated Definitions

Much of the clinical syndrome classically associated with sepsis is caused by a nonspecific inflammatory response, not necessarily the infectious organism. Many terms have been coined referring to this response and associated syndromes and processes. A set of definitions were described in 1991 by the American College of Chest Physicians and the Society of Critical Care Medicine.[3] Briefly, the systemic inflammatory response syndrome (SIRS) refers to a systemic inflammatory response, irrespective of the inciting cause, which results in at least two of the following four clinical manifestations: fever; tachycardia; tachypnea or hyperventilation; and leukocytosis, leukopenia, or relative increase of circulating immature neutrophils. When SIRS occurs in response to a confirmed infectious process, the process is termed *sepsis* (see Chapter 11). Infection refers to the invasion of normally sterile host tissue by microorganisms or the inflammatory response generated in response to said organisms. The presence of viable bacteria in the blood is termed *bacteremia*, and the presence of other viable pathogens in the blood is described similarly (i.e., viremia, fungemia, etc.). When sepsis is associated with organ dysfunction, hypoperfusion, or hypotension, the event is termed *severe sepsis*. Septic shock is defined by sepsis-induced hypotension that persists despite adequate fluid therapy and is accompanied by hypoperfusion

abnormalities or organ dysfunction. Manifestations of organ dysfunction can include coagulopathy in addition to classic examples of renal, gastrointestinal, hepatic cardiovascular, or pulmonary dysfunction.[4] The multiple organ dysfunction syndrome (MODS) describes alteration of organ function in an acutely ill patient such that homeostasis cannot be maintained. Multiple organ dysfunction syndrome can occur either as a primary event (i.e., as a direct result of trauma) or secondary to a host response. A syndrome of immunosuppression caused by an overpronounced systemic antiinflammatory response resulting in increased circulating levels of antiinflammatory mediators, leukocyte anergy, or increased susceptibility to infection has been termed the *compensatory antiinflammatory response syndrome* (CARS). The mixed antiinflammatory response syndrome (MARS) applies to fluctuation between episodes of SIRS and CARS.[5]

Endotoxin plays a critical role in the pathophysiology of septic shock in gram-negative sepsis,[6,7] which is common in foals.[2,8-10] Septic foals can have decreased gene expression of tumor necrosis factor alpha (TNF-α) and beta (TNF-β) and increased expression of interleukin-8 (IL-8) relative to healthy foals[11] or increased gene expression of IL-4 and toll-like receptor 4 (TLR4),[12] among other possible abnormalities.

Predisposing Factors and Routes of Infection

Many events can predispose an equine neonate to infection, including maternal illness, alterations in gestational length, partial or complete failure of passive transfer, poor sanitary conditions, improper umbilical care, and others. In short, these can be summarized as prenatal (or maternal) and postnatal factors.

Maternal factors include dystocia, premature placental separation, placentitis, and various nonurogenital maternal conditions such as colic; these have been reported in 24% of bacteremic foals.[13] Complications associated with parturition (i.e., dystocia) have also been associated with neonatal disease.[14] Many of these factors are interrelated. For example, premature placental separation often occurs secondarily to the primary problem of placentitis. In utero infection of the fetus secondary to placentitis typically occurs as the result of an ascending infection and often results in premature delivery.[15] Because chronic placentitis in the mare often results in precocious fetal maturation, a premature foal born to such a mare has a greater chance of being septic, but a higher probability of survival than a foal born at a similar gestational age to a mare without placentitis or other chronic stimulation.

Most postnatal risk factors are very much intertwined with possible routes of infection. The main exception to this is failure of transfer of passive immunity (FPT). Because the foal is relatively immunologically naïve at the time of birth, one would reason that an absence of this natural provision of protection would lead to an increased risk of postnatal infection. A number of studies have documented a close relationship between the foal serum immunoglobulin G (IgG) concentration and incidence of disease.[16-19] Colostrum administration via nasogastric tube was associated with disease in one report,[14] which supports the notion that route and timing of transfer are likely relevant, along with the potential for bacterial challenge. Farm management is particularly important, including general cleanliness, stocking density, exposure to disease, nutrition, and prepartum vaccination and deworming programs. In particular, one study demonstrated that foals with partial FPT were not at any greater risk of disease than those with adequate transfer on a well-managed Standardbred farm.[20]

Postnatal routes of infection include the umbilicus, gastrointestinal tract, and respiratory tract. Although the umbilicus has traditionally been regarded as the most important site for bacterial pathogen entry into the foal, the gastrointestinal tract plays a vital role as well.[21] The foal does not fully discriminate between maternal immunoglobulin and other macromolecules, and absorption of macromolecules occurs through specialized cells via pinocytosis. Absorption of macromolecules peaks shortly after birth, and declines to less than 1% by 20 hours.[22] Unlike in other species, absorption of immunoglobulins does not appear to be Fc-receptor mediated in the foal. The foal will selectively absorb IgG and IgM over IgA.[23] In neonatal pigs and lambs, deprivation of milk or colostrum can delay intestinal permeability to immunoglobulins by up to 5 days, whereas this can be hastened by feeding a large volume of colostrum or milk shortly after birth.[24,25] In the foal, alternatively, intestinal permeability to immunoglobulins cannot be delayed through withholding of macromolecules.[26] It is not known if premature closure can be induced by the feeding of macromolecules immediately after birth in foals.

Other postnatal factors that may predispose to neonatal sepsis include gestational age and environmental conditions. Foals with exceptionally short or long gestational lengths may be at risk for development of sepsis.[27] Unsanitary environmental conditions can result in an increased bacterial load to the neonatal gastrointestinal tract, especially during the initial periods of udder seeking.[21]

Clinical Signs and Diagnosis

Physical Examination Findings

Initial clinical signs can be vague and vary widely. Some of the most frequently reported signs include decreased or absent suckling from the mare, diarrhea, and lethargy, which may progress to recumbency. For those foals considered normal at any point prior to onset of illness, lethargy and anorexia are often the first signs noted.

Examination of the foal should always include examination of the mare's udder for fill; depressed foals will often stand with their head underneath the mare and can have dried streaming milk on their foreheads. Dehydration becomes a more significant problem as time progresses from lack of intake. Tachycardia and tachypnea are common but not always present. Oral, conjunctival, and vulvar mucous membranes can become hyperemic, injected, and/or petechiated. Occasionally, petechiae are noted along the internal pinnae of the ears, and hyperemia can be noted along the coronary bands. Capillary refill time may be rapid in hyperemic foals or substantially delayed in those that have become hypovolemic. Other signs of hypovolemia include decreased borborygmi, poor peripheral pulses, cool extremities, and decreased or absent urine output. Rectal temperature may be normal or mildly increased, and sepsis should not be ruled out on the basis of a normal rectal temperature. Hypothermia can be associated with advanced sepsis or moderate to severe prematurity. If untreated, these early signs can progress to septic shock and often death.

Septic foals may have additional localizing signs associated with specific foci of infection. Diarrhea is common and may be the first clinical sign observed. Other localizing signs may include uveitis, seizures, joint effusion, lameness, physeal swelling, respiratory disease or distress, subcutaneous abscesses, patent urachus, and omphalitis.

Physical examination of the mare and placenta are considered an extension of the foal's physical examination. Any indication of placental or maternal abnormality should raise suspicion for neonatal illness. Finally, not all histologically evident placental abnormalities are obvious on gross inspection.

Clinicopathologic Findings

Clinical signs and historical information alone are often sufficient for suspicion of sepsis, but laboratory data may be supportive. Leukopenia, characterized by neutropenia, is the most common hematologic finding associated with acute sepsis. In one study, septic foals less than 1 week of age had lower total white blood cells (WBCs), neutrophils, and lymphocytes and higher bands and monocytes than healthy age-matched controls.[28] An important differential diagnosis is the premature or dysmature foal that commonly has a decreased neutrophil count in the absence of sepsis. Septic foals typically have a degenerative left shift and evidence of toxicity (Dohle bodies, toxic granulation, and vacuolization), whereas these findings are not typical of uncomplicated prematurity. Thus a microscopic examination of the blood smear is an extremely important part of the complete blood count (CBC) in any equine neonate. In older septic foals (8-14 days), the total WBC, neutrophils, and bands were higher than in age-matched controls.[28] A high fibrinogen concentration at or shortly after birth should raise the suspicion of in utero infection.[29]

Abnormal serum glucose concentrations are common in septic foals. Hypoglycemia (<100 mg/dL) is common initially, especially in foals less than 24 hours of age.[29] Although hypoglycemia is predominantly related to decreased intake, endotoxemia can contribute to hypoglycemia by decreasing hepatic gluconeogenesis and increasing peripheral glucose uptake. In the initial phase of treatment, one should carefully monitor the rate of supplementation because many foals subsequently develop hyperglycemia in response to dextrose infusion. Other biochemical abnormalities common in septic foals include azotemia and hyperbilirubinemia.[2]

Common arterial acid-base abnormalities include acidemia and hyperlactatemia.[29,30] Arterial hypoxemia (<70 mm Hg) was extremely common in early reports,[29] but arterial oxygen tensions of 90 mm Hg (mean)[31] and 64 mm Hg (median)[13] have been reported more recently. One should note that a decrease in PaO_2 is common following a change from standing or sternal recumbency to lateral recumbency.[32] Foals with gram-negative enteric bacteremia were noted to be more likely to have an elevated $PaCO_2$ than other bacteremic foals.[13]

The coagulation and fibrinolytic systems of the septic newborn are often abnormal, with clinically relevant decreases in antithrombin III and elevations in prothrombin time (PT), activated partial thromboplastin time (APTT), fibrinogen, fibrin degradation products[28] and D-dimer concentrations.[33] Detectable plasma endotoxin but not blood culture result was significantly correlated with abnormal PT and PTT in one report.[28] Some patients may develop active hemorrhage and/or thrombosis, which can include thrombosis of the aorta or iliac, femoral, or brachial arteries.

Endocrine adaptations to illness, including sepsis, can also occur in the neonatal foal. Increased concentrations of adrenocorticotropic hormone (ACTH) and cortisol have been documented in both septic and nonseptic hospitalized neonates.[34-39] Data on the stress response and survival are conflicting; some septic foals are capable of a stress response, whereas relative adrenal insufficiency appears present in others. Nonsurvival has been associated with both higher and lower cortisol concentrations and a high ACTH:cortisol ratio.[34,35,37,39] Thus evaluation of basal total cortisol, ACTH, and ACTH stimulation can provide additional information regarding hypothalamic-pituitary-adrenal (HPA) axis status in a given septic foal.[36] A more thorough discussion of endocrine adaptation in the foal is available elsewhere.[40]

Definitive Diagnosis

Blood culture is the gold standard for diagnosis of systemic bacterial infection. Identification of a causative organism allows for directed antimicrobial therapy, as well as determination of patterns in infection. Samples for culture should be collected from a large vein (usually jugular or cephalic, but other sites such as the saphenous can be used as well) after surgical clip and aseptic preparation. The sample should be collected into a sterile syringe without anticoagulant and immediately placed into appropriate media. Sample collection from a venous catheter is acceptable, provided it is done directly from the catheter at the time of placement without compromise of sterile technique. For those foals receiving antimicrobial therapy prior to sample collection, an appropriate medium with resins may improve microbial recovery.[41] Regardless of the media used, care should be taken to infuse the recommended volume of blood to promote optimum recovery.

Two main limitations hamper the ability of blood cultures to be useful from a diagnostic standpoint. First, positive results are usually not available for at least 48 hours following submission. Second, a positive blood culture, while extremely specific, does not confer optimal sensitivity. Many foals with histologic evidence of sepsis at necropsy have historical evidence of a negative blood culture. This can result from a number of reasons, including prior antimicrobial therapy and low circulating bacterial population. In one study, only 40% of *Escherichia coli* infections were successfully identified by blood culture relative to those organisms obtained from culture at necropsy.[42] Thus a means of identifying at-risk foals would be a valuable tool for the attending clinician.

The first scoring systems for sepsis were adopted and modified in the 1980s, with a stated aim of predicting whether a foal would be septic prior to return of blood culture results.[43,44] The modified "sepsis score" currently used in many hospitals is calculated on a number of historical findings, physical findings, and laboratory data and had a reported sensitivity and specificity of 92.8% and 85.9%, respectively.[44] The sepsis score has not been as accurate at other institutions. Recent data have shown a false negative rate of 48% in blood culture positive foals in Ohio.[13] In a study at the University of Georgia examining foals with either a sepsis score ≥11, a positive blood culture, or ≥3 foci of infection, 43/247 had a sepsis score <11 but at least one of the other criteria and 46/250 had a sepsis score ≥11 without either of the other criteria.[45] In a Virginia study, the modified[44] and original sepsis scores[43] each produced a positive predictive values of 84% with negative predictive values of 55% and 53%, respectively.[31] Results from these studies stress the importance of regional and institutional variability in the use of such scoring systems.

The modified sepsis score was reevaluated at the University of Florida, the same geographic population for which it was originally generated, obtaining a similar sensitivity (89%) but lower specificity (67.5%) using positive blood culture alone as a gold standard, rather than including evidence of specific foci of infection at necropsy as well (Sanchez and Lester, unpublished observations, 2003). Due to the heavy weighting of historical information and related problems, moderate to severely premature foals often can have a positive sepsis score without positive blood culture. But, because many of the maternal problems resulting in prematurity can also lead to systemic sepsis, this crossover is easily predictable. The problem with clinical application of these scoring systems is their relatively low specificity and negative predictive value of these systems. Thus, although a "positive" score is supportive of sepsis in a suspected animal, a "negative" score alone should not be used to withhold antibiotic therapy from an at-risk foal. Similarly, the use of a positive score alone, without complimentary culture results or necropsy findings, should be used cautiously to confirm a diagnosis of sepsis for retrospective studies.

Causative Organisms

Several retrospective studies have evaluated the most common organisms isolated from both blood culture and necropsy specimens in septic foals over the years. A summary of reported bacterial isolates is presented in Table 6-1. Whereas gram-positive organisms predominated in the 1940s through 1950, *E. coli* has remained the predominant organism isolated from septic foals in recent studies regardless of clinic location or methodology.[8,13,29,42,45-47] As far as the next most prominent isolate, however, era and geographic location appear to play a major role. In Pennsylvania in the late 1990s, gram-positive bacteria (*Enterococcus, Streptococcus, Staphylococcus* spp.) cumulatively played a major role in disease pathogenesis,[8] whereas *Actinobacillus* spp. accounted for approximately 30% of all isolates at Ohio State University in the late 1990s.[13] A Georgia study reported a dramatic decrease in the percentage of *E. coli* isolates between 1986-1990 and later 5-year sampling periods (1991-1995 and 1996-2000).[45] The predominant organisms with increased percentages over the same period were *Enterococcus* and *Staphylococcus* spp. When evaluating trends by decade (1982-1989, 1990-1999, 2000-2007) in a Florida population, *E. coli* remained the predominant isolate; *Actinobacillus* spp. were more common in the 1980s relative to the 1990s and 2000s, *Salmonella* spp. were isolated less frequently in the 2000s relative to other decades, and enteric gram-negative organisms were less frequently isolated in the 2000s relative to the 1980s.[10]

Systemic fungal infections can also occur in neonatal foals. The most commonly implicated organism is *Candida albicans*, a dimorphic fungus, although other organisms may play a similar role.[48,49] These infections have typically been associated

Table 6-1 Summary of Reported Frequency of Bacterial Isolates

	Wilson[42]	Koterba[29]	Raisis[46]	Gayle[77]	Marsh[8]	Stewart[13]	Henson[45]			Corley[9]	Russell[47]	Sanchez[10]		
Location	CA, USA	FL, USA	NSW, Australia	TX, USA	PA, USA	OH, USA	GA, USA			CA, USA	NSW, Australia	FL, USA		
Number of foals	47	27	24	29	155	101	250			85	110	423		
Blood cultures only?	No	Yes	No	Yes	Yes	Yes	No			Yes	Yes	Yes		
Admission only?	No	No	No	NS	No	Yes	No			No	Yes	No		
Years of study	1978-87	1982-83	1989-92	1988-95	1991-98	1993-2000	1986-90	1991-95	1996-2000	1995-2004	1999-2004	1982-89	1990-99	2000-07
Number of isolates	85	29	24	38	203	130	214	112	126	109	124	113	192	249
E. coli	30.6	58.6	50	36.8	18.7	30	59	29	26	40.3	31.4	39.8	29.7	28.1
Enterobacter spp.	3.5	3.4	12.5	18.4	12.3		18	8	9	1.8	8.1	5.3	6.2	5.2
Klebsiella spp.	12.9	6.9		10.5	3.9		16	15	7	4.6	0.8	7.1	8.3	5.6
Salmonella spp.		3.4	12.5	18.4	2.9		17	1	3			6.1	5.7	1.2
Actinobacillus spp.	18.8	6.9	12.5	2.6	8.9	23.1	11	8	7	19.3	6.5	8.8	1.6	2.4
Pasteurella spp.		3.4			1.5							1.8	6.8	7.2
Pseudomonas spp.	4.7	3.4		5.3	4.9							0.9	2.6	1.2
Enterococcus spp./Group D Streptococcus					9.4		0	2	19	6.4	12	2.6	5.7	8.4
Streptococcus spp.	8.3		8	7.9	9.4		33	15	8	9.2	13	8	8.8	11.2
Staphylococcus spp.	3.5	3.4		5.3	9.8		7	8	15		9.7	3.5	3.6	2.4
Clostridium spp.	2.4	3.4									1.6	3.5	2.5	2.8
All gram-negative	75.3	93.1	91.7	78.9	62.6	72.3	77	69	58	74.3	57.3	77	67.2	63.9
All gram-positive	17.6	3.4	8.3	21.1	32.5	23.1	23	31	42	21.1	40.3	19.5	24.5	30.5
All anaerobe	2.4	3.4			3.4	4.6				4.6	2.4	3.5	6.8	2.8
All fungal/yeast					1.7							0	1.6	2.8
Overall survival (%)	31.9	25.9	70.8	48.3	NS	55	44			67	74.5	48	55.9	71.4

Data are expressed as a percentage of the total isolates from each study.

Number of foals: Number of foals from which bacteria were cultured.

Blood cultures only: Yes = Samples restricted to culture of blood only; No = Samples included blood or infected tissue collected at necropsy.

Admission only: Yes = Samples restricted to those obtained within 24 hours of a foal's admission to the hospital.

NS, Not stated.

with prolonged hospitalization with invasive monitoring techniques[49] or immunodeficiency.[48] Prolonged antimicrobial therapy and administration of parental nutrition have been suggested as risk factors for the development of candidiasis. A common clinical sign is a fever unresponsive to antimicrobial therapy. Most foals with systemic infection will also develop thrush (white plaques on the lingual surface) either concurrently or prior to showing clinical signs of systemic infection, thus a daily oral examination is recommended for all hospitalized foals. Antifungal therapy should be strongly considered in any presumed septic foal that develops thrush and clearly indicated in any animal with a confirmed isolate.

Therapy

Antimicrobial Therapy

Antimicrobial therapy is the definitive therapy for treatment of septic foals. Initially, broad-spectrum bactericidal antibiotics must be used with specific choices based on previous experiences and cost. Antimicrobial therapy should begin immediately in any foal in which sepsis is suspected and should not be delayed pending blood culture results, as sensitivity data typically require 3 to 4 days. Therapy can be altered if necessary when these data become available. A minimum therapeutic course of 2 weeks is recommended for bacteremic foals without localizing clinical signs. If localizing signs, such as pneumonia or septic arthritis, are present, a minimum course of 4 weeks is recommended.[27] Recommended dosages for commonly used antimicrobials are listed in Table 6-2.

Few published veterinary reports discuss antimicrobial sensitivity of organisms isolated from septic neonatal foals. Geographic variability is evident, and a summary of selected antimicrobial susceptibility profiles published since 2000 are listed in Table 6-3. In some reports, a slightly lower percentage of gram-negative isolates are sensitive to gentamicin relative to amikacin.[2,8,45,50] In 1994, it was reported that 95% and 91% of gram-negative isolates were sensitive to amikacin and cefotaxime, respectively, while sensitivity to gentamicin and trimethoprim-sulfa was much lower.[2] Some organisms, such as *Enterobacter, Acinetobacter, Enterococcus,* and coagulase-positive *Staphylococcus* spp. have demonstrated substantial resistance.[8] Few studies have evaluated developing antimicrobial resistance. But a Florida study revealed that no group of organisms became more resistant to any drug or drug class over time between the 1980s and 2007.[10]

Thus, based on available data, a recommended initial therapeutic approach involves combining amikacin or gentamicin with penicillin or ampicillin. Alternatively, ceftiofur can be

---

Table 6-2 Recommended Antimicrobial Dosages*

Agent	Preparation	Route	Frequency (hr)	Dosage (/kg)	References
Amikacin	Sulfate	IV, IM	24	21-25 mg	92,93
Gentamicin	Sulfate	IV, IM	36	12-15 mg	94
Ampicillin	Sodium	IV, IM	6	25 mg	
Ampicillin	Trihydrate	IM	12	25 mg	
Penicillin G	Potassium	IV	6	22,000-40,000 IU	
Penicillin G	Procaine	IM	12-24	22,000 IU	
Cefotaxime	Sodium	IV	6	40 mg	51,95
Ceftiofur	Sodium	IV, IM	12	5 mg	96
Ceftiofur	Crystalline free acid	SQ	72	6.6 mg	97
Cefpodoxime	Proxetil	PO	6-12	10 mg	56
Trimethoprim-sulfamethoxazole		PO	12	30 mg	

IV, Intravenous; *IM*, intramuscular; *SQ*, subcutaneous; *PO*, orally.

* These represent recommendations only. Label indications and national or international rules regarding off-label usage of antimicrobials remain the responsibility of the provider.

Table 6-3 Reported Antimicrobial Susceptibility (%) Patterns of Microorganisms Isolated from Equine Neonates*

Isolates	Marsh[8] *Escherichia coli*	Henson[45] GP	Henson[45] GN	Russell[47] GP	Russell[47] GN	Russell[47] All	Sanchez[10] GP	Sanchez[10] NEGN	Sanchez[10] EGN	Sanchez[10] All
Amikacin	90	55	90	0	100	42	45.8	77.8	97.9	84.3
Gentamicin	80	50	75	34	74	56	62.0	79.2	92.1	83.6
Ampicillin	57	74	63	54	63	59	72.7	69.5	49.4	57.8
Penicillin		72	21	47	38	45	67.1	18.2	3.1	29.5
Ceftiofur	80	73	73	37	75	60	50	76.0	85.5	76.6
Ceftazidime							52.9	85.7	98.9	90.5
Chloramphenicol		90	75	73	83	78	92.2	94.4	84.6	87.5
Tetracycline		77	73	61	74	69	70.9	90.1	76.4	77.7
Trimethoprim-sulfamethoxazole	57	37	79	62	71	67	79.7	90.0	80.4	81.9
Enrofloxacin		100	100	37	93	70	74.6	94.5	97.6	91.8
Imipenem							86.7	82.1	100	94.9
Penicillin + gentamicin						72	84.1	78.9	92.1	88.0
Penicillin + amikacin							79.5	77.8	96.3	89.3
Ceftiofur + gentamicin						68				
Ampicillin + gentamicin							89.8	82.7	91.4	89.4
Ampicillin + amikacin							87.5	81.3	97.1	92.1

EGN, Enteric gram-negative isolates; *NEGN*, nonenteric gram-negative isolates; *GP*, gram-positive isolates; *GN*, gram-negative isolates.

* Antimicrobial susceptibility is expressed as a percentage of all isolates for which susceptibility to a given antimicrobial was reported. See Table 6-1 for key to study details.

used alone or in combination with an aminoglycoside. If a foal is severely hypovolemic and azotemic, amikacin should be avoided; a safer initial choice would likely involve a third-generation cephalosporin. If amikacin is used, therapeutic drug monitoring is recommended to ensure appropriate individual dosing. An additional recommendation includes serial creatinine monitoring every 2 to 3 days and/or serial urinalyses, including sediment examination to monitor for potential renal adverse effects. Cefotaxime is a good choice for foals with gram-negative meningitis[51] or those with unresponsive pneumonia.

Unfortunately, the range of oral antibiotics is limited in horses. Because of significant resistance, trimethoprim/sulfamethoxazole combinations should not be used in septic foals without documented sensitivity and then only as a long-term option following initial parenteral therapy. Several aminobenzyl penicillins (amoxicillin and ampicillin) and first-generation cephalosporins (cefadroxil and cephradine) have good bioavailability in young foals (in contrast to older foals and adult horses) but have a limited gram-positive spectrum of activity.[52-55] Cefpodoxime proxetil, a third-generation cephalosporin available for oral administration, was recently shown to be effective against 90% of *Klebsiella* spp., *Pasteurella* spp., and β-hemolytic streptococci.[56] An increase in the frequency of administration would likely increase the effectiveness of this drug against *E. coli*. Fluoroquinolones, such as enrofloxacin, have an excellent spectrum of activity against gram-negative and some gram-positive organisms but have been associated with arthropathy in foals.[57,58] Thus use of this agent should be reserved for those cases with documented resistance to other antimicrobial agents and informed owner consent.

Antiendotoxin Therapy

Not surprisingly, many septic foals have detectable plasma endotoxin concentrations.[28] In vitro work has shown that β-lactam antimicrobials appear more likely than aminoglycosides (alone or in combination with ampicillin) to induce endotoxemia and TNF-α activity during treatment of *E. coli* sepsis.[7] Agents commonly used in the treatment of endotoxemia include flunixin meglumine, pentoxifylline, and polymyxin B sulfate.[59-61] None of these agents has been critically evaluated for the treatment of endotoxemia in foals, thus recommendations are extrapolated from work in vitro and in adult horses. Flunixin meglumine and polymyxin B are potentially nephrotoxic, thus they should be used with caution. Flunixin meglumine also has the potential for causing or exacerbating gastric ulceration. Pentoxifylline has been shown to reduce mortality without adverse effects in septic neonates[62] but not adults.[63]

Antifungal Therapy

Attempted medical treatment options for systemic candidiasis include fluconazole, itraconazole, miconazole, and amphotericin B.[49,64] Fungal sensitivity profiles may help direct therapy if available. Pharmacokinetics of these drugs have not been determined in foals. Amphotericin B has been administered at a range of 0.1 to 0.5 mg/kg intravenous (IV) once a day, starting therapy at the lower dose and increasing by 0.1 mg/kg increments per day.[49] Since this drug can cause potentially life-threatening nephrotoxicity, serum creatinine, urine production, and urinalysis should be monitored closely. Fluconazole has previously been administered at 4 to 10 mg/kg orally (PO) every 24 hours. This agent is cheaper, easier to administer, and has far fewer side effects. Miconazole has also been used at a dose of 1 mg/kg IV every 8 hours.[49] Voriconazole has also been used to treat pulmonary aspergillosis.[65]

Cardiovascular Support

Cardiovascular support is critical in foals with hypovolemia, septic shock, or hypotension. In-depth discussions of fluid therapy[66] and the use of inotropes and vasopressors[67] in the neonatal foal have been reported. When a foal presents in septic shock, fluid resuscitation is critical. Initial choices commonly include a combination of crystalloid and colloid (such as hydroxyethyl starch) preparations. Arterial or venous lactate concentration, systemic blood pressure, cardiac output, and central venous pressure can provide additional information regarding volume status and estimation of tissue perfusion.[68] Once normovolemia is restored, neonates typically require approximately 80 to 100 mL/kg/day (5 L/day for a 50 kg foal) to maintain adequate hydration. Clinicopathologic variables to continuously monitor in septic foals include arterial or venous blood gas (depending on pulmonary status), electrolytes (especially sodium and potassium), and glucose. Physical parameters of importance include careful examination for the development of edema (conjunctiva, prepuce, ventrum, distal limbs, etc), urine output, vital signs, and temperature of the distal limbs. Derangements in any of the monitored parameters should be addressed as they arise. One should be particularly mindful of sodium load in the neonate, as requirements and sodium tolerance can differ widely between foals, and specific care should always be taken to avoid fluid overload.[66]

Antacid Therapy

Although uncommon, sick foals can develop gastric ulcers in the glandular region of the stomach. The use of prophylactic antacid therapy is controversial and highly dependent on clinician preference. Gastric pH in critically ill foals can differ greatly from that seen in healthy foals.[69,70] Severely ill, predominantly recumbent patients frequently have alkaline gastric pH patterns, and sick foals capable of acid production respond more variably to IV ranitidine administration than their normal cohorts.[70] Thus glandular ulcer disease in sick neonates is likely not strictly an acid-related problem, and factors, such as alterations in mucosal blood flow, may contribute. In addition, gastric alkalinization can contribute to bacterial translocation.[71] Recently, the use of antiulcer medications (ranitidine, omeprazole) has been associated with an increased risk of diarrhea in a large multicenter retrospective study.[72] In that report, antiulcer medications did not appear to protect against ulcer development in a small number of foals in which ulcers were detected. Should one choose to use them, options for acid suppression include ranitidine, omeprazole, and pantoprazole.[69,70,73-75] Sucralfate remains a possible alternative for ulcer prophylaxis, especially in foals receiving nonsteroidal antiinflammatory drugs (NSAIDs), without altering intragastric pH.

Additional Therapy

In light of the relative adrenal insufficiency identified in some septic foals, low-dose corticosteroid therapy has been suggested for a subset of the septic foal population. But, given the wide variability seen in the septic foal population, more data are needed before such therapy is recommended. Neonatal foals have relatively low glycogen stores at birth, and nutritional support is critically important for foals that are not suckling effectively. This support may be provided enterally or parenterally. Meticulous nursing care is essential for all critically ill foals, especially those that are recumbent and unable to rise.

Focal Infection and Potential Sequelae

Signs consistent with a secondary focus of infection, such as pneumonia, septic arthritis, osteomyelitis, omphalitis, or meningitis, may also occur. In-depth discussions of the various complications are provided in detail in the chapters relating to the relative body systems.

Respiratory Involvement

The lungs are a very common location of focal infection in the septic foal, with a reported incidence of pneumonia ranging from 28%[13] to 50%.[76] Respiratory rate and effort, thoracic auscultation, and rectal temperature can often alert the clinician to the possibility of pneumonia in a given animal. Respiratory function is best assessed in septic foals via arterial blood gas analysis.[2,68] Thoracic radiographs can provide an estimation of disease severity and distribution. In addition to hematogenously acquired pneumonia, septic foals can be at risk for aspiration of either meconium or milk. Directed antimicrobial therapy and maintenance of an acceptable arterial oxygen tension with intranasal oxygen insufflation are the most commonly provided forms of therapy. In those foals with severe hypercapnia in addition to hypoxemia, mechanical ventilation may be necessary.

Gastrointestinal Involvement

Diarrhea and/or enteritis are very common in septic foals, with reported incidence between 16% and 38%.[13,27,76,77] Conversely, approximately 50% of neonates with a primary complaint of diarrhea are bacteremic.[78,79] Thus sepsis should be suspected in any diarrheic neonatal foal. In one report, foals with *Actinobacillus* spp. bacteremia were six times more likely to have diarrhea than those with other isolates[13]; in another report, gram-negative enteric bacteremia was positively associated with diarrhea.[10] With or without enteritis, septic foals can also display signs of ileus and/or colic. Most of these problems resolve with symptomatic treatment and systemic improvement. One must carefully monitor fluid, electrolyte, and acid-base status in foals with diarrhea and account for ongoing losses. Analgesic therapy in colicky foals is somewhat limited, and flunixin meglumine should be used cautiously because of the potential for gastric ulceration. Interestingly, diarrhea was positively correlated with survival to discharge in one report of bacteremic foals.[10]

Umbilical Involvement

Omphalitis refers to infection of umbilical structures. Umbilical remnant infections are considered to be a common source of continued bacterial shedding. Ultrasonographic evaluation of these structures is critical because external signs (pain, heat, swelling) may not be evident. Treatment options include long-term antimicrobial therapy or surgical resection. The reported incidence in septic foals has ranged from 9%[10] to 21%.[77] In one report, diarrhea, rectal temperature, sepsis score, and year of admission were positively correlated with omphalitis, whereas packed cell volume (PCV), serum sodium concentration, enteric gram-negative organisms, and gram-positive organisms were negatively correlated with omphalitis.[10] Many septic foals will develop a patent urachus without involvement of other structures. This problem will often resolve with continued antibiotic therapy, with or without topical therapy.

Uroperitoneum occurs in approximately 2.5% of hospitalized neonates, and those foals with uroperitoneum and a positive sepsis score are less likely to survive than those foals with uroperitoneum and a negative sepsis score.[80] Presumptively septic foals receiving fluid therapy were typically older and less likely to have the classic electrolyte abnormalities associated with uroperitoneum. This suggests that the presumptively septic foals were diagnosed earlier, but the condition occurred later in life. Thus ischemia and subsequent necrosis of the bladder and/or urachus may account for uroperitoneum in the septic population. Because of these risks, routine ultrasonographic assessment of the umbilical structures is recommended in all hospitalized neonates in whom sepsis is either confirmed or suspected. The frequency of repeat ultrasound exams depends on the individual foal's clinical progression.

Septic Arthritis and Osteomyelitis

Orthopedic infections are common in septic foals and represent one of the most important life-threatening and performance-limiting complications. The reported incidence of septic arthritis ranges from 13% to 33%[10,13,77,81] and that of osteomyelitis from 6% to 12%.[10,77,81] Clinical signs include lameness and joint effusion; thus daily palpation of every joint in all hospitalized neonates is imperative. Any lameness and/or joint effusion in a neonate should be considered septic until proven otherwise.

Bone infections normally occur at the epiphysis of long bones, the metaphyseal side of growth plates, costochondral junctions, and the articular facets of vertebral bodies. In one report, septic arthritis and enteric gram-negative organisms were positively associated with osteomyelitis, whereas osteomyelitis and age at admission were positively associated with septic arthritis.[10] In that report, septic arthritis was negatively correlated with survival to discharge from the hospital. Detailed discussion of the diagnosis, treatment, and prognosis associated with orthopedic infections is provided elsewhere in this text.

Meningitis

Meningitis is a rare but extremely serious complication. Major clinical signs include seizures and severe depression, although this is somewhat difficult to assess in a severely compromised foal. Other signs include head tilt, strabismus, nystagmus, and extensor rigidity, depending on the areas in the central nervous system (CNS) that are involved. Cerebrospinal fluid (CSF) typically provides a definitive diagnosis; pleocytosis (normally neutrophilic) is the typical abnormality. Prognosis for foals with meningitis is poor to grave, but if therapy is attempted, third-generation cephalosporins (such as cefotaxime) have been recommended.[51] The major differential diagnosis for neurologic abnormalities in a septic neonate is neonatal encephalopathy (NE). Typically, foals with NE present within 24 to 48 hours following birth, whereas the age of foals with meningitis is more variable. One report noted that foals with gram-negative bacteremia were less likely to have seizures than those with other isolates,[13] whereas in another report, 0/11 bacteremic foals with meningitis survived to discharge from the hospital.[10]

Ocular Involvement

The most common ocular complication in the septic foal is corneal ulceration, noted in up to 12% of bacteremic foals.[10] Ulceration can occur as the result of entropion in a dehydrated foal or, more commonly, trauma. Because foals do not always show clinical signs of corneal ulceration, a daily ophthalmic examination, including fluorescein staining, should be performed in all hospitalized foals. Uveitis can also occur as an ocular extension of systemic disease. Further information regarding the diagnosis and treatment of uveitis is available elsewhere in this text.

Coagulopathy

Disorders of coagulation can occur in septic foals, manifested clinically by either hemorrhage or thrombosis. Probably the most common abnormality is jugular venous thrombosis at the site of an indwelling venous catheter. Other areas of thrombosis include the brachial artery, digital artery, metatarsal and metacarpal arteries, diffuse vascular thromboses throughout the distal limb, the aortic termination, the lungs, and the colon.[28,82-85]

Prognosis/Outcomes

Survival rates for neonatal foals with sepsis have increased from the 25% reported in the early 1980s.[29] More recent retrospective studies report short-term survival rates ranging from 45% to 55%.[13,45,77,86] Others have reported survival as low as 32%[28] and as high as 70% to 72%.[46,76,87] Given the overall advances in neonatal care, it is not surprising that year of admission was positively correlated with survival in a University of Florida report (with an overall survival of 60%) from 1982-2007.[10]

Several factors have been associated with survival in retrospective studies. A study in Georgia in 1998 demonstrated that foals infected with gram-negative organisms were more likely to die than those with gram-positive infections.[28] In a Texas study published that same year, duration of illness prior to admission was inversely related to survival and a foal's ability to stand on admission was positively correlated with survival.[77] In the Georgia study, foals were more likely to survive if they had a sepsis score less than 11, a negative blood culture at admission, blood glucose greater than or equal to 60 mg/dL, body temperature greater than or equal to 100° F [37.8° C], total carbon dioxide (TCO_2) greater than 15 mmol/L, or a low or normal plasma fibrinogen concentration.[45] In a Florida study published in 2008, age at admission, presence of septic arthritis, band neutrophil count, and serum creatinine concentration were negatively associated with survival, whereas year of admission, diarrhea, rectal temperature, neutrophil count, and arterial blood pH were positively associated with survival to discharge in bacteremic foals.[10] In an Ohio State study published in 2002, foals with multiple blood culture isolates had longer periods of hospitalization but not decreased survival.[13] In 2005 a study of foals in Virginia demonstrated that normal arterial lactate concentration either at admission or 18 to 36 hours after admission was a good predictor of survival, whereas increased lactate concentration was not a good predictor of nonsurvival.[30]

Few studies have addressed the long-term survival and performance of septic foals. In one report of Thoroughbred foals with bacteremia, there was no significant difference in percentage of starters, percentage of winners, or number of race starts, relative to a control group of maternal siblings. But foals with positive blood cultures had a lower number of wins, total earnings, and Standard Starts Index relative to control maternal siblings.[10] This is similar to that reported for overall University of Florida Neonatal Intensive Care Unit (NICU) survivors, where the percentage of starters was lower than the control population, but performance over a 2-year period was not different in those animals able to make at least 2 starts.[87] Also, NICU treatment was found not to significantly affect sales performance.[88] Similar findings have been reported for foals with neurologic disease and those with *Rhodococcus equi* pneumonia.[89,90]

Preventive Strategies

Clearly, given the wide range of potentially devastating problems associated with sepsis, efforts to minimize the incidence of disease is critical. Not surprisingly, methods of prevention coincide with the documented risk factors and routes of infection previously discussed. The following suggestions are a basic guide one can offer to clients. Although many of the presented options make sense, none have been proven to reduce the incidence of sepsis. Thus the decision to implement some or all of these practices will depend on the individual farm situation.

1. Maintain a Clean Environment

Although this is one of the most basic concepts in all of medicine, its importance cannot be overemphasized. With specific reference to the foaling situation, foaling stalls should be thoroughly cleaned and disinfected between mares. For each inhabitant, the stall should be cleaned at least daily, if not twice daily, and plentiful clean, dry, fresh bedding should be provided for the mare and foal.

2. Reduce Potential Bacterial Load Introduced During Udder Seeking

The mare's hind quarters, perineum, and udder should be thoroughly cleaned with soap and water prior to the foal's introduction.[21] The key feature to this step that is often overlooked is that the mare must also be dried. This should be done just outside the stall, rather than in the stall to prevent contamination of the foal's new environment. This step requires a great deal of commitment on the part of the farm because it is fairly labor intensive.

3. Ensure Rapid Gastrointestinal Intake

The volume, quality, and timing of colostrum administration are all likely important, rather than just the quality. The ideal scenario involves feeding 6 to 8 ounces of good quality colostrum as soon as the foal develops a good, strong suckle reflex. One of the main concerns with this recommendation is the risk of milk aspiration when untrained individuals are trying to bottle feed newborn, potentially weak foals.

4. Ensure Adequate FPT

Traditionally, FPT to the foal has been considered to be the most important factor in disease prevention. Other factors clearly play a role, however, adequate immunoglobulin transfer should still be assessed and treated, if necessary. A complete discussion on treatment of FPT is included in most equine medical texts.

5. Ensure Appropriate Umbilical Care

Appropriate umbilical care is followed by most horse owners, from the backyard client to the large breeding operation. No published studies in foals have critically evaluated the different preparations used for routine umbilical care. In human neonates, surprisingly few randomized, double-blinded clinical trials have broached this issue. In a recent review of published studies, 4% chlorhexidine was a popular choice and consistently reduced the risk of umbilical and periumbilical infections.[91] This concentration of chlorhexidine is also commonly used for foals, and thus appears to be a better alternative to previously used povidone-iodine solutions.

6. Monitor Foals Closely and Treat Suspect Foals Quickly

When identified early, sepsis can often be treated effectively on the farm with few complications. Thus, when prevention fails, early intervention is critical. Any foal with a fever, diarrhea, lethargy, or inappetence should be thoroughly evaluated and treated appropriately.

Summary

Neonatal infection remains a leading cause of morbidity and mortality in the equine industry despite advances in prevention and treatment. Many factors can influence a foal's risk for the development of sepsis in the peripartum period. Peripartum mare and foal management strategies are likely to be very important in decreasing the likelihood of sepsis. Affected foals require early and aggressive treatment to ensure optimum chance for survival.

The complete reference list is available online at www.expertconsult.com.

Skin Infections

Julia A. Conway, Pamela E. Ginn, and Dawn Logas*

Skin infections, especially contagious dermatologic diseases, include some of the most common causes of equine skin disease. In one report, approximately 25% of all dermatologic diagnoses made over a 21-year period were infectious in origin.[1] For the clinician, it is important to diagnose these conditions quickly to prevent spread to other horses and potentially their human companions. Many of these infectious agents are discussed in detail elsewhere in this book. The purpose of this chapter is to provide an overview that assists the clinician in differentiating, diagnosing, and treating conditions given the appropriate historical information, clinical presentation, and laboratory data.

General Comments

A detailed history is an extremely important component of any dermatologic workup (Box 7-1). The age at time of onset, time of the year, presence of itching, and any other notable detail not generally observed during a short examination can assist physical diagnosis. Concurrent medical conditions or any other noncutaneous signs of illness are important to note and consider. Additional questioning should include whether any topical medications, home remedies, or systemic medications have been used. Response to medications (independent of season) and time to relapse (if a response occurred) are valuable pieces of information to assist diagnosis.

The environment is a causal or predisposing factor for many diseases of the skin. A detailed description or personal inspection of the environment is needed along with a complete travel history. Chronic exposure to moisture, such as wet bedding, constant rain, or muddy pastures, can contribute to the original condition and prevent response to therapy. A basic physical examination should be performed on every patient that exhibits skin disease. Many infectious diseases of the skin reflect the underlying health, nutrition, and immune status of the horse. This can help differentiate primary from secondary conditions. In addition, it is important to determine if the skin lesions reflect the primary condition of the skin. Often, the clinician's first examination is performed after many other therapies have been attempted. Primary lesions consist of pustules, vesicles, nodules, papules, and macules. Most secondary lesions consist of crusts, erosions, ulcers, scales, and alopecia. Noting the presence or absence of pruritus will rule out (or rule in) many diseases. It is important to note if the lesions occur singly or in multiples and whether lesions are confined to haired skin or also involve mucocutaneous locations. Determining what structures are involved should also be part of the physical diagnosis (in addition to confirmation by biopsy).

Dermatologists have a basic and straightforward diagnostic armamentarium that differentiates most diseases. Skin scrapings are essential for diagnosis of parasitic infections (see Chapter 54). Punch biopsies of skin are quick and inexpensive and can yield much needed information. In many cases, the surface crusts are important in making a definitive diagnosis so only minimal preparation of the site, such as clipping of long hair, should be performed. It is important to include surface crusts with the tissue biopsy specimen. Collection of a sterile biopsy for culture is necessary for bacterial and some fungal infections. When disease is global and long-standing, a wedge biopsy may yield more information regarding the primary etiology. Accurate histopathologic assessment with appropriate knowledge of equine-specific diseases is essential and usually requires evaluation by a pathologist with special interest in skin diseases. Special stains for bacteria, fungi, and oomycetes should be pursued when appropriate.

Although many therapies for skin disease in the horse are palliative, etiology-specific treatment should be pursued rather than overuse of broad-spectrum antibiotics. As an example,

---

Box 7-1 Questions for Dermatologic Problems

- Where and when did the lesion start?
- What was the initial appearance of the lesion?
- Which occurred first, pruritus or the lesion?
- Is the condition seasonal or nonseasonal?
- Are other animals or humans affected?
- Is the horse receiving drugs or feed supplements?
- Have any topical therapies been attempted?
- What does the horse eat, and have there been any dietary changes?
- Has the source of the feed been changed?
- Are horses stabled or pastured?
- What is the travel history of the horse?
- Is the horse exhibiting any other signs of illness?
- Has this horse had previous dermatologic conditions?
- What treatments have been used and what was the response?

*The authors acknowledge and appreciate the original contributions of these authors, whose work has been incorporated into this chapter.

neutrophils can be part of noninfectious primary skin condition such as pemphigus foliaceus in which the use of antibiotics is not warranted. Understanding which conditions require antibiotics will save time and money and will be safer for equine patients and owners. An accurate diagnosis will also clarify the prognosis for a cure and set reasonable expectations for the owner.

Crusting/Scaling Dermatoses

Bacterial Etiologies

Crusting/scaling dermatoses affect primarily the epidermis and upper levels of the dermis and have many causes. Often, these dermatoses start as small papules that quickly progress to crust and scale. In addition, clinical signs may include small papules, erosions, excoriations, alopecia, and varying degrees of pruritus (Boxes 7-2 and 7-3).

Bacterial folliculitis is most often caused by coagulase-positive staphylococci (*Staphylococcus aureus, S. intermedius, S. hyicus*).[2,3] Other bacteria infrequently associated with folliculitis include *Streptococcus equi* subsp. *equi*, *Streptococcus equisimilis*, and *Corynebacterium pseudotuberculosis*.[4-6] Dermatophilosis is another bacterial crusting/scaling dermatosis in the horse (see Chapter 30).

Clinical Findings

Most cases of folliculitis start in the spring or summer. The lesions start as small follicular papules that can develop into transient pustules that rupture to form the secondary lesions of crusts (Fig. 7-1). Small foci of alopecia with scaling develop in areas of infected follicles, leading to a moth-eaten appearance

of the hair coat. In severe cases, lesions may enlarge, ulcerate, and have a purulent or serosanguineous discharge. If complicated by furunculosis, nodules and fistulous tracts may be present. Papular lesions can be more painful than pruritic. Most of these lesions start in the tack areas and are associated with friction, high temperature and humidity, excessive sweating, poor grooming practices, and possibly biting insects. Horses also develop staphylococcal folliculitis of the caudal aspect of the pastern and fetlock, which is considered to be one of the causes of "grease heel." If left untreated, lesions of folliculitis may become widespread.

Diagnosis

Diagnosis is made by cytologic evaluation of lesions (pustules, crusts), culture of lesions, and histopathology. Samples for culture are best obtained from fresh papules or pustules. If these are not available, the exudate from underneath a crust is acceptable. The histopathologic findings of bacterial folliculitis are characterized by a suppurative luminal folliculitis (neutrophils fill follicular lumens) and epidermal acanthosis with variable degrees of folliculocentric neutrophilic pustules and serocellular crusting. Follicular distention with rupture and resultant pyogranulomatous dermatitis may be present. Bacteria may or may not be detected within the lesions.

Therapy

Treatment consists of systemic antibiotics, topical therapy, and improved grooming practices and attempts to eliminate other predisposing factors. Antibiotic selection should be based on results of culture and sensitivity testing. This is especially true now that methicillin-resistant *Staphylococcus aureus* (MRSA) infections that potentially can be transferred to horse personnel are being diagnosed more frequently in horses[7-9] (see Chapter 29). Antibiotic therapy should last at least 3 to 4 weeks or 7 to 10 days beyond clinical cure. Topical therapy may consist of chlorhexidine or benzoyl peroxide shampoos. Benzoyl peroxide has the most antibacterial activity but may dry and bleach the coat. Therefore the frequency of topical application depends on

---

Box 7-2 Pruritic Crusting/Scaling Dermatoses

Noninfectious
- Chorioptic mange
- Sarcoptic mange
- Psoroptic mange
- Pediculosis
- Cutaneous onchocerciasis
- Culicoides hypersensitivity
- Atopy
- Food allergy

Infectious
- Dermatophytosis
- Dermatophilosis
- Staphylococcal folliculitis
- Corynebacterial folliculitis
- *Malassezia* dermatitis
- Besnoitiosis

Box 7-3 Nonpruritic Crusting/Scaling Dermatoses

Noninfectious
- Trombiculiasis
- Idiopathic seborrhea
- Pemphigus foliaceus

Infectious
- Dermatophytosis
- Dermatophilosis
- Staphylococcal folliculitis
- Corynebacterial folliculitis
- *Malassezia* dermatitis
- Poxvirus

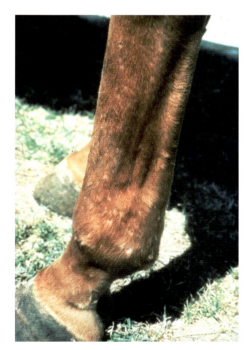

Figure 7-1 Folliculitis of distal limb that cultured positive for *Staphylococcus* spp.

the severity of disease and the topical agent used. For most cases, starting with bi-weekly and decreasing to once-weekly and then every-other-week application is adequate.

Prevention

Improved hygiene is required both for prompt resolution of infection and for prevention of recurrences. All blankets should be thoroughly cleaned with hot water and bleach. Tack should be kept as clean as possible. Cleaning of equipment should be continued on a routine basis. The horse should not be ridden while lesions are active. After the lesions have improved, the horse should be cooled properly and rinsed well after each ride. The horse should be bathed once or twice weekly in hot weather and should always have a clean saddle blanket each time it is ridden.

Fungal Etiologies

Dermatophytosis is a common cause of crusting and scaling (see Chapter 50). *Trichophyton equinum* and *T. mentagrophytes* are the primary causes of ringworm in horses, although *Microsporum gypseum*, *M. canis*, and *T. verrucosum* have been reported. Malassezia has recently been associated with crusting/scaling dermatitis in the horse.[10] *Malassezia pachydermatis* is a lipophilic, nonmycelial, saprophytic yeast often found on normal and abnormal skin of various mammals, including the horse. A novel *Malassezia* spp., *Malassezia equina*, also inhabits normal horse skin. As in the dog and cat, *Malassezia* in the horse tends to be associated with heat, humidity, friction and sometimes other dermatologic diseases, including atopy, insect bite allergy, food allergy, and dermatophytosis. Chronic steroid use and/or immunosuppression may increase risk of infection.

Clinical Findings

The clinical lesions associated with dermatophytosis consist of scales, patchy alopecia, and variable numbers of pustules, folliculocentric papules, and crusts. There may or may not be pruritus. Lesions occur most often on the face, thorax, or girth.

Lesions associated with *Malassezia* dermatitis consist of greasy to waxy crusts, erythema, thickening of the skin, and scales with a foul odor. Pruritus ranges from negligible to severe. The lesions usually start in the intertriginous areas (axilla and groin) but can become generalized.

Diagnosis

The diagnosis of dermatophytosis requires light microscopic identification of plucked hairs colonized by dermatophytes or a biopsy with identification of dermatophytes with concurrent consistent pathologic changes or positive culture in conjunction with either of the aforementioned assessments. Histopathologic changes associated with dermatophytosis include epidermal and follicular hyperkeratosis and a lymphocytic mural folliculitis or suppurative luminal folliculitis. There may also be furunculosis and associated pyogranulomatous dermatitis.

The diagnosis of yeast dermatitis is confirmed by finding numerous *Malassezia* organisms on skin surface cytology. Histopathologic changes of *Malassezia* dermatitis in the horse have not been specifically described. In other species, *Malassezia*-associated dermatitis is characterized by epidermal acanthosis and hyperkeratosis with parakeratotic crusts. Yeasts are detectable in high numbers within the keratin. Inflammation is mild and consists of mixed leukocytes within the dermis.

Therapy

Successful treatment includes management of predisposing conditions and specific antifungal therapy. Ketoconazole, miconazole, clotrimazole, and selenium sulfide all have good activity against *Malassezia*. These antifungal agents are available in a variety of mainly small animal shampoo, rinse, and cream preparations. Many are available in gallon containers and can be used on horses. The affected areas should be kept as dry as possible, as should the horse's environment.

Parasitic Etiologies

Besnoitiosis is a rare coccidian protozoal infection caused by *Besnoitia bennetti* (see Chapter 60). It has been reported throughout the world in both wild and domestic animals. The definitive host for some species of *Besnoitia* is the domestic cat. Sporulated oocysts shed in the feces of the definitive host release sporozoites when ingested by susceptible intermediate hosts such as the horse. Parasitic replication and migration throughout the connective tissues of the intermediate host leads to parasitic cyst formation in many tissues. Numerous cysts can be found in the dermis and subcutaneous tissues and are visible clinically as papules or nodules to the naked eye. Ingestion of infected tissues from the intermediate host leads to infection of the definitive host.

Clinical Findings

Lesions start as small papules in glabrous (hairless) areas. When papules do occur in haired regions, the initial presentation is tufting of the hair coat. These papules spread to cover the entire ventrum, perineum, and face and may become generalized. The nasal, oral, and pharyngeal mucosa may also be affected. As the lesions mature, they become thick and crusted. Alopecia and pruritus are common, and affected horses may be febrile, depressed, and weak.

Diagnosis

Diagnosis of besnoitiosis is made by biopsy. Histopathologically, the dermis and subcutis contain many large (300-650 µ), round cyst-like structures filled with crescent-shaped protozoal bradyzoites. Cysts are actually parasitized, hypertrophied fibroblasts that are surrounded by a thick, hyalinized, collagenous wall. There is a perivascular mononuclear infiltrate and marked epidermal hyperplasia with hyperkeratosis. Mature cysts often lack surrounding inflammation unless they rupture.

Therapy

Successful treatment of besnoitiosis has not been reported in the horse, although trimethoprim-sulfamethoxazole was effective in a miniature donkey.[11]

Viral Etiologies

Poxvirus

Poxvirus infections in horses are rare and have several clinical forms, not all of which are completely characterized or clearly identified as separate conditions. Poxviruses have been associated with relatively benign localized disease to highly contagious generalized papular skin disease. Poxvirus infections have been associated with an exudative dermatitis of the flexor aspects of the hind pasterns (another possible cause of "grease heel"). A mucocutaneous form of poxviral infection affects the muzzle and buccal cavity and can spread to the face and other parts of the body. A third type of equine poxvirus infection associated with generalized papular eruptions is referred to as *equine papular dermatitis*, seen in the United States and Australia. In Africa, a generalized poxviral disease caused by an orthopoxvirus, called *Uasin Gishu disease*, is characterized by generalized papules that become large papillomatous proliferations over time. Recently, in southern Brazil, 14 Crioulo mares and foals had an outbreak of severe cutaneous disease associated with an orthopoxvirus.[12] *Molluscum contagiosum virus* has been associated with poxviral lesions in the horse.[13]

Clinical Findings

Most poxviral infections have a distinctive developmental sequence. Lesions of poxvirus infection begin as erythematous macules that quickly become papular, leading to a transient vesicular stage that gives rise to a pustule and then a crust. If the lesion is on a mucous membrane, vesicles form, leading to ulcer formation. Healing with scar formation is typical.

In equine papular dermatitis, horses develop firm papules up to 0.5 cm in diameter. Lesions begin on the lateral neck, shoulders, and thorax and eventually become generalized. Equine papular dermatitis is highly contagious and spread by direct contact and fomites. In haired areas, a fine, powdery scale may form. Affected horses may show various systemic signs, including pyrexia, lameness, ptyalism, and depression. The symptoms are self-limiting and last 20 to 30 days.

Diagnosis

Diagnosis of a poxviral infection is made by biopsy. Histopathologic changes vary with stage of the lesion. The cells of the epidermal stratum spinosum often show cytoplasmic swelling, leading to keratinocyte rupture and vesicle formation. The dermis is edematous with variable degrees of perivascular mononuclear cell and neutrophil infiltration. Neutrophils migrate into the epidermis to form pustules, which rupture to form crusts. The epidermis becomes extremely hyperplastic. Intracytoplasmic inclusions typical of poxvirus infection may be evident. Specific characterization of the virus causing the lesion may require ancillary studies such as electron microscopy, culture, immunohistochemistry, polymerase chain reaction (PCR), or other molecular biologic techniques.

Molluscum Contagiosum

Etiology

Molluscum contagiosum is a rare proliferative poxviral disease in horses caused by a molluscipoxvirus.[13] The disease is mildly contagious between horses, and transmission occurs by direct skin-to-skin contact and indirect contact with fomites. Molluscum contagiosum has been described in horses, humans, chimpanzees, macropod marsupials, dogs, and several avian species. Equine molluscum contagiosum is potentially an anthropozoonosis.

Clinical Findings

The clinical and histopathologic changes of molluscum contagiosum are identical to those seen in horses with Uasin Gishu disease. However, the causative agent of equine molluscum contagiosum cannot be grown in culture, whereas the agent of Uasin Gishu can be cultured. Lesions usually begin in one area, such as the chest, shoulders, neck, or limbs, then become widespread, with some affected animals having hundreds of lesions. Occasionally, lesions of molluscum contagiosum may remain localized in areas such as the muzzle, axillae, inguinal area, or genitalia. Lesions start as papules that become hyperplastic with thick crusts and horny projections. Papules may become umbilicated with a central pore, often containing a caseous plug.

Diagnosis

Diagnosis of molluscum contagiosum is made by biopsy and is characteristic of the disease. Discrete foci of endophytic epidermal hyperplasia form pear-shaped lobules in the superficial dermis. Keratinocytes are greatly swollen and contain large intracytoplasmic inclusions known as *molluscum bodies*. Affected keratinocytes slough through a pore that forms in the stratum corneum and enlarges to become a central crater. The dermis is not inflamed. Molluscum bodies are readily identifiable with cytology.

Therapy

Treatment of poxvirus infections consist of supportive care and prevention of secondary bacterial infections. Topical therapy with antibacterial shampoos, clean blankets, and dry stalls all help to prevent secondary infection. No reported treatment, including an autogenous bacterin, has been successful for treatment of molluscum contagiosum. Horses may remain covered with hundreds of lesions for several months to years. In some cases, many of the lesions will regress over time, although the regression of all lesions has not been reported. Occasionally, horses will have small numbers of incidental and self-limiting lesions. The clinical course of disease is usually slow and progressive and of little systemic impact on the animal or economic impact on a herd.

Papulonodular Dermatoses

Papulonodular dermatoses have deeper lesions that extend into the lower layers of the dermis (Box 7-4). These lesions consist of multiple or large papules to nodules that may ulcerate, drain, and crust over.

Bacterial Etiology, Diagnosis, and Treatment

Bacterial furunculosis is merely a progression of folliculitis. The most prominent lesions are often seen in the saddle region and include furuncles, draining tracts, and ulcerations. Diagnosis, histopathologic findings, and treatment are the same as discussed for folliculitis. Antibiotic choice should always be based on culture and sensitivity results, and systemic antibiotic therapy should continue for at least 6 to 8 weeks instead of 3 to 4 weeks. If only a few lesions are present, 2% mupirocin ointment can be tried instead of systemic antibiotic therapy.

Papillomavirus

Papillomatosis in the horse is caused by several different deoxyribonucleic acid (DNA) papovaviruses (see Chapter 25). Lesions begin as small, smooth, white-to-gray papules that grow into pedunculated lesions with multiple frondlike keratin projections. Diagnosis is made by histopathology; viral papillomas are characterized by an exophytic, extremely hyperkeratotic and hyperplastic epidermis supported by thin dermal cores. The

---

Box 7-4 Papulonodular Dermatoses

Noninfectious
- Fly bites
- Collagenolytic granuloma
- Tick bite granuloma
- Hypodermiasis (warbles)
- Demodectic mange
- Axillary nodular necrosis
- Straw itch mites
- Unilateral papular dermatosis

Infectious
- Poxviruses
  - Equine molluscum contagiosum
- Papillomaviruses
- Bacterial furunculosis
  - Staphylococcal
  - Streptococcal
  - Corynebacterial
- Leishmaniasis

keratinocytes of the spinous and granular layers have ballooning degeneration and may have intranuclear, pale, basophilic viral inclusion bodies. The stratum granulosum has large and irregularly shaped keratohyaline granules.

Equine papillomavirus type 2 has recently been associated with a case of widespread papilloma formation on the penis of a horse and has been identified in cases of equine penile squamous cell carcinoma tissue suggesting a possible causal relationship between papillomavirus infection and the development of penile squamous cell carcinoma.[14,15]

Leishmaniasis

Etiology

Leishmania, an intracellular protozoal parasite of the mononuclear phagocyte system, can cause papulonodular skin disease in horses.[16,17] Cutaneous leishmaniasis in horses is seen primarily in South America but has been reported in horses residing in the United States. Endemic foci of leishmaniasis exist in Texas, Oklahoma, and Ohio. The majority of cases reported in the United States have been in the dog. Equids (horses, mules and donkeys), cats, and opossums are susceptible to leishmaniasis but are considered secondary, accidental hosts. Leishmaniasis is caused by *Leishmania braziliensis*, a protozoal parasite transmitted by the sandfly. Lesions consist of papules and nodules that become ulcerated and crusted. Common locations for lesions include the muzzle, periocular region, pinnae, scrotum, neck, and legs. Recently, in central Europe, a *Leishmania* spp. was identified in cutaneous lesions of horses that was not classified as Old World or New World *Leishmania* spp. This species exhibited a close phylogenetic relationship to *Leishmania siamensis*.

Diagnosis

Histopathology is usually diagnostic for leishmaniasis, and lesions consist of a superficial and deep granulomatous dermatitis. Inflammation can be diffuse or organized as distinct granulomas (Fig. 7-2). Leishmania amastigotes (Leishman-Donovan bodies) can be identified within macrophages, giant cells, or occasionally within endothelial cells or fibroblasts or free in the interstitium. Organisms are best visualized with a Giemsa stain.

Therapy

Few reports of treatment of leishmaniasis in horses have been published. Lesions in some horses may undergo spontaneous regression. One horse was successfully treated with sodium stibogluconate. This drug is specific for the treatment of leishmaniasis and is a systemic therapy. Many potential adverse effects are associated with this medication, including pain with intravenous injection. Dysrhythmias occur in humans, and the drug is contraindicated in pregnant women and patients with renal disease.

Large Nodular/Mass Dermatoses

Etiology

Nodular/mass dermatoses form a single mass lesion or several large nodular lesions grouped together and have many different etiologies (Box 7-5). These lesions affect primarily the deep dermis and subcutaneous tissue. Eventually, the underlying muscle tissue may also be involved. The overlying epidermis may be completely normal or may contain multiple draining tracts and ulcers.

Subcutaneous bacterial abscesses in the horse can be caused by any bacterium that is inadvertently inoculated into the skin or subcutaneous tissue. *Staphylococcus aureus* in particular but also other staphylococcal species are frequently cultured from these lesions (see Chapter 29). *Streptococcus* spp. (see Chapter 28), *Actinomyces* spp., *Nocardia* spp. (see Chapter 45), *Pseudomonas aeruginosa*, and *Mycobacterium* spp. (see Chapter 45) have been reported less frequently. *Corynebacterium pseudotuberculosis* causes particularly deep-seated abscesses (see Chapter 45). The typical presentation is a solitary, large abscess on the ventral chest, although multiple lesions anywhere on the body can be seen. Insect bites have been proposed as the means by which *C. pseudotuberculosis* is inoculated into the subcutaneous tissue.

Subcutaneous mycoses in the horse can be caused by a myriad of ubiquitous soil saprophytes that are inadvertently inoculated into viable tissue. Eumycotic fungi, such as *Pseudallescheria boydii*, form granules or grains in the tissue.[18] These are normally solitary lesions that may or may not have draining tracts. The grains in the exudate may be dark or white, depending on the particular fungus involved. Phaeohyphomycotic fungi form pigmented hyphae in tissue but not granules. These fungi normally form multiple, nonulcerative nodules. Zygomycotic fungal infections are characterized by nonpigmented,

---

Box 7-5 **Large Nodular Dermatoses/Mass Lesions**

Noninfectious
- Cutaneous habronemiasis
- Primary screwworm
- Blowfly
- Squamous cell carcinoma
- Sarcoid
- Mast cell tumor

Infectious
- Bacterial
  - *Staphylococcus*
  - *Corynebacterium* (pigeon breast)
  - *Nocardia*
  - Actinomycetes
  - Mycobacteria
  - Glanders
- Fungal
  - Eumycotic mycetomas
  - Phaeohyphomycosis
  - Zygomycosis
  - Sporotrichosis
- Oomycetes
  - Pythiosis

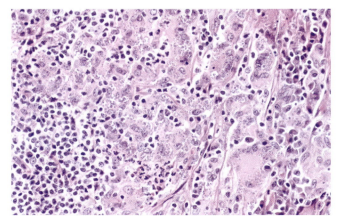

Figure 7-2 *Leishmania* infection in horse. Changes consist of granuloma containing giant cells.

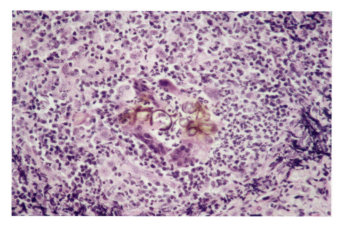

Figure 7-3 Pyogranuloma with phaeohyphomycotic fungi.

poorly staining hyphae in the tissue. These fungi usually cause solitary, ulcerative, granulomatous masses (see Chapter 51). *Sporothrix schenckii*, a dimorphic fungus (see Chapter 48), and *Pythium insidiosum*, an oomycete (see Chapter 51), cause lesions similar to those just described.

Diagnosis

Diagnosis of bacterial infections is made by cytologic examination with culture and sensitivity testing of the exudate. If the abscess does not mature, open, and drain, histopathology and tissue culture may be needed to make the diagnosis. Diagnosis and differentiation of subcutaneous fungal infections is best accomplished by histopathology with tissue culture and sensitivity. Most subcutaneous mycoses are characterized by a nodular to diffuse, granulomatous to pyogranulomatous, deep dermatitis and panniculitis (Fig. 7-3). Lymphocytes and plasma cells may be numerous, and microabscesses may be present. The fungal organism can usually be identified within the areas of inflammation. The overlying epidermis may be acanthotic or ulcerated. Fungal hyphae are best visualized with Gomori methenamine silver stain (GMS) and the periodic acid–Schiff (PAS) reaction.

Therapy

Treatment of bacterial subcutaneous infections is best accomplished by using heat or poultices to promote drainage. Once mature, the abscess should be surgically incised, drained, and lavaged. This therapeutic approach is much more effective than systemic antibiotic therapy. Systemic antibiotics should be reserved for cases in which the abscess does not mature or cannot be drained. Antibiotic selection should be based on culture and sensitivity results. Treatment of fungal infections consists mainly of complete surgical excision. These fungi are notoriously resistant to antifungal drugs. However, specific antifungal therapy may be beneficial in treatment of sporotrichosis (see Chapter 48).

Pastern Dermatitis

Equine pastern dermatitis (EPD) is a multifactorial disease in the horse with a typical cutaneous reaction pattern variously known as "scratches," "mud fever," "grease heel," and "cracked heels."[1,19-23] This disease is highly variable in terms of etiology, duration, and response to therapy (even during sequential outbreaks in the same horse). Etiologic agents responsible for EPD include *Staphylococcus aureus*, *Dermatophilus congolensis*, and *Chorioptes* spp. mites, dermatophytosis, and others.[19-23] A recent case reported in the literature described concurrent infection with intradermal spirochetes and *Pelodera strongyloides*.[19]

A severe form of pododermatitis, verrucous pastern dermatitis, has been described in Draft horses.[20,21] This disease may be staged based on severity and degree of histopathologic change. An increased risk of disease is associated with poor hygiene in the stable and poor quality of the pasture on which horses are managed. However, others have hypothesized an autoimmune etiology for this condition.

Clinical Features

Equine pastern dermatitis can affect any breed of horse, although it is most often described in Draft breeds. Feathering over the pasterns is a likely predisposing factor. This disease has no age or gender predilection but is reported more frequently in adult horses.[1,19-23] Dermatitis affects the caudal aspect of the pasterns, especially in the hindlimbs. The lesions occasionally spread dorsally and anteriorly, involving the front of the pastern and fetlock areas. The condition is frequently bilateral and symmetric, although a single limb may be affected in some horses. Lesions are most common on the nonpigmented areas of the pasterns. If left untreated, lesions coalesce and may produce large areas of ulceration and suppuration.

Equine pastern dermatitis is not usually associated with systemic clinical signs, and the general health of the animal is unaffected. If the disease is severe, secondary distal limb edema and fever may occur. Ultimately, the disease can progress to severe ascending cellulitis. Lameness is variable and can be quite severe.

Diagnosis

Diagnosis of EPD is frequently made solely on the basis of clinical signs. If pustules are present, contents may be obtained for Gram stain of smears, bacterial culture, and antibiotic sensitivity testing. Punch biopsy, obtained with sterile technique, is the appropriate sample for culture. Other noninfectious causes of pastern dermatitis, especially allergic contact dermatitis, photosensitization, and vasculitis need to be ruled out and primary or contributing factors identified. Results of a biopsy interpretation and careful consideration of location of the lesions in terms of sun exposure and pigmentation need to be taken into consideration in some cases. The lesions of photosensitization are not limited to the posterior aspect of the pastern or fetlock regions and only involve areas that lack pigmentation.

Therapy

It may be necessary to heavily sedate or anesthetize an affected horse for initial therapy because lesions can be quite painful. The affected area(s) should be clipped and washed well with an antiseptic solution (e.g., povidone-iodine, benzoyl peroxide). Application of an astringent, such as aluminum acetate solution (Domeboro, Bayer), may be helpful. An appropriate antimicrobial ointment is then applied twice daily. Systemic antibiotic therapy is rarely, if ever, indicated. In severely affected horses, therapy with injectable procaine penicillin may be considered. Broad-spectrum antibiotics or those with a predominantly gram-negative spectrum may be indicated based on culture results.

The complete reference list is available online at www.expertconsult.com.

Reproductive Tract Infections

8

Ahmed Tibary, Lisa K. Pearson, and Cheryl L. Fite*

Infections of the reproductive tract cause a myriad of clinical disorders manifesting primarily as infertility, abortion, and birth of septic foals. This chapter discusses the etiology, pathogenesis, clinical manifestations, treatment, and prevention of these diseases in the mare and stallion. Infectious processes of the reproductive tracts may be divided into venereal and opportunistic. The venereal diseases present important economic and regulatory issues and are reviewed separately in this chapter.

Reproductive Tract Infection in Nonpregnant Mares

Infection of the reproductive tract in the mare, especially endometritis, is the leading cause of infertility in horses and results in substantial annual losses. The female reproductive tract possesses a variety of mechanisms to protect itself against infection. These include physical barriers (vulva, vestibulovaginal sphincter, cervix), local immune mechanisms, and the physical ability to eliminate products of inflammation. Uterine infections, reported in 25% to 60% of barren mares,[1,2] become established when one or several of these natural defense mechanisms fail or become overwhelmed. Bacterial infections result in infertility, early embryonic loss, placentitis, birth of septic foals, and postpartum metritis. Salpingitis, cervicitis, and vaginitis may be part of the clinical presentation of acute or chronic reproductive tract infections in the mare.

Uterine Infections

Etiology

Infectious endometritis is a major cause of infertility and early pregnancy loss[1-12] and is estimated to affect 25% to 60% of broodmares.[13,14] These infections become established when normal defense mechanisms fail to clear potentially pathogenic organisms after they are introduced into the uterus.[2,14] The most common sources of uterine contamination include coitus, parturition, artificial insemination, and aseptic genital examination and manipulation.[9,15,16] The mare's age, parity, number of barren years, and uterine biopsy grade influence the likelihood of persistence of infection.[17-19]

The organisms most frequently isolated from mares with endometritis are *Streptococcus equi* subsp. *zooepidemicus*, *Escherichia coli*, *Pseudomonas aeruginosa*, and *Klebsiella pneumoniae*.[9,16,20,21] Infections caused by *P. aeruginosa* or *K. pneumoniae* are often considered venereal diseases because the organisms are often introduced during coitus, insemination with infected semen, or genital manipulations. *K. pneumoniae* capsule types 1, 2, and 5 are highly pathogenic.[22] Commensal bacteria, such as *Actinomyces pyogenes*, *Proteus* spp., and *Staphylococcus*

spp., are occasionally isolated from mares with endometritis. They are considered likely to be the causative organisms of endometritis if the diagnosis is supported by cytologic or histopathologic evidence of concurrent inflammation. Alphahemolytic *Streptococcus*, *Enterobacter* spp., and *Staphylococcus epidermidis* are rarely causes of equine endometritis and should be considered simple contaminants.[23] *Corynebacterium* spp. and anaerobic bacteria, such as *Bacteroides fragilis*, may occasionally cause endometritis in horses.[20] Anaerobes are most often isolated from postpartum and foal-heat samples.[12] *Taylorella equigenitalis* is the causative agent of a highly contagious venereal metritis, contagious equine metritis (CEM) (see Chapter 38).

The pathogenicity of bacteria depends on their ability to adhere to the endometrium, preventing their removal by normal uterine clearance mechanisms. Adhesive proprieties of *S. equi* subsp. *zooepidemicus* are probably mediated by fibronectin-binding proteins and hyaluronic acid capsule.[24-27] Attachment of *K. pneumoniae* to endometrial cells is facilitated by pili and capsule.[28] Persistent colonization by *P. aeruginosa* is assisted by the secretion of an adhesive matrix that forms a biofilm.[29] These biochemical proprieties also are important in resistance of bacteria to opsonization, phagocytosis, and the action of antimicrobials.[27,30-32] Resistance to phagocytosis is often observed with *S. equi* subsp. *zooepidemicus* and *K. pneumoniae* and is probably mediated by antigenic variation, antiphagocytic M-like proteins, hyaluronic acid capsule, or polysaccharide and Fc receptors.[27,31] Bacterial toxins promote deterioration of complement and exacerbate uterine inflammation.[33]

Candida and *Aspergillus* spp. are the most common fungal organisms isolated from the uterus of mares with endometritis.[16] The incidence of fungal infection in mares with endometritis is estimated to vary between 0.1% and 5%.[34-38] Fungal organisms isolated from the equine uterus include *Aspergillus* spp., several *Candida* spp., *Cryptococcus neoformans*, *Fusarium* spp., *Hansenula anomala*, *Hansenula polymorpha*, several *Rhodotorula* spp., *Scedosporium apiospermum*, *Saccharomyces cerevisiae*, *Trichosporon beigelii*, and *Torulopsis candida*.[34,35,38-42]

Prolonged antibiotic therapy may be a predisposing factor for yeast overgrowth.[38] Transmission of fungal organisms from stallions has not been demonstrated, although fungi have been cultured from the urethra (*Mucor* spp.), fresh semen (*Absidia* spp.), and extended semen (*Candida* spp.) of stallions.[43]

Mycoplasma spp. have been isolated from the external genitalia and semen of clinically normal and infertile stallions, but their exact role in uterine infection is not well established.[44-46] In a study in Denmark, no *Mycoplasma* spp. were isolated from semen samples from 80 stallions.[47] *Mycoplasma equigenitalium*, *M. subdolum*, and *Acholeplasma* spp. are associated with infertility, endometritis, vulvitis, and abortion in mares and with reduced fertility and balanoposthitis in stallions.[44,48-50] *Mycoplasma equigenitalium* and *M. subdolum* were isolated from the genital tract of mares (5%-34%) and aborted equine fetuses (7%); however, the presence of *Mycoplasma* is not always correlated with reduced fertility.[44,48-51]

*The authors acknowledge and appreciate the original contributions of these authors, whose work has been incorporated into this chapter.

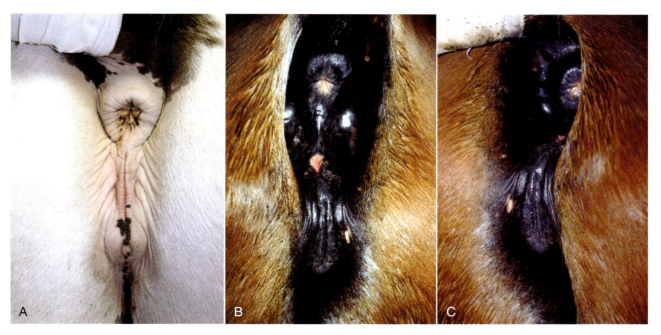

Figure 8-1 A, Normal conformation of vulva in the mare. **B,** Abnormal conformation with parting of vulvar lips at dorsal commissure. **C,** Abnormal conformation with tilting of vulvar lips.

Pathogenesis

Physical Barriers

The uterine cavity is protected from ascending infection by several anatomic structures.[52] The first line of defense is provided by the seal of the normal vulvar labia. Evaluation of vulvar and perineal conformation should be included in all prebreeding examinations or evaluations for infertility. The vulva should be in a vertical position aligned with the anal opening (Fig. 8-1, A). The labia should be tight, with most of its length below the tuber ischii. The vulvar lips may become parted as a consequence of previous traumatic injuries or lesions (Fig. 8-1, B). In older multiparous mares, there is a tendency for extreme relaxation of the vulvar lips, particularly during estrus, as well as tilting of the dorsal aspect of the vulva caused by relaxation of the perineal body. In this situation the vulva becomes horizontal as it is pulled cranially over the tuber ischii (Fig. 8-1, C). These anatomic changes predispose the mare to pneumovagina (windsucking) and pneumouterus, ultimately causing urine to pool in the cranial vagina and contaminate the uterus when the cervix is open. Contamination with fecal material adds to the increased risk of infection.

The second physical barrier in the prevention of contamination of the vagina and eventually the uterus is the vestibulovaginal sphincter. In a normal mare the vestibulovaginal area remains sealed even when the vulvar labia are parted. Compromised vestibulovaginal sphincter function is suspected when air is sucked into the vagina or if the examiner is able to visualize the vaginal cavity directly after parting the vulvar lips. The vestibulovaginal sphincter may become compromised secondary to rectovaginal tears and other foaling injuries.

The third important anatomic barrier to infection is the cervix. The cervix is open during estrus, late gestation, and in the immediate postpartum period. However, compromised cervical function is observed in some mares, and this entity may remain open during anestrus and even diestrus. The most common cause of cervical incompetence is a cervical lesion consequent to dystocia.

A plan for treatment and prevention of uterine infection should include a plan to reestablish normal barrier function.

Surgical procedures, such as episioplasty, vestibulovaginoplasty, and rectovaginal tear repair, should be considered if indicated.

Immunity and Uterine Defense

The concept that mares may be innately "resistant" or "susceptible" to uterine infection was introduced in the 1960s based on the ability of mares to clear experimentally induced or naturally acquired bacterial endometritis.[53,54] Young mares experimentally inoculated with S. equi subsp. zooepidemicus clear infection within a few hours,[53] whereas barren mares inoculated with S. equi subsp. zooepidemicus and P. aeruginosa have a delayed elimination of bacteria.[54] These observations led to further investigation into uterine defense mechanisms to clarify the role of local immunity, neutrophil function, opsonization, and phagocytosis in the prevention and clearance of uterine infection.

Immunoglobulins

The predominant immunoglobulins in uterine secretions are IgG and IgA produced within the endometrium. Uterine immunoglobulin concentration does not differ between mares susceptible and resistant to endometritis, suggesting that this is not a major factor in susceptibility to infection.[55-60] In fact, susceptible mares tend to have slightly higher concentrations of intrauterine immunoglobulins than do resistant mares, but susceptible mares are less efficient at opsonizing streptococci during acute infection.[55]

Neutrophils

Neutrophil chemotaxis is induced by bacteria, endotoxin, spermatozoa, semen extenders, and even sterile water and saline. A massive influx of neutrophils into the uterine lumen occurs in both susceptible and resistant mares[55,61] after local exposure to foreign proteins.[61-64] In some mares, this stimulation elicits a persistent inflammatory response after breeding that has been termed persistent mating-induced endometritis (PMIE). Neutrophils play an important role in this phenomenon, and their effects are exacerbated if bacteria are present.[65,66]

The events leading to PMIE are initiated by a local reaction to the primary antigen, with local production of inflammatory mediators, especially prostaglandin E_2 (PGE_2), and neutrophil influx.[67] Increased vascular permeability resulting from proinflammatory mediators exacerbates the neutrophil influx and leakage of serum proteins into the uterus, peaking as early as 4 hours after inoculation.

This response is primarily mediated by inflammatory mediators such as leukotriene B_4 (LTB_4) and PGE_2.[62,68,69] Mares susceptible to PMIE have a higher expression of proinflammatory cytokines (interleukin-1 beta [IL-1β], IL-6, and tumor necrosis factor alpha [TNF-α]) during estrus and IL-1β and TNF-α during diestrus.[70] It is unclear whether chemotactic responsiveness differs between PMIE-susceptible mares and nonsusceptible mares.[71-73] A second influx of inflammatory fluid is seen 12 hours after insemination. Resistant mares are able to eliminate most fluid by 12 hours in response to the effects of oxytocin and prostaglandin on the myometrium. Susceptible mares fail to eliminate fluid, often because of inherent endometrial or myometrial pathology that renders uterine contractions less efficient at uterine clearance.

The phagocytic activity of neutrophils is thought to be enhanced on entry into the uterine cavity.[69,73] Phagocytic activity is higher in ovariectomized mares treated with estrogens,[74] suggesting that neutrophil phagocytic activity may be highest during estrus. Phagocytic activity of circulating neutrophils is no different between susceptible and resistant mares; however, phagocytic activity and life span of uterine neutrophils are significantly reduced in susceptible mares.[69,75-77] Susceptible mares are more likely to have uterine clearance problems and accumulate more fluid, which may contribute to a reduction in the viability of neutrophils. Differences in neutrophil function between mares susceptible and resistant to endometritis have been demonstrated.[56,71,72]

Opsonizing activity in the uterus peaks 8 hours after inoculation with streptococci.[78] Studies using heat-treated uterine fluid suggest that complement is not a primary opsonizing factor in the uterus.[78,79] Complement is cleaved in uterine fluid, reducing its opsonizing ability within the uterine environment.[79,80] The uterine environment of endometritis susceptible mares seems to be hostile to complement.[61,69,79,81] In contrast, the opsonizing capacity and degree of serum complement activity does not differ between susceptible and resistant mares.[61,79,80,82,83] These observations provide a rationale for the use of intrauterine serum infusion for the treatment of endometritis.[80,84]

Physical Clearance of Infection

Physical clearance of pathogens and inflammatory debris from the uterus plays a major role in the prevention of persistent infection and is most effective during estrus.[85-95] Younger mares are able to eliminate both antigenic (*S. equi* subsp. *zooepidemicus*) and nonantigenic (microsphere) particles more quickly than older mares.[96] Mares susceptible to infectious endometritis are unable to eliminate bacteria from the uterus in the immediate postovulatory period.[97-99]

The effect of uterine pathology on susceptibility to endometritis has been demonstrated.[100] Gross anatomic changes, such as large pendulous uteri, defective myometrial activity, pendulant broad ligaments, and degenerative changes to the vascular and lymphatic drainage of the uterus, are also involved in delayed uterine clearance and the pathogenesis of endometritis.[101-103] Microscopic alteration of the endometrium (ulceration, degeneration, or lack of cilia) may be involved in failure of mucociliary clearance.[24,100,104-106]

Myometrial contractions are less frequent and of shorter duration and intensity in susceptible mares,[107,108] perhaps because of increased fibrosis or biochemical factors affecting uterine contractility. Uterine contractions are reduced in the presence of nitrous oxide (NO), which is found in high concentration in susceptible mares.[85] The role of prostaglandin secretion in PMIE remains unclear despite numerous investigations, possibly reflecting variation in factors inherent to the endometrium that cannot be easily controlled in experimental studies.[109-111]

Diagnosis

Uterine infection may be suspected on the basis of a history of infertility, recurrent endometritis, mucopurulent vaginal discharge, predisposing anatomic features, early embryonic loss, or observation of fluid accumulation on examination of the uterus by ultrasonography. Clinical signs may include vaginal discharge. Confirmation of the diagnosis of uterine infection requires endometrial cytology and uterine culture.[112,113] Uterine biopsy remains the gold standard in the diagnosis of endometritis.

Accumulation of large quantities of fluid during estrus or postbreeding is a good indication of mare susceptibility to endometritis (Fig. 8-2). Resistant mares eliminate mating-induced endometritis within 6 to 12 hours after breeding, whereas susceptible mares may retain variable amounts of fluid for several days. Accumulation of fluid in the uterus is associated with decreased pregnancy rates. All mares should be evaluated 24 hours after breeding and treated if a pocket of fluid remains within the uterine cavity.[89,114-116] Mares with a history of infertility or that are known to be susceptible to endometritis should be evaluated or treated as early as 6 hours after breeding.[117]

Several methods for collection of uterine cytology samples have been described. These include the use of double-guarded swabs, uterine cytology brushes, and low-volume uterine flushes.[86,112] Uterine cytology brushes and small-volume uterine flushes provide the best specimens for endometrial cytology (Fig. 8-3).[118] Swabs are often reliable if there is fluid in the uterus or if the swab is wetted with a sterile saline solution before sampling.

Interpretation of uterine cytology samples may be challenging because of the lack of standardized methodology for evaluation. The most common staining technique for uterine cytologic specimens is a rapid Wright-Giemsa stain (Diff-Quik). Interpretation is based on evaluation of the types of cells and organisms observed[86,112,118,119] (Fig. 8-4). Quantitative methods for the interpretation of equine endometrial cytology have been reviewed recently.[86] Diagnosis of endometritis may be based on the number of neutrophils per number of high-power microscopic fields examined, as a ratio of neutrophils to epithelial cells, or as a percentage of all cells. Endometrial cytology may provide an important clue to fungal infection (Fig. 8-5). Cytology may be negative if infection is recent.[34] Endometrial swabs should always be submitted for anaerobic and aerobic bacterial, as well as fungal, culture. Blood agar plating may be used in the initial fungal culture, but specific culture techniques are required for more precise diagnosis.[34] Chromogenic agar offers good accuracy and ease of use for the identification of bacterial isolates from endometritis in veterinary practices.[4]

Endometrial biopsy is an important and highly accurate method for the diagnosis of uterine inflammation. Special staining techniques, such as Gomori's methanamine silver, are particularly helpful for the diagnosis of fungal endometritis from fixed tissue sections.[120]

Interpretation of diagnostic results may be challenging at times. A diagnosis of endometritis is established if culture is positive and cytology shows more than two neutrophils per 400× field.[121] However, mares with endometritis may have a negative culture and a positive cytology or vice-versa.[122] Sensitivity of culture is improved if small volume lavage is used. Cytology was found to underreport inflammation if only the presence of neutrophils is considered. However, the rate of false negatives decreased substantially when the efflux was also evaluated for presence of debris or cloudiness as sign of

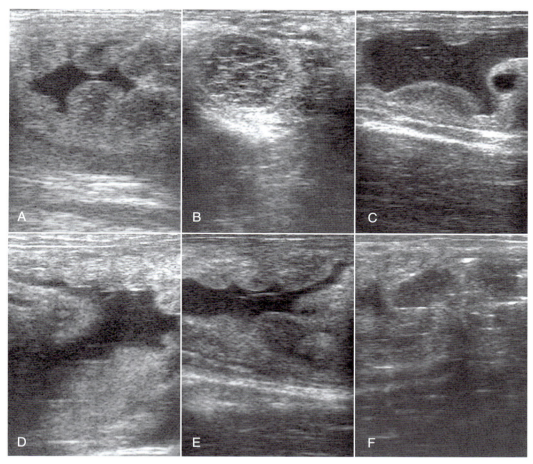

Figure 8-2 Persistent mating-induced endometritis (PMIE). **A, C,** and **D,** Ultrasonograms of uterus at 6, 12, and 18 hours after insemination, respectively. **B,** Corpus hemorrhagicum. **E** and **F,** Uterus after initiation of oxytocin therapy.

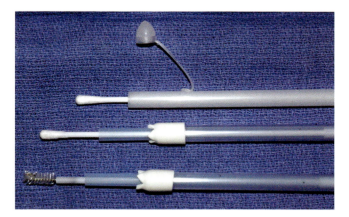

Figure 8-3 *Top,* Single-guarded uterine swab with "pop-out" cap that can be used to collect material of endometrial cytology. *Middle,* Double-guarded swab for endometrial culture and cytology. *Bottom,* Double-guarded endometrial brush for cytology.

inflammation.[112,123] Culture from uterine lavage efflux is particularly helpful in the detection of *E. coli* infection. A large clinical trial involving 2123 mares showed a superiority of uterine cytology compared to uterine culture for the diagnosis of endometritis.[121] The pregnancy rate at 28 days was 60% for mares with 0 to 2 neutrophils per 400× field and only 36% and

23% for mares with 2 to 5 neutrophils and more than 5 neutrophils, respectively.[121] Bacteriologic culture and cytology from endometrial biopsy are most accurate (high sensitivity and positive predictive value) for diagnosis of endometritis. The sensitivity of bacteriologic culture from endometrial biopsy is 82%; diagnosis based on cytologic and bacteriologic examination of endometrial swabs has a sensitivity of 77% and 34%, respectively.[41,122]

Therapy

Treatment of equine endometritis may include local or systemic antimicrobial therapy, uterine lavage, plasma infusion, and colostrum infusion. Most treatment recommendations are made on the basis of clinical experience, with limited evidence for comparative efficacy within the veterinary literature. The authors most frequently recommend treatment of uterine infections with uterine lavage to remove debris and other products of inflammation that may reduce antimicrobial activity, followed by antimicrobial therapy for 5 to 7 days.

Uterine Lavage

The goal of uterine lavage is to "clean" the uterine cavity of organisms, dead neutrophils, cell debris, and products of inflammation before local antimicrobial therapy.[124-126] Uterine lavage may enhance uterine contractions and clearance as a result of transient irritation of the endometrium.[127] Uterine lavage is performed using warmed, balanced electrolyte solution (e.g., lactated Ringer's, physiologic saline) with or without added

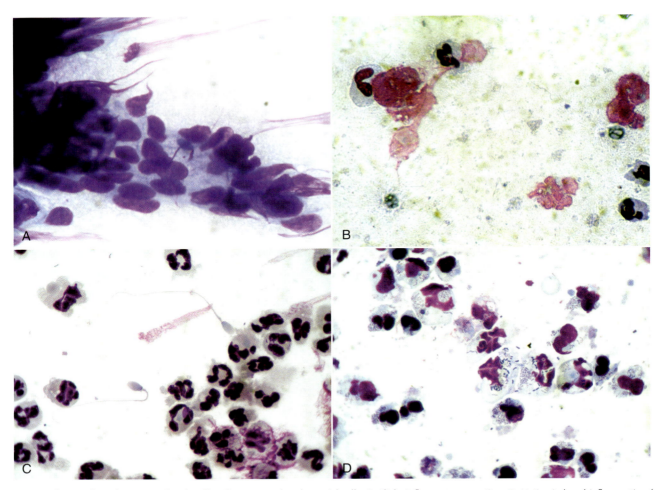

Figure 8-4 Endometrial cytology stained with Diff-Quik. **A,** Normal endometrial cells. **B,** Slight inflammatory reaction. **C,** Mating-induced inflammation (note sperm cells). **D,** Severe infectious inflammation consisting of neutrophils and some mononuclear cells. Intracellular bacteria are present.

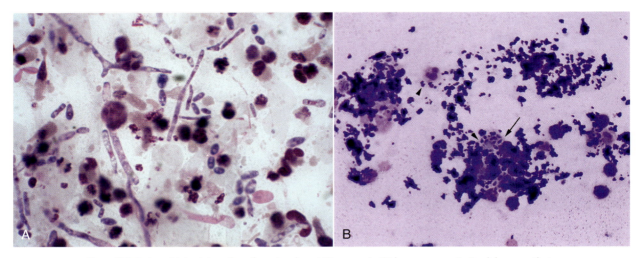

Figure 8-5 Endometrial cytology from fungal endometritis cases. **A,** *Trichosporon* spp. **B,** *Candida parapsilosis*.

antiseptics. A solution specifically formulated for flushing of the equine uterus (Equine Uterine Flush, Bioniche Animal Health, Pullman, WA) is adjusted to appropriate pH and osmotic pressure and contains surfactants to aid in the removal of organisms and debris. Uterine lavage is preferably performed using a large Foley catheter in the same manner as for embryo collection (Table 8-1).

The addition of antiseptics, such as povidone-iodine or chlorhexidine, to uterine lavage fluid is occasionally recommended for the treatment of equine endometritis. At high concentration, however, antiseptics may cause severe inflammation (necrosis) and irreversible damage to the endometrium, with evidence of discomfort at the time of infusion.[128] Povidone-iodine solution may be used at a concentration of 0.05% (5 mL

Table 8-1 Guidelines for Uterine Flushing and High-Volume Uterine Lavage

Uterine Flushing	High-Volume Lavage (Postpartum)
Indications	
Chronic endometritis, pyometra	Partial or total placental retention
Endometritis	Metritis
Persistent mating-induced endometritis	After obstetric manipulations/ fetotomy
	After uterine prolapse
Equipment	
Silicone Foley long catheter (37 or 34 French, 100-mL cuff)	Nasogastric tube; make sure that tube has several side openings (1-1.5 cm in diameter)
Flushing bag (2.5 L)	Bucket
	Nasogastric tube pump
Mare Preparation	
Sedation if needed	Sedation often needed
Wrap tail in plastic sleeve	Wrap tail in plastic sleeve
Palpation per rectum to evacuate feces	Palpation per rectum to evacuate feces
Clean perineal area and vulva	Clean perineal area and vulva
Place catheter using sterile sleeve and lubricate	Place nasogastric tube deep into uterine cavity (within chorioallantoic cavity if placenta is retained)
Insert catheter into cervix and inflate balloon, making sure it is snug against anterior cervical os	Protect side openings of tube by cuffing hand around it
Fluid Choice	
Warm saline (least preferred)	Warm saline
Warm lactated Ringer's solution (LRS)	Warm distilled water preferred
Proprietary fluid (e.g., Equine Uterine Flush lavage solution)	Warm LRS (may be too expensive)
	Warm tap water with 5 mL of 10% povidone-iodine solution and 8.5 g of table salt per liter
Fluid Delivery and Monitoring	
Gravity using flushing bags	Pumped directly into uterine cavity
Volume varies from 500 mL to 2 L	Up to 15 L (depends on size of uterus)
Palpate transrectally to make sure that both uterine horns are sufficiently distended before emptying	Flush twice a day if mare has retained placenta or mare is systemically ill
Repeat flushing until return is clear	Repeat flushing daily as needed (until retained placenta is passed)
Monitor fluid retained by ultrasonography or measuring fluid collected	Monitor by transabdominal ultrasound
Evacuation Help	
Before and after flushing: oxytocin (10-20 IU IV and/ or IM	Retained placenta: oxytocin (20 IU every 4 hours [q4h] IM in the first 12 hours postpartum)
Postbreeding flushing should be started no earlier than 4 hours after breeding	Exercise mare

IV, Intravenous; *IM,* intramuscular.

of 10% povidone iodine solution in 1 L of balanced salt solution) to facilitate elimination of bacterial infection. Adverse reactions are observed in mares after infusion with solution at a concentration of 1% or more.[129] Uterine lavage with 0.05% solution of povidone-iodine solution 4 hours after breeding did not adversely affect pregnancy rates.[130] Uterine lavage with a 1% solution of povidone iodine on days 0 and 2 following ovulation does not induce histologic changes in normal mares but reduces expression of endometrial progesterone receptors.[131]

Use of chlorhexidine diacetate is contraindicated in mares.[132] Chlorhexidine gluconate may cause vulvar inflammation and vaginal straining at concentrations as low as 0.5% and endometrial inflammation at concentrations of 0.25%.[133]

Biofilm is a complex matrix produced by infections with some gram-negative bacteria, yeast, and fungi. Antimicrobial therapy is often unsuccessful in the presence of biofilm,[134,135] possibly because of inactivation of the drug, reduction of its penetration ability, or by the maintenance of a small population of multidrug resistant microorganisms. The most common isolates that produce biofilm are *P. aeruginosa, Staphylococcus epidermis, E. coli, E. cloacae,* and several species of yeast and fungi.

Mares with chronic uterine inflammation or infection associated with biofilm-producing microorganisms do not respond to uterine flushing followed by antimicrobial treatment because uterine exudate and mucus interfere with antibiotic penetration. Mucolytics, such as dimethylsulfoxide (DMSO) and *N*-acetylcysteine, may be useful for treatment of these mares. Intrauterine infusion of 30% DMSO saline solution has been associated with improved biopsy grade and pregnancy rate.[112,136,137] Intrauterine infusion of 0.6% solution of *N*-acetylcysteine used in combination with conventional treatment of endometritis the cycle before breeding or 48 hours before breeding may help eliminate biofilm and inspissated secretions, as well as reduce viscosity of mucus and improve sperm transport.[112,138,139]

Pretreatment of the uterus with buffered chelating agents, such as tris-EDTA, may help to dissolve biofilm and improve antimicrobial activity.[112] Lavage with tris-EDTA (1.2 g Na EDTA and 6.05 g Tris/L of H_2O, titrated to pH 8.0 with glacial acetic acid) 3 hours before infusion of antibiotic has been recommended for treatment of persistent uterine infection with *Pseudomonas* spp. Ethylenediaminetetraacetic acid (EDTA) is thought to bind calcium in bacterial cell walls, making cell walls permeable to antibiotics and bacteria more susceptible to bactericidal activity of antibiotics.[140]

A third-generation buffered chelating agent (Tricide) increases the activity of antifungal drugs in vitro. This effect has been attributed to alteration of the cell wall by removal of divalent cations necessary for maintenance of polysaccharides in the wall. Current recommendations are to infuse 250 to 500 mL of Tricide, or tris-EDTA, into the uterus, then lavage the uterus 24 hours later. The treatment is repeated a second time if the efflux is cloudy. Antimicrobials are infused in utero starting on the third day and continued for a minimum of 5 days.[112]

Antimicrobials

The aim of local uterine infusion of antimicrobials is specifically to eliminate the causative organism[16,141-144] (Table 8-2). The choice of antibiotic is dictated by results of endometrial culture and sensitivity, predicted antimicrobial efficacy in the uterine environment, and consideration of possible adverse uterine effects. Nonbuffered or precipitating solutions should be avoided. *Streptococcus equi* subsp. *zooepidemicus* and *E. coli,* two of the most common bacterial causes of endometritis, are sensitive in vitro to amikacin and gentamicin.[21] The selection of antimicrobials for intrauterine infusion should take into account the pH and solubility of the drugs, as well as the solution used for infusion. Some antibiotics, such as ceftiofur, will lose most of their activity if diluted in a saline solution.[145] The volume of infusion should be sufficient to treat the entire uterine cavity, usually between 60 and 120 mL. Mares are preferably treated during estrus and up to 3 days postovulation. Duration of treatment varies from 3 to 5 days. Aqueous solutions of sodium benzylpenicillin, neomycin, polymyxin, and furaltadone are generally safe and useful for treatment of horses with acute endometritis.[116,145] Aqueous solutions of penicillin, ampicillin,

Table 8-2 Antimicrobials for in utero Treatment of Endometritis in Mares

Drug	Dose*	Comments
Gram-Positive Bacterial Infections		
Penicillin sodium or potassium salt	5 million units (U)	Very effective for *Streptococcus* spp.; economical
Ampicillin	1-3 g	Can be very irritating; use at high dilutions; sodium salt precipitates on endometrium that remains in uterus for prolonged period
Carbenicillin	2-5 g	Reserved for persistent *Pseudomonas* infections (synergistic efficacy with aminoglycosides); usually given on alternate days with aminoglycosides; slightly irritating
Gram-Negative Bacterial Infections		
Gentamicin sulfate	500-2000 mg	Highly effective; generally nonirritating when mixed with an equal volume of $NaHCO_3$ and diluted in saline
Amikacin sulfate	2 g	Use for *Pseudomonas* spp., *Klebsiella* spp., and persistent gram-negative infections
Kanamycin sulfate	1 g	Toxic to spermatozoa; do not use close to breeding
Polymyxin B	1 million U	Particularly effective against *Pseudomonas* spp.
Neomycin sulfate	2-4 g	Use for sensitive *E. coli*; can be irritating; do not use near time of breeding
Gram-Positive and Gram-Negative Bacterial Infections (Broad Spectrum)		
Cephazolin sodium	1 g	
Ticarcillin	1-6 g	Effective for treatment of *Pseudomonas* spp.; not for *Klebsiella* spp. infections. Minimum volume 200 mL
Ticarcillin-clavulanic acid	3-6 g	Effective against *Enterobacter* spp., *S. aureus*, *B. fragilis*. Minumum volume 200 ml
Ceftiofur sodium	1 g	Can become ineffective if diluted with saline
Chloramphenicol	2-3 g	Can be irritating
Fungal (Yeast) Infections		
Nystatin	0.5-2.5 million U	Primarily for yeast (e.g., *Candida albicans*) in the growing phase; insoluble, suspend in 100-250 mL sterile water and vigorously mix immediately before infusion
Amphotericin B	100-200 mg	For infections with *Aspergillus*, *Candida*, *Mucor*, or *Histoplasma*; dilute in 100-250 mL sterile water, a relatively insoluble suspension
Clotrimazole	500-700 mg	For yeast infections (*Candida* spp.); crushed tablets mixed with 40 mL sterile water
Fluconazole	100 mg	For *Candida* spp. infections. Need to adjust the pH to avoid acidic nature
Miconazole	200-700 mg	Most effective for yeast infections (*Candida* spp.) and some resistant fungal infections; infuse once daily for up to 10 days; dilute in 40-60 mL sterile saline before infusion

carbenicillin, ticarcillin, ticarcillin and clavulanic acid, kanamycin, and neomycin have also been recommended. Low-pH antimicrobials, such as gentamicin and amikacin, should be buffered with an equal volume of 7.5% sodium bicarbonate before infusion.[132,143,146,147]

In one study, uterine infusion of enrofloxacin was an effective treatment for endometritis in 80% of 17 mares.[148] This must be pursued with caution since a recent study showed that in utero infusion of the commercial preparation Baytril at a dose of 2.5 mg/kg causes acute endometrial ulceration, necrosis, and hemorrhage.[149] Antimicrobial concentrations in endometrial tissues were greater than the minimum inhibitory concentration (MIC) for most bacterial pathogens for up to 24 hours after intrauterine infusion of enrofloxacin at a dosage of 2.5 mg/kg.[150] Moderate endometrial inflammation was observed 24 hours after infusion but resolved progressively within 2 weeks.

Treatment of fungal endometritis requires large volume uterine flushes followed by intrauterine therapy with antimycotic drugs for 7 to 10 days. Treatment for a longer duration may be required for some mares. The drugs most often used are polyene antimicrobial agents (e.g., amphotericin B, nystatin, natamycin), which alter membrane permeability, and imidazole derivatives (e.g., clotrimazole, econazole, ketoconazole, fluconazole, itraconazole), which interfere with nutrient exchange across the fungal cell wall and cell membrane.[35,142] The prognosis for fertility after treatment of fungal endometritis remains generally poor because of the histologic changes resulting from the chronic inflammation.[38]

Lufenuron, a benzoylphenyl urea derivative and inhibitor of chitin synthesis, used for flea control in dogs and cats, has been recommended for treatment of mares with *Candida parapsilosis*, *Candida paratropicalis*, and *Aspergillus fumigatus* uterine infections. The inhibition of fungal growth is thought to be caused by disruption of the chitin-rich cell wall that surrounds these organisms. Intrauterine infusion is performed with lufenuron (540 mg) suspended in 60 mL of sterile saline solution.[151]

Systemic antimicrobials (e.g., amikacin,[152] gentamicin,[153] ticarcillin,[154] procaine penicillin G, ampicillin, potentiated sulfonamides,[132] ceftiofur sodium,[155,156] and enrofloxacin[157]) may be used for the treatment of endometritis, but little is known about drug concentrations obtained within the endometrium or treatment efficacy after systemic administration (Table 8-3). Systemic treatment has the advantage of preventing inadvertent recontamination of the uterus and repeated trauma to the vagina and cervix in mares. Ciprofloxacin (2.5 g/day) and probenecid (1 g/day) were recommended for systemic treatment of *Pseudomonas* infection.[147] Although an oral dose of ciprofloxacin of 0.5 mg/kg has been used by some practitioners,[158] pharmacokinetic studies have shown that bioavailability of the drug is not very high.[159] Fluoroquinolone antibiotics, such as enrofloxacin and ciprofloxacin, reach therapeutic concentrations in endometrial tissue after intravenous (IV) administration.[160,161] Endometrial concentrations of metronidazole were very low after systemic treatment for 4 days.[162] Enrofloxacin was used systemically for the prevention and treatment of endometritis.[157]

Plasma Infusion

Intrauterine infusion of autogenous plasma (100 mL) anticoagulated with heparin or sodium citrate is suggested to enhance neutrophil function in endometritis-susceptible mares.[61,80] Some clinical trials showed significant benefit with this approach,[80,84,124,163] whereas others were unable to show enhanced bactericidal activity after plasma infusion.[126,164,165] Infusion of plasma with leukocytes may improve pregnancy rate compared with infusion of plasma alone.[166] The discrepancies between results may be caused by several factors, including the strain of bacteria and the amount and type of antibodies present

Table 8-3 Antimicrobials Used for Systemic Treatment of Uterine Infection in Mares

Drug	Dose	Remark
Antibacterials		
Amikacin sulfate	10 mg/kg, IV or IM, SID	Gram negative coverage
Ampicillin Na	29 mg/kg, IV or IM, BID	Gram positive coverage and to treat *E. coli* infections
Ceftiofur	2.5 mg/kg, IM, BID or SID	Broad spectrum
Gentamicin	6.6 mg/kg, IV, SID	Slow infusion. Effective to treat *Enterobacter* spp., *E. coli*, *Klebsiella* spp., *Proteus* spp., *Serratia* spp., *P. aeruginosa*, *S. aureus*
Enrofloxacin	5.5 mg/kg, IV, SID	Slow IV infusion; Effective against Gram-negative infections caused by susceptible bacteria resistant to alternative antibiotics
Penicillin G (Potassium)	25,000 IU/kg, IV, QID	Effective against *S. equi* subsp. *zooepidemicus*
Penicillin procaine	25,000 IU/kg, IM, BID	
Trimethoprim-sulfonamides	30 mg/kg, PO, BID	Effective against *S. aureus*, *E. coli*, *Klebsiella* spp., *Proteus*
Meteronidazole	15-25 mg/kg, PO, BID	Effective against *Bacteroides fragilis* metritis
Antifungals		
Amphotericin B	0.3-0.9 mg/kg, IV, SID	Slow IV infusion
Fluconazole	14 mg/kg loading dose; then 5 mg/kg IV or PO SID	
Itraconazole	5 mg/kg IV or PO, SID or BID	

in plasma. Infusion of serum from horses hyperimmunized against specific strains of *S. equi* subsp. *zooepidemicus* is reportedly more effective in increasing phagocytosis than the infusion of nonimmune serum.[167]

Colostrum Infusion

The goal of colostrum infusion is to enhance the local uterine defense mechanisms by increasing the concentration of immunoglobulins in the uterine cavity. This treatment is reported to be successful in uncontrolled studies.[168,169]

Prevention

Prevention of uterine infection is accomplished by decreasing the likelihood of contamination and by early recognition and treatment of PMIE. Contamination of the uterus can be prevented by correcting vulvar conformation and observing strict hygiene during breeding and genital manipulation. Susceptible mares should be monitored before breeding and bred using minimum-contamination breeding techniques.[170] The purpose of this monitoring is to reduce the chance of contamination of the uterus by bacteria and to eliminate the products of the inflammatory reaction caused by semen.

The primary mechanism for prevention of fluid accumulation in the uterus is contraction of the uterine musculature in response to oxytocin. Oxytocin release is observed in mares after mating, teasing, genital manipulation, and infusion of fluid into the uterine cavity.[92,171,172] Oxytocin injection improves uterine defense by promoting uterine fluid evacuation.[116,164,173,174] Administration of 20 IU of oxytocin intramuscularly (IM) induces uterine contraction for up to 90 minutes.[88] Oxytocin administration to mares susceptible to PMIE at 4 hours after breeding aids in the elimination of excess fluid and improves fertility.[114,116,175] The standard dose for an average mare is 10 IU IV or 20 to 25 IU IM.* Large doses may decrease uterine contractions.[88,176] Oxytocin therapy may be repeated every 6 hours for 24 to 48 hours after breeding.[89,117] A 7% increase in pregnancy rate is reported with a single injection of oxytocin (25 IU IM) within 72 hours of breeding.[116] Oxytocin does not interfere with ovulation or gamete transport if administered no earlier than 4 hours after breeding.[88,177] A long-acting synthetic oxytocin analog, carbetocin, has a half-life of 17 minutes, which is 2.5 times that of oxytocin.[178,179] Carbetocin may be used in place of oxytocin if more prolonged uterine contractions are desired.[180]

Prebreeding and postbreeding uterine lavage may be indicated in mares that tend to accumulate a substantial amount of fluid during estrus.[129,130,181,182]

Prostaglandin $F_{2\alpha}$ ($PGF_{2\alpha}$; 5-10 mg IM) or its analog, cloprostenol (250 µg IM), is recommended for the treatment of mares with PMIE because of its ecbolic properties.[89,94,177,183] Cloprostenol induces weaker but more sustained uterine contractions than oxytocin and is helpful when excessive uterine edema is present.[184] Repeated administration of cloprostenol should be avoided because it has been associated with transient reduction of circulating progesterone levels during diestrus.[89,177]

Prophylactic in utero administration of antibiotics to PMIE-susceptible mares after breeding has been suggested. A combination of oxytocin treatment and intrauterine infusion of broad-spectrum antibiotics increases pregnancy rates in susceptible mares.[116,185] However, such an approach may pose some risk of development of antimicrobial resistance.

Recurrent intrauterine fluid accumulation may be due to cervical abnormalities. This is often the case in old maiden mares that have a very tight cervix. Fluid accumulation prebreeding and postbreeding predisposes these mares to the development of endometritis. Application of the synthetic prostaglandin E1 (PGE1), misoprostol (1 to 2 mg), to the cervix promotes cervical dilation and helps with uterine drainage.[186-188]

Modulation of the immune response of the uterus may be helpful in prevention of postmating endometritis in some mares and mares suffering from metabolic disorders (i.e., equine metabolic syndrome). It is unclear whether administration of corticosteroids (10-50 mg dexamethasone IV[189,190]) after ovulation or insemination will improve pregnancy rates in mares with a history of postbreeding fluid accumulation in the uterus. Although repeated administration of dexamethasone during estrus has been associated with luteinizing hormone (LH)-surge suppression and increased ovulation failure rate,[191] a single treatment does not seem to have any negative effect on ovulation or polymorphonuclear neutrophil (PMN) function.[192,193] Improvement in pregnancy rates has been observed in PMIE-susceptible mares following administration of acetate 9-alpha-prednisolone (0.1 mg/kg, twice a day [BID]) for 4 days starting 48 hours before breeding.[194] It is important to keep in mind that these treatments are an adjunct to prevention of endometritis and steroids should not be used to control inflammation in mares that already have an established uterine infection.

Mares with a history of PMIE may benefit from administration of nonsteroidal antiinflammatory drugs before and after

*References 88, 110, 111, 116, 117, 176.

insemination.[195] A variety of immunomodulators have also been used in attempts to increase pregnancy rates in mares.[70,196-199]

Alternative complementary techniques used to prevent or treat chronic endometritis include electroacupuncture, which has been reported to improve uterine tone and drainage of fluid. However, further research is needed in this area.[200]

Preventive therapeutic measures used preinsemination and postinsemination are often not sufficient. Some mares should undergo extensive surgical correction of the perineal conformation (i.e., urethral extension, episioplasty). A laparoscopic uteropexy technique to restore normal position and improve uterine clearance in mares with a pendulous uterus has been described recently.[201]

Pyometra

Uterine infection may progress toward chronic pyometra, particularly in older mares and mares with severely compromised cervical function (cervical adhesions), vaginal adhesions, or with poor perineal conformation and recurrent urine pooling.[202] Pyometra may develop as the result of severe vaginal adhesions following lengthy obstetric manipulations.[203,204] Isolates from pyometra are similar to those described for infectious endometritis.[202] Systemic signs are rare, although some mares may have intermitent mild colic. Various amounts of vaginal discharge may be observed. The nature of discharges varies from watery to caseous (Fig. 8-6). Many cases of pyometra with complete vaginal or cervical occlusion will only be discovered

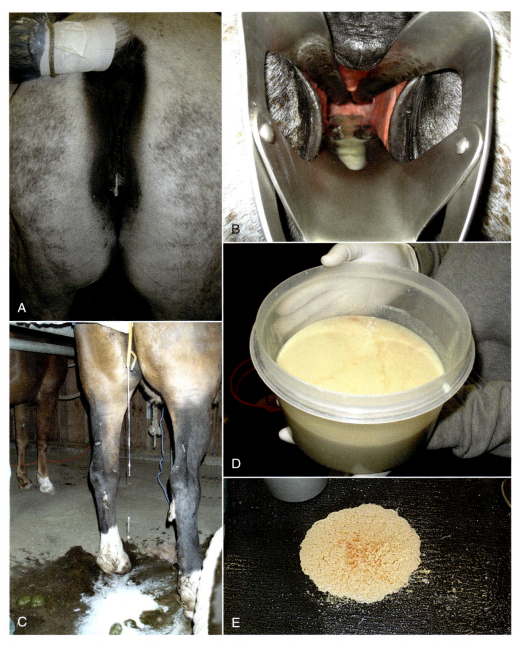

Figure 8-6 Vaginal discharge in mares with endometritis/pyometra. **A,** Discharge may be intermitent and very discrete. **B,** Discharge may not be evident until vaginoscopy. **C,** Discharge may be liquid or extremely thick **(D).** Uterine lavage with a solution of acetylcysteine is often required to liquify very thick uterine content **(E).**

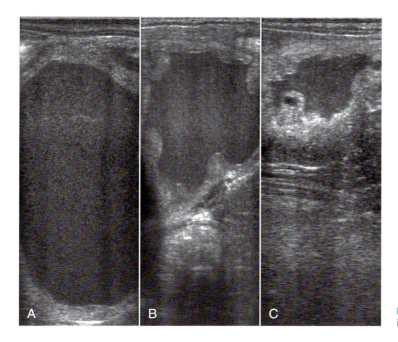

Figure 8-7 Ultrasonogram pyometra. **A,** Body of the uterus. **B,** Miduterine horn. **C,** Tip of the uterine horn.

by transrectal palpation or ultrasonography (Fig. 8-7). Mares with severe chronic pyometra have a very poor prognosis for carrying a pregnancy to term and treatment is often unrewarding. Ovariohysterectomy is often the best approach and should be attempted after uterine lavage with antiseptics.[205-207]

Postpartum Metritis

Postpartum uterine infections are of particular importance because of their severity and effect on the general health of the mare. Septic postpartum metritis accounts for 8% of postpartum emergencies.[208] It is often a result of nonhygienic manipulation during foaling, obstetric manipulations, or retained placenta. Postpartum septic metritis is often associated with gram-negative bacteria such as *E. coli* and *K. pneumoniae*.[209] Mares with postpartum metritis may present with severe systemic complications of endotoxemia and laminitis.[210] Treatment consisting of daily large-volume uterine lavage with warm fluids, systemic antimicrobial therapy (potassium penicillin 22,000 IU/kg, every 6 hours [q6h] IV and gentamicin sulfate 6.6 mg/kg q24h IV), and appropriate therapy for systemic inflammatory response syndrome (see Chapter 11).[208,210-212]

Other Infections of Nonpregnant Mares

Infectious vaginitis and cervicitis may occur as part of the uterine infection process or as a result of local irritation or laceration. Vaginal injuries secondary to breeding or parturition may lead to necrotic vaginitis, abscess formation, and adhesions.[213-217]

Infectious inflammation of the ovaries (oophoritis) with abscessation and peritoneal adhesions may occur after abdominal surgery or peritonitis (Fig. 8-8). Oophoritis may also occur as a consequence of repeated transvaginal ultrasound-guided follicular aspiration.[218] Affected mares may present with abdominal pain, anorexia, fever of unknown origin, and weight loss. Transrectal ultrasonography may help in the diagnosis of these infections. Confirmation of the diagnosis and evaluation of the extent of the lesions may be achieved by laparoscopy. Ovariectomy is usually required for treatment of this condition.[219,220]

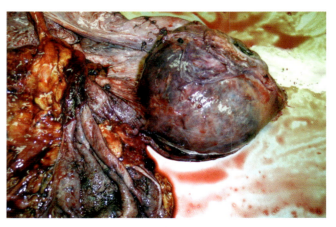

Figure 8-8 Ovarian abscess and adhesions.

Salpingitis is rare in the mare but may result from ascending infection from the uterus after parturition.[219] Salpingitis has been described in mares with contagious equine metritis (CEM)[221] (see Chapter 38). Bilateral salpingitis results in sterility.

Infectious Causes of Abortion

Causes of equine abortion in several countries have been extensively reviewed (United Kingdom,[222-225] United States,[226-232] France,[233-235] Egypt,[214] India[236]). One-third to half of all equine abortions are estimated to be the result of infection.[224] Numerous organisms have been associated with infectious abortion, including viruses, bacteria, and fungi.[234] The prevalence of each organism differs geographically. In England, equine herpesvirus abortion predominates.[224] In France, 79% of infectious abortions are caused by bacteria and 21% by viruses.[233,234] However, the epidemiology of infectious abortion is constantly changing due to introduction of new vaccines and biosecurity measures and emerging infectious diseases.

Bacterial Abortions and Placentitis

Placentitis is a significant cause of equine late-term abortion, premature delivery, and neonatal death. It is implicated as a cause of abortion in as many as 50% of all mares that abort.[224,226-228,237-241] Placentitis is diagnosed in approximately 157 cases of fetal loss each year in Kentucky (approximately 30% of all submitted fetuses).[241] It may be caused by a variety of bacterial, fungal, viral, and protozoal organisms.[222,223,234,242] Bacterial placentitis is most common; fungal placentitis is reported in fewer than 10% of horses with placentitis.[224,227,228,234]

Placentitis is generally classified as three types: ascending, diffuse, and focal mucoid.[241] With the exception of *Leptospira* spp. and nocardioform infection, most bacterial or mycotic placentitis of mares is the result of an ascending infection.[232,243]

Ascendant Placentitis

Ascending placentitis is the most common type of placentitis in horses.[238,241,242] Bacteria isolated from the placenta are comparable to those isolated from the uterus of mares with endometritis.[241,244,245] *Streptococcus equi* subsp. *zooepidemicus*, *E. coli*, *P. aeruginosa*, *Enterobacter* spp., and *K. pneumoniae* are the most frequent isolates.*

In a retrospective study of 954 cases of equine abortion, placentitis was recognized in 24.7% of all submissions.[227] A bacterial or fungal organism was isolated in 68.6% of placentitis cases, and 57.4% of cases yielded bacteria from both the placenta and the fetal organs. Similarly, in a recent retrospective study on 1822 abortion submissions in France, fetoplacental infection represented 64% of the diagnoses with 80% caused by bacterial infection and only 1.8% caused by fungal infection.[234] The most common microorganisms isolated included *S. equi* subsp., *zooepidemicus*, *E. coli*, *Leptospira* spp., nocardioform *Actinomyces*, *P. aeruginosa*, *Streptococcus equisimilis*, *Enterobacter agglomerans*, *K. pneumoniae*, α-hemolytic streptococci, *Staphylococcus aureus*, and *Actinobacillus* spp.[214,233,234] Other bacteria isolated include *Proteus mirabilis*, *Citrobacter diversus*, and fecal and environmental contaminants.[227] Abortions resulting from hematogenous infection with *Actinobacillus equuli*[247] and *Corynebacterium pseudotuberculosis* have been reported.[236,248] A new species of *Arcanobacterium* (*A. hippocoleae*) has been isolated recently from a case of placentitis and stillbirth in a mare in the state of Tennessee in the United States.[249] Placentitis and funisitis caused by *Dermatophilus congolensis* has been described in one case of abortion at 9 months of gestation in a mare.[250] Isolation of more than one bacterium from cases of placentitis is not uncommon, and the most common combinations are *S. equi* subsp. *zooepidemicus* with either *K. pneumoniae* or *E. coli*.[234]

There is a wide geographic variation in the frequency of specific bacterial and fungal isolates associated with equine placentitis and abortion. The incidence of mycotic placentitis varies from region to region because of climate and other environmental factors.[234,238,251,252]

Except for placentitis caused by *Leptospira* spp. or the nocardioform actinomycetes, most equine placentitis occurs in two forms: (1) acute diffuse placentitis with infiltration of neutrophils in the intervillous spaces or (2) focal necrosis of the chorionic villi. Placentitis from abortions before midgestation are chronic, focal, or focally extensive at the cervical area and characterized by necrosis of chorionic villi, presence of eosinophilic material on the chorion, and infiltration of mononuclear inflammatory cells in the intervillous spaces, stroma of villi, chorion, allantois, and vascular layer. Lesions may be either acute or chronic.[227]

Bacterial placentitis most often induces abortion between 6 and 9 months of gestation. Placentitis resulting from *E. coli*

tends to cause later abortion and more stillbirths. Placentitis from *S. equi* subsp. *zooepidemicus* tends to be acute and focal or diffuse. In acute bacterial placentitis, the fetus is generally expelled before 8 months of pregnancy. Acute or diffuse placentitis may not be easy to recognize on gross examination of the placenta. Histologic evaluation of the allantochorion may reveal bacterial emboli with necrosis of chorionic villi or infiltration of neutrophils in the intervillous space. Chronic or focal placentitis typically results in birth of premature or weak foals or late-term abortions. Lesions tend to be located at the cervical star, where discoloration and thickening are observed (Fig. 8-9).

Escherichia coli placentitis is usually acute in mares that abort before 7 months of gestation but is more likely to be chronic and focally extensive, involving the cervical star, in mares that abort after 9 months of gestation. Placental edema and the presence of a white mucoid exudate on the chorion and fetal surface are common findings after abortion caused by *E. coli* placentitis (Fig. 8-10).

Pseudomonas aeruginosa placentitis causes abortion between 6 and 9 months of gestation. It is usually acute and may be either focal or diffuse with a thickened and discolored cervical star. Histologically, the primary abnormality is ulceration of the chorion with infiltration of neutrophils in the villi, chorionic stroma, and vascular layer.

Gross and histologic features of mycotic placentitis were described in detail by Hong et al.[227] Mycotic placentitis and abortion are most likely to occur in the late gestational period. Fungal organisms associated with equine abortion include *Aspergillus* spp.,[228,234,236,253,254] mucoraceous fungi, *Histoplasma caspulatum*,[226,232,241,255,256] *Candida* spp.,[40,241,257] *Mucor* spp.,[234,236] *Coccidioides* spp.,[258-260] and *Cryptococcus neoformans*.[42,261,262]

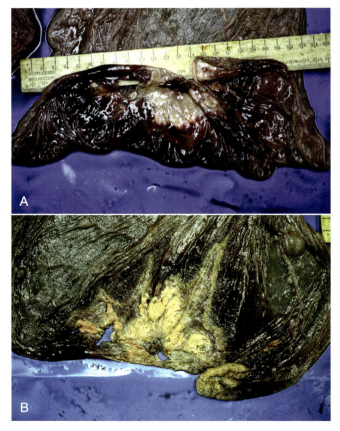

Figure 8-9 Placenta showing severe ascendant placentitis. **A,** Allantoic surface. **B,** Chorionic surface.

---

*References 225, 230, 240, 242, 244, 246.

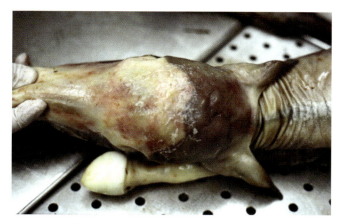

Figure 8-10 *Escherichia coli* abortion. White mucoid exudate on surface of fetal head.

Focally extensive placentitis is usually observed at the cervical star and adjacent area as a thick, leathery area. Histologically, except for histoplasmosis and candidiasis, the fungi induce a chronic, extensive placentitis characterized by extensive necrosis of the chorionic villi; neovascularization in the chorionic stroma; infiltration of neutrophils, mononuclear cells, or mixed inflammatory cells in the villi and chorionic stroma; and presence of fungal hyphae in the necrotic debris. Adenomatous hyperplasia with or without squamous metaplasia of the chorionic epithelium is frequently observed.[227] *Histoplasma capsulatum* caused a multifocal granulomatous placentitis and abortion in one mare in the seventh month of gestation and in three mares in the tenth month. Four newborn foals died from severe granulomatous pneumonia within a few days of birth, and a weanling Thoroughbred developed granulomatous pneumonia and lymphadenitis at 5 months of age.[263]

With *Candida* spp. infection, placentitis is generally diffuse, necrotizing, and proliferative with extracellular, yeast-like spores in the chorionic epithelium. Chronic, focally extensive placentitis is most common, with expulsion of the foal late in gestation.[227]

Hematogenous Multifocal or Diffuse Placentitis

Multifocal or diffuse placentitis is less common than acute, focal placentitis and is usually a result of hematogenous spread of microorganisms to the uterus. This occurs with leptospirosis, salmonellosis, histoplasmosis, and candidiasis. A special focal mucoid form of placentitis, nocardioform placentitis, is emerging as common in several U.S. regions.[227]

Leptospira spp. Placentitis

Leptospira spp. placentitis is characterized by diffuse lesions secondary to hematogenous spread (see Chapter 32). In one retrospective study, *Leptospira* spp. were isolated in 16% of 364 cases of placentitis.[240] Leptospirosis as a cause of placentitis seems to be more frequently diagnosed in Kentucky and South America[227,241,264,265] than in other regions of the world.[225,234,237,266-268] An outbreak of leptospiral abortions has been described on a Thoroughbred farm in California after a flood.[269] In North America the most common isolate is *L. interrogans* serovar *Pomona* type *kennewicki*, which is carried by several wildlife species, including the striped skunk, raccoon, whitetail deer, and opossum.[270] *Leptospira interrogans* serovar *Bratislava* has been reported as a possible cause of abortion without systemic illness in Brazil.[271,272]

Most leptospiral abortions occur between 6 and 9 months of gestation. The affected placenta is thick, heavy, edematous,

hemorrhagic, and occasionally covered with a brown mucoid material on the chorionic surface. Occasionally the affected placenta lacks detectable gross lesions. Green discoloration or cystic adenomatous hyperplasia of the allantois is observed in some cases. Funisitis, inflammation of the umbilical cord, has also been described in leptospiral abortion.[268,273] The fetus may present with mild to moderate icterus and liver enlargement. Fetal histopathologic lesions may include various degrees of nephritis and hepatitis.[266,268] Fetal antibodies against *Leptospira* spp. may be detected in foals by microagglutination test.[227] Spirochetes are present in large numbers in the placental sections.[266] Several serovars of *Leptospira* have been isolated from aborted equine fetuses.* Organisms may also be identified by immunohistochemistry or by PCR.[266,270] High-titer agglutinating antibody (>6400) may be observed in mares, but interpretation of serologic tests remains difficult without confirmation of infection by culture and isolation. Antibiotic treatment (oxytetracycline 5 mg/kg IV once a day [SID] or penicillin G 20,000 IU/kg IM BID) for 5 to 10 days has been reported to help prevent abortion during an outbreak.[269,281] *Leptospira* spp. have been detected by polymerase chain reaction (PCR) in ejaculates of a stallion. This observation merits further investigation on potential legal and health implications.[282]

Nocardioform Placentitis

Nocardioform placentitis is a distinct type of equine placentitis first described in the United States in the late 1980s. Over the past 15 years an increasing number of cases of equine nocardioform placentitis have been diagnosed in Kentucky.[226,228,240,241,283] Nocardioform placentitis may result in abortion, stillbirth, or birth of term weak foals. Some mares may exhibit premature mammary gland development and lactation before abortion.[240,284]

Nocardioform actinomycetes induce a chronic placentitis that results in late-term abortion, stillbirth, or premature birth. The lesion is an extensive and severe exudative, mucopurulent, and necrotizing placentitis centered on the junction of the placental body and horns rather than the cervical pole.[227] Infection of the placenta is generally thought to be a sequela of the hematogenous spread of the microorganisms from a primary port of entry.[283,285] The fetus is often severely underdeveloped as a result of placental insufficiency and does not show any remarkable gross or histologic lesions.[240] The placental lesion is focally extensive (15-30 cm) and frequently located at the base of the uterine horns or at the junction between the body and horns of the placenta. The affected area is thickened, and its chorionic surface is covered with brown, necrotic, mucopurulent exudate and dotted with white or yellow granular structures. Underneath this mucoid material, the chorionic surface is reddish white, mottled, and roughened. Villous necrosis and adenomatous hyperplasia of the allantoic epithelium and hyperplasia with or without squamous metaplasia of the chorionic epithelium are frequently observed.[227,286]

Various groups of gram-positive, filamentous, branching bacteria have been implicated as etiologic agents in mares with nocardioform placentitis, including *Nocardia* spp., *Rhodococcus rubropertinctus*, and *Amycolatopsis* spp.[228,285,287,288] However, most severe infections of this type are caused by the actinomycete *Crossiella equi*.[289]

During the 2002 and 2003 foaling seasons, *Cellulosimicrobium (Cellumonas) cellulans* (formerly *Oerskovia xanthineolytica*) was isolated from fetal tissues or placentas from cases of equine abortion, premature birth, and term pregnancies in Kentucky. Significant pathologic findings included chronic placentitis and pyogranulomatous pneumonia. In addition, microscopic

---

*References 226, 228, 241, 248, 264, 267-269, 274-280.

and macroscopic alterations in the allantochorion from four of seven cases of placentitis were similar to those caused by *Crossiella equi* and other nocardioform bacteria.[290] A review of placentitis cases from Kentucky showed that some bacterial isolates (*Pantonea agglomerans*, *Cellulosimicrobium cellulans*, *Pseudomonas* spp., *Enterobacter* spp., *Enterococcus* spp., and *Staphylococcus* spp.) produce placental gross lesions indistinguishable from nocardioform placentitis.[240]

Pathogenesis and Diagnosis of Placentitis

Because of the importance of placentitis in the pathogenesis of bacterial abortion, experimental models for the study of ascendant placentitis have been used to gain insight into the pathogenesis of disease and provide a method to optimize diagnostic and treatment recommendations.[291-297] Bacterial infection of the chorioallantois induces an increase in expression of proinflammatory cytokines (IL-6 and IL-8) in placental tissue.[298] Subsequent release of PGE_2 and $PGF_{2\alpha}$ into the allantoic fluid leads to premature delivery.[292,293,296,299] The premature delivery of the fetus is most likely caused by acceleration of the fetal maturation process induced by changes in placental function. The resulting endocrine changes lead to increased uterine contractures and intrauterine pressure, causing dilation of the cervix and induction of labor. A premature increase in maternal plasma progestins may be an indication of accelerated fetal maturation or fetal stress. Foals may survive if they are near term (>305 days).[292,298,300,301]

Clinically, placentitis is suspected in mares with premature udder development or lactation and vaginal discharge. However, most mares with placentitis do not show any outward signs of infection.[241,292]

Placentitis may be diagnosed by transrectal and transabdominal ultrasound examination.[112,241,302-304] Measurement of the combined thickness of the uterus and placenta (CTUP) by transrectal ultrasonography is particularly helpful in the diagnosis and monitoring of ascendant placentitis.[303,305-311] The measurements are obtained 2.5 to 5 cm cranial to the cervical-placental junction using a 5- or 7.5-mHz linear transducer. The area measured should be on the ventral aspect of the uterine body just above the middle branch of the uterine artery (Fig. 8-11). Normal CUPT for light horses is less than 8 mm between 271 and 300 days of gestation, less than 10 mm between 301 and 330 days of gestation, and less than 12 mm from 330 days of gestation to term.[305-307,310,312] These measurements are slightly higher in Warmblood and Draft horses and lower in ponies.[302,305,312] Placental malfunction has been associated with CUPT of greater than 15 mm in horses and greater than 12 mm in ponies after 310 days of gestation.[292,302] In a study on 106 thoroughbred mares over 3 seasons, routine transrectal evaluation showed abnormal CUPT in 15% of the pregnancies despite absence of any outward sign (vaginal discharge, premature lactation), which allowed early initiation of treatment and improvement of outcome.[313]

During ultrasonographic evaluation, other features of infectious placentitis may be identified. These include placental separation, accumulation of purulent hyperechoic heterogenous fluid between the endometrium and the placenta, and increased echogenicity of fetal fluid. Increased echogenicity of fetal fluid is caused by meconium, inflammatory debris, and hemorrhage.[292]

Transabdominal ultrasonographic evaluation allows assessment of fetal well-being, as well as areas of the placenta near the body and the uterine horns. Fetal biophysical profile should include fetal heart rate at rest and during activity, quality of fetal fluid, and placental membrane integrity. Features of placentitis include increased CUPT, increasing areas of placental edema or separation, fetal tachycardia (>130 bpm) or bradycardia (<50 bpm), fetal cardiac dysrhythmia, decreased fetal activity and tone, and increased fetal fluid echogenicity (cellular debris and meconium staining).[302,303,314,315]

Endocrinologic evaluation may also help in determining placental pathology and risk for abortion. The most important hormones evaluated are progestins, which are relatively stable during a normal pregnancy. A change in serum progestin concentration (increase or decrease) by more than 50% or a value that is constantly out of the laboratory reference range signals placental pathology or fetal stress.[292,316] Total progestins tend to decrease in aborting mares within 7 days, whereas an increase is observed in chronic cases.[317] Levels of total estrogens below 1000 pg/mL between day 150 and 280 days of pregnancy are associated with a higher risk of abortion.[318]

After abortion or premature birth, most cases of chronic placentitis are easily recognized on gross examination, but microscopic histologic examination is important to determine

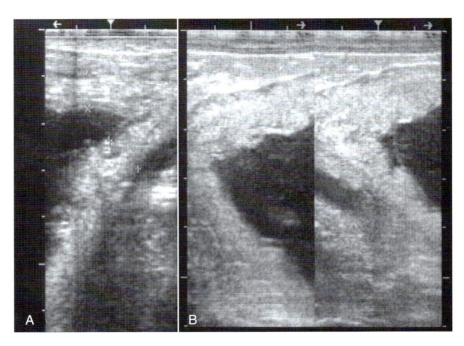

Figure 8-11 Ultrasonogram showing area of measurement of combined uteroplacental thickness. **A,** Normal. **B,** Slightly thickened.

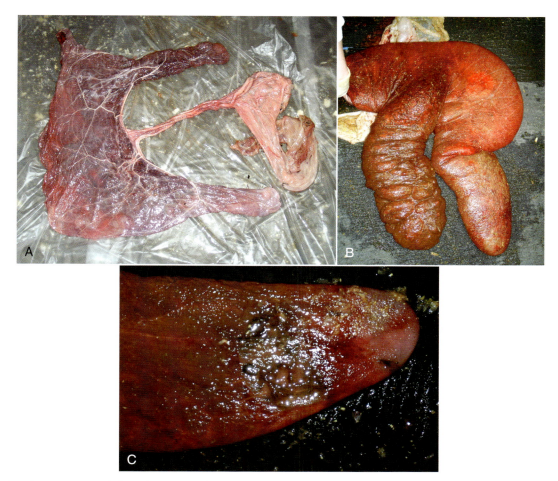

Figure 8-12 Equine placenta. **A,** Normal allantochorionic membrane (fetal side). **B,** Normal allantochorion, uterine side (after distention with water). **C,** Necrotic changes in allantochorion caused by placentitis.

the presence of acute placentitis[224] (Fig. 8-12). In acute placentitis, the infection may be contained within the placenta, and the fetus is usually sterile. Some foals may be born alive with neonatal septicemia.[224]

Treatment of Placentitis

The ultimate goal in treatment of equine placentitis is to maintain gestation for as long as possible to enhance foal viability.[241,295] Treatment recommendations include tocolytic drugs to reduce uterine contraction, antiinflammatory drugs to block the production of cytokines and prostaglandins, and antimicrobial therapy to control growth of bacteria.*

Antimicrobial therapy should be based on culture and sensitivity patterns of bacteria isolated from vaginal discharge or cervical swabs. Pharmacologic studies have shown that potentiated sulfonamides, gentamicin, potassium penicillin, and ceftiofur can cross the placenta and reach MICs sufficient to control *S. equi* subsp. *zooepidemicus* (penicillin G 22,000 IU/kg q6h IV) and *E. coli* or *K. pneumoniae* (gentamicin 6.6 mg/kg q24h IV).[292,321,322] Trimethoprim-sulfamethoxazole (30 mg/kg q12h orally [PO]) presents an excellent choice for the treatment of placentitis caused by susceptible organisms because of its good uterine penetration.[292,319,321-323]

Antiinflammatory therapy is recommended for mares with placentitis to diminish the effects of proinflammatory cytokines and prostaglandins. The most frequently used medications are nonsteroidal antiinflammatory drugs (NSAIDs) such as flunixin meglumine (0.5-1.1 mg/kg BID PO or IV). Pentoxifylline has also been recommended (8.5 mg/kg q12h PO).[292,295,299,319,324]

Induction of uterine quiescence is obtained by administration of progestins to interfere with upregulation of prostaglandin and oxytocin and reduce myometrial activity. The oral synthetic progestin, altrenogest, is used at the label dose (0.044 mg/kg PO q12-24h) or two times the label dose (0.088 mg/kg PO q24h).[241] Alternatively, progesterone in oil can be administered at 300 mg IM q24h.[292,295,319] Long-acting progesterone formulations (one injection lasting 12 or 30 days) are available through compounding pharmacies but have not been thoroughly evaluated for use in mares with placentitis.[325]

In a report on 29 cases of mares with placentitis, 55% of the foals were born healthy but small between 311 to 347 days of gestation while the remaining 13 foals were compromised at birth (pregnancy length ranging from 299 to 355 days). In an Australian study of foals admitted to an intensive care unit, foals from mares with placentitis were significantly more likely to be born at less than 320 days gestation and be diagnosed with perinatal asphyxia syndrome but had similar survival rates and discharge time as others.[326] In another study of 108 foals from mares with placentitis, treatment as outlined previously reduced the risk for development of neonatal encephalitis, neonatal nephropathy, and neonatal enteropathy.[327]

---

*References 112, 292, 295, 303, 319, 320.

Diagnostic Approach for Equine Abortion

A precise diagnosis should be pursued in any case of abortion, premature birth, or birth of a compromised or septicemic foal. Diagnosis of the cause of abortion or in utero infection can be made in most cases with proper history, clinical observations, and collection and submission of all required samples. In one study, only 7.7% of equine abortions, stillbirths, or neonatal foal loss remained undiagnosed when the fetus, placenta, and serum from the dam were submitted.[224] The undiagnosed cases were associated with extensive damage to tissues by scavengers, as well as absence of placenta or early abortion. Samples from the dam should include serum and vaginal or uterine swab.

The importance of placental examination in the diagnosis of abortion, stillbirths, or premature births cannot be overemphasized. Normal and abnormal characteristics of the placenta and descriptions of proper examination of the equine placenta and its pathology have been described elsewhere.[239,328-331] Clients should be instructed to obtain the placenta for proper examination as soon as possible after each foaling. Weight of the placenta should be determined; normal placental weight is approximately 11% of the foal weight. The placenta is usually expelled inside out with the allantoic surface exposed (see Fig. 8-12). It should be gently cleaned of any bedding material, grass, or dirt with cold water, then laid out flat and all surfaces examined. The umbilical cord should be of normal length. The amniotic sac and chorionic surface (red velvety surface) is examined from the cervical star to the tips of the horns on all sides. Samples should be obtained from areas of grossly normal and abnormal placenta and submitted for histopathology, immunohistochemistry, and culture. Some morphologic characteristics of the placenta may allow immediate exclusion of infectious causes of abortion (e.g., umbilical cord torsion, body pregnancy, twin pregnancies). Chronic infectious inflammation is generally easy to detect because of the thick, leathery nature of the placenta. Lesions of placentitis appear tan or brown and thick and may have overlying tenacious, fibrinonecrotic exudate. Cytologic evaluation of a contact smear may reveal inflammatory cells and responsible organisms. Lesions of ascending placentitis are usually located on the cervical star, whereas hematogenous placentitis, as in leptospirosis, may cause diffuse lesions. Nocardioform placentitis has characteristic lesions on the cranial ventral uterine body.

Although it is possible to perform fetal or neonatal necropsy in the field when necessary, it is preferred that the entire carcass be sent to a diagnostic laboratory if possible. If fetal necropsy is performed in the field, proper precautions should be taken to document lesions, prevent contamination, and obtain appropriate samples. Fetal blood samples, as well as pleural and peritoneal fluids, should be obtained. Stomach contents provide an excellent sample for bacteriology. Tissue samples from any abnormal-appearing tissues and from all major organs (e.g., liver, lung, kidney, adrenal gland, placenta, heart, thymus, brain, spleen, small intestine) should be submitted for histopathologic evaluation.[16]

Viral Causes of Abortion

Equine Herpesvirus

Despite the widespread use of inactivated and live herpesvirus vaccines, equine herpesvirus (EHV) remains a common cause of equine abortion[332-335] Herpesviruses and the diseases they cause in horses are discussed in detail in Chapter 14. Equine herpesvirus type 1 (EHV-1) abortion storms continue to be reported in various areas of the world.[16,333,335-339]

The most common cause of equine herpesvirus abortion is EHV-1, although EHV-4 has also been isolated from some equine abortion cases. Both viruses cause similar lesions in the liver and lung; evaluation of the spleen is particularly useful for identification of red pulp necrosis caused by EHV-4.[340] Traditionally, abortions have been attributed primarily to nonneuropathogenic EHV-1; however, recently, neuropathogenic strains of EHV-1 have been detected in association with abortion.[341,342] Other equine herpesviruses (EHV-2 and EHV-5) have also been reported in a few cases of equine abortions.[343] Regardless of which herpesvirus is involved, the pathogenesis of abortion is attributed to vascular necrosis.[332,334,344-347] Viral nucleic acid can be demonstrated in endothelial cells of endometrial arterioles, within endometrial glands, and within placental microcotyledonary infarctions.[335,348] Transplacental transfer of the virus may result in a virus-positive fetus, or severe endometrial vascular pathology (vasculitis and multifocal thrombosis) may result in abortion of a virus-negative fetus.[335,347] Abortion occurs most often during the last third of pregnancy. In utero infection near term may result in the birth of a live infected foal that usually dies a few days later.[335]

For confirmation of herpesvirus abortion, antigen detection in combination with virus isolation, immunohistochemistry, or PCR on fetal lung, liver, spleen, and thymus is recommended. Virologic and serologic investigation of the mare is also recommended.[349-351]

It is important to realize that EHV-1 abortion may occur despite regular vaccination.[333] Causative factors include the mare's individual immunity, level of contamination, virulence of the viral strain, and the performance of available vaccine.[332,352] Therefore, for maximum protection, vaccination strategies should be combined with appropriate biosecurity measures to minimize the likelihood of exposure of pregnant mares to EHV.[332,353]

Vaccines for the control of respiratory diseases caused by EHV-1 have been available for several decades, and currently, more than a dozen commercial vaccines are available throughout the world.[335,354] There are also several vaccines that claim protection against abortion caused by EHV-1. These vaccines should be administered according to the manufacturer's label instructions, usually at 5, 7, and 9 months of gestation.

Management practices that should be part of an EHV abortion prevention program include maintenance of small groups of horses segregated by age and by immune and physiologic status (pregnancy status and stage). Foaling mares should be segregated from the rest of the herd. Particular attention should be given to the risk of mixing equids from different species that may carry different susceptibility or strains of EHV.[332] The most important epidemiologic risk is posed by introduction of new horses onto the farm. If introduction of new animals cannot be avoided, a 21-day quarantine is recommended.

An outbreak of EHV mandates early diagnosis of infected animals and interruption of viral transmission using strict sanitary measures for movement of personnel and animals between stables and paddocks, as well as use of disinfectants. Particular attention should be given to disposal or shipping of fetuses and placenta to appropriate diagnostic laboratories. Mating activities should preferably be halted during an active outbreak.[332]

Equine Viral Arteritis

Equine viral arteritis (EVA) is a venereal disease of horses that can result in abortion (see Chapter 15). Abortion storms have been reported as part of the clinical presentation of the disease.[355-364] Abortion rates can approach 60% in a naïve population[364] as the result of direct impairment of placental function and severe fetal infection.[355,358,365] Diagnosis can be made by viral isolation, immunohistochemistry, PCR, or serology.[366-368] Commercial enzyme-linked immunosorbent assay (ELISA) tests have proved to have very poor sensitivity (26%)

compared to the virus neutralization test, which is considered to be the gold standard for serology.[369] Aborted fetuses may show subcutaneous edema, petechial hemorrhages in the pleura and epicardium, and increases in pleural fluid volume. However, these changes are not necessarily present in all EVA abortions. Gross pathologic changes have also been reported in a few affected placentas, including placentitis and full-thickness necrosis. Other nonpathognomonic histopathologic lesions in the fetus may include vasculitis and perivasculitis in the heart, lung, and spleen; pneumonia and hemorrhage in alveoli; and inflammatory changes in the liver, spleen, and placenta. Control of the disease is based on detection of the shedding stallion(s) and vaccination.[370] The role of persistent infection in stallions in recent outbreaks in France and the United States demonstrated the importance of testing all nonvaccinated stallions before breeding or shipping of semen for artificial insemination.[371,372] The possible transmission of EVA by transfer of embryos obtained from mares inseminated with semen from pesistently infected stallions has been suggested. It is important to note that transmission of the virus was possible despite embryo washing and trypsin treatment.[373] Techniques to "clean" semen from virus-shedding stallions have been described and rely primarily on a combination of density gradient centrifugation and swim-up protocols.[125,374,375] These techniques need further evaluation and may be useful for contaminated frozen-thawed semen for in vitro production of embryos. Vaccination may be safe for healthy pregnant mares up to 3 months prior to foaling, but there is a significant risk for abortion if mares are vaccinated in the last 2 months of pregnancy.[376]

Parasitic Causes of Abortion

Abortion in mares has been associated with a variety of protozoa, including *Trypanosoma evansi*,[377] *Trypanosoma equiperdum*,[378,379] *Babesia* spp. (*Babesia caballi* and *Babesia equi* now named *Theleiria equi*),[16,380,381] and *Neospora* spp.[382] However, studies on the pathogenesis of abortion caused by these parasites are scarce. Vertical, transplacental transmission of *Theleiria equi* has been demonstrated.[383,384]

Neospora caninum, an apicomplexan protozoan parasite, has been isolated from aborted equine fetuses.[385,386] Although not statistically significant, a higher prevalence of antibodies against *N. caninum* has been reported in mares with a history of reproductive failure than in mares with normal fertility.[387] *Neospora caninum* deoxyribonucleic acid (DNA) was detected in three fetal brains, two fetal hearts, and one placenta.[382] Other studies have also suggested a relationship between fetal loss and *N. caninum* infection.[388] The identification of *N. caninum* sequences in fetal tissues is interesting, but the role of *N. caninum* in equine reproductive failure and abortion can only be speculative at present and must be further evaluated.[382,389]

Other Infections Causing Abortion

Chlamydophila

Genital chlamydiosis of horses is reported to result in mild chronic salpingitis,[390] decreased reproductive rates,[391,392] poor ejaculate quality,[393] and occasional abortion.[251,343,394-396] Detection of *Chlamydophila* organisms in aborted equine fetuses ranges from 20% to 55%.[68,396-398] However, other infectious organisms were isolated from many of the same cases, and it was not possible to determine the primary cause of abortion. Chlamydial organisms that have been isolated from horses include *Chlamydophila pneumoniae*, equine biovar, associated with respiratory diseases, and *C. abortus* and *C. psittaci*, which were identified in equine abortion cases.[343,395]

Mycoplasma

The significance of acholeplasmas and mycoplasmas in equine abortion is undetermined. *Mycoplasma* (*M. equigenitalium* and *M. subdolum*) have been isolated from the lung or liver of aborted equine fetuses.[44,48,399] *Mycoplasma bovigenitalium* was isolated from an aborted equine fetus.[400]

Other Infectious Organisms

Abortions have been associated with *Salmonella abortus equi* in horses[233,235,236,241,401-403] and donkeys,[402,404] *Shigella* spp.,[236] *Brucella abortus*,[405-407] *Brucella melitensis*,[398] and *Brucella suis*.[408] However most of these studies have been based on serology rather and lack strong scientific evidence. *Neorickettsia risticii* can be transmitted transplacentally and has also been identified as a cause of fetal resorption, abortion, and birth of weak foals in horses[409-415] (see Chapter 40). Abortion from *Aeromonas hydrophila*, a bacterium found in stagnant water, has been reported in a few horses.[416,417]

An unusual case of abortion in a 6-year-old mare has been associated with a spirochete *(Borrelia parkeri–B. turicatae)* transmitted by ticks in California.[418] The spirochete was isolated from the fetus, suggesting transplacental transmission.

During the mare reproductive loss syndrome (MRLS) outbreak in Kentucky in 2000 and 2001, isolation of nonhemolytic *Actinobacillus* spp. and α-streptococci was a common feature in tissues of aborted fetuses.[419] MRLS was characterized by two types of pregnancy loss: early fetal loss between 40 and 80 days with a few losses up to 140 days and late fetal losses between 10 months and term. Early fetal losses were characterized clinically by increased echogenicity of fetal fluids. Late pregnancy loss lesions included placentitis, funisitis, and perinatal fetal pneumonia.[420] Some authors hypothesized that the pathogenesis of MRLS implicated hematogenous spread to the fetoplacental unit of bacteria carried from the oral cavity and intestinal tract by the setae, or stiff bristle-like barbed hairs, of the exoskeleton of the Eastern tent caterpillar.[421,422]

Mastitis

Mastitis is a relatively infrequent infection in horses.[423,424] An incidence of 5% has been reported in one study.[425] It may be clinical or subclinical. Infectious organisms colonize the mammary gland tissue via hematogenous, percutaneous, or ascending routes.[425] Mastitis is generally seen in heavy-milking mares at the time of weaning but can occur in nonlactating mares and immature fillies.[426] Establishment of the infection and production of a disease state depends on the virulence of the organism and the effectiveness of the local defense mechanisms (local immunity, drainage).[427,428]

Hematogenous infection is generally a sequela of septicemia. Bacteria may also colonize the mammary gland via the teat canal or via a breach in the mammary gland integument (e.g., cutaneous neoplasia, cutaneous habronemiasis, lacerations, or insect bites).[429] Accumulation of milk in the gland predisposes it to ascending infections. Abscesses can be caused by complications of mastitis or penetrating wounds. Abscesses caused by hematogenous spread of *Corynebacterium pseudotuberculosis* have been reported.

Clinically, mastitis may be suspected when mares refuse to let the foal suckle or if the foal is losing weight. Isolation of the same organism from sick foals suggests either transmission from the foal or vice-versa.[429,430] In acute cases, mammary gland enlargement is evident and the mare may show hindlimb lameness or a stiff gait. Leukocytosis with neutrophilia and hyperfibrinogenemia may be seen in some cases. Palpation reveals a

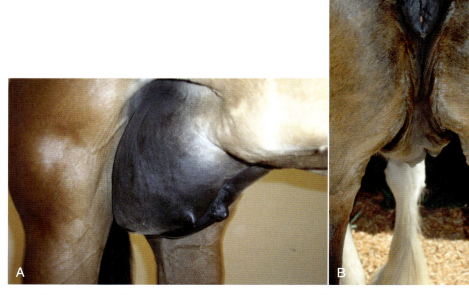

Figure 8-13 Clinical mastitis. **A,** Acute mastitis in a 12-day postpartum mare showing swelling of the mammary gland and ventral edema. **B,** Chronic in a nonlactating mare.

painful, firm udder. Ultrasonographic evaluation of the parenchyma may help identify localized lesions (i.e., abscesses). Mammary secretions may be serous, serosanguineous, hemorrhagic, or purulent. Subclinical mastitis is asymptomatic.[431] Peracute mastitis may cause an endotoxic syndrome[432] (Fig. 8-13).

The most common bacterial isolates in mammary gland mastitis include *S. equi* or *S. equi* subsp. *zooepidemicus*, *Staphylococcus aureus*, *Staphylococcus epidermis*, *Klebsiella* spp., *Pseudomonas* spp., *Corynebacterium* spp., and *E. coli.*[424,430,433-437] *Staphylococcus* infections are associated with a recurrent granulomatous mastitis (botryomycosis).[438]

Fungal (*Aspergillus* spp. and *Coccidioides immitis*) and parasitic (strongyle larval migrans and cutaneous habronemiasis) mastitis have also been described.[439,440]

Diagnosis is confirmed by examination of the mammary gland secretion. Milk may be serous to thick, flocculent, purulent, or hemorrhagic. Cytologic evaluation is important because bacteriology is negative in up to 30% of cases.[428] An increase in degenerated and nondegenerated neutrophils, as well as necrotic debris is noted in the case of mastitis (Fig. 8-14). Infectious agents may also be visualized on cytologic evaluation. Samples should be submitted for bacterial and fungal culture and sensitivity.[435,441,442]

Treatment depends on the extent of the lesions. In acute cases, systemic antiinflammatory and antibiotic therapy is warranted. Hot packing and/or hydrotherapy may help with local swelling. Frequent stripping of the mammary gland helps to eliminate infectious organisms and inflammatory products. Although intramammary infusion of lactating cow intramammary preparations has been reported, this is often difficult to perform in the mare because of the peculiar anatomy of the mammae.* Surgical drainage and flushing with antiseptic may be required in some cases. Severe cases may require unilateral or total mastectomy.[428,445]

---

*References 424, 428, 431, 435, 437, 443, 444.

Reproductive Tract Infection in Stallions

Infections of the reproductive system in stallions can present in one of two main forms: (1) infections that produce clinical signs that may incapacitate the stallion or reduce his fertility and (2) infections that are asymptomatic and may be transmitted venereally to mares (via coitus or direct semen deposition) where they produce clinical signs such as endometritis, infertility, abortion, or systemic disease.[446]

Infectious Diseases of the Prepuce and Penis

Acute inflammation of the prepuce (posthitis) and inflammation of the penis (balanitis) may occur secondary to several infectious diseases. Balanoposthitis is most often caused by coital exanthema (EHV-3 infection), dourine, or parasitic infestation (e.g., *Onchocerca* spp., *Setaria* spp., habronemiasis).[447]

Preputial abscesses may occur subsequent to bacteremia (*S. equi* subsp. *equi* or *Corynebacterium pseudotuberculosis*). In some areas of the world, *C. pseudotuberculosis* abscesses may have a seasonal incidence that parallels the increase in arthropod (vector) population[448,449] (see Chapter 45). Factors, such as a high concentration of horses and *Habronema* spp. infestation, are predisposing factors for these abscesses.[447,450,451] Treatment is generally limited to medical or surgical management of the abscess because systemic antimicrobial therapy is often unsuccessful.[449]

Several infectious diseases may cause lesions on the penis, including dourine, coital exanthema, EVA, and equine infectious anemia. Nonspecific balanitis is generally caused by superinfection with bacteria or fungus (Fig. 8-15).[447,452] Predisposing factors include increased accumulation of smegma or overzealous cleaning of the penis with disinfectants. Excessive use of antiseptic solutions may promote the destruction of the normal flora of the penile mucosa and the selection of some bacteria (e.g., *P. aeruginosa*, *K. pneumoniae*).[452,453] Treatment of nonspecific balanitis requires sexual rest and local application of an antimicrobial ointment.

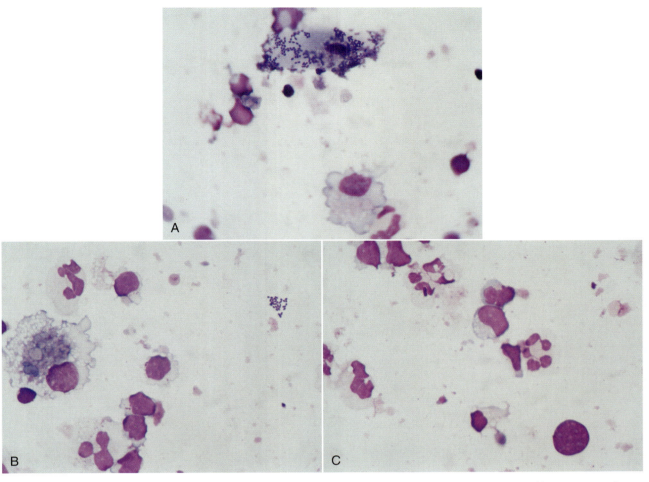

Figure 8-14 Cytology from a case of acute mastitis caused by *Streptococcus equi* subsp. *zooepidemicus*. Note the presence of bacteria, macrophages, and neutrophils.

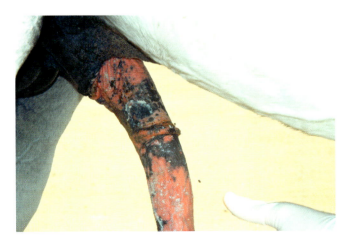

Figure 8-15 Severe nonspecific balanitis.

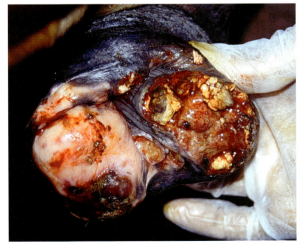

Figure 8-16 Stallion penis with habronemiasis lesions.

Coital exanthema (EHV-3) and dourine (see Chapter 60) are specific infectious processes that involve the penis and are discussed in the section on venereal diseases.

Cutaneous habronemiasis (summer sores) is characterized by granulomatous lesions caused by larvae of *Draschia megastoma, Habronema muscae,* and *Habronema microstoma*[447,452,454] (see Chapter 57 for detailed discussion). Occurrence of this disease has declined with regular use of avermectin anthelmintics.[447,455] Lesions are generally observed at the level of the glans penis or urethral process. Yellow caseous masses composed primarily of eosinophils and larvae are present within the lesions (Fig. 8-16). These lesions should be differentiated from sarcoids or squamous cell carcinoma.[447,452,456-458]

Confirmation of the diagnosis is easily made with histo-pathologic evaluation of a biopsy of the lesion or by contact smears. Prevention of habronemiasis should include protection of genital lesions with insect repellant,[459] regular cleaning of the external genitals, and regular use of ivermectin, especially during the peak of fly season.[447]

Infections of Testes and Epididymis

Orchitis

Orchitis may be caused by bacteria, viruses, or parasites. Bacterial orchitis and periorchitis are relatively rare in stallions.[460] Infection may be ascendant, secondary to trauma, or hematogenous.[447,460,461] Hematogenous infection with *S. equi* subsp. *zooepidemicus*, *S. equi* subsp. *equi*, *Actinobacillus equuli*, *Pseudomonas mallei*, *Salmonella abortus equi*, *Brucella abortus*, and *C. pseudotuberculosis* may occur.[447,460-462] Infections caused by *Streptococcus* spp., *Staphylococcus* spp., and *E. coli* occur secondary to peritonitis.

Systemic clinical signs may include fever, abdominal pain, and poor libido. Local signs may include increased scrotal size, scrotal edema, and increased sensitivity of the scrotal area. Scrotal/testicular ultrasonography may identify areas of liquefaction of the testicular parenchyma or development of granulomatous lesions[438,447,463,464] (Fig. 8-17). Horses with chronic orchitis may have adhesions between the tunica vaginalis and subcutaneous tissue, azoospermia, high numbers of neutrophils in the ejaculate, a high percentage of sperm abnormalities, and poor motility.[447,461,465]

Differential diagnosis should include all other causes of increased scrotal size,[464,466] including inguinal hernia,[460,464] hematocoele,[467,468] hydrocoele,[447,469] testicular cord torsion,[464,470] spermatic artery thrombosis,[471,472] and testicular neoplasia.[447,473] Neutrophilia, fever, and hyperfibrinogenemia without cardiovascular signs suggest orchitis rather than inguinal hernia with intestinal incarceration.[460,464,474]

Treatment of bacterial orchitis may be attempted with systemic antibiotics and NSAIDs, as well as local hydrotherapy, but is generally unrewarding. Unilateral infections are usually best managed by hemicastration. When bacterial orchitis responds to antimicrobial treatment, the affected testicle will progressively atrophy and become fibrotic.[475] Infection may be limited to the scrotal skin and surrounding tissue (periorchitis). These infections may appear following penetrating trauma or insect bites.[464,476] Periorchitis can become complicated with a secondary peritonitis.[477,478]

Viral orchitis has been reported in some horses with equine infectious anemia, EVA, and influenza.[357,447] Orchitis has also been described in horses with granulocytic erhlichiosis.[479]

Parasitic orchitis may be caused by migratory larvae (larval migrans) of *Strongylus edentatus*.[480-484] The nematode *Setaria equina* has been identified in a stallion with chronic orchitis.[485]

Epididymitis

Infections of the epididymis are rare in stallions and are generally accompanied by orchitis. Therefore the same bacteria and parasites associated with orchitis are associated with epididymitis in the stallion.[462,474,486-491] *Pseudomonas aeruginosa* is the most common isolate from bacterial epididymitis in stallions.[492]

Acute epididymitis is very painful and often accompanied by local swelling and fever. Colic signs may be present even in horses with chronic epididymitis. Periorchitis and peritesticular adhesions and sperm granulomas may develop following rupture of the epididymis. Systemic signs and palpable changes are often suggestive of the diagnosis. Azoospermia is possible. Ejaculates may show oligospermia, hypasthenia, and increased numbers of

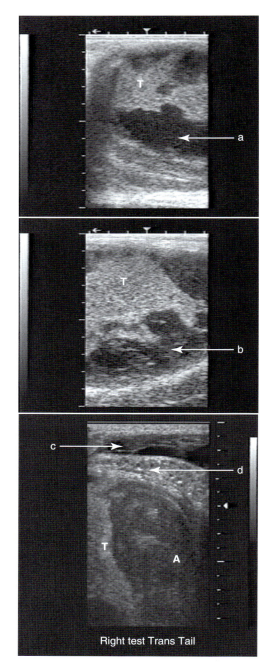

Right test Trans Tail

Figure 8-17 Ultrasonogram of testicle of stallion with orchitis caused by *Corynebacterium pseudotuberculosis* infection. *T,* Testicular tissue; *a* and *b,* abscessed areas; *c,* thickened scrotum with fibrin; *d,* periorchitis; *A,* abscess in testicle.

decapitated sperm cells with increased numbers of neutrophils in the ejaculate.[486,487,490-493] Prognosis for fertility is poor in horses with bilateral epididymitis.[474]

Infections of Accessory Glands

Infections of the stallion accessory sex glands are relatively rare.[494,495] Seminal vesiculitis is the most common.[496-500] Bacterial isolates from stallions with seminal vesiculitis include *P. aeruginosa*, *K. pneumoniae*, *Streptococcus* spp., *Staphylococcus* spp., *Proteus vulgaris*, *Acinetobacter calcoaceticus*, and *Brucella abortus*.[496,497,499-506] Both ascendant routes, from the urinary system, and hematogenous routes of infection are possible. Seminal vesiculitis may be associated with infection of the ampullae of the ductus deferens (ampullitis).[496]

Clinical signs of seminal vesiculitis are variable. Chronic infection may occur without any systemic signs. Acute infection is characterized by pain during ejaculation or transrectal palpation. Seminal vesiculitis may be suspected in stallions with hemospermia, pyospermia, or infertility.* The ejaculate may appear brown or reddish in color and contain a high number of red blood cells and neutrophils.[496,500,507,508]

Diagnosis of seminal vesiculitis requires evaluation of the gland by transrectal ultrasonography and urethroscopy.[447,463,509] The inflamed seminal vesicle increases in size and becomes very soft and easily palpable. In some cases the gland may show lobulation and irregular contours.[495,506,507] On ultrasonography, the gland is two to three times the normal size and its content is densely hyperechoic (normally anechoic).[502,506,510] Endoscopic examination of the colliculus seminalis may reveal localized inflammation[447,507,508,511,512] (Fig. 8-18). Chronic seminal vesiculitis may not show any changes on endoscopic examination.[496] The examination of the gland itself is possible with a small-diameter endoscope (Fig. 8-19). Culture and cytology of fluid obtained directly from the gland by endoscopic aspiration of the ejaculatory duct allow confirmation of the diagnosis.[447,495,511] Microbiologic evaluation may also be performed on samples obtained from preejaculate and postejaculate urethral swabs or sperm.[508]

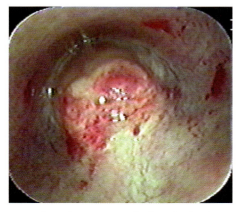

Figure 8-18 Videoendoscopic view of inflamed colliculus seminalis.

*References 447, 495, 496, 500, 502, 506, 507.

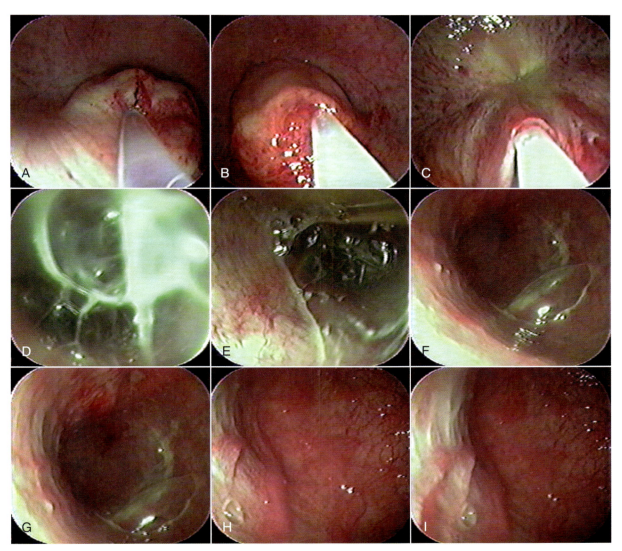

Figure 8-19 Videoendoscopic catheterization of seminal vesicle **(A-C)**, seminal vesiculitis, and seminal vesicle before **(D-F)** and after **(G-I)** flushing.

Treatment of seminal vesiculitis is very difficult because the majority of antimicrobials cannot reach the gland in sufficient concentration.[496,507,508] Broad-spectrum antimicrobials with a high volume of distribution, such as trimethoprim-sulfonamide combinations, may be used systemically.[507] Enrofloxacin reportedly reaches adequate concentration in the seminal vesicles after parenteral administration.[508] Direct flushing and local infusion of antimicrobial drugs into the glands are the preferred method of treatment.[447,452,497,502,513] Local lavage with amikacin and oral treatment with trimethoprim-sulfonamides for 8 days have been successful for the treatment of a stallion with seminal vesiculitis from *Proteus vulgaris*.[497]

The use of minimum-contamination breeding techniques may be indicated in difficult cases of seminal vesiculitis.[170,501] Infusion of an extender containing a specific antimicrobial into the uterus of a mare before breeding, combined with post-breeding uterine lavage, helps prolong the survival of semen and control bacterial growth.* If artificial insemination is an option, collection of the sperm-rich fraction and dilution with an extender containing the proper antimicrobials is indicated.[502]

A radical treatment of seminal vesiculitis consisting of surgical excision of the affected glands has been described. However, such a surgical technique is complicated and often leads to ejaculatory disorders.[505]

Equine Venereal Diseases

The most common equine venereal diseases are CEM (see Chapter 38), coital exanthema (see Chapter 14), EVA (see Chapter 15), and dourine (see Chapter 60). Some bacteria responsible for endometritis in the mares, such as *P. aeruginosa* and *K. pneumoniae*, are also considered venereal. Some of these diseases are subject to strict regulatory guidelines in several countries, and the veterinarian should be aware of the proper procedures for reporting positive or suspect cases.[446,452]

Venereal Transmission of *Pseudomonas aeruginosa* and *Klebsiella pneumoniae*

Pseudomonas aeruginosa and *Klebsiella pneumoniae* endometritis can be spread between horses by venereal transmission.[22,493,501,515-521] Bacteriologic studies should be routinely performed on recently introduced mares and stallions to prevent such infection. Culture is also indicated if there is an increased incidence of endometritis on a stud farm.[453,495,522-525]

Routine washing of the stallion penis with antiseptic solution before and after breeding is contraindicated because it may disturb the normal bacterial flora of the penile surface and promote growth of pathogenic bacteria such as *P. aeruginosa* and *K. pneumoniae*.[453,526,527] Washing the penis with sodium hypochlorite solution (5.25%) or dilute hydrogen chloride (HCl, 0.2%) has been suggested for the treatment of stallions with a positive culture of *P. aeruginosa* or *K. pneumoniae*.[493,522,528,529]

Contagious Equine Metritis

Contagious equine metritis is still a big concern for the equine breeding industry as demonstrated by the 2008 outbreak in the United States.[270] The disease is primarily caused by *Taylorella equigenitalis*, although some have reported isolation of *T. asinigenitalis* from stallions.[446,530,531] The disease is asymptomatic in stallions but causes catarrhal endometritis, cervicitis, vaginitis, and infertility in mares. Several states in the United States require testing of all stallions for CEM before shipping semen. Samples for CEM testing should be taken from the urethral fossa, preejaculation and postejaculation urethral swabs, and semen. Samples from asymptomatic mares should obtained from the clitoral fossa.[531]

Coital Exanthema

Coital exanthema is a very contagious, self-limiting venereal disease caused by equine herpesvirus type 3 (EHV-3). The disease is also known as genital horse pox, eruptive venereal disease, equine venereal vulvitis and balanitis, and coital vesicular exanthema.[532] It is characterized by the development of painful pustular lesions on the external genitalia of stallions and mares.[533,534] The direct effect of this disease on fertility remains a subject of debate. The disease is transmitted by coitus, infected artificial insemination equipment, or gynecologic instruments.[535-539] Mechanical transmission by stable flies has been suggested. Genitonasal contact (behavioral nuzzling/sniffing) has been associated with transmission of the virus and presence of lesions on the lips and nostrils.[540]

The stallion plays an important role in the epidemiology of coital exanthema. The viral replication is limited to the stratified epithelium of epidermal tissue of the skin or the mucocutaneous margins. Clinical signs are the consequence of the lytic viral infection and the local inflammatory response. The lesions develop within a week of infection and consist of multiple circular red nodules on the vulva, vaginal mucosa, clitoral fossa, and perineum in mares and on the surface of the penis in the stallion. The lesions increase in size to 10- to 15-mm circular vesicles, which eventually rupture and become coalescent ulcers (Fig. 8-20). The ulcerative lesions are very painful.[541] Infected stallions may show some discomfort during erection and loss of libido. Anorectal lymphadenopathy was described in mares with EHV-3 infection, but it is not clear whether it is a direct consequence of the viral infection or the result of a secondary bacterial infection.[542]

Medical management of horses with EHV-3 consists of sexual rest until the disease runs its clinical course. Broad-spectrum antibiotic therapy has been advocated by some

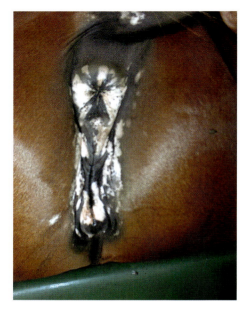

Figure 8-20 Perineal area of mare showing old lesions of equine herpesvirus type 3 (EHV-3) infection (coital exanthema).

*References 129, 130, 143, 170, 181, 501, 514.

clinicians for cases with secondary bacterial infection but is not routinely done. Daily cleansing of the genitalia with an antiseptic solution, particularly in stallions, and local application of creams containing astringents, antiinflammatory agents, and antimicrobials may help with extreme cases of secondary infection.[543] Topical treatment with antiviral cream (5% acyclovir) has been used successfully in a few cases.[544]

Prevention of coital exanthema requires examination of mares before breeding or use of artificial insemination. Clinical signs are easily recognized in both stallions and mares. Confirmation of the diagnosis is made by virus isolation from the lesions or histopathologic examination looking for characteristic inclusion bodies.[537,538] Serology has been used to demonstrate recent exposure. Viral isolation or detection is the gold standard for diagnosis. Samples should be obtained by scraping or vigorous swabbing from the edges of fresh, active lesions and submitted in 2 to 3 mL of viral transport medium on ice.[545] A highly sensitive and specific PCR test for the detection of virus has been recently described.[541,546] Postexposure immunity to reinfection is a subject of debate. The disease may develop in consecutive breeding seasons in exposed horses. However, the clinical signs are milder and the duration and intensity of shedding are lower. Spontaneous reactivation and shedding has been reported in some horses.[532,547] Reactivation of the virus has been produced experimentally in mares with low levels of circulating antibodies treated with corticoisteroids.[548] The importance of possible reactivation and the need for high vigilance in theriogenology practice is well illustrated by a recent report of an outbreak in a large embryo transfer facility in Argentina.[542]

Dourine

Dourine is defined by the Office International des Epizooties (OIE) as a "chronic or acute contagious disease of breeding solipeds that is directly transmitted from animal to animal during coitus." Dourine is probably the oldest equine venereal disease known. It is caused by the only trypanosome that is not transmitted by an invertebrate vector, *Trypanosoma equiperdum* (see Chapter 60). It affects primarily horses and to a lesser degree donkeys.[549] Dourine has been eradicated from North America and most of Europe. It is still reported in Africa (Botswana, Ethiopia, Namibia, South Africa) and Asia (Kyrgyzstan, Mongolia, Pakistan, Russia, Turkmenistan, Uzbekistan), with suspected cases reported in Germany and the Middle East.[379,550-553] A recent report suggest that the disease may be more widespeard in Europe, Italy in particular, than originally thought.[554]

Horses with dourine typically present in one of three clinical phases. Initially, infected horses exhibit edema and fluid accumulation in the genital area starting about 2 weeks after infection. This is followed by development of the characteristic cutaneous lesions from which the disease derives its name, "dourine." The lesions are circular elevated plaques of thickened skin ranging from 1 cm to 10 cm in diameter and resembling money, or "douros." These plaques are observed mostly on the neck, hip, and ventral abdomen. Progressive nervous system compromise leads to paralysis of the hindlimbs, paraplegia, and death.

Clinical signs are highly suggestive of the disease. Dourine can be confirmed by a wide variety of laboratory tests. Complement fixation test (CFT) developed in the early twentieth century remains the internationally recommended test.[555] However, recent studies have shown that this test cannot distinguish among *T. equiperdum*, *T. evansi*, and *T. brucei*.[550,551,556,557] These cross-reactions are important from an epidemiologic point of view because some clinical signs of infection with *T. evansi* may resemble those of dourine.[550,551,558,559] Recently, the trypanocidal molecule (bis(aminoethylthio)

4-melaminophenylarsine dihydrochloride) has been shown to be effective against *T. equiperdum* in chronically infected horses and may be an additional control method in endemic regions.[560] However, many consider that *T. equiperdum* is not curable, and some strains have been shown to develop resistance to the available trypanocidal drugs.[561]

Conclusion: Biosecurity in Breeding Operations

Biosecurity on horse farms and in veterinary hospitals is essential to prevent introduction and spread of infectious diseases. The general approach to biosecurity and disease outbreak control is covered in depth in Chapter 62.

General principles of biosecurity for breeding farms include strict separation of transient and resident horse populations, routine quarantine of all new arrivals on the farm, and segregation of horses according to age and breeding status. Prebreeding uterine culture and cytology should be required for all visiting mares, particularly those that have remained barren in the previous season. Stallions should undergo complete semen evaluation and microbiologic examination of preejaculation and postejaculation urethral swabs, as well as semen. Interpretation of microbiologic evaluation of penile surface swabs, urethral swabs, and semen may be difficult because of the large variety of saprophytic bacterial and fungal flora present.[562] However, isolation of a pure culture from these samples should be considered a siginificant risk for transmission of infection.

Breeding hygiene should be strictly observed to avoid transmission of contaminants to mares. The surface of the penis can harbor several organisms that may be potentially pathogenic.[43,563,564] If artificial insemination is used, particular attention should be paid to the origin of the semen and the health certificate of stallions at collection.[517,524,565] Addition of antibiotics to semen extender may help reduce bacterial loads if the antibiotics are carefully chosen and used at the proper concentration and under specific conditions of incubation.[566-569] Many countries require the addition of specific antibiotics, such as amikacin or ticarcillin, to the extender for the control of *T. equigenitalis*.[570] Antibiotic-containing extenders do not eliminate risk of transmission of organisms.[571] Quality control of semen processing, particularly shipped cooled semen, is often lacking. A study on microbial quality of frozen semen from different European origins showed a high variability in microbial load with an average of 1.4×10^{401} colony forming units per milliliter (cfu/mL).[572] Health importation requirements for frozen semen should be verified for each country of origin and adhered to strictly.[573] The stallion status with regard to EVA and CEM is of particular importance.[359,452] Guidelines are available for use of stallions that shed EVA virus[574] (see Chapter 15). The risk of transmission of infectious diseases by embryo transfer in horses has not been thoroughly evaluated.[575] Proper screening of the stallions, donor mares, and recipients is therefore very important. Advanced reproductive technologies, such as intracytoplasmic sperm injection (ICSI), cloning, gamete intrafallopian transfer (GIFT), and in vitro fertilization, are becoming accepted in the equine breeding industry and need to be evaluated for risk of disease transmission.

On large stud farms, foaling mares should be grouped by gestational stage. They should be monitored daily for rapid mammary development, premature lactation, or abnormal vaginal discharge. High-risk pregnancy mares should be monitored regularly by transrectal and transabdominal ultrasonography. Paddocks should be checked regularly for abortion.

A contingency plan should be elaborated for action to take in cases of abortion. This plan should include proper handling (prompt submission to laboratory) of biologic tissues (placenta and abortus) and measures to isolate the aborting mare from the rest of the herd. On large farms, personnel working with pregnant and parturient mares should have no contact with other horses.

The foaling team should be educated in recognizing abnormal peripartum situations requiring urgent veterinary attention. Hygiene should be emphasized for all personnel attending or assisting in foaling.

On an individual mare level, prevention of reproductive loss from infectious diseases should focus on early diagnosis of sporadic infections that may cause permanent damage to the reproductive tract. Mares that are known to be susceptible to endometritis should be bred using minimum-contamination breeding techniques and monitored for PMIE and treated appropriately. Corrective surgery should be performed on all mares with abnormal perineal conformation.

The potential for disease transmission by visitors should not be underestimated. Visitor contact with animals should be limited or discouraged, particularly for high-risk animals (pregnant mares and stallions). Access to a herd by the general public should be disallowed.

Prevention of introduction of diseases into the herd should also take into account other vector animals (insects, birds, rodents), as well as proximity to other species (e.g., donkeys, wildlife). Pest control may be difficult but should not be overlooked. Regular cleaning and disinfection of the barns and common areas are critical to eliminating disease agents that contaminate housing, feeding, and equipment to minimize spread of disease by humans and other fomites.

The complete reference list is available online at www.expertconsult.com.

Urinary Tract Infections

9

Dana N. Zimmel

Etiology

Urinary tract infection (UTI) is caused by microbial colonization of the kidney, ureter, urine, or proximal urethra. The incidence of UTIs in the horse is low.[1-5] UTIs can be divided anatomically into upper UTI, involving the kidney and ureters, and lower UTI, involving the bladder and urethra. Ascending infections are the most common method of bacterial colonization, with the exception of septicemia-associated nephritis in neonatal foals.[6] Upper UTIs occur less frequently and can occasionally be life threatening.[4] Lower UTI is generally caused by abnormal urine flow. Urolithiasis and partial obstruction are often the cause of both upper and lower UTI in horses.

The most frequently reported bacteria in UTI include *Escherichia coli*, *Proteus* spp., *Klebsiella* spp., *Enterobacter* spp., and *Pseudomonas aeruginosa*.[7] *Streptococcus equi* subsp. *zooepidemicus* and *S. equisimilis* were the two most common *Streptococcus* spp. isolated from renal tissues in both adult horses and foals.[8] Gram-positive infections in horses are less common, but *Staphylococcus* and *Corynebacterium* spp. have been isolated as causes of UTI.[9] *Enterococcus* spp. have been identified in horses with abnormal urine flow or horses that were instrumented with a urinary catheter. Isolation of more than one organism from the urine is common. Neonatal foals receiving broad-spectrum antimicrobials can develop infection with the fungus *Candida* spp. in the lower urinary tract.[4]

The most frequent predisposing factors for development of UTI in the horse include bladder paralysis (Fig. 9-1), urolithiasis (Fig. 9-2), and trauma to the urethra.[4] Urethritis can result from urethral damage in geldings and stallions secondary to neoplasia, habronemiasis, or trauma to the penis or sheath.[10,11] Any alteration or obstruction to urine flow can predispose to infection. Mares are more likely to develop UTI than male horses because of their shorter urethra and the potential for fecal contamination from poor perineal conformation. In addition, mares may

sustain damage to the urethra from trauma associated with foaling.

Cystitis may occur secondary to bladder paralysis, bladder neoplasia, or urolithiasis. Neurologic disease, such as equine protozoal myeloencephalitis or equine herpesvirus type 1 (EHV-1), and trauma can result in bladder paralysis. Consumption of Sudan grass and Johnson grass has resulted in ataxia and urinary incontinence in the southwestern United States from sublethal intoxication with hydrocyanic acid in the plants.[7,12,13]

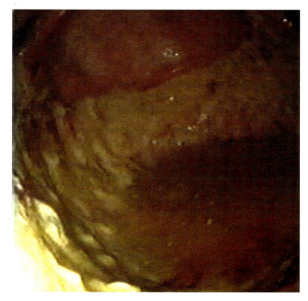

Figure 9-1 Endoscopic image of urinary bladder of 8-year-old Quarter Horse mare with bladder paralysis and recurrent bacterial cystitis secondary to administration of alcohol tail block.

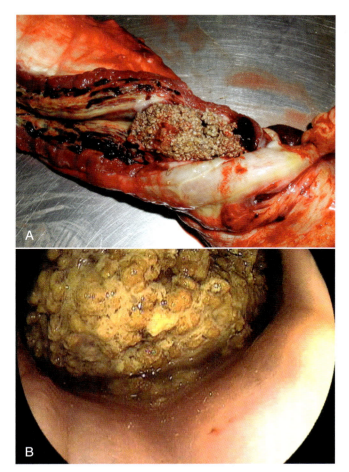

Figure 9-2 Urolithiasis in horses may be associated with concurrent bacterial infection of the urinary tract. **A,** Large urolith in urethra of horse. **B,** Large stone in urinary bladder of horse.

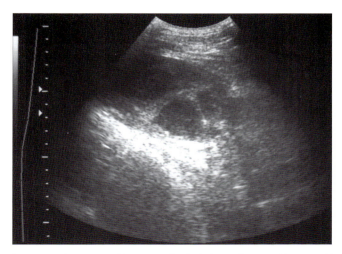

Figure 9-3 Ultrasonographic image of right kidney of 8-year-old mare with pyelonephritis; the lesion was confirmed at necropsy.

Conditions that inhibit bladder emptying at regular intervals encourage the growth of bacteria. Urolithiasis in the bladder can damage the mucosal lining, destroying normal defense mechanisms against microbial colonization. Obstruction of the renal pelvis, ureter, or urethra with urinary calculi may result in UTI. Unlike small animal patients, horses rarely develop UTI secondary to urinary catheterization, with the exception of sick neonatal foals.[13,14]

Because of the high mineral content in the urine and under conditions of urine retention, the equine bladder is prone to developing sabulous cystitis.[15,16] This condition is considered to be secondary to a neurogenic or anatomic inability to empty the bladder for a period of time. Sabulous cystitis is characterized by the presence of a very viscous cystitis with thick mucous sludge that is difficult for horses to void. Frequently, the bladder is colonized with various opportunistic bacteria.

Pyelonephritis is rare in horses[2-4] (Fig. 9-3). The ureters attach dorsally on the bladder, providing a physical barrier to vesicoureteral reflux, which is responsible for ascending infection. Problems that disrupt this normal barrier include ectopic ureter, enlargement of the bladder from paralysis, or obstruction of urine flow from urolithiasis.[13]

Pathogenesis

Urinary tract infections are the result of pathogenic bacteria colonizing the urethra and then migrating to the bladder, where they multiply.[13,17] Fecal bacteria and other opportunistic bacteria can adhere to the uroepithelial cells of the urethra when normal flora is altered by turbulent urine flow.[18] After the pathogenic bacteria colonize in the distal urethra, they must rapidly reproduce between micturition to migrate through the proximal urethra and bladder, which do not have protective flora.

Bacterial virulence properties and host defense mechanisms play a role in the development of UTIs. For example, pathogenic *Escherichia coli* has surface adhesins that can bind to specific glycolipid receptors on uroepithelial cells.[13] Host defense mechanisms include normal flora, normal anatomy, and normal micturition. An intact mucosal defense system includes glycosaminoglycan coating of uroepithelial cells and immunoglobulins in the urine.[18-20] Normal flora of the UTI can be protective against pathogenic bacteria unless urine flow or an anatomic defect compromises the environment. It has been hypothesized that women with recurrent UTI have decreased immunoglobulin A (IgA) in their urine.[21] Glycosaminoglycan can coat the uroepithelium, providing a barrier for bacterial attachment. If this layer is damaged by uroliths or neoplastic cells, infections are more likely to occur. Glycosaminoglycan production is directly influenced by estrogen. Prepubertal and postmenopausal women are at an increased risk of UTI because of a decrease in estrogen.[22] Currently, there is no evidence to support an increased risk of UTI in fillies or pregnant mares.

In the past 10 years, there have been several reports describing surgical treatment of urolithiasis. Culture of urinary calculi from horses frequently yields bacterial growth, however there is limited information regarding the biochemical analyses and bacterial etiology of this condition.[23,24]

Upper UTI in the horse is uncommon and if present, can be from either hematogenous or ascending infection. Although relatively uncommon, nephrolithiasis and ureterolithiasis may predispose to renal infection.[23,24] Infection of the ureter and kidney can occur with compromise of the protective valve, which inhibits vesicoureteral reflux secondary to ectopic ureter, bladder distention, or urethral obstruction. These conditions lead to dilated ureters and vesicoureteral reflux with contaminated urine. The renal cortex is much more resistant to bacterial infection than the renal medulla, decreasing the possibility of hematogenous spread.[18]

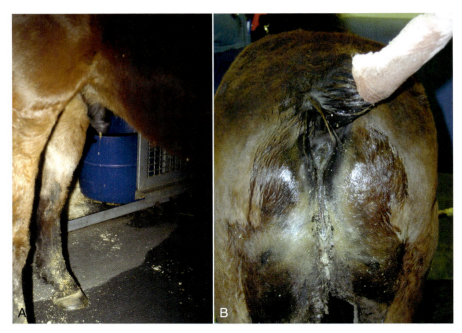

Figure 9-4 Urinary incontinence with secondary urine scald on dorsal aspect of distal hindlimbs in gelding **(A)** and perineal region of filly **(B).**

Clinical Findings

Clinical signs of lower UTI may include dysuria, pollakiuria, stranguria, and incontinence. Urine scalding on the perineum in mares or on the dorsal aspect of the hindlimbs in geldings or stallions may indicate chronic UTI (Fig. 9-4). Hematuria occurs with disruption of the mucosal lining associated with accumulation of sabulous urine sediment or urolithiasis. If hematuria is present only at the end of urination, this suggests that the origin of the problem is the bladder or proximal urethra. If a urolith completely obstructs urine flow, abdominal pain may be the presenting complaint.

Clinical signs of pyelonephritis include fever, weight loss, anorexia, depression, and, in some cases, mild abdominal pain. Often, upper UTI occurs in conjunction with lower UTI. More frequently, pyelonephritis is accompanied by dysuria manifested as pyuria or hematuria. It is difficult to determine if renal insults result in the formation of uroliths or if the uroliths are the source of the infection.[13]

Rectal examination may indicate the cause of a lower UTI. Common problems detected include a large distended bladder, flaccid bladder, thickened bladder wall, and presence of a bladder mass (neoplasm or cystic calculi). A dilated ureter may be palpable in the caudal abdomen and traceable to the kidney in upper UTIs. An abnormally large or small left kidney may aid in the diagnosis but should be confirmed with ultrasonography.

Diagnosis

Analysis of urine confirms the diagnosis of UTI. A sample of urine should be collected by sterile catheterization or collected midstream during urination. The urine sample should be collected in a sterile container and examined within 30 minutes of collection. Cytologic analysis and a bacterial culture and sensitivity should be performed. If urine is allowed to remain at room temperature, bacteria may multiply, and sediment evaluation and quantitative culture results will be inaccurate.[25]

If there is any delay in submission, the sample must be immediately refrigerated.

Interpretation of results varies with the collection method. A normal reference range for horses for a midstream free-catch sample is less than 5 bacteria per high-power field (hpf) on sediment evaluation and less than 20,000 organisms per milliliter (mL). A catheterized urine sample in normal horses has less than 4 bacteria/hpf and less than 300 organisms/mL.[26] Bacterial flora isolated from normal horses mimics the bacteria isolated in horses with UTI. This fact makes bacterial counts critical to determine the presence or absence of infection. Calcium oxalate and calcium carbonate crystals are normally observed in equine urine and are not correlated with the presence of uroliths.

A complete blood count (CBC) and chemistry profile are unremarkable in most horses with lower UTI that does not involve obstruction of urine flow. A neutrophilic leukocytosis is common in horses with upper UTI. Chronic UTI may be characterized by increased total protein concentration and hyperglobulinemia. Horses with bilateral upper UTI may develop azotemia, low urine specific gravity, and casts in the urine sediment.[4,13]

Ultrasonography of the kidneys can aid in the diagnosis of upper UTI caused by calculi, abscess, or neoplasia (see Fig. 9-3). Ultrasound-guided renal biopsy may be necessary to confirm the diagnosis. Transrectal ultrasonography of the bladder can detect a thickened bladder wall or a bladder mass. Evaluation of dilated ureters may also be possible using transrectal ultrasonography.

Endoscopic evaluation of the urethral mucosa, bladder, and ureteral openings is helpful in diagnosis of UTI (see Fig. 9-1). Advantages of endoscopy include identification of small cystoliths that could not be palpated and visualization of the mucosa. In addition, each ureter can be evaluated by observing urine flow and the diameter of the ureteral opening. If only one ureter and kidney are infected, bacterial culture of that side is indicated. Catheterization of the ureter may be performed endoscopically through the biopsy chamber using a polypropylene catheter.[27] The risks of endoscopic evaluation are minimal when sterile equipment is used.

Therapy

Treatment of UTI consists of correcting the underlying problem and initiating antimicrobial therapy. Factors to consider when choosing an antimicrobial for treatment of UTI should include the concentration of the antimicrobial in the renal tissue and urine, ease of administration, expense, toxicity, activity of antimicrobial at different pH levels, and drug interactions. Many antimicrobials are present in high concentrations in the renal tissue and urine as the result of renal excretion. If the organism is susceptible to an antimicrobial agent, it should be effective if the antimicrobial is excreted in the active form and if renal function is normal. Many antimicrobials may be resistant in vitro but achieve adequate concentrations in the urine to be effective. However, the opposite may also be true; for example, Enterococcus spp. are susceptible to trimethoprim-sulfonamide in vitro but are often resistant in vivo.[28]

Trimethoprim-sulfonamide combinations are the most frequently used antimicrobials for treatment of lower UTI in horses. The spectrum of activity includes both gram-positive and gram-negative bacteria. Trimethoprim-sulfonamide combinations are easy to administer and inexpensive. Combinations containing sulfamethoxazole may be problematic; one study suggests that this form is metabolized to an inactive product before urinary excretion.[29] Sulfadiazine is excreted largely unchanged in the urine and may be a better choice for treatment of equine lower UTI.[4,29] For upper UTI infection, therapeutic levels targeted at systemic and tissue levels are appropriate.

Ampicillin and penicillin are effective in the horse when given parenterally for treatment of both upper and lower UTI from gram-positive infections. Penicillin is effective against susceptible Corynebacterium spp., Streptococcus spp., and some Staphylococcus spp. Ampicillin is highly concentrated in the urine and is effective at treating some isolates in the Enterobacteriaceae family despite resistance in vitro. Ampicillin is also appropriate for treatment of Enterococcus spp.[4,30]

Aminoglycosides, such as amikacin and gentamicin, should be used with caution in horses because they are nephrotoxic. They should be used selectively for resistant lower UTI or severe upper UTI.[31] Pharmacokinetic monitoring is indicated for long-term therapy.

Cephalosporins are often used to treat UTI in other species.[18] Ceftiofur is concentrated in the urine and has broad-spectrum antimicrobial activity. Tetracyclines and chloramphenicol are metabolized in the liver and largely excreted in the bile; if high serum concentrations are obtained, however, adequate concentrations may be achieved in the urine to be effective against susceptible bacteria.[4]

Enrofloxacin given at doses as low as 2.5 mg/kg orally every 12 hours can achieve adequate concentrations in renal tissue and urine to be effective against susceptible organisms.[4,32] The duration of antimicrobial therapy for UTI depends on the site of infection. Most cases of lower UTI in horses respond with 7 days of appropriate antimicrobial therapy. Horses with recurrent infection or upper UTI may require 2 to 6 weeks of antimicrobial therapy.[4] In ideal circumstances the urine should be rechecked for bacterial growth 2 to 4 days after the start of therapy and 7 to 14 days after discontinuation of treatment.

The goal of supportive therapy in recurrent lower UTI is to increase urine production, increase water intake, and promote acidification of the urine in cases of cystitis or urolithiasis. Water intake can be increased by offering warm water in cold weather and increasing fiber in the diet. Supplementation with salt (50-75 g) in the feed can increase water consumption.[12] Urine-acidifying agents, such as ammonium chloride, can be administered orally at 60 to 520 mg/kg/day.[33-35] The taste is not palatable and often necessitates passage of a nasogastric tube, making this therapy impractical for long-term administration. In addition, effects on urine pH appear to be only temporary. Vitamin C administered at 1 to 2 g/kg/day orally, methionine (1 g/kg/day), and ammonium sulfate (175 mg/kg/day) decrease urine pH to less than 6 in some horses.[36] Treatment for sabulous urolithiasis may also include bladder lavage.[37] Copious amounts of sterile polyionic fluid should be placed in the bladder in 3-L to 4-L aliquots to flush out debris until all the material is removed.

Additional therapies for treatment of upper UTI are available but not readily accessible in all locations. In some horses with unilateral kidney disease, a nephrectomy may be performed if the other kidney is reasonably functional. Transendoscopic holmium:yttrium-aluminum-garnet (Ho:YAG) laser lithotripsy[38,39] and extracorporeal shockwave therapy[40] have proved to be effective ways of removing calculus in some horses.

The complete reference list is available online at www.expertconsult.com.

CHAPTER

10 Ocular Infections

Caryn E. Plummer, Carmen M.H. Colitz,* and Vanessa Kuonen*

Infectious ocular diseases in horses can occur as a primary condition or as a manifestation of a systemic disease. As a general rule, surface ocular diseases are primary in origin, whereas intraocular diseases are either primary or secondary. This chapter discusses the infectious diseases that affect equine eyes, beginning with surface structures and progressing to intraocular structures. For more detailed information on the specific ocular conditions mentioned in this chapter, please consult an ophthalmology textbook and the recent literature.

Ocular disease can have a tremendous impact on a horse's utility and quality of life. Given the horse's predilection for

*The authors acknowledge and appreciate the original contributions of these authors, whose work has been incorporated into this chapter.

ocular trauma and the environment in which they live, ocular infections are unfortunately all too common. It behooves the farm manager and attending veterinarian to diligently monitor eyes and intervene promptly if signs of ocular discomfort develop or if there are even subtle changes in the appearance of the orbits, eyelids, or globes. Early detection and treatment can in many cases prevent progression of disease that might otherwise be sight or globe threatening. Unfortunately, an animal cannot be counseled to avoid injury, so the responsibility for preventive care falls on the caretakers. Diligent and regular monitoring of the barn and field environment for potential dangers (i.e., nails sticking out of a stall door, the uncovered "J" hooks on water buckets, tree debris, etc) is critical, as is insect control. Many of the agents that can infect the ocular tissues primarily or secondarily are transmitted via insect vectors, and some of the infectious agents that cause systemic disease (and subsequent ophthalmic disease) are either transmitted by or harbored by small mammalian or avian hosts. Keeping the barn free of flies and the feed and tack rooms clean and free of debris that might attract rodents and limiting standing water on the farm can decrease the risks of opportunistic, vector-borne infections. Fly masks are an excellent way to limit exposure of the ocular tissues to flying insects. It is critical, however, that the masks be removed and replaced daily so that the eyes can be inspected and so that problems do not go undiscovered because they are hidden by the mask. Ceiling fans and open breezes may also decrease the incidence of insect transmission of infection.

For most types of infectious ocular disease, there are no major predilections for age or breed. All sizes, ages, and breeds of horse may be affected by ophthalmic disease; however, certain subsets of the horse population may be at greater risk than others. Racing animals that have dirt and debris flung at their faces during competition are at greater risk for corneal wounds than retired animals out at pasture. Fractious animals prone to quick and careless movements are often injured more frequently than more staid and sensible individuals. Any open corneal wound is potentially susceptible to secondary infection. Older animals or those that have intercurrent systemic disease may be slower to heal, thus a higher likelihood of developing secondary infections and complications. Appaloosas and European Warmbloods have a greater incidence of equine recurrent uveitis, suggesting some genetic predisposition for this as yet poorly understood immune-mediated disease. Prevention, aside from stable hygiene as mentioned, can be difficult to achieve. Active vigilance, early recognition of signs, and aggressive treatment are necessary to limit morbidity associated with ocular infections in horses.

Ocular Flora

Bacterial Isolates from Normal Eyes

Normal ocular microflora are predominantly nonpathogenic gram-positive organisms, although some gram-negative and fungal organisms are also present, but these vary, depending on various environmental and management practices.[1] Gram-positive organisms cultured from healthy equine eyes consist of *Bacillus cereus, Streptococcus equi* subsp. *equi, S. equi* subsp. *zooepidemicus,* other streptococci, *Corynebacterium* spp., *Staphylococcus aureus,* and *Staphylococcus epidermidis.*[1-6] Gram-negative organisms isolated from healthy equine eyes include *Moraxella* spp., *Neisseria,* and *Acinetobacter.*[1,3,4] Fungi are commonly isolated from at least 95% of equine eyes consisting of *Aspergillus* spp. and *Cladosporium* spp., unidentifiable and dematiaceous molds, *Chrysosporium* spp., and *Alternaria* spp.[4,6,7] Fungal organisms may contribute to pathology when the corneal epithelium is ulcerated or eroded.[1,7,8]

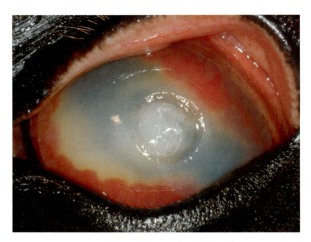

Figure 10-1 Equine eye with lateral paraxial middle to deep stromal malacic corneal ulcer with white blood cell and fungal infiltrates. The remainder of the cornea has diffuse cellular infiltration and edema. The furrow around the ulcer is approximately three-quarters the depth of the stroma. Corneal vascularization has nearly reached the edge of the ulcer but has not invaded the ulcer bed. In addition, there is conjunctival hyperemia; the pupil is hard to appreciate due to the corneal opacity. Fibrin and hypopyon are present in the anterior chamber.

Bacterial Isolates from Diseased Eyes

Consistent with the variability found in normal microflora of the equine eye, the literature describes much variability in the bacterial isolates associated with ulcerative keratitis. In one study, *Pseudomonas aeruginosa* was a highly common isolate, followed by *Enterobacter* spp., *Serratia* spp., and *Citrobacter* spp.[9]; other studies have demonstrated mostly gram-positive organisms consisting of *Streptococcus* spp., β-hemolytic streptococci, and *Staphylococcus* spp.[10] *Pseudomonas* spp. on the other hand were the least common isolate from 17 eyes (13.8%). These papers taken as a whole indicate that bacterial culture is likely of great value in assessment of horses with ocular disease. Although gram-negative bacteria are often perceived as causing severe corneal infection, *Staphylococcus* and *Streptococcus* infections are also capable of causing severe corneal disease.[10-12]

Fungal Isolates from Diseased Eyes

Fungal keratitis appears to be most common in the summer and fall,[10,13-22] although this may vary by geographic location. Fungal keratitis is a vision-threatening disease, with reported maintenance of vision in only one-half to one-third of affected horses[15-18] (Fig. 10-1); *Aspergillus* and *Fusarium* spp. are the typical etiologic agents (Fig. 10-2). Nonetheless, most veterinary ophthalmologists consider prognosis for vision favorable with aggressive surgical and medical management.[13,14]

Primary Ocular Infectious Diseases

Blepharitis

Blepharitis is defined as inflammation of the eyelids, and infectious blepharitis may occur secondary to bacterial, viral, fungal, or parasitic infection. Irrespective of cause, horses with blepharitis present with swollen inflamed eyelid(s). In the horse, bacterial blepharitis is the second most common type of blepharitis after trauma and presents as a unilateral and subacute disease, with mucopurulent discharge or abscess formation.[23] *Moraxella* spp.[24] and *S. equi* subsp. *equi* are most commonly isolated. Viral

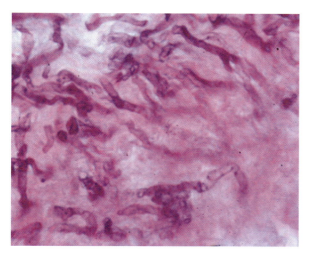

Figure 10-2 Photomicrograph of keratectomy sample with numerous fungal hyphae in stroma (hematoxylin-eosin stain, 600×). *(Courtesy Carmen M. H. Colitz.)*

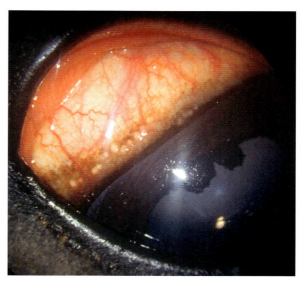

Figure 10-3 Equine eye with numerous lymphoid follicles in perilimbal region appearing as tiny vesicles.

blepharitis most commonly caused by papovavirus and horse pox can cause unilateral or bilateral blepharitis, chronic papillomas, or pustular dermatosis.[25] Numerous fungal organisms cause a blepharitis that is usually unilateral, with chronic alopecia, scaling of the skin, granulomas, draining tracts, or granulation tissue. Specific organisms include *Trichophyton* spp., *Microsporum* spp., *Cryptococcus mirandi*, *Aspergillus* spp., *Rhinosporidium seeberi*, *Histoplasma farciminosus* (epizootic lymphangitis), and phycomycosis.[23,25-28]

Parasitic blepharitis may be unilateral or bilateral with pruritus and can have a gritty caseous discharge. Aberrant migration of the larvae of *Habronema muscae*, *H. microstoma*, or *Draschia megastoma* can result in periocular or eyelid lesions with a raised, irregular, yellow appearance often referred to as "sulfur granules."[29] Biopsy of the affected area can aid in diagnosis to rule out other causes of ulcerative skin lesions such as neoplasia, proud flesh, and bacterial or fungal granulomas.[30] An eosinophilic infiltrate within a fibrous stroma will be evident histologically.[31] Other parasites that can cause blepharitis include *Demodex* spp. and *Thelazia* spp.[25] Parasitic ocular manifestations are discussed in more detail later in this chapter.

Conjunctivitis

Primary conjunctivitis in the horse is uncommon but associated with numerous infectious etiologies (Box 10-1). Clinical signs associated with conjunctivitis are nonspecific to the underlying cause and include conjunctival hyperemia and chemosis. Other clinical signs may include follicle formation, which is often a manifestation of chronicity (Fig. 10-3); mucopurulent discharge; and depigmentation of the lateral aspect of the bulbar conjunctiva. Differentiation of primary conjunctivitis from secondary conjunctivitis resulting from other diseases (e.g., dacryocystitis, keratoconjunctivitis sicca, keratitis, uveitis, glaucoma) is very important.[25] A thorough ophthalmic examination will help with this determination.

Keratitis

Infectious corneal disease in horses most often occurs secondary to corneal trauma but can also be a manifestation of primary ocular disease or systemic disease. Normal, uncomplicated corneal epithelial wound healing in the horse occurs at an average rate of 0.6 mm/day.[32] This rate of reepithelialization

---

Box 10-1 Potential Causative Agents Associated with Conjunctivitis

Bacteria and Bacteria-like Organisms
Streptococcus equi subsp. *equi*
Moraxella equi
Chlamydophila spp.
Mycoplasma spp.

Viruses
EHV-1, EHV-2
Adenovirus
Equine viral arteritis

Fungi
Histoplasma farciminosum
Aspergillus spp.
Rhinosporidium seeberi
Blastomyces spp.

Parasites
Thelazia lacrimalis
Onchocerca spp.
Habronema spp.
Ophthalmomyiasis (various genera and species)
Trypanosoma evansi

---

may be significantly delayed in the face of an infectious process. Every slow healing corneal wound, even those without obvious inflammatory cellular infiltrate, should be considered potentially infected. Microbial culture and sensitivity and corneal cytology are therefore indicated. Healing of corneal stromal wounds is more complicated and involves collagen remodeling and proteoglycan synthesis, eventually resulting in restoration of tensile strength.[33] The rebuilding of corneal stromal tissue is facilitated by the ingrowth of blood vessels. An infectious process in the corneal tissues will very often stimulate the vascularization process; however, some infectious agents (especially fungal agents) may elaborate antiangiogenic factors that delay vessel proliferation.[34,35] Corneal vascularization may be delayed by the use of topical and/or systemic steroids and non-steroidal antiinflammatory drugs (NSAIDs).

The prominent anatomic location of equine eyes and the normal opportunistic bacterial and fungal periocular flora predispose equine corneas to infectious keratitis.

Infectious keratitis caused by trauma may or may not be ulcerative and may be caused or exacerbated by opportunistic bacterial or fungal organisms, or a combination of these.[36] Occasionally, viral agents may be responsible for corneal disease.

Viral Keratitis

Primary infectious keratitis may be caused by equine herpesvirus (EHV) and other respiratory viruses (e.g., adenovirus, influenza, Borna virus). Each of these diseases is discussed separately elsewhere in this text. EHV keratitis typically presents as superficial punctate or dendritic lesions secondary to EHV-2 infection.[34,37-39] Acute cases will be quite painful (blepharospasm, serous epiphora) with chemosis and conjunctival hyperemia.[34] Recurrent cases may exhibit corneal vascularization. The superficial or punctuate lesions of EHV can be identified by rose bengal stain but not always with fluorescein stain. EHV keratitis can also present as anterior stromal or epithelial punctate opacities without ulceration. This makes diagnosis difficult, and other differential diagnoses should be considered, including fungal keratitis and immune-mediated keratitis.[34] Diagnosis of EHV keratitis is difficult, but cytology early in the course of disease may be helpful.[40] Cytology will usually reveal the absence of bacterial or fungal agents and lymphoplasmacytic inflammation.

Therapy for EHV keratitis includes topical antiviral and NSAID therapies. Idoxuridine (0.1%) and trifluridine (0.3%) limit viral replication but do not kill the virus; therefore they should be used between 4 and 12 times daily for 3 to 5 days until the condition stabilizes, then 3 to 6 times daily thereafter. A newer antiviral, 0.5% cidofovir, is effective in cats and requires only twice daily dosing, but its use in horses has not been reported. Some formulations of these medications can be irritating to the eye and most require compounding. If defects in the corneal epithelium are present, the additional use of a broad-spectrum topical antibiotic agent (e.g., neomycin-polymyxin-bacitracin [Neo-Poly-Bac], chloramphenicol) is indicated to prevent secondary bacterial infection. Topical NSAIDs include 0.03% flurbiprofen and 0.1% diclofenac and are helpful for secondary uveitis and inflammation, but they should be used with caution because they may cause recrudescence of viral keratitis in human patients. Topical corticosteroids should be avoided in horses with EHV keratitis, as well as most horses with keratitis. Oral L-lysine is a useful adjunctive therapy in human and feline patients with herpetic keratitis because it limits replication of the virus as a result of its competitive antagonism with arginine.[34] There are no dose guidelines for L-lysine in horses, but empiric supplementary doses of 10 to 30 g once daily indefinitely have been suggested. Viral keratitides that are not associated with EHV are uncommon in the United States but can be treated similarly to EHV keratitis with topical antiviral and NSAID therapy.

The greatest incidence of viral keratitis is in younger animals that travel and are exposed to other animals frequently. Co-mingling and the stress that usually accompanies their performance schedules can predispose them to infection and the development of clinical signs. Recurrence is common, especially when stress is high.

Bacterial Keratitis

Aerobic bacteria are the most common bacterial pathogens; however, anaerobic bacterial infections have been noted. Most cases of bacterial keratitis will be ulcerative in nature and will present with variable degrees of white-to-cream-to-yellow cellular infiltrate within or surrounding the ulcer bed, which may have varying degrees of stromal loss. Prior to applying anything to the ocular surface, a sample should be taken for aerobic culture and sensitivity. Topical anesthesia may then be applied so that a sample for cytology and gram staining can be obtained, which will guide the choice of empiric antibiotics.

Fungal Keratitis

Fungal keratitis is incredibly common in the horse, particularly in certain geographic regions (i.e., southeastern United States). It can occur and has been reported all over the world, however. Fungal infections of the cornea can present with a variety of clinical manifestations ranging from superficial punctate nonulcerative keratitis to deeper stromal defects and melting corneal ulcers to deeper stromal abscesses. *Aspergillus* and *Fusarium* spp. are perhaps the most commonly implicated agents, but a variety of other genera and species have been reported to cause or complicate corneal disease in the horse. Fungal keratitis in most of its forms is associated with prolonged healing times, guarded to poor prognoses, and often great expense for therapy. Fungal virulence factors may inhibit corneal vascularization[34,35] and reduce neutrophil infiltration and cell-mediated phagocytosis,[41] impeding healing and necessitating aggressive medical and surgical intervention.

Nonspecific signs of keratitis include pain (blepharospasm, photophobia, epiphora), serous to mucopurulent ocular discharge, corneal edema, variable corneal vascularization, loss of stromal integrity (melting or keratomalacia), and secondary anterior uveitis (aqueous flare, hypopyon, miosis). Diagnostic evaluation of infectious ulcerative keratitis may include evaluation of corneal cytology, culture and sensitivity, and histopathology. Nonulcerative keratitis is difficult to assess by cytology and culture and sensitivity because of the intact corneal epithelium. Recent reports have described the use of confocal microscopy in the standing horse to assess the depth of fungal keratitis. As this technology becomes more practical, microscopic assessment may aid in better assessment of response to treatment, clearing of the fungal organisms, and prognostication. Definitive diagnosis of both these disorders can often be obtained at surgery by biopsy of the infected tissue. A rapid diagnostic test is quantitative polymerase chain reaction (PCR) for fungal deoxyribonucleic acid (DNA). This assay can also be performed on formalin-fixed, paraffin-embedded tissues for retrospective analysis and may ultimately provide a more rapid and precise identification of corneal pathogens.[42]

Horses with infectious ulcerative keratitis will have loss of corneal epithelium and variable stromal loss. Full-thickness loss of corneal stroma that breeches Descemet's membrane will usually be plugged with fibrin and iris prolapse, with or without aqueous leakage (Fig. 10-4). This is a surgical emergency, and an ophthalmologist should be consulted. Horses with infectious nonulcerative keratitis will have an intact corneal epithelium, but cellular infiltration will be evident within the corneal stroma, that is, corneal abscess (Fig. 10-5). In horses with progressive or perforated corneal ulceration, keratectomy with a conjunctival pedicle flap may provide diagnostic, therapeutic, and prognostic benefit to the patient. Stromal loss that has progressed beyond three-quarters depth may be treated with placement of a synthetic or heterologous corneal graft and a conjunctival pedicle flap (Fig. 10-6) or amniotic membrane transplantation to stabilize the wound and speed healing.

Infectious ulcerative keratitis that has not progressed beyond one-third of the stromal depth can be treated medically. All horses with corneal ulceration should be treated with topical cycloplegics (e.g., atropine, every 6-24 hours [q6-24h], depending on the severity of the reflex uveitis), oral NSAIDs (e.g., flunixin meglumine) for pain and secondary uveitis, and topical antibacterial medications (e.g., Neo-Poly-Bac, neomycin-polymyxin-gramicidin, chloramphenicol, ciprofloxacin, etc, q1-6h), to prevent opportunistic bacterial growth. The

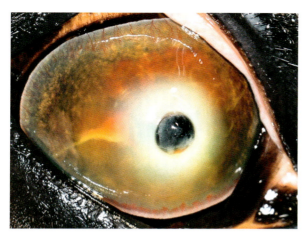

Figure 10-4 Equine eye with axial ruptured descemetocele with iris prolapse. In addition, there is conjunctival hyperemia, corneal vascularization and edema, and fibrin in the anterior chamber.

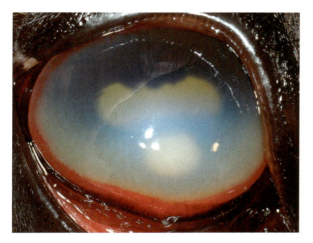

Figure 10-5 Equine eye with creamy yellow-white, ventral paraxial, corneal stromal abscess secondary to small corneal puncture with plant material that had epithelialized, leaving fluorescein-negative lesion. There is also corneal vascularization and edema, severe conjunctival hyperemia, and epiphora. The pupil is miotic and fibrin and hypopyon are present in the anterior chamber. Secondary uveitis is often the most significant clinical manifestation of corneal stromal abscesses. This abscess was fungal in origin, specifically *Fusarium* spp.

frequency of administration of topical antibiotics will depend on the severity of the lesion, its depth, and response to therapy. The clinician should be prepared to alter the antibiotics used if culture and sensitivity indicate a change is necessary. Cytology and gram staining can guide the initial choice of agents used. Depending on the underlying cause, topical antifungal medications (e.g., miconazole, natamycin, itraconazole with dimethylsulfoxide [DMSO], voriconazole, q4-6h) and oral antifungal medications (e.g., fluconazole, itraconazole) may be necessary.[43] If frequent topical therapy is necessary or if the individual is difficult to treat, placement of a subpalpebral lavage should be considered to facilitate therapy. If the horse is rubbing or traumatizing the globe because of discomfort, a hood or face mask can provide considerable protection to the fragile healing eye.

Melting corneal ulcers can rapidly become surgical emergencies and should be treated aggressively (Fig. 10-7). The underlying infectious causes of melting corneal ulcers include many different genera and species of bacteria (e.g., *Pseudomonas* spp., β-hemolytic streptococci) and fungal infections. Neutrophilic infiltrates and previous corticosteroid use can predispose to melting corneal ulcers. Medical management should include compounds with antiproteolytic activity, in addition to the medications just listed, and appropriate antibacterial medications for the specific bacteria and antifungal medications if warranted based on the results of diagnostics or geography. Several antiproteases have been recommended for treatment of melting corneal ulcers, including 0.2% ethylenediaminetetraacetic acid (EDTA), 5% to 10% *N*-acetylcysteine, autologous serum or plasma, and topical or oral tetracycline or doxycycline, and initial therapy with these agents should be instituted hourly.[44] In many instances, the collagenolytic process will be severe enough to warrant the use of more than one antiprotease medication. As the cornea starts to normalize or become more "firm," the frequency of treatment may be slowly decreased. If a member of the tetracycline family is used topically, because of its bacteriostatic nature, its administration should be staggered with the bactericidal antibiotic used by at least 1 hour. Most horses with melting corneal ulcers should be examined by a veterinary ophthalmologist and will likely require surgical intervention.

Nonulcerative infectious keratitis usually takes the form of either multifocal subepithelial foci of inflammatory cells (usually of fungal or viral etiology) or of deeper stromal abscesses, which are usually the result of a fungal infection. Superficial lesions usually respond to medical therapy (topical antimicrobial agents, atropine and systemic NSAIDs), whereas

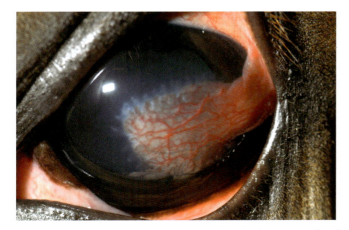

Figure 10-6 Equine eye with conjunctival pedicle flap that has integrated well into the lesion. The eye has no residual inflammation, and the graft will usually be trimmed 6 weeks postoperatively. *(Courtesy Carmen M. H. Colitz.)*

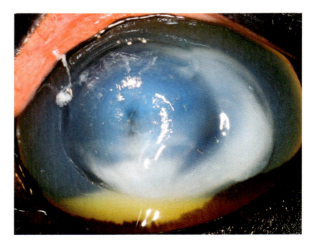

Figure 10-7 Equine eye with large melting ulcer. The entire cornea is edematous, and there is diffuse cellular infiltrate throughout the cornea. Miosis and hypopyon are present as well indicating concurrent uveitis.

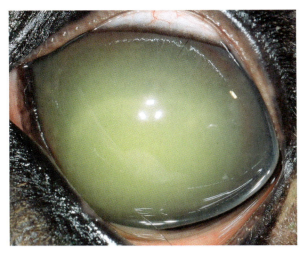

Figure 10-8 Foal's eye with uveitis, secondary to *Rhodococcus equi* infection. There is epiphora, diffuse conjunctival hyperemia, diffuse corneal edema, and fibrin filling the anterior chamber.

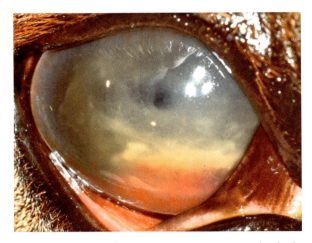

Figure 10-9 Equine eye with acute equine recurrent uveitis (ERU). There is severe conjunctival hyperemia, mucopurulent ocular discharge, diffuse corneal edema, and enophthalmos. The intraocular structures are difficult to see because of the corneal edema. *(Courtesy Carmen M. H. Colitz.)*

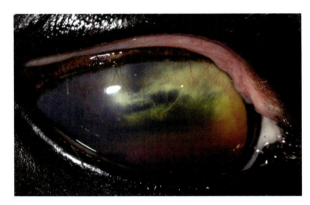

Figure 10-10 Equine eye with equine recurrent uveitis (ERU). There is conjunctival hyperemia, diffuse corneal edema and vascularization, a miotic pupil, and fibrin in the anterior chamber.

deeper fungal abscesses may require surgical removal and replacement of the resultant defect with a synthetic or heterologous corneal graft. A veterinary ophthalmologist should be consulted promptly to determine if surgical therapy is indicated or will be necessary.

Topical corticosteroids should be avoided in all horses with ulcerative keratitis and in any horse with nonulcerative keratitis suspected to be of infectious origin. Indolent or nonhealing corneal ulcers should be managed by debridement and topical antimicrobial and cycloplegic medications, as well as oral NSAIDs. Grid or punctate keratotomy should be avoided because of possible underlying fungal infection.[45]

Uveitis

Uveitis is inflammation of the uveal tract, which includes the iris, ciliary body, and choroid. Anterior uveitis refers to inflammation of the iris and ciliary body, posterior uveitis refers to inflammation of the choroid, and panuveitis refers to inflammation of all components of the uvea. Infectious systemic causes of uveitis include viruses, bacteria, protozoa, and parasites.[46] Specific viral causes of uveitis include equine influenza virus, EHV-1, equine viral arteritis, and equine infectious anemia virus. Bacterial causes include *Leptospira* spp., *Brucella* spp., *Streptococcus* spp., *Rhodococcus equi* (Fig. 10-8), and *Escherichia coli*.[47,48] *Toxoplasma gondii* may cause uveitis in horses. Parasitic etiologies include *Onchocerca* spp. and *Strongylus* spp. More detailed information regarding ocular manifestations of these organisms can be found later in this chapter.

Equine recurrent uveitis (ERU) is an immune-mediated disorder that is the leading cause of blindness in horses. Although the recurrent episodes of ERU are not directly caused by reinfection with microorganisms or parasites, numerous bacterial, viral, protozoal, and parasitic organisms have been implicated in initiating the syndrome (see Chapter 32 for discussion of the association of leptospirosis with ERU).[49]

Clinical signs of active uveitis are nonspecific and include pain (blepharospasm, photophobia, epiphora, ocular discharge), conjunctival hyperemia, scleral injection, corneal edema, keratic precipitates, aqueous flare, hypopyon, hyphema, fibrin in the anterior chamber or vitreous, iris color change, and miosis (Figs. 10-9 and 10-10). Chronic changes include atrophy of the corpora nigra, cataract, fibrosis of the iris, endothelial scarring, phthisis bulbi, and glaucoma. Treatment of uveitis, regardless of

cause, is aimed at decreasing inflammation in the eye, minimizing long-term damage to ocular structures, and preserving vision. Because this disease frequently has an immune-mediated basis, corticosteroids and other antiinflammatory drugs are important for treatment. Systemic and local antimicrobial therapy is also often implemented. Other therapy should be aimed at treatment of possible underlying systemic disease. Lack of response to therapy or recurrence should prompt the attending clinician to consult with a veterinary ophthalmologist in a timely fashion. The long-term prognosis for vision and sustained comfort in a chronically uveitic eye is guarded to poor. Surgical implantation of a slow-release cyclosporine implant may slow the progress of deterioration.[50-54] There are recent reports of the promising use of other immunomodulating agents, such as intravitreal rapamycin, for the treatment of chronic uveitis in horses, although long-term success rates and complications are yet unknown.[55]

Neuro-Ophthalmic Infectious Diseases

Vestibular Disease

Vestibular signs may result from either peripheral or central nervous system (CNS) diseases. Peripheral disease causes

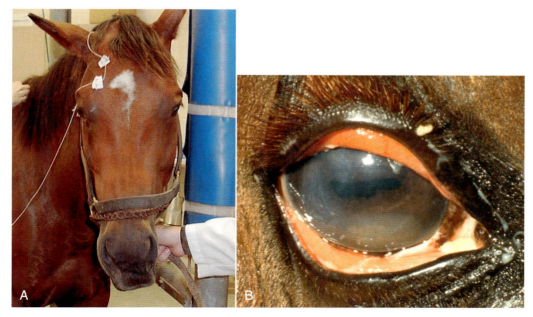

Figure 10-11 **A,** Horse with facial nerve paralysis. The eye developed an infected corneal ulcer as a result of lagophthalmos. Note the dropped ear and lip. **B,** Same horse's eye. There is a dry ocular surface, a corneal ulcer, mucopurulent ocular discharge, corneal vascularization, chemosis and conjunctival hyperemia, and enophthalmos.

ipsilateral head tilt, horizontal or rotary nystagmus with the fast phase occurring away from the side of the lesion, falling, circling, and asymmetric ataxia without conscious proprioceptive deficits or weakness.[56,57] Common causes of peripheral vestibular dysfunction include trauma, otitis media, temporohyoid osteoarthropathy, and guttural pouch disease.[58-61] Facial nerve paralysis (Fig. 10-11) and Horner's syndrome can occur with peripheral disease because of the facial nerve and sympathetic nerve proximity to the petrous temporal bone.[57,60,61]

Central (CNS) vestibular disease presents similarly, although conscious proprioceptive deficits, generalized weakness, and involvement of multiple cranial nerves may be present.[57] Nystagmus may be rotary, horizontal, vertical, diagonal, or disconjugate (different in each eye). The direction of the nystagmus may change with head position in central vestibular disease.[56,57] Paradoxic central vestibular disease may occur with a destructive lesion near the caudal cerebellar peduncle, resulting in clinical signs contralateral to the lesion.[57] Bilateral vestibular disease is difficult to differentiate from generalized cerebellar disease; these horses do not have nystagmus or vestibular eye movements and usually exhibit a symmetric ataxia.[57] Central vestibular dysfunction is often associated with tumors or abscesses but may also be secondary to protozoal, viral, bacterial, or parasitic encephalitides.[62,63]

Diagnostic techniques for determining the underlying cause of vestibular disease in the horse should include radiographs of the skull, endoscopy of the pharyngeal region and guttural pouches, and magnetic resonance imaging (MRI) or computed tomography (CT) scan of the head. Cerebrospinal fluid (CSF) cytology and ancillary testing for viral or protozoal antibodies are indicated if CNS disease is suspected.[60,61] Caloric testing can be performed, although the test is not always reliable, and most horses will resist the procedure. In caloric testing the ear canal is irrigated with cold water, and a normal response is induction of horizontal nystagmus away from the tested side. A decreased or absent reaction indicates the side of the lesion. Brainstem auditory-evoked responses are also useful in demonstrating damage to the cochlea and cranial nerve (CN) VIII and can be

used to differentiate between central and peripheral disease.[64,65] This procedure is reliable in the sedated horse. Treatment and prognosis should address the primary disease process.

Horner's Syndrome

Horner's syndrome is caused by damage or denervation along any portion of the efferent pupillomotor sympathetic nervous system. The sympathetic nervous system originates in the hypothalamus, where the central sympathetic fibers form the tectotegmentospinal tract (first-order neurons).[56] This tract descends ipsilaterally through the brainstem and lateral funiculus of the cervical spinal cord to synapse with the preganglionic cell bodies of the first to third thoracic vertebrae (T1-T3) or T4. These preganglionic sympathetic neurons (second-order neurons) leave the spinal cord through the segmental ventral roots to the paravertebral sympathetic chain, continue through the brachial plexus, and travel with the vagosympathetic trunk until they synapse in the cranial cervical ganglion caudomedial to the tympanic bulla. The postganglionic fibers (third-order neurons) join the tympanic branch of CN IX (glossopharyngeal nerve) within the middle ear and pass over the caudodorsal aspect of the guttural pouch. After the fibers exit the middle ear, they enter the cavernous sinus and join CN V (trigeminal nerve) and continue rostrally as the nasociliary nerve to innervate the orbital smooth muscles, the eyelids (including the third eyelid), and the ciliary body, iris dilator, and iris sphincter muscles.

Horner's syndrome in horses is most frequently seen secondary to guttural pouch disease.[56] Injury to the cranial thoracic spinal cord, brachial plexus avulsions, and traumatic lesions or masses involving the mediastinum, periorbital tissues, or cervical structures may also cause clinical signs of Horner's syndrome.[66-69] Iatrogenic Horner's syndrome can result from surgical ligation of the carotid artery. Other causes unique to the horse include polyneuritis equi syndrome, equine protozoal myeloencephalitis (EPM) affecting the cervical spinal cord, basisphenoid trauma, esophageal rupture, and intravenous injection with various drugs, including phenylbutazone.[70-72] Clinical signs of Horner's syndrome in horses include ptosis, relative enophthalmos, subtle miosis, regional hyperthermia, and excessive sweating on the ipsilateral side of the face.[66,73-75] Cervical sympathetic nerve damage will cause sweating of the neck, congested conjunctival and nasal mucous membranes, and inspiratory stridor.[56,74,75]

The location and cause of the lesion will determine which clinical signs are present, and the location will determine what diagnostic tests should be performed. Often, location may provide the prognosis. Phenylephrine (2% or 10%) or 1:1000 epinephrine are more readily available for the pharmacologic localization of efferent sympathetic lesions. Phenylephrine or epinephrine are direct-acting sympathomimetic drugs that will result in mydriasis within 5 to 8 minutes in postganglionic lesions caused by denervation hypersensitivity of the effector cells.[56] This test can effectively distinguish between preganglionic and postganglionic lesions during the first few weeks of clinical signs.[57] One drop of phenylephrine or epinephrine is applied to each eye (the normal eye is used for comparison), and care should be taken to use the same amount in each eye because the response is dose dependent. Mydriasis, retraction of the third eyelid, resolution of the enophthalmos, and ptosis are all positive responses to the phenylephrine test and indicate a postganglionic or third-order lesion. If a lesion localizes to the postganglionic arm of the pathway, endoscopy of the pharynx and guttural pouch should be performed. Alternatively, CT is another diagnostic option when available.

Systemic Diseases with Ocular Manifestations

Viral Diseases

Many viral diseases affect the eye either directly or indirectly (Table 10-1). The viruses, including the herpesviruses and those responsible for the viral encephalitides among others, that infect the equine may require direct ocular management. Other infections mediate disease primarily through cranial nerve neuropathy, and management is secondary.

Bacterial Diseases

Any systemic bacterial infection has the potential to affect the eyes. Certain specific bacterial diseases, such as tetanus or botulism, may have their own distinctive ophthalmic signs, but most bacterial infections, especially when sepsis has developed, can be associated with ocular inflammation. Please see Table 10-2 for further specifics.

Fungal Diseases

Cryptococcosis

Cryptococcus neoformans is a pathogenic fungus that may cause systemic infection in horses and other mammals (see Chapter 53). Ocular signs are not usually reported in horses with cryptococcosis, although there is one report of a frontal sinus granuloma with a retrobulbar mass causing exophthalmos, periorbital

---

Table 10-1 Viral Systemic Diseases with Ocular Manifestations

Disease	Primary or Secondary Ocular Clinical Signs	Clinical Signs	Treatment	Chapter Reference
Alphavirus (EEE, WEE, VEE)	Secondary (primary clinical signs are of neurologic disease)	Nystagmus, strabismus, pupillary dilation, blindness	Support of neurologic signs	Ch. 20
Equine viral arteritis	Secondary	Mucoid ocular discharge, conjunctivitis, corneal opacity, photophobia, periorbital edema	Symptomatic support: topical lubricants and antiinflammatory medications	Ch. 15
Equine infectious anemia	Secondary	Thrombocytopenia and anemia may result in conjunctival and intraocular hemorrhage	Intraocular hemorrhage results in uveitis, which should be treated with topical and/or systemic antiinflammatory medication	Ch. 23
Rabies	Secondary	Prolapse of third eyelid, blindness, nystagmus, strabismus	Supportive care until euthanasia	Ch. 19
African horse sickness	Secondary	Bulging of supraorbital fossa (considered hallmark of this disease) caused by retrobulbar edema and increased vascular pressure, chemosis	Supportive care: topical lubricants and/or antiinflammatory medication	Ch. 16
Equine herpesvirus type 1	Secondary	Blindness, optic neuritis, retinal detachment, posterior uveitis, anterior uveitis	Support of systemic and neurologic signs; systemic and topical antiinflammatory medications	Ch. 14
Equine herpesvirus type 2	Primary	Blepharospasm, serous to mucopurulent ocular discharge, conjunctival hyperemia, chemosis, superficial punctate corneal opacities and ulcers, dendritic corneal ulcers, corneal edema, corneal vascularization	Topical antivirals, topical NSAIDs	Ch. 14
Adenovirus	Secondary	Serous to mucopurulent ocular discharge (associated with bronchopneumonia), conjunctivitis, panuveitis	Topical and systemic antiinflammatory medications	Ch. 17
Equine influenza	Secondary	Serous to mucoid ocular discharge, conjunctivitis	Topical lubricants and antiinflammatory medication	Ch. 13
West Nile virus	Secondary	Unilateral or bilateral facial paralysis and subsequent exposure keratitis, absent or decreased menace response, keratitis, protrusion of third eyelid, blindness	Symptomatic support: topical lubricants and broad-spectrum antibiotics, partial tarsorrhaphy; topical and/or systemic antiinflammatory medication if uveitis, chorioretinitis or optic neuritis develop	Ch. 21

EEE, Eastern equine encephalitis; *WEE*, western equine encephalitis; *VEE*, Venezuelan equine encephalitis; *NSAIDs*, nonsteroidal antiinflammatory drugs.

Table 10-2 Bacterial Systemic Diseases with Ocular Manifestations

Disease	Primary or Secondary Ocular Clinical Signs	Clinical Signs	Treatment	Chapter Reference
Bacterial sepsis	Primary and/or secondary	Conjunctivitis, conjunctival hemorrhage, corneal edema and vascularization, anterior uveitis, posterior uveitis, intraocular hemorrhage, endophthalmitis	Topical and/or systemic antiinflammatory medications	Ch. 6 and 11
Tetanus	Secondary	Retraction of globes, bilateral prolapse of third eyelids, ventrolateral strabismus, fixed and dilated pupils with normal vision	Supportive care	Ch. 44
Botulism	Secondary	Enophthalmos (secondary to retractor bulbi spasm), ptosis, mydriasis, sluggish PLRs	Supportive care	Ch. 43
Lyme disease	Secondary	Conjunctivitis, keratitis, anterior uveitis, panuveitis, retinal hemorrhage, retinal detachment, papilledema, facial paralysis and subsequent exposure keratitis; has been implicated in cases of chronic uveitis (ERU)	Topical and systemic antiinflammatory medications	Ch. 33
Equine granulocytic ehrlichiosis	Secondary	Icteric sclera, conjunctival petechial, uveitis	Topical antiinflammatory medications	Ch. 39

PLRs, Pupillary light reflexes; *ERU,* equine recurrent uveitis.

swelling, and optic neuritis.[76] Diagnosis is based on histopathologic evidence of fungal hyphae in tissue samples or on cytology, as well as a positive culture.

Epizootic Lymphangitis

Epizootic lymphangitis, caused by *Histoplasma farciminosum,* a fungal agent found mainly in Africa (see Chapter 53), is manifested as nodules and draining lesions of the subcutaneous lymphatic system.[77] A conjunctival form of this disease results from deposition of the organism on the ocular mucous membranes by the biting flies of the *Musca* and *Stomoxys* species. Ocular signs include serous to mucopurulent discharge, blepharedema, and conjunctival papules.[77] Disease progression leads to ulceration of the papules, which may result in obstruction and erosion of the lacrimal duct or secondary keratitis. Diagnosis is mainly by cytology and culture, although serologic assays are also available.[78] Amphotericin B is the treatment of choice, and a vaccine is available for horses in endemic areas.[77,79]

Aspergillosis

Aspergillus spp. are considered opportunistic fungi that rarely cause systemic disease in nonimmunocompromised horses (see Chapters 52 and 53). Aspergillosis is a cause of guttural pouch mycosis; ocular manifestations can include Horner's syndrome, facial nerve palsy, and blindness resulting from ischemic optic neuritis secondary to extension of disease.[80] These organisms are ubiquitous in the environment, and horses are frequently exposed. Treatment with systemic antifungal agents may be attempted; however, the prognosis is always guarded, depending on the underlying disease process and the severity of the lesions.

Equine Leukoencephalomalacia

Equine leukoencephalomalacia (ELEM), also called *blind staggers* or *moldy corn disease,* causes central blindness when the midbrain is affected (see Chapter 53). Severe multifocal neurologic signs, including ataxia, agitation, and seizures, may accompany the blindness associated with ELEM.[81] Chronic ingestion of moldy corn infested with *Fusarium moniliforme* and its associated mycotoxin, fumonisin B1, results in liquefactive necrosis of the white matter.[81] If one horse on the farm is affected, other horses have likely been exposed, and feed should be checked for the mold. Hepatic enzyme activities are often increased in horses exposed to the toxin and may be used as a screening test.[81] Once neurologic signs have developed, the prognosis is poor. If attempted, treatment should consist of supportive care, fluids, and administration of activated charcoal to decrease absorption of the toxin.

Parasitic Diseases

Equine Protozoal Myeloencephalitis

Sarcocystis neurona is the primary etiologic agent of equine protozoal myeloencephalitis (EPM), which is one of the most common neurologic disorders of horses in North America (see Chapter 55). A few reports suggest that *Neospora hughesi* may cause an identical clinical syndrome.[82] Neurologic signs of EPM vary greatly, depending on the area of the CNS that is affected. If CN VII and CN VIII are affected, horses may present with signs of facial nerve paralysis or vestibular disease, respectively.[82-84] Ocular signs associated with facial nerve paralysis include ptosis and absence of the palpebral reflex. If the parasympathetic nucleus of CN VII is affected, neurogenic keratoconjunctivitis sicca will occur, predisposing the cornea to ulceration and secondary infectious keratitis. EPM affecting the cervical spinal cord may cause Horner's syndrome. Pupillary abnormalities and strabismus associated with EPM have been reported.[85] There are no published reports of EPM-induced blindness. Diagnosis, treatment, and prognosis for horses with EPM are discussed in Chapter 55.

Babesiosis (Piroplasmosis)

Piroplasmosis is a hemolytic disease of horses caused by the tick-borne protozoa *Babesia caballi* and *Theileria equi* (see Chapter 56). Ophthalmic signs of babesiosis include serosanguineous ocular discharge, distention of the supraorbital fossa, blepharedema, icteric conjunctiva and sclera, and petechiae and ecchymoses of the conjunctiva.[29,86,87] Diagnosis, treatment, and prevention of piroplasmosis are discussed in Chapter 56.[88,89]

Toxoplasmosis

Toxoplasma gondii is a protozoa that can infect the horse, although clinical disease is rare.[90] One study examined three separate horse populations in India and found that in the few horses with ocular lesions, there was no correlation with positive titers for *T. gondii.*[91] Another serologic study of 71 horses with ocular lesions associated with ERU found no correlation with positive titers for *T. gondii.*[92] There are sporadic case reports of horses with ocular lesions associated with toxoplasmosis. *Toxoplasma gondii* DNA was isolated from the retina, choroid, and sclera of both eyes of a 17-year-old pony from the United Kingdom; however, the presence or absence of ocular lesions or visual deficits was not noted.[93] There is one report of peripapillary and partial optic nerve atrophy in a horse with toxoplasmosis.[94] In a study of seven horses with chorioretinitis, five had *T. gondii* titers of 1:64.[95] One of these horses became acutely blind 4 days before presentation and had diffuse, chronic chorioretinitis in the right eye and acute chorioretinitis in the left eye. At presentation the titer was negative, although 16 days later the titer was 1:64. Postmortem histologic examination of the brain found intracytoplasmic *Toxoplasma* bodies.

Onchocerciasis

Onchocerca cervicalis is spread by *Culicoides* spp. and is a common cause of dermatitis in horses (see Chapters 57 and 59, respectively). It is thought that microfilariae migrate along vessels through subcutaneous tissue to the eyelids, then into the conjunctiva, cornea, and uvea.[96,97] Ocular microfilariae have been reported in horses, and the prevalence varies by geographic location.

The most common ocular lesion evident is depigmentation of the conjunctiva at the temporal limbal region.[96-99] Similar to systemic onchocerciasis, ocular disease is usually caused by an inflammatory reaction to the antigens of dead parasites releasing antigens. Other ocular manifestations include conjunctivitis, peripheral keratitis, and anterior and posterior uveitis.[96,97] Conjunctivitis and keratitis are characterized by chemosis, conjunctival follicles, corneal edema and vascularization, and subepithelial yellow-to-white corneal opacities. Keratitis is typically seen at the temporal limbus but can extend axially and may be accompanied by temporal conjunctivitis and anterior uveitis. Clinical signs of uveitis include epiphora, blepharospasm, miosis, and aqueous flare.[96,97] Signs of posterior uveitis can include peripapillary chorioretinitis and chorioretinal scarring. Although onchocerciasis is often implicated in the pathogenesis of ERU, it is difficult to ascertain the true significance of the association because of the prevalence of the parasite in the normal horse population.[100]

The goal of treatment for onchocerciasis is to reduce ocular inflammation and destroy the microfilariae.[97] Ivermectin is effective at killing microfilariae, but it will not kill the adult parasites.[97,101] Systemic therapy (e.g., flunixin meglumine or phenylbutazone) and topical antiinflammatory therapy is warranted. Topical corticosteroid and NSAID therapy should not be used if a corneal ulcer is present, except under advisement of a veterinary ophthalmologist. Treatment may initially worsen clinical signs, and the disease may recur. Lesions are nonseasonal, and older horses are more likely to be affected than younger horses.

Habronemiasis

Cutaneous habronemiasis, also known as *summer sores*, is caused by aberrant intradermal migration of the larvae of *Habronema* or *Draschia* spp., which are normally found in the stomach (see Chapter 57). Lesions usually develop during the summer months in traumatized skin and are caused by a hypersensitivity reaction to dying larvae. Granulomas with necrotic centers are typically seen on the lower limbs, the urethral process, or the eye. Mineralized larvae can often be observed in the center of the lesion.

Common ocular locations for habronemiasis include the medial canthus, eyelid, conjunctiva, lacrimal caruncle, nasolacrimal duct, and third eyelid.[30,96,102-105] Periocular or eyelid lesions have a raised, irregular, yellow appearance often referred to as *sulfur granules*. The granulomatous lesions are often covered with an exudate and are painful when touched. When the nasolacrimal system is involved, a circular lesion may develop below the medial canthus. Biopsy of the affected area should be performed to aid in diagnosis and to rule out other causes of ulcerative skin lesions. Histopathologically, central cavitations (some with nematode larvae) are surrounded by degenerate and degranulating eosinophils and granulomatous inflammation.[30]

Treatment of habronemiasis consists of an adequate deworming program that includes ivermectin, debridement of the lesions, topical and systemic antiinflammatory therapy, and adequate fly control. In severe cases, systemic corticosteroids may substantially lessen the granulomatous reaction.[30,96,106]

Thelaziasis

Ocular disease caused by *Thelazia lacrimalis* is uncommon. This filarid parasite is a commensal organism that lives in the lacrimal gland, conjunctival fornices, and nasolacrimal duct. It can cause mild blepharoconjunctivitis and dacryocystitis.[107] Diagnosis of thelaziasis is confirmed by identification of the parasite in conjunctival fluid or nasolacrimal flushes.

Setariasis

Setaria digitata and *S. equina* are nematodes normally found in the stomach. Aberrant migration of *Setaria* spp. into the eye can occur in horses, resulting in severe intraocular inflammation.[108] Clinical signs include photophobia, epiphora, corneal edema, hypopyon, aqueous flare, and miosis.[83,109-111] Successful surgical removal of the nematode from the anterior chamber has been reported.[110] In a pilot study, treatment with diethylcarbamazine decreased microfilaremia in horses.[57] Antiinflammatory therapy should be instituted in conjunction with antiparasitic agents.

Dirofilariasis

Intraocular migration of *Dirofilaria immitis* is less common in horses than in carnivores, although successful removal of the nematode from the anterior chamber of a horse has been reported.[96]

Echinococcosis

Echinococcus granulosus is a small tapeworm that causes hydatid disease (see Chapter 60). Dogs are the definitive hosts, and horses are considered intermediate hosts. Exophthalmos, blindness, and head shaking caused by retrobulbar cysts are the only reported ocular manifestations of hydatid cyst disease in the horse.[112,113] The only definitive treatment is surgical excision, although treatment with albendazole can decrease the size of the cyst.[112] Diagnosis is based on positive histopathologic or cytologic identification. Cysts are usually an incidental finding at necropsy, but they are of particular concern because they can cause severe disease in humans, another intermediate host.

The complete reference list is available online at www.expertconsult.com.

11 Systemic Inflammatory Response Syndrome

Katharina L. Lohmann and Michelle H. Barton*

Etiology

The systemic inflammatory response syndrome (SIRS)[1] is the clinical manifestation of dysregulated immune responses to infectious or noninfectious stimuli. The term *SIRS* was coined in recognition of the fact that many clinical signs of systemic inflammation are common to different etiologies and that an infectious cause cannot always be identified. In addition to bacterial infection, recognized underlying causes of SIRS, at least in human patients, include viral infections, fungal infections, severe trauma (including surgical trauma), and ischemia. Apart from the potential role for endogenous inducers of inflammation (see later), cases of SIRS associated with primarily noninfectious conditions, such as severe trauma, may be explained by translocation of bacteria or bacterial products from the intestinal lumen. Translocation occurs through compromise of the mucosal barrier, which is most pronounced with severe inflammation and ischemia, but is also suggested to occur with severe shock states, severe trauma, malnutrition, and strenuous exercise.[2-6] Mechanisms of gut barrier compromise under these conditions may include reduced intestinal blood flow, resulting in ischemia; hypoxemia; and increased body temperature. Apoptosis may compound translocation in septic patients.[7] The occurrence and relevance of translocation has not been investigated sufficiently in horses; however, it may serve to explain the occurrence of systemic inflammation in compromised patients without primary infection or intestinal disease.

Initiation of an inflammatory response requires the presence of inducers, sensors, mediators, and effectors.[8] Inflammation is an indispensable mechanism in the defense against invading infectious organisms, but it is more difficult to understand the origin and role of inflammation with regard to noninfectious stimuli. The 'danger model'[9] proposes that the immune response is initiated by endogenous signals of damaged or stressed cells rather than exclusively by exogenous (or foreign) signals, and the importance of pattern recognition receptors (PRRs)[10] in innate immune responses is now well recognized. Pattern recognition receptors are "hard-wired"[10] receptors of the innate immune system, which recognize 'danger-associated molecular patterns' (DAMPs)[8] that may be of exogenous or endogenous origin. Exogenous or pathogen-associated molecular patterns (PAMPs) include endotoxin, lipoteichoic acid, or viral deoxyribonucleic acid (DNA), which represent molecules that are consistently present in certain types of pathogens and are structurally conserved. Endogenous DAMPs are referred to as "alarmins" and represent molecules, such as heat-shock proteins (HSPs), that are released in connection with trauma, burns, ischemia, hemorrhage, or other sources of cell stress and damage.[8] The Toll-like receptors (TLRs) are an important, albeit not the only, family of PRRs that may be present on the cell surface or intracellularly and in their entirety cover a broad spectrum of DAMPs (Table 11-1). TLR signaling ultimately results in the increased expression of cytokines and other inflammatory mediators, which are responsible for many of the clinical alterations observed in patients with SIRS.

Endotoxin is the major structural component of the outer membrane layer of the gram-negative bacterial cell wall (Fig. 11-1) and can be regarded as the prototypic PAMP. Much of the equine literature and therefore much of this chapter is focused on the immune response to endotoxin and the clinical syndrome of endotoxemia. Sources of endotoxin relevant to equine medicine include gram-negative infections, as well as gram-negative bacteria that are part of the normal intestinal, especially cecal, microflora. Endotoxin molecules have lipopolysaccharide (LPS) structure and consist of three distinct portions: the O-polysaccharide (or O-chain), core oligosaccharide (divided further into inner and outer core), and lipid A (Fig. 11-2). Lipid A represents the biologically active portion of LPS, is well conserved among pathogenic gram-negative bacteria, and as it anchors the endotoxin molecule in the cell membrane, is not available for interaction with inflammatory cells until endotoxin is released from the bacterial cell.[11] This release occurs on cell division and cell death but also on bacterial killing from antimicrobial treatment.[12]

Table 11-1 Toll-Like Receptor (TLR) Ligands

Receptor	Microbial and Synthetic Ligands
TLR1	Triacyl lipopeptides, bacterial lipoproteins
TLR2	Bacterial lipoproteins, lipopeptides, peptidoglycan, yeast zymosan, lipoteichoic acid, atypical lipopolysaccharide (LPS), lipoarabinomannan, high-mobility group box protein-1 (HMGB-1)
TLR3	Double-stranded RNA
TLR4	LPS, Taxol, heat shock proteins (HSPs), HMGB-1, viral F-protein (e.g., respiratory syncytial virus)
TLR5	Flagellin
TLR6	Diacyl lipopeptides, bacterial lipoproteins, yeast zymosan, lipoteichoic acid
TLR7	Imidazoquinoline, loxoribine, single-stranded RNA (viral)
TLR8	Imidazoquinoline, single-stranded RNA (viral)
TLR9	CpG DNA, CpG oligonucleotides
TLR10	Not identified
TLR11*	Ligands derived from uropathogenic bacteria
TLR12*	Not identified
TLR13*	Not identified

Modified from Horner AA, Redecke V, Raz E: Curr Opin All Clin Immunol 4:6, 555–561, 2004; DeFranco AL, Locksley RM, Robertson M: The Toll-like receptor family of innate immune receptors. In Immunity: the immune response in infectious and inflammatory disease, London, 2007, New Science Press.

*Note that TLR11-13 have only been identified in mice to date.

*The authors acknowledge and appreciate the original contributions of these authors, whose work has been incorporated into this chapter.

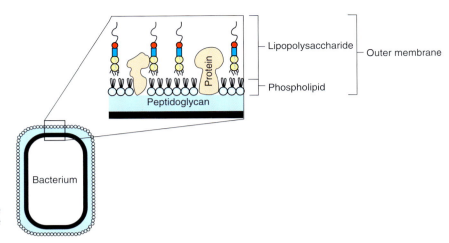

Figure 11-1 Lipopolysaccharide (LPS, endotoxin) is the major component of the outer membrane layer of the gram-negative bacterial cell wall.

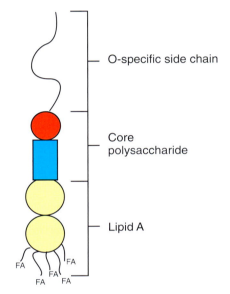

Figure 11-2 Structure of LPS (endotoxin). *FA,* Fatty acid.

For the purpose of case definition in human clinical trials, SIRS is often defined by the presence of at least two characteristic findings, including hypothermia or hyperthermia; tachycardia, tachypnea, or hypocapnia; and leukocytosis, leukopenia, or an increased number of immature leukocyte forms.[1] Use of the term *SIRS* in equine medicine may be appropriate[13] and is becoming more common, although specific diagnostic criteria have not been agreed on to date. Additional definitions applicable to human patients include sepsis (SIRS caused by demonstrable infection, whether localized or in the form of bacteremia), severe sepsis, and septic shock (sepsis-induced hypotension, persisting despite adequate fluid resuscitation, along with the presence of hypoperfusion abnormalities or organ dysfunction).[1] Multiple organ dysfunction syndrome (MODS) is defined as insufficiency of two or more organs, which may manifest as clinical changes or may be diagnosed based on clinicopathologic data. Interestingly, recognition that the above definition of sepsis (and therefore SIRS) may be too restrictive for clinical purposes has led to the proposal of a broader definition that allows inclusion of general variables (e.g., fever, tachycardia, hyperglycemia), inflammatory variables (e.g., leukopenia, presence of band neutrophils, levels of C-reactive protein), hemodynamic variables (e.g., hypotension, hypoxemia), indicators of organ dysfunction (e.g., oliguria, ileus) and tissue perfusion variables (e.g., hyperlactatemia).[14] A staging system that takes into account *P*redisposition, nature of the *I*nsult, markers of the inflammatory *R*esponse, and measures of *O*rgan dysfunction (*PIRO* system) was also proposed and may ultimately allow for more distinct differentiation between morbidity arising from the primary infection and the response to infection. Although it is nearly impossible to discuss SIRS without discussing aspects of sepsis, this chapter focuses on the immune responses to infection and other stimuli, rather than specific aspects of the infection itself, which is specifically addressed in the chapter devoted to sepsis in Chapter 6.

It has to be emphasized that SIRS and even sepsis are clinical terms that do not directly relate to specific diseases or specific pathophysiologic or cellular events.[15] For example, experimental endotoxin challenge models in horses create very similar clinical alterations to a "natural challenge" of gram-negative infection, but one cannot necessarily assume that interventions found to alleviate experimental endotoxin challenge will have the same effect in natural disease. Much work in human medicine has been directed at the neutralization of specific mediators of inflammation, and very few of these interventions have ultimately become established in clinical medicine. Without detracting from the value of studies discussed in this chapter, clinicians must therefore be cognizant of the limitations of experimental work, and well-designed clinical trials will ultimately be needed to address important questions regarding therapy and prognosis of patients with SIRS and sepsis.

Epidemiology

Notwithstanding neonatal sepsis, which is still considered the most common cause of foal deaths in intensive care settings, the frequency of sepsis in horses has not been reported and estimates for the occurrence of SIRS are to date based on detection of endotoxemia. Endotoxemia affects horses and ponies of either gender and of all breeds and ages, including neonatal foals. Studies performed at referral institutions have found that 10% to 40% of horses presented for colic[16-19] and 50% of septic neonatal foals[20] had measurable circulating endotoxin concentrations. The number of colic patients testing positive for endotoxin was increased in some studies when only horses with conditions requiring exploratory surgery were investigated. Interestingly, a recent study found no difference in systemic endotoxin concentrations between horses with medical or surgical colic; those with large intestinal, small intestinal or other lesions; or between horses with strangulating or nonstrangulating lesions, respectively.[19] In the same study, measurable blood endotoxin concentration in horses with colic was not associated with survival.

In other species, including humans, presence of certain gene polymorphisms has been associated with a reduced sensitivity to inflammatory challenge ("hyporesponders") and may also be associated with disease susceptibility and outcome. Investigation of gene polymorphisms is an area of great interest because it may provide the basis for a more individualized approach to patient assessment and therapy. Gene polymorphisms are defined as allelic variants that exist stably in a population and occur in frequencies ($\geq 1\%$) not attributable to new mutations.[21] Polymorphisms most often occur as single-nucleotide polymorphisms (SNPs) and may affect coding, as well as noncoding, regions of genes. Single-nucleotide polymorphisms within coding regions (exons) that result in altered amino acid sequence presumably affect protein function. For example, SNPs in the coding region of the human TLR4 gene are associated with impaired signal transduction in response to LPS stimulation,[22] and a suggested association with poor outcome of sepsis[23,24] may be attributable to a reduced immune defense against infection. Similarly, a polymorphism in TLR2 may be associated with staphylococcal infections.[25] Changes in noncoding regions (introns) or in gene promoters may alter transcription rates and messenger ribonucleic acid (mRNA) stability or may serve as "markers" for certain traits if they are in linkage with biologically active SNPs in other gene regions.[21] For example, a polymorphism in the human tumor necrosis factor alpha (TNF-α) gene promoter[26] may affect the magnitude of TNF-α expression on cell stimulation and may be associated with outcome of septic shock. A polymorphism in the promoter region of the human interleukin-6 (IL-6) gene decreases cytokine production *in vitro* and was found to be associated with an improved outcome of sepsis.[27] Similarly, IL-10 cytokine expression may vary in response to several polymorphisms and may affect outcomes of sepsis.[28-30] It should be noted that study results concerning the relevance and impact of polymorphisms in human sepsis have at times produced incongruent findings.

The biologic significance of SNPs in the equine TNF-α gene promoter[31,32] and other immune response genes[33] has not been determined. One study using whole blood stimulation with LPS reported no association of TLR4 polymorphisms with cytokine production in vitro.[34]

Pathogenesis

Inflammatory Cell Activation

Activation of inflammatory cells resulting in altered cell function is a central event in the inflammatory response and the development of SIRS. As mentioned previously, PRRs include the TLRs, of which 13 have been identified in mammals to date (see Table 11-1). Additional PRRs include the transmembrane receptor for advanced glycation end products and the cytosolic nucleotide-binding domain, leucine-rich repeat-containing proteins, and retinoic-acid inducible gene I-like receptors.[8]

With specific regard to endotoxin-induced signaling, LPS molecules in solution tend to aggregate and form micelles based on their amphipathic nature. In plasma, individual LPS molecules are removed from these micellar aggregates by LPS-binding protein (LBP)[35] and transferred to the surface of inflammatory cells, where binding to a specific receptor complex elicits cell activation. Aside from TLR4, which has been identified as the PRR for endotoxin,[36] the receptor complex includes the cluster of differentiation antigen 14 (CD14) and myeloid differentiation factor-2 (MD-2), a small protein that interacts with the extracellular portion of TLR4. Although all three proteins appear to be required to provide a high sensitivity of cells

to endotoxin, TLR4 is the only protein with a transmembrane domain and therefore deserves particular recognition when investigating cellular stimulation by endotoxin. Toll-like receptor 4 is a 92-kilodalton (kDa) type I transmembrane receptor that is expressed constitutively on neutrophils, monocytes, macrophages, and dendritic cells but also on epithelial and endothelial cells. Expression levels vary among individuals and are regulated in a tissue-specific manner by LPS and cytokines (e.g., TNF-α). The cluster of differentiation antigen 14 is a 60-kDa protein that is constitutively expressed on myeloid cells, including monocytes, macrophages, and neutrophils, as well as B lymphocytes and several other cell types.[11] A soluble form (sCD14) in plasma may further be able to transfer LPS to non–CD14-bearing cells (e.g., endothelial cells) and render these cells endotoxin responsive.[37] Conversely, high concentrations of sCD14 may have 'detoxifying' effects by scavenging LPS and preventing it from interacting with inflammatory cells. Other LPS-binding proteins, including LBP, lactoferrin, lysozyme, hemoglobin, and surfactant proteins may also be able to mitigate LPS interaction with inflammatory cells and the development of SIRS.[38] Toll-like receptor 4, in association with MD-2, represents the actual signaling portion of the LPS receptor complex.[36,39] Myeloid differentiation factor-2 is a small, secreted glycoprotein that associates with the extracellular domain of TLR4 and is most likely required for proper receptor function. Myeloid differentiation factor-2 may also be involved in ensuring proper glycosylation and transport of TLR4 to the cellular surface.

Toll-like receptors signal via four adapter proteins, namely myeloid differentiation primary-response protein 88 (MyD88), TIR-domain-containing adapter protein (TIRAP), TIR-domain-containing adapter protein-inducing interferon gamma (IFN-γ; TRIF), and TRIF-related adapter molecule (TRAM).[40] Intracellular signaling pathways resulting in activation of nuclear factor kappa B (NF-κB) are of major significance for inflammatory cell activation. In effect, cell-signaling events culminate in the translocation of transcription factors to the cell nucleus, with a resulting increase in gene transcription and protein expression. Translational and posttranslational processes may also be activated, such that the regulation of protein expression in response to TLR ligands is a complex event offering multiple targets for regulation and potential therapeutic influence.

Inflammatory Mediators

Mediators of systemic inflammation include cytokines, chemokines, growth factors, components of the complement, coagulation, fibrinolytic and kallikrein-kinin systems, lipid mediators, neuromediators, enzymes, reactive oxygen species (ROS), and reactive nitrogen species (RNS). Table 11-2 summarizes the origin, regulation, and biologic effects of some of the major inflammatory mediators. Release and activity of inflammatory mediators is not a linear but rather a complex, interconnected and interdependent process, which is insufficiently represented by a discussion of individual components in isolation.

Cytokines play a particularly important role because they not only exert pathophysiologically relevant effects but also regulate the release of other mediators. Proinflammatory cytokines (e.g., TNF-α, IL-1) are central to the initiation and maintenance of an inflammatory reaction, and development of SIRS has classically been attributed to an uncontrolled overproduction of these proinflammatory mediators.[41] In recent years, however, studies have increasingly investigated cytokines with mostly antiinflammatory activity, such as IL-10, IL-4, IL-13, IFN-α, and transforming growth factor beta (TGF-β), which are produced along with their proinflammatory counterparts and may serve to contain and attenuate inflammation after an invading pathogen has been eliminated. Downregulating effects on the inflammatory cascade are further attributed to soluble

Table 11-2 Important Mediators of the Systemic Inflammatory Response to Endotoxin

Mediator	Origin	Effects
Tumor necrosis factor alpha (TNF-α)	Macrophages	Synthesis of TNF-α, IL-1, IL-6, prostaglandins, PAF, phospholipase A2, HMGB-1, endothelin, and GM-CSF
	Monocytes	Neutrophil activation, adhesion molecule expression
	Neutrophils	Endothelial activation, enhanced procoagulant activity, iNOS expression
	CD4+ T cells	Activation of coagulation and fibrinolysis
	Natural killer cells	Activation of complement and contact systems
		Catabolic state
		Insulin resistance
		Pyrogen (direct and via IL-1 induction)
Interleukin-1 (IL-1)	Activated macrophages	Pyrogen via central release of PGE2
	Endothelial cells	Release of prostaglandins, leukotrienes, and PAF
	Fibroblasts	Neutrophil activation and chemotaxis, adhesion molecule expression
	Dendritic cells	Endothelial activation, enhanced procoagulant activity, iNOS expression
	Lymphocytes	Activation of coagulation and fibrinolysis
	Keratinocytes	Activation of complement and contact systems
		Acute-phase response
		Increases activity of lipoprotein lipase
		Mobilizes amino acids
		Induces muscle proteolysis
Interleukin-6 (IL-6)	Activated tissue macrophages	Acute-phase response
	Fibroblasts	Stress response
	Keratinocytes	Weak pyrogen
	T lymphocytes	Antiinflammatory effects via induction of IL-10, soluble TNF receptor, IL-1 receptor antagonist, cortisol production
Interleukin-8 (IL-8)	Macrophages	Neutrophil activation and chemotaxis
	Endothelial cells	
Interleukin-10 (IL-10)	T helper (Th) cells type 2	Inhibition of macrophage activation
	Monocytes	Inhibition of synthesis and release of cytokines from T cells and macrophages
	Epithelial cells	Suppresses function of antigen-presenting cells
Interleukin-12 (IL-12)	Macrophages	Induces IFN-γ production
Interleukin-17 (IL-17)	Th-17 cells	Enhances production of other cytokines (e.g., IL-1, IL-6, TNF-α)
Macrophage migration inhibition factor (MIF)	Preformed in leukocytes	Activation of macrophages and T cells
	Anterior pituitary, hypothalamus, adrenals	Enhances production of cytokines, NO, prostaglandins
	Lungs, skin, GI and genitourinary tract	Links immune and endocrine systems
High-mobility group box protein-1 (HMGB-1)	All nucleated cell types	Increases proinflammatory effects of other cytokines (e.g., IL-1), enhances immune cell migration
		Contributes to disruption of epithelial barriers
		Acts as an alarmin in nonseptic inflammation
Thromboxane A2 (TxA2)	Platelets, neutrophils, macrophages, monocytes	Vasoconstriction
		Platelet aggregation
		Bronchoconstriction
		Leukocyte adhesion
Prostaglandin E2 (PGE2)	Most nucleated cells	Vasodilation
		Platelet aggregation
		Pyrogen
		Antiinflammatory effects (e.g., inhibition of neutrophil functions)
Prostaglandin I2 (PGI2)	Vascular endothelial cells	Vasodilation
		Inhibits platelet aggregation
Prostaglandin F2α (PGF2α)	Most nucleated cells	Vasoconstriction
		Luteolysis
Platelet-activating factor (PAF)	Macrophages	Platelet aggregation
	Monocytes	Activation of macrophages and neutrophils
	Platelets	Hypotension
	Neutrophils	Vasoconstriction, increases vascular permeability
	Mast cells	Leukocyte recruitment
	Eosinophils	Visceral smooth muscle contraction
	Endothelial cells	Negative inotrope, arrhythmogenic
		Ileus
Leukotriene B4 (LTB4)	Neutrophils	Chemoattractant
	Monocytes	Promotes neutrophil interaction with endothelial cells
	Alveolar macrophages	Neutrophil activation
		Increases vascular permeability
Leukotrienes C4, D4, E4 (SRS-A)	Eosinophils	Increases vascular permeability
	Monocytes	Bronchoconstriction
		Vasoconstriction
Kinins	Produced from serum precursors	Increases vascular permeability
		Vasodilation (via NO production)
		Smooth muscle contraction
		Pain

Table 11-2 Important Mediators of the Systemic Inflammatory Response to Endotoxin—cont'd

Mediator	Origin	Effects
Complement components (C3a, C5a)	—	Neutrophil activation and chemotaxis Synthesis and release of cytokines (TNF-α, IL-1, IL-6, IL-8) C5a enhances phagocytosis in early stages, contributes to immune suppression in later stages Smooth muscle contraction Mast cell degranulation Release of histamine and serotonin Vasodilator and increased vascular permeability
Oxygen-derived free radicals Nitric oxide (NO)	Macrophages Neutrophils Immune cells Vascular cells (endothelium)	Cell membrane and tissue damage Enzyme inactivation Local vasodilation Slows local blood flow Modulates neutrophil migration Alters epithelial tight junctions (tissue damage)
Granulocyte-monocyte colony-stimulating factor (GM-CSF)	—	Rebound neutrophilia

iNOS, Inducible NO synthase; *IFN-γ,* interferon gamma; *GI,* gastrointestinal; *SRS-A,* slow-reacting substance of anaphylaxis.

cytokine receptors (e.g., soluble TNF receptor), "decoy" receptors (e.g., IL-1 receptor type II) and cytokine receptor antagonists (e.g., soluble IL-1R antagonist), which inhibit cytokine effects at the level of the inflammatory cell. This compensatory antiinflammatory response syndrome (CARS) may be important for a return to normal homeostasis following an insult, but excessive production of antiinflammatory mediators, which has been referred to as *leukocyte re-programming*,[42] may also result in immune suppression and increased risk of infection. The paradigm of "immunologic dissonance," as proposed by Bone,[41] provides a more comprehensive and flexible view of inflammatory responses during inflammation and infection than an isolated view of proinflammatory or antiinflammatory responses. According to this paradigm, every severe insult produces a response consisting of both proinflammatory and antiinflammatory components, and it is the relative balance (or lack thereof) of these components that determines outcome in the form of reestablishment of homeostasis or disease progression toward shock. Recent evidence suggests that it may not be possible to neatly categorize inflammatory mediators as purely proinflammatory or antiinflammatory and that their activity may vary with the type of insult, the timing of exposure, or even the concentration of the mediator, further suggesting that a more global view of the inflammatory response is needed.[8]

As mentioned earlier, SIRS can arise from localized insults if "spillover" of inflammatory mediators into the systemic circulation occurs once a critical concentration has been reached at the local site.[41] Interestingly, it has been proposed that antiinflammatory responses may dominate outside localized sites of inflammation, and that indeed plasma behaves as an immune-suppressive milieu to prevent spread of inflammation and the occurrence of SIRS.[43,44] Research studies and clinical evaluations of inflammatory mediator production should therefore ideally pursue sampling of local organ milieus in addition to blood sampling. In horses, this has been done to some extent with regard to the respiratory tract and peritoneal fluid, but additional work is no doubt needed.

Endothelial Dysfunction, Hemodynamic Changes, and Shock

Septic shock is generally classified as "distributive shock" and is largely attributable to peripheral vascular dysfunction resulting in maldistribution of blood flow and perfusion deficits. Inflammatory mediators, such as prostacyclin and nitric oxide (NO), cause widespread vasodilation and vasoplegia, leading to blood pooling in the periphery and a reduction of effective circulating volume.[45] In addition, cardiac function is compromised by decreased coronary blood flow and the release of myocardial depressant factors; circulating volume is reduced by increased vascular permeability; and tissue oxygen extraction is impaired. Initially, tachycardia and increased cardiac output, as well as increases in central venous pressure and pulmonary arterial pressure (hyperdynamic phase), may have a compensatory effect.[45] However, disease progression is characterized by the development of systemic hypotension and ultimately perfusion deficits of vital organs.

In addition to its role in vascular failure, endothelial dysfunction promotes the development of microvascular thrombosis, thereby contributing to the development of organ failure. Loss of the normal endothelial surface with its antithrombotic properties favors thrombus formation by exposing subendothelial tissue factor and allowing platelet aggregation to occur. Endothelial damage is primarily neutrophil mediated by a mechanism involving neutrophil-derived enzymes (e.g., elastase), hydrogen peroxide molecules, endothelial enzymes (e.g., xanthine oxidase), and endothelial cytosolic iron. Free radicals, predominantly HO$^-$ (hypochlorite), which are formed in endothelial cells, directly cause cell damage; neutrophil-derived matrix metalloproteinases (MMPs) and direct effects of cytokines (e.g., TNF-α, IL-1) also contribute. Constitutive production of NO may afford some protection against radical-mediated endothelial cell damage; however, overproduction of NO by the inducible NO synthase (iNOS) enzyme has detrimental effects and compounds tissue damage.

Neutrophil Activation

Neutrophil activation during bacterial infection generally serves to promote extravasation into infected tissues and increase the cells' bactericidal capacity. Activated neutrophils express adhesion molecules for interaction with endothelial cells, exhibit an increased capacity for phagocytosis and respiratory burst, and release lysosomal enzymes and inflammatory mediators.[46] Neutrophil margination and extravasation occur in three phases, characterized by the expression of different adhesion molecules on neutrophils and endothelial cells. The first phase of neutrophil tethering and rolling is mediated by P-selectin and E-selectin on endothelial cells, which interact with P-selectin glycoprotein ligand-1 (PSGL-1) and sialylated Lewis-X–like structures on leukocytes. Firm adhesion of neutrophils to the endothelium during the second phase results from the interaction between endothelial intercellular adhesion molecule-1 (ICAM-1) and neutrophil integrins leukocyte function–associated antigen-1 (LFA-1) and Mac-1. The third phase of neutrophil transmigration depends on expression of platelet/endothelial cell adhesion molecule-1, located at the intercellular junction of endothelial cells.

Neutropenia is an early finding during experimental endotoxin administration and may be the only specific clinicopathologic evidence of acute sepsis or endotoxemia.[47] Neutrophil margination is observed, particularly within the lung vasculature,[48] and neutrophils are important players in the development of acute lung injury after endotoxin administration. Mechanisms of neutrophil-mediated lung injury may include vascular endothelial damage, neutrophil migration into airways, expression of proinflammatory cytokines (e.g., IL-1, TNF-α), and oxidant-induced injury resulting in loss of epithelial integrity.[49] In some cases, these events may culminate in the development of a "shock lung,"[50] and pulmonary failure remains the leading cause of sepsis-related death in human patients. In cases of recovery, reentry of marginated neutrophils into the circulation leads to rebound neutrophilia; however, it is questionable whether these neutrophils exhibit normal cellular function and signify a recovery of normal immune responses. Increased release of neutrophils from the bone marrow caused by stimulation of myeloid cell proliferation by granulocyte-macrophage colony-stimulating factor (GM-CSF) also contributes to rebound neutrophilia.

Coagulopathy

Development of coagulopathy in SIRS and sepsis can be attributed to simultaneous activation of coagulation and fibrinolytic cascades, as well as impairment of regulatory mechanisms. Development of coagulopathy has been documented in horses with colic,[51-53] as well as in septic foals,[20,54] and microthrombosis may play a role in the development of organ failure.[55,56]

Activation of coagulation is by both the intrinsic and the extrinsic pathways, which converge at factor X and culminate in thrombin-mediated conversion of fibrinogen into fibrin. The tissue factor (extrinsic) pathway is the dominant pathway in vivo.[8] Endotoxin directly activates the intrinsic coagulation pathway through the contact system comprising factor XII (Hageman factor), prekallikrein, and high-molecular-weight kininogen. Activation of the extrinsic pathway results from exposure of subendothelial tissue factor after endothelial damage and stimulation of tissue factor expression on activated mononuclear phagocytes and endothelial cells. Increased expression of monocyte tissue factor (also referred to as *procoagulant activity*) was significantly associated with poor prognosis in equine colic patients,[57] and tissue factor expression by peritoneal macrophages may favor the development of intraabdominal adhesions in colic patients undergoing exploratory laparotomy.[58]

Thrombin is formed initially on tissue factor–bearing surfaces and cells and subsequently stimulates amplified thrombin production on the platelet surface.[59] Thrombin stimulates platelet adhesion and activation and amplifies the coagulation cascade through feedback activation of factors V, VIII, and XI. Platelet aggregation is also favored by increased release of thromboxane A_2 (TxA_2) from activated vascular endothelial cells and release of TxA_2 and platelet-activating factor (PAF) from activated platelets. A predominant role for PAF rather than TxA_2 in endotoxin-induced platelet aggregation has been suggested.[60,61]

Endothelial dysfunction leads to decreased activation of protein C and decreased expression of antithrombin III (ATIII), thereby affecting important regulatory components of coagulation. Activated protein C (APC) is important for the anticoagulant properties of normal endothelium and acts in concert with protein S by inactivating clotting factors Va and VIIIa, as well as plasminogen activator inhibitor (PAI).[62] Production of APC depends on thrombin interaction with thrombomodulin on the vascular endothelium, such that decreased thrombomodulin expression by damaged endothelial cells decreases APC formation. This results in further reduction of APC because of consumption and decreased production in the liver. Reduced APC levels in human patients with sepsis are associated with an increased mortality. Antithrombin III inhibits multiple components of both the intrinsic and the extrinsic coagulation pathway, including clotting factors IIa, IXa, Xa, XIa, XIIa, VIIa/tissue factor, and kallikrein.[63]

Regulation of fibrinolysis occurs at the level of both plasminogen and plasmin, the actual fibrin-degrading enzyme. Increased fibrinolysis leads to an accumulation of fibrin degradation products (FDPs), which inhibit platelet aggregation, thrombin formation, and fibrin polymerization and thereby enhance bleeding tendency. Fibrin degradation products also play a role in increasing vascular permeability. Cytokines such as TNF-α and IL-1 activate fibrinolysis by increasing expression of both tissue-type (tPA) and urokinase-type (uPA) plasminogen activator. These cytokines, however, also stimulate synthesis of PAI, which opposes fibrinolysis. Increased plasma concentrations of PAI were observed in horses with colic,[64,65] suggesting that inhibition of fibrinolysis and therefore further increased procoagulant tendency may be the predominant abnormality in these patients.

In the most severe cases, these changes result in consumptive coagulopathy and disseminated intravascular coagulation (DIC).[66] More frequently, however, coagulopathy is subclinical or is recognized by an increased thrombotic tendency (e.g., jugular venous thrombosis) or an increased bleeding tendency (e.g., following venipuncture or nasogastric intubation). Diffuse microthrombosis may contribute to tissue ischemia and the development of organ failure. Evaluation of coagulation parameters to detect subclinical disease is an important step in patient assessment.

The recognition of positive-feedback loops between coagulation and inflammatory pathways[67] has provided novel insights into the pathophysiology of inflammation during SIRS and sepsis. Coagulation components, such as fibrinogen and high-molecular-weight kininogen, are increased as part of the acute phase response,[38] and activation of coagulation results in endothelial cell activation and expression of inflammatory cytokines, such as IL-6 and IL-8, thereby contributing to leukocyte activation and endothelial adhesion.[59,68] Thrombin formation increases generation of TNF-α, IL-1, and IL-6 and leads to generation of complement component C5a, which in turn increases tissue factor expression. Treatment of human patients with severe sepsis with recombinant APC initially showed beneficial effects,[69] which were attributed to decreased endothelial injury and vascular dysfunction, antiinflammatory effects via blockade of NF-κB activation, diminished neutrophil activation, and an increased expression of antiapoptotic genes.[38,59] However, a major follow-up study failed to show beneficial effects, and the drug was recently withdrawn from the market.[70]

Complement Activation

Complement activation in response to infection serves the purpose of enhancing phagocytosis and pathogen destruction, inducing bacterial cell lysis through formation of a membrane attack complex, and promoting and regulating inflammation through individual complement components such as C3a and C5a.[8] The three pathways of complement activation are the classical, lectin, and alternative pathways.

Endotoxin activates the alternative pathway by direct interaction with complement components. Complement activation further occurs on bacterial surfaces, by acute-phase proteins, and by immune complexes.[71] Plasmin and kallikrein, produced during activation of coagulation and fibrinolysis, also activate C3 and C5, which cause vasodilation and increase vascular permeability by activation of mast cell degranulation (anaphylatoxins). The cleaved fragment, C5a, further acts as a chemotaxin and increases leukocyte migration, promotes neutrophil adhesion to endothelial cells, stimulates enzyme release from phagocytic cells and superoxide anion production by neutrophils, and activates leukotriene production in neutrophils and monocytes. This component also has inhibitory effects on neutrophil function and contributes to a procoagulant state. Blockade of C5a generation or C5a receptor blockade during the onset of sepsis improves survival in experimental models.[71]

Acute-Phase Response

During acute inflammation, production of a number of proteins by the liver is increased, possibly to counteract and contain inflammatory responses.[72] This acute-phase response is primarily initiated by IL-1 and IL-6 and is limited to the first 24 to 48 hours after an insult. Acute-phase proteins identified in horses include fibrinogen, haptoglobin, ferritin, transferrin, ceruloplasmin, coagulation factor VIII:C, serum amyloid A, C-reactive protein, α_1-acid glycoprotein, and phospholipase A_2.[73] Hepcidin, a protein involved in regulation of iron metabolism, has also recently been suggested as an acute-phase protein.[74] Fibrinogen is the acute-phase protein most frequently evaluated in horses, and the capacity for fibrinogen production often outweighs increased fibrinogen consumption in clinical or subclinical DIC.[75]

Clinical Findings and Diagnosis

Classically, diagnosis of SIRS is based on alteration of body temperature (hypothermia or hyperthermia), heart rate (tachycardia), respiration (tachypnea or hypocapnia), and leukocyte parameters (leukocytosis, leukopenia or an increased number of "band" neutrophils).[1] These criteria have been adopted in the equine literature.[76,77] Additional parameters thought to be associated with sepsis include delayed capillary refill time, abnormal mucous membrane color, decreased urine production, and hypotension.[77]

The clinical signs of SIRS can be replicated by experimental administration of endotoxin in horses, and endotoxin infusion models have been used widely in the evaluation of inflammatory parameters and therapeutic interventions. Severity of signs depends on the dose and length of infusion of endotoxin, and additional signs, such as depression, anorexia, sweating, muscle fasciculations, decreased intestinal sounds, and signs of abdominal discomfort, are observed. Response to endotoxin infusion is often divided into an early "hyperdynamic" phase with hyperemic mucous membranes and an accelerated capillary refill time and a later "hypodynamic" phase in which mucous membrane color changes to brick red or purple and congestion, a periapical "toxic line," and a prolonged capillary refill time are observed[47] (Fig. 11-3). With continued endotoxin infusion, depression and anorexia worsen and diarrhea may develop, whereas abdominal pain usually subsides (Fig. 11-4). Shock is characterized by decreased pulse pressure and reduced venous filling, cool extremities, diffusely gray or purple mucous membranes, and

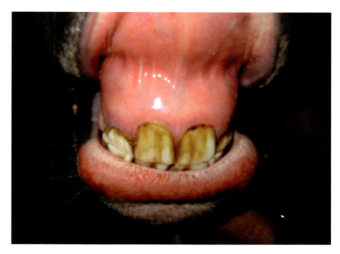

Figure 11-3 Congested and hyperemic mucous membranes in a horse with endotoxemia. *(Courtesy Dr. Clare Ryan.)*

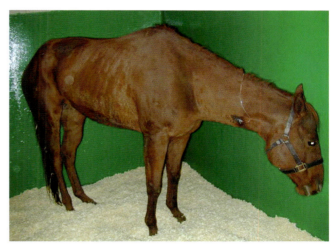

Figure 11-4 Obtunded mentation is often observed in horses with SIRS or endotoxemia. *(Courtesy Dr. Clare Ryan.)*

reduced body temperature. A "muddy" mucous membrane color and diffuse scleral reddening (Fig. 11-5) indicate vascular endothelial damage and increased capillary permeability.

In clinical patients, additional findings may include those of underlying disease processes and complications. Coagulation abnormalities may be identified as thrombosis at catheter placement sites (Fig. 11-6), petechiae or ecchymoses (Fig. 11-7), and an increased bleeding tendency (e.g., following venipuncture or nasogastric intubation). Spontaneous gross hemorrhage in the form of epistaxis may occur in severe cases that have progressed to overt DIC.[78] Clinical signs of organ failure can vary greatly because any body system can be affected but may include those of renal failure (e.g., oliguria, anuria), respiratory failure (e.g., dyspnea, abnormal lung sounds), hepatic failure (e.g., icterus, hepatic encephalopathy), or cardiac failure (e.g., dysrhythmias). Laminitis should be regarded as a type of organ dysfunction in horses, and horses should be monitored through assessment of gait, hoof wall temperature, digital pulse strength, sensitivity to hoof tester pressure, and radiographic assessment (Fig. 11-8). Laboratory evaluation should be included to detect subclinical organ dysfunction such as renal dysfunction, myocarditis, or myonecrosis.[79-81] Abortion should be considered a potential

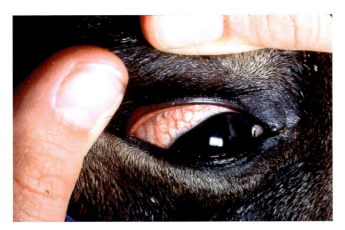

Figure 11-5 Marked scleral injection secondary to endotoxemia. *(Courtesy Dr. Clare Ryan.)*

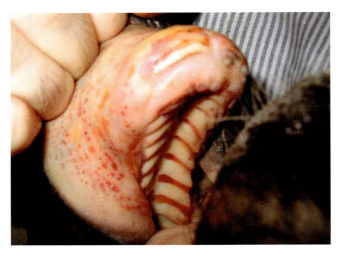

Figure 11-7 Petechial hemorrhages of oral mucous membranes in a neonatal foal with gram-negative sepsis. *(Courtesy Dr. Clare Ryan.)*

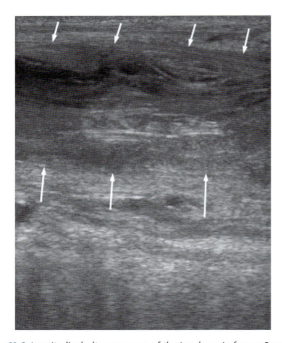

Figure 11-6 Longitudinal ultrasonogram of the jugular vein from a 3-year-old Thoroughbred colt that developed septic jugular thrombosis after surgery to correct colon torsion. Three weeks after onset of signs, the large heterogenous thrombus *(between arrows)* has become very echogenic, with central linear echoes reflecting fibrosis as thrombus begins to resolve. *(Courtesy Dr. Celia Marr.)*

complication in pregnant mares and may be caused by increased prostaglandin $F_2\alpha$ ($PGF_2\alpha$) production and reduced progesterone concentration.[82,83]

Some of the research concerning endotoxemia specifically has focused on measurement of plasma endotoxin concentrations. The Limulus amebocyte lysate (LAL) assay[84] is commercially available in form of a multisample assay kit, but its use has mostly been restricted to research purposes.[85] The performance of the LAL assay in proteinaceous biologic fluids has been questioned because endogenous plasma proteins can inhibit the Limulus reaction.[86] An alternative chemiluminescent endotoxin assay[87] may be more useful for stallside use in

equine patients,[88] but it requires special equipment in the form of a luminometer.

Fibrinogen concentration will often be increased as an indicator of the acute-phase response. A coagulation profile should be evaluated in horses with severe SIRS and should include a platelet count, clotting times (prothrombin time [PT], activated partial thromboplastin time [aPTT]), and ATIII and FDP concentrations. In a report of horses with acute gastrointestinal (GI) disease, coagulation profiles showed abnormalities in 28 of 30 horses,[52] indicating the high prevalence of subclinical coagulopathies. Reported abnormalities include increased concentration of FDPs and soluble fibrin monomer, prolonged PT indicating factor VII consumption, prolonged aPTT indicating factors VIII:C and IX consumption, prolonged thrombin time, decreased ATIII activity, thrombocytopenia, and decreased protein C and plasminogen activities. A diagnosis of DIC may be made if three or more coagulation parameters are abnormal; however, some clinicians prefer to reserve the diagnosis of DIC for horses with overt clinical signs of hemorrhage and thrombosis.[53] Prognostically, decreased ATIII concentration reflects most closely the risk of death in mature horses with colic.[52] Persistent abnormalities or worsening of coagulation parameters on repeated evaluation probably should be regarded as a negative prognostic indicator.

Several studies have evaluated the potential prognostic value of specific cytokine concentrations in patients suffering from SIRS or sepsis. In septic human patients, the magnitude of increase in TNF-α and IL-6 concentration is correlated with the severity of sepsis, whereas concentrations of IL-1 are often undetectable and show poor correlation with disease severity.[89] In horses, plasma activity of TNF-α is positively correlated with mortality in patients with acute GI disease and in septic neonates.[16,90,91] Increased IL-6 expression may be associated with poor prognosis in septic foals[92] and IL-10 correlated with non-survival in sick foals, although there was no difference in gene expression between healthy and sick (including both septic and nonseptic) foals.[93]

Therapy

Given the complexity of the inflammatory cascade, the presence of feedback loops among types of inflammatory mediators, and the redundancy in the effects of many mediators, it is

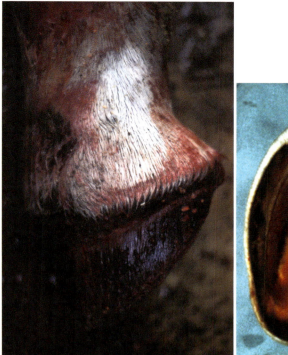
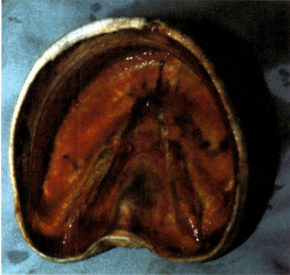

Figure 11-8 Sloughed hoof capsule and left hind digit of a 5-year-old Thoroughbred stallion that developed widespread arterial thrombosis in the metatarsal region secondary to enterocolitis associated with quinidine toxicity. *(Courtesy Dr. Celia Marr.)*

unlikely that interruption of the inflammatory process at one site will suffice to treat SIRS. A common approach is to address multiple aspects of inflammation, which may include cell activation, mediator production, and mediator effects. Additional major objectives in the management of horses with SIRS are treatment of any underlying conditions and general supportive care. In human medicine, the "Surviving Sepsis Campaign"[94] provides internationally accepted guidelines for treatment of severe sepsis and septic shock based on the available evidence; however, even these rather detailed guidelines cannot replace the clinical decision-making process for individual patients.

Source Control

An obvious necessity for the treatment of SIRS is correction of the underlying cause, thereby reducing the amount of inflammation inducers available for cell interaction. If bacterial infection is suspected as the inciting cause of SIRS (sepsis), the site of infection, identity, and antimicrobial susceptibility pattern of the offending organism should be identified by clinical examination and adjunctive tests as deemed necessary. To this end, diagnostic tests may include thoracic or abdominal radiography and ultrasonography, abdominocentesis or pleurocentesis, serial blood culture, fecal cultures, urinalysis, and urine culture. Blood culture is especially important in neonatal foals with suspected sepsis; the umbilicus (external and internal structures) and joints should further be given special consideration as potential septic foci in foals. With specific regard to gram-negative infections, the release of endotoxin on bacterial death[95] needs to be considered and *in vitro* studies suggest that the magnitude of endotoxin release may depend on the type and dose of the antimicrobial drug.[12] Endotoxin release was inversely related to antimicrobial drug concentration, which suggests that adequate dosing based on the patient's body weight is imperative. Some clinicians suggest combining antimicrobial therapy with

endotoxin-binding drugs (see later) during the initial treatment phase.

In addition to early appropriate antimicrobial therapy, removal of infected tissues or fluids is indicated where possible. For horses in which SIRS results from translocation of bacteria or bacterial products, every effort should be made early to identify whether intestinal compromise warrants surgical exploration (e.g., strangulation obstruction) or demands medical therapy (e.g., acute colitis). In the absence of a definitive diagnosis, exploratory laparotomy is indicated in patients showing persistent abdominal pain and deterioration of cardiovascular parameters, including heart rate, pulse pressure, mucous membrane color, and capillary refill time. Resection of compromised bowel serves to limit translocation; however, clinical impression suggests that translocation may be transiently increased after correction of strangulating lesions and restoration of blood flow. Administration of LPS scavengers, such as polymyxin B, before intestinal manipulation may therefore be useful.[96] Relatively little research has been devoted to the medical control of translocation. In patients with primary intestinal disease, systemically administered antiinflammatory drugs, such as flunixin meglumine or dimethylsulfoxide (DMSO), may decrease intestinal inflammation and aid reestablishment of mucosal barrier function. Topical medications, such as bismuth subsalicylate, have a coating effect and possess antiinflammatory properties; however, it is questionable whether these compounds maintain their medicinal activity by the time they reach the small intestine and especially the large intestine. Prokinetics promote intestinal motility and may decrease contact time with the compromised mucosa. Lidocaine (initial bolus of 1.3 mg/kg followed by a constant-rate infusion at 0.05 mg/kg/min) is often used for its antiinflammatory, analgesic, and "indirect prokinetic" properties and may inhibit cytokine production and hemodynamic changes in response to endotoxin.[97] In a recent study,[98] lidocaine reduced the clinical score and TNF-α concentration in serum and peritoneal fluid of horses with experimental endotoxemia but did not prevent infiltration of inflammatory cells into the peritoneal cavity. Treatments aimed at reestablishing normal mucosal barrier function include the use of misoprostol and experimentally, glutamine and acetylcysteine.[99,100] Misoprostol is a synthetic PGE_1 analog[101] and may speed intestinal healing by improving intestinal blood flow in cases of nonsteroidal antiinflammatory drug (NSAID)-induced GI ulceration and right dorsal colitis. Misoprostol decreased basal acid secretion in horses;[102] however, its effectiveness in treating colonic disease has not been evaluated. Important side effects of misoprostol, including colic, diarrhea, and abortion in pregnant mares, need to be taken into account before administration.

Lipopolysaccharide Scavengers

In the early stages of endotoxemia, removal of endotoxin from the circulation may be achieved by antiendotoxin antibodies or endotoxin-binding drugs. Antibodies that bind LPS are thought to provide steric blockade against lipid A interaction with inflammatory cells and to increase LPS and bacterial clearance by opsonization and complement activation.[103-105] A vaccine for protection against endotoxemia in horses is commercially available (Endovac-Equi, Immvac, Columbia, MO); experimentally, vaccination with bacterin-toxoid vaccines prepared from "rough" mutants of *Salmonella typhimurium* and *S. enteritidis* provided protection against homologous and heterologous endotoxin challenge and carbohydrate overload.[106,107] Despite these encouraging results, most research and clinical application have focused on passive immunization with plasma or serum products obtained from hyperimmunized horses. Antibodies against endotoxin are generally raised against the core region of LPS to ensure cross-reactivity among LPS from different sources. To expose the core region, mutant bacterial strains producing LPS with a reduced or absent O-chain, so-called rough LPS, are used. Mechanisms proposed to allow protection by anticore LPS antibodies against smooth LPS present in natural infections include serum enzymatic factors that allow unmasking of shared antigenic sites, incomplete LPS assembly during infection, and partial disruption of bacterial cells by other host defense mechanisms and by antimicrobial treatment.[108] Studies evaluating the efficacy of anti-LPS antibodies in horses have yielded conflicting results. Several authors have reported protective effects in experimental endotoxemia, clinical endotoxemia, clinical cases of enterocolitis and peritonitis, and prophylactically in foals and surgical colic patients.[109-111] Conversely, other studies failed to show beneficial effects of an *Escherichia coli* O111:B4 (J5) antiserum in an experimental endotoxemia model[112] or of equine plasma containing antibodies raised against "rough" *E. coli* O111:B4 (J5) and *Salmonella minnesota* Re595 cells in a clinical study of endotoxemic foals.[108] Hyperimmune plasma was not significantly more effective than "nonimmune" plasma in the foal study,[108] whereas a clinical study of adult horses with endotoxemia caused by intestinal insults demonstrated a significant benefit of hyperimmune over "preimmune" plasma.[110] One experimental study in foals reported adverse effects of *S. typhimurium* antiserum in the form of increased respiratory rates and increased serum activities of IL-6 and TNF-α after endotoxin challenge; this observation may have been attributable to a priming effect of minimal LPS contamination of the serum, as identified by the LAL assay.[113]

Currently available anti-LPS antibody products for use in horses include hyperimmune plasma obtained from horses vaccinated with a rough strain (J5) of *E. coli* (Equiplas-J, Plasvacc USA Inc., Templeton, CA) and serum containing antibodies against a rough *Salmonella typhimurium* strain (Endoserum, Immvac). Hyperimmune plasma without specific antiendotoxin

antibodies is available from several sources (Hi-Gamm Equi, Lake Immunogenics, Ontario, NY; Equiplas Plus, Plasvacc USA) and may aid in treatment of endotoxemia, especially if coagulopathy is present, by providing complement components, fibronectin, clotting factors, and ATIII.

Polymyxin B is a polycationic antibiotic that is able to bind and neutralize endotoxin by interaction with the anionic phosphate substitutions of the lipid A backbone. As opposed to anti-LPS antibodies, polymyxin B binds endotoxin molecules based on their charge, such that antigenic differences among bacterial strains have less impact on the efficacy of this drug. Assuming that the underlying cause of endotoxemia can be corrected, the benefit of administering polymyxin B is likely limited to the first 24 to 48 hours of treatment, and prolonged use is not expected to provide additional advantages.[96]

Polymyxin B at doses of 1000 and 10,000 units per kg body weight (U/kg) was able to significantly reduce *ex vivo* TNF-α production for 3 to 6 and 12 to 24 hours, respectively, although a demonstrable effect on endotoxin binding was only observed for the higher dose.[114] In horses with experimentally induced endotoxemia, pretreatment with polymyxin B at a dose of 6000 U/kg was effective in suppressing cytokine production and clinical signs of endotoxemia.[113] In another endotoxin infusion experiment, pretreatment with polymyxin B (1000 and 5000 U/kg), as well as treatment 1 hour after the start of LPS infusion (5000 U/kg), significantly reduced clinical signs of endotoxemia, leukopenia, and plasma TNF-α activity.[115] The dose-dependent effect observed in these studies is likely attributable to the 1:1 binding stoichiometry of polymyxin B to LPS molecules; therefore individual clinicians may choose to vary the dose of polymyxin B depending on the perceived severity of disease. The 6000 U/kg dose was found to achieve biologically effective serum concentrations for at least 8 hours.[116]

Current recommendations suggest intravenous (IV) administration of polymyxin B at 1000 to 6000 U/kg every 8 to 12 hours.[96] Repeated administration (5 doses at 6000 U/kg each) was not associated with significant adverse effects in healthy horses[116]; however, one study in healthy ponies reported neurologic signs (ataxia, hypermetria, apnea, head shaking) after administration of 18,000 to 36,000 U/kg every 6 hours for a total of 48 hours.[117] Because of its nephrotoxic and neurotoxic properties, caution is advised when administering polymyxin B to dehydrated, hypovolemic, or azotemic patients. In human patients, toxicity of polymyxin B was increased when the drug was used concurrently with aminoglycoside antibiotics or was given soon after anesthesia.[118] A polymyxin B-Dextran-70 conjugate may reduce toxicity in horses.[119]

Blockade of Inflammatory Cell Activation

As mentioned earlier, the body's own antiinflammatory mechanisms include production of soluble cytokine receptors (e.g., soluble TNF receptor), "decoy" receptors (e.g., IL-1 receptor type II) and cytokine receptor antagonists (e.g., soluble IL-1R antagonist), and beneficial effects of polyclonal IV immunoglobulin in human patients may in part be attributable to these components.[38,120] Use of monoclonal antibodies specifically against TNF-α and use of recombinant IL-1R antagonist, on the other hand, did not improve outcomes in clinical studies.[121,122] Use of "atypical" LPS molecules as specific endotoxin antagonists[123] has also been evaluated; curiously, recognition of LPS molecules as agonists or antagonists depends on the host species and is likely attributable to the TLR4 and/or MD-2 portion of the LPS receptor complex.[124-127] The TLR4 blocker, E5564 (Eritoran, Eisai Inc, Boston, MA) may have potential as a LPS antagonist for use in horses, although at this is point, evidence is limited to in vitro studies.[128]

Nonsteroidal Antiinflammatory Drugs

Interference with the production and effects of inflammatory mediators represents a mainstay of treatment of SIRS in equine medicine. NSAIDs are used frequently in the treatment of colic, as well as for septic and inflammatory conditions, with the goals of suppressing prostanoid production, reducing fever and inflammation, and relieving pain. Additional beneficial effects include iron chelation and scavenging of oxygen-derived free radicals; however, these may only be achieved at doses high enough to increase the risk of side effects.[129] All NSAIDs exert their effects by inhibiting cyclooxygenase (COX) and reducing eicosanoid production, and although beneficial effects have been demonstrated for all commonly used NSAIDs in horses,[130-132] flunixin meglumine may be used most frequently for treatment of endotoxemia and SIRS. Numerous studies using experimental models of endotoxemia have demonstrated that flunixin meglumine improves clinical signs, reduces cytokine release, improves blood pressure and maintains tissue perfusion, prevents hypoxemia and lactic acidosis, reduces endothelial damage, reduces the risk of pregnancy loss in mares, and increases survival.[83,130,133-138] A dose-dependent effect of flunixin meglumine on eicosanoid production has been demonstrated, and a reduced dose of the drug (0.25 mg/kg every 8 hours)[139,140] appears to be used widely.[141] Until comparative clinical studies are performed, choice of the "full" dose (1.1 mg/kg once or twice daily) or a reduced dose may depend on the individual case and clinician preference. With regard to adverse effects, including GI ulceration and renal papillary necrosis, flunixin meglumine ranges between phenylbutazone and ketoprofen, although doses higher than those generally used in clinical cases were evaluated.[142]

Corticosteroids

The rationale for using corticosteroids in the management of shock, including septic shock, has been based on their global antiinflammatory action involving multiple pathways and cell types and their ability to maintain homeostasis and organ function. Clinical studies on the use of corticosteroids at antiinflammatory "high" doses (>30 mg/kg of methylprednisolone or 2-4 mg/kg of dexamethasone daily) in human patients failed to show significant survival benefit in most patients with sepsis and septic shock.[143] More recently, relative adrenal insufficiency and peripheral corticosteroid resistance have been identified in septic human patients, resulting in recommendations to use "low-dose" corticosteroids (e.g., 200-300 mg hydrocortisone daily) in the treatment of septic shock.[143] In addition to replacement therapy, low doses of corticosteroids in human patients with septic shock promote shock reversal and reduce shock mortality.

A limited number of studies have evaluated the effects of corticosteroids in experimentally induced equine endotoxemia. Dexamethasone (2 mg/kg) and prednisolone (10 mg/kg) were less effective than flunixin meglumine in reducing cytokine production, hemoconcentration, and hemodynamic changes.[133,144] Dexamethasone did inhibit TNF-α production by LPS-stimulated equine peritoneal macrophages *in vitro*; however, the required concentration was much higher than that achieved by currently recommended doses.[145] A cosyntropin (adrenocorticotropin hormone [ACTH]) stimulation test for evaluation of the hypothalamic-pituitary-adrenal (HPA) axis in neonatal foals has been proposed,[146] and low response to administered cosyntropin was associated with development of MODS and shock in hospitalized foals in that study. A short course of low-dose hydrocortisone therapy in healthy foals was associated with reduced cytokine gene expression following *ex vivo* cell stimulation but did not alter neutrophil function and did not affect response to ACTH stimulation *in vivo*.[147]

Other Mediator-Directed Therapies

Antioxidants may reduce tissue damage by scavenging reactive oxygen radicals that are released from activated neutrophils and other cell types. The most commonly used antioxidant in horses is DMSO, and surveys show that it is frequently used in the treatment of endotoxemia.[141] In horses with colic, antioxidants have been suggested for treatment of reperfusion injury after periods of bowel ischemia; however, experimental studies have largely failed to show beneficial effects,[148-151] and the role of oxidative processes in the development of ischemia and reperfusion injury in the equine colon has been questioned.[152] Because mucosal loss was increased when large colon ischemia and reperfusion were treated with a higher dose (1 g/kg) of DMSO,[150] a lower dose (0.1 g/kg) has been proposed and is used by many clinicians. Dimethylsulfoxide is typically administered IV as a 10% solution in fluids, however, administration by nasogastric tube as a 10% to 20% solution is also possible.

Allopurinol exerts antioxidant effects by inhibiting xanthine oxidase, an enzyme produced from xanthine dehydrogenase during periods of ischemia, which catalyzes formation of superoxide radicals on reperfusion.[153] Experimentally, allopurinol afforded protection against endotoxin challenge in horses,[154] although a protective effect against reperfusion injury was not observed.[149]

Several studies have addressed the approach of selectively suppressing the production or biologic effects of specific inflammatory mediators. In experimentally induced endotoxemia, beneficial effects have been demonstrated for PAF receptor antagonists,[155] inhibitors of TNF-α production, and antibodies directed against TNF-α.[156] Despite its ability to inhibit TNF-α activity *in vitro*, a polyclonal anti–TNF-α antibody was unable to improve clinical and hematologic parameters when given shortly after an *in vivo* endotoxin infusion.[157] Clinical studies on the use of these drugs in equine patients are lacking, and based on the human literature, targeted mediator suppression can probably not be expected to offer an overall survival benefit.[71]

Pentoxifylline is a methylxanthine derivative and phosphodiesterase inhibitor that can alter neutrophil function and inhibit production of various cytokines, including TNF-α and IL-6, as well as IFNs, thromboxane B_2 (TxB_2), and thromboplastin.[158] Experimentally in horses, pentoxifylline reduced the effect of endotoxin infusion on rectal temperature and respiratory rate at individual time points but had no effect on cytokine production, heart rate, or blood pressure.[159] Added benefit may be achieved by combining pentoxifylline with flunixin meglumine.[160] A common dosage recommendation for pentoxifylline in horses is 8 mg/kg orally every 8 hours, although higher dosing at less frequent intervals (10 mg/kg orally every 12 hours) has also been suggested.[161] Because of its rheologic properties, that is, its ability to increase red blood cell deformability and improve microvascular blood flow, pentoxifylline may further be useful for the treatment of horses with or at risk for laminitis. Contrary to human studies, however, pentoxifylline did not reduce aggregation of equine platelets.[162]

Supportive Care

Supportive care is a crucial aspect of the management of patients with SIRS or sepsis. Important considerations include reestablishment of intravascular volume and hydration, maintenance of electrolyte and acid-base homeostasis, pain control, and nutrition.

General principles of fluid therapy apply; rapid resuscitation may be necessary in patients presenting in shock. For initial resuscitation, isotonic solutions (e.g., lactated Ringer's solution, 10-20 mL/kg/hr) or a small bolus of hypertonic saline (7.2%

sodium chloride, 4 mL/kg) may be used. Hypertonic saline administration transiently increases plasma osmolality and results in fluid shifting from the interstitial and intracellular space into the vasculature, thereby restoring circulating volume. Hypertonic saline must be followed with isotonic solutions to restore total body fluid volume. In horses administered endotoxin experimentally, treatment with hypertonic saline increased cardiac output and decreased total peripheral resistance and was superior to administration of an equal volume of normal saline.[163] Because of the possible risk of hypernatremia and hyperchloremia, serum electrolyte concentrations should be monitored in horses given hypertonic saline, especially if renal excretion may be compromised. Heart rate, pulse quality, mucous membrane color, and capillary refill time can be used to monitor patient response to fluid therapy; measurement of blood pressure is indicated in shock patients but is often not practical. Failure of dehydrated horses to urinate once fluid volume has been restored should prompt careful evaluation of renal function. Specific electrolyte abnormalities reported in horses undergoing experimental endotoxin challenge include hypocalcemia, hypomagnesemia, hypokalemia, and hypophosphatemia.[164,165]

Hypoproteinemia and hypoalbuminemia are not only frequent concerns in patients with significant intestinal inflammation but also in horses with body cavity effusions and in patients with acute renal failure. In addition to gross protein losses, vascular endothelial damage may result in leakage of fluid and protein into the interstitium, leading to tissue edema formation and contributing to organ dysfunction and fluid losses. Colloids help to maintain plasma colloid osmotic pressure and reduce edema formation; plasma may have the additional benefit of exerting immunomodulatory effects and providing coagulation factors. Administration of plasma to maintain serum total protein concentration above 4.2 g/dL has been suggested[166]; however, large volumes of plasma required to achieve this goal may sometimes be unavailable or prohibitively expensive.

Of the synthetic colloids, hetastarch (hydroxyethyl starch) is most often used in horses; in hypoproteinemic horses given hetastarch at a dose of 8 to 10 mL/kg, a significant colloid oncotic effect was maintained for 24 hours.[167] Hetastarch should be administered at 5 to 15 mL/kg by slow IV infusion and should be accompanied by an equal or greater volume of isotonic crystalloid fluids.[168,169] Possible adverse effects of hetastarch treatment include the development of coagulopathies, and its use in horses with established coagulation parameter abnormalities should be preceded by careful evaluation of the risks and benefits. In one study, effects of hetastarch on coagulation parameters of treated horses were evident at higher doses (20 mL/kg) and appeared to be caused by a decrease in von Willebrand factor antigen (vWF:Ag) activity,[170] whereas another study did not report the occurrence of bleeding abnormalities.[171] One study comparing small volume (hypertonic saline plus hetastarch) to isotonic fluid resuscitation of horses with experimentally induced endotoxic shock did not report differences in basic coagulation parameters between horses[165]; however, the severity of the model may have outweighed any potential effect of hetastarch on coagulation. In the same model, small volume resuscitation failed to significantly improve hemodynamic responses in treated horses but ameliorated the effect of endotoxin on hypocalcemia.[165,172] In human patients, hetastarch use has been associated with prolonged aPTT, decreased factor VIII activity, and decreased serum fibrinogen concentration.[173]

Inotropic and vasopressor support should be considered in patients with evidence of inadequate tissue perfusion after restoration of circulatory fluid volume. For human patients with septic shock, current recommendations include the use of norepinephrine or dopamine as the vasopressors of choice and dobutamine to increase cardiac output.[94,174] Norepinephrine has been evaluated in hypotensive critically ill foals and was found to increase mean arterial pressure and urine output at a dose of up to 1.5 μg/kg/min concurrently with dobutamine.[175] Doses for dobutamine of 1 to 2 (up to 5) μg/kg/min as a continuous infusion are recommended for use in horses.[176] Monitoring parameters for horses or foals treated with vasopressors and inotropes should include heart rate and rhythm as well as blood pressure.

Management of Coagulopathies

Successful management of the underlying disease process is likely the most appropriate way to prevent and treat coagulopathies. In the horse with SIRS or sepsis, however, treatments specifically directed at interruption of coagulation and fibrinolytic cascades may be useful. Because most coagulopathies in these patients are subclinical, management and monitoring must be based on the evaluation of coagulation parameters as discussed previously.

Common anticoagulants for use in horses include heparin and aspirin; alternative medications have also been reviewed in the literature.[177] The effects of heparin depend on adequate concentration of ATIII and include inhibition of thrombin; facilitation of ATIII-mediated inhibition of clotting factors IX, X, XI, and XII; release of tissue-factor pathway inhibitor; and inhibition of platelet activation.[178,179] Because of the need for adequate ATIII concentrations, administration of heparin in plasma may be useful, especially if endogenous ATIII concentration is low. One study evaluating DIC in horses with colic found no significant survival benefit if horses were treated with heparin alone[75]; however, patient numbers in this study were relatively small. One recommended dosing regimen for heparin includes an initial administration of 80 to 100 U/kg, followed by 40 to 80 U/kg three times daily or a continuous infusion of 5 to 25 U/kg/hr.[166,179] Horses treated with heparin should be monitored for increased bleeding tendency; in addition, heparin may result in thrombocytopenia and anemia from erythrocyte agglutination. Use of low-molecular-weight heparin to avoid these complications has been recommended[180]; suggested doses for horses are 50 to 100 U/kg q24h subcutaneously for dalteparin and 40 to 80 U/kg subcutaneously for enoxaparin.[179,181,182] At a dose of 50 U/kg once daily in colic patients, dalteparin elicited fewer side effects than unfractionated heparin, which was associated with jugular vein changes, transiently decreased hematocrit, and prolonged clotting times.[183]

Aspirin (acetylsalicylic acid) irreversibly inhibits COX activity in platelets, thereby preventing platelet aggregation and reducing the occurrence of microthrombosis. The currently recommended dose is 10 to 30 mg/kg orally every 48 hours. Increased bioavailability after rectal administration has been reported recently, and lower doses may be adequate if the drug is administered by this route.[184] An oral dose of 300 mg acetylsalicylic acid in healthy horses[185] resulted in prolonged bleeding time and reduced blood viscosity. However, the benefit of aspirin treatment in endotoxemic horses has been questioned after findings that aspirin did not inhibit endotoxin-induced platelet aggregation in vitro.[60,61] Clopidogrel was recently shown to reduce adenosine diphosphate (ADP)-induced platelet aggregation in vitro[186] and could have therapeutic applications.

Fresh-frozen plasma products can be used to replenish coagulation factors and ATIII; platelet-rich plasma may further be indicated in patients with thrombocytopenia. As an alternative to commercially available products, collection of platelet-rich plasma using platelet collection kits and two-speed centrifugation techniques has been suggested.[179] The volume of plasma administration depends on the severity of coagulation abnormalities; however, a minimum of 1 to 2 L should probably be administered to an adult horse.

Future Therapeutic Directions

Inhibitors of apoptosis or programmed cell death have shown beneficial effects in experimental models of sepsis and multiorgan apoptosis is thought to contribute to sepsis morbidity.[187] Specifically, inhibition of lymphocyte apoptosis, which may contribute to immunosuppression, and inhibition of intestinal epithelial cell apoptosis, which may promote endotoxin and bacterial translocation, improved survival in animal models.[188,189] Increased lymphocyte apoptosis may be one mechanism by which critically ill patients are predisposed to sepsis[189] and may contribute to the immune suppression and mortality of sepsis.[187] Increased apoptosis was also found in lung epithelial cells[190] and vascular endothelial cells[191]; the latter may contribute to microvascular dysfunction and organ failure in septic patients.[192] The observed increase in apoptosis during sepsis may be caused by an acceleration of physiologic processes[189] and may be mediated by cytokines such as TNF-α.[71] In addition to reducing available immune cells, apoptosis may indirectly induce immune tolerance because phagocytosis of apoptotic cells increased release of antiinflammatory cytokines while it suppressed production of proinflammatory mediators.[193,194] Conversely, necrotic cells had immunostimulatory effects. This immunomodulating effect of apoptotic and necrotic cells, respectively, may be mediated by IFN-γ.[189]

Adenosine receptor ligands have been suggested as modulators in inflammatory diseases. Agonists for the adenosine A1 and A3 receptor and antagonists for the A2A receptor appear most promising based on experimental models of sepsis[195]; however, the role of the A2A receptor is insufficiently understood and antagonists, as well as agonists, have shown benefits in different experimental models.[195] Preliminary work in horses suggests a potential role for adenosine A2A agonists in endotoxemia.[196-198]

Ethyl pyruvate inhibits binding of NF-κB to DNA and subsequent transcription of inflammatory genes including TNF-α, IL-1β and IL-6, and also functions as an antioxidant and free radical scavenger.[199] Experimental evidence suggest that ethyl pyruvate reduced cytokine production following LPS exposure of cells *in vitro*.[199,200]

Omega-3 fatty acids (FAs) have been evaluated for their potential to alter composition of cell membrane phospholipids and alter production pathways of inflammatory mediators. Omega-3 FA incorporation into cell membranes reduces the availability of arachidonic acid (an omega-6 FA) for cleavage by COX and shifts eicosanoid production from the 2-series prostaglandins and 4-series leukotrienes to their 3- and 5-series equivalents.[201] These latter mediators have reduced biologic activity and therefore may reduce the severity of inflammatory responses. In addition, omega-3 FAs may be able to reduce LPS-induced cellular activation by preventing upregulation of CD14 on monocytes by endotoxin.[202] Experimentally, IV infusion of omega-3 FAs was able to alter cell composition of membrane phospholipids,[203] and endotoxin-induced expression of tissue factor, TxB_2, and TNF-α *in vitro* was reduced significantly in horses fed omega-3 FAs in the form of linseed oil for several weeks.[204,205] However, no significant clinical benefit was observed in horses on an omega-3 FA–rich diet when they were given endotoxin *in vivo*.[206] Infusion of a phospholipid emulsion reduced experimentally induced endotoxemia[207] but caused dose-dependent hemolysis.[208] Phospholipids are thought to interact with LPS and cellular receptors and reduce cell activation.

Summary

The inflammatory response to infectious and noninfectious stimuli is very complex, and strict regulation normally ensures removal of offending stimuli and return to homeostasis without harm to the host. SIRS is the clinical syndrome in which the immune response becomes dysregulated and "spirals out of control," which can ultimately result in shock states and multiple organ failure. An understanding of the components of the inflammatory response is important to identify potential therapeutic targets; however, addressing individual aspects of inflammation in isolation is unlikely to effectively reduce the global effects of SIRS. Although experimental studies provide crucial information, properly designed clinical trials will ultimately be necessary to identify strategies that improve treatment outcomes for our patients.

The complete reference list is available online at www. expertconsult.com.

Laboratory Diagnosis of Viral Infections

12

Melissa Ann Bourgeois and J. Lindsay Oaks*

Introduction

The purpose of this chapter is to provide a basic description of the methods most often used in contemporary diagnostic virology laboratories, including the key advantages and disadvantages of the tests and concerns about interpretation. When appropriate, figures illustrate the use of a test with specific equine viral diseases. Each chapter in this section provides pathogen-specific sampling and testing.

The ability to diagnose viral infections is important for equine clinicians. Accurate and timely laboratory confirmation of a viral infection allows more effective supportive clinical management, earlier detection of complications, more accurate prognosis, more effective isolation protocols, evaluation of vaccination programs, detection of vaccination failures, and probably in the future, selection of appropriate antiviral drugs.

Unfortunately, clinically timely, sensitive, and specific laboratory assays for the diagnosis of viral infections have traditionally been challenging. Viral infections generally are detected either directly by demonstration of the virus in clinical samples or indirectly by detection of antiviral antibodies in serum or other fluids. However, the pathogenesis of the virus and the host immune response must often be taken into account and can make testing for viral infections difficult. In most viral infections, viremia is usually only present for a short period of time, the virus itself may be unculturable, antibodies can take weeks to develop, and detectable antibody responses often decrease with time.

Classic methods of direct virus detection, including isolation in cell culture or in laboratory animals, detection of viral antigens by immunolabeling, and electron microscopy, form the foundations of diagnostic virology. Although they are still very good tests, clinical utility has often been constrained by expense, extended time for results, and low sensitivity. Serologic testing has often had problems with sensitivity or specificity, as well as difficulties in distinguishing recent from past infection or between infection and vaccine titers. The application of molecular biology techniques to diagnostic virology has greatly improved the clinical utility of virus testing. The most reliable and rapid format for nucleic acid detection is polymerase chain reaction (PCR), whereas for protein antigen detection, immunohistochemistry (IHC) and the enzyme-linked immunosorbent assay (ELISA) formats are economical to perform and are often very sensitive and specific. For serologic assays, newer testing formats, such as the ELISA, as well as the ability to produce highly purified and defined recombinant viral proteins or peptides for use as antigen targets, have

greatly improved the sensitivity, specificity, and accuracy of antibody tests.

Viral evolution is an important but underappreciated consideration that continually alters the accuracy and success of viral diagnostics. Viruses are constantly changing to evade the host immune response and adapt to new environmental niches. Newly developed drugs and vaccines create selective pressures and resultant new viral clades with resistance. If viruses change rapidly, then the specificity of a current test may be affected if the appropriate conserved elements of the virus are not targeted. The most extreme consequence of this could be incorrect diagnoses from false negatives on diagnostic tests. These mutational events can also lead to decreased effectiveness of the host immune response and vaccines, such as occurs when equine influenza virus (EIV) mutates the viral hemagglutinins (genetic drift) or even sometimes "switches" hemagglutinin (genetic shift). Mutations in viruses can also lead to the appearance of new or more severe clinical syndromes: a recent example is the increased neuropathogenicity associated with a point mutation in the polymerase gene of equine herpesvirus type 1 (EHV-1).[1] Despite the dramatic advances in methodology, however, many of the traditional caveats about test validation and the interpretation of results remain the same. Assumptions about the performance characteristics of any new test or testing method should not be made. Newer tests are not automatically better tests, and the sensitivity and specificity of any new test or testing method must be evaluated individually and with respect to the performance of the previous test and, where available, a gold standard. For example, PCR assays are often assumed to be more sensitive than virus isolation, but this is not always true. Irrespective of the method used for detection, the significance of a result in a clinical sample must always be interpreted in the context of the patient, the pathogenesis and epidemiology of the disease, and the host responses to that disease.

Usually, the diagnostic laboratory will select the test(s) for a specific disease based on the available facilities and the current optimal test for a given virus. However, the clinician still needs to be aware of the inherent advantages and limitations of any given test and to interpret the results of the test accordingly. Moreover, understanding the various testing options may allow a clinician to select a laboratory based on the type of test offered. Appropriate sample collection and transport is critically important for accurate laboratory results. Communication with the laboratory is extremely important. The ability of the laboratory to provide good service is enhanced with good clinical histories, differential diagnoses, and specific testing requests. The laboratory is also a valuable source of information about sample collection and transport, testing methodology, and interpretation of results. For the diseases in which the assay can be performed by the clinician, such as an antigen ELISA test for influenza, full responsibility for interpretation and performance of the test rests with the clinician.

*The authors acknowledge and appreciate the original contributions of these authors, whose work has been incorporated into this chapter.

Detection of Virus or Viral Components

Isolation of Live Virus

Cell Culture, Egg Culture, and Animal Inoculation

The isolation of a virus in cell culture is the original virus detection assay and gold standard of viral diagnostics.[2] Viruses cannot live independently outside a cell, thus the clinical specimen is inoculated onto living cells and then the cells are examined daily to detect and identify any viruses that propagate. Living cell cultures are first established in plastic wells or Petri dishes. Clinical samples are homogenized in cell culture growth media, centrifuged or filtered to remove larger debris and bacteria, treated with antibiotics to remove contaminating bacteria that may infect and destroy the cell cultures, and then inoculated onto the cells. Viral growth in the cells is detected by characteristic changes in the infected cells, called the *cytopathic effect* (CPE), caused by the virus (Fig. 12-1). When viral CPE is suspected in a cell culture, the presence of a virus as well as its identity is confirmed by additional tests such as fluorescent-labeled antiviral antibodies, PCR for viral nucleic acids, or electron microscopy. Occasionally, clinical samples are inoculated into laboratory animals for isolation of viruses, for example, into the brain of suckling mice for isolation of alphaviruses (e.g., eastern and western equine encephalitis viruses)[3] or into embryonated eggs for isolation of equine influenza virus.[4] Depending on the virus or virus strain and the specific cells being used for isolation, viral growth may not cause any visible changes and is called *noncytopathic*. For these viruses, screening for the presence of virus must be done in all inoculated cell cultures by some other method such as immunofluorescence for viral antigens or PCR for viral nucleic acids.

One of the primary advantages of virus isolation in cell culture is its potentially high sensitivity and excellent specificity. Because inoculated cell cultures are generally passaged serially two or three times before being called "negative," there is usually significant amplification of any virus present in the sample. This initial amplification also may still be required for many PCR tests. However, virus isolation requires that viable virus be present in the sample. Viability may be adversely affected by sample collection and storage, timing of sample collection, postmortem interval, and sample transport. This is particularly true for fragile viruses such as herpesviruses and other enveloped viruses. Therefore good sample collection and transport are critical for successful virus isolation. Sensitivity is also affected by the type of cells used for isolation. Different cell types vary in their ability to propagate different viruses and thus in their sensitivity of detection.[4] Most laboratories have the ability to use specific types of cultured cells or animal inoculation systems for different suspected viruses to optimize cell culture success rates. The clinician is required to communicate the suspected differential diagnoses, which provides some guidance at the initiation of ancillary diagnostic testing.

Another advantage of cell culture is that an isolate of viable virus is acquired for evaluation of biologic properties such as virulence, antigenic variation, and possibly, susceptibility to antiviral drugs.[2] Fortunately, with most of the common equine viral diseases, this additional information is not essential in the short-term for effective clinical management of individual cases. More and more, the ability to characterize viral isolates, especially those of EHV-1, for viruses such as EIV or African horse sickness (AHS), the ability to type a virus or detect changes in antigenicity may explain vaccine failures or lead to changes in vaccine type.[5,6]

Virus isolation is also a relatively nonselective method of virus detection, which is important for the identification of new viruses. A search for a new virus is usually based first on unexplained viral pathology or clinical features that suggest a viral etiology. Whether the disease is caused by a change in the epidemiology of a recognized viral disease or the appearance of a new virus, the associated investigations generally become research projects and have different goals than the routine detection of recognized equine viral pathogens.

The key disadvantages of virus isolation, in addition to the need for samples with viable virus, as previously noted, are cost and time. Maintaining cell cultures requires highly specialized facilities, equipment, reagents, and trained personnel. Virus isolation and confirmation of the identity of the virus is also labor intensive. Consequently, there is considerable expense involved with this assay, and even for diagnostic laboratories that provide services at a subsidized cost, these expenses are becoming prohibitive for routine diagnostic testing. Turnaround time is also a primary concern since isolation and confirmatory identification often takes a minimum of a week or longer to obtain results. This time frame is often not very useful for short-term

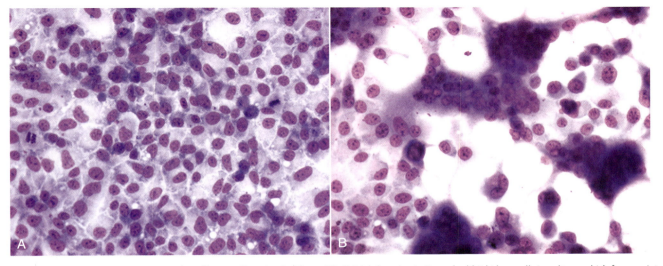

Figure 12-1 Photomicrograph of viral cytopathic effect in cells stained with modified Wright's stain. **A,** Normal rabbit kidney cells in culture, which form an intact monolayer. **B,** Rabbit kidney cells infected with equine herpesvirus type 1 (EHV-1), showing the resultant visible cytopathic effect. Changes include loss of cells seen as holes in the monolayer, stringing of cytoplasm between the cells, and multinucleated cells. Magnification for both panels, 400×.

clinical decision making and biosecurity. These limitations in particular are key reasons for replacing virus isolation with the molecular methods described next.

Detection of Viral Nucleic Acids

Polymerase Chain Reaction, Real-Time Polymerase Chain Reaction, and Nested Polymerase Chain Reaction

Nucleic acid amplification by PCR is now one of the most common assays used to detect the presence of a virus directly in clinical samples. Polymerase chain reaction assays have been developed for a variety of equine viral pathogens from a wide array of sample types[4,5,7-17] (Fig. 12-2).

In conventional PCR, total deoxyribonucleic acid (DNA) or ribonucleic acid (RNA), including viral DNA or RNA if present, is extracted and purified from the sample. For RNA viruses, isolated RNA is converted to complementary DNA (cDNA) in a separate reaction by the enzyme reverse transcriptase (RT); therefore PCR for RNA targets is referred to as *RT-PCR*. A

heat-stable DNA polymerase is then used in a series of cyclic reactions to amplify exponentially any viral DNA or cDNA sequences. The reaction is initiated and driven by two oligonucleotide primers (usually about 15-25 nucleotides in length) that are synthetically produced and complementary to a desired target sequence in the viral genome. This target sequence is selected to be unique for the virus, preventing the primers from binding to and initiating amplification of nonviral sequences in the genome of the host or other pathogens. When the primers bind to the target DNA, they allow the DNA polymerase to initiate copying of the target sequence. The amplicons are generated through successive rounds of annealing, denaturing, and extension. This reaction can be modified to enhance fidelity and also automated to allow for rapid and high-throughput resulting of sampling. Because amplification is exponential, the final result of the PCR assay is a very large number of amplified DNA fragments of a specific length (i.e., the distance between the primers). The amplicon products of PCR amplification can then be detected in several ways. The most common method is agarose gel electrophoresis, which separates DNA fragments based on size (Fig. 12-3). Positive reactions are identified by the detection of DNA bands of the correct size or that hybridize to sequence-specific probes.

Several variants of the PCR assay are designed to decrease the time necessary to perform the assay, minimize manipulations of reactions, and improve sensitivity. Decreased manipulations not only save time and labor, but more importantly, reduce the amount of amplicon contamination that inevitably occurs when opening and closing finished reactions and transferring reaction products to new tubes or analytical gels. Contaminant amplicons are notorious for their ability to get into reagents and other samples, leading to false-positive results. To avoid reaction manipulations, some assays for RNA viruses now use one-step protocols or polymerase enzymes with both RT and DNA polymerase activities, eliminating the need for

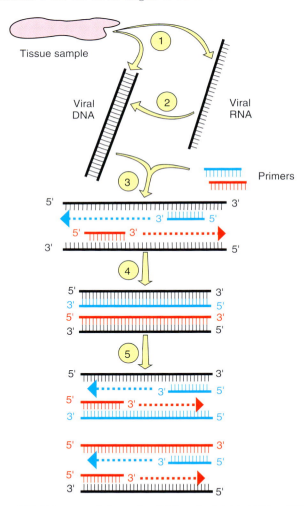

Figure 12-2 Polymerase chain reaction (PCR) method. *1,* Viral DNA or RNA is extracted and purified from tissue or blood samples. *2,* Because the PCR method only amplifies double-stranded DNA, RNA targets are converted to DNA by the enzyme reverse transcriptase. *3,* The double-stranded DNA is denatured with heat; primers are added to the reaction along with nucleotides and with a DNA polymerase such as Taq. Primers bind to complementary sequences in the viral sequences, if present, and initiate copying reactions from the 3′ end of the primers. *4,* After one round of amplification, each original viral target DNA is copied, resulting in two copies of the target. *5,* The process is repeated, which results in exponential amplification of the original target sequence. *DNA,* Deoxyribonucleic acid; *RNA,* ribonucleic acid.

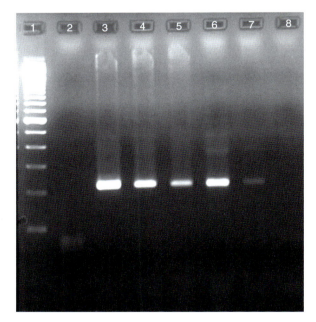

Figure 12-3 Gel analysis of PCRs for equine infectious anemia (EIA) virus. Following PCR, the reaction products are electrophoresed through an agarose gel and stained with ethidium bromide, which allows visualization with ultraviolet light by causing the amplified DNA to fluoresce and appear as white bands in the gel. *Lane 1* is a size standard included with each gel to determine the size of the amplified DNA products. *Lane 2* is a negative control. Lane 3 is a positive control. *Lanes 4 to 8* are test samples, with positive samples in lanes 4 to 7 and a negative sample in lane 8.

separate reactions.[17-19] An important variant is "real-time" PCR, in which amplification of either the target DNA or the cDNA is detected by the formation of a fluorescent signal in the tube, and the level of fluorescence is measured by the PCR machine during each cycle.[7,17,20] This not only eliminates the need for opening amplified reactions for gel analysis, but also allows positive and negative tests to be determined as the reaction proceeds, thus in "real time."

The sensitivity of PCR assays can be maximized by "nested" PCR.[4,8] This modification uses two sets of virus-specific primers. The first set of primers is used for an initial round of amplification as previously described. Some of this reaction product is transferred to a second PCR assay with a second set of primers that will bind to the first amplicon. Because there are two rounds of amplification, this modification allows detection of very low levels of virus. However, because of the extreme sensitivity of nested PCR, this assay is prone to false-positive results from minute levels of amplicon contamination that are very difficult to control in most laboratories.

Other recent variants of PCR used in human laboratories include the ligase chain reaction, strand-displacement amplification, transcription-mediated amplification, and microarray analysis.[2,20] However, these assays are not yet in widespread use for the detection of equine viruses. Nonetheless, these last assays include real-time methods that may be useful for detection of rapidly evolving viruses. The key advantages of PCR assays are speed, cost, sensitivity, ability to detect nonviable virus, and in some cases, safety. Typical PCR reactions can be completed in 4 to 6 hours, allowing for results to be obtained very quickly. Although there are some initial high capital costs for equipment, most of the key steps for PCR can be performed with commercially available kits that are effective, reliable, and relatively inexpensive on a per-test basis. Thus the cost for PCR assays is usually quite reasonable compared with virus isolation. Additional setup costs for control, reagents that are required for each run, regardless of the numbers of samples tested. Consequently, unless there is a communicated need for urgency, most laboratories will accumulate some number of samples before running a test and may report results periodically.

PCR assays are generally quite sensitive because of logarithmic amplification of the target and are often comparable in sensitivity to virus isolation. PCR is especially useful for viruses that are slow, difficult, or unable to be propagated in cell culture such as many of the gamma herpesviruses (e.g., equine herpesvirus types 2 and 5), papillomavirus, EIV, and rotavirus. PCR is also very useful to detect viruses that are fragile and prone to loss of viability during sampling or transport such as many enveloped viruses. Diagnostics using PCR for viruses that are zoonotics, such as West Nile virus (WNV) and Eastern equine encephalitis virus (EEE), is preferable to cell culture techniques that require propagation of live virus. This technology can also be performed on DNA or RNA extracted from formalin-fixed, paraffin-embedded tissues.[15] This option provides not only good laboratory safety but also allows a diagnosis to be made when fresh tissue samples are not available.

Although PCR is considered inherently more sensitive, this not automatically true, and the performance of PCR must be assessed for each pathogen and disease. Problems with both sensitivity and specificity compared to gold standards have been demonstrated. One issue is the tendency for laboratory contamination with amplicons, and the resultant false-positive results are significant issues for the diagnostic laboratory. Laboratories that perform PCR routinely must have extensive and specific protocols, as well as facility design, to prevent contamination. Negative controls should be performed with each run to detect contamination if it does occur. False-positive results from nonspecific amplification may also occur if there are closely related genetic sequences either in the host genome or in other microorganisms. Good primer design, test validation, and controls usually minimize this problem. False-negative results occur because either the sample has too few targets in which the target can be detected against the background of host nucleic acids. False-negative reactions are also caused by inhibitors that remain present in the sample even after isolation of nucleic acids.

False-positive reactions, the lack of a viable virus isolate, detection of virus that may not be clinically relevant, and the inability to detect new or poorly characterized viruses are disadvantages. PCR does not result in the recovery of a viable isolate of the virus, which can be a disadvantage if biologic information about the virus is needed. However, as noted in the section on virus isolation, this information is rarely needed to manage clinical cases. Another potential problem with PCR is the detection of viruses that are not clinically relevant. This limitation is not unique to PCR, and detection of a virus in a clinical sample by any method should not automatically be assumed to be clinically relevant. For example, many adult horses may periodically shed equine herpesvirus subclinically in nasal secretions, and detection of these viruses by either virus isolation or PCR may or may not be important.[16,21] Inactive viruses may also be detected by PCR. Interpretive problems can be in part alleviated by sample selection based on knowledge about the pathogenesis of the disease. For example, the detection of EHV type 1 or type 4 (EHV-1 or EHV-4) in nasal secretions probably indicates shedding and is much more likely to be significant than detection in neural or lymphoid tissues that may harbor latent infections.[22,23]

PCR tests can also be designed through target selection to discriminate between latent and replicating virus, for example, by detection of viral messenger RNA (mRNA) for structural genes that are only present during active virus replication. The tendency to over interpret a positive virology result is somewhat compounded by PCR because of its ability to reliably detect viruses that in the past were difficult to detect. For example, EHV type 2 (EHV-2), a lymphotropic gamma herpesvirus, is poorly documented as a cause of any clinical disease. However, this virus is also ubiquitous in the horse population, and testing with a highly sensitive test such as PCR is likely to give a positive result from any tissue with lymphocytic inflammation, regardless of the etiology.[12] The clinician should be aware that mammals have a normal "flora" of viruses, as well as bacteria and other microbes, and the significance of virus detection must be critically evaluated, especially for viruses with a high background prevalence and that may cause subclinical infections.

Another disadvantage of PCR is that it requires existing genetic information about the virus in question to design primers. Fortunately, this is no longer a significant issue for the major equine viral pathogens, most of which have been extensively studied. However, this may cause false-negative results when there is undetected genetic variation within the primer binding sites of different strains of virus, as in equine infectious anemia (EIA) virus (J. Lindsay Oaks, unpublished data). The need for prior genetic knowledge also makes PCR inherently poor for the detection of new viruses unless highly conserved regions of the genome are targeted. The assays also must be designed to optimize isolation of viral nucleic acids for other methods of confirmatory detection of the presence of a new virus.

Viral Characterization

Advances in genetic sequencing that have made this PCR technology rapid and cost-effective for routine diagnostic virology have also provided a powerful tool for the rapid characterization of new viruses. In this application, primers are designed to bind to highly conserved regions within a virus family or genus and amplify a portion of the genome that is variable and unique for the virus. The sequence of this unique region can then be determined and used for comparison to genetic databases, and it may either identify a well-characterized virus in an unusual disease entity or determine that the virus is a previously undescribed equine virus.

Although specific genetic information about the equine virus is not necessary, some clue as to the general identity of the virus is needed. This is most often accomplished by observing electron microscopic features, reaction with group-specific antibodies in immunofluorescence or IHC assays, or suggestive inclusion bodies within lesions. For example, this approach allowed the rapid characterization of the Hendra virus, a novel virus that fatally infected horses and humans in Australia in 1994,[24] and several new gamma herpesviruses associated with pneumonia in donkeys.[25]

Additional advances that combine biotechnology, molecular biology, and bioinformatics are poised to revolutionize the detection and characterization of new viruses in both humans and animals, as recently demonstrated by a sequence-independent, single-primer amplification protocol that identified two new bovine parvoviruses.[26] It should be noted that these viruses were detected as "proof of principle" rather than in the context of identifying an etiologic agent of disease, which should emphasize that advances in our ability to detect new viruses bring a greater need to critically assess the clinical relevance of these viruses.

There are a number of sequencing methodologies that exist for infectious disease diagnostics, and all use PCR for its basic reaction. The traditional method of Sanger sequencing involves replication (PCR) of the DNA sequence of interest using all four deoxynucleotide bases (A, C, T, and G) and one known di-deoxynucleotide (ddA, ddC, ddT, or ddG). Newer technologies with Sanger sequencing that are now more commonly used include dye terminator sequencing. In this methodology, di-deoxynucleotides are fluorescently labeled, streamlining the process into one reaction. The reaction occurs "real-time," as the incorporation of the fluorescently labeled di-deoxynucleotides emits a fluorescent signal that is read by a computer. These techniques are used both in the research setting and in clinical diagnostics. Recent examples in equine medicine include M-protein typing during *Streptococcus equi* outbreaks, identification of influenza virus subtypes and phylogenetic tracing, and the diagnosis of dermatophytosis outbreaks.[27-29]

Newer, high-throughput, next-generation sequencing methodologies are also being applied to diagnostic testing. Next-generation sequencing produces clonal PCR reactions in microreactors and measures the output (fluorescence or pH change) using specialized equipment. In this way, whole genomes of organisms can be sequenced in short periods of time. In infectious disease diagnostics, these methodologies are particularly useful in new pathogen discovery, tracing pathogen evolution (natural evolution and drug resistance), and in diagnosis in which pathogens are unknown or multiple pathogens may be involved. The latter is possible since many of these techniques involved do not use specific primers. Instead, the sequences of interest are replicated using generic probes and primers that are ligated on to the ends of the DNA strands to be sequenced.

The major drawback to all of the sequencing methodologies, as well as PCR, is the possibility of contamination. Amplification of contaminating sequences can interfere with identification of the infectious agents, so care must be taken when collecting the samples. Another major concern, especially with next-generation sequencing techniques, is the sequence output. Sequence output can be so large that annotation of the genetic information is a major impediment and requires use of specialized programs and expertise. However, the advantages to both dye terminator and next-generation sequencing are so great that their use will most likely continue to increase in clinical diagnostics.

In Situ Methods: Detection of Virus in Tissue Sections

Histopathology

Routine histopathology on formalin-fixed, hematoxylin-eosin–stained tissue sections of biopsy or necropsy samples often provides strong supporting evidence that a lesion or disease is viral. Although rarely definitive, the distribution of lesions or necrosis and the patterns and types of inflammation are often strongly suggestive of a viral etiology. Inclusion bodies, if present, are often highly characteristic of certain viruses. For example, adenoviruses cause karyomegaly and intensely basophilic intranuclear inclusions. Most alpha herpesviruses, such as EHV-1, EHV-3, and EHV-4, cause eosinophilic to basophilic intranuclear inclusions without karyomegaly. Paramyxoviruses cause both intranuclear and intracytoplasmic inclusions. Some viruses, such as lentiviruses and rotaviruses, do not typically result in inclusions in vivo. Thus, in cases in which tissue samples are obtained for diagnosis, histopathology should not be overlooked for the diagnosis of viral infections. In addition, formalin-fixed, paraffin-embedded tissue samples can be used for PCR analysis, electron microscopy, and IHC.

Immunofluorescence and Immunohistochemistry

Immunofluorescence and IHC use antiviral antibodies to detect viral antigens in tissue sections. The assays technically differ only in the method used to detect bound antibody. Immunofluorescence uses a fluorescent label, usually fluorescein, conjugated either to the antiviral antibody itself (direct immunofluorescence) or to an anti-antibody (indirect immunofluorescence), and viewed with ultraviolet light (Fig. 12-4, *A* and *B*). Immunofluorescence is usually performed on frozen tissue sections fixed in acetone or methanol.

The antiviral antibody is referred to as the primary antibody and can be either immune serum from a known-infected horse or antiviral antibodies generated in laboratory animals, usually mice, rabbits, or goats. The type of primary antibody used in a test is based on the amount of viral protein expected to be in a lesion (sensitivity) and the cross-reactivity of the antibodies with nonviral antigens in the host or in unrelated pathogens (specificity). As a general rule, monoclonal antibodies are highly specific, but because they only recognize one epitope and thus fewer antibodies are able to bind to each target molecule, they may be limited in sensitivity. In contrast, polyclonal antisera usually provide good sensitivity because they react with multiple epitopes on multiple viral proteins, but their polyclonal composition also makes them more likely to be cross-reactive and have problems with specificity. Fluorescent label directly or indirectly is conjugated to the antiviral antibody, and when placed on the tissue, the virus is detected by a fluorescent microscope. An important advantage of immunofluorescence is that it can be performed rapidly. Another advantage is that it demonstrates antigen in association with lesions or affected tissues, which is supporting information that suggests the virus is relevant to the lesion. The detection of viral proteins is usually indicative of active replication, as opposed to latent infections.

The major disadvantage with immunofluorescence assays of tissues is that frozen sections have poor morphology, making visualization of lesions difficult. In addition, fluorescent assays on tissues can be technically challenging to read. Finally, most immunofluorescent assays have limited sensitivity and specificity compared with contemporary immunohistochemical methods.

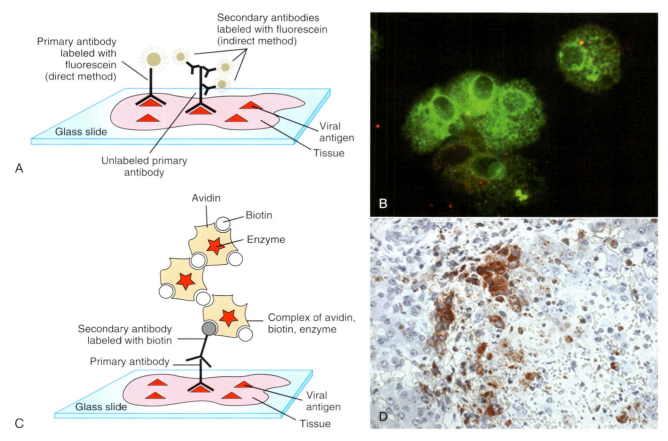

Figure 12-4 Immunostaining methods for the detection of viral antigen in tissue samples mounted on glass slides. **A,** Immunofluorescence method, including direct and indirect protocols. **B,** Photomicrograph of equine alveolar macrophages infected with equine infectious anemia virus and detected by indirect immunofluorescence. The primary antibody is a mouse monoclonal antibody against equine infectious anemia virus; the secondary antibody is an anti-mouse IgG labeled with fluorescein. Viral antigen is indicated by the bright green fluorescence emitted from the fluorescein when the stained tissue section is observed under ultraviolet light. Magnification, 630×. **C,** Avidin-biotin immunohistochemical method. **D,** Photomicrograph of equine fetal liver from a case of equine herpesvirus type 1 (EHV-1) abortion stained for EHV-1 antigen by immunohistochemistry. The primary antibody is rabbit polyclonal antisera against equine herpesvirus type 1; the secondary antibody is an anti-rabbit IgG labeled with biotin. The signal is amplified by complexes of avidin and biotin that also contain horseradish peroxidase that then reacts with a chromogen to form a red-colored precipitate. Viral antigen is indicated by the red-stained precipitate in the cytoplasm of infected cells in a necrotic focus in the liver. Magnification, 400×.

Immunohistochemistry is very similar to immunofluorescence but, instead of fluorescent labels, uses enzymes that are conjugated to a secondary antibody for detection of bound primary antibody. The enzyme reacts with a colorimetric substrate to cause a colored precipitate that can be viewed with standard light microscopy (Fig. 12-4, C and D). Immunohistochemistry is usually performed on formalin-fixed, paraffin-embedded tissue sections, which have much better tissue morphology than frozen sections, and this allows better detection of lesions and correlation of lesions with viral antigen. Formalin-fixed, paraffin-embedded tissues are also easier to process, and the chromogenic reactions are technically easier to read than immunofluorescence. More importantly, significant advances in detection systems have greatly amplified the signal generated by each bound primary antibody. For example, many standard IHC assays now use a secondary antibody conjugated to biotin, then use an avidin molecule conjugated to more biotin and the enzyme. Haines and Chelack[30] provide a detailed overview of IHC techniques (see Fig. 12-4).

Other variations also may be used, but all are designed to amplify significantly the signal generated by each bound primary antibody.[31] The effect is to make the IHC tests very sensitive. Because of signal amplification, fewer primary and secondary antibodies are required for the assay, which decreases nonspecific binding and improves the test specificity. Test specificity has also been improved by recombinant protein technology, which allows greater control over the antigens used to produce the primary and secondary antibodies. Finally, in addition to being able to be performed quickly, the cost on a per-test basis is low compared to virus isolation. For these reasons, IHC is a common and effective method for the detection of a number of equine viral infections.[32-37]

Microarray Detection of Viruses

Most microarrays are used in a research setting, although their application in clinical diagnostics is becoming more common, especially for detection of unknown viruses.[38] A microarray is a collection of microscopic spots of DNA (probes) printed onto a flat surface such as glass or nylon. These probes correspond to a gene of interest such as a unique known sequence for a virus. Nucleic acids from a clinical sample of interest are labeled with a dye (fluorescent Cy3 or Cy5 or silver) and hybridized to the array. If the sample contains virus with a sequence complementary to one of the probes, the sample will bind to that specific probe. The array is then read using specialized scanners, and the sample is considered positive for the infectious agents.

There are a number of arrays currently in use for infectious disease diagnostics, all varying slightly in their approach to detection. These include arrays with probes targeted to known infectious agent sequences (Virochip, GreeneChip, Lawrence Livermore Microbial Detection Array), arrays with point mutated probes (resequencing pathogen microarrays), and arrays containing randomly generated sequences (universal detection arrays).[38] Many arrays are available commercially for use in human medicine. Although veterinary microarrays for infectious disease diagnostics are mostly limited to research use, their usefulness can be seen in diagnostic assays ranging from detecting and typing fecal organisms, such as *Salmonella* and *Clostridia*, to detecting genetic mutations that may lead to increased disease susceptibility.[39,40] The primary advantage of microarray technology for infectious disease diagnostics is the ability to screen for a large number of pathogens. This is particularly important when screening for novel pathogens or if there is a limited amount of sample. Newer microarray technologies like beaded microarrays allow for higher throughput sample processing. However, microarrays do have their disadvantages in the costly equipment to produce and use them. Furthermore, microarray use requires a good deal of expertise and training, although with newer technologies and time, they should become easier to use.

In Situ Hybridization

In situ hybridization detects viral DNA or RNA in tissue sections with a labeled DNA or RNA probe that is complementary to and thus binds to the target viral sequence. In most other respects, in situ hybridization is very similar to IHC. In situ hybridization is typically performed on formalin-fixed, paraffin-embedded tissue sections. The DNA or RNA probes are usually labeled with a molecule such as digoxigenin, which is then detected by IHC as previously described, using a primary antibody that binds to the digoxigenin. In situ hybridization assays can be very sensitive and specific and have most of the same advantages as immunofluorescence and IHC. However, in situ hybridization is technically more complex and relatively expensive to perform. Thus, although this method is used in research laboratories,[33,41,42] it is unlikely to be offered as a common diagnostic test.

Detection of Virus in Clinical Samples

Enzyme-Linked Immunosorbent Assay (Indirect ELISA)

Rapid tests for viral antigen can be performed using ELISA formats that detect antigen. For this type of test, an antiviral antibody is immobilized on either a membrane or the well of a plastic plate. The test sample is then added, and if viral antigen is present, it is bound by the antibody and thus immobilized. Bound antigen is detected with a different antiviral antibody that binds to another part of the viral antigen and is visualized by generating a colorimetric reaction, as described for IHC (Fig. 12-5). The most common equine viral diseases that can be diagnosed using antigen ELISA include intestinal rotavirus infection[43,44] and EIV.[6,45] In most cases, these tests are human kits that detect group-specific antigens that cross-react with the equine viruses. An antigen ELISA has also been described for the rapid diagnosis of AHS.[46]

The key advantage of antigen ELISA tests is that they are fast, with results available in minutes. They generally are also easy to use, require minimal equipment, and are even amenable to being used stall side. In general, although ELISA tests may have reasonable sensitivity and specificity, they are often lacking in both these parameters relative to other tests, and both false-positive and false-negative results should be expected.[6,47] Studies of the rotavirus test in cattle[47] and the influenza test in horses[6] have shown that different products may vary in sensitivity and specificity. Also, the influenza tests may detect viral antigen from horses given intranasal immunizations, which is also a problem for PCR.[48]

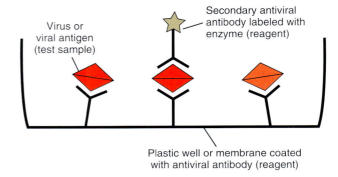

Figure 12-5 Enzyme-linked immunoabsorbent assay (ELISA) method for the detection of antigen. Antiviral antibodies are coated onto and fixed to either plastic wells or membranes. The test samples are processed and added to the wells or membranes. If viral antigen is present, it is bound to and thus also fixed to the plastic or membrane. Following washes, another antiviral antibody labeled with an enzyme is added. This second antibody typically binds to a different viral antigen to prevent competitive inhibition of binding by the first antiviral antibody. Following washes to remove any unbound second antibody, a chromogen that reacts with the enzyme to form a color change is added. Color changes (i.e., positive reactions) can only occur if viral antigen is present in the sample.

To optimize the sensitivity of antigen ELISA tests, it is important to sample animals at times when viral shedding is maximal; keep in mind that this is likely to be early in the course of disease and may only be of short duration. The predictive value of tests should be maximized by careful selection of cases with appropriate supporting epidemiology, clinical signs, and laboratory evidence, and animals should not be shedding vaccine virus. Also, when the validity of the results is a concern, confirmatory tests should be considered.

Electron Microscopy

The direct visualization of viral particles in clinical specimens is another rapid test for the presumptive diagnosis of viral infection. In general, electron microscopy is of low sensitivity and requires large numbers of virions to be present for reliable detection. However, the characteristic ultrastructural appearance of different viruses gives this test good specificity for diagnosis to the level of virus family. Diagnostic electron microscopy is used routinely for diagnosis of viral enteric diseases, such as rotavirus,[43,44] in which animals with clinical disease tend to shed large amounts of virus. Electron microscopy is also used occasionally to detect unusual viral infections[49] or to support other laboratory findings.[50] Electron microscopy is also used in the laboratory as a rapid method for the presumptive identification of cell culture isolates[51,52] and can be particularly useful for selecting PCR primers that bind to family-specific or genus-specific conserved regions for genetic sequence analysis.

Detection of the Serologic Response

Testing for the presence of antiviral antibodies in serum or plasma is a classic method for the indirect detection of viral infections. Despite some limitations with interpretation, serology can still be a reliable and useful diagnostic tool. One major advantage is that collection of serum from horses is simple and relatively noninvasive, can be obtained antemortem, and lends itself to testing large numbers of animals. Serology is particularly useful for detecting infections in which virus is not easily detected by other means, as with WNV,[53] EIA virus, and EEE virus.

Over the years, a wide variety of testing methods have been used to detect antiviral antibodies, including virus neutralization (VN), agar gel immunodiffusion (AGID) and other immunodiffusion tests, hemagglutination inhibition (HI), indirect immunofluorescence (IFA), complement fixation (CF), Western blot (WB), radioimmunoassay (RIA), and most recently ELISA and its variants. Despite the wide array of testing formats, all of these tests use some type of viral antigen as a reagent to capture antibody, if present, from a test serum sample, and then use some type of detection system to indicate that antibody has bound to the antigen. These tests can vary widely in their sensitivity, specificity, complexity, and cost. The two most common serologic test formats for equine viral diseases are the VN and ELISA tests, and only these are discussed in detail here.

Virus Neutralization

The VN test detects antibodies capable of neutralizing the infectivity of the virus. Serial dilutions of serum are mixed with a reference strain of viable virus (in this case the antigen) and incubated to allow any antibody present to bind and neutralize the virus, and then dilutions are inoculated onto cells. The presence or absence of viral growth is observed. The highest dilution (i.e., the least amount of antibody) that neutralizes infectivity is the titer. A variant of the VN test is the plaque reduction neutralization (PRN) test. This test is sometimes used for viruses that form distinct plaques of CPE in cell cultures, with each plaque representing a single infectious unit. The end point is defined as the dilution of serum that reduces the number of plaques by some statistically significant level (often set at >50%-90%).

Advantages of the VN or PRN tests are that they are usually highly sensitive and very specific. Neutralizing antibody can be used to differentiate viruses at the strain level. The main disadvantage is that the generation of neutralizing antibody has a slower onset and rise in the primary immune response. Furthermore, since many horses have been vaccinated for these diseases or have had previous field exposure, paired samples are necessary to confirm recent infection. These tests require living cell cultures, production and maintenance of titered virus stocks, and highly trained personnel, and they are labor intensive. Thus these tests tend to be costly and potentially cumbersome and the minimum turnaround time is 48 hours with most taking at least 1 week. These tests also require working with viable virus, which may present a laboratory hazard when testing for viruses that also infect humans.

Enzyme-Linked Immunosorbent Assay

One of the most common serologic tests currently offered is ELISA. The general principle of ELISA is that the viral antigen is bound to either a well in a plastic plate or a membrane. The test serum sample is added, and any antibody against the antigen becomes bound to the plate or membrane. After washing away unbound antibody, a secondary antibody against antibody (e.g., anti-equine immunoglobulin G [IgG] or immunoglobulin M [IgM]) conjugated to an enzyme (e.g., horseradish peroxidase) is added and will bind to any equine antibodies still present. This complex is visualized by the addition of a colorimetric substrate that reacts with the enzyme to create a visible color change. The color change is compared to controls either visually or spectrophotometrically (Fig. 12-6).

The primary advantages of ELISA are that it is relatively rapid and easy to perform and can be quite sensitive and specific. The sensitivity and specificity of the assay can also be manipulated by selection of antigens[54,55] and use of secondary antibodies selective for either IgG or IgM.[56,57] One of the major disadvantages of ELISA is that the results are often simply

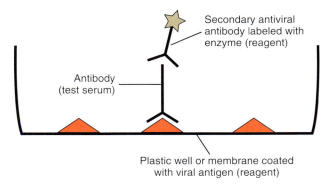

Figure 12-6 Enzyme-linked immunoabsorbent assay (ELISA) method for the detection of antibody. Viral antigen is coated onto and fixed to either plastic wells or membranes. The test samples, generally serum, plasma, or whole blood, are added to the wells or membranes. If viral antibodies are present, they bind to and thus also become fixed to the plastic or membrane. Following washes, a secondary antibody against the isotype of the antibody being detected in the test sample (e.g., anti-equine IgG and/or IgM, and labeled with an enzyme) is added. Following washes to remove any unbound second antibody, a chromogen that reacts with the enzyme to form a color change is added. Color changes (i.e., positive reactions) can only occur if antiviral antibodies are present in the sample.

reported as positive or negative and not quantitatively to detect changes in titer. As discussed next, for diseases in which the background seroprevalence is high, fourfold or greater changes in titer are necessary to determine recent exposure. In these cases, the ELISA titer must be determined for acute and convalescent sera to demonstrate recent exposure.[58-61]

Agar Gel Immunodiffusion

The AGID is used to detect antibodies to viral antigen. A known viral antigen is placed into a center well in agar. Unknown sera samples and positive controls are placed in surrounding wells. The sera samples and the antigen are allowed to diffuse toward each other. If antibodies to the antigen are present in the sample, then a line of precipitation will form, indicating that the horse has been exposed to that antigen. This test is often used (along with the ELISA) to screen horses that are positive for EIA virus. The ELISA is a faster test, taking approximately 4 hours, whereas the AGID test takes approximately 24 hours. The AGID is the required format by some regulatory bodies for the Coggins test.[62]

Hemagglutination Inhibition Assay

The hemagglutination inhibition (HI) assay is used to titrate the antibody response to a viral infection. The HI assay takes advantage of some viruses' ability to hemagglutinate (bind) red blood cells, therefore forming a "lattice" and preventing the red blood cells from clumping. In the HI assay, twofold dilutions of the sera to be tested are made in 96 well plates. A known titer of the virus is added, and the plate is incubated for 30 minutes at room temperature. Red blood cells are then added and the plate incubated for a further 30 minutes at room temperature. If antibodies are present in the sera sample that cross-react with the virus, the antibodies will bind to the virus and prevent the virus from hemagglutinating the red blood cells. In this way, the exact titer of the antibodies in the sera can be determined. This assay is the standard for equine influenza diagnostics.[63]

This assay has the advantage of being quick and easy to perform, especially if there is a predominant virus subtype that is suspected. However, the HI assay may not detect antibodies in samples that are not cross-reactive to the virus being tested (i.e., are against different subtypes of influenza virus). Thus all the possible different viruses and viral subtypes should be tested, which is not always feasible. In addition, immunity to the virus may involve other aspects of the host response, including t-cell responses and antibodies against other components of the virus besides the hemagglutinating protein. The HI assay will not detect these aspects of the host immune response. In this regard, plaque reduction neutralization tests would be more comprehensive.

Serologic Interpretation

Regardless of the test format used, there are some common themes for interpretation of serologic results. This is related in part to the biology of the disease and in part to the sensitivity and specificity of the assay. Only in selected diseases is a single positive or negative antibody result informative. A single positive or negative result is diagnostic only for persistent infections in which a positive test is synonymous with infection such as EIA.[64] Conversely, a negative test indicates there is no infection, although the possibility remains that an animal in the early stages of infection may not yet have seroconverted. Thus, if there is a high index of suspicion that an animal is infected, a retest at a later time will be indicated. For diseases such as equine viral arteritis, in which only a proportion of animals are persistently infected (e.g., approximately 30%-60% of infected stallions), a seronegative result is good evidence for lack of infection. However, a positive test may or may not indicate persistent infection and would be an indication for additional testing such as virus isolation.[65]

Because IgM is the initial antibody isotype formed transiently in a primary immune response, single antiviral IgM antibodies by ELISA may be used as a marker for acute infection and thus recent exposure,[57,58,66-68] although some individuals may have persistent IgM titers.[58] Single increased titers are also sometimes correlated to acute infection, as in EHV-1 infections. Although it is likely that either past vaccination or infection leads to more modest titers (e.g., <1:128), the natural variation in host immune responses can easily lead to overinterpretation of single titers. This type of result should at best be considered suggestive and add to the index of suspicion. Single titers may also be useful in samples from sites where no antibody should be present, except through local infection and production, such as in cerebrospinal fluid (CSF) for neurologic infections. However, the presence of serum antibody caused by leakage across the blood-brain barrier associated with inflammation or necrosis needs to be ruled out by measuring albumin quotients and IgG indices as indicators of blood contamination.[56,69]

For most viral infections, reliable detection of acute infection (i.e., recent exposure) requires demonstrating a fourfold or greater increase in titer between acute and convalescent serum samples. This applies to many of the common equine viral diseases in which there is a high background seroprevalence either from previous natural infections or from vaccination. Because most serologic tests do not distinguish vaccination and natural titers, accurate vaccination histories are also necessary to interpret serologic findings. Fourfold decreases may also indicate recent exposure.[58] However, decreasing titers as an indicator of recent infection are often unreliable because most viruses lead to titers that persist for months to years, and antibody decay curves are more prolonged and much less predictable than antibody production curves.

Another important concept regarding interpretation of serology is the difference in utility of screening tests versus confirmatory tests. No test is 100% sensitive and specific, and designing tests to achieve 100% sensitivity will invariably lead to loss of specificity and false-positive results; conversely, tests that have 100% specificity will lose sensitivity and are likely to have false-negative results.[70] These parameters are often set intentionally, depending on the disease in question. To test for diseases in which infected animals should not be missed, the primary serologic test will be a screening test that has very high sensitivity and that is expected to lead to false-positive results. The predictive value of a positive (or negative) test result is also a function of the prevalence of the disease in the population being tested.[70] For example, with a low-prevalence disease, there is a high statistical probability that positive results are false and that negative results are true. Therefore positive results obtained from screening tests should be verified by a confirmatory test, which is usually a test with higher specificity and lower sensitivity. It is inappropriate to take action based on a positive test result of a screening test without confirmation, especially for a low-prevalence disease.

The sensitivity and specificity of antibody testing has been enhanced by the use of recombinant viral proteins or peptides as antigens in serologic tests. One example is testing for EIA virus, in which replacement of whole-virus antigen preparations with recombinant viral proteins has improved the sensitivity and specificity of the AGID (Coggins) and ELISA tests.[71-73] The improvement in specificity is especially important because EIA in the United States is now a low-prevalence disease.

The complete reference list is available online at www.expertconsult.com.

13   Equine Influenza Infection

Grabriele A. Landolt, Hugh G.G. Townsend, and D. Paul Lunn

Etiology

Influenza A viruses are members of the family *Orthomyxoviridae*, which contains enveloped viruses with segmented, single-stranded, negative-sense ribonucleic acid (RNA) genomes (Fig. 13-1). The *Orthomyxoviridae* comprise five genera: influenza A, B, and C viruses; Thogotoviruses; and isavirus. Influenza A viruses can be distinguished from type B and C based on the antigenic nature of their nucleoprotein (NP) and matrix (M) proteins. In contrast to influenza A viruses, which can be isolated from a wide variety of species (including horses), influenza B viruses appear to infect primarily humans. Influenza C has been isolated mostly from humans, although they have also been shown to infect pigs and dogs.[1-3] Whereas influenza A and B contain eight separate segments of single-stranded RNA, influenza C viruses possess only seven.[4]

The virions of influenza A include a host cell–derived lipid envelope and are 80 to 120 nm in diameter. Embedded in the lipid envelope are the virus-encoded glycoproteins hemagglutinin (HA) and neuraminidase (NA)[5,6] and the integral M2 protein, which functions as an ion channel. The HA serves as the viral receptor–binding protein and is responsible for fusion between the virion envelope and the host cell. The receptor-binding site is located on the globular head portion of the molecule and forms a pocket that is inaccessible to antibodies. Thus the amino acid residues creating the pocket are largely conserved among viruses.[6-10]

The HA is the major target of the host immune response, and there are five antigenic sites on the HA molecule, covering much of the surface of the globular head portion. Immune pressure is the driving force in the selection of mutants with amino acid substitutions in these antigenic sites, allowing the mutant virus to escape neutralizing antibodies (antigenic drift).

The NA is the second large surface glycoprotein. It is a type II integral membrane glycoprotein[5,10] and is responsible for the cleavage of the α-ketosidic linkage between a sialic acid molecule and an adjacent sugar D-galactose or D-galactosamine.[11] The NA facilitates the mobility of the influenza virus virion by removing sialic acid residues from viral glycoproteins and infected cells, therefore assisting in the release of the budding virus particles.[12-14] As with the HA, the NA is a major antigenic determinant and undergoes substantial antigenic variation.[15,16]

The most abundant virion protein is the viral matrix protein (M1), which likely underlies the envelope, serves as the major structural protein of the virion, and associates with the ribonucleoprotein (RNP) complexes of the virus. The eight separate RNPs of influenza A have the appearance of flexible rods[17] and are speculated to consist of a segment of RNA loosely encapsidated by several NP molecules. Located at the end of each RNP are the three viral polymerase proteins PB1, PB2, and PA. The segmented nature of the viral genome is a critically important feature of the influenza A virus structure. In the event that cells are infected with two (or more) different viruses, the exchange of RNA segments between the viruses allows the generation of progeny viruses containing novel combinations of genes. This phenomenon is referred to as *genetic reassortment*[18,19] (Fig. 13-2). In theory, random incorporation of RNA segments could lead to the creation of 254 new gene combinations from two parental viruses. Nonetheless, the identification of selective packaging

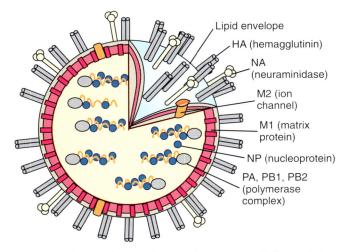

Figure 13-1 Schematic diagram of structural components of influenza A virus. Three integral membrane proteins—hemagglutinin (*HA*), neuraminidase (*NA*), and the ion channel protein (*M2*)—are embedded in the lipid envelope of the virion. The matrix protein (*M1*) is thought to underlie the lipid envelope. Associated with the viral ribonucleic acid (vRNA) is the viral polymerase complex, consisting of *PA*, *PB1*, and *PB2*. The viral nucleoprotein (*NP*) encapsidates the vRNA segments.

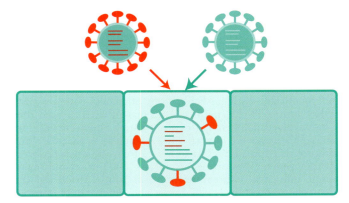

Figure 13-2 Schematic diagram illustrating genetic reassortment. In the event that cells are infected with two (or more) different viruses, the exchange of RNA segments between the viruses allows the generation of progeny viruses containing novel combinations of genes. In theory, random incorporation of RNA segments could lead to the creation of 254 new gene combinations from two parental viruses.

signals within the 3' and 5' coding regions of the influenza virus genes suggests that the incorporation of RNA segments into the virion is only partially random.[20]

Influenza A viruses can be divided into subtypes based on antigenic properties of their HA and NA envelope glycoproteins. To date, seventeen HA subtypes and ten NA subtypes have been recognized. All but one of the HA and NA subtypes have been recovered from aquatic birds.[3,21-24] These birds play a particularly important role in influenza epidemiology because they provide a vast global reservoir of viruses of the majority of subtypes. Phylogenetic analyses have indicated that viruses from aquatic birds were the ancestral source of the current lineages of mammalian viruses.[21,25-27] In contrast, only a limited number of subtypes of influenza viruses have been associated with infection of mammalian species. In humans, only viruses of H1, H2, H3, N1, and N2 subtypes have circulated widely in the population[3,26,27]; only H1, H3, N1, and N2 subtypes have been consistently isolated from pigs[28-30]; and apart from occasional reports of horses infected with viruses of subtypes H1N1, H2N2, and H3N2 (usually in association with human infections),[31] equine influenza infections have been restricted to viruses of H7N7 (A/equine/1) and H3N8 (A/equine/2) subtypes.[32-35]

Outbreaks of a disease resembling influenza have been reported as early as 1751, although the etiologic agent was not isolated until 1956.[32,33] The virus, designated A/Equine/1/Prague/56, was isolated during an outbreak of influenza in Czechoslovakia and was characterized as H7N7.[36] H7N7 influenza viruses have not been detected in the horse population since the late 1970s.[21,37,38]

In contrast, equine H3N8 viruses, first isolated in the United States in 1963 (A/equine/2/Miami/1/63), continue to circulate in large parts of the world, except Australia, New Zealand, and Iceland.[37,39,40] In August 2007, equine influenza infection was confirmed for the first time in Australia. The virus appears to have been introduced into the Australian horse population by importing horses from Japan, a country that was also experiencing an outbreak of the disease at the same time.[41,42] However, by employing stringent quarantine procedures, movement restrictions, and vaccinations, the outbreak was contained with no new cases reported after December 2007.[43] In December 2008, 12 months after identification of the last clinical case, Australia regained its equine influenza free status in accordance with the OIE Terrestrial Animal Health Code.[44,45]

Despite intensive vaccination programs, equine H3N8 influenza infections have remained a serious health and economic problem throughout most parts of the world. In the late 1980s, severe widespread influenza outbreaks were observed in horses in South Africa,[46] in India,[47,48] and in the People's Republic of China,[49-51] where equine influenza viruses were not known to be circulating. The H3N8 virus of the South African outbreak was most likely introduced by importation of infected horses from the United States or Europe.[37,52] The outbreaks in the People's Republic of China were caused by both conventional strains of equine H3N8 virus and viruses that were antigenically and genetically distinguishable from other circulating equine H3N8 viruses. Phylogenetic analysis of said virus showed that it had evolved independent of the existing equine lineage. Its genetic features were of avian lineage, indicating that the virus had probably spread directly to horses from the avian reservoir without genetic reassortment.[49] In late 2003, a second major equine influenza outbreak occurred in South Africa and the outbreak was most likely also due to a breakdown in biosecurity measures.[53]

Since the early to middle 1980s, the equine H3N8 influenza viruses have diverged into two distinct evolutionary lineages, Eurasian and American.* While both lineages initially circulated

*References 7, 27, 39, 40, 54, 55.

centered largely on the geographic region of origin,[7] the American lineage strains since appear to predominate with only rare isolation of the Eurasian lineage strains.[56,57] Continued genetic divergence has resulted in the formation of three American-like sublineages with distinct antigenic characteristics: a South American lineage, a Kentucky lineage (newly also referred to as the classic American lineage), and a Florida lineage.[39] The Florida sublineage strains have spread across Europe, and the majority of viruses isolated in Europe since 2003 belong to this sublineage.[56,58,59] Further genetic evolution of the Florida sublineage has resulted in the formation of two groups of viruses (referred to as *Florida sublineage clades 1 and 2 viruses*) with divergent HA sequences. The viruses isolated from the 2003 South African and the 2007 Japanese and Australian outbreaks were closely related to Florida sublineage clade 1 viruses and were most likely of North American origin.[41,56] Although the genetic and antigenic evolution of H3N8 equine influenza viruses is significant in terms of immunization, when compared to human influenza viruses, equine strains have demonstrated relatively little genetic diversion.

Epidemiology

Influenza is the most frequently diagnosed and economically important cause of viral respiratory disease of the horse.[36,60-62] Outbreaks of this disease have occured regularly throughout the world. New Zealand and Iceland may be the only countries where outbreaks of the disease have not occurred.

All ages and breeds of *Equidae* may be infected with the virus.[63-65] Natural disease occurs in individual foals,[63,64,66,67] but in endemic countries only one outbreak of influenza among young foals (3-6 months of age) has been reported to date.[67] Longitudinal studies of North American racehorse populations, before the availability of highly efficacious vaccines, showed that the highest incidence of disease was observed in 2- and 3-year-old horses,[62,68] likely caused by commingling of animals that lacked previous exposure to viral antigen.[69]

With the exception of occasional outbreaks in naïve populations, equine influenza is of greatest importance in large populations, where the disease is endemic and movement of animals among regions is routine. In addition to age and commingling of susceptible animals, influenza-specific serum antibody concentration is a highly specific correlate of protection against infection and disease. Animals with high concentrations of homologous antibody are almost always protected against experimental challenge.[70-74] During a 3-year study of a large population of racehorses, animals with high concentrations of serum antibody had 10 to 40 times lower odds of developing disease than did horses with no detectable antibody.[68] Horses exposed to viral antigen within the past 6 to 12 months through natural infection[75,76] or administration of a potent killed vaccine[77] or an intranasal, temperature-sensitive, modified live vaccine[78] may show evidence of reduced clinical signs and decreased viral shedding in the presence of little or no detectable antibody.

Equine influenza has a short incubation period. Experimentally infected animals experience fever and begin to shed large quantities of virus in nasal secretions within 48 hours of infection.[78-81] Secondary bacterial infections of the respiratory tract, largely resulting from proliferation of β-hemolytic streptococci, are routinely observed[69,82-85] and are considered important in the pathogenesis of bacterial pneumonia of horses.[86-88] Influenza morbidity rates within susceptible groups of horses may be as high as 60% to 90%.[47,89,90] Mortality rates are usually less than 1%,[50] although a 1998 outbreak caused by a newly emergent strain of the virus in China was associated with a mortality rate of 20% in some herds.[49] Morbidity rates within large groups of horses with varying degrees of previous exposure to influenza antigen may range from 20% to 37%.[60,91] Outbreaks of equine influenza may occur at any time of the year, although seasonal outbreaks have been reported,[60,74] probably related to the yearly convergence of component causes (risk factors) resulting in disease at regular intervals within individual sites or geographic locations.

After natural infection, ponies were reported to be resistant to infection for 32 weeks, with partial clinical protection persisting for more than 1 year.[75] Similar data are not available for horses, although a longitudinal study of a large population of racehorses showed that horses present during an outbreak of respiratory disease in one season were significantly less likely to show clinical signs of disease during an outbreak in the following year.[68] Efficacious vaccines against equine influenza are available, and their widespread use is having a significant impact on the epidemiology of the disease. Although vaccination does not generally provide sterile immunity or full protection against clinical disease for more than a few months, the vaccination of populations of horses is reducing the frequency of disease outbreaks and the frequency and severity of clinical signs when outbreaks occur among vaccinated animals.[74,84,92-95]

Outbreaks of equine influenza occur most often when susceptible animals are congregated and kept in close contact with each other (e.g., racetracks, horse shows, sales yards, airplanes). Human studies show that spread is through direct-contact transmission with infected subjects, droplet transmission (contagious droplets greater than 10 μm and capable of being projected over moderate distances by coughing), and airborne transmission (infectious droplets less than 5 μm, capable of wide dissemination in confined environments and of reaching the lower respiratory tract of susceptible individuals).[96] No experimental studies have shown that transmission occurs through fomites, although human epidemiologic studies provide indirect evidence.[97,98] Among horses, rapid and effective spread is enhanced by a 2-day incubation period, high concentrations of virus in nasal secretions, an explosive cough, the practice of housing horses in confined spaces, and possibly, the ability of the virus to survive in wet environments (e.g., water bowls) for 72 hours and on dry surfaces (e.g., clothing, grooming equipment, vehicles, feed) for 48 hours.[97]

Anecdotal evidence suggests that disease spreads very quickly in small groups of confined animals and that all susceptible horses may become infected within 2 to 3 days. However, outbreaks occurring in large groups or populations, comprised of animals with varying histories of exposure and immunity, may last for 3 to 4 weeks,[60] thus providing at least some opportunity to institute procedures to limit the extent and severity of such outbreaks.

Several studies show that after experimental infection, horses typically shed virus for 6 to 7 days.[52,78-80] Although a carrier state does not occur, subclinical infections and viral shedding are probably common, particularly after infection of partially immune animals. Partial immunity is likely in animals that have not been recently exposed or vaccinated or may be caused by mismatching of vaccine strains and circulating field virus.[84,93,99] These animals are likely important in the spread of the disease within and between groups of horses[37,100,101] and, along with fomites,[102-104] provide a rational explanation for disease outbreaks among horses that have not experienced direct exposure to clinically diseased animals. The international transport of subclinically affected horses has been the suspected cause of many reported outbreaks of the disease in countries or regions with large numbers of susceptible animals.[103]

Outbreaks of equine influenza in naïve populations, such as those occurring in recent years in South Africa, India, and Australia, present a different picture than those occurring in the endemic populations in North America and Europe. Data collected during the 2007 outbreak in Australia, cases clustering around large urban centers[105] with their high concentration of horses and premises but spreading over a total area of 300,000 km^2 and infecting an estimated 9360 properties and 70,000 horses has provided new information on the epidemiology of the disease in naïve populations.[105-108] The outbreak followed a classic epidemic curve, peaking in 6 and lasting 18 weeks. The initial distant spread was due to transport of infected horses within 10 days of release of virus.[105-107] Local spread within 5 to 10 km of infected premises was related to direct horse to horse contact, aerosol droplets from coughing horses, and indirect contact (fomites and human assisted).[63,106-109] The contribution of airborne virus in the spread of the epidemic is unknown.[107,110] Commonly, 75% to 100% of horses on infected properties showed clinical signs of disease within 5 to 9 days.[63,111] Mares on Thoroughbred studs were most severely affected.[90] Signs in foals and yearlings were generally mild. Despite one cluster of fatalities in foals, death caused by influenza was extremely uncommon.[112]

Spread of disease across the entire country was prevented through restricted movement of horses, augmented by biosecurity and vaccination protocols.[106,108,109] Strict biosecurity was associated with a significant decrease in the odds of a premise becoming infected.[113] Vaccination with a highly efficacious vaccine was implemented after the peak of the epidemic. Its impact on disease occurrence in the general population has not been determined.[106]

Pathogenesis

Influenza A viruses replicate and induce pathologic changes throughout the entire respiratory tract, with the most significant pathology present in the lower respiratory tract.[3] The primary targets of low pathogenic strains of influenza A viruses in mammalian species are the airway epithelial cells. After exposure of the upper airway mucosa to virus, infection is initiated by binding of the influenza virus HA to sialic acid residues on target cells located in the upper respiratory tract. However, for the virus to gain access to the cellular receptors, the virion first has to penetrate a mucus layer that forms a protective barrier over the cell surface. The viral NA promotes virus access to respiratory epithelial cells by destroying mucous glycoproteins[15] and removing decoy receptors present on mucins, cilia, and cellular glycocalix.[16]

After viral attachment, the virion is taken up into the cell through receptor-mediated endocytosis. After internalization and acidification of the endosomal compartment, the HA protein undergoes a conformational change,[114,115] which leads to the insertion of the hydrophobic fusion peptide into the endosomal membrane and ultimately to the fusion of the viral and cellular membranes. After membrane fusion and release of the RNPs into the cell's cytoplasm, the RNPs are actively transported into the nucleus,[116] where messenger RNA (mRNA) synthesis is initiated. During virus replication, the virus-encoded nonstructural protein (NS1) inhibits cellular protein synthesis by inhibiting the maturation of cellular mRNAs. The NS1 protein is multifunctional, and apart from inhibiting both polyadenylation and splicing of cellular pre-mRNAs, it also counteracts interferon (IFN)-dependent and IFN-independent antiviral responses.[76,117,118]

In polarized epithelial cells, low pathogenic influenza viruses assemble and bud from the apical surface of the cells.[76,119,120] Interaction between the cytoplasmic tails of the HA and NA proteins and the internal proteins (most likely M1) are thought to be the main driving force behind the formation of the budding particles.[121,122] By removing carbohydrate chains from the virion and the cell surface, NA enzymatic activity is thought to be required to release the newly formed influenza virus virions completely from the cell.[12-14]

The virus spreads quickly throughout the respiratory tract, damaging the respiratory epithelial cells, particularly in the trachea and bronchial tree.[104,123] Virus replication leads to cell death, largely through virus-induced apoptosis,[124-126] and subsequent desquamation and denudation of respiratory epithelial cells. Histologic evaluation of infected respiratory epithelium reveals vacuolization and swelling of the columnar ciliated cells, accompanied by clumping and subsequent loss of cilia.[127] Consequently, tracheal mucociliary clearance is impaired, predisposing affected animals to the development of secondary bacterial infections.[34,123,128,129] Within 1 day after the onset of clinical signs, focal erosions of the respiratory cells down to the basal layer are evident. Viral antigen can be demonstrated predominantly in the respiratory epithelial cells and only rarely in the basal cell layer.[130] The disruption of the superficial cell layers allows opportunistic bacteria to invade the respiratory epithelium of both the upper and the lower respiratory tract, leading to bacterial bronchopneumonia and other complications.[3,104,130] Submucosal edema and hyperemia occur with peribronchial and peribronchiolar infiltration by neutrophils and mononuclear cells.[3,37,127] About 3 to 5 days after onset of illness, regeneration of the epithelium begins, characterized by the appearance of mitotic figures in the basal cell layer.[3] In uncomplicated cases, complete resolution of the epithelial damage takes a minimum of 3 weeks.[129,131]

Complications of equine influenza virus infections include secondary bacterial pneumonia, myositis, myocarditis, and limb edema; in rare cases, neurologic disease may be observed.[35,128,130,132] Attempts at virus recovery from the heart or brains of affected horses have been unsuccessful to date, although a recent study demonstrated a mild, transient increase in cardiac troponin I in ponies experimentally inoculated with equine influenza virus and supports a direct relationship between influenza infection and myocardial damage.[133] Yet, based on the lack of evidence for virus replication in these tissues, it has been speculated that myocardial damage is caused indirectly, such as through an increase in the expression of inflammatory mediators (e.g., nitric oxide).[134] Finally, it has been suggested that influenza infection might predispose horses to the development of recurrent airway obstruction (RAO) and exercise-induced pulmonary hemorrhage (EIPH).[35,104,128]

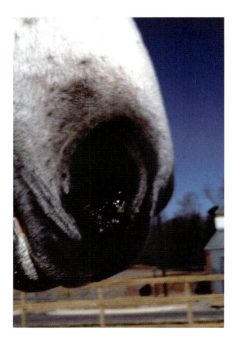

Figure 13-3 Serous nasal discharge typical of horse with acute influenza virus infection. *(Courtesy Dr. John Barneso.)*

Clinical Findings

Clinical signs of influenza virus infection were extensively described after its first discovery,[128] and the same clinical findings are still observed almost 40 years later. Signs of disease are typically seen 48 hours and sometimes as early as 24 hours, after exposure in natural or experimentally infected horses. Pyrexia is typically the first clinical sign, with temperatures sometimes exceeding 106° F (41.1° C), peaking at 48 to 96 hours after infection. The increase in rectal temperature may be biphasic with a second peak of pyrexia observed around day 7 after infection. Nasal discharge follows, initially serous (Fig. 13-3), but typically becoming mucopurulent by 72 to 96 hours after infection. Coughing, sometimes paroxysmal, typically develops during this same period. Retropharyngeal lymphadenopathy is a variable but common finding, as is tachypnea. Most affected horses become anorexic at the time of the initial pyrexia, although this typically resolves in 1 to 2 days. Weight loss is well documented after influenza virus infection. Clinical signs typically resolve in 7 to 14 days in uncomplicated cases, although

coughing may persist for 21 days. In severe infections, lung sounds become increased in amplitude, with adventitial sounds sometimes detected. Ultrasonographic imaging of the thorax has been used to demonstrate pulmonary consolidation; pneumonia is a common sequela between 7 and 14 days after infection.[135] Persistent respiratory disease can occur beyond 14 days after infection and is thought to be the result of secondary bacterial infection.

Morbidity can approach 100% in outbreaks in susceptible populations. Mortality is typically low, although neonatal infection can be fatal,[66] resulting in severe bronchial and interstitial pneumonia. The effects of influenza virus infection in donkeys and mules is typically more severe than in horses and can result in mortality.[136] It is also important to recognize that subclinical disease with viral shedding may be common in previously vaccinated horses and represents an important source of contagion.[136] The effects of influenza virus infection can be significantly exacerbated by even moderate exercise, resulting in increased weight loss and other clinical signs.[135]

Immunity

Equine influenza virus infection generates a broad range of adaptive immune responses in systemic and mucosal compartments,[81] and infection also stimulates important innate immune responses.[137] In the horse, many investigators have demonstrated that antibody responses are strongly associated with protection. A protective immune response, such as that following infection, is characterized by induction of influenza virus–specific immunoglobulin G isotype a and b (IgGa, IgGb) and immunoglobulin A (IgA) antibodies in both the circulation and the nasopharyngeal secretions, with the IgG isotype responses predominating in the circulation and IgA in the respiratory tract.[81,138,139]

Nasal IgA is an important mediator of protective immunity to influenza virus infection in other species,[140,141] through neutralization of viral particles at the respiratory epithelium and in the intracellular compartment.[142-144] Nasal IgA responses are a characteristic of the protective immunity that follows equine influenza infection,[138,139] and influenza virus–specific IgA-producing B lymphocytes have been detected in mucosal lamina propria and lymph nodes draining the nasopharynx of the horse.[81] Virus-specific IgG antibodies can also contribute to immune exclusion at the respiratory epithelium in a mouse model, although the lack of specialized mechanisms for transporting IgG to the respiratory surface means that its role is less important.[145] In the horse, there is evidence for local production of influenza virus–specific IgGa and IgGb at respiratory mucosal surfaces after infection,[81,146] and indirect evidence that virus-specific nasal IgGb antibody responses can contribute to a reduction in nasal shedding of influenza virus.[147] However, IgG antibody responses tend to be more short-lived in equine respiratory secretions than IgA responses.[148,149]

In the circulation, IgGa and IgGb are thought to be the principal protective IgG subisotype responses to influenza virus,[81,139] whereas IgG(T) responses are not associated with protection.[139] Circulating antibody has been measured in a number of ways in horses, including conventional hemagglutination inhibition (HI) assays, single radial hemolysis (SRH) assays, virus neutralization (VN) assays, and enzyme-linked immunosorbent assay (ELISA).[139,150] Of these techniques, SRH and ELISA may have the greatest sensitivity and utility, and it appears that SRH results correlate closely with IgGb ELISA results (Lunn and Townsend, unpublished data). Much attention has focused on the correlation between levels of circulating antibody measured by SRH tests and protection from influenza virus infection.[74] This tool has proved very useful, and SRH responses are often used to measure vaccination effect and predict protection. However, after circulating antibody responses to a prior influenza virus infection have waned, horses can remain protected against a further challenge.[75] In addition, circulating antibody responses measured by SRH to a cold-adapted, modified live influenza vaccine are almost undetectable, although this vaccine provides long-lasting protection from challenge infection.[78,151] Taken together, these observations illustrate that although circulating antibody responses are an important predictor of protection against influenza virus protection, a lack of antibody does not invariably predict susceptibility.

The role of cellular effectors in resistance to equine influenza virus infection is less well investigated. Virus-specific cytotoxic T lymphocytes (CTLs) are important for protection from influenza virus infection,[152,153] and there is a single description of the measurement of major histocompatibility complex (MHC)-restricted CTL responses to equine influenza virus.[154] The lack of other CTL studies reflects the difficulty in detecting this equine immune response to influenza virus using available methods. Currently, influenza virus–specific lymphoproliferative responses and interferon gamma (IFN-γ) gene expression may be the best available measures of virus-specific cellular immune responses in the horse. Production of IFN-γ is an indicator of T-helper 1 (Th1) cell-mediated immunity and can contribute to immunologic protection of humans from influenza virus infection and disease.[141] Furthermore, several studies indicate an association between IFN-γ production and the concomitant generation of antigen-specific CTL responses.[155,156] A number of studies have demonstrated the development of equine IFN-γ responses to influenza virus consequent to either infection or vaccination.[81,157,158] Similarly, influenza virus–specific lymphoproliferative responses have also been associated with protective immunity.[81,146,157]

The importance of HA-specific immune responses in protection from influenza virus infection is well known, and vaccination studies in horses using deoxyribonucleic acid (DNA) vaccination and recombinant vaccines expressing the HA gene all confirm the importance of the HA antigen for protection.[147,157,159] Studies using modified vaccinia Ankara vector vaccines have demonstrated that NP-specific equine immune responses can also result in reduced clinical disease after challenge infection, although the degree of protection was inferior to that induced by HA vaccination.[157] Influenza virus NP is an internal viral structural protein, and therefore NP-specific antibodies are not capable of virus neutralization and do not control virus shedding in the horse[157] or other species.[160] NP typically serves as an important target antigen for cellular immune responses and can elicit cross-protective immunity to heterologous strains of influenza virus.[161] In the equine vaccination studies conducted to date, NP-specific immune responses included both lymphoproliferative and IFN-γ responses, and it is possible that NP-specific immune responses could make a significant contribution to equine immunity to influenza virus infection.

Diagnosis

In a group of susceptible horses, a presumptive diagnosis of influenza virus infection can be made based on the rapid spread of an acute, febrile respiratory disease characterized by a dry, hacking cough.[104] However, laboratory diagnosis is required to confirm and differentiate influenza from other respiratory pathogens. The methods presently used for diagnosis of equine influenza virus infections include virus isolation, antigen detection by fluorescent antibody and ELISA testing, reverse transcriptase–polymerase chain reaction (RT-PCR)–based assays, and serologic analyses.[104,162-165] However, many of these methods have one or more disadvantages, such as lack of sensitivity, long turnaround time, prohibitive costs, or the need for a high degree of technical expertise in the laboratory. Thus, to institute optimal control measures, it might be necessary to combine several of these diagnostic tools to identify the etiologic agent accurately and rapidly. The World Organization for Animal Health (OIE) publishes the Manual of Diagnostic Tests and Vaccines for Terrestrial Animals at their Web site (http://www.oie.int/), which provides an extremely useful resource for current testing methodology.

Antigen Detection

Virus Isolation

Virus isolation from clinical samples is critical for epidemiologic investigation and vaccine production and is generally carried out in embryonated chicken eggs or cell culture. In the naïve horse, by the third or fourth day after infection, large amounts of virus are shed into the secretions of the respiratory tract.[34,165] Therefore the best results for virus isolation can often be achieved by collecting nasal swab samples (Fig. 13-4) within the first 24 to 48 hours after onset of clinical illness.[35] In partially immune animals the length of virus shedding is often shorter, decreasing the diagnostic sensitivity of virus isolation. Therefore it is useful to sample the more immunologically naïve horses in a group to increase the likelihood of demonstrating infectious virus.[104] Nasal swab samples are best collected using polyester-tipped swabs. Cotton swabs should be avoided because influenza viruses can adhere to the cotton fibers, decreasing the likelihood of isolating virus from the sample. The swabs should be placed in sterile viral transport medium and kept on ice until further analysis.

Traditionally, embryonated chicken eggs have been the biologic system of choice for isolating influenza viruses. The robust yield of virus from eggs has led to their widespread use in research laboratories and for vaccine production. However, their use may be of limited value for diagnostic laboratories.

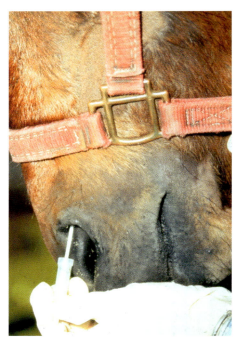

Figure 13-4 Technique to obtain nasal mucosal swab for antigen detection or virus isolation. Short, polyester-tipped (noncotton-tipped) swab is most appropriate for sample collection. Virus isolation from a nasal mucosal swab is most sensitive for detection of equine influenza virus if obtained during the first 24 to 48 hours of fever.

Depending on the virus strain, amount of virus present in the sample, sample quality, and handling, detection of the presence of infectious virus by egg inoculation can take a minimum of 2 or 3 days. In horses with mild or subclinical infections, viral titers in nasal secretions are often low, sometimes requiring several passages before sufficiently high viral titers are produced to allow detection using conventional HA assays.[165]

Alternatively, equine influenza virus can be propagated in cell culture. Although the virus can infect a variety of primary and continuous cell lines, many of these do not support productive viral replication.[166-169] The most widely used cells are Madin-Darby canine kidney (MDCK) epithelial cells. Unfortunately, the use of cell culture for influenza virus isolation also has several limitations. For example, depending on the protocol and cell lines used, substantial differences in influenza recovery rates from clinical samples can occur.[170] In addition, MDCK cells are generally considered less permissive than embryonated chicken eggs for equine influenza viruses.[171] Other, less frequently used cell lines include mink lung epithelial cells (Mv1Lu) and chick embryo fibroblasts. Mv1Lu cells in particular might provide a useful alternative system for the isolation of influenza A viruses from clinical samples. Recent studies found that Mv1Lu cells and mixtures of MDCK and Mv1Lu cells supported the replication of a wider range of influenza A virus than MDCK cells alone.[172,173]

Immunoassays

A number of ELISAs using monoclonal antibodies to detect the viral NP in nasal swab samples have been developed as a more rapid alternative to virus isolation. Although influenza A viruses can differ substantially in their HA and NA genes, the sequences of the internal genes, such as the M, NP, and the NS genes, are highly conserved among all subtypes and strains of influenza A viruses.[4] As such, a diagnostic test aimed at the detection of NP is likely to be capable of identifying a wide variety of influenza

A viruses from different host species. An additional advantage of ELISA-based assays over virus isolation is that these tests are able to detect virions that have lost their infectivity during sample handling, storage, and transport to the laboratory.

Originally intended for the diagnosis of human influenza infections, an antigen-capture ELISA has been adapted for the detection of equine H3N8 viral antigen.[174,175] Briefly, to detect viral antigen, a "capture" antibody, directed against the influenza NP, is linked to a 96-well plastic plate. The clinical sample is added to the wells, and if viral antigens are present, they will be bound to the immobilized antibody. Subsequently, bound viral antigen is detected by use of a second enzyme-linked antibody. The antigen-capture ELISA was evaluated during an outbreak of equine influenza in the United Kingdom in 1989 and, when used in combination with virus isolation, was found to enhance the virus detection rate by 44%.[176] Moreover, the test was shown to be particularly useful for detection of viral antigen in samples heavily contaminated with bacteria.[104,165]

Commercial development of optical immunoassay (OIA)-based test kits (e.g., Flu OIA assay [Biostar, Boulder, CO], Directigen Flu-A assay [Becton Dickinson Microbiology Systems, Cockeysville, MD), designed to detect the NP of human influenza A viruses, has facilitated the widespread use of this procedure. Many investigators found such commercial diagnostic kits to be useful, and frequently, these assays were considerably more sensitive than traditional virus isolation.[177-181] Furthermore, these OIAs proved to be highly specific and rapid, whereas virus isolation in embryonated chicken eggs required up to three passages before hemagglutination became evident.[177-179,181] Yet, while these test kits were able to identify infected horses consistently at the peak of virus shedding, they may not be sensitive enough to detect low levels of virus shedding reliably.[7] Therefore, whenever possible, horses with severe clinical signs are preferable for testing during a suspected influenza virus outbreak to increase the likelihood of obtaining positive results.[179]

Immunofluorescence

Employing influenza virus–specific fluorochrome-labeled antibodies, immunofluorescence (IF) is based on the immunodetection of virus-infected cells obtained from nasal scrapings or tracheal washes. Although the assay was reported to be highly sensitive and rapid,[165,182] IF requires substantial sample preparation and handling. Briefly, samples are centrifuged to separate the cells from respiratory mucus. The cells are washed, spotted onto glass slides, acetone fixed, and incubated with influenza-specific antibodies. Antigen-positive cells are detected by use of a secondary fluorochrome-labeled antibody.[104,165,182] A study comparing the detection of influenza viruses by IF to a commercially available OIA for diagnosis of influenza virus infections in humans found that the IF had a significantly higher sensitivity than the OIA.[182]

Reverse Transcriptase–Polymerase Chain Reaction

During the past decade, advances in PCR technology and other DNA amplification techniques have resulted in these methods becoming key tools in diagnostic laboratories.[183-185] By choosing appropriate oligonucleotide primers, a selected region of the viral genome can be amplified. In vitro DNA synthesis is catalyzed by a special DNA polymerase isolated from thermophilic bacteria that is stable at high temperatures. PCR is extremely sensitive and can theoretically detect a single-copy of DNA in a sample. Trace amounts of RNA can be detected in the same way by first transcribing them into DNA with RT.

RT-PCR–based assays have been used successfully for the detection of a broad range of influenza A virus subtypes from clinical samples.[164,172,182,186,187] In contrast to virus isolation, RT-PCR does not require the presence of viable virus,[188] and therefore the sensitivity of RT-PCR methods is often substantially higher than for virus isolation. Despite these advantages, the technique can also have a number of shortcomings. Because of the assay's high sensitivity, the greatest problem facing the diagnostic application of PCR is the production of false-positive results. These are often attributable to contamination by nucleic acids, particularly from previously amplified material (carryover). Any contaminant, even the smallest airborne remnant, may be multiplied and produce a false-positive result. In fact, a recent study reported that even administration of an inactivated whole-virus influenza vaccine at time of nasal swab samples collection resulted in the contamination of the sample with the vaccine virus and in the creation of a false-positive RT-PCR result.[189] Contamination of the nasal swab sample most likely occurred through aerosolized vaccine, contaminated fomites, or inadvertent sample handling.[189] False-negative results might also be encountered when employing RT-PCR–based testing and can result from the nature of the sample tested. Ribonucleases (RNases) are present in various quantities in specimens collected from the respiratory tract, and these enzymes can gradually digest viral RNA.[190,191] This may reduce the sensitivity of RT-PCR–based tests in clinical samples that contain large amounts of RNases and a low concentration of viral RNA. In addition, PCR assay inhibitors (e.g., lactoferrin, hemoglobin) can represent a substantial problem in diagnostic PCR-based assays.[192,193] The presence of PCR inhibitors have been reported in about 2% of samples from the respiratory tract.[194]

In diagnostic laboratory settings the use of RT-PCR can be limited by cost and the availability of adequate test sample volume. To overcome these shortcomings, multiplex PCR assays have been developed. In multiplex PCR, more than one target sequence can be amplified by including more than one pair of primers in the reaction. Multiplex PCR has been shown to be a valuable and cost-effective tool for monitoring the emergence of new variants and subtypes of influenza A viruses.[195,196] In addition, multiplex PCR has also been used successfully to screen clinical samples simultaneously for multiple equine respiratory pathogens.[197] In contrast to conventional PCR methods, real-time PCR does not require post-PCR processing steps (e.g., gel electrophoresis and determination of fragment size) and can therefore generate results within 4 to 5 hours. By employing a target-specific fluorescent probe, real-time PCR is a highly sensitive and specific method for the detection of equine influenza virus in clinical samples and can also be used for quantification of virus.[198-200] Based on these advantages, real-time RT-PCR–based assays are now widely used in routine diagnostic settings.

Antibody Detection

In the past, serologic tests have been the key tool by which influenza infections were diagnosed. Most serologic assays are fairly easy to perform and cost-effective. In addition, a large number of samples can be collected and tested simultaneously, facilitating large-scale herd surveillance. Because many horses have been vaccinated, however, diagnosis of influenza infection can often be made only by testing paired samples (acute and convalescent titers) collected 10 to 21 days apart and demonstrating at least a fourfold increase in antibody titer over a period of several weeks (seroconversion). Therefore serologic testing often provides only retrospective information, and subclinical infections, which may not be accompanied by seroconversion, might not be detected.[201] In addition, because of the inherent variability of immunoassays, paired samples always should be run by the same laboratory. To diagnose influenza infection, seroconversion should be demonstrated, and therefore baseline (acute) samples must be collected early in the

course of infection. The tests commonly used to detect influenza-specific antibodies include HI, VN, complement fixation (CF), SRH, and ELISA-based testing.

Hemagglutination Inhibition

Hemagglutination inhibition tests are simple, sensitive, inexpensive, and rapid and therefore are often the method of choice for assaying antibodies to influenza A virus. The test relies on the hemagglutination activity of the influenza HA and the ability of HA-specific antibodies to inhibit the virus from agglutinating erythrocytes (Fig. 13-5). Briefly, dilutions of serum are incubated with virus, and erythrocytes are added. After incubation, the HI titer is read as the highest dilution of serum that inhibits hemagglutination. A fourfold or greater increase in HI antibody titer is regarded as evidence of infection.[165,202] Hemagglutination inhibition antibodies define subtype-specific antigens on the virus particle, thus allowing the differentiation of equine influenza H3N8 and H7N7 subtypes.[203] In addition, HI assays have found wide application in the analysis of antigenic differences between strains in equine and human influenza surveillance. One of the main shortcomings of the HI test is interlaboratory variation. Although a study comparing the sensitivity of HI and SRH tests on human sera found that both tests had similar sensitivity, the interlaboratory reproducibility of HI was significantly lower.[202]

Single Radial Hemolysis

For SRH tests, sheep erythrocytes, which have previously been incubated with influenza virus, are mixed with guinea pig complement and incorporated in agarose gels (Fig. 13-6). Heat-inactivated serum samples are then added to wells cut into the gel, and the antibody titer is determined based on the zone of hemolysis induced by diffusion of the antibody-positive sample

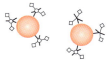

1) Prepared test antigen: RBCs with adsorbed virus

2) Add patient serum

+ (anti-influenza Ab)   − (no specific Ab)

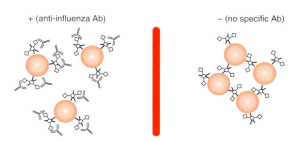

Antibody blocks hemagglutinin: no RBC agglutination   Hemagglutinin not blocked: RBC agglutination

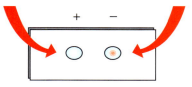

+   −

Figure 13-5 Schematic diagram of hemagglutination inhibition (HI) assay. Chicken red blood cells *(RBCs)* agglutinate in the presence of influenza virus, but this can be inhibited by the addition of influenza virus–specific antibody *(Ab)*. HI results in cells coating the bottom of a round-bottomed test plate, whereas lack of antibody allows for clumping of cells into a pellet.

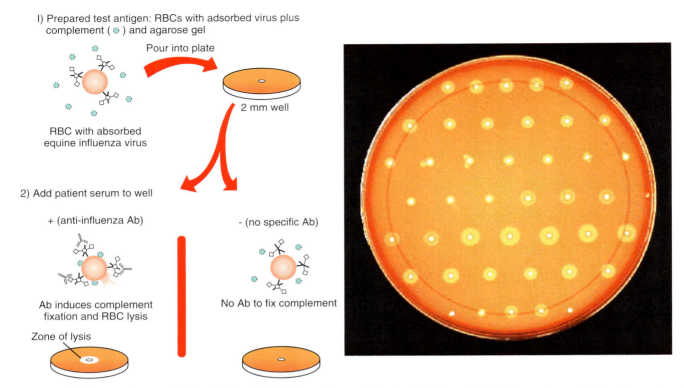

1) Prepared test antigen: RBCs with adsorbed virus plus complement (⊛) and agarose gel

Pour into plate

RBC with absorbed equine influenza virus

2 mm well

2) Add patient serum to well

+ (anti-influenza Ab)

\- (no specific Ab)

Ab induces complement fixation and RBC lysis

No Ab to fix complement

Zone of lysis

Figure 13-6 *Left,* Schematic diagram of single radial hemolysis (SRH) assay. Sheep red blood cells *(RBCs)* coated with influenza virus and guinea pig complement are mixed with molten agar and poured in a plate. Test equine serum and control serum can be added to individual wells cut in the agar, and the zone of hemolysis corresponds to the amount of influenza virus–specific complement-fixing antibody *(Ab)* present in the test equine serum. *Right,* Typical result.

from the well.[138,204,205] An increase of 50% or 25 mm^2 is considered evidence of recent infection.[202] Although more labor intensive than HI assays, SRH tests have been shown to be more reproducible than HI tests.[202] Since it was found that the level of antibody measured by SRH after vaccination correlates well with the level of protection, SRH may also be used to predict the level of antibody-mediated immunity and determine the need for revaccination.[72,73,165]

ELISA-Based Assays

ELISAs detecting antibodies to equine influenza H3 HA have been developed as an alternative method to traditional HI tests and were found to be sensitive, rapid, and reproducible.[206] For example, an assay employing an HA protein produced in a baculovirus expression system demonstrated broad reactivity with serum antibodies generated after infection with heterologous H3N8 influenza virus strains.[207] Because conventional serologic tests do not provide information as to whether existing antibodies were produced in response to infection or vaccination, an ELISA aimed at the detection of antibodies to the NS1 protein has been developed.[208] Because antibodies to NS1 can be demonstrated only in influenza virus–infected horses,[209] and NS1 is antigenically and genetically highly conserved across influenza A viruses,[210] NS1 is a good candidate for a differential diagnostic marker, capable of differentiating between infected and vaccinated animals (DIVA). Subsequent testing of horses that were either experimentally infected with A/equine/Kentucky/1/81 (H3N8) and A/equine/La Plata/1/93 (H3N8) or vaccinated with inactivated influenza H3N8 and H7N7 virus demonstrated that the NS1-based ELISA was a useful tool to distinguish postvaccination antibody titers from those generated by recent infection.[208] A slightly different approach to differentiate between infected and vaccinated horses was taken in the 2007 equine influenza outbreak in Australia. During the

process of selecting a vaccine to limit the spread of infection, an important consideration was that the vaccine, in combination with an appropriate serologic test, would provide DIVA capacity.[211,212] Consequently, the canarypox-vectored vaccine (Recombitek, Merial, Duluth, GA) was chosen, because it induces an antibody response only to the influenza HA protein. Coupled with a blocking ELISA (bELISA) detecting serum antibodies to the influenza NP, this strategy allowed vaccinated horses to be distinguished from infected horses with high diagnostic sensitivity (approximately 97%), and this testing strategy was used extensively during the Australian equine influenza control and eradication effort.[213,214]

Pathologic Findings

Given the limited mortality associated with equine influenza infection, there are few reports of gross pathologic findings, although an early publication summarizes the original studies performed when equine influenza virus infection was first recognized.[128] Subacute inflammatory disease of the nasal mucosa, pharynx, larynx, and trachea is observed. Pulmonary changes include bronchitis, peribronchitis, and perivasculitis, with subacute interstitial pneumonia, edema, and focal bronchopneumonia. Myocarditis is a variable finding. Neonatal infection with equine influenza virus can result in severe fatal bronchointerstitial pneumonia accompanied by pulmonary congestions, tracheitis, bronchiolar and alveolar necrosis, and squamous metaplasia,[215-217] although such occurrences are rare.

Hemogram findings in equine influenza virus infection include a moderate normocytic, normochromic anemia.[128] The leukogram typically shows a leukopenia, which results from both neutropenia and lymphopenia of 3 to 5 days' duration[128,218];

neutropenia is not a consistent finding, and the neutrophil/lymphocyte ratio is often increased during this period.[16,128] Monocytosis during early convalescence is a variable finding.[127,128]

Therapy

Medical Therapy

Symptomatic treatment is the primary form of therapy for equine influenza virus infection and should include rest in a nonstressful environment. It is important to ensure adequate hydration, and nonsteroidal antiinflammatory drugs (NSAIDs) may reduce morbidity caused by pyrexia and myalgia. Affected animals should be monitored for development of complications such as pneumonia or myocarditis, and any horse exhibiting signs of respiratory disease beyond 10 days postinfection should be considered at high risk of secondary bacterial infection. The duration of adequate convalescence is difficult to gauge but is typically much longer than owner's expectations. Estimates for the period before horses should be returned to athletic activity vary from 50 to 100 days,[219] to a week for each day of fever.[136]

Antiviral Therapy

Vaccination is the best option for the control of equine influenza, and limitations inherent to influenza immunoprophylaxis (e.g., lack of vaccine coverage or protective immunogenicity) have stimulated an interest in the use of antiviral therapy in the horse. Moreover, in contrast to vaccines, antivirals can be rapidly employed to combat an influenza virus outbreak. Despite this, use of antiviral drugs to combat equine influenza infection should be carefully deliberated. As a large body of evidence indicates that the use of antiviral drugs can result in the development of antiviral resistance among influenza A viruses, indiscriminate use of antivirals could potentially reduce the effectiveness of treatment during an outbreak.[220-222] Two classes of influenza antiviral drugs are currently licensed for the prophylactic and therapeutic use against influenza A virus in humans: the M2 ion channel blockers and the NA inhibitors.

Amantadine (1-aminoadamantane hydrochloride) and rimantadine (methyl-1-adamantanemethylamine hydrochloride) target the transmembrane domain of the M2 ion channel protein. Both drugs inhibit virus replication by blocking ion channel activity of the M2 protein through allosteric inhibition. Amantadine and rimantadine have antiviral properties against all subtypes of influenza A virus.[222] Their primary antiviral action results from blocking the flow of H+ ions from the acidified endosomal compartment into the interior of the virion, a process necessary for release of the viral RNPs. A second effect of both drugs is to block maturation of the HA during transport from the endoplasmic reticulum to the plasma membrane.[223,224]

Influenza virus inhibitory concentrations of amantadine and rimantadine range from 0.03 to 1.0 µg/mL,[225] with rimantadine about fourfold to tenfold more active than amantadine.[226] In humans, amantadine and rimantadine have good oral bioavailability and very large volumes of distribution.[161,227] In horses, oral administration of amantadine was associated with substantial interanimal variation in bioavailability, ranging from very low (~10%) to a maximum of 70%, and was not substantially affected by prior fasting of the horses.[228] Therefore oral administration of amantadine in horses, although effective in some animals, might fail to produce effective plasma concentration in others. In contrast, intravenous (IV) administration of amantadine at doses ranging from 10 mg/kg every 8 hours (q8h) to 5 mg/kg every 4 hours (q4h) was suggested to be sufficient to maintain effective plasma concentrations.[228] Amantadine is

excreted primarily unmetabolized in urine, and therefore the dosage must be adjusted in patients with renal insufficiency to reduce the risk of adverse effects.[229] The most common adverse effects observed as a result of amantadine therapy are central nervous system (CNS) effects.[229,230] At high doses (>15 mg/kg), the drug was reported to produce acute seizures and even death in horses.[228] In humans the concurrent use of antihistamines, anticholinergics, and psychotropic drugs is thought to enhance the neurotoxic effect of amantadine.[226] When administered orally to healthy humans and horses, rimantadine was much less frequently associated with adverse CNS effects than amantadine.[229,231] Moreover, the bioavailability of rimantadine after oral administration in horses appeared considerably more uniform than the oral bioavailability of amantadine. The administration of 30 mg/kg of rimantadine every 12 hours (q12h) resulted in sufficiently high plasma concentrations without causing observable signs of adverse effects.[231]

Clinical trials conducted with influenza virus–infected humans and horses suggest that amantadine and rimantadine are equally effective in reducing the severity and duration of illness.[231-234] In addition, oral administration of rimantadine reduced virus load in nasal secretions, although the duration of nasal virus shedding was similar to that in the untreated controls.[231] The potential benefits associated with the administration of M2 ion channel blockers during an influenza virus outbreak may be limited by the rapid development of drug resistance. Amantadine and rimantadine resistance can develop as early as one day after start of treatment.[235] Such resistant viruses may then spread to susceptible contacts and cause disease, indicating that acquisition of drug resistance is not associated with attenuation of the virus.[236,237] Resistance can pose a major problem when these drugs are used in close-contact environments.[238,239] In recent years, the incidence of naturally occurring amantadine-resistant seasonal human-influenza virus has increased significantly around the world. Amantadine-resistant strains were found to have spread extensively around the world, including to some countries where the use of the M2 channel inhibitors was minimal.[240]

The NA inhibitors zanamivir and oseltamivir block the activity of the viral NA protein, therefore inhibiting the release of virions from the infected cells.[241,242] Both zanamivir and oseltamivir have demonstrated antiviral activity against a number of equine influenza viruses in vitro, with inhibitory concentrations generally ranging from 0.015 to 0.09 µM.[243] Because of its low oral bioavailability, zanamivir is administered in nasal sprays or drops, a nebulized mist, or a dry-powder aerosol.[241] To date, the drug's clinical effectiveness has not been tested in horses. In contrast, oseltamivir phosphate (OP) is well absorbed from the equine gastrointestinal tract and rapidly metabolized to oseltamivir carboxylate (OC).[244] Oral administration of OP at a dose of 2 mg/kg body weight resulted in OC plasma concentration well above the equine influenza virus inhibitory concentrations found in vitro.[244] In humans, oseltamivir has a long duration of action, thus dosing is typically recommended at twice daily for treatment and once daily for prophylaxis.[241] In contrast, OC is rapidly eliminated from horse plasma. Therefore, to maintain effective plasma concentrations, it was suggested that oseltamivir dosing intervals should be less than 10 hours in the horse.[244] In humans, oseltamivir is generally well tolerated. The most frequent adverse effect is nausea and less frequently, vomiting.[241] In a recent study, no clinical or serum biochemistry abnormalities were observed in horses receiving 6 mg/kg of oseltamivir every 12 hours for 5 days.[244] While oseltamivir has been shown to be effective for prevention and early treatment of influenza infection in humans, there are limited data on the drug's clinical efficacy in horses. Oral administration of 2 mg/kg of OP prior to (prophylaxis) and soon after experimental inoculation (treatment) was found to reduce the magnitude of nasal virus shedding and severity of clinical signs.[245] In addition, researchers found that bacterial counts of *Streptococcus equi* subsp. *zooepidemicus* in bronchoalveolar lavage fluids collected 7 days after inoculation with influenza were significantly lower in horses receiving OP compared to the placebo-treated control horses.[245]

As with the M2 ion channel inhibitors, emergence of NA inhibitor-resistant variants is a major concern. While oseltamivir resistance has not been documented for equine influenza strains, the prevalence of drug-resistant seasonal human H1N1 viruses has rapidly increased since the late 1990s and exceeded 90% in the 2008-2009 influenza season.[221,246-248]

Prevention

Vaccination

Vaccination against equine influenza virus infection is a common and important practice for the control of disease, and a wide variety of vaccine formulations are available. Inactivated vaccines remain the most common type of vaccine in use around the world, although both modified live and recombinant vaccines are commercially available. Many publications have documented the ability of inactivated equine influenza vaccines to protect against homologous viral challenge, which also demonstrates a correlation between protection and prechallenge antibody level.[71,72,249,250]

The value of inactivated equine influenza virus vaccines critically depends on the quality and quantity of viral antigen and the choice of adjuvant.[201,251] Some of the most successful inactivated vaccines have used adjuvants such as ISCOMS or carboxypolymer-based compounds (carbomer, carbopol),[71,249] and a recent North American study showed a clear advantage to carbomer-based products.[77] The use of some adjuvants, such as alum, have been associated with induction of nonprotective immune responses.[139]

Another critically important consideration is which strains of virus are used for preparation of the vaccine. The inclusion of the equine H7N7 virus is no longer considered necessary for equine influenza vaccines. Moreover, as no Eurasian H3N8 viruses have been isolated in recent years, the OIE expert panel on equine influenza vaccine composition no longer deems the inclusion of these viruses in vaccines necessary. However, further evolution of the American lineage H3N8 virus continued to result in failure of killed vaccines in outbreaks in 2003,[252] and ongoing evolution of this lineage into two new clades with distinct antigenic identity poses new challenges to vaccine formulations.[57] Ongoing surveillance and inclusion of viral antigens representative of contemporary circulating viruses will remain a priority.

An intranasal, cold-adapted, modified live equine influenza virus vaccine based on a Kentucky 1991 H3N8 virus is available in North America and provides protection for up to 12 months after a single administration, although only a 6-month claim is made on the product data sheet.[78,151] Intranasal vaccine administration is generally well tolerated in horses.[253] At the time of its introduction, this vaccine was found to protect against both European and American lineages, despite including only an example of the latter.[254] It is now some years since there were reports of the efficacy of this vaccine against contemporary circulating viruses.[77] A recombinant canarypox vector-based equine influenza vaccine has shown excellent performance against even the most recent circulating viral lineages, including those that have overcome modern inactivated vaccines.[159,200] These examples illustrate the increasing role and potency of novel equine influenza vaccines not based on conventional inactivated formulations. Experimentally, there are a number of

reports of alternative successful vaccination strategies, including the use of DNA vaccination,[81,146,147,255,256] and the development of a modified vaccinia Ankara (MVA) vaccine vector.[157,158] The use of the MVA vector had the particular advantage of generating nasal mucosal influenza virus–specific IgA. More recently, commercial vaccines using ISCOM-matrix formulations have been described.[257,258]

Recommendations for equine vaccination are available from a variety of sources.[259,260] General recommendations are not to vaccinate in the presence of maternal immunity in foals before at least 6 months of age.[261] Vaccination of mares with inactivated vaccines that are known to generate high-titer antibody responses 2 to 6 weeks before parturition is likely to provide protection of foals through passive transfer of immunity. Initial vaccination series for inactivated vaccines should include three doses, and this approach is recommended even when data sheets only recommend two initial doses. The timing of these initial vaccinations is important. An interval of 3 to 4 weeks between the first and second dose is recommended, but a longer interval of 3 to 4 months between the second and third dose is preferred. This results in the third dose of the initial series being administered when the antibody response to the second vaccine dose has waned, and the amplitude of the antibody response to the third dose is consequently much greater.[77] This regimen of three initial doses of vaccine, with intervals of 1 month between the first and second doses and with 3 to 4 months between the second and third vaccine doses, is recommended independent of the recommendations present on data sheets. Contemporary inactivated vaccines with established protective efficacy are likely to perform well if this approach is taken, and subsequent booster vaccinations should be given at 6-month intervals in high-risk populations. The modified live cold-adapted vaccine only requires a single initial dose and is recommended for booster doses at 6-month intervals. If a known period of high risk of infection is anticipated, a booster vaccination should be given even to well-vaccinated horses 1 to 2 weeks before the risk period.

Husbandry

Control of equine influenza virus infection can be substantially addressed by adequate husbandry procedures. It is informative to review the OIE qualifications for influenza-free countries.[262] If the same criteria are met for horses entering an equine establishment, it is likely that influenza virus infection can be excluded. Specifically, horses should be isolated for 4 weeks before introduction into the horse population, horses should be fully vaccinated before admission to the isolation facility, no clinical signs of influenza should be detected during the isolation period, and no new animals should be introduced into the isolation facility during the isolation period. Some countries also perform influenza virus diagnostic testing at the beginning of the isolation period, using tests such as the Directigen ELISA (Becton, Dickinson, Franklin Lakes, NJ). The recent outbreak of equine influenza virus in Australia, a country previously free of infection, was a result of a breakdown in these quarantine procedures.[43] During this outbreak and the subsequent eradication of equine influenza virus to reestablish Australia's equine influenza virus free status, new experience was gained in the use of a variety of diagnostic techniques for managing and controlling the spread of major outbreaks.[263]

Although the OIE criteria may be too demanding for most horse owners, adequate vaccination and 2 weeks of full isolation on the facility could be regarded as an excellent compromise. Frequently, even this standard is difficult to achieve, and we remain heavily dependent on vaccination for protection. Nevertheless, other husbandry procedures, including segregating equine populations on horse facilities, can be valuable. This allows for potential containment of disease outbreaks because infection moves slowly through large facilities where horse populations are segregated.[60] Shared grooming equipment and tack may increase the risk of contagion.[68]

Monitoring of vaccine response by serology has been reported to help in prevention and control of influenza virus outbreaks, and the SRH test can be used for this purpose.[74,264] Surveillance for detection of influenza virus is routinely practiced in some areas with large equine populations and offers the opportunity for early detection of outbreaks and for detection of new virus strains that may not be controlled by vaccine.[265]

Public Health Considerations

Influenza A viruses have partial host range restriction, meaning that viruses from one species can occasionally transmit to infect another species. However, biologic barriers exist that limit such spread. Human volunteers were found to be susceptible to infection with H3 equine-lineage viruses,[266] although phylogenetic analyses suggest that exchange of influenza virus genes between horses and other species is limited. This has led to the hypothesis that horses may be "dead-end" hosts for influenza A viruses. However, this notion has been challenged by at least four separate natural transmission events of equine H3N8 influenza virus to dogs that occurred in the United States,[267] the United Kingdom,[268,269] and in Australia.[270] In addition to these naturally occurring cross-species transmission events, equine influenza virus has also been found to spread from an experimentally infected horse to a dog that was housed in the same stall.[271] However, despite this seeming susceptibility of dogs to infection with equine H3N8 influenza virus, with the exception of the transmission event in the United States where the equine origin virus has become established in the canine population, there is no evidence of widespread circulation of H3N8 influenza in dogs in the United Kingdom[57] or Australia.[270] Moreover, recent experimental inoculations of horses and ponies with two different canine H3N8 influenza isolates did result in only mild clinical signs and minimal nasal virus shedding, suggesting that the canine isolates may have reduced infectivity for horses.[272,273]

The complete reference list is available online at www.expertconsult.com.

14

Equine Herpesviruses

Josh Slater

The equine herpesviruses (EHVs) are highly successful pathogens of all members of the Equidae family worldwide.[1-4] Of the nine EHVs characterized thus far, five types (EHV-1 to EHV-5) infect the domestic horse, and EHV-6 to EHV-9 are associated with infections in wild equids,[5] including asses and zebra.[6-9] The EHVs are ubiquitous in both domestic and wild equid populations, and it is likely that the enduring success of the EHV as pathogens results from ancient co-evolution with the Equidae family and adaptation of the virus life cycle to ensure efficient spread within the equid population.

The equid herpesviruses, as with other herpesviruses that infect animals and humans, have sophisticated life cycles adapted to exploit the host animal population and ensure virus persistence. Their life cycles involve infection of multiple cell types in different tissues, with different mechanisms for evasion of the host immune response. Latency, in which recovered horses carry virus in a quiescent (asymptomatic) form for extended periods, is central to the success of these viruses. First, latency provides a mechanism not only for the maintenance of virus in the infected herd but also for the introduction of virus into new herds through the movement of latently infected horses. Second, latently infected horses form a reservoir of transmissible infection through reactivation, resulting in infection of new, susceptible, in-contact horses.

In domestic horse populations the most important and most studied of the EHVs are the alpha herpesviruses EHV-1 and EHV-4. These respiratory pathogens are also responsible for abortion and neurologic disease. EHV-3 is an uncommon venereal pathogen and is not discussed in this chapter (see Chapter 8). The clinical importance of the gamma herpesviruses EHV-2 and EHV-5 is less clearly defined, although some evidence suggests that EHV-2 and EHV-5, in certain situations, may be clinically important as respiratory and ocular pathogens (see Chapter 10). There is growing evidence that EHV-5 is associated with a progressive nodular interstitial fibrotic pulmonary disease known as *equine multinodular pulmonary fibrosis* (EMPF), although causality has yet to be established.[10-12] There has been speculation that these viruses may act as immunosuppressive agents, predisposing to other viral infections, or may be involved in persistent, chronic fatigue syndromes.

The EHVs have a major economic and welfare impact on all sectors of the horse industry worldwide through their direct clinical effects on the horse, including respiratory disease, abortion,[13,14] and paralysis,[15] and through their effects on the horse industry, including interference with horse movement for breeding and competition. The first equine herpesviruses to be described were EHV-1 and EHV-4.[16-18] These viruses are closely related but genetically and phenotypically distinct and were originally designated as subtypes 1 and 2 of EHV-1.[19-23] These two viruses have been the subject of a major international research effort over the past 5 decades. This research has produced a wealth of fundamental virologic and immunologic knowledge about their pathogenesis and the interactions between these viruses and the horse.[3] This information in turn has allowed effective management control programs to be devised. These are embodied in the United Kingdom in the

Horserace Betting Levy Board's Code of Practice (www.hblb.org.uk) and in North America in the American College of Veterinary Internal Medicine (ACVIM) consensus statement on EHV-1[24] and the Control Guidelines for Infectious Disease published by the American Association of Equine Practitioners (AAEP) (www.aaep.org/control_guidelines_intro.htm). From the outset, EHV research has been directed toward vaccine development; the first EHV-1 vaccines were used in 1961,[25] and there are now a variety of killed and live commercial EHV vaccines available in Europe and North America.

This chapter concentrates on EHV-1 and EHV-4 and reviews current understanding of their virology, epidemiology, pathogenesis, clinical disease, treatment, and prevention.

Etiology

Advances in the understanding of the molecular biology and virology of the equine herpesviruses have greatly improved our understanding of their pathogenesis,[1,3] the immune responses required to control virus replication and spread in the host,[26] and the identification of key immunologic viral targets.[27,28] This information is a prerequisite for effective vaccine design.

Virology Overview

EHV-1 and EHV-4 are alpha herpesviruses (members of the *Alphaherpesvirinae* subfamily) and belong, along with bovine herpesvirus-1, suid herpesvirus-1, canine herpesvirus-1, felid herpesvirus-1, and Marek's disease virus (MDV), to the *Varicellovirus* genus, the prototypic virus of which is the human pathogen varicella-zoster virus (VZV).[29] The varicelloviruses share some similarities with the herpes simplex viruses (HSV-1 and HSV-2), the cause of cold sores and genital herpes, respectively, but are genetically and phenotypically distinct. Indeed, the varicelloviruses are sufficiently different to merit care in extrapolation of data from the simplex viruses to the EHVs, as with the use of the antiviral agent acyclovir to treat EHV-1 neurologic disease (see section on Treatment).

Each of the *Alphaherpesvirinae* has a restricted host range, typically infecting a single target species, although laboratory animal models have been employed to study many of these viruses, including EHV-1, -2, and -5, with varying success. The varicelloviruses all share common genome structure and are of broadly similar genome size.

EHV-1 and EHV-4 are closely related[30,31] but genetically and antigenically distinct with different disease profiles. EHV-1 is principally a pathogen of the domestic horse, but there is serologic evidence of occasional infection of domestic cattle and captive camelids and cervids. In contrast, EHV-4 is an exclusive pathogen of the domestic horse. In the laboratory, some aspects of EHV-1 pathogenesis can be modeled with limited success in mice[32-34] and hamsters,[35,36] but this has not proved possible for EHV-4.

Within the *Varicellovirus* genus, there is a spectrum of cellular tropism from principally neurotropic viruses (e.g., VZV) to viruses that are principally lymphotropic (e.g., MDV). EHV-1 and -4 lie midway along this spectrum, being both neurotropic and lymphotropic during their life cycle (see section on Pathogenesis). A key feature of the life cycle of EHV-1, distinguishing it from EHV-4, is that it efficiently infects a variety of cell types,[37] including respiratory epithelial cells,[38] endothelial cells,[39] neuronal cells,[40] and lymphoid cells.[41,42] The EHV-4 virus, on the other hand, has a tropism principally restricted to epithelial and neuronal cells and has limited potential for infection of endothelial and lymphoid cells.

The gamma herpesviruses EHV-2 and EHV-5 are primarily lymphotropic, establishing functional latency in these cells.[43,44] Although viral deoxyribonucleic acid (DNA) has been detected in trigeminal ganglia,[45] reactivation from this site has not been demonstrated. EHV-2 and EHV-5 have typical *Gammaherpesvirinae* genome structures, with close similarity to saimiri and Epstein-Barr viruses.[46] They have different disease profiles from EHV-1 and EHV-4 and share no cross-protective antigens with these viruses.

Viral Genomes

In the short time since EHV-1 and EHV-4 were completely sequenced,[47,48] partial or complete virus genomes can now be sequenced comparatively easily allowing rapid sequencing of entire genomes of EHVs of interest, enabling comparative genomics of large numbers of EHV-1 isolates to be assessed. The availability of genome sequences, together with the molecular techniques and reagents to manipulate individual genes or groups of genes, has revolutionized understanding of EHV-1 gene function and regulation. The genomes of several EHV-1 isolates, including high-virulence and low-virulence strains, have been cloned as bacterial artificial chromosomes into *Escherichia coli*, providing a greatly improved means of studying viral gene function.[49-51] Transposon mutagenesis, a well-established technique in microbial genetics, has been successfully applied to EHV-1, providing a rapid means of screening the entire genome for virulence genes.

Virus genetics have major clinical implications for EHV-1 immunology and control programs. Identification of virulence-associated genes provides targets for live attenuated vaccines, and a complete understanding of viral gene expression and regulation provides essential insight into viral antigen targets for the immune system, a prerequisite for protein or DNA vaccination strategies.

EHV-1 and EHV-4 possess linear double-stranded genomes and share the same overall genome conformation with a unique long region (U_L) joined to a unique short region (U_S) that is flanked by an identical pair of inverted repeat regions, the terminal repeat (T_R) and internal repeat (I_R) regions[47,48] (Fig. 14-1). Genes located in the repeat regions are thus represented twice in the genome. Both genomes are of similar size and share extensive sequence homology but are genetically (and phenotypically) distinct viruses. The EHV-1 genome is 150 kilobases (kb) in size and encodes 76 open reading frames (ORFs; genes), of which 63 are located in the U_L, nine in the U_S, and four in the repeat (I_R) regions. The EHV-4 genome is slightly smaller (145 kb) with 76 genes, each of which has a direct positional and sequence counterpart in EHV-1. The EHV-2 genome is larger (184 kb) and contains 79 ORFs, of which 77 are predicted to code for proteins.[46]

Both EHV-1 and EHV-4 possess five unique genes (numbers 1, 2, 67, 71, and 75) that have no homologs in other sequenced herpesviruses and have been the subject of considerable research in the expectation that their products play pivotal roles in pathogenesis. Although the roles of these unique genes have not been completely elucidated, studies in vitro and in mice have failed to identify distinctive roles in pathogenesis.[52,53]

Viral Replication

The key feature of the molecular biology of EHV-1 and EHV-4 is that gene expression is tightly ordered into a highly controlled cascade.[54] The result is that the horse's immune system is exposed to virus gene products in a sequential fashion, providing specific opportunities for immunologic intervention. One complete cycle of virus replication (the lytic cycle) takes approximately 20 hours, during which a well-ordered

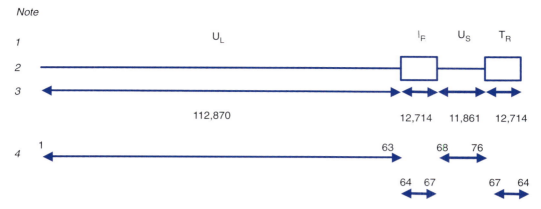

Figure 14-1 Genome organization of equine herpesvirus type 1 (EHV-1). The genome is 150 kb in length and is predicted to encode 76 open reading frames (ORFs; genes). *Note 1:* The genome contains two unique regions; the unique long region (U_L) and the unique short region (U_S). U_S is flanked by a repeat region creating identical, but inverted, repeats: the internal (I_R) repeat and terminal repeat (T_R) regions. *Note 2:* Schematic representation of the different genome regions. *Note 3:* Length of the different regions in base pairs. *Note 4:* Genes contained in the different regions. U_L contains genes 1 to 63; U_S contains genes 64 to 67; I_R contains genes 68 to 76; and T_R contains genes 67 to 64.

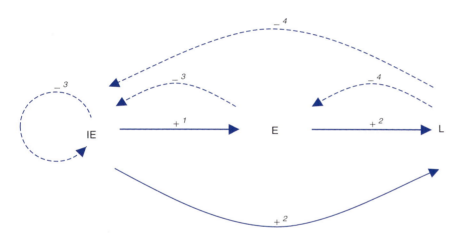

Figure 14-2 Regulation of equine herpesvirus type 1 (EHV-1) gene expression during lytic infection. Gene expression is coordinately regulated into three phases: immediate early *(IE)*, early *(E)*, and late *(L)*. *Note 1:* The IE protein transactivates (upregulates expression of) promoters of the E genes. *Note 2:* The IE and E proteins (EICP 22 and 27) transactivate L genes. *Note 3:* The E protein EICP 0 downregulates IE; the IE protein downregulates (autoregulates) its own promoter. *Note 4:* The L proteins downregulate expression of E genes and the IE gene.

progression of events occurs: attachment to the host cell membrane, membrane fusion and penetration, translocation of viral DNA to the nucleus, viral DNA replication, viral protein synthesis, capsid assembly, egress from the nucleus, envelopment and egress from the cell, and death (lysis) of the cell as progeny virions are released. During these different stages of infection, viral gene transcription and regulation is sequentially regulated into three distinct phases: immediate early (IE), early (E), and late (L) (see section on Virus Proteins).[54-57] Gene products from each phase have regulatory roles that, acting in concert with host cell proteins, upregulate ("switch on") expression of other phases while downregulating ("switching off") their own phase (Fig. 14-2).

Lytic and Latent Infection Cycles

On entry to host cells, the virus enters either a lytic cycle or latent cycle of infection. These two pathways appear to be independent, to occur simultaneously, and to diverge immediately after viral entry in the cell. Virus replication is not required for the establishment of latency. The lytic cycle, as previously described, results in release of new virus particles from the infected cell. During the latent cycle of infection, viral DNA translocates to the nucleus, but the transcription and translation cascade of all gene classes is blocked, with the exception of limited transcription in the region antisense to the IE gene. This results in expression of the EHV latency-associated transcript (LAT).[58-60]

The mechanisms that control entry into lytic and latent infection cycles are not well understood. In the nervous and lymphoid systems, it appears that the two infection cycles occur in parallel, principally within neurons of the trigeminal ganglion and CD8+ T lymphocytes.[40,61,62] Although the genetic mechanisms responsible for suppression of gene transcription and translation in latency have not been fully elucidated, it seems unlikely to be entirely caused by antisense repression of IE gene transcription by LAT messenger ribonucleic acid (mRNA).

During latency, the genome exists in multiple copies in a continuous (circular) episomal form in the nucleus of infected cells. Latently infected cells do not express viral antigens and are thus not detectable immunologically. Latently infected cells represent a subset of neurons and CD8+ lymphocytes.[63]

The numbers of latently infected neurons within the trigeminal ganglion has not been determined; in the circulation, latently infected lymphocytes are rare and are estimated to occur at a frequency of 1 in 10^4 or 10^5. The number of latently infected lymphocytes declines over time but is increased during reactivation episodes or by exposure to new infections. The population of latently infected neurons is assumed to be stable because these are long-lived cells. It is not known whether repeated reactivations increase the number of latently infected neurons.

Periodically, the latent genome undergoes reactivation, during which a "reverse trip" occurs in which unenveloped virus capsids are assembled within latently infected cells before translocation to the respiratory epithelial surface, where they undergo envelopment and become infectious virus particles. Once delivered to the respiratory epithelial surface, virions undergo one of two fates: (1) neutralization by local mucosal immunity or (2) establishment of infection and a repeat of the events that occurred during primary infection, with shedding of infectious virus in respiratory tract secretions and possibly development of viremia[64] (Fig. 14-3). The precise details of this reverse trip from neurons of the trigeminal ganglion[40] and circulating T lymphocytes[63] are not fully understood. It is assumed that the transfer of reactivating virus from lymphocytes to the respiratory epithelium involves expression of viral proteins on the surface of reactivating lymphocytes to allow cell-cell fusion and direct virus transfer. This process may also occur within the uteroplacental unit and the central nervous system (CNS), providing a mechanism for disease recurrence with reactivation.[3]

At a cellular level the molecular, cellular, or other events that control the switch from latency infection to reactivation are unknown. Reactivation involves a switch from latent to lytic cycle that is initiated by transcription and translation of the IE gene, inducing the lytic gene cascade as seen during primary infection. It is not known whether initiation of transcription requires a specific trigger, possibly transactivation of the IE promoter by viral, cellular, or exogenous factors, or whether it occurs spontaneously. The IE promoter can be transactivated by a variety of viral and cellular proteins, including proteins encoded by EHV-2,[65] although the biologic significance in relation to reactivation is not known.

Whatever the mechanism of reactivation, it is likely that the outcome of most reactivation events, which may occur frequently at the cellular level, is neutralization of reactivating virus by mucosal immune responses, and thus prevention of virus shedding from the respiratory tract and development of viremia. Reactivation only becomes detectable at horse level, by nasal shedding or viremia, when the host immune response is compromised either by treatment with corticosteroids[64] or other immunomodulatory compounds or by a variety of management stressors,[66] including transport, illness, and hospitalization. It is not known how frequently horse-level reactivation and shedding actually occurs, but it is sufficiently frequent to maintain these viruses in the global horse population.

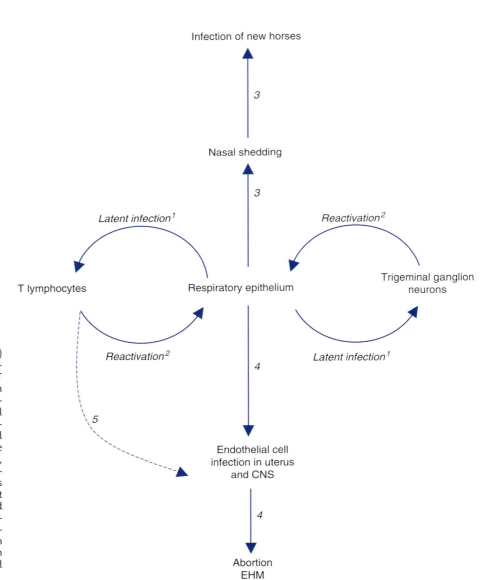

Figure 14-3 Equine herpesvirus type 1 (EHV-1) latency and reactivation. *Note 1:* Latency is established in trigeminal ganglionic neurons and in T lymphocytes. *Note 2:* Reactivation from both sites delivers virus back to the respiratory epithelium. *Note 3:* Dependent on the ability of local (mucosal) immune responses to neutralize reactivated virus, reactivation may result in nasal shedding and infection of new, susceptible horses. *Note 4:* Within the reactivating horse, replication of reactivating virus in respiratory epithelium may seed a viremia (mirroring events during primary infection), with subsequent endothelial cell infection in the uterus and central nervous system (CNS), resulting in abortion or equine herpesvirus myeloencephalopathy (EHM). *Note 5:* It is possible that reactivation may occur locally within the uterus or CNS, with direct transfer of reactivating virus to endothelial cells in these sites.

Viral Proteins

The virus encodes a single IE gene, 55 E genes, and 20 L genes. The 76 gene products have a variety of different functions, giving the EHV surprising complexity and comparatively sophisticated life cycles, features that greatly complicate attempts to understand pathogenesis and devise control measures. Functions have been assigned to the majority of viral proteins. At least 30 are associated with the virion, of which 6 form the capsid,[67] 12 are associated with the tegument[68,69] (located between the capsid and the envelope), and a further 11 are glycoproteins[70] anchored to and projecting from the envelope. The remaining proteins are involved with viral replication functions, including DNA replication enzymes; regulation of the viral gene cascade; and virus egress from infected cells. The regulation of the sequential cascade of viral genes into IE, E, and L phases[54] is controlled by six genes whose gene products act as transactivators and transcriptional regulators/suppressors: the IE gene (gene 64), four E genes (EICP 22, 27, 0 and TR2), and one L (ETIF) gene. Five of these genes (IE, EICP22, EICP27, TR2, and ETIF) are essential for virus replication in vitro.

The single IE protein is extremely important from an immunologic perspective because it is the first virus expressed by infected cells and, in some horses at least, contains a dominant cytotoxic T lymphocyte (CTL) epitope, making it a key vaccine target.[28,54,55,71-78] For example, in experimental studies, vaccination with the IE protein reduced clinical disease, nasal shedding, and magnitude of viremia,[79] although the CTL response to IE is MHC/ELA restricted and is greatest in the A3/B2 haplotype.[23,80] The 1487 amino acid IE protein, essential for virus replication, is a vital regulatory protein,[81] repressing its own promoter and transactivating expression of early and late gene promoters. It possesses different functional domains, including a DNA-binding domain responsible for binding its own promoter, a domain responsible for translocation of the IE protein to the infected cell nucleus, and a domain that binds transcription factor IIB (TFIIB) from the infected cell.[82-84]

Four E proteins (EICP 22, 27, 0, and TR2) have regulatory activities. EICP22 and 27 (gene 5) function synergistically with the IE protein to transactivate E and L genes, and EICP0 (gene 63) is also a powerful transactivator but is antagonistic to the IE protein and competes for the cellular transcription factor TFIIB.[51,56,83,85-91]

The late protein regulatory protein ETIF[57,92] is the product of gene 12 and is the EHV-1 equivalent of the HSV alpha transinducing factor (α-TIF), a key transactivator that binds upstream of the IE gene and transactivates the IE promoter. ETIF is required for cell-to-cell spread; ETIF mutants produce small plaques in cell culture, and although capsids are produced, envelopment in the cytoplasm does not occur.

Glycoproteins

The 11 envelope-anchored surface glycoproteins of EHV-1 and EHV-4 play key roles in pathogenesis, including host specificity and cellular tropism.[62,93] They mediate viral attachment to and entry into cells as well as fusion of infected cells and direct cell-to-cell spread of virus. They are the principal viral immunogens, at least for humoral immunity, and are the major targets for virus-neutralizing antibody. Five glycoproteins (gB, gD, gH, gK, gL) are absolutely required for virus replication in tissue culture and are termed essential. The remaining six (gC, gE, gG, gI, gM, gp300) are not required for replication in vitro and are termed nonessential, a designation that does not translate to the in vivo situation because deletion mutants in these glycoproteins are viable but less virulent. Although convalescent horse sera recognize all 11 glycoproteins, 3 (gB, gC, gD) are "immunodominant," that is, they are the principal viral antigens

recognized by the equine host. Further features of gB, gC, and gD that have made them prime vaccine candidates are (1) they are protective in mice; (2) gB, gC, and gD deletion mutants are nonpathogenic in mice; (3) gB and gD are involved in cell-cell fusion and spread of virus; (4) gC is involved with binding to host cell receptors; and (5) gD[94] is involved with virus entry into cells and appears to be responsible for cellular tropism and host cell specificity.[95-109] The functions of the other glycoproteins are less well characterized: gE and gI are involved in cell-cell spread of virus with gE deletion mutants proposed as potential vaccine candidates[110]; gG interferes with neutrophil chemotaxis[111]; gK is implicated in cell-cell spread and virus egress; gM is likely involved in cell penetration and cell-cell spread[50,72]; and gH is essential for virus replication, plays a role in integrin-independent cell-to-cell spread,[112] and is partially protective in mice.[113] Novel B cell epitopes for EHV-1 and EHV-4 are present in gH and form the basis of a commercial enzyme-linked immunosorbent assay (ELISA) test differentiating the immune response to the two viruses.[114,115]

Taken together, it is clear that the glycoproteins are important epitopes for the humoral immune response; recombinant gD, for example, has been shown to elicit humoral responses similar to commercial vaccines in the horse.[116] It is therefore likely that they will be included in future protein, subunit, recombinant, or DNA vaccines for the EHVs. Glycoproteins do not appear to be important CTL epitopes, however, and vaccines based on these glycoproteins alone are unlikely to induce efficient cellular immune responses.

Epidemiology

The principal reservoir of infection for EHV is latently infected horses. Environmental transmission is of most importance during outbreaks when horses are kept in close confinement and probably plays a minor role in maintenance of these viruses in the horse population. Environmental persistence of EHV is short, estimated to be less than 7 days in most conditions, with a maximum survival of 35 days.[117] The viruses are labile and easily inactivated by heat and disinfectants. Serologic surveys suggest that most adult horses have been exposed to EHV-1, -2, -4, and -5. Epidemiologic studies of stud farms suggest that infection is acquired within the first few weeks or months of life, generally before or just after weaning, from adult mares that asymptomatically shed virus[118-121] (Fig. 14-4).

It is not clear whether the maintenance of endemic infection is caused by cycles of subclinical infection within the mare population or reactivation of endogenous latent infection in individual mares. The life cycles of the EHV share four main features: (1) early and widespread infection of young horses, (2) a widespread carrier (latent) state in adult horses, (3) transmission from latently infected adults to new generations of young stock, and (4) widespread "silent" adult-adult, adult-foal, and foal-foal endemic infection cycles of transmission.

Spread of Infection

Infection is spread by direct horse-to-horse contact, as well as indirectly by fomites and personnel. The most common transmission route is through the respiratory tract by aerosolized droplets of respiratory tract secretions. Infection can also occur by ingestion or inhalation of droplets from surfaces. All horses with clinical disease and reactivating horses are considered to be contagious by the respiratory route, although shedding adult horses may show no overt clinical signs. Aborted foals, fetal membranes, and placental fluids contain large quantities of infectious virus and are particularly hazardous.

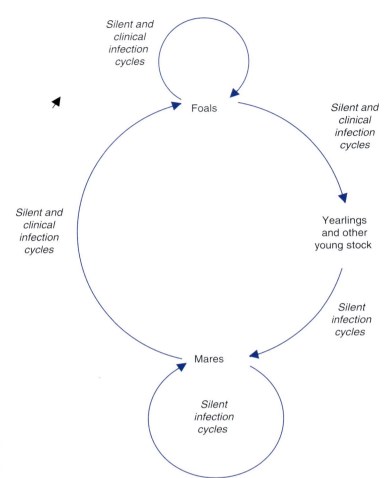

Figure 14-4 Transmission of equine herpesvirus type 1 (EHV-1). EHV-1 is transmitted through "silent" (subclinical) and "clinical" infection cycles. Adult horses (principally mares) infect foals early in life; infection is transmitted between foals and young stock. Endemic infection is maintained in mares by contact with younger stock and by subclinical transmission between mares. In all age groups, reactivation of latent virus provides the source of infectious virus to maintain endemic infection.

Latency

Latency and reactivation are key features of the epidemiology of EHV-1 and EHV-4 infections and are responsible for the ubiquitous distribution of these viruses in the horse population. The large majority of recovered horses carry latent EHV infections for extended periods, possibly for life.[61,62] Latency almost certainly also plays a key role in the biology of EHV-2 and EHV-5, since the majority of adult horses and almost all foals harbor latent infection in circulating lymphocytes. EHV-1 and EHV-4 enter into a latent state in the lymphoreticular system, in circulating and lymph node CD8+ T lymphocytes, and in neurons within the trigeminal ganglia.[40] EHV-2 and EHV-5 establish functional latency in circulating lymphocytes and trigeminal ganglia, from which virus can be reactivated in vitro.[122,123] Viral DNA can also be detected in other locations,[124] including the trigeminal ganglia,[45] but it is not clear whether virus is capable of undergoing reactivation from these other sites. These latently infected cells form, by means of periodic reactivations that result in shedding of infectious virus from the host, a transmissible reservoir of infection that maintains all the EHVs in the horse population.

Reactivation from Latency

Periodically, latently infected horses experience reactivation episodes, during which infectious virus is shed into respiratory tract secretions, with the potential for infecting other, susceptible horses. Reactivation of latent EHV-1 and EHV-4 infections from horses has been observed in field situations after transport,

handling, rehousing, and weaning, and reactivation has been achieved experimentally in horses by treatment with high doses (10 times therapeutic doses) of corticosteroids.[40,125] The frequency with which reactivation occurs in response to the stresses imposed by the modern horse industry is unknown. Reactivation is generally asymptomatic, resulting in "silent" shedding of virus, thus providing a mechanism for maintenance of endemic infection cycles and the apparently unexplained appearance of disease in closed populations of horses.

Abortion or neurologic disease may be the result of local reactivation of virus, that is, reactivation of EHV-1 within blood vessels of the uterus, placenta, or CNS, resulting in endothelial cell infection and thrombo-ischemia in those organs.[126-129] In this situation, disease occurs without prerequisite respiratory infection, nasal virus shedding, or viremia. Regardless of the sites from which reactivation occurs, it is likely that latency and reactivation are important in the epidemiology of EHV-1 abortion and neurologic disease. The majority of natural EHV-1 abortions occur singly,[130] rather than as "abortion storms,"[131] implying that abortion may have resulted from reactivation of endogenous latent virus rather than from a newly acquired respiratory infection. Such reactivations of latent EHV-1 may also explain abortions that occur many weeks or months after infection, beyond the period of viremia that follows. It is not clear whether latency is also important in the epidemiology of neurologic disease. However, it is logical to assume that endogenously reactivated virus may be responsible for isolated neurologic cases or for seeding virus into groups of horses where outbreaks of neurologic disease occur.

Pathogenesis and Pathologic Findings

Respiratory Tract

Following inhalation of virus or contact with infected fomites, both EHV-1 and EHV-4 replicate in upper respiratory tract epithelial cells. After experimental infection, virus can also be transiently recovered at low titer from lower respiratory tract (tracheal and bronchoalveolar) lavage samples. Virus replication causes death of epithelial cells, resulting in epithelial erosions. EHV-1 quickly spreads to cells in the underlying lamina propria, with infected (viral antigen-expressing) endothelial cells, lymphocytes, and monocytes detectable in respiratory tract–associated lymph nodes within 48 hours.[132,133] From these sites, virus-infected lymphocytes enter the circulation, resulting in a CD8+ T lymphocyte–associated viremia that disseminates virus widely, including into the uterine and CNS vascular endothelium.[134,135] In parallel, EHV-1 also rapidly gains access to neurons of the trigeminal nerve, reaching the trigeminal ganglion by 48 hours after infection, establishing latency in trigeminal ganglionic neurons.[40] Experimentally, EHV-1 shedding occurs from the respiratory tract for up to 14 days, and viremia persists for up to 21 days.[136] Using real-time polymerase chain reaction (PCR) methods, virus DNA shedding from the nasal cavity can be detected for longer periods.[137] In the field, however, shedding and viremia may be transient and intermittent, making detection difficult in the later stages of infection.

The detailed pathogenesis of EHV-4 infections has not been elucidated. The initial mucosal phase probably closely parallels that of EHV-1, with infection of the respiratory tract and its associated lymphoid system. Persistent EHV-4 nucleic acids have been demonstrated in the trigeminal ganglion[138] and circulating lymphocytes[62] after recovery from infection, but infectious virus has not successfully been reactivated from these sites in vitro. Most isolates of EHV-4 have low endotheliotropism, do not establish viremia, and therefore do not cause abortion or neurologic disease.[37,139] The duration of nasal shedding of EHV-4 is usually more transient than for EHV-1,[137,140] even when measured by sensitive methods such as real-time PCR.

Viremia

Viremia disseminates virus to the uterus[141] and CNS and is therefore a prerequisite for these diseases. However, not all viremic pregnant mares abort, and only a very small minority of viremic horses develop neurologic disease. Local reactivation can also be responsible for these diseases without detectable viremia (see section on Latency and Reactivation). Viremia also delivers virus to other organs, detectable by PCR assays, but does not result in clinically apparent organ dysfunction. Viremia is cell associated, primarily within CD5+/CD8+ T lymphocytes,[142-144] and free virus is rarely detected in the blood. Lymphocytes do not support lytic infection in vivo; virus can be liberated from these cells using only co-cultivation (in vitro reactivation) assays. Lymphocytes are susceptible to infection in vitro only after mitogen stimulation,[145] which also increases the efficiency of reactivation in vitro.[63] Genotypically neuropathogenic isolates of EHV-1 induce higher magnitude and longer duration viremia than genotypically nonneuropathogenic isolates, which may explain why endothelial cell infection in the uterus and CNS is more likely to occur following infection with neuropathogenic isolates.[146] Viremia seldom occurs with EHV-4 infection, although some "high-virulence" isolates capable of inducing viremia exist, and EHV-4 DNA can be transiently detected in circulating lymphocytes after infection but is detected only briefly and at low frequency after infection even by real-time PCR.[140,147]

Uterus

The pathogenesis of EHV-1 abortion involves virus translocation from the circulation into the placental unit and induction of uterovascular lesions.[148] Infection of endothelial cells in the pregnant uterus causes a vasculitis that affects small arteriolar branches in the glandular layer of the endometrium at the base of the microcotyledons.[129] If these endometrial vascular lesions are widespread, the fetus may be aborted before detectable transplacental spread of virus has occurred.[149,150] Virologically negative abortions[151] in earlier EHV-1 challenges had been assumed to be caused by maternal stress or pyrexia, and the incidence of this type of abortion after spontaneous field infections is not known. However, in a survey of 241 abortions in the United Kingdom between 2001 and 2003,[150] 9 were "typical" EHV-1 abortions (i.e., placenta and fetus were virus positive), whereas 6 were "atypical," and there was no detectable fetal infection by either PCR or immunohistochemical methods.[151] The susceptibility of uterine endothelial cells to infection with EHV-1 is low in early pregnancy compared with late pregnancy, and any potential association of EHV-1 infection with early embryonic death and resorption has not been investigated. Historically, "high-virulence" EHV-1 isolates have been regarded as causing both abortion and neurologic disease. However, recent experimental comparison between such strains has shown that this is not the case: certain genotypically defined neuropathogenic strains (e.g., OH03) have low abortigenic potential, whereas others (e.g., Ab4) have high potential for both abortion and neurologic disease.[152]

The pathogenesis of abortion caused by less-virulent isolates of EHV-4 is not as clear[153] because these isolates appear to have a reduced affinity for endothelial cells; however, abortion is also caused by vascular lesions and thrombo-ischemia. The rare cases of abortion that follow infection with EHV-4 are also likely to involve the capacity of certain isolates of EHV-4 for replication in uterine and fetal endothelial cells.

Central Nervous System

The pathogenesis of EHV-1 neurologic disease also involves vasculitis and thrombo-ischemia following endothelial cell infection.[154] In vitro models have been developed to study interactions between peripheral blood mononuclear cells infected with EHV-1 and brain endothelial cells, which suggest that infection of brain endothelium occurs via direct cell-cell transfer of virus.[155] There is little evidence for lytic virus infection of neurons or direct viral neuropathology,[156] and virus has rarely been isolated from the CNS. Affected horses demonstrate sites of vasculitis with virus antigen expression in the brain and spinal cord, with or without local hemorrhage and thrombo-ischemic necrosis.[157,158] Neurologic clinical signs therefore result from ischemic death of nervous tissue, and the virus thus causes a myelopathy, encephalopathy, or myeloencephalopathy, depending on which regions of the CNS are affected. EHV-1 neurologic syndromes are therefore generally referred to as equine herpesvirus myeloencephalopathy (EHM).

Virulence

There are wide variations in virulence among different isolates of EHV-1 and EHV-4. High-virulence EHV-1 strains, such as Ab4 and Army-183, are endotheliotropic, efficiently cause viremia, are abortigenic, and after experimental inoculation of horses, cause high rates of abortion and neurologic disease. Other isolates, such as V592, are less virulent, have reduced endotheliotropism, cause only "low-level" viremia, and rarely cause abortion or neurologic disease.[37,153] The availability of genome sequences for different EHV-1 strains has allowed identification of sequence variations that correlate with specific phenotypes. Small differences at genome sequence level account for marked phenotypic differences. For example, Ab4 and V592 exhibit only 0.1% difference in sequence (150 bases in 150,000). These are mostly single-base changes, causing coding changes in 31 genes. Gene 68 (U_S2) shows the highest variation rate (2%) and is now used as a phylogenetic marker for epidemiologic analysis. However, no relationship appears to exist between the phylogenetic groups generated by this method and the pathogenic potential of strains.

Dimorphism in the sequence of gene 30 (encoding DNA polymerase) does, however, provide a means of genotypically identifying some paralytic strains of EHV. A single-base change, substituting G for A at positions 2254, resulting in an amino acid change from N (asparagine) to D (aspartate) at amino acid position 752, correlates with paralytic potential. The majority of nonparalytic strains possess N at position 752, whereas the majority, but not all, of paralytic viruses possess D at position 752.[159] It is not clear whether dimorphism in this gene is a surrogate marker for other virulence determinants because virulence may intuitively be expected to be determined multigenetically. The real-time PCR assay[137] detecting this dimorphism has been widely employed in experimental and clinical settings, including epidemiologic studies, and as part of outbreak control measures.[160] Several studies have reported the prevalence of latent "neuropathogenic" EHV-1 infections as between 7% and 24% in populations of horses in the United States, South America, and Europe,[161,162] with suggestions that the prevalence has increased over time. Initial experimental infections of horses with N_{752} or D_{752} EHV-1 mutants suggested a strong association between with neuropathogenicity and D_{752}, with the D_{752} mutant inducing higher magnitude viraemia.[163] However, the significance of these data remains uncertain, and field data has emerged suggesting that neuropathogenicity is indeed a multifactorial characteristic, with evidence that host responses to the virus, as well as virus genotype influence the outcome of infection[164] and that virus genotype may not be particularly closely associated with neuropathogenicity. Epidemiologic studies have found that significant proportions of EHM cases (24%-65%) are not associated with the D_{752} variant, whereas D_{752} is associated with an increasing prevalence of abortions.[165-167]

Immunology

Natural or experimental infection induces a solid but transient protective immune response to EHV that protects against reinfection for 3 to 6 months. During this time, there is clinical protection and sterile immunity (i.e., exposure to virus does not induce nasopharyngeal virus shedding or viremia). Exposure of mares early in gestation protects them from abortion in the later, susceptible stages of gestation. Furthermore, mares that have aborted in 1 year usually do not abort in subsequent years.[168]

The life cycle of EHV-1, and to a lesser extent EHV-4, is complex and involves infection of multiple cell types.[3] The initial mucosal colonization and replication phase of infection is rapidly followed by an invasion phase, during which virus enters the lamina propria and gains entry into blood vessels and lymphatics through endothelial cell infection, and a distribution phase, in which infected lymphocytes disseminate virus throughout the horse. In parallel, latency is established. It is now clear that immune control of pathogenesis requires an integrated, multicomponent immune response, and that there are unlikely to be simple correlates of protective immunity. This is in marked contrast to "hit and run" virus pathogens with comparatively simple pathogenesis, exemplified by equine influenza viruses, for which measurement of the humoral immune

response provides a simple and accurate measure of disease susceptibility and resistance.

For the EHVs, humoral immune responses alone do not provide protective immunity. An effective immune response to the EHVs requires a combination of mucosal and systemic humoral and cellular immune responses. Much of these data have come from experimental infections, and information from field infections or naturally occurring outbreaks is still scarce. The techniques and reagents required to study the cellular immune response to EHV infection have recently become available, allowing rapid progress to be made in this complex area of immunology. Although not completely elucidated, viral epitopes that drive cellular immune responses have been identified, and the relationship between major histocompatibility complex (MHC [ELA]) haplotype and virus antigen recognition by CTL is being unraveled.

Infection induces strong systemic humoral immune responses characterized by an initial, rapid, but short-lived (<3 months) immunoglobulin M (IgM) response, followed by a slower-onset but longer-lived (>12 months) immunoglobulin G (IgG) response (see section on Diagnosis). The principal IgG isotypes produced are IgGa, IgGb, and IgGc. Only small quantities of immunoglobulin A (IgA) are found in the circulation in convalescent sera. In diagnostic laboratories, these responses are measured using the complement fixation (CF) test for the short-lived (IgM) antibody response and the virus neutralization (VN) test for the longer-lived (IgG) antibody response. Systemic humoral immune responses alone are not sufficient to protect horses from infection. VN antibody titers do not correlate with protection from infection. High VN titers are associated with reduced nasal virus excretion but do not influence the duration of viremia or the frequency of viremic cells in the circulation,[169] presumably because viremic cells express few, if any, virus antigens and are therefore not recognized as targets by the immune system.[170] Infection induces mucosal immune responses characterized by mucosal IgA production. In contrast to VN antibody, mucosal IgA titers do correlate with protection from infection.[171] The IgA response is short lived after a single infection but persists longer with subsequent infections. Mucosal IgA is an important first line of defense against EHV-1 infection. It is known to be neutralizing in vitro, although its function in vivo has not been fully characterized.

Infection induces both tissue (mucosal and lymphoid) and circulatory cellular immune responses mediated by CD8+ CTLs.[172-174] Understanding of the cellular immune response has advanced rapidly in the last 10 years, and there is abundant evidence that CTL responses are not only central to recovery from infection but also provide a correlate of protective immunity.[26,175] CTLs are the effector arm of the cellular immune response and kill infected cells that present virus antigens on their surface in the context of MHC class 1 (ELA-A) molecules; that is, CTL responses are MHC-1 (ELA-A) restricted. The CTL response is directed by "professional" antigen-presenting cells (dendritic cells and macrophages). These cells are also MHC-1 restricted and work in concert with the Th1 subset of CD4+ T helper cells and an associated panel of cytokines, including interleukin-2 (IL-2), interferon-gamma (IFN-γ), and tumor necrosis factor alpha (TNF-α).[28,176] The polymorphic nature of ELA-1 molecules in the horse means that individuals vary in their CTL responses to particular virus antigens. As with other herpesviruses, MHC-1 expression is downregulated on the surface of infected cells, thus providing a means of immune evasion by the virus.

EHV-1 and EHV-4 infections cause changes in leukocyte populations in infected horses characterized by leukopenia followed by leukocytosis. The initial leukopenia consists of lymphopenia and neutropenia, with an initial depletion in CD8+ cells, and occurs between days 7 and 13 after infection. This is followed by a leukocytosis, consisting principally of a lymphocytosis, that continues to day 21 to 28 after infection. EHV-1, but usually not EHV-4, infection induces a cell-associated viremia that is associated mainly with infection of CD8+ cells, although a small proportion of monocytes and possibly CD4+ cells also become infected. In vitro, these cells are refractory to infection unless stimulated by mitogens. Both CD8+ and CD4+ cells release IFN-γ, an indirect marker of cytotoxic activity, in response to EHV-1 infection in vitro, suggesting both cell types are responsive to EHV-1.[28,176] IFN-γ assays have been widely employed to study cellular immune responses to EHV-1, including the generation of protective immunity by experimental and commercial vaccines as alternatives to the more laborious methods required to measure CTL activity directly.[42,177]

CTL responses to EHV were initially measured using a bulk lymphoproliferative assay.[173] Although lymphoproliferative responses increased after infection, there was no clear correlation with protection. The assay was refined by measuring the frequency of CTL precursors (CTLp) by limiting dilution analysis (LDA).[175] For the first time, this provided a correlate of protective immunity: high numbers of CTLp correlated with protection, whereas horses with low CTLp numbers were susceptible to infection. High frequencies of circulatory CTLp also correlate with protection from abortion in the face of EHV-1 challenge.[26]

The EHV-1 antigens that act as CTL targets have been mapped, providing valuable information on which virus antigens stimulate cellular immune responses. A variety of viral proteins have been mapped, including IE, several glycoproteins (e.g., gB, gC, gD), structural proteins, and proteins involved in replication. The IE protein, the first virus protein to be expressed in infected cells, is the most efficient CTL epitope. However, the ability of this protein to induce CTL responses varies with MHC haplotype; efficient responses are seen only in horses with the ELA-A3.1 haplotype.[27,79,80] A universally immunodominant CTL epitope, the functional equivalent of gB, gC, and gD for the humoral immune response, seems unlikely, but a panel of viral proteins constructed around the IE protein may fill this role.

Immune Evasion

The changes that occur in blood and pulmonary leukocyte populations after EHV-1 infection, including the lack of viral antigen expression on the surface of infected leukocytes, have led to the recognition that EHV-1, as with many of the herpesviruses, modulates the horse's immune response. Because cytotoxicity against EHV-1 proteins is MHC-1 restricted, it is not surprising that EHV-1 produces proteins that interfere with MHC-1 presentation of virus antigens as a means of evading the horse's immune response to infection.[178] Whether this immunomodulation represents immunosuppression is an area that requires further investigation. EHV-1 causes specific but incomplete downregulation of MHC-1 on the surface of infected cells that is mediated, by an unknown mechanism, by the IE, or possibly E, proteins of EHV-1.

Clinical Findings

The clinical disease syndromes associated with EHV-1 and EHV-4 infection are well recognized. These viruses cause respiratory disease, abortion, and neurologic disease. EHV-1 is associated with all three syndromes, although the virulence of individual isolates shows considerable variation (see section on Virulence). EHV-4 is principally a cause of respiratory disease, although some highly virulent endotheliotropic, abortigenic isolates exist.

The role of EHV-2 and EHV-5 in clinical disease is uncertain. In most cases the virus is isolated from nasal and blood samples of apparently healthy foals and adult horses.[10,122,123,179] EHV-2 and EHV-5 are universally present in horse populations and in surveillance studies highly age associated.[180] The viruses can be detected (by the presence of DNA and recovery of virus from leukocytes) in 60% to 80% of adult horses and almost 100% of foals. EHV-2 is detected less frequently in nasal swabs in adult horses, but longitudinal surveys suggest the virus is frequently shed from apparently healthy foals. EHV-2 has been isolated from cases of keratoconjunctivitis in foals and weanlings[181] and is a presumed etiologic agent of some chronic superficial keratopathies in adult horses, although the evidence for this is weak (see Chapter 10). EHV-2 has been implicated in respiratory disease in foals and weanlings and isolated from the lungs of a stillborn foal. Both EHV-1 and EHV-5 have been inferred as a cause of abortion based on finding DNA from these viruses in aborted fetuses, however, any causal relationship has not been proved. Both EHV-2 and EHV-5 have been suggested as causes of equine fatigue and poor performance syndromes, although little evidence exists to support this.[182] Some have suggested that EHV-2 may act as an immunosuppressive agent in foals predisposing to other infections,[183] including other respiratory viruses and *Rhodococcus equi*.[184] The actual association of EHV-5 to a specific lung disease is still based on various case reports of horses with multinodular fibrosis.[12] In a retrospective study of a large collection of tracheal and bronchoalveolar fluid samples, EHV-5 was detected overall in less than 2% of samples, although the virus was not detected in any fluids from healthy horses. In those samples in which EHV-5 was detected, a specific clinicopathologic character.[180,182,185] The more detailed disease descriptions that follow relate to EHV-1 and EHV-4.

Respiratory Disease

Accumulated evidence indicates that EHV-1 is an uncommon cause of clinically apparent respiratory disease.[186-189] Several large epidemiologic surveys in Thoroughbred populations in Europe and North America have failed to associate EHV-1 with respiratory disease. EHV-4, however, is associated with respiratory disease. Both viruses generally cause self-limiting upper respiratory tract disease. In neonatal, immunocompromised, and other naive young animals, these viruses can cause severe lower respiratory tract disease (viral pneumonitis) and can lead to secondary bacterial bronchopneumonia. These foals show progressive disease with marked depression, pyrexia, tachypnea, and dyspnea. Horses experimentally infected with EHV-1 or EHV-4 show a short (1-3 days) incubation period before respiratory signs appear.[134,190] In the field, longer incubation periods of up to 10 days have been observed, presumably caused by differences in strain virulence, infective dose, and host immunity. In previously infected horses, clinical respiratory signs may be of minimal severity and of short duration,[41,132,191] or they may be completely inapparent in older horses. This applies particularly to pregnant mares and mature horses with neurologic disease; these animals usually show no respiratory clinical signs before abortion or onset of paralysis.[192] This is also the case during reactivation of latent EHV-1 or EHV-4, which usually results in asymptomatic virus shedding and viremia.

Primary infection in naive foals infected with virulent strains of EHV-1 results in clinically obvious upper respiratory tract disease.[134,136] Depression and anorexia are associated with a biphasic pyrexia of 8 to 10 days' duration, which peaks on days 1 to 2 after infection and again on days 6 to 7. Initially there is serous nasal discharge, conjunctivitis, and serous ocular discharge. The character of the nasal discharge progresses rapidly to mucoid and then mucopurulent by days 5 to 7, which is

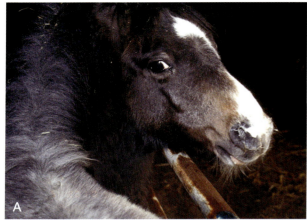
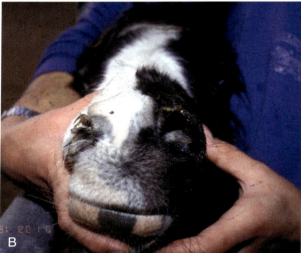

Figure 14-5 A and B, Foals and young horses infected with equine herpesvirus type 1 (EHV-1) may develop clinically apparent respiratory disease. Nasal discharge is initially serous but quickly becomes mucopurulent.

usually attributed to secondary bacterial infection (Fig. 14-5). There is progressive lymphadenopathy, principally of the mandibular lymph nodes, although occasionally the retropharyngeal lymph nodes become sufficiently enlarged to become palpable. Lymph nodes reach maximum size between 7 and 10 days after infection and can remain enlarged for many weeks. There is a biphasic change in both the circulating and the pulmonary leukocyte population consisting of an initial leukopenia caused by both lymphopenia and neutropenia, for the first 5 to 7 days after EHV-1 infection. This is followed by a leukocytosis, consisting principally of a lymphocytosis.[134,191] Coughing, in contrast to equine influenza virus infections, is not a major clinical sign in EHV infection but may be more prominent where management practices are substandard, especially with poor stable air hygiene and failure to rest the horse from training or performance activities.

On recovery from EHV-1 or EHV-4 upper respiratory tract disease, some horses may develop a "poor performance syndrome," which may be associated with nonspecific bronchial hypersensitivity and a syndrome resembling inflammatory airway disease in young horses and recurrent airway obstruction in older horses. Thus the economic losses associated with respiratory disease are associated not only with the costs of veterinary care and lost days training during the acute stages of infection but also with the longer-term, detrimental effects on athletic performance.

A recently described nodular fibrotic interstitial pulmonary disease called *equine multinodular pulmonary fibrosis* (EMPF) has been linked to infection with the gamma herpesvirus EHV-5. EMPF mainly affects middle-aged to old horses and is characterized by progressive replacement of pulmonary tissue by multiple fibrous masses,[12] which contain EHV-5 DNA, and clinical signs, which include depression, weight loss, pyrexia, and lower respiratory tract signs. The majority of horses do not recover. Causation has not been demonstrated, however, and the ubiquitous distribution of the equine gamma herpesviruses in the global equid population confounds attempts to demonstrate epidemiologic links to EMPF.[185]

Abortion

Pregnant mares infected with EHV-1 usually abort in the last third of pregnancy and appear refractory to abortion if virus is encountered earlier (<120 days) in gestation.[141] There are usually no warning signs, and abortion occurs precipitously.[149] Specifically, there are usually no respiratory signs before abortion occurs. Mares often abort standing up, and the foal is usually expelled within the intact amnion and may be expelled within the intact allantochorion. Occasionally, a live foal is born that dies shortly after birth.[4,13] EHV-1 abortions are rare events and generally occur sporadically in individual mares.

"Abortion storms" are now extremely uncommon, presumably a reflection of the improved management measures that have been implemented as part of EHV-1 control measures on studs. However, devastating abortion storms have been recorded and remain a constant threat if scrupulous hygiene precautions are not followed.[193]

Most mares conceive successfully shortly after the abortion and foal normally the following year. Mares rarely abort from EHV-1 infection in successive years but may eventually become reinfected and abort again. Abortion is occasionally caused by "high-virulence" isolates of EHV-4,[194] with phenotypes resembling EHV-1. These isolates exhibit endotheliotropism, lymphotropism, and an ability to invade the allantochorion, causing placental and fetal ischemia.[37]

Other Reproductive Syndromes

Neonatal Foals

Neonatal EHV foal disease is rare. It is associated primarily with EHV-1 infection[15] and occasionally with EHV-4. It is not clear whether affected foals are infected in utero or whether infection is acquired, presumably from the dam, immediately after birth. Affected foals are born live but are sick at birth or become ill within 1 to 2 days. They show marked and rapidly progressive lower respiratory tract signs (dyspnea and tachypnea) caused by primary viral pneumonitis that leads to respiratory distress, hypoxia, and death. Secondary bacterial bronchopneumonia develops in foals that survive more than 2 or 3 days. These foals may survive for 10 to 14 days but eventually die from respiratory disease and a complex combination of other complications, including generalized lymphoid depletion and profound leukopenia. Occasionally, EHV-4 has been associated with neonatal foal disease and mortality.[195]

Stallions

Stallions infected with EHV-1 may develop scrotal edema, loss of libido, a reduction in sperm quality, and shedding of infectious virus (through infected leukocytes) into semen, which may continue for 3 weeks after infection.[196-198] It is not known whether these changes affect fertility or whether venereal shedding plays a role in epidemiology, in a manner analogous to equine viral arteritis (EVA).

Neurologic Disease

EHM is sporadic and uncommon but is a potentially devastating manifestation of EHV-1 infection[199] and has been recognized clinically for many years.[200] EHV-4 neurologic disease is rare, but isolated cases have been identified. Anecdotal field evidence suggests that the neurologic disease is becoming increasingly common, leading to speculation that viruses with increased neurovirulence are circulating and this is supported by some molecular epidemiologic data.[167] Although the apparent increase in prevalence may be caused by increased awareness and improved sampling of suspected clinical cases, it does seem likely that, in North America at least, EHM is an increasing problem to the horse industry.[201] EHM is not restricted by pregnancy, age, or gender and can occur in foals, yearlings, geldings, stallions, and both barren and pregnant mares.[202] Transmission is assumed to be through the respiratory route, and contagious transmission occurs from clinical cases that can result in large outbreaks of disease.[203,204] In index cases the source of infection may be newly acquired infection from other clinical cases[205] or reactivating virus or may be endogenous reactivating virus.

Clinical signs appear during or toward the end of the viremic phase of infection, similar to the pathogenesis of abortion. The interval between infection and subsequent onset of neurologic disease is usually between 6 and 10 days but may be as short as 1 day. There are invariably no premonitory clinical signs of respiratory disease, and pyrexia is likely to be the only warning clinical sign.[203,205] Cases are often sporadic, but large outbreaks can occur, affecting 30% to 40% of horses on the premises, and in North America, epizootics of disease have occurred affecting several states from point sources of infection at shows and competitions.[201,206-208] Affected horses should be assumed to be contagious, and strict biosecurity precautions taken to prevent spread to other horses on the premises. These precautions should be based around isolation, ideally in a separate air space, and should aim to prevent aerosol spread, as well as indirect spread via fomites. Precautions should be implemented for a minimum of 14 days after the onset of clinical signs in each affected horse.[203,205]

The presentation and severity of clinical signs are highly variable and depend on the extent and location of the neurologic lesions[192,209] (Fig. 14-6). The caudal segments of the spinal cord and sacral plexus are affected most often, although outbreaks have been described in which horses develop acute-onset paralysis with cerebral signs, followed by rapid death. Clinical signs usually appear suddenly and reach their peak intensity within 2 to 3 days of onset. Neurologic dysfunction ranges from temporary ataxia and paresis to complete paralysis. The hindlimbs are usually the most severely affected, although quadriplegia has been observed. Bladder dysfunction, characterized by atony with incontinence or urinary retention, and cutaneous perineal and limb sensory deficits result from sacral nerve involvement. Some affected horses develop a head tilt.

The prognosis for nonrecumbent horses is favorable, but it is poor for recumbent horses, which frequently develop fatal complications (e.g., extensive myopathy, pneumonia, intussusception, bladder rupture) and require euthanasia.

Diagnosis

History and Clinical Signs

Although a thorough history should be taken and a detailed clinical examination performed, it is usually not possible to diagnose any of the diseases associated with infection by EHV with certainty on clinical grounds alone. Except for infections in foals and young horses, EHV infections generally do not cause clinically apparent respiratory disease, and even then, there is little to distinguish EHV respiratory disease from that caused by other viral and bacterial pathogens. In particular, EHV-1 seldom causes obvious respiratory clinical signs in adult horses, and a common misconception is that monitoring for respiratory disease provides warning of impending abortion or EHM.

Abortion and neurologic disease (EHM) generally occur without any premonitory clinical signs apart from pyrexia, which, unless the horse is being closely monitored, is unlikely to be detected. Sudden abortion in the last third of pregnancy with the fetus still contained in the allantochorion is suggestive but not diagnostic of EHV-1 abortion. Abortion storms raise suspicion of EHV-1 infection in a herd, but these are rare. A presumptive diagnosis of EHM can sometimes be made with more confidence based on clinical signs, especially if more than one horse is affected, but diagnosis of individual cases on clinical grounds is difficult.

Because of these difficulties, further investigations are always required to confirm EHV disease, either by direct demonstration of virus (virus isolation, virus antigens, or nucleic acid) or indirect evidence of infection (serology). During outbreaks in particular, it is important to select rapid, sensitive, and specific diagnostic tests to enable rapid implementation of biosecurity measures and limit disease spread. In practice, the usual approach of diagnostic laboratories is to make an initial, perhaps preliminary, rapid diagnosis, followed by more time-consuming tests for confirmation (Table 14-1).

Case Selection

Correct selection of cases for sampling within an affected group is vital to gain the best-quality information from clinical pathologic investigations. Virus shedding from the respiratory tract, especially from adult horses, is generally short lived (<10 days), may be intermittent, and is most reliable soon (<5 days) after infection. All samples for direct demonstration of virus should therefore be collected from early clinical cases whenever possible. This generally means identifying in-contact horses with pyrexia but probably few or no other clinical signs because these appear later in the course of disease. Early sampling is especially important in suspected EHM cases because clinical signs appear toward the end of the viremic phase of infection, by which time virus shedding is waning or may have ceased. Diagnosis of EHV-1 abortion is perhaps the most straightforward because this is achieved using the aborted foal and placenta.

Selection of early clinical cases is also extremely important for indirect demonstration of infection using serology. Cases should be selected carefully, especially for aborting mares and EHM, because the delay between infection and appearance of obvious clinical signs may mean that the first of the paired serum samples already contains maximum titers of antibody, and a further rise on the second paired sample will therefore not occur. Although in these situations it is possible to infer evidence of infection on the basis of a falling titer, this can be misleading.

Direct Demonstration of Infection

Immunofluorescence

Direct immunofluorescence (IF) tests are very rapid (hours), simple tests with acceptable sensitivity and specificity that are used as the front-line diagnostic test for demonstration of virus antigens in nasal or nasopharyngeal swab samples or in frozen (cryostat) sections from aborted fetal and placental tissues. Although IF detects virus antigens expressed on the surface of infected cells and therefore does require live virus to be present in the sample, it is important to remember that its sensitivity approaches, but does not exceed, that of virus isolation.

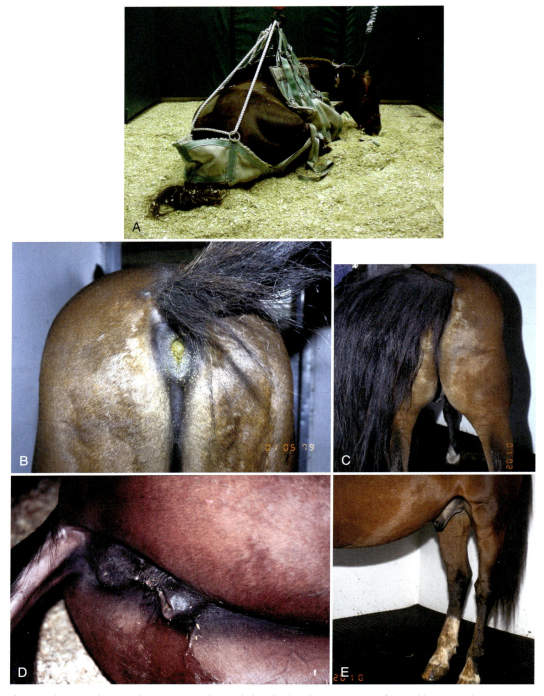

Figure 14-6 Clinical signs in horses with equine herpesvirus myeloencephalopathy (EHM) vary in severity from mild ataxia and proprioceptive deficits to severe ataxia and recumbency requiring extensive supportive care **(A)**. Other clinical signs may include loss of anal tone **(B)**, flaccid paralysis of the tail **(C)**, and urinary incontinence **(D)** with secondary urine scald on the hindlegs **(E)**. *(A, Courtesy Dr. Chris Sanchez, University of Florida.)*

Polymerase Chain Reaction

Several PCR tests have been devised for the detection of nucleic acid (DNA) of the EHVs,[52,124,138,210-216] with different type-common and type-specific primers capable of distinguishing between the different EHVs.[62,217] PCR is an enzymatic exponential DNA amplification technique that, in optimum conditions, is extremely sensitive, capable of detecting as few as 10 to 100 copies of target viral DNA.[218] However, the sensitivity of PCR tests in clinical samples is reduced, probably from

the presence of inhibitors of the polymerase enzyme, other impurities within the DNA, and degradation of the viral DNA target. As for IF techniques, the sensitivity of PCR approaches that of virus isolation. PCR tests can be performed on respiratory tract swab or lavage samples, blood, or fresh, frozen, or fixed tissue samples.

The original PCR tests were nonquantitative and were incapable of estimating the amount of virus DNA present in the sample. Recently, quantitative ("real-time") PCR techniques have been devised for EHV-1 and EHV-4 that allow estimation

Table 14-1 Diagnostic Tests for Equine Herpesvirus Type 1 (EHV-1)

Diagnostic Test	Rapid Test?	Sample Required	Comments
Immunofluorescence (IF)	Yes	Airway swabs or frozen sections; fresh blood samples (for viremia)	Useful initial screening test; highly specific; false negatives occur; blood samples may be transiently IF positive
Polymerase chain reaction (PCR)	Yes	Airway swabs or lavages; blood; frozen or fixed tissue samples	Highly specific test; can differentiate between different EHVs; qPCR allows estimation of virus load and presumptive differentiation of lytic and latent infection; D/N752 qPCR used to identify viruses with neuropathogenic potential; good sensitivity; false negatives occur
Virus isolation	No	Airway swabs and lavages; fresh blood, fetal and placental tissue samples	"Gold standard" for diagnosis; time-consuming; highly specific; false negatives occur
Histopathology	No	Fixed tissue samples	Definitive diagnosis of abortion and EHM, especially if used with ISH
Hematology	Yes	Whole blood in EDTA	May provide nonspecific evidence of virus infection
Serology	No	Serum (clotted blood samples); take two samples 10-14 days apart to demonstrate rising antibody titers	Highly specific test, although CF and VN tests do not differentiate EHV-1 from EHV-4, but EHV-1 gG ELISA is type specific (allows differentiation); provides indirect retrospective evidence of infection; early case selection important

EHM, Equine herpesvirus myeloencephalopathy; ISH, in situ hybridization; EDTA, ethylenediaminetetraacetic acid; qPCR, quantitative PCR; CF, complement fixation; VN, virus neutralization.

of virus load in samples.[137,219] These tests have quantified virus in respiratory tract and blood samples after experimental infection. They may have clinical application in the identification of latently infected horses, which is not currently possible, by measurement of virus load in leukocytes because virus copy number in latently infected leukocytes is between two and three orders of magnitude less than that in lytically infected cells.[220-222]

Virus Isolation

Virus isolation remains the "gold standard" for laboratory diagnosis of EHV infections and provides unequivocal evidence of the presence of infectious virus in clinical samples (respiratory tract, blood, fetal, and placental tissue samples). The technique involves demonstration of typical cytopathic effect (CPE) in susceptible cell cultures inoculated with the supernatant from the sample, which can be followed by immunoassays or PCR tests to confirm the identity of the isolated virus, if required. EHV-induced CPE is normally detectable within 5 to 7 days of culture. Although false-negative results occur because the technique requires the presence of infectious virus, virus isolation has higher sensitivity than both IF and PCR assays in clinical samples.

Histopathology

Histopathology is an essential method for confirming EHV infection in aborted fetuses and samples collected postmortem from horses with EHM.[223] Characteristic pathologic changes include eosinophilic inclusion bodies in airway epithelial and hepatic cells from aborted fetuses and vasculitis, often thrombosis, of CNS blood vessels. Immunohistochemistry (IHC) can be performed on paraffin-embedded, formalin-fixed tissue sections to demonstrate virus antigen expression by infected epithelial and endothelial cells and provides valuable confirmation of the cause of vasculitis in the CNS and fetal tissues and placenta.

Viral nucleic acids (DNA) can also be detected in fixed tissue sections by in situ hybridization (ISH) techniques. In principle, ISH provides additional sensitivity over IHC because, whereas all virus-infected cells contain viral DNA, only a proportion express viral proteins. Although DNA-DNA ISH has the potential to detect both lytically and latently infected cells, experimental evidence suggests that the technique is insufficiently sensitive to detect the low copy number of virus genomes present in latently infected cells and that the more sensitive RNA-DNA hybridization techniques must be employed for this purpose. Practically, this means that ISH-positive cells can be

taken as direct evidence for EHV infection without the need to distinguish latent and therefore possibly irrelevant cells from lytic infection.

Indirect Evidence of Infection

Hematology

Practitioners typically collect blood samples for hematologic analysis (total and differential white blood cell counts) from horses with suspected EHV disease. At best, these samples provide nonspecific indication of a viral infection but are not diagnostic of EHV infection. Experimentally, EHV-1 and EHV-4 infections induce a biphasic change in total and differential white blood cell counts. There is an initial transient leukopenia with lymphopenia in the first 7 to 10 days after infection, which is replaced by a leukocytosis with lymphocytosis up to day 21 after infection. During the second (leukocytosis) phase, the increase in lymphocyte numbers reverses the normal ratio between neutrophils and lymphocytes (approximately 2:1) and can be regarded as a nonspecific indication of viral infection. In reality, however, the variation in hematology parameters among normal horses and the difficulties in correctly timing the collection of samples significantly limit the value of hematology, especially on single samples, to gain supportive evidence of EHV infection.

Serology

Serology can be used to gain a retrospective diagnosis of EHV-1 or EHV-4 infection and forms a valuable part of longitudinal surveillance. After infection there is an initial rapid increase in IgM antibody, detectable at 4 to 5 days, peaking at about 20 to 30 days, and decreasing to baseline values between 60 and 80 days.[224] There is a later but more sustained increase in IgG antibody, detectable 8 to 10 days after infection, peaking at 30 to 40 days, and persisting for many (>9) months. These antibodies can be measured by CF, measuring principally IgM antibodies[225]; VN, measuring principally IgG antibodies; and ELISA, which detects type-specific antibodies directed against EHV-1 and EHV-4 gG and hence distinguishes between the two viruses. CF titers rise immediately after infection, peak rapidly, and then decay, whereas VN titers show a more gradual rise but remain elevated for extended periods. Rising CF titers on paired samples 10 to 14 days apart provide unequivocal evidence of EHV infection and can be useful during outbreaks of disease[137] when longitudinal sampling is possible. Significant increases in antibody are interpreted by most diagnostic laboratories to be a threefold to fourfold increase. A high CF titer in a single serum sample provides good preliminary evidence of infection and is a valuable initial diagnostic test in suspected EHM cases. The type-specific (EHV-1/EHV-4) gG ELISA has been proposed as rapid screening tool for the initial diagnosis of suspected EHV cases.[115]

The longevity of VN antibodies means they are not useful for investigation of acute cases. They can be used, however, for disease prevalence surveys because they indicate historical exposure to infection. One drawback of CF and VN tests is that these antibodies are generated against epitopes common to both EHV-1 and EHV-4 and therefore do not allow differentiation between infection with the two viruses. Both type-common and type-specific ELISA tests are commercially available, although the type-specific assay, measuring antibody directed against EHV gG,[226,227] is the more useful because it differentiates between infection with EHV-1 and EHV-4.[228] As discussed earlier, appropriate case selection for serologic diagnosis is essential, and the clinician should remember that previous vaccination and maternal antibodies confound the interpretation of serologic investigations.

Cerebrospinal Fluid Analysis

Cerebrospinal fluid (CSF) from horses with EHM may have increased total protein (principally albumin) concentration without a concomitant increase in nucleated cell count. CSF may also show xanthochromia (yellow discoloration, Fig. 14-7) caused by increased protein concentrations and red blood cell breakdown. These CSF changes, in conjunction with characteristic clinical signs, are suggestive but not diagnostic of EHM. Antibodies against EHV-1 in the CSF may be the result of leakage from the circulation secondary to EHV-1 endothelial cell infection and vasculitis, or other causes of vasculitis, rather than local production within the CNS and, although indicative of exposure to EHV-1, are not necessarily conclusive of EHM.

Diagnosis of Latent Infection

The ability to identify latently infected horses with accuracy would greatly assist control programs because these animals form the reservoir of transmissible EHV infection and are responsible for maintenance of infection in the horse population. Diagnosis of latent infection antemortem is a considerable challenge both clinically and in the laboratory. Latently infected horses cannot be identified with certainty using any of the currently available diagnostic methods (Table 14-2). There are several reasons for this: (1) latently infected horses are "silently" infected, exhibiting no clinical signs of disease; (2) latently infected cells express no virus-encoded proteins and thus escape immune detection; (3) the latent virus genome is transcriptionally silent, except for limited transcription from the region antisense to the single IE gene; (4) latently infected cells harbor a relatively small number of virus genomes; and (5) latently infected leukocytes form only a small subset of the total leukocyte population, making them comparatively rare cells. These observations mean that the standard diagnostic tests previously described do not readily differentiate between lytic (acute) and latent infection cycles and that, with the exception of PCR and possibly VN assays, latently infected horses are generally negative using most current diagnostic tests. Leukocytes harbor detectable, latent EHV DNA for many months, possibly years, after infection and provide the only means presently available of identifying latently infected horses (the presence of VN antibodies indicates previous exposure to virus but not necessarily that latent infection has been established). Latently infected horses are more readily detectable during reactivation episodes because they shed infectious virus, often become viremic, and seroconvert.

Presumptive diagnosis of latent infection can be made in a horse that has (1) negative respiratory tract samples by IF, PCR, and virus isolation and negative blood samples by IF; (2) negative or positive blood samples by virus isolation (co-cultivation); (3) positive blood samples by PCR; and (4) detectable serum VN titers. It should be remembered that detection of viral DNA by

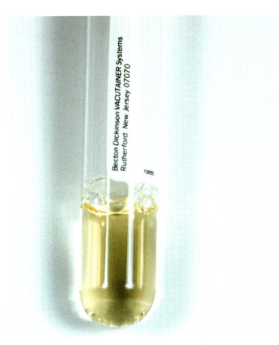

Figure 14-7 Xanthochromic cerebrospinal fluid sample from a horse with equine herpesvirus myeloencephalopathy (EHM). *(Courtesy Dr. Chris Sanchez, University of Florida.)*

Table 14-2 Diagnosis of Latent and Lytic Infection Cycles Using Common Commercial Diagnostic Tests

Sample Site	Diagnostic Test	Latent Infection[a]	Lytic Infection
Airway	Immunofluorescence	Negative	Positive
	Virus isolation	Negative	Positive
	PCR	Negative[b]	Positive
Whole blood	Immunofluorescence	Negative	Positive (transiently)[c]
	Virus isolation	Negative[d]	Positive
	PCR	Positive[e]	Positive[e]
Serum	Serology	Positive or negative[f,g]	Positive[g]
Tissue[h]	Immunofluorescence	Negative	Positive
	Virus isolation	Negative[d]	Positive
	PCR	Positive[e]	Positive[e]

PCR, Polymerase chain reaction.

[a]Results for all assays during reactivation would be same as during lytic infection.

[b]Real-time PCR assays generally fail to detect virus in airway samples from latently infected horses.

[c]There is brief expression of virus antigens during viremia.

[d]Direct virus isolation from fresh blood or tissue is negative during latent infection, but co-cultivation techniques are positive.

[e]Estimation of virus load by qPCR allows presumptive differentiation into lytic and latent infection (higher virus load indicates lytic infection).

[f]Serum viral neutralization (VN) titers remain raised for many months, but in the absence of periodic reactivation, latent virus is likely to persist for longer than the duration of detectable VN antibody.

[g]During lytic infection and reactivation, complement fixation (CF) and VN antibody titers increase.

[h]Postmortem fresh, frozen, or fixed samples of lymph nodes and trigeminal ganglia.

PCR is not unequivocal evidence for the presence of latent infection (i.e., a functional virus genome that is capable of reactivation) because the assay detects a fragment of one virus gene, and "residual" or fragments of virus DNA in host cells will produce positive results with PCR tests. For this reason, the search for markers of "functional" latency (i.e., latent virus genome that is capable of undergoing reactivation, leading to production of infectious virus) has been a research priority. Initial optimism that LATs might provide such a marker has now diminished because of technical difficulties in its detection and the realization that LATs are not universally present in cells carrying functional HSV-1 latent infection. These problems notwithstanding, the advent of quantitative PCR methods[140] has allowed presumptive differentiation of lytic and latent infection cycles in leukocytes based on estimation of virus copy number in infected cells.[160] This has improved the utility of PCR assays and provides a comparatively rapid and simple method for the diagnosis and differentiation of acute disease and latent infection.

Diagnosis of latent infection postmortem is more straightforward, although estimation of viral load by qPCR and the relative ease by which this method allows detection of multiple classes of genes, including those associated with transcriptional activity or latency, provides useful information about latent versus lytic infection and likely sites of functional latency.[160] Viral DNA is detectable by PCR assays in most tissues, including respiratory tract, respiratory tract drainage lymph nodes, spleen, other lymphoreticular organs, and CNS. Co-cultivation (an in vitro test of reactivation) is the "gold standard" test for latent infection because it provides unequivocal evidence of functional (reactivatable) latent infection. Latently infected tissues do not yield infectious virus on direct culture (homogenization followed by sonication and titration of tissue supernatant on monolayers of susceptible cells) but do yield infectious virus when dispersed, viable tissue cells are cultured, perhaps for extended periods (up to three passages), with monolayers of susceptible cells. The sensitivity of this assay can be increased for latently infected leukocytes by stimulation with T-cell mitogens. Perhaps not surprisingly, only a subset of PCR-positive tissues, for both EHV-1 and EHV-4, are also positive by co-cultivation. Overall, it appears that EHV-1 establishes functional latency in the lymphoreticular system (principally CD8+ T lymphocytes) and the CNS (neurons of the trigeminal ganglion). Latent virus can be detected in fixed tissue sections using RNA-DNA ISH to detect virus genome and RNA-RNA ISH to detect EHV LATs, although these are research techniques that are not available commercially.

Treatment

Respiratory Disease

Horses with EHV respiratory disease are contagious and should be isolated (see Chapters 66 and 67). Exposed, in-contact horses should also be isolated. It is generally necessary to establish "clean" and "dirty" areas to separate unaffected horses from the affected horse(s) and in-contacts. Yard staff must be briefed about barrier nursing, and biosecurity precautions (which at their minimum should include the use of gloves, dedicated boots, and overalls) must be implemented. Affected horses should not be worked until at least 7 days after clinical signs have resolved and should be kept in stables with good air hygiene (dust free with low concentrations of allergens, bacteria, and irritants).

Respiratory disease is generally mild and self-limiting and does not require specific treatment. Broad-spectrum antibiotics are often administered but seldom indicated to prevent secondary bacterial infections. The beta-2 sympathomimetic clenbuterol stimulates mucociliary clearance and may assist in reducing airway contamination but is usually not required. Mucolytics (e.g., Dembrexine) could also be considered but again are not usually indicated. Occasionally, horses fail to recover at the expected rate or may develop persistent postviral syndromes, and immunomodulation therapy may be beneficial in these cases (see Chapter 66).

Abortion

Abortion occurs without warning. There is no evidence that treatment of in-contact mares with antiviral agents (e.g., acyclovir or other nucleoside analog antiviral agents; see later discussion) assists with prevention of abortion. Once abortion has occurred, rigorous biosecurity measures should be implemented (see section on Control and Chapter 62). The affected mare should be examined to ensure that the entire placental unit has been expelled, which is invariably the case. In the rare cases in which this does not occur, the mare should be treated for retained fetal membranes.

Ocular Disease

Cases of suspected EHV keratoconjunctivitis or chronic superficial keratitis have been treated empirically with antiviral compounds, mainly idoxuridine[43] and acyclovir[15,208] (see Chapter 10). Little pharmacologic basis exists for the use of these compounds in horses, although they have been successfully used to treat HSV keratopathies in humans. Horses with nonulcerative chronic superficial keratitis respond well to corticosteroid and cyclosporine treatment, suggesting that pathology is immune mediated, rather than directly virus induced.

Equine Herpesvirus Myeloencephalopathy

Horses with confirmed or suspected EHV-1 neurologic disease may be contagious and should therefore be subjected to the same rigorous biosecurity measures as aborting mares. Strict hygiene precautions and barrier housing are necessary because virus can be transmitted by both direct (aerosol) and indirect (fomites) means within stable yards and equine hospitals (see Chapter 62). These measures do create additional difficulties for nursing affected horses, especially those with more severe clinical signs, but are required to prevent disease spread within the hospital. Affected horses should be stabled in isolation or a geographically separate part of the yard. This may not be possible for recumbent horses, for which stables with specialized overhead equipment may be required for sling attachment. Dedicated footwear, gowns, and gloves must be worn when attending affected horses. Equipment and utensils should not be shared with other horses.

The stable should contain sufficient bedding to prevent trauma to the horse, and the environment should be quiet to prevent excitement. Recumbent horses can be successfully nursed in slings (e.g., Anderson sling), but scrupulous attention must be paid to welfare and secondary complications (e.g., skin trauma, decubital ulceration, impaction colics). An indwelling Foley catheter is required in horses with bladder paralysis, urinary retention, and overflow. Application of petroleum jelly to the perineum and an extension line to direct urine away from the perineum help to prevent urinary scalding. Urinary catheters should be maintained in a sterile fashion, but cystitis is a common complication, and prophylactic broad-spectrum antibiotics should be considered. Water intake must be carefully monitored because horses may be unable to drink the 50 to 70 mL/kg daily required to maintain hydration. Intravenous (IV) fluid therapy is indicated for horses that are unable to drink, especially horses in slings. Attention must be paid to food intake, and a palatable high-energy, high-protein gruel should be offered. The addition of oil to the gruel can make a valuable contribution to energy intake.

Treatment of horses with neurologic disease is largely empiric because little experimental or clinical evidence exists to support many of the drugs used. No controlled studies have compared treatments in affected horses, partly because the sporadic and uncommon nature of the disease makes controlled studies in the field difficult. Based on pathologic observations that the nervous system lesion is a thrombo-ischemic injury secondary to virus infection of endothelial cells, many clinicians treat affected horses with nonsteroidal antiinflammatory drugs (NSAIDs) and antiviral drugs.[229] Dimethyl sulfoxide (DMSO 1 g/kg diluted 1:10 in saline and given IV once daily for 3-5 days), corticosteroids (dexamethasone 0.1 mg/kg IV once daily for 3 days), and NSAIDs (flunixin 1.1 mg/kg IV twice daily for 3-5 days) are believed to aid recovery. Concern has been expressed that corticosteroid treatment may exacerbate disease by allowing continued viral replication or viral reactivation; however, this is without foundation. Although reactivation has been induced experimentally by dexamethasone treatment, this was achieved with doses tenfold higher than those used clinically. Similarly, dexamethasone treatment, even at 1 mg/kg IV, did not increase the duration or titers of virus replication during experimental challenge, whereas the T-cell immunomodulator cyclosporin-A increased both titers and duration of shedding.

Herpesvirus antivirals are nucleoside analogs that interfere with virus replication by preventing viral DNA synthesis in virus-infected cells.[230,232] Nucleosides are the building blocks of DNA, consisting of a base (adenine, guanine, thymine, cytosine, or uracil) linked to a sugar (ribose in RNA or deoxyribose in DNA). They are called adenosine, guanosine, cytidine, thymidine, or uracil, depending on which sugar they contain. Before they can be incorporated into a new strand of DNA, nucleosides have to be "activated" by the sequential addition of three phosphate groups to the carbon in the 5' position of the carbon ring of the sugar to form triphosphate nucleotides. This process is known as phosphorylation and is carried out by enzymes called kinases. In addition to the 5' phosphate group, the sugar ring also carries a hydroxyl group on the 3' carbon. The new DNA strand is formed as the enzyme DNA polymerase links nucleotides together to form a polymer by sequentially adding sugars through their 5 phosphate group to the free 3' hydroxyl group on the end of the DNA strand. Nucleoside analogs are similar in structure to nucleosides and can be incorporated into growing DNA strands but they act as chain terminators and stop viral DNA synthesis.

Work has progressed assessing the nucleoside analogs for in vitro efficacy and pharmacokinetics against both neurologically and fetally derived EHV-1.[231,233-242] Veterinarians may still choose acyclovir for treatment of EHV-1 based on its lower cost compared to the newer nucleoside analogs and its published use in outbreaks and individual horses.[232,234,208,243,244] Nonetheless, orally administered acyclovir will not be efficacious due to its poor bioavailability which has been demonstrated in multiple independent studies.[231,235-240] In a hamster subcutaneous infection mortality model, ACV given at 100 mg/kg orally (PO) for 5 days afforded poor protection against death, with mortality rates of 70%.[232] In contrast, pencyclovir administered at doses as low as 2 mg/kg PO provided complete protection in this model. Clinical cases of EHV-1 neurologic disease have been treated with ACV at a dose of 10 mg/kg PO five times daily, which would produce mean peak plasma concentrations of 0.287 μg/mL (range, 0.226-0.869 μg/mL),[233] a value significantly below the lowest estimate of the required inhibitory concentration for EHV-1. In contrast, an IV infusion of 10 mg/kg ACV produced peak plasma concentrations of 13.7 ± 5.9 μg/mL, suggesting that the IV route, not the oral route, is capable of achieving effective ACV concentrations in

the horse. Valacyclovir, a prodrug of acyclovir was developed to improve the bioavailability issues of acyclovir that has also been problematic in humans and various studies have examined the absorption and distribution of valacyclovir in the horse.[235-240] Work by Maxwell et al (2008)[239] indicates that the bioavailability of acyclovir is indeed higher if derived from valacyclovir (Maxwell 2008).[239] Based on this work, valacyclovir would be administered with a loading regimen of 27 mg/kg every 8 hours for 2 days followed by a maintenance dose of 18 mg/kg every 12 hours. In the Garre et al (2009)[240] study where 40 mg/kg of valacyclovir was administered three times daily to EHV-1 experimentally infected ponies demonstrated no differences in the severity of respiratory signs, plasma virus load, and nasal virus shedding.

Bioactivity is also a potential problem for EHV-1 antivirals. In a study comparing several analogs, ganciclovir was the most potent for reducing plaque size in the highest variety of isolates.[234] In vitro testing of abortigenic and neuropathogenic isolates of EHV-1 found no difference in the susceptibility to ACV, although all isolates were more sensitive to ganciclovir than to ACV.[234] The pharmacokinetic work of Carmichael et al[235] indicated that an initial dose of 2.5 mg/kg intravenously administered every 8 hours for 24 hours followed by oral administration of this same dose every 12 hours would maintain effective serum concentrations of ganciclovir in horses. Ganciclovir had superior blood levels when compared to valganciclovir.

Vaccination

Effective vaccines against the EHVs must satisfy a difficult series of demands: a safe and efficient delivery route and induction of a multilayered immune response, consisting of long-lived systemic and mucosal immune responses producing serum and mucosal VN antibody, together with high frequencies of CTLp and memory B cells. This is further complicated by the influences of MHC haplotype on CTL recognition of virus antigens. Virus strain variation may have an effect, and the horse's immune status and preexisting latent infection are also likely to influence the response to vaccination. It is not surprising therefore that each of the currently available EHV-1 vaccines induces some but not all of the desired components of the immune response against EHV-1, and none produces complete protection. A general feature of all current commercial vaccines is that they induce high titers of VN antibody in adult horses, which are presumably primed by previous exposure to the EHV, but induce weaker or perhaps undetectable responses in immunologically naive animals, especially foals. There is little evidence that existing vaccines induce significant cellular immune responses.

Vaccination has been used, in combination with management measures, to control EHV-1 infection for more than 40 years.[25,236] It is difficult, however, to assess the impact of vaccination on the control of EHV disease because of a lack of randomized, controlled field studies. The first EHV-1 vaccination program was carried out in Kentucky in 1961 using a live hamster-adapted strain that protected horses for 3 months against respiratory disease. Field data also suggested a reduction in abortion frequency in vaccinated mares. A commercial vaccine (Pneumabort-K) was subsequently used extensively in Kentucky and was credited with reducing abortions; in a 3-year period, 140 of 20,223 nonvaccinated mares aborted (0.69%) compared with 14 of 6806 vaccinated mares (0.18%). An inactivated vaccine was credited with reducing abortion rates from 6.8 in 1000 to 1.6 in 1000.[245] Over a 20-year period, commercial vaccines reduced the incidence of abortion in Kentucky by almost 75%.[246] Vaccination assisted in this reduction, but the vigorous implementation of hygiene measures undoubtedly had a major impact by reducing the spread of virus and thus the occurrence of multiple abortion storms.

More recently, a randomized control study has been carried out to assess the efficacy of a commercial inactivated combined EHV-1/EHV-4 vaccine.[247] Vaccination did not reduce respiratory clinical signs or influence viremia but did reduce nasal shedding of virus and did appear to decrease abortion. There are no data on the ability of current vaccines to prevent EHV-1 neurologic disease, and the relative rarity of this disease makes it unlikely that such data will be forthcoming. Similarly, no data are available on the use of these vaccines in an outbreak of EHV disease (respiratory, abortion, or neurologic), although from first principles it is unlikely that any of the current vaccines would induce a sufficiently rapid immune response to intervene in pathogenesis, especially for neurologic disease. There is a clinical suspicion that frequently vaccinated horses may be at increased risk of developing neurologic disease, and some veterinarians therefore believe that vaccination during an outbreak of neurologic disease is contraindicated. Vaccination of pregnant mares does not appear to be effective at blocking the cycle of silent transmission of either EHV-1 or EHV-4 on large studs.

There are currently 10 killed commercial EHV vaccines available (8 in United States and 2 in Europe) and 2 live vaccines (1 in United States and 1 in Europe). These vaccines induce high titers of CF and VN antibody and appear to offer some protection against respiratory disease. They reduce the duration and titer of nasal virus shedding of virus, but there are contradictory reports of the ability of killed and live vaccines to reduce viremia and hence abortion, with some demonstrating reduction in viremia by whole killed-virus vaccines and others demonstrating reduction in viremia by modified live-virus vaccines.[248,249] The effect of vaccines on abortion in the field is less clear[250-253] because again the rarity of field abortions makes these studies difficult. There are no experimental or field studies that provide data on the ability of any of the commercial vaccines to protect against neurologic disease because of the difficulties in reproducing this disease experimentally and the relative rarity of naturally-occurring cases. These vaccines therefore assist with disease control and are not intended, or marketed, to provide complete protection from disease. The reasonable expectation of current vaccines should not be to produce sterile immunity but rather to reduce the severity of clinical disease and limit virus shedding from infected horses, thus reducing contagion. Vaccines should therefore be used to supplement hygiene control measures, which have a central role in reducing exposure to virus.

Extensive research continues to develop improved vaccines against EHV-1 and EHV-4. Thus far, the other EHVs have received little attention because they are less clinically and commercially important. Attention is currently focused on recombinant vaccines, using baculovirus and canary pox as vectors to deliver EHV-1 glycoproteins gB, gC, and gD, and on DNA vaccines, delivering the same glycoproteins together with candidate CTL epitopes. Efficient humoral immune responses are generated by vector vaccines or by combined approaches using DNA vaccination to prime and a protein vaccination to boost, but generation of high-frequency CTL responses remains problematic. Other research challenges are the construction of sufficiently attenuated yet immunogenic modified live-virus vaccines and the identification of appropriate adjuvants and delivery routes.

Control

The control of EHV disease is by a combination of management and hygiene measures supplemented by vaccination.[207,254,255]

Worldwide, EHV-1 disease control programs have three common goals: (1) prevention of disease entry onto premises; (2) limiting the extent of spread and severity of clinical disease once EHV-1 enters the premises or appears in the herd; and (3) limiting the spread of disease to adjacent premises during an outbreak. In the United Kingdom, these measures are formalized into a voluntary code of practice (hblb.org.uk) that has greatly assisted in disease control. Guides to infectious disease control are published by the AAEP (www.aaep.org) and the American College of Equine Internal Medicine has published an expert consensus opinion on EHV-1 control.[24]

Prevention of disease entry onto premises is not straightforward because the majority of adolescent and adult horses carry latent EHV infections. Diagnosis of latent infections is not straightforward (see section on Diagnosis), and in any event, exclusion of latently infected horses is impractical. To reduce the risk of disease entry into premises, new arrivals should ideally have been vaccinated before arrival and should be kept isolated from other horses until sufficient time has passed for disease to become apparent. On studs, newly arrived and "walk-in" mares should be kept strictly separate from resident in-foal mares for 56 days after covering. Mares arriving at studs to foal should be transported at least 28 days before the foaling due date. Horses that have arrived from sales or markets are at particular risk, as are any animals whose background, health, and vaccination status is uncertain. In yards with no pregnant mares, new arrivals should be kept isolated for at least 21 days and preferably 28 days after arrival because virus shedding may occur after reactivation. Minimizing management stress in resident horses, including transport, disruption of established social groups, and weaning, should assist in reducing the frequency of reactivation. If clinical respiratory or neurologic disease occurs in a new arrival, the horse should be isolated for at least 28 days from the onset of clinical signs.

Limiting the extent of spread of disease on the premises is greatly assisted by simple stock management measures (see Chapter 62). Different age groups should not be mixed, and group size should be kept as small as practicable. Pregnant mares should be isolated from other horses on the premises and should be subdivided into small groups to reduce the risk of large-scale outbreaks. Mares in the last third of pregnancy (the highest risk period for EHV-1 abortions) should ideally be housed and managed individually. Isolation areas should be rigorously maintained and located in a geographically separate area of the premises, and staff should understand and be able to apply the principles of barrier housing. As soon as disease is suspected on clinical grounds (e.g., respiratory clinical signs, abortion, stillborn foals, neonatal foal death, onset of neurologic disease), the horse should be isolated and appropriate clinical samples immediately submitted to a diagnostic laboratory (see section on Diagnosis). Any in-contact horses should ideally be isolated and carefully monitored for signs of disease. If the in-contact group is large, it should be subdivided. If the in-contact group cannot be isolated, it should not be moved, and horses from the group should not be mixed with horses from other groups.

Because the virus can persist in the environment, even though this is for limited periods, all discharges from the affected horse should be removed and the area disinfected using Virkon or other approved disinfectants. This is especially important after an abortion; the large volumes of infectious allantochorionic and amniotic fluids, fetal membranes, and the aborted foal present a high contagion risk. Bedding should be disinfected before disposal or destroyed by burning. Vehicles and equipment should be disinfected. If EHV-1 is confirmed, the aborted mare and exposed or in-contact horses should be kept isolated for 28 days and not mixed with pregnant mares for 56 days. Mares can be safely covered on their second estrus after abortion. Pregnant in-contact mares should not leave the premises until after foaling. Horses with neurologic disease should be kept isolated for a minimum 14 days,[203] although longer periods of up to 28 days have been recommended to account for the maximum possible duration of viremia. Movement of all horses on and off the premises should stop for a period of 28 days.

Limiting spread of disease to adjacent premises requires efficient and open communication among the attending veterinarian, the premises' owners, and other parties working with the affected premises. Owners of horses that have come into contact with animals on the affected premises should be informed. Care must be taken with vehicles and other fomites to avoid transmission, and these should be rigorously disinfected. Personnel should be aware that they can indirectly transmit virus. Horse movements on and off the premises should stop for at least 28 days, but pregnant mares should not leave until after they have foaled. Affected horses, especially neurologic cases, should be tested (by nasopharyngeal swabs) to make sure they are no longer contagious and are free from disease before leaving the premises.

Event management is especially difficult and an increasingly important risk factor especially for North American events. For many U.S. states, outbreaks of neurologic or abortion disease caused by EHV-1 are not reportable, thus detection of EHV-1 on an original premises to prevent movement of horses to other events or farms is unlikely to occur in the near future. Coupled with common long-distance travel to events in the United States, these outbreaks now involve several states, many premises, and a high degree of work hours required for tracing and quarantine of horses. A typical example is one of the latest incidents that occurred in the United States in 2011. Horses competing in a national cutting horse event were confirmed positive for EHV-1 resulting in a 10 state outbreak. Horses were exposed at this event in Utah and then were traced back to Arizona, California, Colorado, Idaho, New Mexico, Nevada, Oklahoma, Oregon, Utah, and Washington after horses dispersed from the facility. Fifty-four of the 90 confirmed cases (either testing positive for EHV-1 or diagnosed with EHM) were horses that participated in the event with the remaining 36 exposed at destination premises. Ten of the 13 deaths were horses that were exposed at the original event and the remaining 3 were those of secondary or tertiary contact at the next facility. A total of 242 premises independent of the original premises were exposed, and 62/242 premises had either suspect or confirmed EHV/EHM cases. Given the widespread movement of horses, identification of sick horses and limiting exposure before dispersal of stock to various locations is essential. Early implementation of case identification, trace-back investigations, testing, and quarantine are the only reliable methods of control. Based on the outbreak events in 2006, 2007, and 2011 in the United States, the quarantine and test procedures in Box 14-1 are highly recommended.

The complete reference list is available online at www.expertconsult.com.

Box 14-1 Management Guidelines for Equine Herpesvirus Type 1 (EHV-1) Outbreaks

I. Define Horses by Risk: Case Definitions
- *Suspect EHV-1 case:* An exposed horse that becomes febrile (rectal temperature greater than 101.5° F) during the monitoring period.
- *Confirmed EHV-1 case:* A suspect EHV-1 case whose infection is laboratory confirmed by virus isolation and/or PCR detection of the virus, or a fourfold change in titer on the serum neutralization test using paired sera.
- *Suspect equine herpesvirus myeloencephalopathy (EHM) case:* An exposed horse exhibiting signs of central nervous system (CNS) dysfunction, including, most commonly, posterior incoordination, weakness, recumbency with inability to rise, or bladder atony.
- *Confirmed EHM case:* A suspect EHM case testing positive for EHV-1 by virus isolation and/or polymerase chain reaction (PCR) assay on nasal swab or blood (buffy coat). In cases of sudden death or when the horse dies as a result of neurologic complications, the postmortem lesions are consistent with those of myeloencephalopathy and EHV-1 has been isolated, detected by PCR, or demonstrated by immunohistochemical examination of the CNS.
- *Nonclinical EHV-1 case:* An exposed horse with no clinical signs (afebrile, nonneurologic) testing positive for EHV-1 by virus isolation and/or PCR assay on nasal swab or blood (buffy coat). (Testing exposed nonclinical horses is not recommended.)

II. Monitoring of Exposed Horses
- Isolation and monitoring are recommended for all premises with exposed horses.
- Exposed horses should initially be monitored for fever and/or neurologic signs for at least 7 days.
- Owners should confirm with their practicing veterinarian or State animal health officials whether any requirements exist for notification to the State Veterinarian.
- Once suspect or confirmed cases are identified on a premises, then all horses on the premises should be managed as described in the next section.
- Suspect and confirmed clinical cases need to be strictly isolated from nonclinical horses.
- Suspect clinical cases should be sampled for laboratory confirmation of EHV-1.

III. Management of Suspect and Confirmed EHV-1 or EHM Cases
- *Management Option 1:* Cases and herd mates isolated for at least 21 days past resolution of clinical signs, then releasing test on all horses on the premises.
  - Confirmed and suspect EHV-1 and EHM cases should remain isolated with no movement of horses in or out of the affected premises for a period of at least 21 days from the resolution of clinical signs in all horses on the premises. Daily monitoring of rectal temperatures for all horses on the premises should continue through the 21-day period, and horses should not be on any nonsteroidal antiinflammatory drugs (NSAIDs) during this time because NSAIDs will mask a fever. If no new suspect or confirmed cases are identified during the 21 days, then sample all exposed horses on the premises using real-time or nested PCR testing of nasal swabs. If all negative results are obtained, the quarantine can be discontinued.
- *Management Option 2:* Cases and herd mates isolated for at least 28 days past resolution of clinical signs with no releasing test.
  - Confirmed and suspect EHV-1 and EHM cases should remain isolated with no movement of horses in or out of the affected premises for a period of at least 28 days from the resolution of clinical signs in all horses on the premises. Daily monitoring of rectal temperatures for all horses on the premises should continue through the 28-day period, and horses should not be on any NSAIDs during this time. If no new suspect or confirmed cases are identified within this 28-day period, then the quarantine can be discontinued with no additional diagnostic testing.

USDA: APHIS: Veterinary Services: Centers for Epidemiology and Animal Health, Center for Emerging Issues: http://www.aphis.usda.gov/animal_health/emergingissues/downloads/ehv1final.pdf. Equine Herpesvirus Myeloencephalopathy: A Potentially Emerging Disease.

USDA, APHIS, Veterinary Services: http://www.aphis.usda.gov/vs/nahss/equine/ehv/ehv_2011_final_sitrep_062311.pdf. Equine Herpesvirus (EHV-1)—FINAL Situation Report, June 23, 2011.

15   Equine Viral Arteritis

Udeni B.R. Balasuriya and N. James MacLachlan*

Equine viral arteritis (EVA) is an infectious disease of equids that is caused by equine arteritis virus (EAV). EAV infection occurs throughout much of the world, although the prevalence of both subclinical EAV infection and EVA varies greatly between countries and among horses of different breeds.[1] The vast majority of EAV infections are inapparent or subclinical, but occasional outbreaks of EVA are characterized by any combination of influenza-like illness in adult horses, abortion in pregnant mares, and interstitial pneumonia in very young foals.[1,2] EAV establishes a carrier state in mature intact male horses (e.g., colts and stallions) but not in mares and geldings or sexually immature colts. The persistently infected carrier stallion plays a central role in maintenance and perpetuation of EAV in the equine population. Importation of EAV carrier stallions and infective semen has been implicated in the introduction of EAV into various countries around the world on numerous occasions. This apparent global dissemination of EAV and rising incidence of EVA likely reflect the progressive increase in national and international movement of horses for competition and breeding, as well as increased recognition of the importance of EAV infection.[3,4]

Etiology

Equine arteritis virus was first isolated from the lung of an aborted fetus after an extensive outbreak of respiratory disease and abortion on a Standardbred breeding farm near Bucyrus, Ohio, in 1953.[5,6] Equine viral arteritis was identified as an etiologically distinct disease after isolation of the causative virus (EAV) and description of characteristic vascular lesions.[7] Equine viral arteritis was distinguished from equine influenza and equine herpesviruses type 1 and type 4 (EHV-1, EHV-4), which potentially cause similar respiratory and reproductive disease syndromes in horses.[5,6] Although it was not definitively confirmed to be a new disease entity until 1953, descriptions of a clinically indistinguishable disease were recorded in the late eighteenth and early nineteenth centuries and referred to as "pinkeye," "infectious or epizootic cellulitis," "influenza erysipelatosa," "Pferdestaupe," "Rotlaufseuche," and "equine influenza."[8-11]

Molecular Properties of Equine Arteritis Virus

Equine arteritis virus is the prototype virus in the family *Arteriviridae* (genus *Arterivirus*, order Nidovirales), a grouping that also includes porcine reproductive and respiratory syndrome virus, simian hemorrhagic fever virus, and lactate dehydrogenase-elevating virus of mice.[12-15] The EAV virion is an enveloped, spherical, 50- to 65-nm particle with an isometric core that contains a single-stranded, positive-sense ribonucleic acid (RNA) molecule. The EAV genome length varies between 12,704 to 12,731 bp among different virus strains and includes a 5' leader sequence (224 nucleotides) and at least 10 open reading frames (ORFs)[16-21] (Fig. 15-1).[16-21] The two most 5'-proximal ORFs (ORF1a and ORF1b) occupy approximately three-fourths of the genome and encode two replicase polyproteins (pp1a and pp1ab). These precursor proteins are extensively processed after translation into at least 13 nonstructural proteins (nsps; nsp1-12, including nsp7 α/β) by 3 viral proteases (nsp1, nsp2, and nsp4).[15,22,23] The greatest variation in the EAV replicase gene occurs in the portion of ORF1a encoding the nsp2 protein, with considerable variation at amino acids 388 to 488.[18,19,21,24]

The structural proteins of the EAV virion include seven envelope proteins (E, GP2, GP3, GP4, ORF5a protein, GP5, and M) and a nucleocapsid protein (N), which respectively are encoded by ORFs 2a, 2b, 3-4, 5a, 5b, and 6-7 that are located at the 3' proximal quarter of the genome.[25-29] These structural proteins are expressed from six subgenomic viral messenger RNAs (sg mRNAs) that form a 3'-co-terminal nested set and contain a common leader sequence encoded by the 5'-end of the genome. Three of the minor envelope proteins (GP2, GP3, and GP4) form a heterotrimer in the EAV particle, and the M and GP5 proteins form a disulfide-linked heterodimer.[28,30,31] All major structural proteins (N, GP5, and M) and four of the minor envelope proteins (E, GP2, GP3, and GP4) are essential for the production of infectious progeny virus. Furthermore, elimination of ORF5a protein expression cripples EAV, leading to progeny virus with small plaque phenotype and significantly reduced virus titer. The amino terminal ectodomain of the GP5 protein contains the known neutralization determinants of EAV (amino acids 49 [site A], 60-61 [site B], 67-90 [site C], and 98-106 [site D]). Heterodimerization of the GP5 and M proteins is critical for the authentic posttranslational modification (glycosylation) and conformational maturation of the neutralization determinants in GP5.[24,32] The M protein may act as an essential scaffold on which the GP5 protein folds to form the epitopes that induce neutralizing antibodies in virus-infected animals.

The greatest sequence variation in the ORFs encoding structural EAV proteins occurs in ORFs 3 and 5, which encode GP3 and GP5, respectively.[18,19,21,33-36] GP5 expresses the major neutralization determinants of EAV, and although considerable variation exists in the sequence of the GP5 protein of field strains of the virus, there is only one serotype of EAV and all strains evaluated thus far are neutralized by polyclonal antiserum raised against the prototype virulent Bucyrus strain.[19,32,35,37-42] However, field strains of EAV are frequently distinguished on the basis of differences in their neutralization phenotype with polyclonal antisera and monoclonal antibodies, and similarly, geographically and temporally distinct strains of EAV can differ in the severity of the clinical disease they induce and in their abortigenic potential.[1,2,43-47] Although strains of EAV from North America and Europe share as much as 85%

*The authors acknowledge and appreciate the original contributions of these authors, whose work has been incorporated into this chapter.

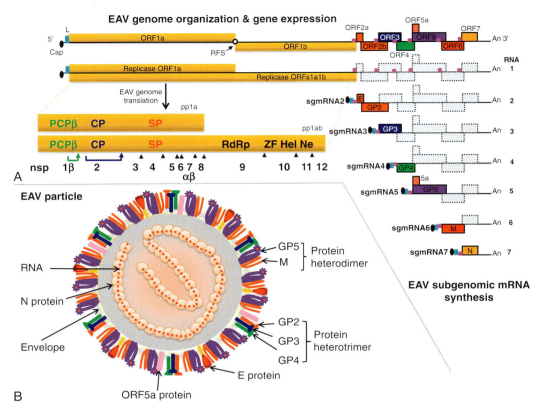

Figure 15-1 Schematic representation of equine arteritis virus (EAV) genome organization and gene expression **(A)** and the virus particle **(B)**. The open reading frames *(ORF)* encoding replicase proteins and viral structural proteins are depicted. The 5′ cap structure, 5′ leader sequence *(L)*, ribosomal frame shift *(RFS)* of the *ORF1a/1b*, and the 3′ poly A tail *(An)* are indicated. The processing of EAV replicase polyprotein 1ab is shown below the genome. The predicted PCPβ and CP cleavage sites are indicated by *green* and *blue arrows*, respectively. The 3CLSP (SP) cleavage sites are indicated by *black arrowheads*. The genes encoding structural proteins are depicted in various colors. *PCP*, Papain-like cysteine protease; *CP*, cysteine protease; *SP (3CLSP)*, 3chymotrypsin-like serine protease; *RdRp*, RNA dependent RNA polymerase; *ZF*, predicted zinc finger; *Hel*, helicase; *Ne*, NendoU; *nsp*, nonstructural protein; *sgmRNA*, subgenomic mRNA.

nucleotide identity,[21,35,46] these viruses generally segregate into either a North American or European group (including European subgroup-1 and European subgroup-2) based on ORF5 phylogenetic analysis.[19]

Using reverse genetics, the virulence determinants of EAV have been mapped to both nonstructural (nsp1, nsp2, nsp7, and nsp10) and structural proteins (GP2, GP4, GP5, and M).[48] However, major virulence determinants appear to be located in the structural protein genes of the virus. The interactions among the GP2, GP3, GP4, GP5, and M envelope proteins all play a major role in determining the CD14+ monocyte tropism, while tropism for CD3+ T lymphocytes is determined by the GP2, GP4, GP5, and M envelope proteins but not the GP3 protein.[49] Combined amino acid substitutions in E, GP2, GP3, and GP4 proteins or a single amino acid substitution in the GP5 protein all lead to persistent infection in cell culture (HeLa cells).[50] However, no specific viral proteins have been identified as critical to establishment of persistent infection in the stallion reproductive tract. In summary, the virulence determinants of EAV appear to be very complex and involve multiple genes encoding both envelope and nonstructural proteins (multigenic), and the viral determinants of persistent infection in stallions are uncharacterized.

Resistance to Physical and Chemical Agents

Equine arteritis virus is readily inactivated by lipid solvents (ether and chloroform) and by common disinfectants and detergents. Equine arteritis virus survives 75 days at 4° C (39.2° F), between 2 to 3 days at 37° C (98.6° F), and 20 to 30 minutes

at 56° C (132.8° F). Tissue culture fluid or organ samples containing EAV can be stored at −70° C (−94° F) for years without significant loss of infectivity. The virus also survives in cryopreserved semen samples and embryos for many years.

Epidemiology

Outbreaks

Since the recognition of EVA in 1953, outbreaks of the disease have been reported from Switzerland,[51,52] Austria,[53,54] Poland,[55,56] Italy,[57,58] the United Kingdom (UK),[59-62] Spain,[63] Netherlands,[64] Canada,[65,66] and the United States.[1,2,45,67-71] At least four major documented outbreaks of EVA have occurred in the United States since the 1953 epizootic[43,68,70,71]; the first outbreak occurred at Standardbred racetracks in Kentucky in 1977.[70] Subsequent epizootics included an extensive outbreak in Thoroughbred horses in central Kentucky during the 1984 breeding season[71] and another in racing Thoroughbred horses in 1993 (>200 clinical cases) that began at the Arlington racetrack in Chicago and then spread to horses at Churchill Downs, Prairie Meadow, and Ak-Sar-Ben.[68] The 1984 outbreak of EVA in Kentucky Thoroughbreds generated widespread interest, publicity, and concern.[4,59,72,73] A well-documented outbreak of EVA occurred on a single Warmblood breeding farm in Pennsylvania in 1996, precipitated by an imported carrier stallion.[2,43] Similarly, the first recorded outbreak of EVA in the UK followed the importation of an Anglo-Arab stallion from Poland.[60,74] There have been a number of recent EVA outbreaks reported from North America and Europe.[59-63,75] These include an extensive multistate occurrence of EVA in the United States in 2006/2007 involving American Quarter Horses (AQHs) and two outbreaks of EVA in France during 2006 and 2007.[18,19,76,77]

Seroprevalence and Breed Predilection

Equine viral arteritis is a disease of the horse, but antibodies to EAV recently have been identified in donkeys in South Africa and Brazil.[78-80] Serologic surveys have shown that EAV infection occurs among horses in North and South America, Europe, Australasia, New Zealand, Africa, and Asia.[1] However, the seroprevalence of EAV infection of horses varies between countries and among equine populations within some countries. Iceland and Japan, for example, are apparently free of the virus. Equine arteritis virus infection is relatively common in horses in a number of European countries; studies conducted in 1973 estimated the seroprevalence of EAV infection at 11.3% of Swiss horses and 2.3% of English horses.[81,82] Similarly, approximately 14% of Dutch horses were seropositive to EAV in surveys done in 1963 and 1975.[81] In German horses, 1.8% were seropositive in a study conducted in 1987, and the seroprevalence increased to 20% in a subsequent survey in 1994.[83] In the United States, the 1998 National Animal Health Monitoring System (NAHMS) equine survey showed that only 2.0% of unvaccinated horses were seropositive to EAV.[84] Similarly, resident unvaccinated California horses had a seroprevalence to EAV of only 1.9%, whereas 18.6% of horses imported into California from other countries (most often European Warmbloods) were seropositive.[85]

The seroprevalence of EAV infection varies not only between countries but also among horses of different breeds and ages, with marked disparity between the prevalence of infection of Standardbred and Thoroughbred horses.[86,87] Equine arteritis virus infection is considered endemic in Standardbred but not Thoroughbred horses in the United States, with 77.5% to 84.3% of all Standardbreds but only up to 5.4% of Thoroughbreds being seropositive to the virus.[1,69,87-90] Similarly, the seroprevalence of EAV infection of Standardbred horses in California was 68.5% in 1991, versus less than 2% in all other breeds tested.[88] The seroprevalence of EAV infection of Warmblood stallions is also very high in a number of European countries, with about 55% to 93% of Austrian Warmblood stallions testing positive for antibodies to EAV.[91] Furthermore, the 1998 NAHMS equine survey showed that only 0.6% of the AQH population was seropositive to EAV.[84] Nonetheless, the extensive outbreak of EVA in 2006-2007 mainly involved AQHs, which likely increased the seroprevalence of EAV within this breed. Consistent with the epidemiology of this outbreak, artificial insemination with infective semen, movement of donor/recipient mares, and embryo transfer have likely favored an increase in seroprevalence of EAV in AQHs.

In addition to management and environmental risk, profound differences in the breed-specific seroprevalence of EAV infection may reflect inherent genetic differences that confer resistance to infection. Recent studies have suggested that there is a genetic difference between stallions that become carriers after exposure to EAV and those that are able to clear the virus and become sereopositive noncarrier stallions. Specifically, this trait was linked to in vitro susceptibility of CD3+ lymphocytes to infection with EAV (see later).[92] Preliminary data from these studies indicate that carrier stallions that have an in vitro susceptible CD3+ T lymphocyte phenotype to EAV infection may represent those that have a higher risk of becoming persistently infected, as compared to stallions that do not possess this phenotype.[93] Finally, the seroprevalence of EAV infection increases with age, indicating that horses may be repeatedly exposed with increasing age.[91,94]

Transmission

Transmission of EAV between horses occurs through either respiratory or venereal routes (Fig. 15-2).[1,6,86,95-97] Horizontal respiratory transmission of EAV occurs after aerosolization of infected respiratory tract secretions from acutely infected horses; high titers of EAV are present in respiratory secretions for some 7 to 14 days during acute infection.[96] However, direct and close contact is necessary for aerosol transmission of EAV between horses.[67,87] Equine arteritis virus can also be transmitted by aerosol from urine and other body secretions of acutely infected horses, aborted fetuses and their membranes, and the masturbates of acutely or chronically infected stallions.[82,91,96,98-101] Venereal transmission of EAV contained in the semen of stallions that are either acutely or chronically infected with EAV is the other important route of natural transmission of the virus.[86,97]

Persistently infected carrier stallions are the essential reservoir responsible for perpetuation and maintenance of EAV in equine populations. Persistent EAV infection that occurs in carrier stallions is highly unusual in that virus is shed only in the reproductive tract; thus 85% to 100% of seronegative mares bred to long-term carrier stallions become infected with the virus and seroconvert within 28 days. Mares are also readily infected by artificial insemination with semen collected from shedding stallions.[45] Mares that become infected following natural or artificial insemination can readily transmit the virus by the respiratory route to susceptible cohorts in close proximity.[95] Recently, it has been demonstrated that under experimental conditions, EAV can be transmitted to naïve recipient mares via embryo transfer from a donor mare inseminated with EAV-infective semen to a naïve recipient mare.[102]

Other, less common modes of transmission of EAV include congenital infection of foals after transplacental transmission of the virus in mares infected in late gestation.[103] The virus is not teratogenic, but congenitally infected foals frequently develop a rapidly progressive, fulminating interstitial pneumonia and fibronecrotic enteritis.[56,103-106] Lateral dissemination of EAV also can occur through contaminated fomites (e.g., personnel, clothing, vehicles, equipment).[1,67,82,87] Importantly, indirect spread from carrier stallion to a susceptible horse has been reported.[43] The virus then rapidly spreads by aerosol to in-contact horses. Similarly, EAV was spread among nonbreeding Lipizzaner stallions in South Africa by the apparent aerosolization of virus shed into bedding in the masturbates of a carrier stallion(s).[107]

Carrier State and Molecular Epidemiology

The asymptomatic carrier stallion is the fundamental natural reservoir of EAV, as described more than 100 years ago when it was noted that healthy stallions could transmit so-called epizootic cellulitis-pinkeye or influenza (which likely was EVA) to mares at breeding.[10,11] The EAV carrier state was poorly defined until the 1984 epizootic in Kentucky when studies unequivocally established the importance of the carrier stallion in the natural epidemiology of EAV infection.[86,97,108,109] These studies confirmed the chronic carrier state in naturally infected Thoroughbred stallions using test matings and isolation of virus from semen. This work demonstrated that 30% to 35% of stallions infected during the outbreak subsequently became long-term carriers.[97]

Persistently infected stallions can be divided into three groups based on the duration of virus shedding in semen.[86,110] The short-term, or convalescent, carrier state lasts only a few weeks after clinical recovery, and the intermediate carrier state lasts for 3 to 7 months in both naturally and experimentally infected animals. The long-term, or chronic, carrier state can last for years and even the entire life of some infected stallions.

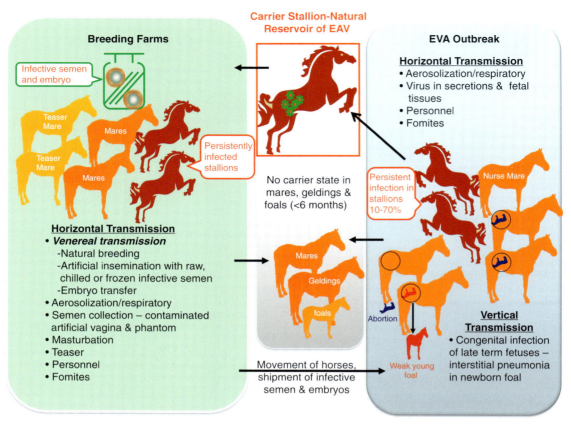

Figure 15-2 Transmission of equine arteritis virus (EAV) between horses and the role of the carrier stallion in the epidemiology of equine viral arteritis (EVA).

Some persistently infected, long-term carrier stallions cease to shed virus after years of persistent infection, with no apparent later reversion to a shedding state. However, the mechanism responsible for this spontaneous clearance of EAV from persistently infected stallions is not clear. There is no convincing evidence that carrier stallions are or can become intermittent shedders of the virus or develop latent infection.

Carrier stallions frequently have moderate to high titers of serum neutralizing antibody to EAV and shed the virus constantly in their semen, but virus is not present in their blood, urine, or other body secretions.[1] Equine arteritis virus appears to be restricted to the reproductive tract during persistent infection of carrier stallions, and highest titers of the virus consistently have been demonstrated in the ampulla of the vas deferens ($>10^5$ pfu/g tissue).[1,109] Virus in semen is associated with the sperm-rich fraction and not with the preejaculatory fluid, and the titers of virus in sequential ejaculates vary little from the same stallion.

The mechanism of persistence of EAV in the male reproductive tract is not clear. However, persistence of EAV in stallions is testosterone-dependent[111,112]; persistently infected stallions that were castrated and treated with testosterone continued to shed the virus in semen, whereas untreated animals ceased shedding virus. Studies in prepubertal and peripubertal colts have demonstrated that EAV replicates in the male reproductive tract of a significant proportion of colts for a variable period (up to 6 months) after clinical recovery in the absence of circulating concentrations of testosterone equivalent to those found in sexually mature stallions.[108] However, long-term persistent EAV infection does not occur in colts exposed to the virus before the onset of puberty. Similarly, persistent infection does not occur after EAV infection of mares, geldings, or

fetuses.[1,112] Thus EAV was not isolated from the reproductive tract of seropositive mares 1 month after infection,[112,113] and convalescent mares did not transmit infection to susceptible stallions during mating or to contact horses.[87,91,114]

The carrier stallion clearly is responsible for generating the genetic heterogeneity that distinguishes individual field strains of EAV. Sequence analyses of the variable ORF5 gene of strains of EAV sequentially present in the semen of carrier stallions showed that EAV behaves as a quasispecies (population of genetically related viral variants) during persistent infection, leading to both genetic and phenotypic divergence of the virus.[21,34,43] Outbreaks of EVA result from the emergence and spread of specific variants of EAV that are present in the quasispecies virus population in the semen of individual carrier stallions; however, the mechanisms involved in selection and emergence of virulent viral variants remain unclear. It is also clear that novel variants with distinct neutralization phenotypes arise during persistent infection of carrier stallions and that the altered neutralization phenotype of these variants correlates with amino acid changes in specific regions of the GP5 envelope glycoprotein.* However, all the variants that arise in the course of persistent infection of carrier stallions are neutralized by high-titer polyclonal equine sera, which suggest that immune evasion is not responsible for the establishment of persistent EAV infection of carrier stallions. There also is no evidence that positive selective pressures are responsible for establishment of persistent EAV infection of stallions.[21,34]

The recent advent of molecular techniques has helped greatly to increase our understanding of the epidemiology of EVA. Investigation of an extensive outbreak of EVA on

---

*References 32, 34, 37, 38, 43, 45.

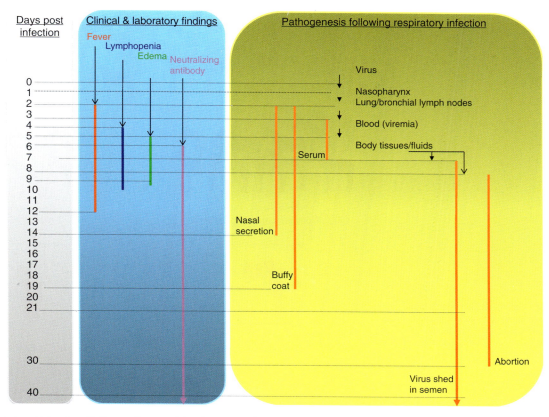

Figure 15-3 Clinical and laboratory findings and sequential pathogenesis of equine viral arteritis (EVA) after experimental respiratory infection. Vertical bars correspond to the chronologic occurrence of the respective clinical or laboratory findings and the distribution of virus in body tissues and secretions.

breeding farms showed that a single virus variant present in the semen of a carrier stallion was selected and then efficiently transmitted by aerosol among other horses on the farm.[43] Thus it appears that the considerable genetic heterogeneity afforded by the viral quasispecies likely facilitates persistence of EAV in the reproductive tract of carrier stallions. However, only some members (variants) within the quasispecies appear to be capable of efficient aerosol transmission to other horses, perhaps because of an enhanced ability to replicate within the respiratory tract. The individual strains of EAV that circulated during a single or small EVA outbreak are generally genetically stable during repeated horizontal and vertical passage in horses, unlike the diverse, quasispecies virus population in the semen of the carrier stallions on the farm. However, molecular characterization of virus strains from the 2006-2007 multistate EVA occurrence that spanned a period of more than 10 months of active circulation of EAV in horses of several breeds, on multiple farms in different states in the United States, showed that genomic variability tended to increase with extensive horizontal and vertical transmission of EAV over an extended time period.[19,115] Moreover, one of the isolates from an aborted fetus had a very distinct neutralization phenotype and was not neutralized by monoclonal antibodies that neutralized the other isolates. Similarly, this virus was neutralized to a significantly lower titer by polyclonal antisera as compared to other isolates.

In summary, genetic divergence of EAV occurs in the course of persistent infection of the reproductive tract of carrier stallions, leading to the emergence of novel strains of EAV, and likely compensating for the minimal virus diversity that is generated during EVA outbreaks when the virus can be transmitted by respiratory and/or venereal routes. Therefore the persistently infected carrier stallion serves as the natural reservoir that

harbors EAV between breeding seasons and also provides the environment in which genetic diversification of the virus occurs.

Pathogenesis

The pathogenesis of EVA has been studied by both the experimental inoculation (intranasal, intramuscular, intravenous) of horses with strains of EAV of different virulence and the careful evaluation of natural outbreaks of EVA.[2,47,95,96,116-122] Quantitative distribution of EAV has differed greatly between individual experiments, which likely reflects the inherent differences in the route of infection, virus dose, strain of virus, and quality of the specimens used for virus isolation.[27] Briefly, following replication in the respiratory tract epithelium, EAV is rapidly spread within the lung and bronchial lymph nodes (within 2 days) after aerosol infection, and then is disseminated throughout the body through the circulation (viremia). Virus can be isolated from the nasopharynx, buffy coat, and serum for a variable time after intranasal exposure (Fig. 15-3). Virus can be isolated from the nasopharynx for 2 to 14 days after infection and from buffy coat for 2 to 19 days. Virus typically is isolated from serum or plasma for 7 to 9 days, and the disappearance of virus from serum coincides with the development of virus-specific neutralizing antibodies. Virus can be isolated from a wide variety of tissues and body fluids of infected horses beginning about 1 to 2 days after infection.[96] Aside from occasional cases in which EAV has been isolated from buffy coat cells for several months after infection and from the reproductive tract of prepubertal colts (<6 months), EAV generally is not isolated

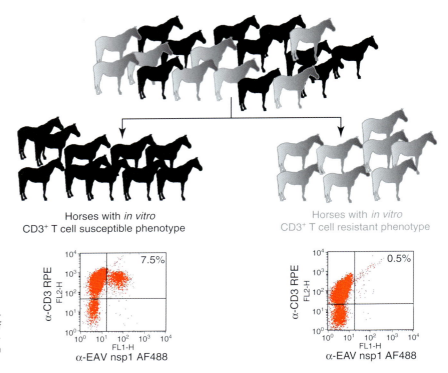

Horses with *in vitro*
CD3⁺ T cell susceptible phenotype

Horses with *in vitro*
CD3⁺ T cell resistant phenotype

Figure 15-4 In vitro infection of peripheral blood mononuclear cells from horses with virulent Bucyrus strain of equine arteritis virus (EAV) divides horses into CD3⁺ T cell–susceptible and CD3⁺ T cell–resistant groups based on dual color flow cytometry analysis.

beyond 28 days after infection except from the semen of carrier stallions.

The pathogenesis of EVA is not clearly defined. Many of the clinical manifestations of EVA result from vascular injury, and death in horses inoculated with the highly virulent, horse-adapted Bucyrus strain of EAV is a consequence of severe vascular damage leading to disseminated intravascular coagulation (DIC). The characteristic vascular lesions of EVA have been compared to those of Aleutian disease of mink and other immune-mediated vascular diseases.[123,124] The lesions of EVA, however, do not appear to be the result of immune-mediated injury because they develop at only 4 to 5 days after experimental inoculation, which is not consistent with an immune-mediated process. Furthermore, arteries larger than 1 mm are affected, and neither immunoglobulin G (IgG) nor complement (C3) are present in the lesions, as would be expected if immune complexes were responsible.

Therefore vascular injury in EVA likely results from direct virus-mediated injury to the lining (endothelium) and walls (media) of affected vessels. Equine arteritis virus infects and replicates in endothelial cells (ECs) and causes extensive damage to the endothelium and the subjacent internal elastic lamina, then gains access to the media of affected vessels. Increased vascular permeability and leukocyte infiltration resulting from generation of chemotactic factors lead to hemorrhage and edema around these vessels.[125,126] In addition to ECs, EAV also replicates in macrophages in infected horses; EAV infection of in vitro cultured equine ECs and macrophages leads to their activation, with increased transcription of genes encoding proinflammatory mediators, including interleukin-1 beta (IL-1β), IL-6, IL-8, and tumor necrosis factor alpha (TNF-α).[127] Furthermore, virulent and avirulent strains of EAV induced different quantities of TNF-α and other proinflammatory cytokines from both infected ECs and macrophages. These studies strongly suggest that cytokine mediators that are produced by ECs and macrophages have a central role in the pathogenesis of EVA. Furthermore, recent studies have demonstrated that the clinical outcome of EAV infection is determined by host

genetic factors. Specifically, based on the in vitro susceptibility of CD3⁺ T lymphocytes to EAV infection, horses were divided into susceptible and resistant groups (Fig. 15-4).[93,128] Subsequently, a genome-wide association study (GWAS) identified a common, genetically dominant haplotype associated with the in vitro susceptible phenotype in the region of equine chromosome 11 (ECA11; 49572804-49643932).[92] Experimental inoculation with EAV into horses with in vitro CD3⁺ susceptibility or resistance showed a significant difference between the two groups of horses in terms of proinflammatory and immunomodulatory cytokine mRNA expression and evidence of increased clinical signs in horses possessing the in vitro CD3⁺ T cell–resistant phenotype.[129] These studies provide direct evidence for a correlation between variation in host genotype and phenotypic differences in terms of the extent of viral replication, occurrence and severity of clinical signs, and cytokine gene expression that result from EAV infection in individual horses.

Abortion after EAV infection of pregnant mares likely is the result of a lethal fetal infection, rather than myometritis or placental damage that impairs progesterone synthesis, leading to fetal expulsion.[118] The tissues of aborted fetuses contain higher titers of virus than those of the dams from which they abort, indicating that substantial virus replication occurs in the fetus itself.[118] The stress that results from fetal infection would be expected to activate the fetal hypothalamic-pituitary axis, thus inducing abortion.

Clinical Findings

The clinical signs observed in natural cases of EVA vary considerably among individual horses and between outbreaks and depend on factors such as the strain of the virus, challenge dose, route of exposure, host factors (genetics, age, and physical condition), and environmental conditions (e.g., management practices).[1,47,82,103] Although there is only one known serotype of EAV, the clinical disease produced by different virus strains

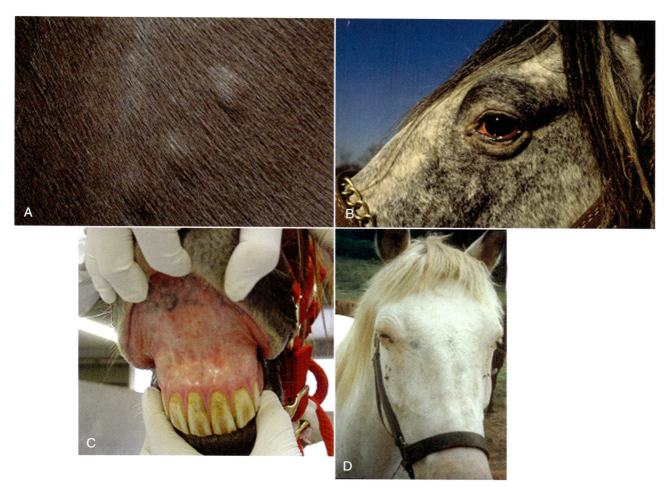

Figure 15-5 Representative example of clinical signs of equine viral arteritis (EVA) after experimental inoculation of horses with virulent strains of equine arteritis virus (EAV). **A,** Urticaria; **B,** conjunctivitis and periorbital edema; **C,** mucosal petechiation; **D,** facial edema; **E,** preputial and hindlimb edema; **F,** scrotal edema; **G,** edema of the mammary gland; **H,** limb edema. (**B, D, F,** and **G** Courtesy of Dr. Peter J. Timoney, Gluck Equine Research Center, Lexington, KY.)

Continued

ranges from severe, lethal infection caused by the horse-adapted Bucyrus strain to clinically inapparent infection.[87,118,130] The vast majority of EAV infections are inapparent, especially those that occur in mares bred to persistently infected stallions.[1,86,97] Regardless of the infecting virus strain, the vast majority of naturally infected horses recover uneventfully from EVA. Very young, old, debilitated, and immunosuppressed horses are predisposed to severe EVA. Outbreaks of clinical disease caused by EAV infection are characterized by one or more of the following: abortion of pregnant mares; fatal infection in neonatal foals congenitally infected with the virus; fulminant infection of neonates, leading to severe interstitial pneumonia or pneumoenteritis; and systemic illness in adult horses, with any combination of leukopenia and pyrexia, respiratory signs with nasal and ocular discharge, peripheral edema, hives, and persistent infection of stallions.[103,105]

With the notable exceptions of abortion and fulminant respiratory disease in foals, mortality rarely if ever occurs in natural outbreaks of EVA. The highly virulent horse-adapted Bucyrus strain of EAV (which causes high mortality in healthy adult horses) is not representative of field strains of the virus and is best regarded as a laboratory aberration.

Clinical cases of EVA are characterized by an incubation period of 2 to 14 days (6 to 8 days after venereal exposure), pyrexia of up to 41°C that may persist for 2 to 9 days (see Fig. 15-3), and any combination of depression and anorexia;

conjunctivitis and rhinitis with nasal and ocular discharge; leukopenia; periorbital and supraorbital edema; edema of the limbs, especially of the hind limbs; midventral edema involving the scrotum and prepuce or mammary glands; urticaria that may be localized to sides of the neck or face or may be generalized over most of the body; and abortion.* Less frequently observed signs include icterus; photophobia; corneal opacity; coughing and dyspnea; abdominal pain and diarrhea; ataxia; petechiation of the nasal mucosa, conjunctiva, and oral mucous membranes; submaxillary and submandibular lymphadenopathy; and adventitious edema in the intermandibular space, beneath the sternum, or in the shoulder region (Fig. 15-5).† The most consistent clinical features of EAV infection are pyrexia and leukopenia.[121,122,134]

Abortion in pregnant mares is not preceded by premonitory signs and may occur late in the acute phase or early in the convalescent phase of the EAV infection.[1,6,65,113,134] Abortions have been documented at 3 months to over 10 months of gestation after natural or experimental infection.[1,6,95,113,125] Abortion rates in outbreaks of EVA have varied from less than 10% to more than 60%.[1] Infections with the strain of EAV that caused the 1984 Kentucky outbreak resulted in an abortion rate of

*References 1, 6, 44, 82, 96, 99, 101, 113, 122, 131.
†References 5, 6, 52, 65, 67, 95, 117, 132, 133.

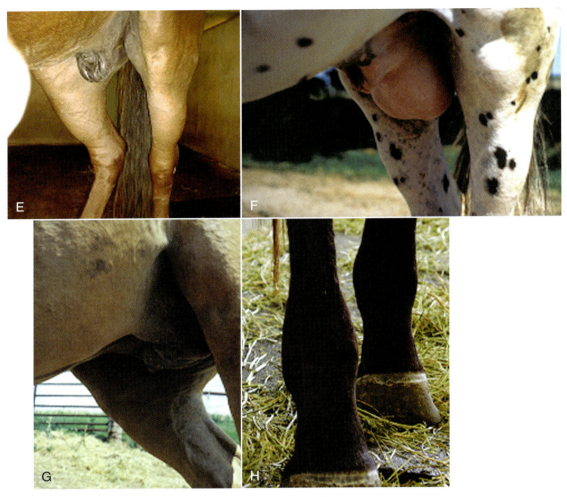

Figure 15-5, cont'd

71%.[95] The abortigenic potential of different strains of EAV has not been adequately compared, but it appears that strains differ in their abortigenic potential as they do in their virulence characteristics.

Stallions may undergo a period of temporary subfertility associated with decreased libido, sperm motility, concentration, and percentage of morphologically normal sperm in ejaculates during acute EAV infection. These changes can persist for 6 to 7 weeks after experimental EAV infection of stallions[1,135] and are considered to result from increased testicular temperature rather than any direct virus-induced pathologic effect. Semen quality is apparently normal in persistently infected stallions, despite active shedding of the virus into the semen. Similarly, venereal infection of mares by persistently infected carrier stallions does not appear to result in subsequent fertility problems.[1]

Diagnosis

Clinical EVA resembles a number of other infectious and noninfectious diseases of horses, and therefore a presumptive diagnosis must be confirmed by laboratory testing of clinical samples.[1,136] The differential diagnosis of EVA includes other viral respiratory tract infections of the horse (EHV-1, EHV-4, equine influenza virus, equine rhinitis A and B viruses, equine adenovirus, and Getah virus), equine infectious anemia, African horse sickness, Hendra, leptospirosis, purpura hemorrhagica, urticaria, and toxicosis caused by hoary alyssum *(Berteroa incana)*. Equine viral arteritis is characterized histologically by a distinctive arteritis that differentiates it from these other diseases, although vasculitis certainly is not pathognomonic of EVA. Importantly, the severity and distribution of vasculitis varies greatly between cases of EVA.

Abortion from EVA can also present a diagnostic dilemma. Differential diagnoses include EHV-1 (or rarely EHV-4), although fetuses are typically expelled without any premonitory signs in EHV abortions. Equine herpesvirus-infected fetuses are expelled fresh and frequently have characteristic gross lesions, whereas those infected with EAV are usually partially autolyzed and lack pathognomonic lesions. Laboratory diagnosis of EVA is currently based on any combination of virus isolation, viral nucleic acid or antigen detection, and serology.

Virus Isolation

The most appropriate specimens for virus isolation (VI) from live horses include nasopharyngeal swabs or washings, conjunctival swabs, and citrated or ethylenediaminetetraacetic acid (EDTA) blood samples for separation of buffy coat cells. Heparinized blood is not suitable for virus isolation because of the inhibitory effect of heparin on the isolation of EAV in cell culture.[137] The sperm-rich fraction of the ejaculate is optimal for virus isolation from equine semen samples.[1] Placenta, fetal fluids, lung, spleen, and lymphoid tissues should be collected for virus isolation to confirm cases of EAV-induced abortion. A wide variety of organs and lymph nodes associated with the alimentary and respiratory tracts should be collected for virus isolation in suspected cases of "pneumoenteric" forms of EVA in young foals.

Specimens should be collected as soon as possible after the onset of clinical signs or suspected EAV infection. Nasopharyngeal and conjunctival swabs should be immediately placed in transport medium (any cell culture medium or balanced salt solution containing 2% to 5% fetal bovine or calf serum) and either refrigerated or, preferably, frozen at −20° C or lower.[1] All other specimens for virus isolation should be packed in dry ice and dispatched by overnight delivery to an appropriate laboratory, except for blood samples, which should be refrigerated.

Cell culture isolation of EAV is usually done in the rabbit kidney-13 (RK-13) continuous cell line, and development of a cytopathic effect in inoculated cells indicates the presence of virus. The identity of the virus isolate should always be confirmed by immunofluorescence or immunoperoxidase staining or by microneutralization assay with EAV-specific antiserum or monoclonal antibodies.

Histopathologic Examination and Viral Antigen Detection

Tissue samples should be fixed and saved in 10% neutral buffered formalin and submitted for histopathologic and immunohistochemical examination at an appropriate laboratory. Indirect immunohistochemistry is a reliable, powerful, and rapid assay to diagnose EAV infection in tissues and occasionally in skin biopsies.[138] An avidin-biotin complex (ABC) for immunoperoxidase staining using monoclonal antibodies to individual EAV proteins has been successfully used to detect viral antigens in formalin-fixed paraffin-embedded samples, as well as in frozen tissue sections.[118,139,140]

Viral Nucleic Acid Detection

Several reverse transcriptase–polymerase chain reaction (RT-PCR) assays (e.g., standard RT-PCR, RT-nested PCR [RT-nPCR], and real-time RT-PCR [rRT-PCR]) for detection of the EAV nucleic acids in cell culture supernatants and clinical specimens have been developed.[141-147] These assays target different genes (ORFs 1b, 3, 4, 5, 6, and 7), and their sensitivity and specificity vary considerably. The sensitivity of RT-PCR–based assays is significantly increased by using either RT-nPCR that incorporate two primers pairs specific for ORF 1b or real-time TaqMan RT-PCR that uses primers and a probe specific for a highly conserved region of ORF7.[148,149] Several potential advantages exist with RT-PCR–based assays over the current VI procedure. VI is currently the OIE-approved gold standard for the detection of EAV in semen and is the prescribed test for international trade. However, it has been demonstrated that at least one of the rRT-PCR assays described in the literature has an equal to or higher sensitivity than VI for the detection of EAV nucleic acid in semen samples.[148]

Serologic Diagnosis

Serologic diagnosis of EVA is based on virus microneutralization and is standardized by the World Organization for Animal Health (OIE) and described in the OIE manual.[150] The assay is performed in the presence of guinea pig complement, and the CVL-Weybridge strain of EAV is used as the challenge virus in most laboratories.[151] Carrier stallions usually have very high titers of serum neutralization antibody. For serologic diagnosis

of acute EAV infection, acute and convalescent sera (paired serum samples) should be collected at a 21-day to 28-day interval, and a fourfold or greater increase in serum antibody titer is indicative of seroconversion (or <4 to ≥1:4 change in antibody titer). Recent investigation demonstrates that the use of specific commercial inactivated EHV-1 vaccines induce serum cytotoxicity that can interfere with accurate interpretation of the virus neutralization test (VNT), although this potential problem currently appears to affect European more than North American horses.[152] Several laboratories have developed and evaluated enzyme-linked immunosorbent assays (ELISAs) to detect antibodies to EAV using whole virus, synthetic peptides, or recombinant viral proteins (e.g., GP5, M, and N) as antigens. Various studies have shown that the source of antigen, as well as the sera evaluated, can markedly influence the results obtained with EAV protein-specific ELISAs and competitive ELISAs. However, none of these ELISAs or a recently described microsphere immunoassay (Luminex) has yet been shown to be of equivalent sensitivity and specificity to the VNT[153-160] so that none has yet gained widespread acceptance. The microneutralization assay remains the "gold standard" for detection of serum antibodies to EAV.

Pathology

Descriptions of the gross and histopathologic lesions of EVA are based on examination of material derived from horses that were experimentally inoculated with the virulent Bucyrus strain of EAV or from natural outbreaks of EVA.* Of great importance, the highly virulent, horse-adapted strain of EAV causes a very severe and often fatal infection that is not representative of the disease caused by field strains of the virus. Common gross necropsy findings in horses inoculated with the Bucyrus strain of EAV include edema, congestion, and hemorrhage in subcutaneous tissues, lymph nodes, and viscera of the thoracic and abdominal cavities, and pulmonary edema and pleural and pericardial effusion can be spectacular in fulminant cases. These gross lesions result from severe panvasculitis, with especially severe histopathologic changes in medium and small muscular arteries throughout the body, including hemorrhage, edema, and necrosis of vessel walls, with accompanying infiltration of lymphocytes and neutrophils. Similar necrosis and accumulation of inflammatory cells occurs in and around thin-walled vessels (veins and lymphatics). Vascular thrombosis and associated tissue infarction may be present in the lungs, adrenal glands, and large intestine, along with extensive lymphoid necrosis in the germinal centers of the bronchiolar and mesenteric lymph nodes. Sinuses of the bronchial lymph nodes may contain unusual, large, pleomorphic cells that resemble reactive histiocytes. Severe, diffuse interstitial lymphocytic nephritis with tubular necrosis has also been described in severe cases of EVA.[139]

The distribution of EAV antigen in infected tissues has been evaluated by both immunofluorescence and immunoperoxidase staining.[104,118,139] Equine arteritis virus antigen was localized to endothelium lining vessels of all calibers and types (Fig. 15-6). Macrophages in lymph nodes and many other organs were also infected. Viral antigen was demonstrated in the tunica media of infected arteries, as well as the renal tubular epithelium.[139] Immunoperoxidase staining of frozen sections of placenta and fetal tissues demonstrated that viral antigen was localized to the cytoplasm of a very limited number of cell types, including endothelial cells in arteries, veins, and lymphatics; trophoblast

---

*References 1, 6, 7, 96, 100, 103, 104, 113, 118, 126, 138-140, 161, 162.

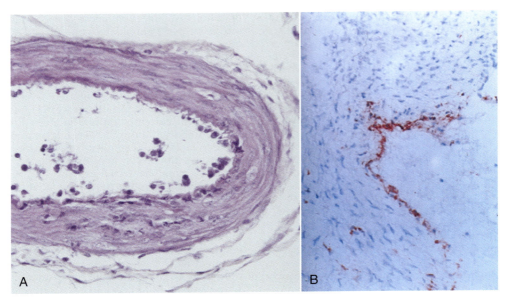

Figure 15-6 A, Medial necrosis of muscular artery, and, **B,** immunohistochemical staining of equine arteritis virus (EAV) antigen in endothelium of vessels in the placenta of EAV-infected fetus.

cells of the chorioallantois; and macrophages in a variety of lymphoreticular tissues.[118,139]

Fetuses aborted after natural or experimental infections of EAV frequently do not show any obvious gross or histopathologic lesions.[5,6,117,125] Fetuses are usually partially autolyzed at expulsion and may have increased peritoneal and pleural fluid, as well as petechial hemorrhages in the mucosal linings of the respiratory and digestive tracts and on the serosal lining of the peritoneal and pleural cavities. The placenta typically is grossly unremarkable and expelled with the fetus. Additional reports[163] described disseminated vascular lesions in the liver, adrenal gland, spleens, kidney, brain, and lymph nodes of two equine fetuses aborted during an outbreak of EVA.[163] The placenta of one fetus had severe vasculitis with necrosis of the arterial walls. Vascular lesions were also described in several tissues of a fetus that was aborted after experimental inoculation of a pregnant mare with the virulent, horse-adapted Bucyrus strain of EAV.[118]

The gross lesions in foals with fatal EVA include diffuse severe pulmonary edema, pleural and pericardial effusion, and petechial and ecchymotic serosal and mucosal hemorrhages in the small intestine.[103,105,106,139] Microscopic lesions include the following[139]:

- Severe interstitial pneumonia with hypertrophic type 2 pneumocytes containing intracytoplasmic EAV antigen, vascular congestion, interlobular and intralobular edema, and extensive infiltration and accumulation of mononuclear inflammatory cells.
- Fibrinoid necrosis of the tunica media of small muscular arteries, associated with EAV antigen in the walls of affected vessels.
- Multifocal hemorrhage and lymphoid depletion in the thymus, spleen, and mesenteric lymph nodes.
- Diffuse, severe edema and multifocal hemorrhages in the intestinal submucosa and serosa.

Lesions have been described in the reproductive tract of prepubertal and peripubertal colts inoculated with EAV.[162] Acute necrotizing vasculitis involving the testis, epididymides, vas deferens, ampullae, prostate, vesicular glands, and bulbourethral glands was present during acute infection (7-14 days after infection). Multifocal accumulations of lymphocytes and plasma cells were present within the ampullae and parenchyma of the reproductive tract after 28 days.

Therapy

As with other animal viral diseases, there is no specific antiviral treatment for horses infected with EAV. Virtually all naturally infected horses recover from EVA uneventfully, although horses with severe clinical signs should be treated symptomatically with nonsteroidal antiinflammatory drugs (NSAIDs), antipyretics to control fever, and diuretics and support wraps to reduce edema.[1,82] Breeding stallions and horses in training should be rested. There is no effective treatment for young foals with EAV-induced interstitial pneumonia or "pneumoenteritis" other than prophylactic administration of antibiotics to counter possible secondary bacterial infections. Also, no consistently effective treatment currently exists to eliminate the carrier state in stallions persistently infected with EAV other than surgical castration. However, the EAV carrier state is clearly testosterone-dependent, and transient suppression of testosterone production in carrier stallions may offer therapeutic promise in the elimination of EAV infection.[1,82,111,164] There are preliminary data to support that gonadotropin-releasing hormone (GnRH) vaccines or antagonists can temporarily limit the shedding of the virus in the semen of carrier stallions. A peptide-conjugated phosphorodiamidate morpholino oligomer (PPMO) targeting the genomic 5' terminus of EAV has been capable of curing HeLa cells persistently infected with EAV under in vitro conditions.[165] The PPMO-cured HeLa cells were free of infectious virus, viral antigen, and EAV nucleic acid as measured by plaque assay, indirect immunofluorescence assay, and rRT-PCR, respectively. These findings demonstrate that PPMOs can be used to eliminate persistent EAV infection in cell culture, although the efficacy of PPMO against EAV in vivo remains to be addressed.

Prevention

Immunity

Both natural and experimental infection of horses with either virulent or avirulent strains of EAV result in long-lasting immunity against reinfection with all strains of the virus, including the most virulent strains.[5,119,132] The humoral immune response to EAV is characterized by the development of both complement-fixing and virus-specific neutralizing antibodies.[166,167] Complement-fixing antibodies develop 1 to 2 weeks after infection, peak after 2 to 3 weeks, and steadily decline to disappear by 8 months, whereas neutralizing antibodies are detected within 1 to 2 weeks after exposure, peak at 2 to 4 months, and persist 3 years or more.[1,121,122,131,167] Foals born to immune mares are protected against clinical EVA by passive transfer of neutralizing antibodies in the colostrum. Neutralizing antibodies appear a few hours after colostrum feeding, peak at 1 week of age, and gradually decline to extinction between 2 to 6, rarely 7, months of age.

The serologic response of horses to the individual structural and nonstructural proteins of EAV varies significantly. Immunoblotting studies have confirmed that infected horses respond to a number of viral structural proteins (N, GP5, and M) and that sera from horses other than carrier stallions most consistently recognized the conserved carboxy-terminal region of the M protein.[168] Similarly, sera from horses experimentally or persistently infected with EAV strongly reacted with nsp2, nsp4, nsp5, and nsp12.[169] However, horses vaccinated with the current modified live virus vaccine did not react with nsp5 and reacted weakly with nsp4. The innate immune response to EAV infection is not fully characterized, but studies have shown that virus inhibits type I interferon (IFN) production in infected cells. Recent studies have demonstrated that nsp1, nsp2, and nsp11 are capable of inhibiting type I IFN activity. Of these three nsps, nsp1 has the strongest inhibitory effect by inhibiting IFN synthesis. The failure to induce type I IFN in EAV infected cells may allow the virus to escape the equine innate immune response.

Minimal information is available on the cellular immune response to EAV in horses. Castillo-Olivares et al[170] described EAV-specific cytotoxic T lymphocyte (CTL) responses using peripheral blood mononuclear cells (PBMCs) from convalescent EAV-infected (experimental) ponies. The data showed that cytotoxicity induced by EAV-stimulated PBMCs was virus specific, genetically restricted, and mediated by CD8+ T cells and that EAV-specific CTL precursors persist for at least 1 year after infection. Further studies are needed to identify the specific viral protein(s) targeted by the CTL response of EAV-infected horses.

Vaccination

A modified live-virus attenuated vaccine (ARVAC, Pfizer Animal Health Inc., Exton, PA) is licensed for use in the United States and Canada for prevention of EAV infection in horses.[1,100,171] A killed-virus vaccine (Artervac, Pfizer Animal Health Inc., Kent, UK) is licensed for use in the UK, Ireland, France, Hungary, and Denmark.

The modified live-virus (MLV) vaccine is administered intramuscularly to horses. A small minority of horses vaccinated with this MLV vaccine develop mild febrile reactions and transient lymphopenia.[172-175] Vaccine virus may be sporadically isolated from the nasopharynx and buffy coat, usually for only about 7 days but rarely up to 32 days after vaccination.[1,100,171] Vaccinated stallions usually do not shed virus in either semen or urine. However, a very low level of virus in the semen of one vaccinated stallion has been recently reported (<1 pfu/mL virus at 4 and 6 days postvaccination [DPV]).[174] Therefore it is recommended not to use semen from first-time vaccinated stallions for artificial insemination purposes before 14 DPV. The MLV vaccine is not recommended for use in pregnant mares, especially during the last 2 months of gestation, or in foals less than 6 weeks of age. Apparent fetal

infections with MLV after vaccination of pregnant mares have been documented but only rarely.[176,177] A recent study has shown that it is safe to vaccinate healthy pregnant mares up to 2 months before foaling and during the immediate postpartum period.[177]

Maternal antibodies to EAV disappear between 2 and 6 months of age[94,178]; thus it is recommended that foals be vaccinated at 6 months of age, before the onset of puberty. Foals can be vaccinated before 6 months of age in high-risk situations, but they should also be revaccinated after 6 months of age. Vaccinated colts are resistant to development of the persistently infected carrier state after subsequent exposure to EAV. The protective immunization of prepubertal colts is therefore central to effective control of the spread of EAV infection.

Virus-neutralizing antibodies are induced within 5 to 8 days after MLV vaccination, and peak antibody titers are achieved by 7 to 14 DPV (maximum mean titer varies between 1:32 and 1:256 occurring during 13 to 14 DPV). Following vaccination neutralizing antibodies will last for at least 2 years.[1,87] Revaccination greatly increases the serologic response of horses, providing protective immunity that persists for several breeding seasons. Although MLV vaccination provides sustained protection against clinical EVA, it does not always prevent reinfection of vaccinated horses or subsequent limited replication of field strains of the virus.[179] Vaccinated mares inseminated with semen from carrier stallions became infected, as evidenced by the transient isolation of virus from buffy coat and nasopharynx, but did not develop EVA. Furthermore, a contact seronegative mare also became infected in this same study, indicating that infectious virus was shed by the vaccinated mares. However, the MLV vaccine has been successfully used to curtail several large-scale outbreaks of EVA in the United States, including the 1984 outbreak in Thoroughbred horses in Kentucky. Since 1984, the MLV vaccine has been extensively used in control programs in several states.

The MLV vaccine is not licensed in either Europe or Japan, and an inactivated (killed) EAV vaccine containing an adjuvant (Artervac) was formulated for use in the UK after an outbreak of EVA in 1993.[180] This vaccine is also administered intramuscularly, and a booster immunization is recommended after 3 to 4 weeks and semiannually thereafter. Although this vaccine induces high titers of neutralizing antibodies, its ability to prevent EVA and persistent infection of stallions is less characterized than that of the MLV vaccine. Experimental EAV vaccines have also been developed recently using recombinant DNA technology, but none of these vaccines have reached the market.[122,181]

Husbandry and Control Programs

There is no established domestic EVA control program in the United States. However, the recent publication from the United States Department of Agriculture (USDA) Animal and Plant Health Inspection Service (APHIS), *Equine Viral Arteritis: Uniform Methods and Rules*, describes the minimum standards for detecting, controlling, and preventing EVA, as well as minimum EVA requirements for the interstate and intrastate movement of horses.[182] The EAV carrier stallion is the essential natural reservoir of the virus and has a pivotal role in the transmission and maintenance of EAV infection in horse populations.[1,86] Therefore outbreaks of EVA can be prevented by the identification of persistently infected stallions and the institution of management practices to prevent the introduction of EAV-infected horses (Fig. 15-7).

All stallions should be tested for EAV antibodies before they are vaccinated with the MLV or inactivated EVA vaccines. A neutralization antibody titer of 1:4 or greater (titer ≥1:4) is

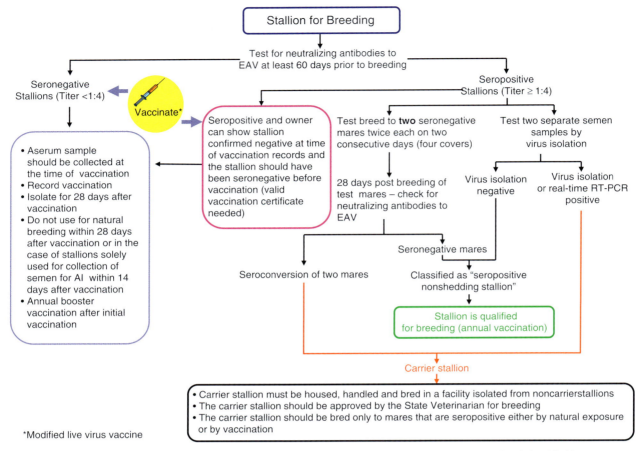

Figure 15-7 Flowchart outlining the guidelines for breeding stallions for the prevention and control of equine viral arteritis (EVA). *(Modified from U.S. Department of Agriculture [USDA], Animal and Plant Health Inspection Service [APHIS]: Equine viral arteritis: uniform methods and rules, effective April 19, 2004.)*

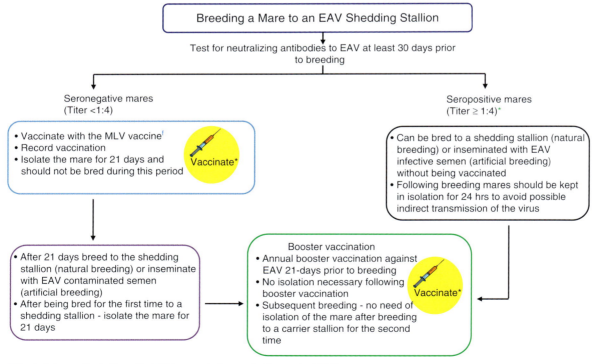

Figure 15-8 Flowchart outlining the guidelines for breeding a mare to an equine arteritis virus (EAV)–shedding stallion for prevention and control of equine viral arteritis (EVA). *(Modified from U.S. Department of Agriculture [USDA], Animal and Plant Health Inspection Service [APHIS]: Equine viral arteritis: uniform methods and rules, effective April 19, 2004.)*

regarded as positive. If seronegative stallions are vaccinated, they should be vaccinated 28 days before the breeding season or semen collection and receive an annual booster. Vaccinated stallions should be isolated for 28 days after vaccination and receive boosters annually. Nonvaccinated seropositive stallions should be tested for virus shedding by VI or rRT-PCR or by test breeding to seronegative mares (at least two) that are monitored for seroconversion at 14 and 28 days after breeding. There is no need for vaccination of stallions that are seropositive as a result of natural infection. Young fillies and geldings benefit from vaccination before going to the track or to any environment with the potential for exposure to EAV. Vaccination of colts 6 to 12 months of age is done to prevent the future establishment of the carrier state in these animals[108,111,164] and thereby reduce the natural reservoir of EAV, which is especially important in breeds in which the infection is prevalent (e.g., Standardbreds, Warmbloods).

Stallions that are confirmed semen shedders and carriers of EAV can be used for breeding purposes provided that stringent requirements are met (Fig. 15-8).[1,3,73,86,183] Carrier stallions should be kept physically isolated and bred only to mares that are seropositive from either previous natural exposure or vaccination (no less than 3 weeks previously). Mares should be kept isolated from other nonvaccinated or seronegative horses for 3 weeks after being bred to a shedding stallion or after insemination with infective semen. It is also critical that carrier stallions be isolated and collected separately to prevent contamination of collection equipment, teasers, and premises with ejaculate because EAV can be transmitted to susceptible horses by indirect aerosol contact. When embryo transfer is used for breeding, it is highly recommended that both donor and recipient mares be vaccinated against EVA if the former are to be bred with EAV-infective semen.[102]

If an outbreak of EVA on a farm is suspected based on clinical signs and history, the state veterinarian should be notified, affected and in-contact horses isolated, movement of horses on and off the farm discontinued, at-risk horses vaccinated, and breeding activity stopped to prevent further spread of the virus. Diagnosis of EVA should be confirmed by laboratory testing as soon as possible. Stalls and equipment on the affected premises should be decontaminated with disinfectants; EAV is susceptible to phenolic, chlorine, iodine, and quaternary ammonium compounds. Quarantine is discontinued when no additional clinical cases of EVA or serologic evidence of infection are observed for 3 to 4 weeks.

Public Health Considerations

Equine arteritis virus (EAV) is a pathogen only of equids. There is no evidence indicating that it can infect humans.

Acknowledgments

The author gratefully acknowledges the advice, assistance, and intellectual input he has received over many years of productive collaborative research with Dr. Peter J. Timoney and the late Dr. William H. McCollum of the Maxwell H. Gluck Equine Research Center, University of Kentucky, and Dr. N. James MacLachlan at the Department of Veterinary Pathology, Microbiology and Immunology, School of Veterinary Medicine University of California, Davis.

The complete reference list is available online at www.expertconsult.com.

CHAPTER

16 African Horse Sickness

Maureen T. Long and Alan J. Guthrie*

African horse sickness (AHS) is a noncontagious, infectious, insect-borne disease of equids caused by African horse sickness virus (AHSV). In horses, the course of the disease is usually peracute to acute, and more than 90% of immunologically naïve animals die. Clinically, AHS is characterized by pyrexia; edema of the lungs, pleura, and subcutaneous tissues; and hemorrhages on the serosal surfaces of internal organs. Mules are less susceptible than horses and donkeys, and zebras rarely show clinical signs of disease.

An Arabic document reports the first known historical reference to a disease resembling AHS occurring in Yemen in 1327.[1] In 1569, Father Monclaro's description of the travels of Francisco Baro in East Africa reported AHS disease in horses imported from India.[1,2] Horses and donkeys, which are nonindigenous to Africa, were introduced to the southern region of the continent shortly after the arrival of the first settlers of the Dutch East India Company in the Cape of Good Hope in 1652.[1] Records of the Dutch East India Company frequently refer to "perreziekte" or "pardeziekte" in the Cape of Good Hope.[2] In 1719, almost 1700 horses died from AHS in the Cape. During the exploration and expansion into the interior of southern Africa, the Voortrekkers reported severe losses among their horses.[1] Exploration of southern, central, and East Africa by Livingstone was complicated by his inability to use horses on some of his journeys.[2] Although horses die as a result of AHS every year in southern Africa, major epizootics before the 1950s occurred about every 20 to 30 years. Severe losses were reported in 1780, 1801, 1839, 1855, 1862, 1891, 1914, 1918, 1923, 1940, 1946, and 1953.[1] The 1854-1855 epizootic was the most severe, with almost 70,000 horses dying, representing more than 40% of the horse population of the Cape of Good Hope.[3]

Initially, AHS was confused with anthrax and piroplasmosis. In the early 1900s, M'Fadyean,[4] Theiler, Nocard, and Sieber[1] all

*The authors acknowledge and appreciate the original contributions of these authors, whose work has been incorporated into this chapter.

succeeded in transmitting the disease with a bacteria-free filtrate of blood from infected horses, confirming disease causation by a virus. The pioneering research of Sir Arnold Theiler, who founded the Veterinary Research Institute at Onderstepoort in 1908, revealed the plurality of "immunologically distinct strains" of AHSV because immunity acquired against one "strain" did not always afford protection against infection by "heterologous strains."[2,5-8] Alexander[9,10] showed that viscerotropic isolates of AHSV became neurotropic but did not lose their immunogenicity after serial intracerebral passage in mice. This work led to the development of the first polyvalent vaccine against AHS in the 1930s.[11,12] Although Pitchford and Theiler[13] proposed in 1903 that AHS may be transmitted by biting insects, it was not until 1944 that Du Toit[14] confirmed that *Culicoides* species were likely vectors of both AHS and bluetongue viruses.

In endemic areas, severe losses caused by AHS have ceased since the development of polyvalent vaccine. However, the occurrence of epizootics in countries outside the endemic regions in Africa[15-17] serve as a warning that AHS may spread to areas traditionally free of the disease. AHS is one of the important diseases to consider when moving equids internationally, but movement can be accomplished safely by following appropriate quarantine and testing procedures.[18,19]

Etiology

AHSV is a member of the genus *Orbivirus* in the family Reoviridae and as such is morphologically similar to other orbiviruses such as bluetongue virus (BTV) of ruminants and equine encephalosis virus (EEV; see Chapter 26).[20,21] The virion is not enveloped and is about 70 nm in diameter. It consists of a two-layered icosahedral capsid composed of 32 capsomeres.[22] The genome comprises 10 double-stranded ribonucleic acid (RNA) segments, each of which encodes at least one polypeptide.[23] The core particle comprises two major proteins, VP3 and VP7, which are highly conserved among the nine AHSV serotypes, and three minor proteins, VP1, VP4, and VP6.[22,24] Together these proteins make up the group-specific epitopes.[25] The core particle is surrounded by the outer capsid, which is composed of two proteins, VP2 and VP5. VP2 is the protein responsible for antigenic variation.[26-28] At least three nonstructural proteins have been identified in infected cells (NS1, NS2, and NS3/3a).[29-31]

Nine antigenically distinct serotypes have been described.[32,33] Although there may be some cross-relatedness between the serotypes, there is no field evidence of any intratypic variation.[32,33] All nine serotypes have been documented in eastern[34] and southern[32,33,35] Africa, whereas serotype 9 is more widespread and appears to predominate in the northern parts of sub-Saharan Africa.[36,37]

Epidemiology

AHSV is biologically transmitted by *Culicoides* spp., of which *C. imicola* and *C. bolitinos* have been shown to play an important role in Africa.[38,39] Recently, other *Culicoides* spp. were investigated for their susceptibility to virus infection and vectorial capacity in addition to *C. imicola* and *C. bolitinos*.[40] In this study, it was shown that vectorial capacity is highly variable and depends on virus strain; season; abundance of vector, in addition to susceptibility of the insect to virus infection; and virus load. Although there was high variability in this capacity, virus was successfully recovered from one additional Avaritia *Culicoides* species and nine other non-Avaritia *Culicoides* species. Although

many of these had low virus titer and overall recovery, for the avian feeder, *C. leucostictus*, the virus could be recovered during different annual cycles at high rates. The disease therefore has a seasonal occurrence, and its prevalence is influenced by climatic and other conditions that favor the breeding of *Culicoides* spp. *C. variipennis*, a midge prevalent in the United States but not present in Africa, has been shown to transmit AHSV under laboratory conditions.[41] Although other insects have been suggested as possible vectors of AHSV, none has been shown to play a role under natural conditions. Biting flies may play a minor role in the mechanical transmission of AHS; however, because the viremia in horses is relatively low and AHSV is susceptible to desiccation and high temperature, this method of transmission is inefficient. AHSV can be transmitted between horses by parenteral inoculation of infective blood or organ suspensions, and it is more readily transmitted by the intravenous than by the subcutaneous route.[1]

A continuous transmission cycle of AHSV between *Culicoides* midges and zebras was shown to exist in the Kruger National Park in South Africa.[42] Under such circumstances, a sufficiently large zebra population can act as a reservoir for the virus.[43-45] Donkeys may play a similar role in parts of Africa with large donkey populations.[46] In view of the high mortality in horses, this species is regarded as an accidental or indicator host. Animals that have been infected with AHSV do not remain carriers of the virus, which explains the failure of the disease to become established outside tropical Africa, despite the occurrence of many outbreaks outside endemic areas.[1]

AHS is endemic in eastern and central Africa[2] and spreads regularly to southern Africa. In endemic areas, different serotypes of AHS may be active simultaneously, but one serotype usually dominates during a particular season. The disease is also reported from time to time in countries in North Africa, from where it has occasionally extended into the Middle East and Spain.[47,48] However, its intrusion into North Africa and countries around the Mediterranean and in Asia is impeded by the Sahara desert.[49] AHS has not been recorded in Madagascar or Mauritius.

AHS was recorded in Egypt in 1928, 1943, 1953, 1958, and 1971[50]; in Yemen in 1930; and in Palestine, Syria, Lebanon, and Jordan in 1944.[47,51-53] In 1959, AHS serotype 9 occurred in the southeastern regions of Iran. This was followed by outbreaks during 1960 in Cyprus, Iraq, Syria, Lebanon, and Jordan, as well as in Afghanistan, Pakistan, India, and Turkey. Between 1959 and 1961, this region lost more than 300,000 equids.[53,54] In 1965, AHS occurred in Libya, Tunisia, Algeria, and Morocco and subsequently spread to Spain in 1966.[55] Between 1987 and 1990, AHS serotype 4 occurred in Spain, with the source of infection being zebras *(Equus burchelli)* imported from Namibia.[16,17] AHS was also confirmed in southern Portugal in 1989 and Morocco between 1989 and 1991, with these outbreaks being extensions of the outbreak in Spain.[16,55] In 1989 an outbreak of AHS serotype 9 occurred in Saudi Arabia.[15] AHS was also reported in Saudi Arabia and Yemen in 1997 and on the Cape Verde Islands in 1999.

AHS can be distributed over great distances if equids incubating the disease are translocated by land, sea, or air.[17,57] Outbreaks have also been reported to result from wind-borne spread of infected vectors.[58]

AHS appears in the northeastern part of South Africa, in December or January and spreads southward. The extent of the southerly spread is influenced by the presence of favorable climatic conditions for the breeding of *Culicoides* midges.[49] Early and heavy rains followed by warm, dry spells favor the occurrence of epizootics. Although parts of the inland plateau of South Africa and most of the Cape Province are usually free of AHS, the disease has sometimes extended into these areas and caused serious losses. Significant losses were reported at

Belfast, a town situated about 2100 meters (8000 feet) above sea level during the severe epizootic of 1923.[59] The first cases of AHS usually occur at the beginning of February, but the most serious outbreaks usually occur in March and April. Following the first frosts, which usually occur at the end of April or in May, the disease disappears abruptly. However, in the northeastern parts of South Africa, where the occurrence of frost is less common, deaths may continue to occur into May and June.[1] In recent years the southerly spread of AHS has been less extensive, probably as a result of the widespread use of a more effective vaccine, which became available in 1974.[49] Approximately 300,000 doses of polyvalent AHS vaccine are sold annually by Onderstepoort Biological Products. It is speculated that immunization of horses in these regions establishes a fairly effective "immune barrier" that seems to impede the southerly spread of the disease.[49] Outbreaks of AHS associated with the introduction of infected animals have been reported in the Cape Peninsula in 1967,[49] 1990,[60] 1999,[61] and 2004.

The emergence and re-emergence of AHSV has caused large outbreaks of disease in new populations since 2005.[62] In Ethiopia, which has 42% of the African equid population, 5.2 million donkeys, 2.8 million horses, and 0.6 million mules reside and are vital for transportation of both people and goods.[62,63] Confirmed outbreaks have occurred in 1999, 2004, and 2008. Prior to 2005, the predominant serotypes were AHSV-6 and AHSV-9 and the outbreak in 2008 consisted of AHSV-2. AHSV-2 and AHSV-7 were associated with the outbreak in Senegal in 2007.[64] Also during 2007, an outbreak reported in Nigeria was caused by AHSV-2. AHSV-9 has been circulating in West Africa, and following an outbreak in 2007, two vaccines using a live-attenuated AHSV-9 were used to vaccinate horses.[65] Recent sampling conducted in 2009 demonstrated 956 of equids were seropositive, and the circulating strain appeared to be 100% similar to a gene segment (2) of the live-attenuated AHSV-9 strain.[65]

AHS affects primarily equine animals. Horses are most susceptible to the disease (mortality of 70%-95%), but mules are less so (mortality of 50%-70%). Most infections of donkeys and zebras are subclinical.[2,47] Generally, horses of all breeds are equally susceptible to AHS, but variation in susceptibility to the same virus in individual horses has been reported.[2] Some indigenous horses in North and West Africa, which descend from animals that have been present there since at least 2000 BC, have apparently acquired natural resistance to AHS.[66] Foals born to immune mares acquire passive immunity by the ingestion of colostrum.[67] This passive immunity progressively declines and is completely lost after about 4 to 6 months. Donkeys in the Middle East appear to be more susceptible to AHS (mortality of 3%-10%) than southern African donkeys.[47] Zebras are highly resistant to AHS and only show a mild fever after experimental infection.[68]

Serosurveys conducted in association with recent outbreaks demonstrate that in vaccinated animals, around 30% of horses and mules remain seropositive while approximately 50% of donkeys are positive reflecting more subclinical infection in donkeys.[63] There is no difference associated with age or sex of animals.[63] Presence of AHS is highly associated with environmental factors that support vector density.[40,69-72] These include warm, moist climates; there are different associations with elevation, depending on the part of Africa and the association of habitat with Culicoides breeding habitat. Each habitat may favor a particular vector. For instance, C. bolitinos, as a vector, allows transmission in cooler, drier climates because it will breed in bovine dung.

Dogs are the only other species that contract a highly fatal form of AHS.[73-76] All reported clinical cases in dogs have resulted from the ingestion of infected carcass material from horses that have died from AHS.[77,78] AHSV-9 has been isolated from the blood of stray dogs in Egypt,[50] and antibodies to AHSV have been detected in the sera of dogs in India[79] and South Africa.[80] However, it is doubtful that dogs play any role in the spread or maintenance of AHSV because Culicoides spp. do not readily feed on them.[80] Besides zebras,[68,81-83] no other wildlife or domestic ruminants have been shown to play a significant role in the epidemiology of AHS.

Pathogenesis

After infection, initial multiplication of AHSV occurs in the regional lymph nodes and is followed by a primary viremia,[84] with subsequent dissemination to endothelial cells of target organs.[85] Effusions into body cavities and edematous changes of various tissues, as well as serosal and visceral hemorrhages, are consistent with endothelial cell damage. In experimental cases of AHS, high virus concentrations are found in the spleen, lungs, cecum, pharynx, choroid plexus, and most lymph nodes by the second day after inoculation. This precedes the onset of fever or detectable viremia. By the third day after inoculation, virus is present in most organs. Virus multiplication at these sites gives rise to a secondary viremia of variable duration. In horses the viremia is generally not higher than 10^5 TCID$_{50}$/mL and lasts 4 to 8 days but does not exceed 21 days. In donkeys and zebras the viremia is lower but may last as long as 4 weeks.[84] In zebras, viremia has been reported in the presence of circulating antibodies.[68]

The factors determining the course and severity of infection are not well understood. Small plaque variants produce severe clinical reactions, whereas large plaque variants of AHSV are less pathogenic.[84] Fully susceptible horses, such as foals that have lost their colostral immunity or horses that have never been exposed to AHSV, usually develop the peracute "pulmonary" form of AHS. Exercise during the febrile stage of the disease may also precipitate this form of AHS.[51,84] During the 1959 Middle East epizootic of AHS caused by serotype 9, severe myocardial lesions with extensive areas of degeneration and necrosis of myocytes, accompanied by a marked inflammatory response, were described in fully susceptible horses, particularly those with the "cardiac" form of the disease.[86] In this form of AHS, heart failure is attributed to hydropericardium[84,87] and myocardial damage.[86] However, most natural cases of AHS are of the "mixed" form, with evidence of both pulmonary and cardiac compromise.[48,84,86] Irrespective of serotype, the main targets for AHSV include heart, lung, and spleen.[88] Within these organs, microvascular endothelial cells and monocytic lineage cells support viral replication. Clinical virulence has been associated with the in vitro ability of the virus to create a cytopathic effect (CPE) in endothelial cells,[89] which includes cell swelling and eventual lysis. In addition, AHSV also induces apoptosis within mammalian cells.[90] The actual virus protein that mediates viral CPE is not known; however, modifications in the NS3 protein can modify virus load and release from the cell.[89] Modifications in these and other gene segments likely come from reassortment of different strains of viruses when the mosquito host is simultaneously infected with two or more strains of virus.[91]

Clinical Findings

The clinical findings of natural and experimental cases of AHS have been described.[17,86,92-94] In experimental cases the incubation period is usually between 5 and 7 days, but possibly as short as 2 days and rarely as long as 10 days. The duration of the incubation period depends on the virulence of the virus and the dose of virus received.

"Dunkop" or "Pulmonary" Form

The "dunkop" or "pulmonary" form is the peracute form of AHS, and recovery is the exception. This form of AHS occurs when AHSV infects fully susceptible horses. In endemic areas, it is also common in foals that have lost their maternally derived passive immunity. Dunkop is also the usual form in dogs that become infected after ingestion of AHSV-infected carcass material.

The incubation period for pulmonary AHS is short, usually 3 to 4 days, and is followed by a rapid rise in temperature over 1 or 2 days, with the body temperature reaching 104° F to 106° F (40° C-41° C). The dunkop form is characterized by marked and rapidly progressive respiratory failure, and the respiratory rate may exceed 50 breaths per minute. The animal tends to stand with its forelegs spread apart, its head extended, and the nostrils dilated. Expiration is frequently forced, with the presence of abdominal heave lines. Profuse sweating is common, and paroxysmal coughing may be observed terminally, often with frothy, serofibrinous fluid exuding from the nostrils (Fig. 16-1). The onset of dyspnea is usually very sudden, and death occurs within 30 minutes to a few hours of its appearance. Sometimes, an apparently healthy horse at work becomes listless, suddenly severely dyspneic, and dies shortly thereafter. Initially, the appetite of affected animals remains good despite the high fever and respiratory distress. The prognosis for horses with the dunkop form is extremely poor (<5% recover). If animals recover, the fever subsides gradually, but the breathing remains labored for several days.

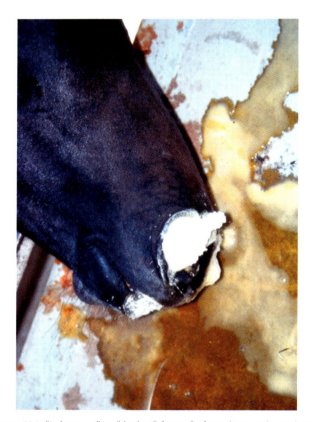

Figure 16-1 "Pulmonary" or "dunkop" form of African horse sickness (AHS), with froth and serous fluid at nostrils caused by severe alveolar edema.

"Dikkop" or "Cardiac" Form

The incubation period in the "dikkop" or "cardiac" form of AHS is longer than the "dunkop" (pulmonary) form, usually 5 to 7 days, followed by a fever of 102° F to 106° F (39° C-41° C) that persists for 3 to 4 days. The more typical clinical signs do not appear until the fever has begun to decline. At first the supraorbital fossae fill as the underlying adipose tissue becomes edematous and raises the skin well above the level of the zygomatic arch (Figs. 16-2 and 16-3). The edema can later extend to the conjunctiva (Fig. 16-4), lips, cheeks, tongue, intermandibular space, and laryngeal region and may extend a variable distance down the neck toward the chest, often obliterating the jugular groove. As the swellings increase, dyspnea and cyanosis may supervene. However, ventral edema and edema of the lower limbs are not observed. Unfavorable prognostic signs include petechial hemorrhages on the conjunctivae and on the ventral surface of the tongue; if they occur, these hemorrhages become evident shortly before death. Some animals may show signs of severe colic, repeatedly lie down, are restless when standing, and frequently paw the ground.

The course of the dikkop form of AHS is always more protracted and milder than in the dunkop form, with mortality greater than 50%. Death usually occurs within 4 to 8 days after the onset of the febrile reaction. In horses that recover, swellings gradually subside over 3 to 8 days. Paralysis of the esophagus may be a complication, particularly in patients with severe edematous swellings of the head, resulting in dysphagia.[94] In severely affected animals, the esophagus becomes distended, and animals may die from foreign body pneumonia. Equine piroplasmosis is a common complication of AHS during recovery.[1,95] In such horses, icterus, anemia, and impaction are evident.

"Mixed" Form

Although the most common form of AHS, the "mixed" form, is rarely diagnosed clinically, it is seen at necropsy in the majority

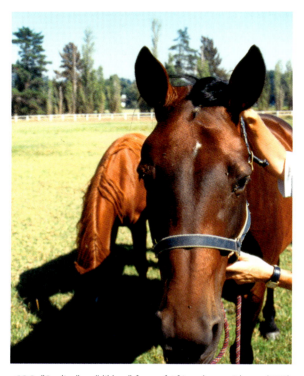

Figure 16-2 "Cardiac" or "dikkop" form of African horse sickness (AHS), with filling of supraorbital fossae.

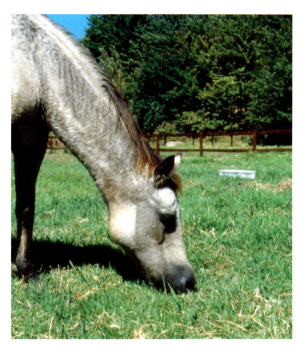

Figure 16-3 Severe edema of head associated with cardiac form of African horse sickness (AHS).

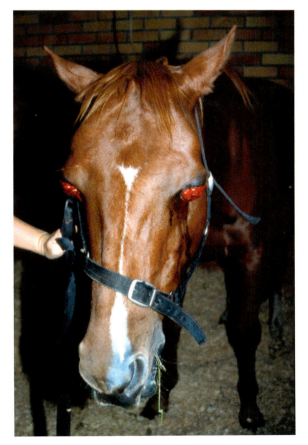

Figure 16-4 Severe conjunctival edema and hyperemia with some hemorrhage in horse with African horse sickness (AHS).

of fatal cases of AHS in horses and mules. Initial pulmonary signs that are mild and not progressive are followed by edematous swelling and effusions, and death results from cardiac failure. More often, the subclinical cardiac form is suddenly followed by marked dyspnea and other signs typical of the pulmonary form. Death usually occurs 3 to 6 days after the onset of the febrile reaction.

Horsesickness Fever

Horsesickness fever is the mildest form of AHS and is frequently not diagnosed clinically. The incubation period is between 5 and 9 days, after which the temperature gradually rises over 4 to 5 days to 104° F (40° C), followed by a drop in temperature to normal, then recovery. Apart from the febrile reaction, other clinical signs are rare and inconspicuous. Some animals may be depressed with partial loss of appetite, congestion of the conjunctivae, slightly labored breathing, and increased heart rate, but these signs are transient. Horsesickness fever is usually observed in donkeys and zebras or in immune horses infected with a heterologous serotype of AHSV.

Diagnosis

Diagnosis of AHS is virtually impossible during the early febrile phase of the disease. Hematologic abnormalities include leukopenia, thrombocytopenia, and elevated hematocrit, erythrocyte count, and hemoglobin concentration. Hemostatic abnormalities include increased concentration of fibrin degradation products and prolonged prothrombin, activated partial thromboplastin, and thrombin clotting times.[96] A presumptive diagnosis should be possible once the characteristic clinical signs have developed. The typical macroscopic lesions of AHS on necropsy are often sufficiently specific to allow a provisional diagnosis of the disease.

The clinical signs of AHS may be confused with those of equine encephalosis (see Chapter 26). Many of the epidemiologic features of the two infections are similar. Horses with swelling of the supraorbital fossae, eyelids, or lips as a result of equine encephalosis cannot be differentiated clinically from the "cardiac" form of AHS. However, mortality from AHS is much higher than from equine encephalosis. Virus isolation and identification are essential to confirm either diagnosis.

The disseminated petechiation associated with the cardiac form of AHS may be similar to that found in animals with purpura hemorrhagica and equine viral arteritis. However, the subcutaneous edema observed in these conditions tends to be more ventral than that observed in animals with AHS. In purpura hemorrhagica the hemorrhages tend to be more severe, numerous, and widespread than in AHS. The early stages of piroplasmosis may occasionally be confused with AHS. AHS may also be complicated by piroplasmosis, and ventral edema may be severe in these horses.

AHS is foreign to almost all countries outside of sub-Saharan Africa and is an Office International des Epizooties (OIE)-listed disease. Suspected cases of AHS must therefore be reported to the State Veterinary Authority and must always be subject to laboratory confirmation. Virus isolation is still the gold standard, although recent work has indicated the reliability of both antigen enzyme-linked immunosorbent assays (ELISAs) and polymerase chain reaction (PCR) to detect AHSV in blood and tissues.[97-104] In May 2012 the World Assembly of Delegates of the OIE amended the Terrestrial Animal Health Code and Terrestrial Manual to accept tests for PCR detection of virus and the competitive ELISA for serology (see http://www.oie.int). Blood samples collected in heparin during the febrile stage of the disease or specimens of the lungs, spleen, and lymph nodes collected at necropsy and kept at 4° C (39.2° F) can be used for virus detection.[105]

Primary virus isolation can be performed using a variety of cell cultures (BHK21, Vero, or MS cells)[50,53,106,107] or by intracerebral inoculation of suckling mice.[105] Cytopathic effects (CPE) characterized by increased refractivity and detachment of cells can appear 3 to 7 days after inoculation of cultures but may only become conspicuous in the second passage. After three passages, advanced CPEs develop within 2 to 4 days.[105] Serotyping of AHSV isolates is performed using virus neutralization (VN) tests employing type-specific antisera in mice[33,108] or more often on various cell cultures.[109,110]

Group-specific antibody to AHSV can be detected by using complement fixation (CF),[35,105,111] agar gel immunodiffusion (AGID),[105,111] indirect fluorescent antibody (IFA),[111,112] and ELISA tests.[16,105,111,113,114] Serotype-specific antibody to AHSV can be detected using serum neutralizing tests.[35,105,111] CF antibody titers are of short duration,[35,51] whereas neutralizing and ELISA antibodies persist for a number of years.[115] The recombinant protein of VP7 is highly conserved across serotype of virus and is a main target for development of rapid ELISAs.[116] Monoclonal antibodies to this target have been used to develop a reliable competitive inhibition ELISA that is now recommended for international trade.[117]

Several PCR assays[118-121] have been described to detect AHSV and to differentiate between serotypes.[122,123] PCR-based assays are rapid, sensitive, and versatile and may supplement or replace some of the older conventional methods. The recent validation of type specific real-time PCR tests has allowed development of high throughput, and these have demonstrated good correlation, sensitivity and specificity compared to virus isolation and virus neutralization testing, even though some assays perform better than others.[124-127] These PCR assays primarily target viral segments 5 or 7. Although these tests detect all of the serotypes, not all genetic variants within a serotype can be differentiated.[127] Furthermore, PCR can be applied to specimens from clinical cases that do not contain live virus such as formalin-fixed and other archived tissues. Antigen-capture ELISAs that detect antigen in mammalian and insect tissue homogenates and cell culture have also been reported.[60,128,129]

Pathologic Findings

Macroscopic Pathology

"Dunkop" or "Pulmonary" Form

The most striking finding in the pulmonary form of AHS is diffuse, severe, subpleural, and interlobular edema of the lungs (Fig. 16-5). The lungs do not collapse on opening of the thorax and are heavier than normal. Severe hydrothorax is common, with the pleural cavity containing several liters of transparent, pale-yellow, gelatinous fluid. Subcutaneous and intermuscular edema is usually absent. Edema may also involve the mediastinum, base of the heart, and the parietal pleura. Serous fluid oozes from the cut surface of the lung. The trachea and bronchi usually contain large amounts of froth and yellow serous fluid (Fig. 16-6). Petechiae and ecchymoses are sometimes present on the mucosa of the trachea. The bronchial and mediastinal lymph nodes are severely swollen and edematous. The spleen is normal in size, with the white pulp more prominent than usual. Moderate, diffuse congestion of the mucosa of the glandular part of the stomach is a consistent finding (Fig. 16-7). Patchy congestion of the serosal surface of the small intestine and scattered petechiation on the intestinal serosa are common. There is usually some degree of ascites.

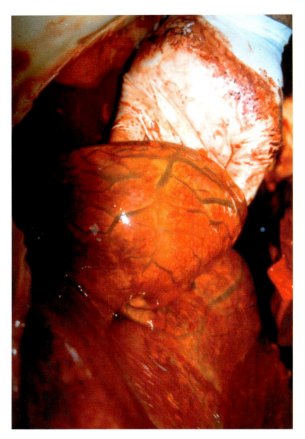

Figure 16-5 Severe septal edema of lungs associated with "pulmonary" or "dunkop" form of African horse sickness (AHS).

"Dikkop" or "Cardiac" Form

The most characteristic finding in the cardiac form of AHS is the presence of distinctly yellow edema of the subcutaneous and intermuscular connective tissues. The edema is particularly severe around the ligamentum nuchae. In mild cases, only the head and neck are involved, but in severe cases the edema involves the lower parts of the neck, the thorax, and shoulders. The eyelids, supraorbital fossae, and lips are often involved. The tongue may have petechiae or ecchymoses on its ventral surface and is occasionally swollen and cyanotic. Severe hydropericardium is almost invariably present. Subepicardial petechiation and subendocardial ecchymoses, particularly over the papillary muscles, are usually present (Fig. 16-8). Pale-gray areas of varying size may occur in the myocardium of horses with severe myocardial damage. The lungs are usually normal or slightly congested, and hydrothorax is rare. The lymph nodes are swollen and edematous. Mild nephrosis may be present. Moderate to severe edema, congestion, and petechiation of the mucosa of the cecum, colon, and rectum are common (Fig. 16-9). In horses with esophageal paralysis, the esophagus is distended with a variable amount of compressed food.

"Mixed" Form

Lesions described for the pulmonary and cardiac forms of AHS and edematous infiltration are found together in animals that die of the mixed form of the disease.

Microscopic Pathology

In horses with pulmonary involvement, widening of the interlobular septa and locally extensive pockets of alveolar edema

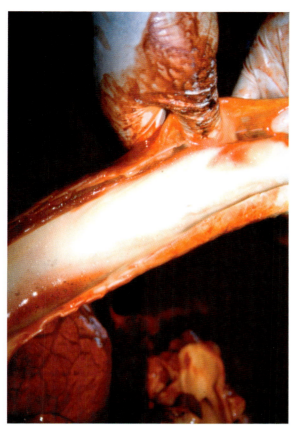

Figure 16-6 Froth and serous fluid in trachea in horse with pulmonary form of African horse sickness (AHS).

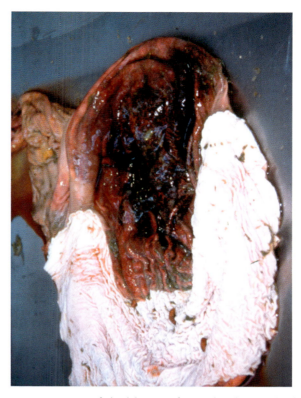

Figure 16-7 Congestion of glandular part of stomach in horse with African horse sickness (AHS).

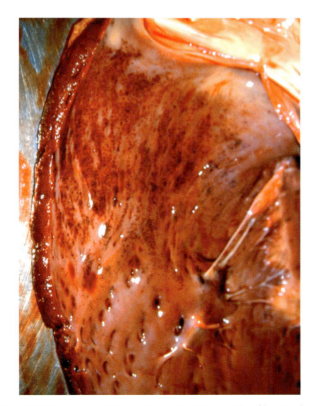

Figure 16-8 Subendocardial hemorrhages in right ventricle of heart in horse with "dikkop" or "cardiac" form of African horse sickness (AHS).

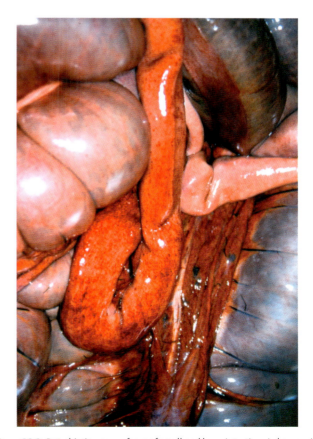

Figure 16-9 Petechiation on surfaces of small and large intestines in horse with African horse sickness (AHS).

are the predominant findings.[86,93,130] Perivasculitis, characterized by edematous separation of the adventitial connective tissue of medium-sized vessels, and focal influx of mononuclear cells are evident in the lungs.[93,130] Type I pneumocytes occasionally separate from the alveolar wall.[93] The microscopic lesions in the heart vary considerably, with the myocardium appearing essentially normal in a large proportion of cases. Changes range from focal myocardial hemorrhage with no myofiber changes to acute degeneration of myocardial fibers with loss of cross-striations and occasional fragmentation of the sarcoplasm. Occasionally, this is accompanied by infiltration of inflammatory cells.[86,130] The germinal centers of most lymph nodes and the spleen show varying degrees of lymphocyte depletion and nuclear karyorrhexis.[93,130] In situ hybridization[130] and immunohistochemical staining[131] have revealed the presence of AHS viral nucleic acid or antigen in endothelial cells in the lung, heart, and spleen. Ultrastructural changes have also been demonstrated in endothelial cells in the lungs.[85]

Therapy

There is no specific treatment for AHS. Affected animals should be provided with supportive therapy, nursed, and rested because the slightest exertion may result in death. Animals that survive should be rested for at least 4 weeks after recovery before being returned to light work. They should also be carefully monitored for co-infections with piroplasmosis which can complicate recovery.

Prevention

Since the demonstration in the early 1930s that AHSV could be attenuated by serial intracerebral passage in mice, the immunization of horses against the disease has been greatly simplified and improved.[10,11,47,132] The first highly effective attenuated vaccine was produced in 1936.[133] Virus attenuation occurs faster during passage in cell culture than in mouse brain.[134] The size of plaques in cell culture has been found to be a marker of the virulence of AHS viruses, and therefore large plaque variants are now selected as candidate vaccine strains.[84,105,135]

In endemic areas, annual vaccination of horses in late winter or early summer is a practical means of control. Unfortunately, prophylactic immunization against AHS cannot be relied on to protect all horses fully against infection or disease. However, horses that have received three or more courses of immunization are usually well protected against AHS. Onderstepoort Biological Products currently produces a polyvalent vaccine containing attenuated strains prepared in two components, one trivalent (serotypes 1, 3, and 4) and the other quadrivalent (serotypes 2, 6, 7, and 8).[135] Immunization consists of the administration of these component vaccines at least 3 weeks apart. Serotypes 5 and 9 are not included in the vaccines because serotypes 8 and 6, respectively, are reported to afford adequate cross-protection after experimental challenge.[136] There has been concern that use of attenuated strains could result in reversion to virulence or recombination of the vaccine strain with wild-type strains to create a new viral variant, but this has not been substantiated.[136] In other countries where AHSV is not endemic the use of a modified vaccine is also of concern for allowing persistence of an attenuated virus in those areas. Thus recombinant vaccines are in development in some of these countries, which include vaccinia or canarypox as a vector.[137-140] In addition, development of a monovalent inactivated and adjuvanted vaccine is underway in Italy.[141]

Generally, immunization has little or no side effects. A slight temperature increase may occur between 5 and 13 days after vaccination as a result of virus replication. Occasionally, individual animals vaccinated for the first time may show a severe vaccine reaction and may develop clinical signs of AHS. The simultaneous administration of several serotypes of attenuated AHS in horses usually results in the production of antibody against each serotype, although the response of individual horses may vary, and in some animals, antibody against one or more of the serotypes may not be detectable by neutralization tests.[67,142] This may be caused by interference between viruses in the polyvalent vaccine or overattenuation of vaccine strains.[33,143] During the outbreak of AHS in Spain, about 10% of animals immunized for the first time with a monovalent, attenuated AHSV-4 vaccine failed to seroconvert. However, at least some of these animals are resistant to challenge.[16]

The antibody acquired from colostrum correlates well with the antibody level of the dam and determines the duration of passive immunity.[67,142] Because of possible interference of passive immunity with response to vaccination in foals born to immune mares, it is recommended that foals should not be immunized before they are 6 months of age. However, some foals acquire low levels of antibody to one or more AHS virus serotypes via the colostrum, and neutralizing antibody to individual serotypes may decline to undetectable levels shortly after birth, with a result that these foals can become susceptible to infection well before age 6 months.[142]

The risk of infection in susceptible horses can be reduced significantly by stabling them before dusk until after sunrise because *Culicoides* spp. are nocturnal and are not inclined to enter buildings.[142] The application of insect repellents and the use of insecticides on animals also reduce the risk of infection.

After a suspected outbreak of AHS in a country previously free of the disease, attempts should be made to limit further transmission of the virus and to achieve eradication as soon as possible. It is important that control measures be instituted immediately. The control measures in epizootic situations include (1) delineation of the area of infection; (2) strict movement controls within, into, and out of the infected area; (3) stabling of all equids at least from dusk to dawn; (4) insect control measures; (5) temperatures of all equids measured for early detection of infected animals; (6) consideration of immediate vaccination of all susceptible animals with an attenuated polyvalent vaccine, pending serotyping, and subsequent use of a relevant monovalent vaccine; (7) identification of all vaccinated animals; and (8) notification of the OIE about the disease outbreak.[19]

The International Animal Health Code provides guidelines for the importation of domestic horses from AHS-infected countries or zones.[19] These include the housing of animals in vector-protected quarantine facilities for at least 40 days and testing for the absence of AHSV or demonstration of a stable or declining AHS antibody titer.

Public Health Considerations

Accidental aerosol infection occurred in four workers packing mouse-brain attenuated strains of AHS vaccine at Onderstepoort Biological Products.[144] They developed nonfatal encephalitis and chorioretinitis, which resulted in partial loss of vision or blindness. These neurotrophic strains have since been removed from the AHS vaccine produced by Onderstepoort Biological Products.

The complete reference list is available online at www.expertconsult.com.

17 Adeno, Hendra, and Equine Rhinitis Viral Respiratory Diseases

C.J. (Kate) Savage, Deborah Middleton, and Michael J. Studdert*

Equine Adenoviruses

Equine adenovirus type 1 (EAdV1) appears as a subclinical infection in most immunocompetent foals and horses. However, there is serologic evidence of widespread infection in equine populations in numerous different countries around the world.[1,2] It causes mild, upper respiratory tract (URT) disease in normal foals but has caused acute URT disease, as well as follicular conjunctivitis in foals that have been experimentally infected. One of these foals was specific-pathogen-free (SPF) and colostrum-deprived but immunocompetent at 6 weeks of age; the other foal was younger, had received colostrum, and sustained decreased clinical signs, despite its age (4 days).[3] Equine adenovirus type 1 is the dominant pathogen in Arabian foals with severe combined immunodeficiency disease (SCID), which is a uniformly fatal, inherited disorder. These foals have a progressive EAdV1 bronchopneumonia, as well as EAdV1-related pathology in many other organs and tissues.

Etiology

Equine adenoviruses are members of the genus *Mastadenovirus*, family *Adenoviridae*. Only a single antigenic type of EAdV1 has been isolated from horses with respiratory disease.[4,5] A second serotype, equine adenovirus type 2 (EAdV2), has been isolated from the feces of foals with diarrhea.[6] The biophysical properties of EAdV are similar to those of adenoviruses of other species. Equine adenoviruses are nonenveloped, 70 to 80 nm in diameter, and the capsid is composed of 252 capsomers; 240 hexamers occupy the faces and edges of the 20 equilateral triangular facets of an icosahedron, and 12 pentamers occupy the corners. The inner core contains the double-stranded deoxyribonucleic acid (DNA) genome, which for EAdV1 is 34.4 kb in length. Restriction endonuclease maps and genome orientation data were published for EAdV1,[7] and genomic sequence data for both viruses were also published.[8,9] Nucleotide sequence data for the EAdV2 genome corroborated at the molecular level that EAdV2 is distinct from EAdV1 and that the two viruses evolved separately.[8] Cavanagh et al[10] recently sequenced the EAdV1 genome. An unexpected finding was the similarity to two other recently characterized bat adenoviruses.[10]

Epidemiology

Equine adenovirus type 1 occurs worldwide, and seroprevalence rates vary from less than 2% to 100%, depending on the serologic test used and the age, breed, activity, and size of the population sample reported.[5] The prevalence of antibody to EAdV1 increases with age so that, in some populations, about 70% of yearlings and 2-year-old horses have EAdV1 antibody. Serologic evidence indicates a high infection rate in the first year of life, but in some populations, 50% of horses under 1 year lack EAdV antibody and are presumably at risk for EAdV disease.[4]

Interestingly, research in California using polymerase chain reaction (PCR), followed by virus isolation if positive, did not demonstrate EAdV1 infection from nasopharyngeal swabs from 47 apparently healthy racehorses, which were in race training at the time. No horses were positive.[11]

All adenovirus infections appear to be followed by a latent carrier status and shedding of the virus; however, this is poorly characterized for EAdV1. Studies in the Pirbright, United Kingdom (UK), pony herd indicated that EAdV1 infections were often subclinical, and that virus may persist in the nasopharyngeal mucus for up to 68 days after primary infection.[12] Equine adenovirus type 1 was isolated from a foal, without clinical signs at the time of isolation, at 3 days of age.[13] It seems that foals may acquire infection from their dams or other horses in their cohort during the suckling period, even in the presence of detectable levels of maternal antibody. Thus, if there is persistent or repeated EAdV infection, the passive immunity of the foal would be converted to an active immunity, probably without significant clinical disease. Disease may develop if primary infection occurred after maternal antibody had declined, or if the foal was unable to produce an active immune response. This overview of the early natural history of EAdV1 is supported by the natural history of EAdV1 in Arabian foals with SCID, in which the transmission pattern and consequences of infection are viewed in the absence of an active immune response.[14]

Equine adenovirus type 2 has been isolated in Australia and New Zealand.[6,15] Sera from horses of diverse breeds and ages were collected from widely separated geographic areas in Australia; 327 horse sera were tested for EAdV2 neutralizing antibody, and 77% of these sera were positive (maximum titer, 1:640). This pattern of infection is likely to occur worldwide.

Pathogenesis

Equine adenovirus type 1 presumably is acquired as a droplet or close-contact respiratory or ocular infection. The virus replicates in epithelial cells throughout the respiratory tract, producing lysis and sloughing of these cells and a hyperplastic response in underlying noninfected cells. It is likely that respiratory disease in foals is more likely to be clinical, if there is total or partial failure of maternal antibody transfer. Recovery from disease caused by EAdV1 alone in immunologically competent horses presumably occurs within a week to 10 days, but mixed infections with other viruses and bacteria may cause more severe and prolonged disease.[12,16] Multiple infections involving various combinations of EHV-1 and EHV-4, equine rhinitis A

*The authors acknowledge and appreciate the original contributions of these authors, whose work has been incorporated into this chapter.

and equine rhinitis B viruses, and equine adenoviruses were recognized in 15 of 69 outbreaks of respiratory disease of horses in the UK.[1] The significance of individual viruses in the pathogenesis of disease cannot be identified in such studies.

Equine adenovirus type 1 may infect cells of the gastrointestinal (GI) tract and may be shed in feces; consequently, it may also be transmitted through a fecal-oral cycle. Equine adenovirus type 1 was isolated from neuritis of the cauda equina in two of three cases, but no adenovirus was detected by immunofluorescence.[17] It was probably an incidental contaminant.[17]

Immunity

Immunocompetent foals develop EAdV1 antibody, recover spontaneously from the disease, and generally do not possess recoverable virus by day 10 after infection.[16] In experimental infections of colostrum-deprived and colostrum-fed foals, the colostrum-fed foals had less severe changes than colostrum-deprived foals.[3,16]

Reinfection by EAdV1 was found to occur frequently in a group of 16 mares and foals, and many of these infections (or reinfections) occurred in the presence of high levels of circulating antibody.[18] Immunoglobulin A (IgA) in nasal secretions is responsible for resistance to reinfection in human infections with adenovirus or rhinoviruses. A similar situation could occur in horses, when rapidly declining levels of nasal antibody after an infection could soon render the horse susceptible to reinfection, despite high serum antibody levels.

After intramuscular (IM) immunization with live EAdV1 and subsequent development of high serum antibody levels, an SPF foal proved resistant to intranasal challenge with EAdV1.[3] There was a greater than twofold increase in serum-neutralizing (SN) antibody after challenge; clinical disease did not develop and virus was not isolated. Immunity was correlated with prior exposure to the virus and high circulating SN antibody levels.

An experimental inactivated EAdV1 vaccine elicited high antibody titers in rabbits, mice, and foals. Using nude mice as a model of T-cell immunodeficiency, it was shown that production of EAdV1 SN antibody and to a lesser extent, hemagglutination-inhibiting (HI) antibody was T lymphocyte dependent.[19] As a measure of cell-mediated immune responses, an EAdV1-specific in vitro lymphocyte blastogenesis assay was developed and evaluated using lymphocytes from four vaccinated and two unvaccinated control horses. The four vaccinated horses showed marked increases in stimulation indices in response to EAdV1 antigen (maximum stimulation indices, 5.3-18.6).[20]

As mentioned, EAdV1 is associated as a dominant pathogen in the uniformly fatal, inherited disease syndrome, SCID.[21,22] When first recognized in the early 1970s, SCID was estimated to cause the death of about 3% of all purebred Arabian foals. Foals are born with a total absence of T and B lymphocytes, and SCID is inherited as an autosomal recessive gene.[23,24] A consistent and dominant feature of SCID is a progressive EAdV1 bronchopneumonia (Fig. 17-1). The virus causes pathology in a wide variety of other organs and tissues in SCID foals, including the GI tract, liver, pancreas, and bladder.

Clinical Findings

Many authors have isolated EAdV1 from nasopharyngeal swabs obtained from horses of varying ages with and without respiratory disease.[3,11,25-27] Clinical signs in immunocompetent horses are likely to be minimal, with EAdV1 infection frequently being subclinical and asymptomatic.[11] In a study of hospitalized and healthy foals and horses in California, Bell et al found that EAdV1 was detected via PCR in nasopharyngeal swabs of hospitalized (6/15) and control (nonhospitalized foals with a normal physical examination [7/12]) foals. No difference in incidence was found (p = 0.34). Four hospitalized foals had

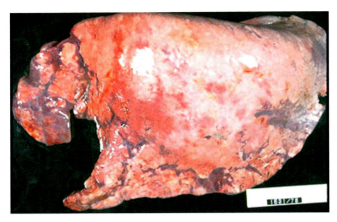

Figure 17-1 Lung of 63-day-old purebred Arabian foal that had severe combined immunodeficiency disease (SCID). There is extensive bronchopneumonia. The lungs have failed to collapse. On the cut surface of the lung, essentially all bronchi are plugged with thick, cream-colored exudate.

respiratory disease—only 50% of these (2/4) were positive on nasopharyngeal swab for EAdV1 via PCR. These two positive foals died, but there was no histologic evidence of infection with EAdV at necropsy. In this study, if PCR were positive, then virus isolation was attempted. One control foal was positive for EAdV1 isolation in cell culture, as were two hospitalized foals. None of the 47 race horses had EAdV1 detected via PCR from nasopharyngeal swabs; however, two (2/12) nonhospitalized mares were positive. Interestingly, their foals were positive control foals as well.[11]

However, despite evidence showing no infection in 2- to 6-year-old racehorses in training at a single point in time,[11] infection can occur in equine populations and may be a cause of undiagnosed respiratory disease in young horses in work. As previously mentioned, it can cause upper respiratory disease with nasal discharge and conjunctivitis. Other clinical signs may include coughing after exercise and enlarged submandibular lymph nodes.[1,5]

Respiratory disease signs were described in a single, experimentally infected SPF foal that was cesarean delivered, colostrum-deprived, and artificially reared in an EAdV-free environment.[3] The foal was healthy and 6 weeks old when infected and had been shown to be immunocompetent. After intranasal infection with EAdV1, clinical signs included mucopurulent nasal discharge, severe follicular conjunctivitis (Fig. 17-2), transient anorexia and pyrexia, and sustained tachypnea. There were no changes in blood leukocyte numbers. Equine adenovirus type 1 was readily isolated from nasal, conjunctival, and rectal swabs and from lung, trachea, bronchial lymph nodes, and small intestine tissue homogenates obtained after necropsy at 6 days after infection.

The clinical response to experimental infection of a 4-day-old foal that received colostrum but was artificially reared from 12 hours after birth in an EAdV1-free environment and that had a 1:320 SN antibody titer and a 1:40 HI antibody titer was similar to that of the previous foal, except fever was not as marked or as sustained, the conjunctivitis was less severe, and nasal discharge was minimal.[3] Equine adenovirus type 1 was readily isolated from nasal and conjunctival swabs and from trachea and lung but not from rectal swabs, small intestine, or bronchial lymph nodes, when a necropsy was conducted 6 days after infection.

Severe or fatal bronchopneumonia has been occasionally recorded in nonimmunodeficient Thoroughbred foals.[27,28] The severity of disease caused by infection with EAdV1 in Arabian SCID foals is well described, including severe bronchopneumonia.

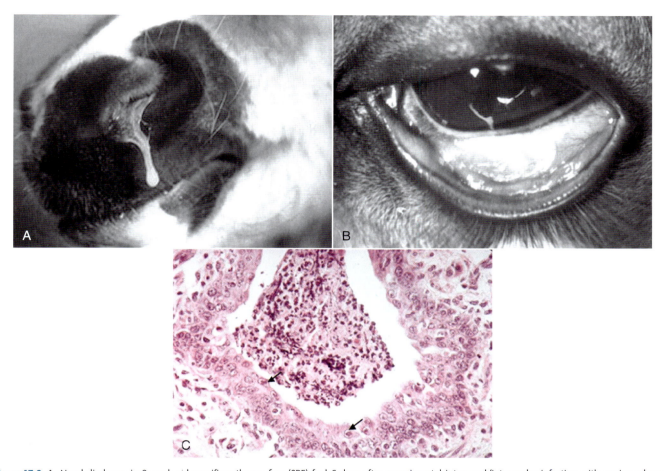

Figure 17-2 A, Nasal discharge in 9-week-old specific-pathogen-free (SPF) foal 6 days after experimental intranasal/intraocular infection with equine adenovirus type 1 (EAdV1).[17] **B,** Conjunctivitis in the same foal 6 days after infection. **C,** Low-power image of bronchiolitis of the same foal. Note proliferation and disorientation of bronchial epithelial cells and the highly cellular bronchial exudate. *Arrows* indicate adenovirus inclusion bodies in nonsloughed bronchial epithelial cells.

The production of soft feces in adult horses, indicative of GI infection, has been reported as a sole manifestation of EAdV infection.[1] Replication of EAdV1 in cells of the GI tract was confirmed after experimental intranasal infection.[3]

Equine adenovirus type 1 was reported as a potential cause of abortion in mares, and abortion was reproduced experimentally after intrauterine inoculation of the virus.[16] However, claims for the natural occurrence of EAdV abortion are unsubstantiated.

Diagnosis

Clinical Laboratory

Virus isolation from nasopharyngeal and conjunctival swabs during the acute phase of infection is possible but not frequently reported. Equine adenovirus type 1 may also be isolated from rectal swabs but would need to be differentiated from EAdV2. Polymerase chain reaction primers have been designed for the detection of both EAdV1 and EAdV2.[29] Detection of adenovirus in negatively stained preparations from fecal samples by electron microscopy (EM) is readily achieved. Immune precipitation, complement fixation, hemagglutination, HI, and SN assays have been extensively used in diagnosis and seroepidemiologic studies. Equine adenovirus type 1 hemagglutinates human blood group O and equine erythrocytes but not those of sheep or chicken.[30]

Virus Isolation

Equine adenovirus type 1 and EAdV2 are highly host cell specific and have been cultivated only in cells of equine origin (e.g., fetal equine kidney)[11] in which both viruses produce a cytopathic effect. On light microscopy and hematoxylin-eosin (HE) staining, intranuclear inclusion bodies are a prominent feature of the cytopathology of adenovirus-infected cells. On thin-section EM, virions assembled in the nucleus form crystalline aggregates.

Serology

Adenoviruses are typed on the basis of SN assays. Most adenoviruses hemagglutinate appropriately chosen red blood cells (RBCs), and HI assays are used for antibody detection. Hemagglutination is mediated by the knob-like tip of the penton binding to receptors on the RBC surface. Type-specific antigenic determinants defined by SN and HI assays are located on the outward-facing surface of the hexamers. Equine adenovirus type 1 possesses the common group-specific Mastadenovirus antigen.[30] An HI antibody to EAdV1, by definition, is type specific.[6,30] Extensive analysis of adenoviruses recovered from horses with respiratory disease, including SCID Arabian foals, indicated that on SN and HI assays, all were a single antigenic type, designated EAdV1.[4,31] On SN assay, EAdV2 is unrelated to EAdV1.[6]

Pathologic Findings

After experimental infection the colostrum-deprived SPF foal showed gross and histopathologic evidence of rhinitis, conjunctivitis, tracheitis, and pneumonia. There was both bronchopneumonia and interstitial pneumonia in affected areas of lung. Duodenal villous atrophy and idiopathic glomerular hyperplasia were also observed. Equine adenovirus antigen was detected by indirect immunofluorescence antibody staining of trachea and lung but not in frozen sections of bronchial lymph node or small intestine. In the SPF foal that received colostrum, gross and histologic evidence of EAdV1 disease was similar but less severe than that observed in the SPF colostrum-deprived foal.[3]

Therapy and Prevention

There are no specific therapies for equine adenovirus infections, and vaccines have not been marketed. For both prophylaxis and therapy, as for other neonatal and perinatal infectious diseases, the provision of supplemental passive antibody either through colostrum or parenterally administered EAdV1 hyperimmune sera should be considered when there is a failure or partial failure of maternal antibody transfer. An accurate diagnosis of EAdV1 would rarely be known, and in most cases, supportive treatment should be used where necessary.

Public Health Considerations

No human public health implications are associated with equine adenoviruses.

Hendra Virus: a Henipavirus

Hendra virus (HeV), formerly known as *equine morbillivirus*, was first recognized in 1994 as the cause of an outbreak of acute respiratory disease. It is a rare infection of horses that is also a lethal zoonosis, and it has been recognized in two states of Australia: Queensland and New South Wales. The initial outbreak affected 20 Thoroughbred racehorses in Hendra, a suburb of Brisbane, Queensland, Australia. Fourteen horses died or were euthanized at the time of the outbreak. The trainer of the horses and a stable hand were infected and became seriously ill with an influenza-like illness, and the trainer died from severe interstitial pneumonia.[32] In the following year, a third human patient was identified, in this case dying from encephalitis that was attributed to HeV infection. Interestingly, exposure of this individual had most likely occurred 13 months earlier when assisting with the necropsy examination of two horses that were retrospectively diagnosed with Hendra disease.[33,34] Since then, numerous sporadic incidents of single or multiple deaths in horses have been reported, as well as infection and/or death of people attending to diseased horses. There is strong epidemiologic evidence of horse-to-horse transmission of HeV in the two largest outbreaks in 1994 and 2008 (Table 17-1). All cases have occurred in northern New South Wales (NSW) or Queensland (QLD).[35-37]

Pteropid bats (flying foxes) are the reservoir host for Hendra virus, as well as for Nipah virus, which belongs to the same genus *(Henipavirus)* as Hendra but found in Malaysia, Cambodia, India, and Bangladesh. Nipah virus caused a major disease outbreak in Malaysia in 1999, where virus spillover from flying foxes led to respiratory disease and febrile encephalitis in domestic pigs and humans; seroconversion of horses was rarely identified. Nipah virus also regularly causes human disease in Bangladesh and nearby India, but with different epidemiologic features; thus human-to-human transmission is commonly reported, with no strong evidence for involvement of domestic animals in the chain of transmission to humans.

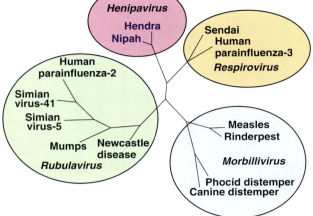

Family Paramyxoviridae

Figure 17-3 Phylogenic relationship of Hendra virus to other members of the family Paramyxoviridae, based on analyses of predicted amino acid sequences of virus matrix proteins. *(Courtesy Linfa Wang, CSIRO Livestock Industries' Animal Health Laboratory.)*

Etiology

Hendra virus is a member of the genus *Henipavirus* in the order Mononegavirales, in the family *Paramyxoviridae*, subfamily *Paramyxovirinae*. Nipah virus and HeV form a distinct clade within the family *Paramyxoviridae*[38] (Fig. 17-3). Virions are enveloped with a nonsegmented, single-stranded, negative-sense ribonucleic acid (RNA) genome that is 18,234 nucleotides in length.[39] In negatively stained electron micrographs, the virus is pleomorphic and approximately 180 nm in diameter. Unusually, the HeV envelope is covered with two kinds of spikes that are 10 nm and 18 nm long and give the particle a "double-fringed" appearance, which is not a feature of previously described paramyxoviruses. These spikes contain the F (fusion) glycoprotein trimers and G (attachment) glycoprotein tetramers. The nucleocapsid is 18 nm wide and has a periodicity of 5 nm.[40] Hendra virus does not agglutinate RBCs from a range of species, including human type O, monkey, equine, porcine, bovine, guinea pig, chicken, and goose, when tested at 4° C, 22° C, and 37° C, or possess detectable neuraminidase activity.

Epidemiology

Flying foxes of the genus *Pteropus*, order *Chiroptera*, are the natural hosts for HeV, and antibodies have been found in all four Australian mainland species, with up to 47% of the bats testing positive.[41,42] However, transmission of HeV from bats to horses is a rare event, and it is not known precisely how this takes place. There is epidemiologic evidence of horse-to-horse transmission, particularly where the outbreak has been centered on a stable complex or veterinary clinic, with transmission opportunity attributed to contamination of surfaces or equipment by infectious fluids from the index case.[43] Transmission by aerosol does not appear to be an important means of spread under natural circumstances, and in general, the infection in horses is not considered to be highly transmissible, with direct droplet contact exposure required. Similarly, the attack rate for humans exposed to potentially infectious equine bodily fluids

Table 17-1 Hendra Virus Outbreak in Australia*

Date/Town	State	Mortality[†]: Horses	Mortality/ Morbidity: Humans	Dogs
August 1994 Mackay	QLD	n = 2	n = 1 (died)	—
September 1994 Hendra	QLD	n = 21	n = 1 (died) n = 1 (ill)	—
January 1999 Cairns	QLD	n = 1	—	—
October 2004 Cairns	QLD	n = 1	n = 1 (ill)	—
December 2004 Townsville	QLD	n = 1	—	—
June 2006 Peachester	QLD	n = 1	—	—
October 2006 Murwillumbah	NSW	n = 1	—	—
June 2007 Peachester	QLD	n = 1	—	—
July 2007 Cairns	QLD	n = 1	—	—
July 2008 Redlands	QLD	n = 5	n = 2 (1 died/1 ill)	—
July 2008 Proserpine	QLD	n = 3	—	—
Aug 2009 Cawarral	QLD	n = 4	n = 1 (died)	—
September 2009 Bowen	QLD	n = 2	—	—
May 2010 Tewantin	QLD	n = 1	—	—
June to July 2011 Boonah	QLD	n = 3	—	n = 1 (seroconverted; dog was euthanized after a second positive antibody test, in line with current government policy)
June 2011 Beaudesert	QLD	n = 1	—	—
June 2011 Logan Reserve	QLD	n = 1	—	—
June 2011 Wollongbar	NSW	n = 2	—	—
July 2011 Macksville	NSW	n = 1	—	—
July 2011 Park Ridge	QLD	n = 1	—	—
July 2011 Kuranda	QLD	n = 1	—	—
July 2011 Hervey Bay	QLD	n = 1	—	—
July 2011 Lismore	NSW	n = 1	—	—
July 2011 Boondall	QLD	n = 1	—	—
July 2011 Chinchilla	QLD	n = 1	—	—
July 2011 Mullumbimby	NSW	n = 1	—	—
August 2011 Ballina	NSW	n = 1	—	—
August 2011 South Ballina	NSW	n = 1	—	—
August 2011 Mullumbimby	NSW	n = 2	—	—
August 2011 Gold Coast Hinterland	QLD	n = 1	—	—
August 2011 Ballina	NSW	n = 1	—	—
September to October 2011 Beachmere	QLD	n = 3		
January 2012 Townsville	QLD	n = 1	—	—
May 2012 Rockhampton	QLD	n = 3	—	—
May 2012 Ingham	QLD	n = 1	—	n = 1 (initial weak positive, clear on subsequent tests, deemed not positive, so euthanasia not performed)
June 2012 Mackay	QLD	n = 1	—	—
July 2012 Rockhampton	QLD	n = 1	—	—
July 2012 Cairns	QLD	n = 1	—	—
September 2012 Port Douglas	QLD	n = 1	—	—
October 2012 Ingham	QLD	n = 1	—	—
January 2013 near Mackay	QLD	n = 1	—	—

QLD, Queensland; NSW, New South Wales.

*The number of horses, humans, and dogs known to be infected with or have seroconverted to Hendra virus in Australia in NSW and QLD, in chronologic order. Town names are given for clarity. All outbreaks were in QLD or NSW.

[†]Mortality refers to animals that died or were euthanized for humane reasons or because they were seropositive or virus—isolation positive.

is estimated at 10%.[44] The presence of antibody to HeV in asymptomatic horses has been confined to disease outbreaks suggesting that the virus is not maintained within the horse population.

Pathogenesis and Pathology

In horses exposed to HeV by the oronasal route and under controlled laboratory conditions, HeV RNA may be recovered from nasal secretions 48 hours after contact with the virus and may persist throughout the incubation period.[45] This suggests that systemic spread of virus is preceded by local replication in the nasal cavity or nasopharynx, as has also been proposed for Nipah virus.[46] Increasing gene copy number is observed in the immediate presymptomatic and symptomatic stages of infection, and at this point, viral RNA is also recoverable from oral cavity

secretions, urine, feces, and blood, suggesting that the greatest transmission risk is posed at this time.[45] This is in accordance with field observations around human infection with HeV.

At necropsy examination the most prominent gross lesion is firm, dark red lungs with dilated lymphatic vessels and hemorrhage and froth in the trachea, bronchi, and bronchioles.[47,48] Fibrin tags may be seen on the pleura (Fig. 17-4). The pericardial sac may contain serous fluid. In some horses with HeV infection, extensive subcutaneous hemorrhages were observed, but these may have been agonal.

The characteristic histologic lesion in both naturally occurring and experimentally induced acute HeV infection is vasculitis with fibrinoid degeneration and necrosis of the vascular wall. This lesion typically involves smaller vessels in lung, brain (including meninges), spleen, lymph nodes, and kidney. However, lesions may also be detected in nasal mucosa, liver,

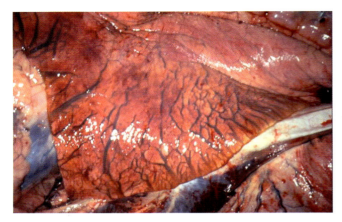

Figure 17-4 Gross lesions in lung of horse experimentally infected with Hendra virus, showing pneumonia and dilation of lymphatics. *(Courtesy CSIRO Livestock Industries' Australian Animal Health Laboratory.)*

heart, stomach, intestine, uterus, and ovary. Severe involvement of the lung is common, with diffuse areas of necrotizing alveolitis and marked fibrinous alveolar exudates accounting for the respiratory signs that are often noted at clinical examination. Syncytial cells may also develop in vascular endothelium and endothelium of lymphatic vessels, as well as in respiratory epithelial and lymphoid cells. Extensive deposits of viral antigen may be seen on immunohistochemical examination of affected tissues.

The few known field cases of HeV that have recovered from acute disease have been euthanized in line with current national policy. Mild to moderately severe, focal, nonsuppurative meningoencephalitis with gliosis and perivascular cuffing has been identified in these animals, and HeV genome has been recovered from the brain. The pathogenesis and significance of these findings is not yet understood.

Experimentally, cats, ferrets, and guinea pigs are susceptible to HeV, and although some pathologic differences exist in these species, the diseases are similar to that observed in horses.[49,50] Rats, mice, and chickens are not susceptible to experimental infection, and only one of two dogs exposed under laboratory conditions developed neutralizing antibody to the virus.[47] However, during 2011 a dog on an outbreak property was identified to have antibody to HeV without having shown signs of disease (see Table 17-1).

Clinical Findings

The incubation period of HeV in horses has been proposed to be 4 to 16 days,[32,51,52] after which horses show severe, acute, febrile respiratory disease sometimes accompanied by facial swelling, ataxia, and terminally, copious frothy nasal discharge as the result of pulmonary edema. More recently, neurologic signs have predominated in some outbreak events, with clinical features comprising hypersensitivity, ataxia, disorientation, facial paralysis, head tilt, circling, head pressing, and stranguria,[43] although there is no evidence that significant viral strain mutation has occurred. The clinical course of disease is generally short, with most horses dying within 48 hours of the onset of signs. Affected horses may also be found dead. Laboratory testing is essential to confirm a diagnosis of HeV infection.

Diagnosis

Hendra virus is classified as a biosafety level 4 (BSL4) agent, and laboratory diagnostic testing should be carried out under the appropriate conditions of biosafety and biocontainment.

Virus Isolation

Hendra virus may be reisolated from clinical specimens using several cell lines—Vero cells are most commonly used.[53] Preferred tissue samples for this purpose are lung, spleen, kidney, and brain.

Quantitative Real-Time Polymerase Chain Reaction

Quantitative real-time PCR has been used extensively to identify acutely infected animals in outbreak investigations, as well as in experimental studies[54,55]; blood and nasal swabs are the specimens of choice for diagnostic confirmation in the live animal.

Serology

Serum neutralization (SNT) and enzyme-linked immunosorbent assay (ELISA) tests have been developed to detect antibodies against HeV, with application primarily to epidemiologic investigations associated with the management of outbreaks. As SNT must be carried out at BSL4, ELISA is usually employed as the first-line screening test.

Antigen Detection

Immunohistochemistry may be used for detection of HeV antigen in clinical specimens and is particularly helpful where formalin-fixed tissues only are available for examination.

Therapy

No specific therapy exists for horses with HeV infection. Because of the serious zoonotic potential of HeV, even supportive therapy should not be undertaken once a diagnosis is confirmed. While exclusion diagnostic testing is being carried out, any interventions necessary for reasons of animal welfare should be undertaken with due consideration of the zoonotic risk.

Prevention

Vaccination

A key strategy for reducing HeV infection risk to people and other susceptible in-contact horses is to remove the virus-shedding horse from the chain of transmission. Conditions that favour spill-over of HeV from bats to horses are not well understood, and this aspect of disease emergence may not be amenable to control in the foreseeable future. Accordingly, immunization of horses holds promise both for protecting the health of horses exposed to HeV-infected bats and, in the event that an immunized horse does become infected, for reducing any viral replication that may occur to a level that prevents on-going transmission.

Efficacy testing of one candidate HeV vaccine has been carried out in laboratory mammals,[56] and in horses. The vaccine is based on recombinantly expressed soluble versions of the G glycoprotein (sG) from HeV[57] that has been formulated for use in horses with a proprietary adjuvant as an inactivated subunit vaccine. Preliminary data gathered after using a prime-boost immunization regime confirmed seroconversion of vaccinated horses, and immunized horses were protected from disease following exposure to an otherwise lethal HeV challenge. In addition, no viral shedding was identified and no viral genome was recovered from tissues (D. Middleton, unpublished observations). Clearly, vaccination of horses against HeV has the potential both to protect the health of horses and to break the chain of transmission of HeV from bats to people. Other vaccine platforms, such as canarypox virus-based recombinant vaccine carrying the glycoprotein (G) gene,[58] may in time provide an alternative product that is also fit for this purpose. In November 2012, Equivac® HeV was released by Pfizer under permit issued by the Australian Pesticides and Veterinary Medicines Authority (APVMA). This vaccine is supplied and administered to horses by veterinarians under strict conditions.

Other Methods

General recommendations have been made to horse owners with the aim of reducing the risk of contact of their animals with potential sources of infection such as flying fox secretions, urine, feces, spats, or aborted fetuses.[41] These include providing feeding and watering locations that are under cover, avoiding feedstuffs (such as fruit) that may be attractive to flying foxes, and relocating horses away from paddocks containing flowering trees at times of flying fox abundance. Outbreaks of the disease currently require immediate quarantine of the premises, controls on the movement of horses within a defined disease control zone, and serologic surveillance to determine the extent of infection. A greater understanding of the virus and the disease, as well as the vaccination of "at risk" horses in the future, may allow less onerous disease control programs to be used. Information on the persistence of the virus in the environment and the possibility that recovered animals may act as carriers and potential sources of infection needs further exploration.

Public Health Considerations

Although transmission of HeV to humans is a rare event, the serious consequences of infection must be considered when examining horses that may be infected with HeV, collecting clinical samples, or undertaking in vitro or in vivo laboratory tests. The known human infections have occurred after contact with the secretions or bodily fluids of infected horses at the time of terminal illness or during necropsy examination rather than directly from bats. Human-to-human transmission has not yet been reported. However, there are many difficulties inherent in making reliable recommendations on reducing risk of transmission from infected horses and in particular, relying on Personal Protective Equipment (PPE) for this purpose. Difficulties include: (1) the propensity for outbreaks to occur in a warm climate where compliance with certain items of PPE may be poor; (2) the emotional attachment of humans to their horses that leads to regular close contact, but where use of PPE is perceived as impractical; and (3) specific knowledge gaps, including lack of definition of occupational exposure limits to HeV, unknown infectious dose (especially by inhalation), and unknown viral load in the air.

Members of the horse industry involved with the care of horses that are in or have travelled from the northern NSW region and from QLD are increasingly developing protocols and procedures for managing the HeV transmission risk posed by routine activities.

In other parts of Australia, a challenge for veterinarians and horse handlers is to remain vigilant for the possibility of HeV, despite the low likelihood of its occurring. However, a horse exhibiting signs consistent with HeV that has recently arrived from QLD or northern NSW must be considered a possible or probable case, depending on the clinical signs. The fact that early signs of HeV resemble many other equine diseases, including colic, pneumonia and pleuropneumonia (travel sickness), makes this problematic. The more distinctive features of HeV, including severe respiratory distress, cardiovascular collapse, and neurologic signs, are manifest after HeV is detectable in secretions. Consequently, if the horse is demonstrating these signs and although they are not pathognomonic for HeV, it is imperative that in-contact people use PPE, biosecurity methods, and test the horse for HeV.

Equine Rhinitis a Virus and Equine Rhinitis B Viruses

Picornaviruses are recognized causes of acute upper respiratory and systemic disease in horses. When first isolated in the 1960s, the biophysical properties of these viruses indicated that they were members of the family Picornaviridae. As the majority of the isolates were acid labile (infectivity destroyed at pH 3), they were classified in the genus *Rhinovirus*, which includes the common cold viruses of humans, and named *equine rhinoviruses*. Both the naming and the classification implied that the biology, including clinical diseases and pathogenesis, would parallel human common cold viruses, which are the prototypic members of the genus *Rhinovirus*.

Despite seroprevalence rates of 20% to 80% for equine rhinitis A virus (ERAV), equine rhinitis B virus type 1 (ERBV1), and equine rhinitis B virus type 2 (ERBV2), these viruses are seldom specifically diagnosed as causes of respiratory disease in horses. Their relative "neglect" may be related to the dominant position of influenza viruses and equine herpesvirus types 1 and 4 (EHV-1, EHV-4) as causes of acute upper respiratory disease in horses but is also related to a lack of sensitive, widely available, and adopted diagnostic tests.

Etiology

Three acid-labile serotypes, called *equine rhinoviruses 1, 2, and 3*, were originally identified. A fourth serotype, termed *acid-stable picornavirus* (ASP), was also isolated. Sequence analysis of the genome of two strains of equine rhinovirus 1 indicated that this virus was most closely related to foot-and-mouth disease virus (FMDV),[59,60] and accordingly, the virus was reclassified in the genus *Aphthovirus*, although as a separate cluster, and renamed equine rhinitis A virus (ERAV).[61] Until that time, FMDV had been the sole member of the genus *Aphthovirus*. Analysis of the sequence of the genome of equine rhinovirus 2 indicated that, although most closely related to "encephalomyocarditis virus,"[60] which is a member of the *Cardiovirus* genus, it was sufficiently distinct from all other picornaviruses to be assigned as the sole member of a new genus *Erbovirus* (erb[o] for equine rhinitis B) and renamed equine rhinitis B virus (ERBV).[61] Some ERBV1 isolates have been shown to be stable at acid pH, and these can also be distinguished from acid-labile ERBV1 by genomic sequence analysis.[62] Sequence analysis of the antigenically distinct equine rhinovirus 3 indicated that this virus was a second serotype (ERBV2) within the genus Erbovirus.[63] Acid-stable picornaviruses have been isolated from the respiratory tract (prototype 4442/75) and oral cavity of horses,[64,65] and it has been shown that they are a third serotype (ERBV3) within the erbovirus genus.

ERAV was first isolated and characterized in the United Kingdom by Plummer.[66-68] Subsequently, ERAV was isolated in many parts of the world.[69] Most isolations of so-called equine rhinoviruses were antigenically similar to the virus (PERV/62) originally isolated by Plummer[66] in 1962 and now designated ERAV. Hofer et al[70] confirmed that there were at least two distinct serotypes of equine rhinovirus. The identity of a second serotype (prototype 1436/71) was confirmed by Newman et al,[71] and after sequencing of the genome[60] and renaming,[61] this virus is now designated ERBV1. Steck et al[72] indicated the existence of a third serotype, and genomic sequencing of the prototype strain of this virus (313/75) confirmed that it was a second member of the genus *Erbovirus*, proposed to be designated ERBV2.[64] Only one other isolation of ERBV2 from a horse with febrile respiratory disease has been reported.[73,74] The so-called acid-stable equine picornaviruses were identified as a distinct serotype[64,65] and as noted, are now designated ERBV3.

Virions measure 24 to 30 nm in diameter. The genome is a single-stranded, positive-sense RNA. Virions are not inactivated by lipid solvents (ether, chloroform) or by nonionic detergents.

Epidemiology

Equine rhinitis A virus, ERBV1, and ERBV2 are spread by contact through nasal secretions and aerosol inhalation.[75,76] Equine rhinitis A virus is also shed in urine for prolonged periods, and urine aerosol is considered to be an important mode of transmission.[77,78] As a coincidental part of a study of the carrier status of equine arteritis virus in male horses, McCollum and Timoney[77] showed that 432 of 2523 (17%) postrace urine samples were positive for ERAV by virus isolation. The frequency of urine shedding was highest in 2-year-old horses (26%) and appeared to decline steadily to 5% in 8-year-old horses, although horses up to 10 years of age shed virus. There were no differences in urine shedding of ERAV between stallions and geldings. Persistent shedding in urine for up to 146 days was demonstrated in individual horses. In a study of 20 young stallions in which both nasopharyngeal and urine samples were examined for ERAV, only 1 of 11 stallions from which virus was isolated was double positive; 5 of the 20 stallions yielded virus from nasopharyngeal swabs and 7 from urine samples. A possible interpretation of these data is that virus shedding from urine is more prolonged than shedding from the nasal cavity. Although the role of fecal and urine shedding in the transmission of ERAV has not been fully elucidated, it appears that urine is an important mode of transmission,[77] presumably by inhalation of a urine aerosol, as also proposed by Powell.[78] McCollum and Timoney[77] did not recover ERBV1 or ERBV2 from urine.

Although labile at pH less than 6.5, ERAV may remain infectious in the environment under favorable conditions for extended periods, perhaps months.[76] Generally, ERAV is most frequently isolated, whereas ERBV1, ERBV2, and ERBV3 appear less frequently isolated. A notable exception to this view was a study of 92 horses with acute respiratory disease in Canada,[79] in which ERBV was isolated from 28 of 64 (44%) nasopharyngeal swabs from horses with acute febrile respiratory disease; of the 28 virus-positive horses, 6 (21%) demonstrated a fourfold increase in ERBV2 antibody titer.

Equine rhinitis A virus, ERBV1, and ERBV2 maternal antibody was present 12 hours after suckling in foals born to antibody-positive dams. By 10 to 12 months, however, ERAV SN antibody was not detected in any of the progeny horses, whereas ERBV1 and ERBV2 SN antibodies were common (83% and 100%, respectively).[80] In a U.S. study, the overall percentage of horses less than 3 years old with SN antibodies to ERAV and ERBV was 73%, whereas 90% of horses older than 4 years were positive.[81] The prevalence of ERAV antibody in Australia indicated a maximum infection rate of 47.9% (170 of 355 serums), and accordingly, at any one time, 50% of the population was susceptible.[75,80] In a study in Japan, paired serum samples were collected from 3012 racehorses that developed pyrexia at two training centers between 1980 and 1986.[82] Seroconversion to ERAV was demonstrated in 102 (3.4%), and the mean age of horses seroconverting was 2.44 years. In a study by Carman et al,[79] 9 of 92 (10%) horses that presented with respiratory disease had a significant rise in ERAV SN antibody, suggesting that ERAV was the cause of respiratory disease in these horses; the corresponding figure as previously noted for ERBV was 6 of 28 (21%) horses.

In a more comprehensive seroprevalence study, 388 serums from 291 horses were tested for SN antibody to ERAV, ERBV1, and ERBV2.[80] The prevalence of ERAV, ERBV1, and ERBV2 SN antibodies was approximately 37%, 83%, and 66%, respectively. One part of this study included serum from 44 Thoroughbred horses obtained when they were newly introduced into a training center and their average age was 23 months, with a second sample obtained approximately 7 months later. Equine rhinitis A virus, ERBV1, and ERBV2 SN antibody was present in 8 (18%), 34 (77%), and 39 (89%) of horses, respectively, when first bled, and in 27 (61%), 34 (77%), and 38 (86%) of horses, respectively, when tested 7 months later. In this study, 19 of the 44 horses (43%) seroconverted to ERAV within 7 months of entering the training stable. For ERBV1 and ERBV2, the percentage of seropositivity between the first and second samples was about the same. Notably, however, 5 (12%) and 4 (9%) of the 44 horses, respectively, seroconverted to ERBV1 and ERBV2, although this rate of seroconversion was offset by the observation that 5 (12%) and 6 (14%) of the horses, respectively, seroreverted (became antibody negative). Among all the horses, the average ERAV SN antibody titer was relatively high (3796), and in contrast, ERBV1 and ERBV2 titers were relatively low (average of 84 and 45, respectively) and often fell to below detectable levels (seroreverted) over time at a rate comparable to seroconversion. In general, Thoroughbred horses 6 to 24 months of age are serologically negative to ERAV and do not seroconvert until after entering training stables. This suggests that most horses are infected with ERAV during the period of training and racing.[76,80,83]

Pathogenesis

After aerosol or indirect transmission, virus replicates in nasal epithelial cells. Viremia is a regular feature of ERAV infection. Virus disappears from the blood after onset of antibody production, although it persists in the pharynx and may be isolated from feces in small amounts (<10 $TCID_{50}/g$) for at least 1 month after infection (samples were not tested beyond this time).[68] Isolation of the virus from feces was considered curious because virus was not isolated at any time from gut, indicating that it must either infect and persist in lower gut cells or be transported from the pharynx through the bloodstream in a manner not detectable by standard virus isolation procedures. The demonstration that ERAV is shed in urine for prolonged periods, up to 146 days in one study but almost certainly longer,[77] led to a view that persistent infection may be established in the urinary tract, possibly in the bladder.

A temporary suppression of cell-mediated immunity in Standardbred horses with decreased athletic performance, in association with symptoms such as intermittent fever and mild pharyngitis, was linked to ERAV infections.[84] In this study, lymphocyte proliferation assays to evaluate cell-mediated immunity and a bioassay for equine type 1 interferon were used as markers for detection of viral infection.

Clinical Findings

Equine rhinitis A virus is generally considered to cause mild to moderate respiratory disease,[69,70,76,79] although clinical signs may be quite variable,[70] and nasal discharge is not invariably present.[76] In many cases, infection is subclinical. The incubation period is 3 to 8 days. Clinical signs in natural outbreaks of disease may include fever (41° C ± 0.5° C), anorexia, and serous nasal discharge that becomes mucopurulent.[85] Of course, secondary bacterial infection may be involved in the production of the latter. There may be coughing and pharyngitis. Recovery in uncomplicated cases occurs within 7 days. Where pharyngitis persists, coughing may continue for 2 to 3 weeks. Although persistent shedding of ERAV in urine and feces is presumably a consequence of prolonged infection, no disease has been linked to nonrespiratory sites of infection.[77]

Plummer and Kerry[68] showed that after experimental infection of horses with ERAV, the incubation period averaged 4.25 days (range: 2-8 days). Illness was characterized by fever (up to 40.6° C), anorexia, nasal discharge, pharyngitis, and lymphadenitis involving at least the submaxillary and pharyngeal lymph nodes. Bronchitis was also recognized. Based on serologic conversions, most authors recognize that subclinical infections occur. Viremia consistently developed on average at 5.4 days (range: 3-7 days) and lasted 4.5 days (range: 4-5 days). The disappearance of virus from the blood coincided with the onset of antibody production.

Equine rhinitis B virus infection of horses may also result in an acute febrile respiratory disease characterized by coughing and lymphadenitis and recovery, although there is persistent infection and virus shedding from the respiratory tract.[64,77,79,83,86] In contrast to ERAV viremia, urine and fecal shedding have not been recognized in association with ERBV infection.

Diagnosis

Clinical Laboratory and Virus Isolation

Equine rhinitis A virus replicates in cultured equine cells, as well as in cells from several heterologous animal species.[76] The cytopathic effect (CPE) was produced in primary cell cultures from horse, dog, rabbit, hamster, and monkey; in a diploid cell line of equine origin; in cell lines that included HeLa and Hep 2 from humans, rhesus monkey, and African green monkey kidney (LLC-MK2 and Vero cells); and in a rabbit kidney cell line (RK13). Of these, RK13 and Vero cell cultures were found to be efficient host systems for some ERAV strains.[67,73,77] The CPE produced occurs at 37° C (98.6° F) and resembles that produced by other picornaviruses in which infected cells round up, shrink, and show marked nuclear pyknosis, becoming refractive and eventually degenerating and detaching from the surface.[81] However, primary isolation and propagation of ERAV in cultured cells have proved difficult in some cases.[67,75] ERAV may replicate in primary equine fetal kidney (EFK), Vero, and RK13 cells without causing obvious CPE, and switching cell lines was necessary to maintain cytopathic ERAV.[87] Similarly, primary isolation of ERBV also seems to be difficult; isolation rates achieved in some studies[70,80] were not matched in other studies.[73,75,88]

These variable success rates correlating acute respiratory disease with rhinitis viruses may simply reflect the real situation at the time the samples are taken. An alternative view is that the noncultivability of the viruses from particular outbreaks may be an important factor. Variation in the susceptibility of the cell lines used for isolation or genetic variation (quasispecies) in the viruses themselves could account for higher success rates of virus isolation in some studies compared with others.

Serology

The demonstration of rising SN antibody titer in paired sera collected about 2 weeks apart will confirm a diagnosis for ERAV or ERBV infection.

Virus Detection

Reverse transcriptase–polymerase chain reaction (RT-PCR) has been developed for the detection of ERAV in nasopharyngeal swabs and other samples collected from horses with acute respiratory disease.[87,89,90] An ERBV-specific nested RT-PCR that amplified a product within the 3D^{pol} and 3′ nontranslated region of the viral genome was developed.[73] This RT-PCR detected all 24 available ERBV1 isolates and one available ERBV2 isolate. The limit of detection for the prototype strain

ERBV1.1436/71 was 0.1 50% tissue culture infectious doses. Using this RT-PCR, DNA was amplified from 6 of 17 nasopharyngeal swab samples from horses that had clinical signs of acute febrile respiratory disease, but from which ERBV was not initially isolated in cell culture. The sequences of these six ERBV-positive samples had 93% to 96% nucleotide identity, with six other partially sequenced ERBV1 isolates and one ERBV2. Equine rhinitis B virus was isolated from one of the six samples at fourth cell culture passage when it was shown that the addition of 20 mg/mL MgCl$_2$ to the cell culture medium enhanced the growth of the virus. The study highlights the utility of PCR for the identification of viruses in clinical samples that may initially be considered negative with conventional cell culture isolation.

Pathologic Findings

No detailed studies on the pathology of ERAV and ERBV infections have been done other than in explant organ cultures infected with ERAV.[91,92] ERAV replicated in cell and organ cultures but was released almost exclusively from nasal turbinate epithelium. On thin-section EM, organ cultures inoculated with ERAV appeared normal, with the exception of rare, island-like lesions in infected nasal turbinate, and virus particles were not seen.

Therapy

There is no specific antiviral therapy for rhinitis virus infection in horses. Therapy should be symptomatic and supportive.

Prevention

Vaccines for ERAV or ERBV have not been developed commercially until the 2012 release of an adjuvanted, inactivated vaccine to protect against ERAV. This new vaccine has a conditional license in the United States; efficacy and potency tests are in progress. An experimental inactivated ERAV vaccine produced primary immune responses in horses, mice (including athymic nu/nu mice), and rabbits.[93] The problem of multiple serotypes recognized for FMDV does not occur because ERAV is antigenically and genomically remarkably stable over time and geographic location.[90] The occurrence of three serotypes of ERBV would need to be considered in any vaccine development.

Public Health Considerations

Evidence indicates that ERAV infects humans after both natural and experimental infection. A human volunteer infected with ERAV developed severe pharyngitis and swelling of the pharyngeal lymph nodes accompanied by fever, and virus was isolated from his blood.[66,67] Based on serologic data, humans may be infected with ERAV by contact with infected horses, but clinical disease or subsequent human-to-human transmission of virus was not recognized in such naturally occurring infections.[66,67,94] Kriegshauser et al[94] tested 137 sera from veterinarians for the presence of ERAV and ERBV1 SN antibody. Four (2.7%) and five (3.6%) human sera had low levels of neutralizing "activity" to ERAV and ERBV1, respectively. The authors concluded that the risk of acquiring ERAV and ERBV1 as zoonotic infections among veterinarians appears low.

The complete reference list is available online at www.expertconsult.com.

Viral Diarrhea

K. Gary Magdesian, Roberta M. Dwyer,* and Marta Gonzalez Arguedas*

Equine Rotavirus

Diarrhea is a frequently encountered medical problem of newborn foals, and rotavirus is the most common cause of foal enteritis in major breeding centers of the United States, Ireland, and England, as well as other countries.[1,2] In a recent study evaluating prevalence of infectious agents in foals with gastrointestinal (GI) disease, rotavirus was the most common agent found in the feces of sick foals (35% versus 3% in healthy foals, $p = 0.0002$) using polymerase chain reaction (PCR).[3] Both single cases of rotaviral diarrhea and severe farm outbreaks can occur. However, with the use of a commercially available vaccine, practical farm management practices, and hygiene measures, this disease can be controlled.

Etiology

The family *Reoviridae* consists of five genera: *Orthoreovirus*, *Orbivirus*, *Coltivirus*, *Aquareovirus*, and *Rotavirus*. These are all double-stranded, ribonucleic acid (RNA), nonenveloped viruses with a diameter of about 80 nm (Fig. 18-1). The genus *Rotavirus* is subdivided into several groups (A-G) based on differences in the group-specific inner capsid protein, VP6. Equine and other animal isolates are in group A; groups B to G cause disease in humans, swine, fowl, and other animals.[4] Further subdivision is made based on serologic assays using neutralizing antibodies to two outer capsid proteins, VP4 and VP7. Strains containing VP4 are referred to as P (protease-sensitive) serotype and strains containing VP7 as the G (glycoprotein) serotype, with many containing both.[5] Strains are named based on the G and P genotypes. At least 7 G serotypes (G3, G5, G6, G8, G10, G13, and G14) and 6 P serotypes (P1, P3 P7, P11, P12, and P18) have been described in horses.[5-10] The G3 serotype has been identified in Kentucky and Japan and has been used in equine vaccine trials.[11-13] The G3P[12] and G14P[12] serotypes are among the most prevalent in foals and are the primary strains circulating in horse populations in many countries.[6,14-16] The G3 type of equine rotavirus has two associated subtypes: G3A and G3B.

Rotaviruses are stable within a pH range of 3 to 7 and are resistant to iodophor, quaternary ammonium, chlorine, and hypochlorite (bleach) disinfectants. Ethanol, phenols (efficacy varies with the specific product), and formalin can inactivate the virus.[17-19] Peroxygen and accelerated hydrogen peroxide disinfectants are also effective against rotavirus.

Epidemiology

Equine rotaviruses have been detected from diarrheic foals in many countries, including the United States, Argentina, Britain, Ireland, Germany, Australia, New Zealand, South Africa, and Japan. In a retrospective study of foals with diarrhea presented to the University of Florida, rotavirus was the most frequently detected infectious agent (20% of cases).[20] Equine rotaviruses only cause clinical disease in foals and are considered primarily species specific; for example, cattle rotavirus affects cattle and not horses or humans. However, a recent report suggested that an unusual equine strain (H-1) may have originated from a porcine rotavirus strain that was transmitted to horses because at least 9 of 11 of its gene segments were found to be of porcine virus origin.[21] No natural reservoir for equine rotavirus has been identified. Mares may shed the virus subclinically, although this is transient and not considered to be as significant in magnitude as from diarrheic foals.[22] Considering the large concentrations of virus shed into the environment (10^{11} particles/g feces) by diarrheic animals, as well as the ability of the virus to remain viable for as long as 9 months,[23] the potential for an outbreak after the first clinical case is very real.

Rotavirus is transmitted by the fecal-oral route through contaminated feces or fomites and is highly contagious. The incubation period is 12 to 24 hours. Adult horses are not clinically affected during outbreaks of foal diarrhea, but some mares with diarrheic foals will seroconvert, indicating subclinical infection.[22] Studies of more than 400 adult horses performed in conjunction with rotavirus vaccination trials in Kentucky, Japan, and Argentina revealed a seroprevalence rate in broodmares approaching 100%.[11-13] However, these studies were conducted in concentrated horse-breeding regions, and seroprevalence in adult horses in other geographic areas may be less.

The average age of foals with rotaviral diarrhea was 75 days, with a reported range of 2 to 155 days in one study.[1] In a retrospective study of referred cases, foals ≥1 month of age were significantly more likely to have rotavirus as compared to foals less than or equal to 1 month of age (odds ratio [OR] 13.3, 95% confidence interval [CI] = 5.3-33, $p < 0.00001$).[20] In this study, the mean age of foals positive for rotavirus was 81 days

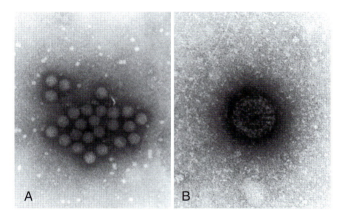

Figure 18-1 Electron micrographs of rotavirus. **A,** Particles magnified at ×135,000. **B,** Single particle magnified at ×300,000. (*Courtesy Ms. Patricia Van Meter, University of Kentucky.*)

*The authors acknowledge and appreciate the original contributions of these authors, whose work has been incorporated into this chapter.

(range 2-253) days. The results of these two studies are in contrast to those of a third study, which found that most diarrheic foals with rotavirus were 5 to 35 days of age, and the majority were in the younger age range.[24] The average duration of diarrhea in affected foals is 3 days (range, 1-9 days), with fecal shedding of rotavirus particles continuing for an average of 3 days after return of normal feces.

With appropriate supportive care, including fluid and electrolyte replacement therapy, rotaviral diarrhea has a low mortality and high morbidity in foal populations. In one study from a referral center, the survival rate of foals with rotaviral diarrhea was 94%.[20] During a 3-year study of rotavirus on multiple central Kentucky horse farms, no foal had a confirmed recurrence of disease after recovery. In another study, fecal shedding of virus was demonstrated in clinically normal foals on 7 of 10 farms undergoing an outbreak of foal rotaviral diarrhea.[1,25] This shedding does not continue after resolution of disease in other foals on the farm.

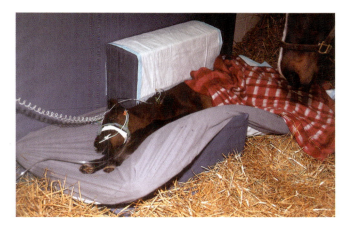

Figure 18-2 Young foals can develop life-threatening dehydration and electrolyte imbalances from rotavirus infection, requiring intensive care.

Pathogenesis

After rotavirus enters the GI tract, it invades and rapidly multiplies in columnar epithelial cells of the villous tips in the duodenum and jejunum.[24] This results in significant blunting of the villi and subsequent villous atrophy. The loss of these epithelial cells results in the absence of disaccharidases, especially lactase, causing transient lactose intolerance and a hyperosmotic solution in the intestinal lumen. This leads to malabsorption and maldigestion of nutrients and acute diarrhea. Intestinal crypt cells are not affected as they are in canine parvovirus infection. Therefore crypt cells continue to replicate, differentiate, and eventually replace the tip cells destroyed by the virus, resulting in a self-limiting disease. Chronic diarrhea (>14 days) is not typical of rotavirus infection.

Clinical Findings

The severity of rotavirus infection varies, depending on the foal's age and immune status, the virulence of the virus, and the quantity of viral inoculum. Foals less than 3 months of age are most severely affected, with neonates exhibiting the highest morbidity and mortality. Approximately 18 to 24 hours after ingestion of infective material, foals show signs of lethargy, decreased suckling, and diarrhea that may vary from "cow pie" to watery consistency. With watery diarrhea, the foals' tails may not be wet or stained with feces because of the projectile nature of the diarrhea. Fever may or may not be present. Anorexia and abdominal pain may also be present.

During farm outbreaks of rotavirus, foals may show severe diarrhea, dehydration, anorexia, fever, and lethargy within 10 days of birth. Younger foals are often more susceptible to severe disease because of their limited ability to self-correct fluid and electrolyte imbalances that accompany severe diarrhea (Fig. 18-2). Electrolyte imbalances may include hypochloremia, hyponatremia, hypokalemia, and acidosis. The hemogram results with rotaviral diarrhea vary and may be normal or reveal evidence of hemoconcentration (e.g., increased packed cell volume) and leukopenia.[26] With treatment, the mortality rate of rotaviral diarrhea is low. In one retrospective study of diarrheic foals presented to the University of Florida, 44/47 (94%) of foals with rotavirus diarrhea survived to discharge from the hospital.[20]

Diagnosis

Field Testing Procedures

Although electron microscopy (EM) for detection of viral particles in feces is widely considered to be the "gold standard" for rotavirus diagnosis, this test is not routinely available and is relatively expensive, and the turnaround time for results may be up to several days.

Commercial diagnostic assays are based on detection of VP6, the most abundant protein in viral particles.[5] Because VP6 is highly conserved across rotaviruses that affect many species, human rotavirus test kits are routinely used in equine practice and veterinary diagnostic laboratories. A fecal sample (1-3 g) or fecal swabs from affected foals should be submitted for rotavirus antigen testing by latex agglutination, immunoassay (enzyme-linked immunosorbent assay [ELISA]),[27,28] or other diagnostic methods described later. Samples that can be tested within 8 hours should be held at room temperature or refrigerated. Veterinarians should contact testing laboratories for recommendations regarding storage and shipment (cooled versus frozen) of samples if testing cannot be performed within 8 hours of sample collection.

Results from latex agglutination rotavirus test kits are available (Virogen Rotatest, Wampole Laboratories, Princeton, NJ) within 10 to 15 minutes of processing the sample (Fig. 18-3). The Virogen Rotatest has 100% sensitivity and 96.3% specificity compared with ELISA for diagnosis of bovine rotavirus infection.[29] Compared with EM for identification of viral particles in pediatric stool samples, the Virogen Rotatest has a sensitivity of 86% and specificity of 95%.[30]

The ImmunoCard STAT! rotavirus test is an immunogold-based, horizontal-flow membrane assay that yields results within 10 minutes. It had a sensitivity of 94% and specificity of 100% in one study of pediatric stool samples[31] and has been found useful for rapid diagnosis of bovine rotavirus infection.[27]

The Dipstick "Eiken" ROTA Dipstick immunochromatography assay was shown to have a sensitivity of 81.9% and specificity of 98.2% as compared to reverse transcription–PCR (RT-PCR) in one study.[32]

In another study, there was very good agreement (kappa = 0.88, 95% CI = 0.81-0.96) between detection of rotavirus by ELISA (Sure-Vue Rota Test, SA Scientific Ltd, San Antonio, TX) and by EM, the latter widely regarded as the "gold standard" for diagnosis.[20] Using EM as the reference, rotavirus ELISA had a sensitivity of 91%, specificity of 98%, and accuracy of 96%.[20] Because none of these assays has a sensitivity of 100%, a negative result should not rule out rotavirus. If suspicion is high despite a negative result, then the test should be repeated. Alternatively a test with higher sensitivity, such as PCR, should be used.

Polymerase chain reaction (reverse transcription; RT-PCR) of feces recently has become commercially available for use in

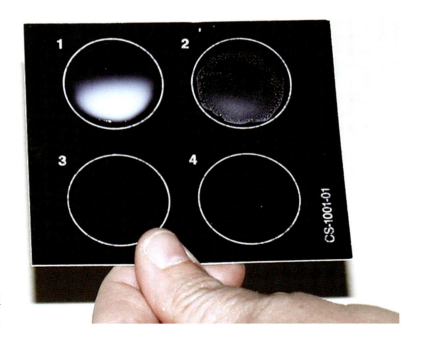

Figure 18-3 Latex agglutination test (Virogen Rotatest) showing homogenous fluid on negative sample (*1, left*) and agglutination of particles and clearing of fluid in rotavirus-positive sample (*2, right*).

foals.[3,33] Until more data correlating PCR results with clinical disease are available, PCR initially should be coupled with ELISA or latex agglutination during an outbreak. After the first case has been diagnosed, PCR alone can be utilized to detect additional cases and foals that are shedding virus subclinically.

Other Diagnostic Options

Other laboratory methods for diagnosis of rotaviral diarrhea include polyacrylamide gel electrophoresis[34] and various molecular techniques,[33,35] all using fecal samples. Rotaviruses are extremely difficult to grow in cell culture, so virus isolation is impractical for clinical use.[4] Serology for diagnostic purposes in foals is unreliable.[22]

As with testing feces for *Salmonella*, a single negative test result is not conclusive for the absence of rotavirus infection. In the author's experience, a minimum of three negative test results on samples properly obtained and stored before testing gives confidence in stating that a foal does not have rotaviral diarrhea.

A separate fecal sample should be obtained to rule out other causes of acute foal diarrhea, including *Salmonella*, *Clostridium difficile* or *perfringens*, coronavirus, *Cryptosporidium*, *Giardia*, and parasites as well as coinfection with these agents. Although concurrent infection with rotavirus and other pathogens, such as coronavirus, is possible, several studies have concluded that rotavirus infections in foals often occur without simultaneous infection with other potential pathogens.[1,2]

Pathologic Findings

Mortality is low in rotavirus infections; foals less than 14 days of age are at highest risk of death. In foals that die from dehydration and electrolyte imbalances, epithelial cells at the tips of intestinal villi are destroyed in the duodenum and occasionally the jejunum. The infection produces little inflammatory response in surrounding tissue.[4]

Therapy

Isotonic fluid therapy to correct electrolyte imbalances is especially important in young foals and those that are significantly dehydrated. Adsorbents and protectants, such as bismuth subsalicylate (0.5-1 mL/kg orally [PO] 2-4 times/day), di-tri-octahedral smectite paste (0.6 mL/kg PO 2 times per/day), and activated charcoal (0.25-0.5 g/kg PO once to once daily) for a few days may help in binding toxins and firming the feces, although owners should be aware that overuse can cause constipation. In addition, smectite and activated charcoal should be staggered with other oral medications to avoid nonspecific binding. Feces of foals treated with bismuth subsalicylate may appear dark in color, similar to the color observed with proximal GI tract hemorrhage. Doses of bismuth subsalicylate should be conservative because foals with compromised GI tracts may absorb salicylate and be subject to systemic effects.

In severely affected animals, parenteral nutrition may be indicated.[26,36,37] Parenteral nutrition allows for "bowel rest" by preventing foals from nursing for a 12- to 24-hour period if diarrhea is severe.

Because of the blunting effects of rotavirus on the small intestinal villi, exogenous lactase should be supplemented in foals with rotaviral diarrhea. A dose of 6000 Food Chemicals Codex U/50-kg foal (120 U/kg), PO every 3 to 8 hours has been recommended.

For uncomplicated rotavirus diarrhea in older foals (>30 days), antibiotics may not be indicated in all cases unless the animal is highly compromised or is in danger of septicemia, in which case broad-spectrum parenteral antibiotics should be used. The presence of neutropenia or fever warrant antibiotic use in these cases. Foals less than 30 days of age routinely should be treated with broad-spectrum antibiotics because of a high prevalence of bacteremia in foals with diarrhea/enteritis (up to 50% at admission in one study).[38] Foals with failure of passive transfer or with hypoproteinemia secondary to diarrhea may benefit from replacement with intravenous (IV) plasma transfusion.[36]

Foals with rotavirus diarrhea may present with mild signs of colic. Pain may be controlled with appropriate doses of nonsteroidal antiinflammatory drugs (NSAIDs) such as flunixin meglumine (e.g., 0.25 mg/kg every 12 hours [q12h] or 0.5-1 mg/kg IV q24h) or butorphanol (0.02-0.05 mg/kg intramuscular [IM] q4-6h). Respiratory rate and character should be monitored if butorphanol is used, as depression may be a side effect. Frequent or prolonged administration or inappropriately high doses of flunixin meglumine increase the risk for gastric ulceration and renal disease in foals.[37] Serum creatinine and albumin or total protein concentrations should be monitored in foals being administered flunixin meglumine.

Diarrhea is a significant risk factor for the development of gastric ulcers in foals.[39] Prophylactic treatment with proton-pump blockers (e.g., omeprazole 2-4 mg/kg PO q24h or pantoprazole 1.5 mg/kg IV diluted q24h) is recommended for most affected foals. Omeprazole oral paste (GastroGard, Merial, Duluth, GA) facilitates healing of equine gastric ulcers and is approved for treatment of foals greater than or equal to 4 weeks of age but has been studied and can be used in younger foals.[40,41] Other antiulcer medications include H2 antagonists such as ranitidine (6.6 mg/kg PO q8h), famotidine (2.8 mg/kg PO q12h), or cimetidine (12-20 mg/kg PO q8h). However, ranitidine has exhibited a blunted duration of alkalinizing response in clinically ill neonatal foals.[42] Ranitidine has some prokinetic properties and should be used with caution in foals with dysmotility. Sucralfate can also be used (20 mg/kg PO q6-8h) to potentially promote ulcer healing. Because sucralfate may inhibit the absorption of other oral medications, it should not be administered at the same time as other drugs.[43]

Supportive care and hygiene are critically important for foals with rotaviral diarrhea to avoid pressure ulcers, scalded perianal skin, and secondary infections. Foals recumbent in soiled surroundings are predisposed to secondary problems such as infected skin wounds and pneumonia. Stalls should be kept as dry and clean as possible and should be heavily bedded. To prevent dermatitis between the hind legs and in the perianal area, baby oil, baby powder, zinc oxide ointment, or commercial diaper rash ointments may be applied. Should the skin become compromised, the area should be cleaned and an antibiotic ointment applied.

Nitazoxanide (NTZ) has been studied for use in human children with rotaviral diarrhea. It is labeled for treatment of diarrhea caused by *Cryptosporidium* and *Giardia* infections in humans older than 1 year of age. A randomized clinical trial showed that NTZ decreased the duration of rotaviral diarrhea in hospitalized pediatric human patients.[44] However, diarrhea and colitis are risks associated with NTZ use in horses, and it should therefore be used with extreme caution until further studied.

Prevention

Vaccination

Since 1996, the Equine Rotavirus Vaccine (Pfizer Animal Health, Madison, NJ) has been marketed under conditional license (U.S. Department of Agriculture [USDA]). The vaccine contains an inactivated strain of a G3 equine rotavirus serotype (H2 strain or G3P[12]) in a metabolizable oil-in-water adjuvant.[11] This vaccine is administered intramuscularly to pregnant mares at 8, 9, and 10 months of gestation to heighten colostral immunity. Each pregnancy requires revaccination with 3 doses. This vaccine has been utilized extensively in equine intensive locales in central Kentucky, Florida, Newmarket in the United Kingdom (UK), and other major breeding centers in the United States, UK, and Ireland. Antirotaviral antibodies are concentrated in colostrum and absorbed by suckling foals.[11,12] In one study, foals of 100 vaccinated and 65 unvaccinated mares were studied. Vaccinated mares had received an inactivated rotavirus (G3P2, G3P12, and G6P1) vaccine at 9 and 10 months of gestation. The morbidity of diarrhea was 30% in foals born to vaccinated mares, in contrast to 80% in foals from unvaccinated mares. Duration of diarrhea was shorter in foals in the vaccinated mare group (1.8 days versus 7.3 days). Importantly, there was 0% shedding detected in the diarrheic foals born to vaccinated mares, as opposed to 80% shedding in the diarrheic foals

of unvaccinated mares.[45] In a second study of 627 mares over 2 years, the vaccine was administered at 8, 9, and 10 months of gestation in a randomized controlled trial. The vaccine was determined to be safe, and antibody titers were significantly higher in foals born to vaccinated mares for up to 90 days postpartum. The incidence of rotaviral diarrhea was decreased in the foals of the study group as compared to controls; however, this was not statistically different. Although beneficial, vaccination should be considered an adjunctive to farm hygiene and meticulous husbandry practices, rather than a replacement for them.

Husbandry/Infection Control

Because rotaviruses are excreted from diarrheic foals in large concentrations (up to 10^{11} particles/g), overcrowding is a significant risk factor for outbreaks of foal diarrhea. Rotavirus can survive for months in the environment.[4] Manure and bedding from stalls of affected foals should be considered a biosecurity threat to unaffected foals. This material should not be spread on pastures but rather composted in an area isolated from horses or disposed of according to local ordinances.

Hygiene of foaling areas is critical for disease prevention. Affected foals should be isolated and released when fecal shedding stops (through repeat fecal PCR testing). Because rotavirus is a nonenveloped virus, it has natural resistance to disinfectants that primarily disrupt the viral lipid envelope. Prevention and control of outbreaks of equine infectious diseases are discussed in Chapter 63. Peroxygen, accelerated hydrogen peroxide, and some phenolic disinfectants have efficacy against rotaviruses.

Public Health Considerations

Rotavirus is not regarded as a zoonotic disease because of species specificity. However, standard barrier precautions of disposable gloves, disinfectant foot baths, use of dedicated equipment, and hand washing should be taken with any equine diarrheic disease.

Equine Coronavirus

Coronaviruses cause a variety of GI and respiratory diseases in a number of veterinary species. Although coronavirus-induced enteritis has been suspected in foals with diarrhea, direct pathogenicity of equine coronavirus (ECoV) in equids has not been definitively demonstrated until recently.[46,47] Traditionally regarded as a pathogen of foals only, investigators have now documented the presence of ECoV in adult horses with fever and enteric disease.[48]

Etiology

Coronaviruses are members of the *Coronaviridae* family, order Nidovirales, all of which are positive-sense RNA viruses.[49-52] The family *Coronaviridae* has two subfamilies: *Coronavirinae* and *Torovirinae*. The subfamily *Coronavirinae* contains three genera: *Alphacoronavirus*, *Betacoronavirus*, and *Gammacoronavirus*. Equine coronavirus is a *Betacoronavirus* similar to human coronavirus OC43, human enteric coronavirus, bovine coronavirus, and canine respiratory coronavirus.[53] The coronaviruses were so named because the unusually large, club-shaped peplomers projecting from the envelope give the viral particle the appearance of a solar corona.[50,52,54] The tubular nucleocapsid is composed of a phosphorylated nucleoprotein and appears to be connected directly to a transmembrane protein, *M*, which spans the lipid bilayer three times. Only a small fraction of its mass is exposed to the external environment.[50,52,54,55] Two types of prominent spikes line the outside of the virion. The long spikes, which consist of the *S* (spike) glycoprotein, are present on all coronaviruses and give them their characteristic "corona" appearance. The short spikes, which consist of the hemagglutinin-esterase (HE) glycoprotein, are present in only some coronaviruses.[50,52,53,55] The other subfamily under family *Coronaviridae* is *Torovirinae*, and within that family is the genus *Torovirus*. Toroviruses are established agents of gastroenteritis in animals, and the type species of the genus is Berne virus (BEV), a chance isolate from a diarrheic horse in 1972.[51,55-58] Torovirus is discussed in more detail later in this chapter.

Epidemiology and Clinical Findings

Coronaviruses are a common cause of disease in humans and domestic animals.[52] They have been identified in mice, rats, chickens, turkeys, swine, dogs, cats, rabbits, horses, cattle, camelids, and humans.[46,50,59,60] They cause respiratory, GI, neurologic, and generalized infections.[55] In horses, it is believed that coronavirus spreads through fecal-oral transmission; however, other routes of transmission, such as respiratory and mechanical, may also be possible but so far unknown.[55,61] Most coronaviruses infect only cells of their natural host species and a few closely related species.[52] In their natural host species, coronaviruses exhibit marked tissue tropism. Virus replication in vivo can be either disseminated, causing systemic infections, or restricted to a few cell types, often the epithelial cells of the respiratory or enteric tract and macrophages, causing localized infections. Coronavirus replication takes place in the cytoplasm of infected cells.[52] Like rotavirus, coronavirus causes damage to the villi of the intestinal mucosa, resulting in loss of absorptive capacity, leading to a malabsorptive diarrhea. The course of disease is typically initiated in the proximal small intestine.

Anzai et al[61] investigated the effect of long-distance transport of 29 racehorses (age 2 years) on serologic evidence of infection with potential respiratory pathogens, including coronavirus. Serum antibody titers to coronavirus were evaluated by serum neutralization (SN) test using bovine coronavirus (BCV), which is closely related antigenically to ECoV.[53,61,62] Two horses were seropositive for BCV 1 month before transportation (titers 10 and 40). These horses were transported in the same vehicle as four horses that were seronegative to coronavirus. The four seronegative horses seroconverted after transportation (titers between 10 and 20 within 1 month), but none developed clinical signs, and a direct relationship between disease and coronavirus infection could not be confirmed.[61] This study suggested that ECoV could possibly spread among horses while they are stabled together or during transport, although this requires confirmation. This hypothesis is consistent with serologic evidence that BCV or its related virus is widely prevalent in horses in Japan.[61,62]

Coronavirus-like particles have been observed by negative-contrast EM in fecal samples from healthy and diarrheic foals,[63-68] from one foal with combined immunodeficiency syndrome and diarrhea,[69] and from adult horses concurrently diagnosed with *Neorickettsia risticii*, the causative agent of Potomac horse fever.[70] Concurrent infections with rotavirus[65,66] and *Cryptosporidium*[69] have also been reported in foals.

In a single case report, a coronavirus antigenically related to BCV was identified in a 5-day-old Quarter Horse foal with enterocolitis.[47] This foal developed severe diarrhea starting on the second day of life, indicating a short incubation period, and had multiple secondary complications, including fungal pneumonia, marked limb edema, and hypoproteinemia. A complete blood count revealed an inflammatory leukogram with a regenerative left shift, anemia, and thrombocytopenia. The foal developed vascular pathology in the distal limbs and eventually had detachment of the hoof wall from the laminar structures and was euthanized. Bacterial cultures from feces were negative for enteric pathogens, and viral particles were not observed on EM. Coronavirus was identified in intestinal tissues of the foal by immunohistochemistry using BCV-specific monoclonal antibodies and in feces using an antigen-capture ELISA designed for BCV detection, indicating a lack of sensitivity of EM in this case.[47,53] The foal's serum antibody titer to BCV increased over an 8-day period from 1:25 to 1:100.[2]

Despite the reports of probable coronavirus infection in foals, there were no definitive descriptions of ECoV isolation from sick horses before 2000.[47,63,64,69,70] The first isolation and characterization was described in 2000 from the feces of a 2-week-old Arabian foal.[53,75] The foal had diarrhea and fever, which persisted for 6 days, after which the foal recovered with medical treatment.

A third case report described coronaviral diarrhea in a 3-day-old Thoroughbred foal that developed diarrhea on the second day of life.[71] This foal had mild anemia, leukopenia with a left shift and lymphopenia, and hyperfibrinogenemia. Interestingly, this foal developed marked hyperglycemia (257-500 mg/dL) and transient diabetes mellitus associated with low insulin concentrations. Coronavirus particles were observed on EM. The foal survived with intensive treatment, including a 26-day course of insulin therapy. The authors speculated whether the coronaviral infection could have played a role in pancreatic injury, resulting in transient diabetes mellitus. Coronavirus has been associated with pancreatic damage in other species.[72,73]

Coronavirus in Adult Horses

Recently coronavirus has been associated with febrile and enteric disease in adult horses.[48] Previously, there was suggestion of a coronavirus-like agent in horses with Potomac horse fever.[70] Aside from that, coronavirus was thought to be an intermittent pathogen of only young foals. In the recent study from Japan,[48] 132/600 draft racehorses that were 2 to 4 years old developed increased rectal temperature and in some, diarrhea of 2 to 4 days' duration. Coronavirus infection was documented through RT-PCR, virus isolation, indirect immunofluorescence, and viral genome sequencing, as well as serology of affected horses.

In 2011-2012, a number of outbreaks of coronavirus disease in adult horses occurred in the United States, including California, Texas, Wisconsin, and Massachusetts.[74] These were diagnosed through RT-PCR of feces, and the virus was sequenced to have 98% to 99% homology to the NC99 strain described by Zhang et al.[75] Eighty six percent of sick horses tested by fecal PCR (38/44) were positive for ECoV. Seven percent (7/96) of clinically healthy horses on the premises were fecal positive.[74] The most common clinical signs were anorexia (88%), lethargy (78%), and fever (73%).[74] Other signs included changes in fecal character (soft-formed to watery) and colic, but these were in a minority of horses. The morbidity ranged from 20% to 57% on affected premises. Clinical signs resolved in most horses within 1 to 4 days. Approximately 6.8% of horses were euthanized because of the severity of clinical signs, including acute neurologic disease or marked endotoxemia. Common hematologic changes included leukopenia with neutropenia and/or lymphopenia. Shedding in feces generally occurred for a few days. In this report, follow-up fecal samples were available for seven horses, and PCR detection of ECoV persisted for 3-9 days.[74]

A recent coronavirus outbreak occurred in Japan, involving 204/650 (31%) horses.[76] Fever was found in 96% of horses, and only 13% developed diarrhea and/or colic. Most horses recovered in 2-4 days, except for those with watery diarrhea which took 5-10 days. Two horses (0.98%) with watery diarrhea and stomatitis died. Two strains were identified, which represented antigenic shift from prior strains.[76]

Diagnosis

Coronavirus infection may be suspected if other etiologic agents of diarrhea in foals or adults have been ruled out, especially in outbreak situations. It can also occur as a coinfection with other enteric pathogens. Coronaviruses are difficult to isolate and propagate in cell culture. The diagnostic method of choice is direct demonstration of coronavirus antigens in biologic samples.[9] Current practical and sensitive means of diagnosis is through fecal RT-PCR.[3,77]

Negative-stain EM can also be used to identify coronavirus-like particles in feces; however, it is not as sensitive as PCR.[53,64-66,69,70,78] If viral particles are not present in sufficient numbers, EM examination may require considerable searching or may be unrewarding.[2,16] Fecal ELISA may also be used, although its sensitivity and specificity for use in horse feces remains to be determined.

Because of the cross-reactivity between BCV and ECoV, detection of neutralizing antibody to BCV in horses provides presumptive evidence of exposure to ECV.[47,53,61,62,64] Because the presence of SN antibodies against BCV in equine sera may be a common finding, acute and convalescent samples should be examined for evidence of increasing titer.[47,61,62] Convalescent serum samples from horses with suspected ECoV infection may be evaluated approximately 10 days after the onset of disease. In human patients, a fourfold increase in titer to coronavirus is indicative of recent active infection. An antemortem diagnostic panel for ECoV can include assay for serum antibody titer to BCV and fecal capture ELISA evaluation for coronavirus antigen.[47] However, RT-PCR of fecal samples is currently more practical (and rapid) for use by practitioners.

Additional studies are needed to determine the prevalence of ECoV infection in healthy and sick horses, the occurrence of mixed infections of coronavirus and other enteric pathogens, and the relative importance of ECoV as a cause of enteric disease in horses.[53]

Husbandry/Infection Control

Horses infected with ECoV should be isolated due to potential for fecal-oral spread. Fortunately, most horses appear to shed the virus only for a few to several days.[74] Optimally horses should be tested negative on fecal PCR prior to being released from isolation. Coronaviruses are enveloped viruses and are therefore susceptible to common disinfectants including sodium hypochlorite, ethyl acohol, povidone iodine, phenols, accelerated hydrogen peroxide, and peroxygen based disinfectants.

However, based on work with human coronaviruses, quaternary ammonium compounds may have variable to relatively poor activity against coronavirus. The presence of organic matter should be a consideration in choice of disinfectant.

Equine Torovirus

Etiology

Equine torovirus (Berne virus) was originally isolated from a rectal swab of a horse with hepatic and GI disease in Berne, Switzerland, in 1972.[79] It is currently classified in the subfamily *Torovirinae* with bovine, human, and porcine toroviruses, within the family *Coronaviridae* and order Nidovirales.[80-82] The enveloped virions are pleomorphic with large protein spikes on the surface, resembling the peplomers of coronaviruses. The nucleocapsid has a tubular appearance with helical symmetry. The positive-sense RNA genome is estimated to be 20 to 25 kilobases in length with six open reading frames (ORFs). Four structural proteins have been identified: spike (S), membrane (M), hemagglutinin-esterase (HE), and nucleocapsid (N) proteins.

Epidemiology

Although originally isolated from a horse with GI disease, a causal link between Berne virus and equine disease has not been established. Limited seroepidemiologic studies indicate that the virus is present in Europe and the United States. Neutralizing antibody is also found in the sera of other ungulates (cattle, sheep, goats, pigs), laboratory rabbits, and at least two species of wild mice (*Clethrionomys glareolus* and *Apodemus sylvaticus*).[83]

Clinical Findings

Despite widespread evidence of exposure to Berne virus, no evidence indicates that this virus is associated with clinical disease in horses. Inoculation of the virus into two foals induced neutralizing antibody without associated clinical signs.[83] Bovine torovirus has been associated with gastroenteritis in calves and possibly pneumonia in older cattle.[82,84] Human and porcine toroviruses are associated with gastroenteritis in people and pigs, respectively.[85-87]

The complete reference list is available online at www.expertconsult.com.

CHAPTER

19 Rabies

Pamela A. Wilkins and Fabio Del Piero*

Rabies virus (RABV) is an enveloped ribonucleic acid (RNA) rhabdovirus that induces lethal polioencephalomyelitis and ganglionitis in infected animals.[1,2] The disease is universally

endemic in mammals and other warm-blooded vertebrates, except in Australia, where other types of zoonotic lyssaviruses transmitted by flying foxes (bats) are present. The disease has been excluded or eradicated from some countries, or parts of them, especially islands (e.g., Great Britain, New Zealand, Iceland). According to the Centers for Disease Control and

*The authors acknowledge and appreciate the original contributions of these authors, whose work has been incorporated into this chapter.

Prevention (CDC), domestic animal species accounted for 8% of all rabid animals reported in the United States in 2010. The number of reported rabid domestic animals has decreased among all domestic species except domesticated cats.

Etiology

Viruses in the *Rhabdoviridae* family known to infect mammals belong to either the genus *Vesiculovirus* (vesicular stomatitis virus serotype New Jersey and serotype Indiana, Chandipura virus, and Piry virus) or the genus *Lyssavirus* (rabies virus and rabies-like viruses).[1,2] Lyssaviruses include six distinct genotypes that can be classified according to their degree of amino acid homology. Genotypes 2 (Lagos bat virus) and 3 (Mokola virus) are the most phylogenetically distant from the vaccinal and classic rabies viruses of genotype 1. Genotypes 4 (Duvenhage virus) and 5 (European bat lyssavirus 1 [EBL1]) are closely related to each other, with the separate genotype 6 represented by EBL2.

Rabies virus virions are enveloped, bullet-shaped, 45 to 100 nm in diameter, and 100 to 430 nm long (Fig. 19-1). Surface projections of the envelope are distinct spikes, dispersed evenly over the whole surface (except for the quasiplanar end of bullet-shaped viruses). The uncoiled nucleocapsid is filamentous, with regular surface structure, and cross-banded. Virions

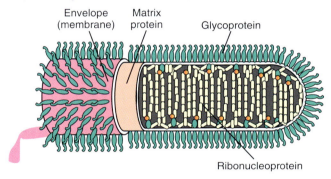

Envelope (membrane)   Matrix protein   Glycoprotein

Ribonucleoprotein

Figure 19-1 Diagrammatic representation of rabies virus. *(Courtesy Centers for Disease Control and Prevention, Atlanta.)*

contain 1% to 2% nucleic acid composed of one molecule of linear, usually negative-sense, single-stranded RNA. Nucleotide sequences of the 3′ terminus are inverted and complementary to similar regions on the 5′ end and are the same for each gene segment in species of the same genus. Virions contain 65% to 75% protein, most of which are structural. RABVs are recognized and classified through panels of monoclonal antibodies against nucleocapsid proteins. The pattern of antiglycoprotein reactivity of the isolates allows identification of the viral subtype.

Epidemiology

Rabies virus is transmitted to warm-blooded animals by bites from infected vectors such as foxes, raccoons, skunks, bats, and vampire bats. In 2003, wild animals accounted for more than 91% of all cases of rabies reported to the CDC.[3] Rabies control programs in the United States, including vaccination programs, have significantly decreased, if not eliminated, rabies in humans caused by canine variants. However, ever-increasing numbers of human cases are attributable to bat variants, a group difficult to target for rabies control by traditional methods.

In the United States, rabies infection of terrestrial mammals occurs in geographically defined regions, and transmission is usually within species, with occasional spillover to other species that rarely maintain intraspecific transmission (Fig. 19-2).[4] Host switching of rabies virus variants does occur, and once established, these variants can perpetuate regionally and become enzootic in new reservoir species. Phylogenetic analysis of circulating variants has suggested that canine rabies virus variants were the probable origins of several circulating wildlife variants of foxes (Texas and Arizona), skunks (California and north central United States), and mongooses (Puerto Rico). The remaining rabies virus variants in the United States (i.e., raccoon, south central skunk, and Flagstaff rabies virus) have been phylogenetically associated with switching from bat-associated rabies virus variants. Circulating independently of RABV variants associated with mesocarnivores are multiple variants associated with several species of bats. More than 30 species of bats have been reported with rabies in the United States, and more than 8 rabies virus lineages have been identified and associated with these bat species. However, in contrast to the circulation

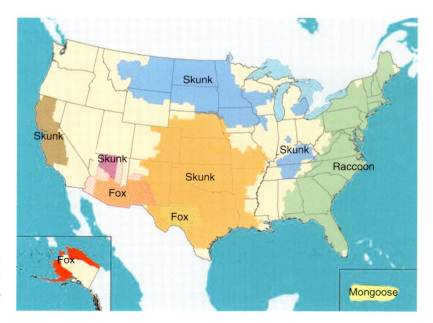

Figure 19-2 Rabies reservoirs. Distribution of major rabies virus variants among mesocarnivore reservoirs in the United States and Puerto Rico, 2010. *(From Blanton JD, Palmer D, Dyer J, Rupprecht CE: Rabies Surveillance in the United States during 2010, JAVMA 239(6):773-783, 2011.)*

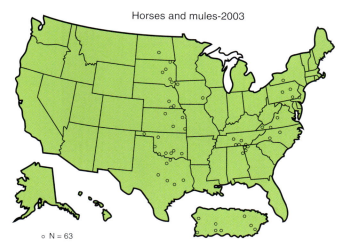

Horses and mules-2003

○ N = 63

Figure 19-3 Distribution of equine rabies cases in the United States and Puerto Rico in 2003. Note Central and Mid-Atlantic to Northeastern distribution in the continental United States. Most cases are caused by the local reservoir type, that is, Central (skunk) and Mid-Atlantic to Northeastern (raccoon). *(Courtesy Centers for Disease Control and Prevention, Atlanta.)*

of rabies in mesocarnivores, the greater mobility and population interactions of bats preclude definitive determination of the distribution of bat rabies virus variants other than the geographic ranges of the implicated host bat species. Recent studies have suggested lower frequencies of cross-species transmission and host shift with increasing phylogenetic distance between bat species. Similarities in biologic barriers and social structures of closely related bat species could account for higher rates of cross-species transmission of rabies virus and may be a factor in the evolution of current bat rabies virus variants. Thirty-seven horses or donkeys were reported as testing positive for rabies in 2010, which is an almost 10% decrease from 2009 (Fig. 19-3). In 2010, Connecticut, Colorado, Michigan, Montana, North Carolina, Nebraska, New Mexico, Tennessee, Virginia, and West Virginia reported one case each; New York reported two; Pennsylvania reported six; Oklahoma reported six, and Texas had the largest number of equine cases with eight.[4] Rabid raccoons and foxes are primarily concentrated in the eastern United States, whereas rabid bats are more widely dispersed, with large numbers located in Texas and Oklahoma. Rabid skunks are concentrated in the northeastern United States, the Mid-Atlantic region, and the Central Midwest, particularly Texas. The majority of rabies in horses occurs in animals with no history of vaccination, although it may be recognized in animals not vaccinated within a year of diagnosis.[5]

Pathogenesis

The primary means of transmission of RABV is through the bite of an infected animal that inoculates saliva containing virus into tissues of a receptive animal. The virus likely replicates in muscle tissue at the site of inoculation. Rabies virus is believed to remain near the site of initial inoculation for most of the incubation period. In 1889, DiVestea and Zagari[6] showed that mortality was greatly diminished by severing the sciatic nerves of experimental animals before virus was inoculated in the footpad. This reduction in mortality is seen even when the nerves are severed several days after inoculation of virus.[7] Delayed progression of infection within muscle cells is thought to be responsible for the long incubation period of clinical rabies.[8]

Eventually, RABV binds to nicotinic acetylcholine receptors at the neuromuscular junction, the major site of entry into neurons.[9,10] The neural cell adhesion molecule, the low-affinity p75 neurotrophic receptor, and perhaps the N-methyl-D-aspartate NR1 receptor may also function as RABV receptors.[11-14] The virus then travels in an ascending fashion through the spinal cord to the brain or from the cranial nerves directly to the brainstem. Once transit in peripheral nerves begins, it progresses rapidly through transsynaptic neuronal spread. Virus can be observed in peripheral nerve myelin late in infection.[15] Clinical signs appear to result primarily from neuronal dysfunction secondary to drastically diminished synthesis of proteins required for maintenance of normal neuronal function.[16] After it reaches the brain, RABV is passed centrifugally to tissues and organs. It reaches the salivary glands and nasal secretions after passage down appropriate cranial nerves.[17]

Clinical Findings

Several authors have described clinical signs of rabies in horses in detail.[5,18-20] These signs range from poor racing performance to bizarre behavior and may include spinal cord, cerebral, and cranial nerve signs; apparent lameness; gastrointestinal signs; and genitourinary signs (Fig. 19-4). Clinical signs are progressive from onset until death, which usually occurs by day 10. Average survival from the onset of clinical signs is approximately 5 days. Clinical chemistry and hematology results are nonspecific and nondiagnostic. Cerebrospinal fluid (CSF) analysis reveals increased protein and lymphocytes but is not diagnostic.

Spinal cord signs are frequently observed in horses with rabies and may include subtle hindlimb lameness or shifting of weight in the hindlimbs, progressing to knuckling of one or both fetlocks. Ataxia or weakness usually follows, with paresis advancing to total pelvic limb paralysis when spinal cord signs are present. Associated signs may be constipation, tenesmus, paraphimosis in males, dribbling of urine from bladder paralysis, and flaccid tail and anus.

The classic description of encephalic signs includes evidence of progressive depression ("dumb" form) or aggression ("furious" form). Depression is often characterized by extreme obtundation, whereas aggression often includes hyperesthesia and self-mutilation. Other accentuated cerebral responses observed in rabies patients are hypersexuality with frequent mounting behavior, localized or generalized pruritus leading to self injury, tremors, seizures, alert eyes and ears despite paralysis or ataxia, blindness, head pressing, bellowing, and opisthotonos. Dysphagia, salivation, and a weak tongue may occur, often accompanied by an inability to drink, which may reflect laryngeal paralysis.

Several common diseases should be considered as differential diagnoses of rabies. In the paralytic form with spinal cord signs predominating, sacral injuries from estrous activities and spinal cord neoplasms or abscesses should be considered. In advanced rabies cases approaching coma, many encephalitides and toxic central nervous system (CNS) diseases should be considered.

Diagnosis

There is no definitive antemortem test for rabies in horses. A minimum protocol for postmortem diagnosis of rabies can be found at the CDC website.* Clinical signs are suggestive but nondiagnostic. CSF from rabies patients may be normal, have

*http://www.cdc.gov/rabies.

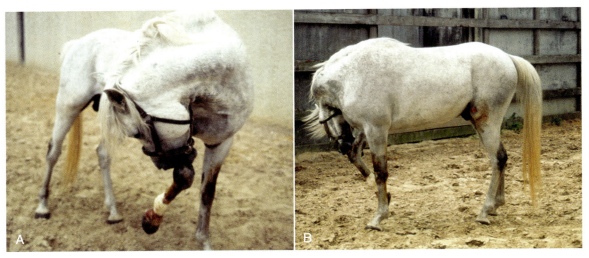

Figure 19-4 Arabian stallion with rabies exhibiting signs of self-mutilation. Aggressive biting behavior led to human injury and rabies virus exposure, with subsequent human prophylactic treatment. *(Courtesy Dr. Ian G. Mayhew.)*

only increased protein values, or have both increased nucleated cells and protein. Most nucleated cells in the CSF of rabies patients are mononuclear cells. However, one report of 21 cases of rabies in horses found mononuclear pleocytosis without increases in protein concentration in five of six horses. No other antemortem tests are potentially helpful to the practicing veterinarian.

The brain from suspect animals must be submitted to a regional laboratory approved by the respective state health department for rabies testing, using CNS tissue smears and direct immunofluorescence with monoclonal antibodies. Other ancillary tests, including enzyme-linked immunosorbent assay (ELISA), reverse transcriptase–polymerase chain reaction (RT-PCR), and peroxidase immunohistochemistry (IHC), are available and reliable but are not considered official diagnostic tools.[5] These latter tests can be used when fresh tissue is not available or as research tools. In a simple, rapid, single-step RT-PCR test of the nucleoprotein (N) gene of RABV, a conserved set of RT-PCR primers is designed to amplify the most variable region in the N gene. The cornea impression smear test using direct fluorescent IHC is not reliable for rabies in animals. Intracerebral murine inoculation is not used as a routine diagnostic tool but can be used to propagate the virus. The fluorescent antibody virus neutralization (FAVN) test is used for the detection of antibodies against rabies virus. This test can be modified by using monoclonal antirabies antibodies and a peroxidase antimouse conjugate, instead of a fluorescent antirabies conjugate, with the results read on an automatic multichannel spectrophotometer. Rabies virus is highly neurotropic but has been also observed in glial cells, epithelial cells of the cornea, hair follicles of carnivores, adrenal medulla, and skeletal muscle.

Pathologic Findings (Figs. 19-5 through 19-13)

Gross CNS lesions of rabies are rare in horses and may consist of focal to multifocal, mild to moderate hemorrhages. Self-trauma or aspiration pneumonia may be seen. Histologic lesions of rabies in horses are similar to lesions in cattle, although with more frequent neuronal vacuolization, and much less frequent Negri body formation.[5,9] There is a clear viral tropism for gray matter, neuronal cell bodies, and glial cells. Less virus antigen is found in animals euthanized early in the disease process.

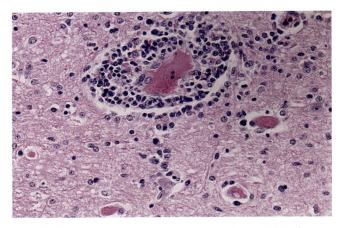

Figure 19-5 Rabies; horse, cerebrum, neocortex. Polioencephalitis characterized by perivascular small lymphocyte cuffs, gliosis *(right)*, and neuronal satellitosis *(below)*. (Hematoxylin-eosin [HE] stain.) *(Courtesy Dr. Fabio Del Piero.)*

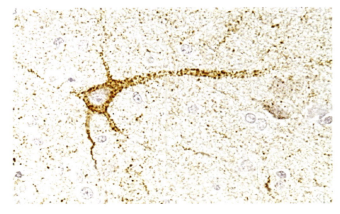

Figure 19-6 Rabies; horse, neocortex. The cytoplasm of this cortical neuron is prominently colonized by rabies virus, which extends within the dendrites and the axon; surrounding fibers are diffusely colonized, and the astrocytes are hypertrophied. (Indirect peroxidase immunohistochemistry [IPIHC] and hematoxylin [He] stain.) *(Courtesy Dr. Fabio Del Piero.)*

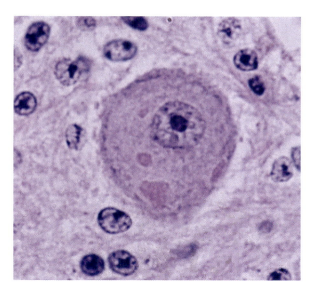

Figure 19-7 Rabies; horse, cerebellum, Purkinje cell. Intracytoplasmic eosinophilic Negri inclusion bodies. (HE stain.) *(Courtesy Dr. Fabio Del Piero.)*

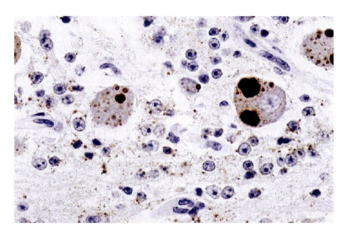

Figure 19-9 Rabies; horse, cerebellum. Purkinje cells and granular cells contain variously sized, round to oval, often prominent, rabies virus aggregates. (IPIHC and HE stain.) *(Courtesy Dr. Fabio Del Piero.)*

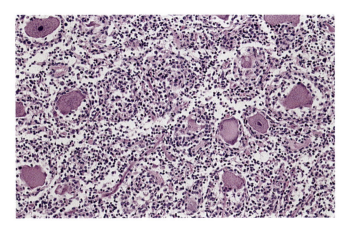

Figure 19-11 Rabies; horse, trigeminal ganglion. Severe, diffuse lymphocytic ganglionitis. (HE stain.) *(Courtesy Dr. Fabio Del Piero.)*

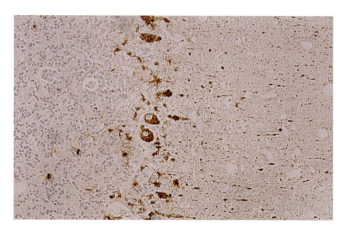

Figure 19-8 Rabies; horse, cerebellum. Abundant intracytoplasmic rabies virus within Purkinje cells, granule cell layer *(left)*, and in particular within the molecular layers and fibers *(right)*. (IPIHC and HE stain.) *(Courtesy Dr. Fabio Del Piero.)*

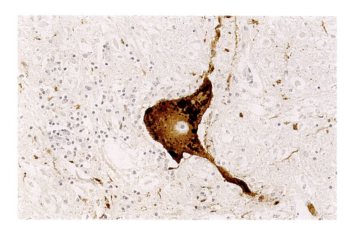

Figure 19-10 Rabies; horse, brainstem. The cytoplasm of this nuclear neuron is heavily colonized by rabies virus, which extends within the visible dendrite and the axon; surrounding fibers also contain rabies virus, and there is moderate focal gliosis *(left)*. (IPIHC and HE stain.) *(Courtesy Dr. Fabio Del Piero.)*

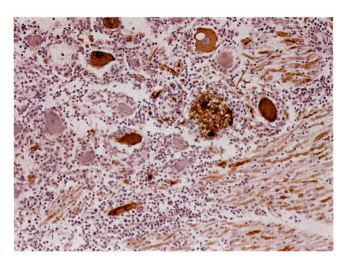

Figure 19-12 Rabies; horse, trigeminal ganglion. Abundant intracytoplasmic rabies virus within ganglial neurons and trigeminal nerve fibers *(right)*; there is a gathering of glial cells replacing a necrotic phagocytized neuron (Nageotte body) and lymphocytic ganglionitis. (IPIHC and HE stain.) *(Courtesy Dr. Fabio Del Piero.)*

Histologic lesions observed in rabid animals, which died or were euthanized, consist of nonsuppurative perivascular encephalomyelitis with ganglionitis. Moderate to severe lymphocytic perivascular inflammation in gray and white matter of cerebral hemispheres with mild lymphocytic leptomeningitis is often present. In the basal nuclei, gray matter of the thalamus, and the brainstem, there is prominent inflammation with diffuse gliosis and the presence of lymphocytes in the neuropil. In these areas and in the hippocampus, neuronophagia, neuronal chromatolysis, microglial cell nodules, and proliferation of rod cells tend to be constant features. Moderate lymphocytic inflammation infiltrates the subependymal tissue of the lateral ventricles and fornix. The cerebellum contains mild perivascular lymphocytic inflammation in the molecular layer, mild lymphocytic leptomeningitis, and moderate inflammation of the white matter. Negri bodies, eosinophilic intracytoplasmic inclusions associated with accumulations of viral and cell protein (see Fig. 19-7), are observed in pyramidal cells of the hippocampus, extensively in Purkinje cells, and infrequently in the neocortex, without inflammatory changes. Mild ring hemorrhages are occasionally observed multifocally. Trigeminal ganglia are affected by severe lymphocytic inflammation with neuronal degeneration, neuronophagia, and formation of Nageotte bodies, which are aggregates of glial cells replacing a neuron (see Figs. 19-11 and 19-12).

Using indirect peroxidase IHC with monoclonal antibodies, RABV can be identified within neural cell cytoplasm and processes.[5] Often the distribution of RABV is prominent, with marked intracytoplasmic immunoreactivity of almost all neurons in every brain area and diffuse granular positivity of the neuropil of cerebral and cerebellar cortices, the thalamus, and the gray matter of the brainstem and spinal cord. Rabies virus forms fine to large granules and 3- to 10-micron inclusion bodies that are single or multiple and distributed homogenously within the cytoplasm. RABV is predominantly observed in neuronal cell bodies, axons, and dendrites, which appear morphologically normal. There is prominent immunostaining of cortical neurons, pyramidal cells, and neurons of gyrus dentatus, as well as nuclei of the thalamus and brainstem. In the cerebellum, RABV is primarily localized within the Purkinje cells and some neurons of the granular and molecular layers. The spinal cord often contains abundant RABV in dorsal and ventral horns, with sparing of the white matter. RABV is also observed in some astrocytes and oligodendrocytes, ganglion cells of the retina and trigeminal ganglia cells, and autonomic ganglia of celiac-mesenteric ganglia. Negri bodies are reported in less than 30% of cases, and their absence should not rule out rabies as a diagnosis.

Therapy

No known therapy is effective for treatment of unvaccinated or vaccinated horses with clinical rabies. Horses presenting with clinical signs of rabies should be isolated to prevent possible human exposure. Healthy, vaccinated horses suspected of being exposed to rabies may be quarantined for a period of observation for development of clinical signs. All species of livestock are susceptible to rabies; horses are among the most frequently infected. Horses exposed to a confirmed rabid animal and currently vaccinated with a vaccine approved by the U.S. Department of Agriculture (USDA) for that species should be revaccinated immediately and observed for 45 days (Table 19-1). Unvaccinated horses should be euthanized immediately. If the owner is unwilling to have this done, the horse should be kept under close observation for 6 months. More than one rabid horse in a herd, or herbivore-to-herbivore transmission, is uncommon. Therefore, if a single animal has been exposed to or infected by rabies, quarantine of the rest of the herd is not necessary.

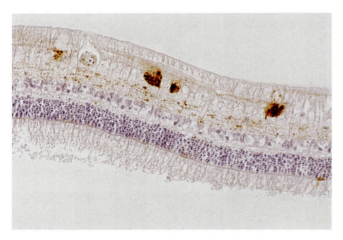

Figure 19-13 Rabies; horse, retina. In absence of histologic lesions, the entire retinal layers contain variable quantity of granular intracytoplasmic rabies virus; particularly colonized are the ganglion cells, the inner plexiform layer, and the outer nuclear layer. (IPIHC and HE stain.) *(Courtesy Dr. Fabio Del Piero.)*

Prevention

The mainstays of rabies prevention are vaccination and exposure avoidance. The American Veterinary Medical Association (AVMA) defines core vaccinations as those "that protect from diseases that are endemic to a region, those with potential

Table 19-1 Approved Rabies Vaccines for Use in Horses (as of 2004)				
Product	**Manufacturer**	**Dose**	**Recommended Booster**	**Route***
Monovalent (Rabies Inactivated)				
RABVAC 3	Boehringer Ingelheim Vetmedica (Lic. #124)	2 mL	Annually	IM
RABVAC 3 TF	Boehringer Ingelheim Vetmedica (Lic. #112)	2 mL	Annually	IM
IMRAB 3	Merial Inc. (Lic. #298)	2 mL	Annually	IM
EquiRab	Merck Animal Health	1 mL	Every 2 years	IM
Combination (Rabies Inactivated)				
Equine POTOMOVAC + IMRAB	Merial Inc. (Lic. #298)	1 mL	Annually	IM

*IM, Intramuscular.

Box 19-1 Rabies Vaccination Protocol*

Adult Horses

Broodmares: Annually, before breeding.
Other adult horses: Annually.

Foals

From vaccinated mares: First dose, 6 months, second dose at 7 months.
Boost again at 12 months, then annually thereafter.
From unvaccinated mares: First dose, 3 to 4 months. Second dose at 12 months, annually thereafter.

*Based on vaccination guidelines of the American Association of Equine Practitioners (AAEP).

public health significance, required by law, virulent/highly infectious, and/or those posing a risk of severe disease. Core vaccines have clearly demonstrated efficacy and safety, and thus exhibit a high enough level of patient benefit and low enough level of risk to justify their use in the majority of patients." The American Association of Equine Practitioners (AAEP) considers rabies vaccine a core vaccination for horses. Parenteral animal rabies vaccines should be administered only by, or under the direct supervision of, a veterinarian. Any veterinarian signing a rabies certificate should ensure that the person administering the vaccine is identified on the certificate and is appropriately trained in vaccine storage, handling, administration, and management of adverse events. This practice ensures that a qualified and responsible person can be held accountable to make certain the animal has been properly vaccinated.

A peak rabies antibody titer is reached within 28 days of primary vaccination. An animal is currently vaccinated and is considered immunized if the primary vaccination was administered at least 28 days previously and vaccinations have been administered appropriately.

Regardless of the age of the horse at initial vaccination, a booster vaccine should be administered 1 year later (Box 19-1). Because a rapid anamnestic response is expected, an animal is considered currently vaccinated immediately after a booster vaccination. Rabies is rare in vaccinated animals. If suspected, such an event should be reported to state public health officials, the vaccine manufacturer, and the USDA Animal and Plant Health Inspection Service (APHIS) Center for Veterinary Biologics.* The laboratory diagnosis should be confirmed and the virus characterized by a rabies reference laboratory. A thorough epidemiologic investigation should be conducted.

Public Health Considerations

Rabies is considered a zoonotic disease. Although the author was unable to find a single case of documented transmission of rabies from horse to human, the possibility is real, and all equine rabies suspects† must be handled as if a significant threat to human health exists. Animals with suspected rabies should only be handled by individuals who have had appropriate rabies preexposure vaccination. A list of all "in-contact" and potential in-contact individuals, including owners and private parties, should be developed and kept current. It is convenient to place a clipboard near the stall housing a rabies suspect and require individuals to sign the list if they enter the stall, handle the patient, or handle biologic material from the patient. If rabies is a differential diagnosis, laboratory personnel handling body fluids obtained for diagnostic purposes should be informed of this potential. This is best accomplished by labeling all specimens obtained as "rabies suspect" on their containers and clearly stating this on any submission paperwork. Details of the CDC postexposure prophylaxis (PEP) protocols can be found on the CDC website.* Rabies remains preventable when proper PEP is administered after an exposure; however, recent cases of recovery after treatment (the Milwaukee Protocol of coma induction and antiviral administration) and abortive rabies virus infection suggest the disease may possibly not be universally fatal.[21,22] Public education should continue to emphasize avoiding exposure to bats and other potentially rabid wildlife and seeking prompt medical attention after exposure to such animals.

Horses suspected of having rabies should be handled carefully, with examiners using protective gear that includes eye goggles, face shields/masks, and gloves during all examinations. Persons performing necropsy examinations on horses with suspected rabies are at increased risk of exposure to RABV, and more extensive protective measures should be considered. Individuals who move the bodies of rabies suspects should wear rubber boots, a scrub suit, double gloves (the outer glove being heavy vinyl with gauntlets), and a face shield for splash protection. Additionally, individuals who decapitate and remove brains of rabies suspects should use the protection of a Tyvek coverall (or surgical gown at a minimum) and a mist mask rated for biohazards (N95 rating or better; routine surgical masks are unacceptable for this purpose). The brain half that is submitted for rabies testing should be placed in a sealed plastic container, the external surface thoroughly cleaned with an appropriate disinfectant, and the container then placed in a second clean plastic container. Samples for rabies testing should be transported in rigid leakproof containers with the sample stabilized within the container by frozen gel packs or similar materials. The outer container should meet the federal standards for transport of diagnostic or dangerous goods.

The carcass and other specimens obtained at necropsy should not be submitted for additional studies until a negative rabies test result is obtained from the appropriate testing facility. If a positive test result is reported, all interested parties should be notified immediately, including the state veterinarian. Exposed individuals should consult their physician and local and state health authorities regarding postexposure treatment, which will vary depending on suspected level of exposure and preexposure vaccination status.

Acknowledgments

The authors would like to acknowledge the assistance of John Krebs, MS, from the CDC, in the preparation of the manuscript. We would also like to acknowledge the CDC for allowing free use of their images.

The complete reference list is available online at www.expertconsult.com.

---

*http://www.aphis.usda.gov/animal_health/vet_biologics/vb_contact.shtml; telephone: 800-752-6255; or e-mail: CVB@usda.gov.
†http://www.aphis.usda.gov/animal_health/vet_biologics/vb_contact.shtml; telephone: 800-752-6255; or e-mail: CVB@usda.gov.

---

*http://www.cdc.gov/mmwr/preview/mmwrhtml/00056176.htm.

Equine Alphaviruses

Maureen T. Long and E. Paul J. Gibbs*

The alphaviruses of North, Central, and South America cause the most severe neurologic diseases of horses and humans on the planet. These viruses continue to cause neurologic disease and death in humans and horses on an annual basis, even though the vaccines are highly protective in horses. The reporting of these diseases (or the suspicion of such) on an international and national basis is a basic duty of all veterinarians to ensure the health and safety of humans and horses. Before the availability of vaccination for equids, hundreds of thousands of horses were affected and died in annual outbreaks. Vaccinations against alphaviruses are considered the core component of immunoprophylaxis for all horses in the United States as outlined by the American Association of Equine Practitioners.

Eastern Equine Encephalitis

Etiology

The first recorded epidemic of eastern equine encephalitis (EEE) virus in horses likely occurred in Massachusetts in 1831, and EEE virus was isolated from a horse 2 years later. The first recorded human case occurred in that state in 1838.[1] The genus *Alphavirus* belongs to the family Togaviridae and includes several viruses that have been isolated from horses with neurologic disease. Of these alphaviruses, EEE, Western equine encephalitis (WEE), and Venezuelan equine encephalitis (VEE) viruses are the most frequently isolated from epidemics of encephalitis in horses and humans in the Western Hemisphere; however, there are others throughout the world that either are known to cause disease in horses or have only been described as pathogenic to humans (Table 20-1).[1-8] The other genus in the family Togaviridae, *Rubivirus*, contains no viruses of known equine significance.

Togaviruses are single-stranded, enveloped, linear positive-sense ribonucleic acid (RNA) viruses measuring 60 to 70 nm in diameter.[9-14] Within the envelope there is a nucleocapsid with icosahedral symmetry composed of peplomers arranged as trimers. Each peplomer is a heterodimer composed of two glycoproteins, E1 and E2.[11] The glycoproteins E1 and E2 are immunodominant proteins that induce neutralizing antibody.[10,12,13,15-17] The E2 glycoprotein induces the strongest neutralizing antibody response (both polyclonal and monoclonal), possesses hemagglutinating properties, and the activity is pH dependent.[15,18-23] Both hemagglutination inhibition (HI) activity and neutralizing specificity have historically been used to differentiate viral species and their antigenic types (Table 20-2). Initial classification frequently employs the common

Table 20-1 Geographic Location, Affected Hosts, and Disease Manifestation of Alphaviruses

Families	Virus	Geographic Location	Affected Host, Disease
Alphavirus	Sindbis	Africa, Australia, India	Birds, subclinical (used in research in rodent models)
	Eastern equine encephalitis (EEE)	North America, South America, Central America/Caribbean	Horses and humans, encephalitis
	Western equine encephalitis (WEE)	North America, South America	Horses and humans; encephalitis
	Ross River	Australia, Papua New Guinea	Humans and horses; endemic polyarthritis
	Semliki Forest	East and West Africa	Rodents and occasionally humans; encephalitis
	O'nyong-nyong	Primarily Uganda	Humans; polyarthritis, rash, and fever
	Chikungunya	Africa Asia with recent outbreaks in Europe	Humans; acute to chronic arthralgia
Rubivirus	Rubivirus	No known pathogenicity in animals	

Table 20-2 North American Alphaviruses Reported to Cause Encephalitis in Equines

Antigenic Complex	Antigenic Subtype	Antigenic Variety	Equine Clinical Syndrome	Distribution
Eastern equine encephalitis (EEE)		North American	Encephalitis	North America, Caribbean
		South American	Encephalitis	South, Central America
Venezuelan equine encephalitis (VEE)	(I) VEE	AB	Encephalitis	South, Central, North America
		C	Encephalitis	South, Central America
		E	Encephalitis	Central America
	(II) Everglades		Unknown	Florida, USA
Western equine encephalitis (WEE)	WEE	Several	Encephalitis	North, South America
	Highlands J		Rare encephalitis	Eastern North America

Modified from Weaver SC, Powers AM, Brault AC, et al: Molecular epidemiological studies of veterinary arboviral encephalitides, Vet J 157:123–138, 1999.

*The authors acknowledge and appreciate the original contributions of these authors, whose work has been incorporated into this chapter.

group-specific antigenic determinants that are still usually defined by serologic techniques such as fluorescent antibody (FA) and virus neutralization (VN).[18,19,25-31] Molecular sequencing and bioinformatics are currently used for reclassification and molecular epidemiologic studies.[32-34]

There is only one known species of EEE virus, but in reality, EEE virus exists as separate North and South American variants.[33] North American (NA) isolates of EEE virus differ by less than 2% in their genomic nucleotide sequence analysis, whereas South American (SA) isolates can be considered more genotypically distinct because nucleotide divergence can be as high as 25%. There are two lineages and five subtypes of EEE virus; lineage I is composed of NA subtype I, and lineage II is composed of SA subtypes II to IV.

For an RNA virus, prone to mutation, alphaviruses evolve relatively slowly.[2,32,35-40] This slow progression reflects adaptation of viruses to multiple hosts, which presumably requires more genomic conservation for maintenance in nature. Despite this lower evolution rate, these viruses have the ability to adapt rapidly to new ecologic challenges and thus result in intense epizootics.

Epidemiology

The general life cycle of alphaviruses involves transmission between birds or rodents and mosquitoes. Extensive work has been performed regarding the field ecology of EEE virus in North America.[41-48] In North America, EEE virus is perpetuated in a sylvatic cycle between avian hosts (passerine birds) and mosquitoes, and historical work indicates transmission in this cycle primarily involves the ornithophilic mosquito, *Culiseta melanura*.[49-53] In general, birds do not develop disease but develop sufficient titer viremia to allow transmission to feeding mosquitoes.[50] The more recently introduced birds, such as European starlings and House sparrows, are more susceptible to mortality from EEE virus infection.[54-65] Recent work in Alabama indicates that the northern cardinal is the primary target for *C. melanura* feeding but that other mosquitoes are capable of feeding on a wider variety of birds, including robins, chickadees, owls, and mockingbirds.[66,67] In addition, mosquitoes, such as *C. erraticus*, could change their feeding habits from avian hosts to mammalian hosts, depending on the year or the timing within the year. These types of vectors could be more important for the cycle of transmission to humans and horses; nonetheless, predicted activity is most aligned with infection rates found during surveillance trapping of *C. melanura*.

Mammalian reservoirs may also be important during years of high EEE virus transmission.[46,57,68-71] Rodents make up 25% of the mammalian species in Florida. Experimental infection of cotton rats, a common type of marshland rat, resulted in virus blood levels just capable of transmitting EEE virus, with juvenile rats developing higher titers and 100% mortality after infection.[72]

Horses and humans are clinically affected but do not develop viremia sufficiently high enough to transmit virus back to vector mosquitoes and are considered "dead-end" hosts. Enzootics of EEE virus are capable of causing outbreaks of disease in multiple species besides horses, including alpacas, llamas, cattle, swine, cats, and dogs.[73-80] Exotic birds are especially susceptible, including emus, the ring-necked pheasant, Pekin ducks, and Chukar partridges.[81-84]

Habitat type is also associated with propensity for EEE virus re-emergence in northern latitudes and probably uninterrupted transmission in southern United States latitudes.[85-87] Freshwater hardwood swamps are the most associated ecologic niche for EEE virus, and in the South, re-emergence within mammalian hosts occurs in "tree farms" that are associated with Florida's inland freshwater swamps. These cultivated swamp edges have the opportunity for comingling of susceptible domesticated species and humans.

Because alphaviruses are transmitted by arthropod vectors, clinical disease occurs during the arbovirus season of late summer and early fall in temperate zones, with year-round transmission possible in the tropics and subtropics. The United States has the highest reported cases in the southeastern states, but infection has been detected in all states east of the Mississippi River and some western states such as Texas.[88] In the South, the most activity is found in Florida.[89] In recent years, intense focal activity has been reported in Michigan, Wisconsin, Ohio, Massachusetts, and New Hampshire.[88,90-93] In 2005, Massachusetts experienced a human case affected rate of over 5 times the rate of the preceding 10 years. Ongoing work by the Centers for Disease Control and Prevention (CDC) indicates that affected people resided within one-half mile of a cranberry bog or a swamp associated with forest habitat. During this epidemic, enzootic activity was also detected in clinically affected horses (9), alpacas (4), emus (2), and llamas (1).[90,94,100]

The question of EEE virus persistence or re-emergence in northern niches remains.[51,95,96] Since 2005, in northern latitudes, EEE virus activity generally reappears in well-known locales in New York, Wisconsin, and Massachusetts.[88,90-93] Also, there can be new emergences such as has been observed in New Hampshire, Michigan, and Maine.[90,92,93,97,98] Although the former indicates that there is likely some type of overwintering mechanism for this virus, reintroduction of EEE virus during migration can occur.[99] Some studies favor new introduction based on comparison of viruses isolated from various location (Connecticut), whereas other areas demonstrate evolution of EEE virus into distinct viruses, indicating geographic persistence (New York and New Hampshire). Recent work in avian species has examined viral persistence in avian hosts with re-emergence with season, but this has not been substantiated.[100] Transovarial transmission of EEE virus does occur in the mosquito host.[51,99] In tropical and subtropical climates, the year-round mosquito/avian cycle likely obviates the need for a period of diapause in mosquito populations, but this may be more important in maintaining northern activity from year to year.

Culiseta melanura, a temperate breeding species of mosquito, does not readily breed in the Caribbean, and EEE is not an endemic disease in this relatively focal region, with all viruses attributable to lineage I.[39] Only sporadic reports or small epidemics of EEE disease in horses have been recorded in these areas, likely through migratory influx of viremic birds providing occasional sources of virus for secondary vectors. These secondary vectors can initiate short-term outbreaks but cannot maintain the disease endemically.

In Central and South Americas, the principle vectors of EEE virus belong to the *Culex (Melanoconion)* spp.[101-103] These vectors feed on birds, rodents, marsupials, and reptiles. As such, SA EEE virus has higher viral loads in cotton rats compared to NA EEE virus.[72] Before 2000, comparatively few epidemics of EEE in horses were recorded in South America, with minimal disease reported in humans.[34,39] Furthermore, there are notable differences in virulence between SA EEE virus strains. More recently, in 2008 and 2009, larger outbreaks have occurred in Central and South America.[104-109] In Northeastern Brazil, 229 horses were affected with a case fatality rate of 73% with similar severity of disease as that of NA EEE virus.[115] This changes our basic understanding of NA and SA EEE virus pathogenesis; more investigation is required to determine if this reflects emergence of more virulent SA strains or better surveillance.

Pathogenesis

The alphavirus genome is 9.7 to 11.8 kb in length and encodes both nonstructural and structural proteins. With a

5′-methylated and a 3′-polyadenylated cap, the nonstructural proteins are encoded at the 5′ end and the structural proteins at the 3′ end of the genome.[110-116] Unlike flaviviruses, which translate the entire genome, only the 5′ end is initially translated in alphaviruses. The resultant polyprotein is subsequently cleaved by a proteinase. Viral RNA-dependent RNA polymerase is formed from two of these proteins, and complementary (negative-sense) RNA (cRNA) is transcribed.[117,118] From this template, full-length viral progeny are transcribed, and a short "subgenomic" portion is transcribed.[119-121] The latter, which has a cap at the 5′ end and a polyadenylated tail, is translated to form a polyprotein that is processed to the five viral proteins: E1, E2, E3, 6K, and C.*

New World alphaviruses attach via the E2 protein to heparin sulfate, which as a receptor enhances neurovirulence.[124,125] Importantly, loss of binding to heparin sulfate decreases neurovirulence but increases lymphoid tropism.[125,126] Lymphoid tropism in these neuroattenuated strains enhances interferon-alpha/interferon-beta (IFN-α/IFN-β) release.[127] Furthermore, other work has demonstrated that nonattenuated strains induce little IFN-α/IFN-β release and are not lymphotropic. Eastern equine encephalitis virus replicates poorly in dendritic cells and macrophages by restriction of translation of EEE virus.[126,128-130] However, EEE virus replicates efficiently in both fibroblasts and osteoclasts. Alphaviruses replicate to high titer in the cytoplasm of infected cells and exit the cell by the budding of preassembled nucleocapsids through the plasmalemma.[131,132] They cause cytopathic effects (CPEs) in a wide range of vertebrate cells in vitro, particularly embryonic avian cells.[133-135] Infection causes complete shutdown of host-cell protein and nucleic acid synthesis. Invertebrate cells, such as C6/36 derived from *Aedes albopictus*, are equally sensitive to infection with alphaviruses, but no CPE is apparent, and cell division is unaffected.[136,137] This attenuation is associated with the ability of the mutant virus to stimulate secretion of IFN-α/IFN-β in mammalian cells but not mosquito cells. Work in mice indicates the T-cell receptor (TCR) is required for protection from lethal encephalitis and survivorship is independent of IFN-γ responses mediated by the absence of an IFN-γ receptor.[138]

Clinical Findings

Eastern equine encephalitis virus is one of the most pathogenic neurotropic viruses of man and horses. In the United States, most cases of EEE disease in horses occur in the northern parts of Florida, the Carolinas, Alabama, and Louisiana. Outbreaks in the northern states occur generally in nonvaccinated horses. In total, several hundred equine cases are confirmed each year, despite the widespread availability of vaccines. In Florida, many horses that succumb to EEE virus are not vaccinated, less than 3 years of age, and stock-type horses (Long, unpublished data).[3,139-143] There is no gender predilection. After experimental inoculation, there is a short febrile response at 2 to 3 days (likely corresponding to viremia).[144] The time to onset of neurologic disease of EEE virus is generally 7 days to 2 weeks (some reports indicate as short as 3 days, but this cannot be verified). In clinical cases, pyrexia is the first clinical manifestation of infection and can be as high as 104° F; in partially vaccinated horses, this may be significantly lower.[31] Temperature has usually abated or is only moderately elevated between 101° F to 102° F by the time encephalitic signs become evident. Clinical signs are progressive in nature but variable with common systemic signs of depression and anorexia. Changes in mentation manifest frequently as severe forebrain disease, including obtunded mentation, blindness, head pressing, and teeth grinding. Early hyperexcitability quickly changes to stupor and, if

---
*References 110, 111, 113, 115, 122, 123.

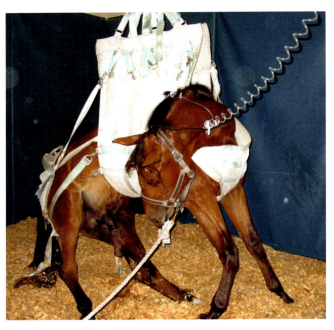

Figure 20-1 Two-year-old Thoroughbred colt profoundly affected with eastern equine encephalitis (EEE) virus. This horse had clinical signs for approximately 36 hours. Initial signs consisted of fever and depression. The horse rapidly deteriorated and by 24 hours after onset was not easily roused. This horse also had persistent priapism, a common clinical sign in male horses with encephalitis.

standing, the head hangs low with drooping ears, the eyelids become slightly swollen and partly closed, the lips become flaccid, and the tongue protrudes from the mouth (Fig. 20-1). Early signs of severe ataxia, staggering, generally progresses to full paralysis and recumbence. Cranial nerve signs include dysphagia and weak tongue. The course of disease in severely affected horses varies between 2 and 14 days, the former is most common in the nonvaccinated horses. Nearly all horses with NA EEE virus die, and in the latest published data, most horses with SA EEE virus die.[107]

Diagnosis

Clinical signs and antemortem clinical pathologic findings are not specific for alphavirus infection. Viral and other encephalitides can cause abnormal cerebrospinal fluid (CSF), and EEE virus is unique in that acute infection frequently results in a neutrophilic pleocytosis (Fig. 20-2). Because high mortality is associated with this disease, identification of a neutrophilic pleocytosis indicates probable EEE infection and offers the veterinarian a chance to prognosticate regarding the horse's survival. The neutrophils in the fluid have toxic changes and frequently are hypersegmented. In more chronic or partially vaccinated horses, the cellular component may be mononuclear.

All alphaviruses are reportable diseases, thus it is paramount to obtain a definitive diagnosis for clinical signs of any encephalitis in the horse.[88] This allows institution of effective control measures because of the risk of these viruses to the health and well-being of both humans and equine livestock. Blood is an inappropriate specimen for virus recovery because usually no circulating virus is present when signs of encephalitis become apparent. In an epidemic situation, however, it might be possible to isolate the virus from nonencephalitic horses in the affected group, particularly if they have increased body temperatures.[145,146]

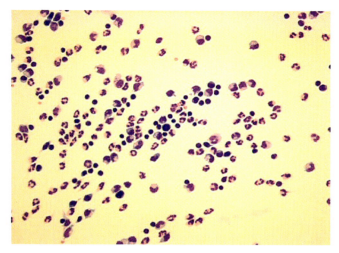

Figure 20-2 Photomicrograph of cerebrospinal fluid (CSF) from horse with eastern equine encephalitis (EEE). This horse had exhibited clinical signs for less than 72 hours when the CSF was obtained. The CSF contains more than 50% nondegenerate neutrophils.

Currently, no reliable antemortem diagnostic tests are available to detect EEE virus in clinically affected horses, and serology provides the mainstay of presumptive antemortem diagnosis. The demonstration of specific immunoglobulin M (IgM) antibody (dilution of 1:400) is a highly specific and sensitive method for diagnosis.[147] The detection of IgM antibody in CSF (if available) is even more conclusive, but horses may succumb before there is an antibody response intrathecally. Rising antibody titers to EEE virus, WEE virus, or VEE virus in the sera of horses that survive can be detected by testing of acute-phase and convalescent-phase sera, but the opportunity to collect a second sample is limited by the high death loss. Even in endemic areas, it is not possible to diagnose or differentiate EEE, WEE, or VEE in the horse with any certainty based on clinical signs and epidemiologic circumstances, and definitive testing must be performed.

The viruses of EEE, WEE, and VEE frequently can be detected after death in brain material of diseased horses by isolation of virus in cell cultures (e.g., Vero cells), through intracerebral inoculation of suckling mice, and by detection of specific nucleotide sequences using reverse transcriptase–polymerase chain reaction (RT-PCR) technology.[28,35,148-155] Rapid real-time PCR assays performed on clinical specimens have been developed to differentiate between alphaviruses and flaviviruses. For alphaviruses, the CDC protocol utilizes two primer sets, which also detect virus in formalin-fixed tissues.

Rabies, hepatic encephalopathy, West Nile virus (WNV), and equine protozoal myeloencephalitis are the major diseases that must be considered in the differential diagnosis in the Western Hemisphere. Other diseases that should be considered in the differential diagnosis are equine herpesvirus type 1 infection of the central nervous system (CNS) and leukoencephalomalacia (a neuromycotoxicosis caused by the ingestion of maize infected with *Fusarium moniliforme*.

Pathologic Findings

In horses, brain lesions are thought to be the direct result of viral replication and are characterized by necrotizing encephalitis with neuronal dysfunction.* No consistent gross lesions are found in horses that die of EEE, WEE, or VEE, except that

*References 75, 78, 144, 149, 150, 156-160.

meninges are frequently congested. This congestion is usually quite pronounced with EEE virus infection. In addition, frequent, focal areas of dark discoloration are found in brain slices and are most prominent in grey matter of cerebrum at the level of the corona radiata. Histologically, neuronal necrosis with neurophagia, marked perivascular cuffing with both mononuclear and polymorphonuclear leukocytes, and focal and diffuse microglial proliferation are evident. The lesions are more pronounced in the gray matter than in the white matter of the brain. Lesions are most marked in the cerebral cortex, thalamus, and hypothalamus, whereas the spinal cord is mildly affected. Severe lesions usually occur more often in the cervical spinal cord than in lumbar cord segments. Organisms may be demonstrated in affected CNS tissues by immunohistochemistry in fixed sections with severe lesions; this assay is highly sensitive, unlike assays for West Nile virus (WNV) where staining is inconsistent and requires examination of several sections.

Therapy

No known antiviral medications demonstrate reliable activity against alphaviruses, and treatment of disease in affected horses is supportive. The survival rate for EEE infection is low compared with other infectious encephalitides. In most cases, horses die 3 to 5 days after onset of signs.

Some clinicians advocate the use of corticosteroids as a component of therapy for horses with neurologic signs consistent with viral encephalitis and neutrophilic CSF. If administered early, corticosteroids (to reduce brain edema) and intravenous (IV) fluids may aid recovery. In human patients, treatment with methylprednisolone (1000 mg/100-kg patient) is often recommended. Administration of flunixin meglumine (1.1 mg/kg every 12 hours [q12h] IV) or other antiinflammatory medications to horses with EEE does not often result in the dramatic response frequently observed in horses with WNV. Mannitol (0.25-2 g/kg q24h IV) may assist in the control of brain edema. Detomidine hydrochloride (0.02-0.04 mg/kg IV or intramuscular [IM]) is effective for prolonged tranquilization.

IV immunoglobin therapy has been used in humans for both its proposed neutralization of virus and immunomodulatory effects.[161] IFN-α is a relatively common therapy; its recommendation is based on anecdotal reports in the human and veterinary literature.[162-166] More data are supporting suppression of type I IFNs in the pathogenesis of EEE virus infection. Limited information regarding the efficacy of IFN-α in the horse is available.

Prevention

Eastern equine encephalitis infection in horses is preventable with proper vaccination.[167,168] Available vaccines are formalin-inactivated preparations, consist of the same virus seed stock, and are multivalent, containing either EEE virus and WEE virus or EEE, WEE, and VEE viruses. In the states most affected by EEE virus, adult horses should be vaccinated a minimum of two times per year. Veterinarians should monitor surveillance data and be aware of areas where EEE virus occurs year after year.

Horses that reside in endemic areas and are aged 4 years or less should receive alphavirus vaccines three times per year. It is essential that all broodmares be vaccinated 1 month before foaling to ensure adequate passive transfer to foals. All foals should be tested for adequate passive transfer 24 hours after birth. In foals from vaccinated dams, vaccination should be performed at 5, 6, and 8 months. In foals in which the dam has not been adequately vaccinated, vaccination should be performed at 4, 5, and 7 months. All yearlings must be vaccinated between January and March within the year after birth, and receive at least two more injections 4 months apart. This vaccination schedule should continue until horses are 4 years of age. All horses arriving in the south from northern states should be vaccinated 30 days before arrival. Imported horses that ship directly to southern states from countries where the vaccine cannot be obtained before arrival are at risk for EEE virus for 2 years after their arrival. It is imperative that these horses receive three initial injections and then continue three times a year for at least 2 years after arriving in the southern United States.

As stated previously in this chapter, the alphaviruses are enveloped and thus are not stable in the environment and are easily inactivated by common disinfectants. Vector control can be achieved through reducing the breeding activities of mosquitoes by implementing appropriate water management systems, although this can be difficult in extensively rural areas.[169-171] The widespread dispersal (usually achieved by aerial spraying) of insecticides has been used successfully, although a number of critical factors need to be considered before embarking on such a step. Concern over indiscriminate spraying of insecticides can be mitigated in some circumstances if the biology of the mosquito vector is well known. For example, in northern Florida, where EEE is endemic, treating the pools of water in which *Cs. melanura* breeds with a larvicide is often practical and economically feasible on those farms with valuable horses. Swamps with soil types that support the breeding of *Cs. melanura* can often be recognized by the nonentomologist by the presence of the loblolly bay tree *(Gordonia lasianthus)*; this broadleaf evergreen tree grows to a height of about 30 feet and can easily be recognized by its white, magnolia-like flowers and serrated leaves.

Public Health Considerations

Eastern equine encephalitis virus is highly pathogenic for humans but usually requires a vector for transmission to occur. The horse does not develop a sufficient level of viremia with EEE and WEE to act as a reservoir or an amplifying host for these viruses. However, EEE virus can be infectious to personnel handling EEE virus–infected tissues (CNS) and fluids (CSF) so efforts must be made to minimize any inadvertent inoculation with sharp instruments. In the laboratory setting, EEE virus must be handled as a biosafety level 2 agent to minimize aerosolization. In experimental models, nasal inoculation causes disease. The alphaviruses are also considered select agents (SE) under the United States Department of Agriculture (USDA) and CDC bioterrorism programs. Handling of these agents requires SE status granted by these respective agencies.

Western Equine Encephalitis

Etiology

Western equine encephalitis virus is also an alphavirus of the family Togaviridae and classified as a group IV positive-sense single-stranded RNA virus. Western equine encephalitis virus is most closely related to EEE virus, and it is theorized that WEE evolved from EEE.[33,172,173] Nucleotide analyses reveals that this virus is a combination of both EEE and Sindbis viral sequences, which has been confirmed by both molecular epidemiology of various isolates and through the complete sequences of WEE, performed in 2000.[33,172-175] Phylogenetic analyses indicate that North and South American WEE lineages appear to have evolved independently over several decades.[36,176-178] Yet within North and South America, the genotypes are relatively homogenous. Variant WEE virus has been reported in several countries in South America (Argentina, Guyana, Ecuador, Brazil,

Uruguay), but only in Argentina has it been associated with human disease and significant enzootics in horses.[175,179-181]

"New World" viruses of the WEE complex include Aura, Highlands J, Fort Morgan, Buggy Creek, and WEE, whereas the "Old World" representative is Sindbis virus. There are mainly two antigenic subtypes of WEE virus and these include WEE and Highlands J viruses.[36,175,182-184] Most infections that occur east of the Mississippi River are caused by the Highlands J (HJ) virus.[176,183,185,186] Although generally considered less pathogenic for mammals than WEE virus, HJ virus has caused natural cases of encephalitis in horses and is pathogenic for domestic turkeys, pheasants, and exotic species of birds.[176,183,185] Other subtypes of WEE virus that may cause disease in North American horses include Fort Morgan and Buggy Creek viruses.[187] Most WEE infections in the western United States are likely the result of infection with one of the several antigenic variants of the actual WEE subtype.[144] This virus is more pathogenic in horses and humans than closely related viruses, although minimal disease has been reported in humans and horses in the last decade. One WEE variant, Y62-WEE, has been identified in Russia.[188] No equine disease has been associated with either Sindbis or Aura viruses, other members of the Alphavirus family.[188]

Epidemiology

Since 1964, WEE has been reported in 639 people with the most recent large outbreak reported in 1975 with 132 cases (http://www.cdc.gov/ncidod/dvbid/arbor/arbocase.htm). The highest number of cases has been reported in Colorado and Texas, followed by Minnesota and California. Historically, large outbreaks of WEE have been described in horses. The virus was first identified in association with a large epizootic that occurred in the San Joaquin Valley of California in 1930. Approximately 6000 horses were affected, with a case-fatality rate of 50%.[145] This outbreak continued and spread to several western states from 1931 to 1934. Within a decade, another 300,000 equid cases were reported, with several thousand human cases. Over the last decade, reports of WEE in horses have been limited and sporadic, possibly reflecting vaccination and protective immunity gained by subclinical exposure.[189,190]

Culex tarsalis is the primary vector that maintains WEE virus in an enzootic cycle with birds, especially nestling passerines.[32,191] *Culex tarsalis* population abundance is favored by a rapid increase in temperature following a cool, wet spring, resulting in the rapid melting of snow and flooding of rivers.[168,192,193] This species of mosquito also has a predilection for irrigated lands as breeding sites.[58] Other ornithophilic mosquitoes become infected as the summer progresses, and the infection eventually spills over to other types of birds, mammals, and possibly reptiles and amphibians. Most, if not all, of these infections are inapparent. This in turn results in the virus becoming established in species of mosquitoes with host preferences other than birds. Horses, even those that are obviously clinically affected, do not produce viremia high enough to infect mosquitoes.[145]

At least two variants of WEE virus (Fort Morgan and Buggy Creek) have been isolated in western North America and are transmitted between birds by swallow nest bugs *(Oeciacus vicarius)*.[185] Neither variant is considered to be pathogenic for humans or horses. A third variant, HJ virus, is mainly found east of the Mississippi River and has been isolated from horses dying of encephalitis.[183,185,186,194] Information is limited on the number of horses infected with HJ virus on an annual basis. Black bears and rodents have been found to be serologically positive to WEE in Florida.[195]

In South America, where *Cx. tarsalis* does not occur, antibody prevalence rates in birds are lower than in North America, and the species (vertebrate and invertebrate) responsible for maintaining the virus on that continent have not been identified.[196,197] *Aedes albasfaciatus* has experimentally transmitted WEE virus to chickens in Argentina.[196,197]

Reservoir hosts for WEE may be variable, but the classic life cycle proposed is cycling of virus between a mosquito vector and avian reservoirs. Birds, snakes, and squirrels have all been experimentally infected.[68,69,198-205] Garter snakes became asymptomatically infected and had sustained viremia for an average of 10 to 12 days. Frogs were also found to be readily susceptible to infection. Both snakes and frogs could be inoculated orally. Birds in general do not have high sustained viremias in WEE infection and also show limited disease. A variety of birds have been inoculated, including chickens, bobwhite quails, and sparrows. Adult chickens and bobwhite quails had low viremias, which made them suitable sentinels because they developed sustained antibody responses. Pigeons develop low viremia but unsustainable antibody responses.[207] When infected with WEE intranasally, squirrels develop disease and also high levels of viremia before death.[70,210,211] Infection with WEE in six species of rodents has been performed; several of these species were susceptible to the virus and some able to mount high and sustained viremias.[212] Although this depended on the strain of WEE virus used, small ground mammals may be important reservoirs for WEE.[58] Like EEE infections in emus, these animals are susceptible to disease and have been part of epizootics as recently as the mid-1990s. Vaccination is recommended for these species.

Pathogenesis

Western equine encephalitis virus is similar to other alphaviruses, EEE and VEE viruses in its neurotropism in horses and humans. As such there is actually limited work directly with WEE regarding its pathogenesis. As demonstrated in rodent models, there is high level of variation between strains of WEE.[212-214] Importantly the strains isolated from South America are more virulent for mice. Like other alphaviruses, WEEV has a predilection for cerebral cortex and midbrain.[215] In hamsters, WEE primarily infects neurons and virus is not detectable in astrocytes or glial cells.[216] In vitro studies demonstrate that the enhanced susceptibility of immature hosts may be due to immaturity of the neuron.[217] Immature neuronal cells are more susceptible to WEEV infection; mature neurons were able to suppress viral replication with exogenous type I interferons. WEEV induces interferon-beta (IFN-β) transcription upon infection of neuronal cells.[217,218] This upregulation is mediated through interferon-response factor-3 (IRF-3) and in fact increase in activity of this signaling cascade will enhance protection against viral infection.

Clinical Signs

Although WEE virus causes less severe signs than either EEE or VEE virus, WEE virus is neuroinvasive across strains, and neurologic signs of disease in horses are similar to these alphaviruses.[139,219] Like its other neurotropic relatives, children and young animals of all susceptible species are more likely than adults to develop clinical CNS disease. After experimental inoculation, there is a short febrile response at 2 to 3 days (likely corresponding to viremia).[144] The time to onset of neurologic disease of WEE is generally 7 days to 2 weeks (some reports indicate as short as 3 days, but this cannot be verified). Inapparent infections in horses are common. In clinical cases, pyrexia is the first clinical manifestation of infection. Temperature has usually abated or is only moderately elevated by the time signs of encephalitis become evident. The course of disease in severely affected horses varies between 2 and 14 days. Most horses fully recover from WEE. The mortality rate (case-fatality rate) is 20% to 30%.

Diagnosis

In initial outbreaks of WEE where extensive evaluation of equals was performed, CSF was composed of a mononuclear cell population primarily consisting of lymphocytes. Protein within the CSF may or may not be elevated, and the average white blood cell (WBC) count was 100 to 200 cells/μL.

As stated earlier, most reliable antemortem testing is based on detection of antibody responses to WEE. Because horses frequently survive infection, VN testing can demonstrate a rising (fourfold minimum change) titer that is confirmatory. Serologic testing for other encephalitides should be performed simultaneously in states where WEE and EEE distributions overlap. The IgM capture enzyme-linked immunoassay (ELISA) test has been a useful format for WEE testing. As of this time, the author has not found any cross-reactivity of EEE virus–positive horses with WEE in the IgM format. If a horse succumbs to infection, then a postmortem examination with antigen detection consisting of either immunochemistry (IHC), real time-PCR, or viral isolation should be performed, especially for public and animal health purposes.

Pathology

Many of the histopathologic changes in the brain of WEE-infected horses are similar in those observed in EEE-infected horses except that there are limited numbers of neutrophils within cellular accumulations.

Treatment

Like EEE virus, treatment of WEE infection is supportive. In a 1933 publication, treatment of horses with plasma from surviving (hyperimmunized) horses was therapeutic.[220] There is experimental evidence in a hamster model of WEE that treatment with IFN increased survival.[164] Other novel antiviral agents may be on the horizon.[221,222]

Prevention

Western equine encephalitis is preventable with vaccination protocols similar to those described indicated in the section on prevention of EEE virus in this chapter.[167,168] Because the incidence of WEE has dramatically declined in the United States, even in sentinel and mosquito testing, it has been recommended by some clinicians that WEE be removed from the multivalent preparations for immunization. This is inadvisable because WEE virus disease in humans and horses still occurs in South America and the possibility will always exist for re-emergence because of the ubiquitous presence of *C. tarsalis* in the western United States. The last reported outbreak was in Brazil in 2006.

Venezuelan Equine Encephalitis

Etiology

The VEE virus complex is composed of six distinct subtypes (I-VI) with several strains within subtypes designated by letter.[29] The "epidemic or epizootic" types of VEE viruses (types IAB, IC, and IE) have been isolated during outbreaks of encephalitis in horses in the Western Hemisphere in the past 20 years. The "endemic or enzootic" types of VEE virus are considered to be of low pathogenicity for equids under most circumstances.[144,223,224] These include ID and IF variants from Central America and Brazil, respectively.[29,225] Type II (Everglades) virus is found in Florida. Type III (Mucambo) virus has three subtypes of potential pathogenicity for the horse.[29,226] The other types are type IV (Pixuna) virus, type V (Cabassou) virus, and type VI virus. These viruses have been isolated in Trinidad, French Guiana, western North America, and Peru. The Pixuna subtype of VEE is associated with febrile illness in horses in Brazil.[29]

Epidemiology

Venezuelan equine encephalitis virus is one of the most important human and veterinary pathogens in the New World.[7] The virus, both historically and very recently, has been responsible for large outbreaks of disease in both humans and horses over large geographic areas. The first recognized outbreak of VEE occurred initially in equids in Colombia and then in Venezuela in 1935 and 1936, although it is speculated to have been active in this area since 1920.[227] Documentation of human disease occurred in a Colombian outbreak in the 1960s, when an estimated 50,000 to 100,000 equids (horses, mules, donkeys) died and 250,000 humans were affected (mainly an influenza-like disease, but some cases of encephalitis and death). It is uncertain whether the 1969–1971 epidemic that was first reported in Ecuador and subsequently spread to Central America, Mexico, and Texas was directly related to this outbreak in Colombia or was caused by the use of an incorrectly inactivated subtype IAB strain vaccine.[225,228-230]

These epidemics reveal the potential for VEE to spread rapidly within an equine population, with a case-fatality rate approaching 90% in some areas; this is confirmed in more recent outbreaks.[142,231,232] The availability of vaccines and active surveillance throughout the Americas since the early 1970s have reduced the overall impact of the disease throughout the Americas.[224] However, outbreaks of VEE continue to occur in the 1990s in Chiapas and Oaxaca, Mexico, Venezuela, and Colombia.[233-237] The geographically extensive outbreak in 1995 had all the initial hallmarks of the 1969–1971 epidemic.[224] Not only did large numbers of horses, mules, and donkeys die, but there were also an estimated 75,000 to 100,000 human cases of disease. VEE viruses isolated in 1995 that caused disease in equids and thousands of people were genetically similar to those associated with disease in the 1960s.[40,175,224,244]

Key to understanding the epidemiology of VEE is recognition of the differences in the basic biology of two transmission cycles, enzootic and epizootic, of this virus[238] (Fig. 20-3). Three basic changes occur in the enzootic-epizootic cycling: (1) the virus mutates closer to the more pathogenic IAB and IC strains, (2) there is a change in reservoir host from the spiny rat to the equine, and (3) there is a change in mosquito vector.[238-242]

Table 20-2 indicates that certain strains of virus are found only in the enzootic cycle. These viruses, subtypes I-E, II, III, and IV, tend to be of low pathogenicity for equids and do not result in high levels of viremia in horses.[18,27,229,243,244] Many theories exist on the origin of epizootic VEE viruses, primarily of the subtypes IAB and IC.[27,245-250] These viruses are associated with variable but often quite high equine mortality (20%-85%).[250] In contrast to most arboviruses in the horse, efficient amplification of the virus by equids is the hallmark of epizootic VEE. Several theories exist regarding the source of IAB and IC strains and how they persist in the environment between outbreaks.[230] Although molecular analyses have been used to address this, a comprehensive understanding of how epidemics in horses originate remains elusive.[251] Isolates that are virulent for horses do not appear to be transmitted in the interepizootic period.[252,253] There is some evidence for circulation of these viruses in the interepizootic period, but no latency is associated with these infections. No evidence suggests that the epizootic strains coexist in the enzootic cycle. Mutation of enzootic strains may allow the emergence of highly pathogenic virus and initiation of epizootics.[240] The enzootic cycle centers around

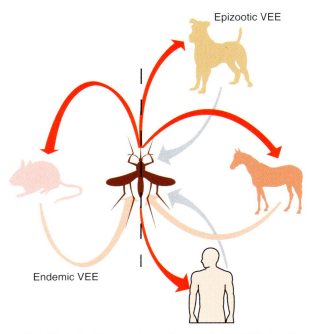

Figure 20-3 Life cycle of Venezuelan equine encephalitis (VEE) virus. During the endemic cycle, VEE is maintained in a sylvatic ecosystem with a rodent reservoir (spiny rat) and mosquito vector, generally *Culex* spp. (*Melanoconion*). On generation of an epizootic strain of VEE, multiple-vector species transmit the virus. The horse generates a sufficiently high-titer viremia to amplify the virus significantly. Several other terrestrial mammals also are susceptible to infection and develop significant viremia (including human and dog).

sylvatic rodents, such as spiny and cotton rats, which have high natural infection rates and can develop viremia high enough to transmit VEE to mosquitoes.[253-257] Even opossums, bats, and shore birds likely are important in dispersal of enzootic virus.[258-260] The importance of equine infection in maintenance of epizootic VEE is evidenced by the observation that human disease has never been demonstrated in the absence of equine disease.[144,146,261] All mammalian hosts are capable of developing a high-titer viremia of approximately 10^5 to 10^7 pfu/mL for up to 5 days, but the horse is likely to be the most important mammalian host in terms of vector capacity.[144,224,262] In contrast to EEE and WEE, in which horses are not considered to be a major source of virus for the vector, in VEE epidemics, horses are the most important amplifiers of virus activity.

Humans usually develop a flu-like illness, with only 4% to 14% exhibiting neurologic signs and symptoms.[149] Case-fatality rate for humans is approximately 1%. Several other species of mammals, including domestic rabbits, small ruminants, and dogs, develop potentially fatal clinical disease after VEE virus infection.[250] During an epizootic, dogs regularly become infected and may be capable of virus amplification.[263,264] Cattle and swine also seroconvert.[265] More than 100 species of birds have been either virologically or serologically associated with transmission of epidemic VEE virus. Shore birds in general and herons in particular appear to be capable of serving as amplifier hosts.[266,267] Birds may develop viremia as high as 10^8 TCID$_{50}$/mL of blood.

The subgenus *Melanoconion* (*Culex cedecci*) is likely to be the most important vector of enzootic VEE.[268] This vector resides in tropical forests and swamps and feeds on small forest mammals at night. Some species of this mosquito have broader feeding patterns. Activity for this vector peaks with high ambient temperature and rainfall. Several species of mosquitoes from at least 11 genera have been determined to be naturally infected with epidemic strains of VEE virus.[242,261,269-274] Virus has also been isolated from *Culicoides* spp. *(Ceratopogonidae)* and blackflies *(Simuliidae)*, but it is not known whether insects in these families are capable of biologic transmission of VEE virus.[273] In addition, ticks, including the species *Amblyomma cajennense* and *Hyalomma truncatum*, may be capable of viral transmission.[203,275-277]

Pathogenesis

Much of the understanding of the pathogenesis of alphaviruses comes from studies comparing the difference in pathogenicity between endemic and epidemic strains of VEE. Virulence of VEE virus correlates with viremia as opposed to specific neurovirulence per se. Low-virulence strains are more susceptible than high-virulence strains of VEE to interferons (IFN-α, IFN-β).[278-282] Comparatively, epidemic and epizootic VEE have similar ability to invade the CSF and when inoculated intracerebrally, have similar pathogenesis, even though there are differences in in vitro growth characteristics.[247,283] Changes in the E2 glycoprotein confer virus replication, resulting in rapid development of CPEs in vitro. However, the relationship between pathogenesis and virus strains is more complex than just viral characteristics; whereas virulent strains of VEE differ in their ability to stimulate endogenous intracellular antiviral functions, ultimately mortality (in experimental models) appears to depend on genetics of the host.

Studies in mice demonstrate that neural invasion is likely to occur secondary to vascular infection or invasion through the olfactory epithelium.[232] After inoculation, there is local viral replication in fibroblasts. In young mice, there is intense replication in osteoclasts of developing bone, possibly explaining that young animals and humans are much more susceptible to severe disease. The reticuloendothelial system is a major target in epidemic VEE infections. The viruses cause encephalitis after hematogenous or neuronal spread.[180,284,285] Immunity, after both inapparent infection and clinical disease as caused by VEE, is long lasting in all species.

Clinical Findings, Diagnosis, and Pathologic Findings

The clinical findings in horses with VEE virus infection are similar to EEE virus except that there can be a wider variation in mortality in horses, ranging from 40% to 90%. Diagnosis and pathologic findings are also similar to the EEE and WEE viruses.

Prevention

Immunization of horses has proved highly effective as an adjunct to other control measures in outbreaks of VEE, in which horses may serve as a source of infection for mosquitoes.[247,286,287] The 1969–1971 VEE epidemic in Central America and the southern United States was controlled partially by immunizing large numbers of horses with an attenuated VEE virus strain, TC-83.[283,283] This vaccine strain was produced by serial passage of an epidemic variant in guinea pig cell cultures. Because of concerns over the presence of low-level viremia in some horses and the possible transmission of vaccine virus between horses by mosquitoes and reversion to virulence, inactivated vaccines against VEE are now available for use in horses. These vaccines are not widely used in North America because they compromise the international movement of horses for competition and breeding.

The distinct possibility exists that VEE outbreaks could be completely prevented if sustained and widespread vaccination with live, attenuated VEE vaccines was performed in Central and South America.[262] Public health and animal industry officials should maintain quantities of the live attenuated TC-83 vaccine. The use of the formalin inactivated vaccine (usually marketed as a multivalent antigen) is discouraged in VEE epidemics because of the need for multiple vaccinations (and thus delayed onset of protection).[262] Formalinized vaccines generally induce short-lived immunity to VEE and this results in a lack of long-term compliance by owners and agricultural officials. In the long run, more rural economies can not sustain multiple annual vaccination protocols. Thus development of safe vaccines that induce long-term protection in equids that is reasonable for agrarian economies is essential for controlling epizootics.

Surveillance for encroachment of alphaviruses in new geographic locales is also paramount to control. Most southern states in the United States have encephalitis testing programs that offer subsidized testing for horses with suspected viral encephalitis; however, with regionalization of testing and enhanced status as a biological threat, surveillance testing has decreased in some states. At the very least, enhanced passive surveillance for alphaviruses should be undertaken when environmental conditions are favorable.

The complete reference list is available online at www.expertconsult.com.

---

21 Flavivirus Encephalitides

Gretchen Henry Delcambre and Maureen T. Long

Infections caused by *Flaviviridae* family viruses have made an impact on human health throughout history. Yellow fever virus (YFV), now eradicated from North America, is a centuries old arthropod-borne virus (arbovirus) that in Africa and South America annually causes morbidity in 200,000 people with an estimated 30,000 mortalities.[1] Seventy-five percent of people who contract hepatitis C virus (HCV) from contact with infected blood will develop severe chronic liver disease.[2] This family of viruses had little documented recent impact on the domestic equine until the debut of West Nile virus (WNV) in the United States in 1999. With significant morbidity and mortality associated with the disease in human, avian, and equine populations, the *Flavivirus* genus has had a large spotlight of interest cast on it in both the clinical and research fields.

Etiology

The *Flaviviridae* family consists of three distinct genera: *Flavivirus*, *Hepacivirus*, and *Pestivirus*.[3] The type species of these genera are YFV, HCV, and bovine viral diarrhea virus 1, respectively. Among the 53 species of *Flavivirus*, there are a number of historically significant and pathologically active viruses responsible for diseases including Japanese encephalitis (JE), dengue fever, tick-borne encephalitis (TBE), and West Nile encephalitis (WNE).[4] Although some of these viruses are transmitted directly or have an unidentified vector, the majority of them have a known tick or mosquito vector. About one-fourth of all flaviviruses are of veterinary importance, and about half of all members of *Flaviviridae* are zoonotic.

The members of the JE serogroup that are most likely to cause overt disease in horses are JE virus (JEV) and WNV. Disease in horses caused by Murray Valley fever (MVF) virus is geographically restricted to the South Pacific and is sporadic in occurrence.[5-7] Several other members of the *Flavivirus* genus have been detected serologically in horses, but with limited reports of clinical disease (Table 21-1). Experimental

Table 21-1 Partial Taxonomic Structure, Primary Vector, Hosts, Geographic Distribution, and Veterinary Significance of Genus *Flavivirus*, Family Flaviviridae*

Serologic, Virus Group	Virus Species	Primary Vector	Amplifying Hosts	Location	Veterinary Diseases
Tick-Borne Viruses					
Tick-borne encephalitis[†]	Kyasanur forest disease	*Haemaphysalis spinigera*	Blanford's rat, striped forest squirrel, house shrew	India	Mortality in nonhuman primates
	Langat	*Haemaphysalis* spp., *Ixodes* spp.	Rats	Russia, Southeast Asia	
	Louping Ill	*Ixodes ricinus*	Sheep, grouse	Iberian peninsula, United Kingdom	Ovine encephalitis and mortality, equine encephalomyelitis, canine central nervous system signs
	Omsk hemorrhagic fever	*Dermacentor* spp.	Muskrats, voles	Russia	Mortality in birds
	Powassan	*Ixodes* spp., *Dermacentor* spp., *Haemaphysalis* spp.	Lagomorphs, rodents, mice, skunks, dogs, birds	North America, Russia	Experimental equine, canine encephalitis
	Royal Farm	Family Argasidae	Small mammals, likely small ruminants	Afghanistan	
	Tick-borne encephalitis	*Ixodes ricinus, Ix. persulcatus*	Small rodents	Asia, Europe, Finland, Russia	Neurologic equine, canine, and primate cases described
Seabird tick-borne	Meaban, Saumarez Reef, Tyuleniy	*Ixodes* spp., Family Argasidae	Sea birds	Africa, Australia, France, Norway, Russia, United States	
Mosquito-Borne Viruses					
Aroa	Aroa		Rodents	Venezuela	
Dengue	Dengue	*Aedes* spp.	Humans, nonhuman primates	Asia; Africa; Caribbean; North, Central, and South America	
Japanese encephalitis	Japanese encephalitis	*Culex tritaeniorhynchus*	Birds, swine	Asia, India, Russia, Western Pacific	Equine encephalitis, Abortion in swine
	Koutango	*Culex* spp.		Senegal, Central African Republic	
	Murray Valley fever	*Culex annulirostris, Aedes normanensis*	Birds, horses, cattle, marsupials, and foxes	Australia, Papua New Guinea	Equine encephalitis[‡]
	St. Louis encephalitis	*Culex* spp.	Birds	North, Central, and South America	No overt clinical signs
	West Nile	*Culex* spp.	Passerine birds (crows, sparrows, robins)	Africa; Middle East; Europe; North, Central, and South America; Australia	Equine, Camelid, Ovine encephalitis
Kokobera	Kokobera	*Culex annulirostris*	Macropods, horses?[§]		
Mosquito-borne	Ilheus, Sepik	*Psorophora ferox, Aedes aegypti, Ae. serratus*	Birds	Central and South America	
Yaoundé	Yaoundé	*Culex* spp.	Birds		
Ntaya	Braganza, Israel turkey meningoencephalitis, Ntaya, Tembusu, Yokose	*Culex* spp.	Birds, small ruminants	Central and South Africa	
Spondweni	Zika	*Aedes.* spp., *Mansonii* spp.	Unknown; nonhuman primates	Africa, India, South Asia	No overt clinical signs

Table 21-1 Partial Taxonomic Structure, Primary Vector, Hosts, Geographic Distribution, and Veterinary Significance of Genus *Flavivirus*, Family Flaviviridae—cont'd

Serologic, Virus Group	Virus Species	Primary Vector	Amplifying Hosts	Location	Veterinary Diseases
Yellow fever	Yellow fever, Banzi, Bouboui, Edge Hill, Uganda S, Wesselsbron	*Aedes* spp., *Haemagogus* spp., *Sabethes* spp.	Humans, nonhuman primates	Africa, Central and South America	Clinical disease in nonhuman primates
No Known Vector					
Modoc	Cowbone Ridge, Jutiapa, Modoc, Sal Vieja, San Perlita	Unknown	Rodents	Western United States	
Rio Bravo	Apoi, Bukalasa, Carey Island, Dakar, Entebbe bat, Rio Bravo, Saboya	Unknown	Bats	United States, Mexico	

Data checked with http://www.publichealthassociate.com. Accessed through the veterinary information network (vin.com).

*There are many classified and unclassified *Flaviviruses* omitted from this table for simplicity. Refer to www.ncbi.nlm.nih.gov/taxonomy to explore the most up-to-date information on taxonomic structure and virus subspecies of the *Flavivirus* genus.

†Data from Dobler G: Vet Microbiol 140(3-4):221–228, 2010.

‡Data from VET Watch, April 2011. Department of Primary Industries, Victoria, Australia. Accessed at http://www.dpi.vic.gov.au/agriculture/pests-diseases-and-weeds/animal-diseases/vetsource/vetwatch/vet-watch-april-2011.

§Serologic evidence only.

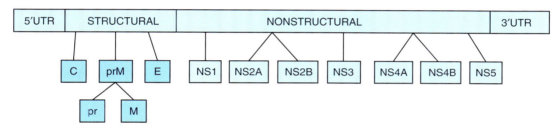

Figure 21-1 Idealized genomic organization of members of the genus *Flavivirus*. This is a positive-sense, single-stranded RNA virus consisting of two structural and seven nonstructural proteins.

reproduction of disease in horses must still be established for many of these viruses. The following discussion emphasizes WNV and JEV.

As with other Flaviviridae members, WNV and JEV are positive-sense, single-stranded ribonucleic acid (RNA) viruses[8] measuring approximately 50 nm in external diameter.[9] The virions are spheric and enveloped and contain a nucleocapsid composed of a capsid protein approximately 120 amino acids in length.[10] Electron microscopy reveals an icosahedral symmetry of the envelope and capsid. An approximately 11-kb genome contains a single open-reading frame (ORF) that is translated in its entirety and cleaved into 10 viral proteins by both cell and viral proteases[11,12] (Fig. 21-1). There are three structural proteins, capsid (C), premembrane (prM)/membrane (M), and envelope (E), and seven nonstructural (NS) proteins. The NS proteins are cleaved after translation into NS1, NS2A, NS2B, NS3, NS4A, NS4B, and NS5 and are required for viral replication and assembly.[11]

The C, M, and E proteins are important in virulence for the JE group.[13-18] Although not understood entirely, C protein is essential in virion assembly,[19] and large deletions in its sequence renders the WNV virus nonvirulent.[20] The M protein is formed from a precursor protein (prM protein), which is modified as immature virions are secreted through the Golgi network of the cell, leaving the C-terminal portion of the protein inserted in the envelope of the mature virion. Among other things, M protein may play a role in viral replication.[21] The E protein is only secreted in its native conformation through association

with the prM protein. This immunodominant viral protein exists in the virion as a β-pleated sheet arranged head to tail, with the distal ends anchored in the membrane. This protein is dimeric, held together with intermolecular disulfide bonds, and lies flat against the lipid bilayer. The large E protein is important in receptor ligand binding and fusion to host cells, the latter being pH dependent. There are three major domains of this protein in WNV. Domain II contains a region important to virus binding in the brain. Domain III is important for vector and host virulence.[22] In WNV, glycolysis of the E protein is strain dependent and associated with virulence. Viral binding to glycosaminoglycan on cells changes virulence in both JEV and WNV.

The NS proteins in flaviviruses are structurally and functionally similar and are involved in synthesis of viral RNA.[23,24] The glycoprotein NS1 is essential for virus function and appears to be important for cell activation as part of viral synthesis.[25-27] The NS1 protein is found on host cell membranes and must interact with NS4A in this process. The proteins NS2A and NS2B are formed by cleavage of full-length NS2. Changes in the C-terminal of this protein results in loss of viral replicative ability. The NS3 protein is highly conserved between flaviviruses and, at the N-terminal, encodes a serine protease. The C-terminal of this protein has sequences typical of RNA helicases and triphosphatases.[28] The NS4b protein appears to block antiviral cytokines.[29] The NS5 protein is essential for viral replication by forming the "cap" at the 5′ end of a genome. Viruses, as opposed to eukaryotic cells, have a type I cap at the end of

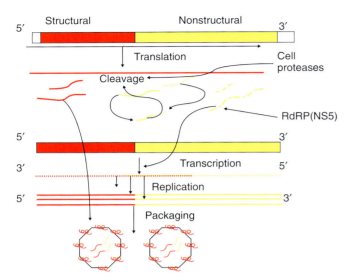

Figure 21-2 *Flavivirus* replication cycle that demonstrates a first round of virus translation to produce proteins that are cleaved by host and viral proteases. Production of a positive-strand virus by viral proteins results in progeny packaged in mature virions. After rounds of translation and replication occur, virus is released by cell lysis or, more often, budding from the infected cell.

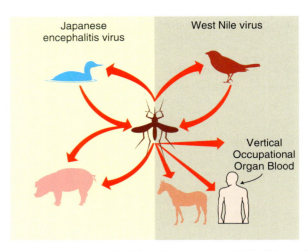

Figure 21-3 West Nile virus (WNV) and Japanese encephalitis (JE) virus life cycle in which the primary transmission cycle is between avian or porcine reservoirs and mosquitoes. Horses and humans are aberrant hosts.

the genome, which in a cytoplasmic virus, such as WNV, must be formed solely by viral proteins. In addition, this is the site of the viral RNA-dependent RNA polymerase (RdRp), an essential protein for formation of negative-strand RNA from the genome of the positive-strand "parent" RNA virus.[29,30]

JE serogroup viruses are thought to infect the cell through glycoprotein receptors that are likely highly conserved by hosts.[30-32] After receptor-mediated endocytosis, there is fusion of the viral membrane with membranes of the endosomal vesicle, and the nucleoprotein is released into the cytoplasm. After translation, the serine protease NS2B-NS3A, along with cell proteases, cleaves the polyprotein at multiple sites to generate viral proteins (Fig. 21-2). The RdRp copies the negative-strand RNA from the genomic RNA template. These negative-strand RNAs become templates for the synthesis of new genomic RNAs. There are likely alternating periods of replication and translation until a sufficient pool of structural proteins has accumulated. Once there is a pool of genomic RNA, virion assembly occurs in the rough endoplasmic reticulum (ER) membranes. Immature virions with the prM protein accumulate in vesicles and are transported through the host secretory pathway, where the E and prM proteins are modified. Virions are transported to the plasma membrane in vesicles and released by exocytosis. Mammalian cells will release progeny virus within 10 to 12 hours after infection.

Epidemiology

Life Cycle and Transmission

Japanese encephalitis serogroup viruses are vector-borne diseases, with transmission occurring to avian and mammalian hosts from blood meal–seeking mosquitoes[33] (Fig. 21-3). Virus is maintained within vector populations by horizontal or vertical transmission. Climate-limited amplification of the virus within a vector occurs in warmer seasons but is minimal during colder temperatures[34,35]; therefore, reservoir hosts are required for amplification and maintenance of the virus year-round. Typical reservoirs include birds such as passerines. For JEV,

Ardeidae (herons and egrets) and swine are also important amplifying reservoir hosts. Horses and humans are "dead-end" hosts and do not amplify the virus in quantities sufficient to infect mosquitoes.

Additional modes of transmission have been identified in the North American WNV encroachment. First, transmission through oral ingestion has been proven in both avian and mammalian hosts, and oral and cloacal shedding has been demonstrated in birds.[36-40] Second, WNV may be transmitted through contaminated blood transfusion or organ transplantation if donors are viremic.[41-44] Third, vertical transmission through placenta and milk has been demonstrated in humans.[42,45] This last feature is important in JE and several JE serogroup virus infections.

Vectors

The spread and yearly incidence of JE serogroup viruses coincides with the availability of vectors and reservoir hosts with transmission potential. Thus, outbreaks are seasonal and reflect mosquito activity. *Culex* spp. mosquitoes are the primary vector for the JE serogroup.[40,44,46-48] WNV has been detected in 64 species of North American mosquito, but the overall vector efficiency (moderate to high) and wide feeding activity range of *Culex* spp. indicate that North American WNV outbreaks are propelled mainly by this genus.[49] Most of the data supporting this conclusion is based on vector efficiency studies under laboratory conditions, experimental feeding studies, and frequency of identification of WNV in mosquito pools.[49,50] In the northeastern United States, more than half of WNV-positive mosquito pools are *Culex pipiens*.[51-55] In the western United States, populations of the highly efficient *Cx. tarsalis* constitute the majority of positive pools, with *Cx. pipiens* the next most frequent.[49,56-58] In the southeastern United States, *Cx. quinquefasciatus* and *Cx. nigripalpus* have the highest WNV infection rates.[59-63] In the southwestern United States, epidemics are most often associated with positive pools of *Cx. quinquefasciatus*, *Cx. tarsalis*, and *Cx. pipiens*.[55,64-67] *Culex restuans*, frequently identified as part of the "*Cx. pipiens*" complex, is often one of the top five positive species.[49,67] Positive vector species incidence is driven by environmental habitat, which may cause variation from these reported common species.[68]

Although *Culex* is important in the epidemiology and spread of WNV, relatively little is known regarding the actual vector of transmission to the horse. Blood meal analysis suggests that

Cx. pipiens mosquitoes are primarily avian feeders. Mammalian feeders include predominantly *Anopheles quadrimaculatus, Coquillettidia perturbans,* and *Aedes albopictus.*[69,70] *Culex salinarius, Cx. (Melanoconion)* spp., *Aedes vexans, Ae. albopictus, Psorophora ferox, Ps. columbiae, Coquillettidia perturbans, Anopheles quadrimaculatus, An. crucians,* and *Ochlerotatus atlanticus* were reported engorged with equine blood in a 2-year surveillance study in south Louisiana.[71] *Culex pipiens, Cx. salinarius,* and *Ae. vexans* are likely the most important bridge vectors, which feed from both reservoir and host.[72-74]

Experimental infection of horses through mosquito transmission studies is accomplished with *Ae. albopictus,* a common mammalian feeder and moderately efficient vector of WNV.[75,76] In studies thus far involving low numbers of horses, 9 of 10 horses become viremic, and all seroconvert to the virus. One out of 11 horses develop neuroinvasive disease. Members of the *Cx. tritaeniorhynchus* group of mosquitoes are the most important vectors for JE and were used in the experimental transmission and reproduction of disease in horses.

Several species of ticks have been investigated for potential to transmit WNV. Transtadial transmission was demonstrated in one study of *Ixodes* ticks but failed to occur in a second study.[77,78] *Carios capensis* can transmit WNV under experimental conditions to ducklings, and *Ornithodoros moubata* can transmit WNV under experimentally to mice.[78,79]

Hosts and Reservoirs

A reservoir host is one in which a pathogen is amplified in vivo so that it can be transmitted to a vector species.[53] A blood meal taken from a mammal containing 10^5 to 10^7 plaque-forming units per milliliter (PFU/mL) of WNV results in infection of 30% to 100% of feeding mosquitoes, respectively. Humans voluntarily infected with the Egyptian strain of WNV developed virus titers of 10^3 to 10^5 PFU/mL.[80] Horses develop titers of 10^1 to 10^3 PFU/mL after experimental infection via exposure to WNV-positive mosquitoes.[81] Dogs and cats experimentally exposed to WNV produce viremias lower than 10^4 PFU/mL, but individual cats can develop titers that would permit virus transmission.[82] Cats can become infected after oral exposure.

Viral titers capable of transmitting JEV are similar to those for WNV transmission. Swine are a notable reservoir host for JE. Primary clinical manifestations include abortion, birth of weak pigs, and limited neonatal survival. Semen from infected boars contains infectious virus and has decreased sperm count and motility.

To date, more than 300 species of WNV-positive birds have been reported to the WNV Avian Mortality Database from the Centers for Disease Control and Prevention (CDC). High levels of viral amplification occur in many bird species, especially Passeriformes (e.g., songbirds) and Charadriiformes (e.g., shorebirds).[39] Modeling of WNV outbreaks has identified some species of birds as "super-spreaders" including of the American robin, followed by the house sparrow, and, where present, the fish crow.[83,84] Corvids (e.g., crows) are known to develop a high viremia (10^{-0} PFU/mL) but with high mortality, which limits their potential as efficient reservoirs or their role in spread of the virus as compared to robins and house sparrows.[36,38,39,85,86]

Although corvid susceptibility has been described as unique to the North American outbreak, early studies with the Egyptian WNV strain produced high mortality in crows.[87,88] The remarkably explosive North American outbreak of WNV has introduced new potential hosts for the virus. Seropositive, free-ranging mammals include the big brown bat, little brown bat, eastern chipmunk, eastern gray squirrel, eastern striped skunk, white-tailed deer, brown bear, rabbit, and raccoon.[40,53,89,90] Serologic evidence of natural infection has been demonstrated

in domestic dogs and cats.[36,37] Neurologic disease has been confirmed as natural WNV infection in gray and fox squirrels but has been difficult to reproduce in experimental infection.[91] New world camelids and sheep develop neurologic disease with natural exposure to WNV.[92-94] Alligators can have an extremely high viremia and may be an important reservoir for WNV in the southeastern United States.[90] There are reports of both farmed and free-ranging alligators with neurologic signs from which WNV has been isolated. In farm-raised alligators, cloacal shedding of virus has been demonstrated, with oral infection likely.

Geographic and Seasonal Distribution

The largest documented outbreak of equine neurologic disease caused by a flavivirus began in 1999 with WNV encroachment into the United States, emerging in New York City. In 2002, an epizootic resulted in 14,571 cases of equine WNE and accompanied an epidemic of 4,156 human cases with 284 resulting deaths.[95] Between 1999 and 2006, nearly 25,000 cases of equine WNE were reported in the United States, with an estimated average 30% to 40% case-fatality rate. Positive equine case reporting has decreased to an average of 300 a year from 2007 to 2010.

By 2005, WNV had been identified in all 48 continental U.S. states[96] (Fig. 21-4). Canadian provinces reporting disease included Quebec, Ontario, Manitoba, Saskatchewan, and Alberta, with New Brunswick and Nova Scotia reporting evidence of WNV-positive birds.[97] Serologic evidence of WNV has been reported in the Latin American and Caribbean countries of the Dominican Republic, Mexico, Guadeloupe, El Salvador, Puerto Rico, Cayman Islands, Jamaica, Belize, Cuba, and the Bahamas.[40,98-103] As early as 2005, the presence of WNV reached as far south as Argentina. From 2006 through 2010, WNV in general appeared to wane in the United States; however, in 2011 an increase in reporting of human cases occurred, with horse cases remaining between 100 to 300 per year. With 5387 human, 654 equine, and 2436 avian cases, all groups had increased reporting during the 2012 season.

Japanese encephalitis virus annually causes 30,000 to 50,000 human encephalitis cases worldwide, with endemic areas including China, the southeast region of the Russian Federation, South and Southeast Asia, and Australia. Exact numbers of horses with clinical JE are difficult to ascertain; however, there are reports of JE isolation from horses in Taiwan, China, Pakistan, and Australia in the literature since the 1980s. Outbreaks in horses have also been reported in India, Nepal, the Philippines, Sri Lanka, and Northern Thailand with the most recent outbreak in Spain in 2010.[104]

Occurrence of disease caused by JEV and WNV in horses and humans reflects vector activity, seasonally in temperate regions and year-round in subtropical and tropical regions. Intense virus activity in the United States begins in July, with a peak incidence in September and October.[59,105-107] Temperature-dependent spatial modeling supports these disease dynamics, with risk increasing from 25% in late August to greater than 75% by the second week of September.[108-110] A drop in ambient temperature with soft frost usually results in a rapid decrease in reporting activity.[111,112] The appearance of disease from JE is highly variable, depending on the locale. Seasonal occurrence of disease in specific locales should be considered to facilitate timing of equine athletic events and to tailor vaccination regimens appropriately.

Intrinsic Risk Factors

Geriatric humans appear more susceptible to neuroinvasive disease from both JEV and WNV. This age bias in reporting

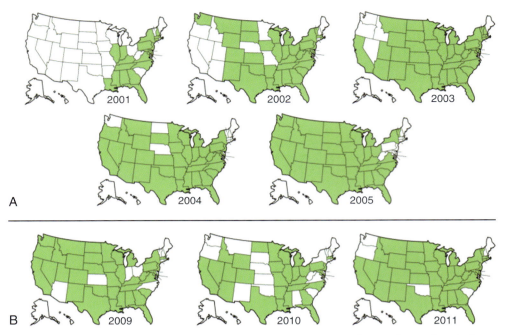

Figure 21-4 A, Serial maps of the United States with green states reporting positive veterinary cases of West Nile virus (WNV). These maps demonstrate the spread of the virus from coast to coast. Veterinary cases are defined as nonavian, nonhuman cases, with horses composing 96.9% of these cases. **B,** Serial compellation of recent WNV-positive veterinary case maps. West Nile virus is an endemic virus.

appears true for WNV in horses.[40,113-117] Although human men are more frequently affected with neuroinvasive diseases, there is conflicting evidence as to whether stallions, geldings, or mares are more likely to die as a result of WNV infection.[118-121] Other factors that contribute to mortality risk in horses include light coat color, nonvaccinated status, pasture-only management, and solid stall walls.[120,121] Additionally, the use of stable fans is positively correlated with WNV infection because the weak air flow does not impede mosquito movement yet can disperse chemical odors emitted from the horse to attract mosquitos.[120]

Pathogenesis

In general, mammalian disease caused by infection with the JE serogroup viruses reflects a predilection for nervous tissue. Neurologic disease in the horse consists of changes in mentation, signs consistent with spinal cord abnormalities, and defects in cranial nerves of the hindbrain.[122-132] Change in behavior likely results from viral infection and pathology induced in the neurons of the thalamus, medulla, and pons, with limited viral load in the cerebrum.[125,126,133] Although the thalamus integrates all sensory input to higher centers, lesions within the midbrain and rostral pons may affect the reticular formation, which has an important role in regulation of consciousness.[132,134] The reticular formation projects to the thalamus, which in turn sends diffuse projections to the entire cortex.[132] This formation also travels directly to the base of the forebrain, which is the source of cholinergic stimulation to the entire cerebral cortex. Disturbances of the reticular formation and the midbrain may induce behavioral changes ranging from severe aggression to somnolence and even coma.

West Nile virus–induced motor deficits are multifocal, asymmetric, and primarily characterized by weakness and ataxia.[124-126,130,133,135,136] These two clinical signs are likely a reflection of brain and spinal cord disease through direct infection of the spinal cord, interruption of motor tracts in the hindbrain, and loss of fine motor control through infection of the large nuclei of the thalamus and the basal ganglia. Ataxia can be attributable to interruption of general proprioception. Although ataxia is commonly detected and can be profound, many horses have difficulty standing, primarily because of profound weakness. These clinical signs are attributable to infection of the gray matter within the midbrain and hindbrain. In the spinal cord, lesions consisting of perivascular cuffing and gliosis tend to increase in frequency and severity caudally, with the most severe lesions appearing in the lumbar cord compared with the cervical cord.[130] Lower motor neuron disease characterized by weakness would be a common clinical sign associated with these spinal cord lesions.

Involuntary skin and muscle fasciculations, tremors, and hyperesthesia, extremely common in WNV disease, likely result from loss of fine motor control, which is regulated mainly by the basal ganglia.[137,138] Movement disorders are observed with flavivirus infection in a long-term Parkinson-like syndrome in rats and experimental infection in monkeys.[138] Infection in the pons and medulla oblongata can explain clinical deficits of cranial nerves VII, XII, and IX.[139]

Like humans, horses also develop signs of flaccid paralysis, which in the quadripedal movement of the horse reflects lower motor neuron disease. These clinical signs likely reflect focal invasion of the lower motor neuron.

Two routes of neuroinvasion are proposed for WNV infection. In the first, WNV causes a low-level viremia, followed by replication in the lymph nodes and entry into the central nervous system (CNS) across the blood-brain barrier.[22] The second proposes transaxonal transmission.[140] In the first theory, it is hypothesized that systemic viral infection results in local cytokine responses that increase the permeability of the blood-brain barrier to viral invasion. In particular, tumor necrosis factor alpha (TNF-α) increases vascular permeability and allows infection of peripheral nerves.[141] Evidence also indicates toll-like receptor 3 (TLR3) plays a role in the entry of WNV into the CNS.[141,142]

Experimental rodent models demonstrate that WNV has a primary predilection for neural tissues of the vertebrate host.[22,143-145] Intraperitoneal injection of WNV (10^2 PFU) into 8- to 12-week-old mice results in dissemination into the CNS by 4 to 6 days after inoculation. The time course of infection in the hamster is similar. Experimental infection of horses results in viremia at days 3 to 5 and clinical signs in 7 to 10 days.[75,146] WNV inoculation into the CNS results in direct infection of nerve cell bodies. In rodent models, initial replication occurs in the basal ganglia, with subsequent dissemination to the cortex, cerebellum, and hippocampus.[147-151] The large neurons of the ventral or anterior horns are infected later in the course of disease. Recent studies in a hamster model supports the transaxonal route of infection when injection of WNV into the sciatic nerve results in transmission of WNV through the peripheral nerve to the cell body of a motor neuron in the CNS.[152-154] In this study, WNV was transported both antero-grade and retrograde, acute flaccid paralysis was induced, and clinical signs were ameliorated by treatment with monoclonal antibody to WNV.

Immune Responses

West Nile virus invades the hosts' innate immune cells like macrophages and myeloid dendritic cells where it is recognized by cytosolic retinoic acid-inducible gene (RIG)-I-like and mela-noma differentiation antigen 5 (MDA5) receptors and endo-somal TLR3 and TLR7.[155,156] Activation of these pattern recognition receptors lead to the downstream production of interferon gamma (IFN-γ), a type I-IFN.[157] Interferons upregu-late major histocompatibility complex class 1 (MHC-1) expres-sion, CD8+ T-cell recruitment, and natural killer (NK) cell activity. Interferon-stimulated genes (ISGs) may hinder RNA translation, viral entry, or viral degredation.[158-160] Mice lacking type I-IFN receptors suffer 100% mortality rates after subcuta-neous WNV infection with increased viral dissemination into typically nonaffected tissues and cell types.[161] Increase in IFN signaling is supported by microarray analysis of gene transcrip-tion in gravely-ill, WNV infected horses.[162] This analysis also demonstrated an increase in genes correlated to interleukin (IL)-15, IL-22, and IL-9 signaling pathways which promote antiviral immune responses.[163-165]

Antigen-presenting cells, including dendritic cells, macro-phages, and NK cells, initiate IFN production, which has down-stream antiviral effects or directly induce cytotoxic effects on infected cells. Macrophage and dendritic cell production of IL-12 induces the differentiation of T-helper cells into Th1 cells, which secrete IL-2 and IFN-γ. Interleukin-4, IL-5, and IL-10 expression by macrophages and dendritic cells drives differen-tiation of T-helper cells into Th2 cells. Th2 cells stimulate B-cell responses and inhibit Th1-cell response, in turn decreasing CD8+ T-cell activity.

The B-cell response is initiated shortly after 1 week postin-fection in horses. These cells produce T-cell dependent immu-noglobulin M (IgM) antibodies early in the disease but will isotype switch to a dominant production of IgG.[166] Antibodies clear viral infection via neutralization, antibody-dependent-cell-mediated cytotoxicity, and complement activation.

Neuronal Injury

Viral invasion into the CNS occurs by disruption of the blood-brain barrier (BBB) via proinflammatory cytokine effects on endothelial cells,[167] direct infection of circulating peripheral mononuclear cells that migrate into the CNS,[168] retrograde transport from peripheral nerves and anterograde spread to other parts of the CNS,[154] or a combination of these.

Chemokine expression by infected neurons is integral in the recruitment of circulating leukocytes into the CNS. These include, CXCR2 for early neutrophil migration, CCR2 for monocyte recruitment; and CXCR3, CCR5, and CXCL10 for CD4+ and CD8+ T cell accumulation.[169-171] Interferon gamma produced by NK T cells, Th1 cells,[171] and CD8+ T cells (positive feedback) also recruits CD8+ T cells.

Although cell lysis occurs with viral replication, WNV also induces apoptosis in neurons, as demonstrated in cell culture and in vivo.[147] In equine and human disease, virus load in neu-ronal tissues is low, indicating the possibility that global bystander injury leads to severe neurologic signs and neuron death. Some suggested mechanisms for neuronal injury and apoptosis include immune responses driven by activated CD8+ T cells,[172] excitotoxicity via glutamate signaling,[162,173-175] and mitochondria-mediated caspase activation.[176] Although CD8+ T cells may be important in long-term protective immune responses, lesions in brains of mice with fatal WNV are pre-dominantly composed of CD8+ T cells.[177,178] Activated CD8+ T cells are responsible for clearance of virally-infected cells by apoptosis-activating mechanisms and are subsequently respon-sible for pathology, particularly, the destruction of motor neurons of the brain and spinal cord. CD8+ T cells may also play a dominant role in inducing BBB permeability.[179]

Clinical Findings

Japanese encephalitis and WNV produce similar clinical signs, except that fatal JEV infection in horses usually results in blind-ness, coma, and death, whereas these signs are relatively limited in WNE horses.[180,181] For both these infections, there is evidence of widespread subclinical infection in both humans and horses. Both exhibit the same disease course based on lineage of virus; clinical neurologic disease develops with neurotropic lineage type I WNV infection, whereas infection with the African lineage type II viruses is predominantly subclinical in nature.[182,183] Kunjin virus, a WNV subtype causes milder clinical disease in horses. Infection with JEV may result in severe clinical disease in naïve horses, but great variation in virulence is seen in JE viruses.

When clinically apparent disease occurs, both systemic and neurologic abnormalities are observed in horses with WNV. A mild to moderate increase in rectal temperature (38.6° C-39.4° C [102° F-103° F]), anorexia, and depression are the most com-mon initial systemic signs.[123] Abdominal pain, which also occurs in people, or a colic episode may be the first clinical presenta-tion.[119,123,125,184] Gait abnormalities, including overt lameness or dragging of a limb, before development of an obvious neuro-logic syndrome have also been reported. Both spinal cord dis-ease and moderate mental aberrations occur. Onset of neurologic signs is frequently sudden and progressive, and the exact course of disease in any one animal is unpredictable.

Irrespective of onset, the literature is rich in descriptions of clinical disease in both humans and horses. While there is ample evidence for a polioencephalomyelitis, one of the initial signs of motor abnormality is a short, slow, stilted gait, described by observers as "lameness" with laminitis being a frequent differ-ential diagnosis at this stage. In human patients, however, bra-dykinesia or slow, deliberate movement is frequently described, and this may be the equine corollary.[116] Spinal abnormalities are characterized by ataxia and paresis that can be asymmetric or involve one or two forelimbs or hindlimbs or by a flaccid paresis that is localized to one or more limbs. This state may be of short duration, or horses may become suddenly recumbent and either die or require prolonged treatment. Horses that become recumbent often need aggressive supportive care.

The major hallmarks of equine WNV encephalomyelitis are muscle fasciculations and changes in personality. Fine and coarse fasciculations of the muscles of the face and neck are common. Fasciculations can be severe and can involve all four limbs and trunk, affecting normal activities such as walking, eating, and interactions with handlers and other horses. Muzzle and eyelid fasciculations are notable. Eyelid activity during this period is enhanced with light, and at times, horses appear photophobic. Many horses have periods of hyperexcitability and apprehension, sometimes to the point of aggression. Frequently, a quiet horse will become hyperexcitable, and an abnormally aggressive horse will become compliant. Interspersed during periods of hyperexcitability, some horses appear to have abnormalities of sudden sleeplike activity resembling narcolepsy. This can occur to the point of cataplexy, and horses may partially or completely collapse for a short period. Some horses show a persistent change of mentation, and a state of nonresponsiveness, resembling coma, results.

Cranial nerves are frequently abnormal for short periods; weakness of the tongue, muzzle deviation, and head tilt are the most common abnormalities reported. Dysphagia has been reported, with esophageal obstruction a possible sequela. Autonomic nervous system dysfunction likely accounts for the respiratory failure and gastrointestinal disturbances.[185] A cauda equina syndrome consisting of stranguria and rectal impaction is infrequently reported.

Overall, the combination, severity, and duration of clinical signs can be highly variable. After initial clinical signs abate, about 30% of horses experience a recrudescence in signs within the first 7 to 10 days of apparent recovery. Overall, about 30% of affected horses progress to complete paralysis of one or more limbs overall. Most of these horses are euthanized for humane reasons or die spontaneously.

Many horses will begin improvement within 3 to 7 days of displaying clinical signs. If the horse demonstrates significant improvement, full recovery within 1 to 6 months can be expected in most of these patients. However, residual weakness and ataxia are common, with long-term loss of the use of one or more limbs infrequently described. Changes in personality have also been reported to persist. Mild to moderate, persistent fatigue on exercise has been observed.[186]

Diagnosis

West Nile Virus

Ancillary diagnostic testing for horses with suspected WNV infection should include complete blood count (CBC), serum biochemistry analysis, and cerebrospinal fluid (CSF) analysis.[187,188] CBC and serum biochemistry profiles of WNV-infected horses are usually normal, but basic blood work can rule out systemic causes of CNS abnormalities such as liver failure. Horses infected with WNV may have a mild absolute lymphopenia. Additionally, they may have elevated muscle enzymes secondary to trauma and prolonged periods of recumbency. A frequent finding is hyponatremia, which has also been described in humans with encephalitis, potentially caused by inappropriate release of antidiuretic hormone.[189,190] Cerebrospinal fluid cell counts and protein concentration may be elevated. Differential cell counts in CSF of WNV-infected horses primarily have increased mononuclear cell populations. Protein concentrations are frequently elevated (N < 70 mg/dL), and the color of the fluid can be mildly xanthochromic.[188]

No pathognomonic signs distinguish WNV infection in horses from other CNS diseases, and a full diagnostic evaluation should be pursued. Infectious CNS diseases that should be considered as differential diagnoses include alphavirus encephalitis, rabies, equine protozoal myeloencephalitis (EPM), equine herpesvirus type 1 (EHV-1), botulism, and verminous meningoencephalomyelitis (e.g., *Halicephalobus gingivalis*, *Setaria*, *Strongylus vulgaris*). Noninfectious causes to consider include hypocalcemia, tremorogenic toxicities, hepatoencephalopathy, and leukoencephalomalacia. In alphavirus encephalitis and rabies, signs of cerebral involvement are characterized by behavioral alterations, depression, seizure, and coma. The appearance of seizure and coma is rare in horses with WNV. Motor function is frequently abnormal in eastern equine encephalitis (EEE) and western equine encephalitis (WEE). In WNV suspects, circling and propulsive walking may occur, but head pressing is rare. Cranial nerve signs common in EEE and WEE are also common in WNV and include head tilt, pharyngeal/laryngeal dysfunction, and paresis of the tongue. Other clinical signs of alphavirus encephalitis that may be observed in horses with WNV infection are muscle fasciculations, hyperesthesia, excitability, blindness, somnolence, and progression to recumbency. Mortality in nonvaccinated horses with EEE is high, approximately 80% to 100% (as in rabies). The incidence of WEE in horses is fairly low in the United States, but mortality and severity of clinical signs would be similar to WNV. Spinal disease caused by EPM is a more difficult differential diagnosis if horses with WNV are not febrile and do not exhibit excessive muscle fasciculations. Both diseases demonstrate hindbrain disease with diffuse spinal cord abnormalities.

Confirmation of WNV infection with encephalitis in horses begins with assessment of (1) whether the horse meets the case definition based on clinical signs and (2) whether the horse resides in an area in which WNV has been confirmed in the current calendar year in mosquito, bird, human, or horse.[135] Serologic testing developed by the National Veterinary Services Laboratory (NVSL) is based on detection of the IgM antibody response that uniformly occurs in acutely infected horses. The preferred test is an IgM antibody-capture enzyme-linked immunosorbent assay (MAC-ELISA).[146] Horses develop a very intense IgM response on exposure to WNV that lasts approximately 6 weeks. This immunologic reaction is much more reliable than in human infection, in which a more persistent IgM response is common. Most diagnostic laboratories utilize the WNV MAC-ELISA for actual confirmation of disease (increases in IgM rarely occur after vaccination). The sensitivity and specificity of this test are 81% and 100%, respectively.[191]

In the nonvaccinated horse, a fourfold change in paired neutralizing antibody titers confirms a diagnosis of WNV infection. The most common neutralizing antibody test formats are the classic plaque reduction neutralization test (PRNT) (Fig. 21-5) for detecting antibody response and a more recently developed microwell format.[122,135,146,192] Vaccination induces formation of neutralizing antibody to the E protein of the virus,[193] which likely confounds interpretation of the PRNT. Since the marketing of equine WNV vaccines in 2001, reliance on the PRNT for serologic confirmatory diagnosis of WNV in horses has diminished. Microsphere immunoassay utilizing recombinant NS1 protein may be useful in detecting antibody response due to natural infection of vaccination.[194]

Other methods for confirmation of a diagnosis of WNV include postmortem detection of WNV by polymerase chain reaction (PCR), culture, and immunohistochemistry (IHC) in CNS tissues. Several methods for detection of WNV nucleic acids in equine tissue have been described. One method is nested PCR targeting the E protein and has demonstrated sensitivity for relatively low viral loads in equine tissues.[195,196] Real-time PCR methodology has been used to detect WNV in equine tissues.[196] Because of the limited viral load, the equine clinician must insist that ancillary testing be performed in several

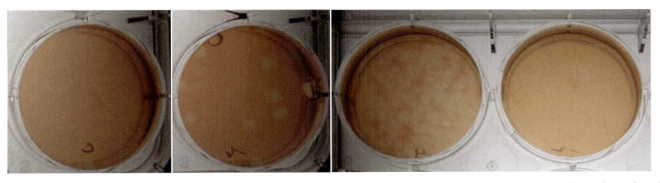

Figure 21-5 Six-well plate exhibiting clearing of monolayer (plaques) of Vero cells as cytopathic effect of West Nile virus (WNV) infection. These plaques form the basis of the "gold standard," the plaque reduction neutralization test (PRNT), for detection of neutralizing antibody to flaviviruses.

sections of brain, especially those with lesions observed by light microscopy.[197]

Serum titers should be evaluated for recent exposure to other encephalitides, including EEE, WEE, and EHV-1. Measurement of titers from paired sera is necessary in vaccinated horses for detecting recent exposure to these diseases. Because WNV can present with asymmetric weakness and ataxia, Western blot testing for EPM should also be performed on serum and CSF. The integrity of the BBB during acute infection is unknown. Initial work indicates little leakage, with most WNV-specific IgM within CSF considered to be of intrathecal origin.[187]

Japanese Encephalitis

Japanese encephalitis should be suspected in horses with compatible clinical signs that reside in an area of virus activity. Diagnostic confirmatory tests include serologic assays such as neutralizing, complement fixation, hemagglutination inhibition, and ELISA tests.[198-200] All single sera testing, including IgM assays, must be interpreted with caution in horses from areas with other endemic flaviviruses such as WNV.[201] In fatal JE cases, viral isolation, PCR assays, and IHC for detection of virus in CNS tissues is confirmatory.

Pathologic Findings

Flaviviruses cause polioencephalomyelitis (inflammation of the gray matter) with lesions that increase in number from the diencephalon through the hindbrain and frequently increase in severity caudally through the spinal cord. The histologic changes within the brain, including inflammatory foci and detectable virus in the thalamus, medulla, and pons, are consistent with changes in behavior.

Gross pathologic findings are limited in WNV infection in the horse. The meninges may be congested. Small to moderately sized foci of hemorrhagic discoloration may be observed in the brain and spinal cord. These areas occur most often in the basal ganglia, rostral colliculus, pons, medulla, and lumbar spinal cord. Edema and softening of tissues are also common findings.

Histopathologic changes secondary to WNV infection are consistent with viral infection and neural cell death.[124] The basal ganglia, thalamus, pons, and medulla have the highest numbers of lesions, with two to several cell layers of predominantly mononuclear perivascular cuffing. Recent IHC has revealed a minor presence of granulocytes (Delcambre, Long, et al, unpublished data). Predominantly confined to the gray matter, glial nodules are present in the brain parenchyma. These lesions are limited in the cortex and cerebellum in the horse. Neuronal damage includes chromatolytic neurons and neuronophagia. Horses with long-standing disease may have areas of neuronal dropout. The spinal cord also has perivascular cuffing, glial nodule formation, and damage to neurons.[124] It is still unknown if these cellular changes are attributable to viral damage or resulting inflammation.

Therapy

No known marketed antiviral medications demonstrate reliable activity against flaviviruses, and thus treatment of disease is supportive.[123,125,202-204] In horses, the survival rate for WNV encephalitis is high compared with other infectious encephalitides. Most horses appear to begin recovery 3 to 5 days after onset of signs, which makes it difficult to assess any pharmacologic intervention accurately, when a feature of analysis is resolving clinical disease. Flunixin meglumine (1.1 mg/kg every 12 hours [q12h] intravenous [IV] given early in the course of the disease) appears to decrease the severity of muscle tremors and fasciculations within a few hours of administration.

To date, much of the mortality in WNV horses results from euthanasia of recumbent horses for humane reasons. Recumbent horses are mentally alert and frequently thrash, sustaining many self-inflicted wounds and posing risk to personnel. Therapy of recumbent horses is generally more aggressive and may include dexamethasone sodium (0.05-0.1 mg/kg q24h IV) and mannitol (0.25-2 g/kg q24h IV). Controversy remains as to whether corticosteroids enhance peripheral and CNS viral load.[205-207] Detomidine hydrochloride (0.02-0.04 mg/kg IV or intramuscular [IM]) is effective for prolonged tranquilization. Low doses of acepromazine (0.02 mg/kg IV or 0.05 mg/kg IM) provide excellent relief from anxiety in both recumbent and standing horses. Until EPM is ruled out or WNV is confirmed, prophylactic therapy with antiprotozoal medications is recommended for horses in geographic areas where *Sarcocystis neurona* infection is prevalent. Other supportive measures may include oral and IV fluids and antibiotics for treatment of infections that frequently occur in recumbent horses (wounds, cellulitis, and pneumonia).

A variety of treatments have been recommended for horses with WNV; however, there is limited evidence at this time to support their efficacy.* The recommendation for IFN-α therapy is based on anecdotal reports in the human and veterinary literature, yet limited information regarding efficacy in the horse

---

*References 97, 116, 199, 203, 208, 209.

is available. In a blinded study in which children with encephalitis caused by JEV were treated with IFN-α, survival was not enhanced. In fact, length of hospitalization was increased in the IFN-α–treated group.

Therapy with WNV-specific recombinant immunoglobulin has also been recommended. In a blinded placebo-controlled trial with low numbers of animals, the risk for development of recumbency was less in horses receiving plasma from horses immunized against WNV (Long, unpublished data). However, plasma treatment did not change outcome and severity of WNV disease. In human patients, high-dose glutamate therapy has been suggested to prevent neuronal cell death. Another experimental therapy in mice is administration of beta-lactam inhibitors, which stimulate GLT1, a chemical that activates glutamate.

Prevention

Epidemiologic and anecdotal evidence exists regarding the effectiveness of vaccination against flaviviruses. Initial epidemiologic studies performed in 2000 established a point source for infection of WNV, demonstrating that outbreaks in horses may be controlled best by vaccination.[146,210,211] This finding was consistent with prior experience with JE, in which vaccines were advocated for horses before the WNV epizootic. The dramatic decrease in WNV cases in the horse likely reflects the success of vaccination.

Currently, three killed vaccines and a recombinant vaccine are licensed for prevention of WNV viremia in the United States, and an inactivated virus vaccine is readily available against JE.[201] Vaccination before the mosquito season is critical. The manufacturer's labeling instructions must be followed for induction of immunity with initial immunization. More frequent vaccination in areas with year-round mosquito seasons is highly recommended. Limited information is available regarding long-term immunity after vaccination especially in the killed vaccines. However, it is not expected that the initial vaccine series will provide long-term protection beyond 1 year.

Where these viruses are endemic, vaccination schedules must be maintained even with a decrease in the incidence of overt disease. Foals must receive three injections of vaccine with time 30 days between with the first and second injections and 60 days time between the second and third injections. Foals should not receive early vaccination if the mare has been vaccinated and should receive the first vaccine at 5 to 6 months of age. Horses that have recovered from clinical disease have long-term immunity and do not require annual boosters.

Public Health Considerations

West Nile virus is considered a zoonotic disease. A bird reservoir maintains the virus in an endemic life cycle in the environment, allowing for transmission by mosquitoes to humans. There is little risk of disease by direct contact with an infected horse, except during postmortem examination with inappropriate handling of infected tissues. Postmortem handling of tissues should be performed with personal protection similar to that for rabies suspect cases (see Chapter 19). The ecology of horse pastures and stables with standing water, a high degree of biologic debris, and "bridge" vectors between birds and mammals likely increase the risk of exposure in that environment. The same types of management tactics for prevention of disease in horses are important for people, except that there is no vaccine. Personal mosquito protection with a DEET-based product is recommended in areas with endemic disease.

The North American epidemic of WNV has demonstrated new modes of transmission, including blood-borne and occupational risks. Blood-borne transmission can occur between viremic hosts. In addition, occupational infection has occurred through necropsy of avian hosts. Veterinarians and horse owners should institute personal protection with appropriate clothing, gloves, and eye protection when coming into contact with animal tissues during the arbovirus season.

The complete reference list is available online at www.expertconsult.com.

Borna Disease

Maureen T. Long, Juergen A. Richt,* Arthur Grabner,* Sibylle Herzog,* Wolfgang Garten,* and Christiane Herden*

Borna disease (BD) is a naturally occurring, infectious, usually fatal, progressive meningoencephalomyelitis, predominantly affecting horses and sheep; less often other Equidae, cattle, goats, and rabbits; and occasionally a variety of other animal species.[1-17] Synonyms used in the past, such as "hot-headed disease" (Hitzige Kopfkrankheit), "brain fever," "subacute meningoencephalitis," and "hypersomnia of horses," reflect the

restriction of the disease to the nervous system. The current name of BD originated from a devastating epidemic among horses of a cavalry regiment between 1894 and 1896 near the town of Borna in Saxony/Germany.[18-20] More sporadic occurrence of equine BD has since been described in different areas of Germany,[3,21-24] Switzerland, Liechtenstein, and Austria.[26] There are reports of equine BD cases in Japan,[27-29] but these could not be confirmed by others. Similar cases of equine encephalitis and/or serologically positive horses have occurred in many other countries, including France,[30-32] Romania, Libya,

*The authors acknowledge and appreciate the original contributions of these authors, whose work has been incorporated into this chapter.

Iran,[33] China,[34-36] and Turkey.[37-39] However, there is still controversy as to whether some reports actually represent endemicity and disease in horses in these and other countries, as well as Australia and the United States.[40-43]

Etiology

BD virus (BDV) is an enveloped virus with a nonsegmented, negative-sense, single-stranded (ss) ribonucleic acid (RNA) genome of 8.9 kilobases, with the characteristic genomic organization of members of the order *Mononegavirales*.[44-47] Some genotypic and phenotypic distinctions of BDV required the classification in the new virus family, the Bornaviridae. During the first decade of the twentieth century, studies of BD focused primarily on defining the etiology, pathology, and pathophysiology of the disease. Final proof for a viral etiology was presented in 1927 by Zwick et al[48] by reproducing the disease with bacteria-free filtrates of brain homogenates from affected horses. Histopathologic studies of the brain revealed massive perivascular infiltrations, reactive astrogliosis, and intranuclear eosinophilic "Joest-Degen" inclusion bodies.[20] The pathologic changes were preferentially localized in the limbic system.[49]

Molecular tools have allowed further identification and addition of the causative agent of proventricular dilation in psittacine birds, which is now designated avian Borna virus (ABV). Several features of BDV replication, such as the nuclear site of replication and transcription, RNA splicing, and the overlap of transcription units, are unique compared with other members of this order.[50-56] BDV particles are spherical, enveloped, and approximately 130 nm in diameter, with spikes 7 nm in length and a nucleocapsid 4 nm in diameter.

On the complementary positive-strand RNA (cRNA), at least six open-reading frames (ORFs) can be identified. ORF I, at the 5′ end of the cRNA, encodes the 357/370–amino acid (aa) nucleoprotein, NP (p38/p39); ORF II encodes the 201-aa phosphoprotein, P (p24); ORF III encodes the 142-aa matrix protein, M; ORF IV encodes the 503-aa glycoprotein, GP; and ORF V (at 3′ end of cRNA) encodes the RNA-dependent RNA–polymerase (RdRp) of BDV, the L protein, which is more than 1600 aa long.[53,58-63] Overlapping with ORF II, the ORF x1 encodes the 87-aa BDV-p10 protein.[61] All of these virus-specific proteins have been detected in BDV-infected material.

Several lines of evidence, including the location on the genome, indicate that the nucleoprotein (NP) and the phosphoprotein (P), together with the L-protein, are part of the ribonucleoprotein (RNP) and therefore part of the functional BDV replication complex. BDV RNPs are infectious after transfection into susceptible cell lines.[64] The BDV-p10 can also bind to the RNP complex, and it is speculated that it may act as a negative regulator of the BDV polymerase activity.[62,65-68] Associated with the BDV envelope are the matrix (M) and the glycoprotein (GP). The BDV-M was thought to be glycosylated, but recent studies demonstrate that it is a nonglycosylated matrix protein, similar to that found in other viruses of the order *Mononegavirales*.[69] Similar to the Filoviridae and Rhabdoviridae, BDV possesses a single surface glycoprotein, BDV-GP, which is posttranslationally modified by N-glycosylation and cleavage by a subtilisin-like protease into two fragments; this is a prerequisite for the invasion of BDV into cells.[70-76]

The RNA transcripts encoding BDV proteins are initiated at three transcriptional start sites and terminated at five transcriptional termination sites. The RNA from the first transcriptional unit codes for the NP.[59,60,77] Alternative initiation at two in-frame AUGs results in the p38 and p39 isoforms of the NP. The RNA from the second transcription unit is bicistronic and codes for the P and p10 proteins. Similar to NP, two isoforms of P have

been detected.[78] RNA transcripts originating from the third transcriptional start site can be terminated at two different termination sites. In both cases, the transcripts may contain up to three introns, and depending on whether intron 1 and/or intron 2 is spliced, the respective mature messenger RNA (mRNA) can code for the M, GP, or L protein.[50,53,58,59,79] It can be assumed that RNA splicing may play an important role in the regulation of BDV genome expression by increasing the versatility of its primary transcripts and by providing the possibility for controlled synthesis of new BDV polypeptides. Lipkin et al recently reviewed the proposed various functions of these proteins in the pathogenesis of BDV.[80]

Epidemiology

The epidemiology and host diversity of BDV infections has been recently reviewed and is presented in Figure 22-1.[81] Borna Disease virus, RNA or protein has been most frequently isolated from horses with clinical disease in European countries including Germany, Switzerland, Liechtenstein, Austria, and Britain.* However, the diagnosis may have been overlooked in other areas because of limited diagnostic resources and focus on BDV. Results from testing with new diagnostic methods that use monoclonal antibodies, reverse genetics, and virus-specific polymerase chain reaction (PCR) technologies suggest that BDV may be more widespread than previously thought so that true prevalence of clinical BD in horses is unclear. Seroprevalence studies demonstrate that BDV infections can occur worldwide.[81,85] Borna disease virus-specific antibodies have been detected in horses from many countries, including several European countries, Turkey, Israel, Japan, Iran, China, Australia, and the United States, but these finding are controversial.† Although Europe has the highest reported incidence of BD and BDV, recently BD has been detected in horses and other animals in North America, Israel, Japan, China, and Iran.[15,35,34,87] Despite the wide geographic range of seropositive horses, clinical disease from BDV has rarely been described outside of Europe.[29,33,43,88-93]

Borna disease has been reported in many other animals such as sheep, cattle, llamas, cats, and dogs,[7,44,94-99] with additional experimental infections in rabbits, ferrets, and primates.[17,100] The identity of the reservoir host has been under speculation for some time, and birds and the white-tailed shrew, *Crocidura leucodon*, are most recently proposed.[101-103] The latter is supported by field studies.

Extensive studies of the seroprevalence of BDV are reported only from Germany, where BD is the most important viral central nervous system (CNS) disease of horses.[3,6,82] These studies demonstrate that the disease occurs predominantly in endemic regions in the central and southern parts of Germany. In contrast to the epidemic course of BD at the end of the nineteenth century, a significant reduction of BD incidence to about 0.3% was noted in an endemic region in central Germany in 1960 and from 1989 to 1996.[131] At present, the incidence in endemic regions in Germany is even lower, approximately 0.02% to 0.04% in Bavaria.[36] Clinical disease in horses is most common in April, May, and June, with a significant decrease in late fall and winter.[82,104]

Most BDV infections appear to be inapparent infections, as indicated by various studies determining BDV seroprevalence. The average seroprevalence of BDV-specific antibodies in clinically healthy German horses varies from 11.5% to 22.5% in

---

*References 1, 6, 20, 22, 26, 82-84.
†References 22, 28, 32, 33, 38, 39, 42, 43, 82, 86.

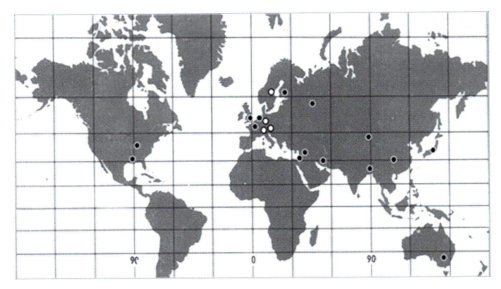

Figure 22-1 Distribution of the reported signs of Borna disease virus (BDV) infection in animals. Countries with antibody, ribonucleic acid (RNA), and/or antigen findings are marked with ● and those where natural neurologic BDV infection has been verified by virus isolation are marked with ○. Countries, such as Italy and the Czech Republic, where the BDV findings are solely based on the controversial triple enzyme-linked immunosorbent assay (ELISA) method, have been omitted. *(From Kinnunen PM, Palva A, Vaheri A, et al: J Gen Virol 94:247-262, 2013.)*

endemic regions.[22] In stables with diseased horses, the prevalence of BDV-specific antibodies is approximately 50%.[3,22] In 72% of horse stables with cases of BD, only individual animals showed clinical signs of BD. Repeated outbreaks of BD in stables are possible, although these are usually observed some time (2 months to several years) after the initial occurrence of BD.[3,22] There is no explanation for the discrepancy between the high seroprevalence and the low incidence of disease; the development of symptomatic disease after BDV infection may depend on the genetic factors, age, and immune status of the host and the genetic characteristics of the virus.

The route of transmission of BDV is uncertain. Investigations in rats showed that BDV can be shed in nasal and lacrimal secretions, as well as in urine, and transmission most likely occurs through open nerve endings in the nasal and pharyngeal mucosa.[105,106] In a few cases, infectious virus could be isolated from the lacrimal and parotid glands of horses with BD (S. Herzog, unpublished results), and virus-specific RNA could be demonstrated in nasal and lacrimal secretions[107] and saliva of such animals; this was also possible in a few seropositive, inapparently infected horses.[100,108] However, there is no evidence of virus replication in lacrimal or parotid gland of inapparently BDV-infected horses (S. Herzog, unpublished results). This indicates that horses infected with BDV, especially with clinical signs of BD, could play a role in the transmission of BDV but horse-to-horse transmission is not likely to play an essential role in spread of disease..

Pathogenesis

Most of the currently available information regarding the pathogenesis of BDV infection is derived from studies of experimentally infected Lewis rats and also from BDV-infected mice.[109-113] In general, it can be assumed that the virus enters the body by intranasal infection through olfactory nerve endings.[105-108] Another possible route is orally, through the trigeminal nerve.[2] After the virus enters the nervous system, it migrates along the axons of the olfactory system to the brain,

where it replicates in neurons and glial cells, preferentially in the limbic system. Over time the virus disseminates throughout the CNS, then spreads to the peripheral nervous system and the neuronal cells of the retina.[112,114,115] Axonal transport, with consequent protection from recognition of foreign antigens by the humoral immune system, may explain the lack of neutralizing antibodies until late in infection. Like rabies, intracerebral spread is likely axonal and transynaptic.[116,117]

In adult rats the virus demonstrates a strict neurotropism with infection of neurons, astrocytes, oligodendrocytes, and ependymal cells.[71,112,113,116-119] Viral antigens and infectivity persist throughout the life of the infected animals exclusively in neural tissues, indicating that BDV causes persistent CNS infection.[120] The occurrence of clinical signs correlates with the appearance of inflammatory lesions in the brain causing a meningoencephalitis involving mainly the limbic system with spread to other areas of the brain during the course of infection.[109,111,121-123] With chronic infection, inflammation decreases despite the presence of viral antigen and infectious virus. This might be caused by a switch from a T helper cell 1 (Th1) to a T helper cell 2 (Th2) immune response in later stages of the disease.[124,125] In contrast, neonatally infected rats harbor infectious virus not only in the CNS but also in parenchymal cells of peripheral organs.[126] When diseased horses and sheep were analyzed for the presence of BDV-specific RNA by the reverse transcriptase–PCR (RT-PCR) technique, the bulbus olfactorius, nucleus caudatus, hippocampus, and cerebral cortex of all animals were positive.[73] RNA was also present in the spinal cord, eye, nasal mucosa, parotid salivary gland, lung, heart, liver, kidney, bladder, and ovaries in some animals. The presence of BDV RNA in tissues of nonneural origin could be caused by virus in nerve endings within these organs. In addition, BDV-specific RNA was detected in conjunctival fluid, nasal secretions, and saliva of two infected animals.[107] Evidence suggests that BDV replication in brain cells and probably other cell types may be controlled by the virus through various strategies such as direct modification of the viral genome, control of transcription, regulation of viral protein expression (e.g., ratios of BDV-N versus BDV-P), or abrogation of BDV glycoprotein synthesis.[58,63,123,127,128] BDV can interfere with various cellular proteins or signaling cascades including neurite outgrowth factor, high mobility group-1(HMG-1), neurotropin signaling (NT), mitogen-activated protein kinase cascade (MRaf/MEK/ERK pathway), activation of nuclear factor-kappa beta (NF-κB) or the induction of the antiviral interferon (IFN) response.[70,129-136] These interactions with host cell function might represent viral strategies to spread, replicate, and persist in the CNS of its host.

Another mechanism of BD pathogenesis is its virus-induced immunopathologic reaction.[137-139] Infection of adult immuno-competent rats results in encephalitis and disease, whereas infection of newborn, athymic, or immunosuppressed animals leads to neither encephalitis nor disease, despite persistent high levels of virus in the CNS of these virus carriers.* BDV-specific antibodies adoptively transferred into immunosuppressed, virus-infected recipients do not induce pathologic alterations or disease.[113] Neutralizing antibodies to BDV are only detectable late, if ever, after infection and might play a role in preventing generalized infection with BDV. Transfer of immune serum into immune-incompetent newborn rats could not prevent persistent CNS infection but did prevent dissemination of the virus from neural tissues to peripheral organs.[142] However, adoptive transfer of immune cells from spleen or lymph nodes of BDV-infected animals is effective in the induction of BD in immunosuppressed virus carriers.[112,113]

In the mouse, the role of virus-specific T cells in the pathogenesis of BD was demonstrated by passive transfer of in vitro established homogenous BDV-specific CD4+ T-cell lines into immunosuppressed virus carriers.[143,144] The recipients consistently developed clinical signs characteristic of acute BD. However, evidence indicates that in addition to virus-specific CD4+ T cells, CD8+ cells are also involved in pathologic alterations.[145-154] These are thought to be a main effector cell in BDV-infection of mice, although there is no lysis of BDV-infected neurons observed in infected mice or rat brains. In rats and mice, BDV-specific CD8+ cytotoxic T lymphocytes (CTLs) are mainly directed against the viral nucleoprotein. The kinetics of CTL induction and subsequent recruitment of these cells to the brain determine the severity of BDV-induced neurologic disease. Downregulation of the functional avidity of virus-specific CD8+ T cells in experimentally infected mice seems to be involved in controlling the inflammatory reaction and facilitating viral persistence. However, immune control of BDV infection could generally be achieved only by antigen-specific immune priming or adoptive transfer of BDV-specific T cells. Taken together, these data indicate that T cells play a crucial role in the pathogenesis of BD. The severe meningoencephalitis with mononuclear infiltrates observed after BDV infection most likely represents a delayed-type hypersensitivity reaction.

As observed in the experimental rat model, brain tissues from various Equidae with spontaneous BD have mononuclear immune cell infiltration with increased expressions of major histocompatibility complex (MHC) class I and class II antigen.[145,149,155-157] The composition of the inflammatory cell infiltrates is similar to that observed in experimentally BDV-infected rats, and therefore a similar pathogenesis of disease in naturally infected Equidae and experimentally infected rats is presumed.

Most research has focused on the detrimental effects of this virus in neurons, as well as infection of astrocytes and activation of microglial cells.[158-163] Even expression of virus-associated proteins (independent of infection) leads to a decrease in synaptic density, with a reduction in brain-derived neurotrophic factor serotonin receptors. Activated microglial cells can induce apoptosis and loss of neurons through apoptosis.[66,164,165]

Clinical Findings

Natural BDV infection can result in peracute, acute, or subacute Borna disease with encephalomyelitis, which leads to death 1 to 4 weeks after onset of initial signs in more than 80% of animals.[2,3,5,22,166] In less severe cases, spontaneous recovery is occasionally observed despite a persistent CNS infection.[2,3,5,22,166] In up to 10% of animals with BD, a chronic, sometimes recurrent course of disease is observed. A mild encephalitis without obvious clinical signs is possible. The incubation period for BD after natural infection is variable, ranging from 2 weeks to several months.*

After experimental infection the average incubation period was 2 to 3 months. More recently, experimental intracerebral infection of three ponies with various doses of BDV resulted in an incubation period of 15 to 26 days.[172] Two ponies were febrile for 3 to 7 days before neurologic signs occurred. The course of BD was dependent on the virus dose used for infection. Two ponies died after rapid onset of CNS symptoms within 28 or 30 days after infection, whereas the third pony survived the infection without residual clinical signs. The major clinical signs were ataxia, head tilt, muscle fasciculation, hindlimb paresis, localized cutaneous hyperesthesia and hypoesthesia, and aggressive behavior, similar to signs of natural BD.

Clinical manifestations of BDV infection may vary among individual animals.[2,3,22,166] Typical clinical signs of BD in horses are simultaneous or consecutive changes in psyche, sensorium, sensibility, and mobility and in the autonomic nervous system.[3,6,95,104] The most common clinical signs are depression with apathy, somnolence, and stupor.[2,3] Alterations in behavior and consciousness can be observed in early stages of BD, and these signs progressively worsen toward the final stages.[2,3,22,166] Slow-motion eating, eating arrest with chewing movements (called *Pfeifenrauchen*, or "pipe smoking") (Fig. 22-2, *A*), and chewing motions without food intake, interrupted by frequent yawns or head pressing, can be present early in the course of disease and are important diagnostic clues. Recurrent fever that is resistant to antipyretic medications may occur in the initial stages of acute BD.[2,3,22,166] Prolapse of the penis without urination; rhythmic repetitive motor activities; disturbances in the mental status with lethargy, somnolence, and stupor; hyperexcitability; fearfulness; and unusual aggressiveness may be observed in variable degrees. These alterations might be caused by impairment of the limbic system, which regulates affective and compulsive behavior.[2,3,22,166]

Hypokinesia and abnormal postures (postural unawareness), as well as decreased skin and deep sensory reactions, are frequently observed, resulting in an impaired reaction to exogenous and nociceptive stimuli and a loss of proprioception (Fig. 22-2, *B*). Early in the course of BD, a deficit of the "cutaneus trunci reflex" and flexor reflex may be noticed. Hyporeflexia of spinal reflexes, head tilt, and hypoesthesia with disturbances in proprioceptive sensory functions are characteristics of more advanced stages of BD. In this stage, horses may exhibit ataxia and imbalance, an abnormal reaction toward exogenous stimuli, and abnormal posture (see Fig. 22-2, *B*).

Impairment of cranial nerve (CN) function as a consequence of inflammatory reactions in the respective CN nuclei, as well as direct effects on CNs, such as the trigeminal nerve (CN V), result in the development of these clinical signs: (1) dysphagia and salivation from pharyngeal paralysis (CNs IX and X), (2) decreased tongue tension and increased tongue movement (CN XII), (3) bruxism and trismus (CNs V and VII), (4) paresis of the facial nerve (CN VII), (5) nystagmus (CNs XI and VII), and (6) strabismus and miosis (CN III).[2,3,22,166]

---

*References 48, 112, 113, 126, 137, 140, 141.

*References 22, 21, 44, 49, 84, 96, 123, 167-172.

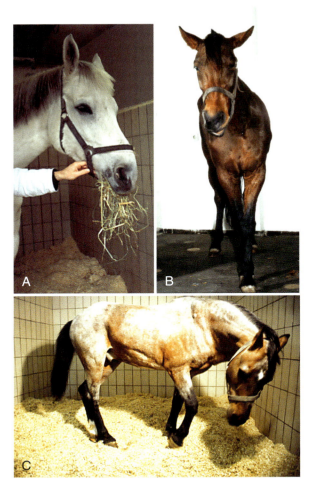

Figure 22-2 Horses with Borna disease (BD). **A,** Seven-year-old gelding affected with somnolence and displaying characteristic arrested eating with chewing movements (called *Pfeifenrauchen*, or "pipe smoking"). **B,** Two-year-old mare affected with disturbances in proprioception (abnormal posture) and paralysis of facial nerve. **C,** Seventeen-year-old Welsh Pony stallion with neurogenic torticollis and compulsive circular walking. *(From Richt JA, Grabner A, Herzog S: Vet Clin North Am Equine Pract 16:579, 2000.)*

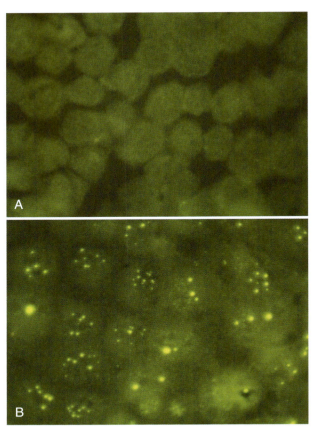

Figure 22-3 Indirect immunofluorescence assay (IFA) of horse sera with Madin-Darby canine kidney (MDCK) cells. **A,** Borna disease virus (BDV)–positive serum incubated with uninfected MDCK cells. **B,** BDV-positive serum incubated with BDV-infected MDCK cells.

In the final stages of BD the horse develops an increased appearance of neurogenic torticollis with torsion dystonia in the neck muscles, in some cases associated with compulsive circular walking (Fig. 22-2, C). A slight tremor in the head area is usually observed, followed by convulsions. Convulsions are regularly associated with head pressing, which is the result of a high cerebrospinal fluid (CSF) pressure caused by the inflammatory reaction in the CNS.[2,3,22,166] Loss of the pupillary reflex and strabismus are often observed at this stage, and affected animals may lapse into a comatose condition. Blindness is often observed in horses with acute BD.

In more than 50% of animals with acute BD, disturbances in chewing and swallowing of food and water develop, which could limit the duration of the disease in some horses.[2,3,22,166] In the final stages of the disorder, food intake ceases, and only 20% of the affected animals are able to swallow small amounts of water. As a consequence of this lack of food intake, a fasting hyperbilirubinemia with icteric mucous membranes develops. Nonneurologic signs, such as recurrent colic, emaciation, and chronic lameness of unknown etiology, as well as behavioral abnormalities such as "head shaking," have also been described.[173] Whether these signs are directly caused by the BDV infection

is not clear, but the disturbed food and water intake might be misdiagnosed as colic.[2,3,22,166]

Diagnosis

Antemortem Diagnosis

Hematologic and biochemical parameters are usually within normal limits in affected horses.[2,3,22,166] Hyperbilirubinemia is frequently observed but is a nonspecific change related to decreased food intake. During the final stages of BD when convulsions occur, a high concentration of lactate may be present in the plasma. In acute disease the quantity of CSF and the concentration of CSF proteins (86.3 ± 14.8 mg/dL; 58 cases) may be increased.[2,3,22,166] The CSF shows a characteristic lympho-monocytic pleocytosis (56.4 ± 32.8 cells/µL) during acute and subacute BD, consistent with the presence of a nonpurulent inflammatory condition.[2,3,22,166] In chronic BD, most CSF parameters are in the normal range, except the CSF lactate concentration, which is usually increased.[2,3,22,166]

Because of the lack of specificity of clinical signs and laboratory abnormalities, Borna disease must be confirmed by the demonstration of BDV-specific antibodies in the serum or CSF of diseased horses,[2,3,166] using Western blot analysis,[43,104,174] enzyme-linked immunosorbent assay (ELISA),[175] or an indirect immunofluorescence assay (IFA)[3,48] (Fig. 22-3). The IFA is acknowledged to be the most reliable method for the detection of BDV-specific antibodies. Antibody titers in sera range between 1:5 and 1:1280 and in CSF between 1:2 and 1:1280.[3,43] No correlation exists between the antibody titers and the clinical signs or the outcome of infection.

Currently, there are descriptions of real-time PCR techniques for BDV and using a highly sensitive technique, the nested RT-PCR, BDV RNA can be detected in cells isolated from the CSF.[176,177] In acute BD, CSF pleocytosis and BDV-specific antibodies can be detected in 100% of affected horses; however, BDV-specific antibodies are often missing in peracute BD, at the beginning of acute BD, or in horses pretreated with corticosteroids.[22] BDV-specific antibodies may be found in the serum, but not in the CSF, of clinically healthy animals.[3,178] The detection of BDV-specific RNA in peripheral blood mononuclear cells (PBMCs) has been proposed as an alternative in the antemortem diagnosis of BD.[25,179] This was not shown to be useful, however, in a study including 175 horses with or without BD.[180]

Because of the multifocal appearance of brain lesions, the resulting clinical signs are not highly specific for BD. CNS infection with a variety of pathogens may result in similar signs. In countries where BD in horses is prevalent, infections with equine herpesviruses, rabies, tick-borne encephalitis, and various bacterial diseases (e.g., botulism, bacterial meningitis) and parasitic diseases (e.g., verminous myeloencephalitis, equine protozoal myeloencephalitis [EPM]) must be considered as differential diagnoses for BD. EPM often has a relatively long incubation period compared with BD. In the Americas, besides these infections, arthropod-borne infections with alphaviruses or flaviviruses, inducing equine encephalitides, and West Nile virus (WNV) infections should be included as important differential diagnoses.

In summary, antemortem diagnosis of BD can be regarded as positive when (1) animals show neurologic signs, (2) BDV-specific antibodies are detectable in the serum and CSF, or (3) CSF and characteristic pathologic changes in the CSF are observed.

Postmortem Diagnosis

The postmortem diagnosis of BD involves histopathology, immunohistochemistry (IHC), and virologic methods, including virus isolation, PCR, and IHC for confirmatory identification of virus. Immunohistochemical analysis can be performed using monoclonal or polyclonal antibodies specific for various BDV proteins[2,178,180] (Fig. 22-4, A). Monoclonal antibodies specific for the BDV nucleoprotein (p38/p39) and phosphoprotein (p24) are frequently used to detect BDV protein in the nucleus and cytoplasm of neurons, neuronal processes, and glial cells.[2,178] The same monoclonal and polyclonal antibodies can be used for the detection of BDV antigen in the CNS of infected horses by Western blot analysis.[20,70] Comparative studies indicate that all three methods, as well as nested RT-PCR, give identical diagnostic results in acute cases of BD.[178,180] The isolation of infectious BDV and the demonstration of virus-specific RNA by in situ hybridization can complete a postmortem diagnosis. These methods, however, are less suitable when the material is in a state of decomposition. In this case, IHC and Western blotting are preferred.[178]

Pathologic Findings

BD manifests as a progressive, severe, nonpurulent meningoencephalomyelitis with a predilection for gray matter. The perivascular and parenchymal infiltration is remarkable (Fig. 22-4, B).[2,109,155,157,178] The pathologic changes associated with BDV infection are similar in all naturally infected animals and are restricted to the CNS (mainly in the gray matter), spinal cord,

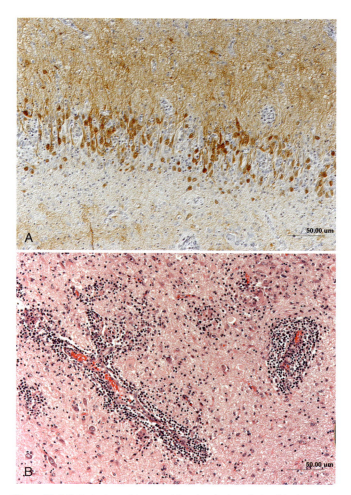

Figure 22-4 Pathologic and immunohistochemical analysis of brain section from horse naturally infected with Borna disease virus (BDV). **A,** Immunohistochemical detection of the BDV nucleoprotein using the monoclonal antibody Bo 18. BDV nucleoprotein is present in the nuclei and cytoplasm of infected neurons and in neuropil. **B,** Photomicrograph revealing nonpurulent meningoencephalitis with mononuclear perivascular and parenchymal immune cell infiltrates.

and retina. The perivascular cuffs consist predominantly of macrophages, T lymphocytes (CD4+ and CD8+), and late after infection, some plasma cells. Degeneration of neurons and neuronophagia are not prominent; however, a loss of pyramidal cells of the hippocampus might be observed, and a reactive astrocytosis can often be observed in all areas with inflammatory lesions. Besides the gray matter of the olfactory bulb, basal cortex, caudate nucleus, thalamus, and hippocampus, the periventricular areas, mainly in the medulla oblongata, can also be affected. No significant lesions are apparent in the cerebellum, and alterations in the spinal cord are inconsistent. In infected neurons, intranuclear eosinophilic (Joest-Degen) inclusion bodies can sometimes be observed preferentially in the hippocampus. If present, they are regarded as pathognomonic for BDV.

A peculiarity of BDV-infected rats and rabbits involves histopathologic changes in the retina, resulting in nonpurulent chorioretinitis with degeneration of rods and cones.[112-114,181] The loss of neurons leads to blindness. Interestingly, such alterations in the retina are not observed in horses, despite occasional observation of clinical signs of blindness. Nevertheless, viral antigen and infectious BDV can be detected in the respective neuronal cell layers in most of the affected horses.[24,178] An explanation for the lack of inflammation and degeneration might be that horses are euthanized before retinopathy can develop. Blindness could also be caused by the severe inflammation observed in the optic region of the thalamus.[24,178]

Therapy

No specific therapy is available for horses with BD despite promising reports several decades ago.[6,104] These early studies are difficult to interpret because the diagnosis of BD was uncertain, and spontaneous recovery of horses has been observed.[2,3,22] A recent report recommends the use of amantadine sulfate (AS), a drug with antiviral activity against influenza A, for treatment of BD in horses.[182] The efficacy of AS for treatment of persistently BDV-infected cell cultures and animals, however, is controversial.[182-184] In a small clinical study, the potential therapeutic effect of AS (2 mg/kg orally) in nine horses with acute BD was analyzed, with no effect in eight animals.[22] After 10 days of AS treatment, one horse showed a significant improvement and recovered from the disease after 6 weeks. From these preliminary data, we cannot conclude whether the recovery of one horse resulted from a potential therapeutic effect of AS or from a spontaneous recovery, as observed in some horses.[166]

A new therapeutic strategy might be CSF filtration to remove cellular and soluble components. CSF filtration was previously used to treat patients with Guillain-Barré syndrome and also in one case of schizophrenia related to "subclinical" BDV encephalitis.[185] This approach was used to filter approximately 400 mL of CSF per day over 5 days. The method was successfully applied in two horses.[2,3,22,166] However, future studies are needed to evaluate its efficacy.

Prevention

For the control of BD on a regional and international scale, veterinarians should constantly be reminded of the need for a careful differential diagnosis of disorders involving the CNS of horses and sheep, and data should be collected by health authorities for continuous survey.

In vaccination experiments, it was found that attenuated virus but not killed vaccines induce protection against BD.[5,186] Immunoprophylaxis with a lapinized live vaccine was practiced for many years in Germany. Because the efficacy of this vaccine was questionable, it was abandoned in 1992.[101] New data from experimental studies applying recombinant parapoxvirus constructs are promising, but their use in naturally infected horses needs further investigation.[187] Nevertheless, in view of the predominant role of cell-mediated immune responses in the development of BD, artificial stimulation of immune reactions carries a risk of exacerbation of disease.

Public Health Considerations

Whether BDV can be described as a zoonotic pathogen is uncertain, but most researchers believe there should be some zoonotic potential.[188,189] In the last decade, it has become obvious that humans can be infected by BDV or a BDV-like agent.[10,85,190-193] BDV-specific antibodies may be detected in a higher percentage of humans who are psychiatric patients than in non-psychiatric patients but the significance of this observation is unclear.[194-200] There is limited evidence for direct transmission of BDV between horses and humans; more likely, a common point source for exposure accounts for the higher seroprevalence seen in humans where infected horses occur.[21,88,188,201,202] Nonetheless, the virus is shed nasally and through lacrimal secretions in BD horses and infected tissues could be a source for personnel handling tissues of animals and horses. Personal protection should be employed when handling horses and animals suspected of symptomatic BD.

The complete reference list is available online at www.expertconsult.com.

Equine Infectious Anemia

Robert H. Mealey

Equine infectious anemia (EIA), also known as "swamp fever," is an infectious disease of horses and other equids characterized by recurrent episodes of fever, lethargy, inappetence, thrombocytopenia, and anemia. The clinical signs of EIA were first described in horses in France in 1843,[1] and the causative agent was shown to be a filterable agent in 1904.[2] This made EIA the first animal disease for which a viral etiology was assigned. During the next 60 years, much descriptive information was obtained in the areas of EIA epidemiology, pathology, and clinical manifestation. However, little progress was made in understanding EIA pathogenesis and immunology, primarily because the virus could not be transmitted to experimental hosts other than the horse and because the virus could not be cultivated in vitro. Not until 1967 was it demonstrated that field strains of the EIA virus could be propagated in equine leukocyte culture,[3,4] and subsequently, several EIA virus strains were adapted to more convenient equine fibroblast culture systems.[5,6] These advancements led to significant gains in the knowledge of the EIA virus, its interaction with host cells, and the immunopathogenesis of EIA. Although the prevalence of EIA is low in many countries, including the United States, persistently infected horses in endemic regions remain a source of infection, and outbreaks continue to occur in areas previously considered free of disease. Thus EIA remains a threat to equine health throughout the world and continues to impact domestic and international equine movement and trade.

Etiology

Equine infectious anemia virus (EIAV) is a lentivirus of the family *Retroviridae* and is closely related to other important lentiviruses, including Maedi visna virus (MVV), caprine arthritis-encephalitis virus (CAEV), bovine immunodeficiency virus (BIV), feline immunodeficiency virus (FIV), simian immunodeficiency virus (SIV), and human immunodeficiency virus (HIV). All lentiviruses cause persistent infections, and most lentiviruses cause slowly progressive disease that frequently results in death. In contrast, EIAV infection results in an acute phase, followed by recurrent clinical disease episodes that eventually subside in most horses. These horses become persistently infected life-long inapparent carriers.

Equine infectious anemia virus has a simple RNA genome that is only 8 kb in length. The genome includes three principal genes (gag, pol, env) and three regulatory genes important for viral replication and pathogenesis. The *gag* gene encodes the structural proteins needed for virus assembly and encapsidation of the genome. These proteins include the nucleocapsid (p11), capsid (p26), and matrix (p15). Gag proteins are the predominant protein components of the EIAV particle.[7] The *pol* gene encodes enzymes required for viral replication (reverse transcriptase) and integration into the host cell genome (integrase). The *env* gene encodes the virus envelope surface unit (gp90) and transmembrane (gp45) glycoproteins.

On encountering a host cell, the gp90 glycoprotein (which projects from the surface of the EIAV envelope) binds to equine lentivirus receptor-1, which is related to the family of tumor necrosis factor (TNF) receptor proteins.[8] After binding, the virus envelope fuses with the host cell membrane and the virion is internalized. Once inside the cell, the EIAV particle uncoats and replication begins with the production of a double-stranded deoxyribonucleic acid (DNA) copy of the ribonucleic acid (RNA) genome, mediated by viral reverse transcriptase. The EIAV DNA is then translocated to the nucleus and viral integrase inserts the viral DNA into the host cell genome where it remains as provirus. The integrated provirus utilizes host cell mechanisms for DNA replication, transcription to messenger RNA, protein production, and assembly of virus particles. Newly assembled virions bud from the host cell, retaining a portion of the cell membrane as the envelope (Fig. 23-1). The replication cycle is repeated as the new cell-free virus particles encounter and infect new host cells.

Incorporation of the provirus into the host cell genome is a principal mechanism of EIAV persistence within the host. In addition, because reverse transcriptase lacks proof-reading ability, mutations accumulate in the viral genome during replication. Consequently, a tremendous number of genetic viral variants ("quasispecies") arise during the course of infection, some of which can escape established immune responses. Antigenic variation and immune escape are therefore major contributing factors to EIAV persistence.

Epidemiology

Prevalence

Equine infectious anemia is a worldwide disease of Equidae, including horses, ponies, donkeys, mules, and zebras. Because EIAV is most commonly transmitted by insect vectors, the prevalence is higher in regions with warm climates. In Brazil, for example, the infection rate in certain horse herds has been as high as 50%.[7] Infection with EIAV is reportable in the United States and to the World Organization for Animal Health (OIE).[9] In the United States, the highest percentage of positive testing horses historically occurs in the Gulf Coast region, which has a favorable climate for vector transmission. Since a reliable serologic test for EIA was developed in the early 1970s[10,11] and identification of reactors and culling of positive horses became possible, the percentage of horses testing positive for EIA in the United States has declined from almost 4% in 1972 to less than 0.003% in 2010.[12,13] Nonetheless, these figures do not necessarily reflect EIA prevalence in the general horse population because they are biased by repeated testing of high-quality horses competing in events that require negative test results. Testing is only required for horses that are entering exhibitions or competitive events, being moved interstate, changing ownership, being imported, or entering auctions or sales markets. The American Horse Council estimates the U.S. horse population at 9.2 million,[14] and according to the U.S. Department of Agriculture Animal and Plant Health Inspection Service (USDA-APHIS), between 1.5 and 2 million horses are tested each year.[12,13] Based on this information, approximately 22% of the U.S. horse population is tested annually. This figure is likely an overestimate because the tests performed in a given year include repetitive testing of an undisclosed number of horses. The USDA National Animal Health Monitoring System Equine 2005 study evaluated 3349 equine operations in 28 states and found that 54.1% of these operations tested at least one horse for EIA during the year and that overall, 37.6% of the horses on all operations were tested.[15] In summary, a large percentage of horses in the United States are not tested and the true EIA prevalence is not precisely known. Annual U.S. EIA testing reports and summaries, distribution maps, and other general information can be found on the USDA-APHIS Web site at http://www.aphis.usda.gov/vs/nahss/equine/eia/index.htm.

In Europe, EIA is endemic in Italy and Romania.[16-18] In Ireland, an EIA outbreak occurred in 2006, and more recently, cases have been reported in France, Germany, and Great Britain.[16-19] The 2006 outbreak in Ireland involved 38 horses and was the first outbreak in Ireland with evidence of transmission.[17,19] The initial cases comprised four foals that were infected iatrogenically by the administration of infected plasma imported without license from Italy.[17] Transmission to the other 34 horses occurred by a combination of iatrogenic means, probable insect vector-borne transmission, and possibly via aerosol.[17,19] The potential aerosol transmission involved 13

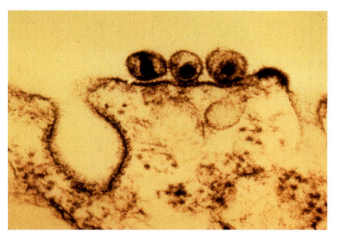

Figure 23-1 Electron micrograph of equine infectious anemia virus (EIAV) particles budding from the cell membrane of an infected macrophage.

horses sharing hospital airspace with an infected mare that had ongoing epistaxis and snorting for 13 hours prior to euthanasia.[19] All infected horses either died or were euthanized, and no further EIA-positive horses have been detected in Ireland since December 2006.[18,20] Government costs associated with control of the outbreak and the successful EIA eradication effort in Ireland have been conservatively estimated to exceed €1 million.[20] At the time of this writing, three EIA cases had occurred in Great Britain since January 2010, and all three infected horses were of Romanian or suspected Romanian origin.[16] The endemic status of persistently EIA-infected horses in countries such as Italy and Romania represents a continual threat for uninfected horses from nonendemic regions traveling in Europe, especially those traveling for competition purposes on 10-day health certificates. Despite the calculated low risk of a horse traveling from an EIA-free country, such as the United Kingdom,[16] to an endemic region and returning to the country of origin and instigating of an outbreak, naïve horses may become infected and pose a risk of transmission because of the time frame of reentry testing. By contrast, in Romania, the EIA threat has likely improved because of European Commission control measures implemented in 2010; these include microchipping horses for trade, requiring health certificates for travel, holding at a premises with no other horses within 200 m (219 yards) for 90 days prior to travel, and requiring premovement EIA testing (twice 90 days apart) and 30 days of isolation postmovement with testing at the final destination.[16] Current EIA information for countries throughout the world can be obtained on the OIE Web site.[18]

Transmission

Blood from infected horses is the most important source of EIAV for transmission to susceptible horses. Transfer of blood via blood-feeding insects is the predominant means of natural transmission. Because the virus does not replicate within insect cells, insects serve only as mechanical vectors, transferring blood on their mouthparts.[21] The most important insect vectors for natural transmission are horseflies and deerflies,[7,21-24] both of which are members of the family *Tabanidae*. Stable flies *(Stomoxys calcitrans)* have also been shown to transmit the virus,[23] but they are less efficient than tabanids as natural vectors. Experimentally, a single horsefly[24] and as few as 6 deerflies[22] or 52 stable flies[22] can transmit the virus from acutely infected horses to susceptible horses. Studies within the last 32 years indicate that mosquitoes do not transmit EIAV.[21,25] Several factors are critical for EIAV transmission by insect vectors. Horses with a high titer viremia and clinical disease are much more likely to transmit EIAV than are inapparent carriers with very low levels of virus in the blood. In one study, horseflies were not able to transmit virus from 10 naturally infected horses with no known history of clinical disease.[26] However, the transfer of 1 mL of whole blood from 7 of these inapparent carrier horses was sufficient to cause infection in susceptible ponies, and 25 horseflies were able to transmit virus from 1 inapparent carrier horse that had an acute clinical disease episode 9 months previously.[26] Vector population and feeding behavior also influence the probability of transmission. For transmission to occur, the vector must find and feed on an infected horse, be interrupted in that feeding, and then find and feed on another horse within a short period of time. Horseflies are not able to transmit EIAV if the subsequent feeding is delayed 4 hours.[24] Tabanids inflict painful bites, contributing to their efficiency as vectors since their feeding is frequently interrupted by defensive movements made by the horse they are biting. Importantly, tabanids have large, slashing mouthparts that sever small vessels, creating a pool of blood. They imbibe blood from this extravascular pool, contaminating their

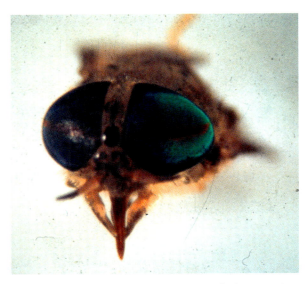

Figure 23-2 Horsefly *(Tabanus fuscicostatus)*. Note the large mouthparts.

mouthparts in the process (Fig. 23-2). As a result, tabanids transfer a relatively large amount of blood when they feed on a subsequent horse.[27] The distance separating infected and susceptible horses is another critical factor for transmission. When tabanids are interrupted in their feeding and released 1 foot (30 cm) from the initial host, 87.5% of them will return to the same horse when other horses are tethered 120 feet (36 m) away.[28] At a separation distance of 160 feet (48 m), 99% of the horseflies would be expected to return to the original horse if interrupted in their feeding. Therefore a 200-yard (180-m) separation distance between horses adequately reduces potential EIAV transmission by tabanids. Finally, transmission is more likely when vectors are present in large numbers, explaining the higher EIAV prevalence in regions with warm climates, as well as the increased incidence during the summer months.[21]

Vertical transmission may occur in utero, at parturition, or following the ingestion of infected colostrum or milk.[29-31] Transplacental transmission appears to be a rare event and is more likely when the mare develops acute clinical disease and high titer viremia during gestation. In one study, 12 of 52 foals from EIAV-infected mares were virus positive (as determined by blood inoculation into susceptible ponies) when tested at 1 week to 6 months of age.[29] Although 7 of the 12 foals were offspring of mares that had clinical signs of EIA during gestation, transplacental transmission was confirmed in only 1 aborted fetus.[29] In other studies, 18 of 20 foals born to infected dams were virus negative (as determined by pony inoculation) at weaning,[32] and 29 of 31 foals from infected mares had no evidence of infection at weaning.[33] In virus-negative foals born to infected dams, EIAV-specific colostral antibody can be detected in serum for 25 to 195 days.[32,33] More recently, of 12 foals born to EIAV-infected mares in a herd of wild horses in Northeastern Utah, none were found to be virus positive by reverse transcriptase–polymerase chain reaction (RT-PCR). However, EIAV-specific colostral antibodies could be detected in the serum from these foals for up to 336 days.[34]

Venereal transmission is possible because semen from infected stallions can result in infection following subcutaneous inoculation.[30] However, breeding EIAV-infected stallions to uninfected mares did not result in transmission except for one possible instance in which a mare sustained a vaginal laceration.[30] Finally, EIAV can be transmitted iatrogenically via transfusion with contaminated blood products and by the use of blood-contaminated materials such as surgical and tattooing instruments, hypodermic needles, and dental equipment. The virus is known to survive for up to 4 days on hypodermic needles held at room temperature.[25]

Pathogenesis

Infection with EIAV can result in a variety of clinical, clinicopathologic, and pathologic abnormalities, including fever, lethargy, inappetence, thrombocytopenia, anemia, splenomegaly, hepatomegaly, lymphadenopathy, weight loss, dependent edema, and hemorrhage.[7,35-37] Clinical disease severity correlates with viral load and thus depends on the level of virus replication. The virus infects macrophages, and most infected macrophages are detected in the spleen.[38] Although peripheral blood monocytes are infected, viral replication occurs primarily in mature tissue macrophages that serve as the predominant source of the high titer viremia during acute infection.[39] Tissue macrophages are also the primary cellular reservoir for EIAV during subclinical infection.[40] Although viral replication is restricted during periods of clinical quiescence, the virus continues to replicate at all times.[40] The spleen contains the highest level of replicating virus during acute infection, but other tissue sites of active infection include the liver, lymph nodes, bone marrow, peripheral blood mononuclear cells, lung, adrenal gland, kidney, and brain.[39-41] During inapparent infection, replicating virus can be detected in most of these same tissues but at much lower levels.[40,41] Endothelial cell infection also occurs in EIAV-infected horses.[42]

Although the immune response to EIAV is critical for the eventual control of viral load and clinical disease, immunologic mechanisms are involved in the development of lesions and clinical disease. The infection and destruction of macrophages and the observation that most of the infectious virus in the serum of infected horses occurs in the form of immune complexes[35,36,43] are important factors in the immunopathogenesis of EIA. Infection of macrophages with virulent EIAV induces the upregulation of TNF-α, interleukin (IL)-1, and IL-6.[44] Elevation in the circulating levels of these proinflammatory cytokines most likely contributes to the fever, lethargy, and inappetence observed during acute disease.[44-47]

Thrombocytopenia

Thrombocytopenia is one of the earliest and most consistent detectable abnormalities in EIAV-infected horses and closely correlates with fever and viremia.[37] The pathogenesis of EIAV-induced thrombocytopenia is multifactorial. An increase in platelet-bound immunoglobulin G (IgG) and IgM during episodes of thrombocytopenia in experimentally infected horses suggests an immune-mediated mechanism.[48] However, foals with severe combined immunodeficiency (SCID) develop the same degree of thrombocytopenia as immunocompetent foals after EIAV infection.[49] Foals with SCID lack functional T and B lymphocytes and cannot mount antigen-specific cell-mediated or antibody responses.[50,51] In addition, platelet production during EIAV infection is significantly reduced in both SCID and immunocompetent foals.[49] These results indicate that suppression of platelet production is likely the predominant mechanism of EIAV-induced thrombocytopenia. Serum activities of potential negative regulators of thrombopoiesis, including TNF-α, transforming growth factor beta (TGF-β), and interferon gamma (IFN-γ), are increased just prior to and at the onset of thrombocytopenia in acutely infected horses.[47] Both TNF-α and TGF-β in plasma from EIAV-infected horses suppress equine megakaryocytes in vitro.[52] Additional work

indicates that platelets become activated but hypofunctional in acutely infected horses, and as a result, platelet aggregates may form, which are then removed from the circulation.[53] This could represent a nonimmune mechanism of platelet destruction in EIAV-infected horses. Finally, infection of endothelial cells could promote platelet adherence and aggregation, leading to thrombocytopenia.[42]

Anemia

Anemia is a consistent clinical abnormality associated with EIAV infection, and its severity directly correlates with the frequency and duration of febrile episodes.[36] Similar to thrombocytopenia, the pathogenesis of anemia is multifactorial and includes immune-mediated erythrocyte destruction, as well as decreased erythropoiesis. Early work indicated that erythrocyte life span is reduced to between 28 and 87 days (normal mean, 136 days) in EIAV-infected horses and that both intravascular and extravascular hemolysis occurs.[54] Immune-mediated destruction is likely initiated by binding of EIAV hemagglutinin subunits to erythrocytes, which then become coated with antibody and bind the C3 component of complement.[35,36,55-57] Erythrocytes might also bind circulating virus-antibody immune complexes.[43] Intravascular hemolysis results from activation of the complement cascade via the classical pathway, whereas extravascular hemolysis occurs as a result of erythrophagocytosis by activated macrophages.[55,58,59] Complement binding requires immune responses (most likely antibody) because EIAV-infected SCID foals, which have an intact complement system, do not have C3 on their erythrocytes.[60] The fact that SCID foals become profoundly anemic indicates that suppression of erythropoiesis is an important mechanism of EIAV-induced anemia.[60] Erythroid progenitor cells are selectively suppressed by EIAV in vitro.[61] Although the exact mechanism by which erythropoiesis is suppressed is unknown, inhibitory cytokines are likely involved. In addition, iron deficiency may play a role during EIAV infection in vivo since plasma iron levels are low, as is the percentage saturation of transferrin.[62]

Immune Control

The precise immunologic mechanisms by which horses control EIAV infection are unknown. The fact that adaptive immune responses are required to terminate plasma viremia is evidenced by the inability of foals with SCID to eliminate the initial viremia following challenge with EIAV, as compared to normal foals.[60] Adoptive transfer of EIAV-specific T and B lymphocytes to a SCID foal results in functional cytotoxic T lymphocytes (CTL) and neutralizing antibody activity and is protective against EIAV challenge.[63]

Neutralizing antibodies are clearly involved in the control of EIAV replication during infection. Early work demonstrated that during periods of viral control (between viremic episodes), serum antibodies develop that neutralize plasma virus derived from previous episodes of viremia and clinical disease but are not capable of neutralizing viral antigenic variants that arise during subsequent viremic episodes.[64-67] Likewise, during episodes of viremia, plasma virus is not neutralized by contemporaneous serum antibodies. Thus recurrent viremic episodes occur when EIAV escapes neutralizing antibody responses, providing evidence that neutralizing antibodies exert a certain level of control, as well as selection pressure, for envelope variation. Amino acid changes primarily occur within the hypervariable V3-V7 regions of the envelope gp90 surface unit (SU).[68] To date, the SU epitopes recognized by equine neutralizing antibodies have not been precisely mapped. However, three linear epitopes recognized by neutralizing murine monoclonal antibodies have been identified, with two in the V3 region and one in the V5 region.[69] The V3 region of EIAV SU is considered to be within the principal neutralizing domain, and relevant to escape from neutralizing antibody, EIAV variants with amino acid changes in the V3 and V4 regions are neutralization resistant.[70] Importantly, neutralization resistance can progressively increase during EIAV infection.[70] However, transition from type-specific neutralizing antibody responses toward more broadly reactive responses occurs during the course of EIAV infection, and these broadly neutralizing antibodies likely play an important role in long-term immune control.[71] Recent studies have shown that passive transfer of immune plasma or purified immunoglobulin containing broadly neutralizing antibody activity can protect against EIAV infection and disease in the complete absence of other adaptive immune responses.[72,73] Finally, studies using an experimental live attenuated vaccine indicated that, although the vaccine could protect horses when the challenge virus had the same envelope, protection against disease decreased as the level of variation in the challenge virus envelope increased.[74] Therefore adaptive immune responses targeting the EIAV envelope, which would include neutralizing antibodies, can be protective. However, the high capacity for envelope variation ultimately limits the protective effects of envelope-specific responses.

Although neutralizing antibodies are undoubtedly important, cellular immune responses are also critical in the control of EIAV. Recrudescence of cell-free viremia and clinical disease occurred in persistently infected inapparent carriers within 6 to 10 days following immunosuppression with either dexamethasone or cyclophosphamide, a time frame in which antibody titers had not changed.[75,76] One of these studies found that the induced viremia was subsequently terminated prior to the appearance of neutralizing antibody.[75] In addition, horses chronically infected with EIAV resisted challenge with heterologous virus, despite the lack of neutralizing antibody to the challenge strain.[77] Other researchers observed that both envelope glycoprotein subunit and inactivated whole-virus vaccines protected horses from challenge with homologous EIAV but not heterologous virus. The observations that vaccination stimulated T-cell–mediated immunity and that protection occurred in the absence of neutralizing antibody led to the conclusion that cell-mediated mechanisms were involved.[78]

As in HIV and SIV, virus-specific CTLs are critically important in EIAV control.[79] The initial plasma viremia in acute EIAV infection is terminated prior to the appearance of neutralizing antibody but concurrent with the appearance of CTLs.[79-81] The early humoral response to EIAV infection is comprised primarily of nonneutralizing antibody,[67] and subsequent episodes of plasma viremia and clinical disease typically resolve prior to the appearance of neutralizing antibody.[64,67,82-84] Cytotoxic T lymphocyte epitopes have been identified in several EIAV proteins, including gag, pol, env, rev, and the protein encoded by the S2 open reading frame.[85-95] Importantly, gag p15 and gag p26 are the most frequently recognized EIAV proteins by CTLs from inapparent carrier horses,[86] occur early in infection, and likely serve as important targets for protective CTL responses.[93] Lastly, the antigenic variants arising during recurrent viremic episodes have been assumed to be the result of selection pressure exerted by neutralizing antibody. However, the fact that recurrent episodes of viremia and clinical disease occur in the face of both neutralizing antibody and CTLs indicates that EIAV variants arise that must escape both neutralizing antibody and CTL responses.[87] Recent work has shown conclusively that adaptive immunity drives the selection of EIAV envelope variants during acute infection.[68] Regardless, virus replication is eventually controlled in inapparent carriers, and this control is likely the result of a broad CTL and neutralizing antibody response.

Clinical Findings

The clinical course of EIA is variable, depending on the dose and virulence of the virus strain and the susceptibility of the horse.[96] Clinical disease may be less severe in donkeys and mules than in horses.[97] Although the distinctions are not absolute, three characteristic clinical stages of EIA have been described.[7,98] Acute EIA occurs following initial infection with a virulent strain of EIAV. Five to 30 days after exposure, pronounced viremia can develop resulting in fever, thrombocytopenia, lethargy, and inappetence. These signs can be mild and are often overlooked. The initial febrile episode usually subsides within a few days, although a small percentage of horses can develop a severe and fatal form of the disease characterized by persistent viremia, severe anemia, and high viral loads in most organs.[99] Following the initial disease episode, a few horses may develop an inapparent infection, but the majority of infected horses experience recurrent episodes of acute clinical disease characterized by viremia, fever, lethargy, inappetence, thrombocytopenia, and anemia. Each episode is associated with an antigenically distinct virus isolate, as defined by neutralizing antibody.[64-67,83,84,100] Clinical episodes typically last 3 to 5 days, and the interval between episodes is variable, ranging from weeks to months. Thrombocytopenia and other clinical signs resolve rapidly with the drop in viral load as each episode is terminated, and infected horses appear normal between episodes. If clinical disease episodes become frequent and severe, the horse develops the classical signs of chronic EIA (a "swamper"), including anemia, thrombocytopenia, weight loss, and dependent edema (Fig. 23-3). Pale mucous membranes, petechiation, icterus, and epistaxis associated with more severe hemolytic anemia and thrombocytopenia can also be observed. Neurologic signs occasionally develop and can include ataxia and encephalitis.[101,102] However, for the majority of infected horses, episodes of clinical disease subside within a year after initial infection, and these horses become inapparent carriers of the virus. These horses are clinically normal and have very low plasma viral loads. Many infected horses never show observable signs of disease and remain inapparent carriers until infection is discovered incidentally by the detection of serum antibody during routine health evaluation. Although the risk of transmission from inapparent carriers is low, they serve as reservoirs of the virus and can transmit it under field conditions.[98,103] Transmission of infection and disease was 100% when 250 mL of whole blood was transferred from seropositive inapparent carriers to susceptible test ponies.[11] Inapparent carriers are infected

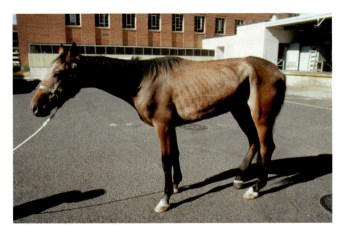

Figure 23-3 An equine infectious anemia virus (EIAV)-infected horse with clinical signs of chronic EIA (a "swamper").

for life, and treatment with immunosuppressive drugs cause recrudescence of plasma viremia and clinical disease,[75,76] indicating that environmental stress could induce a clinical episode.

Diagnosis

Equine infectious anemia should be ruled out in horses showing the clinical signs of acute or chronic EIA, including recurrent fever, thrombocytopenia, anemia, petechiation, weight loss, or ventral edema. Many infected horses have no clinical signs and/or no history of clinical signs. Other abnormalities in the complete blood count and serum biochemistry panel are inconsistent but can include monocytosis, leukopenia or leukocytosis, hypergammaglobulinemia, hyperbilirubinemia, hemoglobinemia, and elevations in liver enzymes.

Definitive diagnosis is made with serologic testing. Because EIAV is a persistent virus that is not cleared by the host, a positive serologic result indicates infection. The agar gel immunodiffusion (AGID) test is one of the official serologic tests approved by the USDA and is the test prescribed by the OIE for international trade. The AGID test, also known as the *Coggins test*, detects precipitating antibody against the EIAV gag p26 protein. The AGID test is the most widely accepted procedure for diagnosis of EIA and is highly specific. However, low levels of antibody can lead to false negative results. The AGID test requires a minimum of 24 hours before results can be reported. Several enzyme-linked immunosorbent assay (ELISA) kits, in both competitive (cELISA) and noncompetitive formats, are also approved by the USDA as official serologic tests. These detect antibodies against p26 and/or gp45 and are more sensitive than the AGID but less specific. Therefore positive ELISA results must be confirmed with the AGID test. Results of ELISA tests can be obtained within an hour. Finally, the Western blot (immunoblot) test for antibodies against EIAV may be conducted by the National Veterinary Services Laboratory as a supplemental test to reach a consensus when other diagnostic tests yield contradictory results. The Western blot is not considered an official test by the USDA.

Early diagnosis may be difficult because serologic tests can be negative 10 to 14 days postinfection.[11] However, most horses seroconvert by 45 days postinfection.[7,37,98] Colostral antibody usually clears by 6 months of age in noninfected foals born to seropositive mares,[98] but recent work indicates that passively acquired maternal antibody can be detected for up to 9 months with the AGID test and for up to 11 months with the cELISA.[34]

Tests that detect and/or quantitate EIAV in the blood are not generally used clinically but are routinely used in research settings. These tests are sensitive and specific and include animal inoculation, virus titration, and quantitative real-time RT-PCR. The animal inoculation test involves the intravenous transfer of 250 mL of whole blood from the suspect horse to a susceptible test pony and monitoring the test pony for seroconversion and clinical signs of EIA. This test is extremely sensitive for detecting infection, including the inapparent carrier state.[11] Virus titration allows quantitation of infectious virus in plasma by titration in cell culture,[67] and real-time RT-PCR allows quantitation of viral RNA in plasma.[87,104] Nested RT-PCR assays (which incorporate a second round of amplification) are highly sensitive. Nested RT-PCR assays allow detection of viral RNA in plasma from inapparent carriers, as well as in plasma from acutely infected horses as early as 3 days postinfection.[105] Despite their sensitivity, these RT-PCR techniques sometimes fail to detect virus in inapparent carriers with very low viral loads. All of the previously mentioned tests that detect virus in blood are expensive and require special expertise and facilities.

Pathologic Findings

In horses with acute disease, necropsy findings can include splenomegaly, hepatomegaly, generalized lymphadenopathy, ventral subcutaneous edema, vessel thrombosis, and mucosal and visceral hemorrhages (Fig. 23-4).[37] Typical tissue lesions include nonsuppurative hepatitis with infiltrates of macrophages and lymphocytes, primarily in the periportal areas (Fig. 23-5).[36] Cellular infiltrates in the kidney and other organs occur in the interstitial areas, primarily in the cortex. These cellular infiltrates are the likely result of specific immune response to viral antigens associated with infected macrophages.[36] This hypothesis is supported by the absence of typical tissue lesions in EIAV-infected SCID foals.[63,106] Glomerulonephritis is characterized by thickened basement membranes with inflammatory cell infiltrates and is associated with immune-complex deposition.[107] In horses with neurologic disease, lesions include lymphohistiocytic periventricular leukoencephalitis,[102] nonsuppurative granulomatous ependymitis, meningitis, encephalitis, and plasmocytic-lymphocytic infiltration of the brain and spinal chord.[101] In inapparent carriers, necropsy results are usually normal and tissue lesions are usually mild or absent.[7,37]

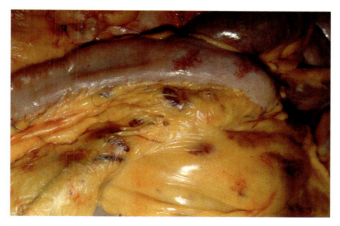

Figure 23-4 Necropsy of an equine infectious anemia virus (EIAV)-infected horse with acute EIA. Note the icteric mesentery and the numerous serosal and mesenteric hemorrhages.

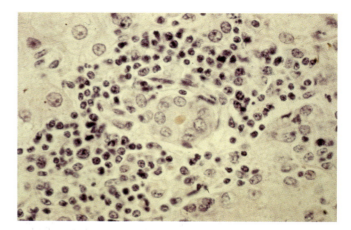

Figure 23-5 Hematoxylin-eosin (H&E)-stained liver section from an equine infectious anemia virus (EIAV)-infected horse. Note the periportal accumulation of lymphocytes and macrophages.

Therapy

There is no specific therapy for EIAV infection. Equine infectious anemia is a reportable disease in the United States, and federal law prohibits interstate travel of infected animals except under special circumstances (see section on Prevention). If elected, supportive therapy would include isolation from other horses; minimizing stress; and providing good nursing care, nonsteroidal antiinflammatory drugs (NSAIDs), leg wraps and hydrotherapy for dependent edema, and blood transfusion for severe anemia and/or thrombocytopenia. Corticosteroids are contraindicated because they will exacerbate viremia and clinical disease.[75,76] Unlike other lentiviruses (HIV, SIV, FIV), EIAV does not cause profound immunodeficiency. However, high levels of viremia can induce transient immunosuppression.[108,109] Therefore antimicrobial drugs may be indicated during febrile episodes to help prevent secondary bacterial infections.

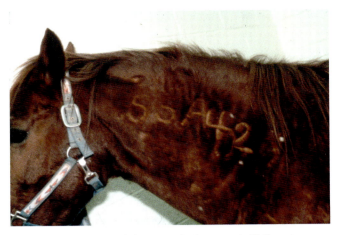

Figure 23-6 A branded equine infectious anemia (EIA) reactor.

Prevention

Equine infectious anemia is an OIE-listed disease and is reportable in many countries, including the United States. There is no approved vaccine against EIA in the United States, thus the USDA control program is designed to maintain a low prevalence by detecting EIAV-infected horses and removing them from exposure to naïve populations, thus decreasing the likelihood of transmission. Although specific procedures and requirements may vary between individual states, the following categories of horses must be tested for EIA using an official test performed by an approved laboratory: (1) horses being imported, horses being entered into exhibitions or competitive events, (2) horses being moved interstate, (3) horses changing ownership, and (4) horses entering auctions or sales markets. When a positive test is obtained, the horse is placed under quarantine and retested for confirmation. Horses that are confirmed EIA positive are called "reactors." All horses that were within 200 yards of the reactor are considered exposed and are also held under quarantine. These horses are tested at 30- to 60-day intervals, and any additional reactors are removed. The quarantine is lifted if all exposed horses are negative at least 60 days after the last reactor was removed.

There are several approved methods for removing an EIAV-infected horse from the general population. Humane euthanasia is most common. The horse could also be moved directly to an approved slaughter facility in a truck or trailer that has been officially sealed. Horses that are not immediately euthanized or shipped to slaughter must be permanently identified with a brand (Fig. 23-6) or lip tattoo. After permanent identification, a positive horse may be quarantined on the premises with a 200 yard separation distance from all other equids. The quarantine area and the quarantined horse must be periodically monitored by regulatory personnel to ensure that the provisions of the quarantine are not violated. Alternatively, the horse may be moved under permit to a federally inspected slaughter facility or a federally approved diagnostic or research facility.

Because the policy in most countries is EIA surveillance with the goal of detection and eradication, vaccination has not been widely used as a means of disease control, and there are no vaccines approved for general clinical use. Regardless, considerable research has been devoted to vaccine development.

Although various inactivated, recombinant protein, subunit, and recombinant vector vaccines have had variable results experimentally, an experimental live attenuated vaccine has shown efficacy against experimental challenge.[74,110,111] In China, where an EIA epidemic reportedly resulted in the slaughter of 424,000 horses, mules, and donkeys, a live attenuated vaccine was developed in the 1970s by serial passage of a virulent virus strain through donkey leukocyte cultures.[112] This vaccine was used in millions of horses between 1975 and 1990 and was credited with controlling EIA in China, leading to discontinuation of the vaccine program.[112-115] Although the precise mechanisms of protective immunity elicited by this attenuated live virus vaccine are still under investigation, it is reportedly effective against several different EIAV strains and no reversion to virulence has been observed,[112-115] which is a concern for persistent viruses with the ability to mutate and recombine.

In the absence of vaccination, there are several recommended procedures for minimizing the risk of EIAV transmission. First, all horses should be tested annually as part of a routine equine health program. This is especially important in areas with increased prevalence, such as the Gulf Coast states of the United States. New horses added to a herd should always be tested, and an EIA test should be part of every prepurchase evaluation. Blood and plasma donors should always be screened for EIAV infection. Needles and syringes should never be used to inject more than one horse, and dental equipment, surgical instruments, stomach tubes, and any other multiple-use equipment should be free of blood contamination and adequately sterilized between procedures. Finally, rigorous environmental and on-animal vector control, especially for horse flies, deer flies, and stable flies, will minimize natural transmission of EIAV.

Public Health Considerations

Equine infectious anemia virus only infects Equidae and therefore poses no public health risk.

The complete reference list is available online at www.expertconsult.com.

24 Vesicular Stomatitis

Brian J. McCluskey

Etiology

Vesicular stomatitis viruses (VSVs) are members of the family *Rhabdoviridae*, which includes viruses that infect vertebrates, invertebrates, and many plant species.[1] The viruses of this family that are known to infect mammals are in the genera *Lyssavirus* and *Vesiculovirus*. Rabies is the most well characterized and most devastating virus of the *Lyssavirus* genus; VSVs are the prototype viruses of the *Vesiculovirus* genus. Vesicular stomatitis viruses are bullet shaped and generally 180 nm long and 75 nm wide.[2] The nucleocapsid, or ribonucleoprotein (RNP) core, and lipoprotein envelope surrounding the RNP core are the two major structural components of VSVs. Spikelike projections extend from the outer surface of the envelope.[1] The genome of VSVs consists of a single strand of negative-sense ribonucleic acid (RNA) and is composed of five genes, *N, P, M, G,* and *L,* representing the nucleocapsid protein, phosphoprotein (a component of the viral RNA polymerase), matrix protein, glycoprotein, and the large protein (a component of the viral RNA polymerase), respectively.[1]

Although there are many members of the *Vesiculovirus* genus, two are of particular interest in the United States, vesicular stomatitis virus–New Jersey (VSV-NJ) and vesicular stomatitis virus–Indiana (VSV-IN). These viruses are similar in size and morphology but generate distinct neutralizing antibodies in infected animals. Thus, although considered distinct viruses, they are often distinguished only by terming one serotype "New Jersey" and the other serotype "Indiana."[3] Other members of the *Vesiculovirus* genus include Cocal, Jurona, Carajas, Maraba, Piry, Calchaqui, Yug Bogdanovac, Isfahan, Chandipura, Perinet, and Porton-S.[1] Cocal and Alagoas are subtypes of VSV-IN and have been associated with disease in animals in South America. Piry, Chandipura, and Isfahan produced only mild lesions in experimentally infected animals.[4] The remaining vesiculoviruses have been isolated from arthropods, mammals, or both but are not associated with disease.[1]

Epidemiology

Disease in United States

The first report of vesicular stomatitis (VS) in the United States was in 1916. However, anecdotal reports from the Civil War period leave little doubt that VS was occurring in horses during that time.[5] In 1926 an extensive outbreak of VS occurred in New Jersey in which approximately 750 cattle on 33 farms were affected, yet the disease appeared in very few horses. The agent was isolated and determined to be distinct from the Indiana strain isolated in the previous year. This new strain of VS was termed "vesicular stomatitis New Jersey strain."[6] Over the next 6 decades, VS occurred sporadically throughout the United States. Only states in New England appear to have been spared incursions of VS.

In the 1990s, three large outbreaks of VS occurred in the southwestern United States and demonstrated the economic impact of surveillance and testing that must be performed to contain VSV. On May 9, 1995, the first case of VS was confirmed in Las Cruces, New Mexico. A "case" was defined as an animal with positive virus isolation or serologic test results, in combination with clinical signs (see Bridges et al[7] for an extensive review of this outbreak). Briefly, 1162 investigations were conducted in 42 states during the outbreak. VS was confirmed in 6 states, including Colorado (165 premises), New Mexico (186 premises), Utah (6 premises), Texas (1 premises), Arizona (1 premises), and Wyoming (8 premises). Overall, 78% of the positive premises housed horses that were positive for VS, 22% of positive premises housed cattle that were positive for VS, and there was one VS-positive llama. All cases where virus isolation was successful were caused by the VSV-NJ serotype.

McCluskey et al[8] have provided a detailed review of the 1997 outbreak in which a large number of cases were identified in the counties east of the Continental Divide in Colorado. The index case for this outbreak in the United States was identified on May 27 in Yavapai County, Arizona, after a report of suspicious vesicular lesions in a horse by a private practitioner. During the 1997 outbreak, 689 investigations for suspect VS occurred in 40 states. Fifty-five percent or 380 premises had animals test positive for VS in four states: Arizona, Colorado, New Mexico, and Utah. Similar to the 1995 outbreak, clusters of cases occurred in the Albuquerque, New Mexico, and Grand Junction, Colorado, areas. Nationwide, 88% of the 802 examinations conducted for suspect VS were on horses, and 97% of 374 positive premises had horses positive for VS. Comparatively, cattle numbered only 10% of these examinations; only 3% of the positive premises had positive cattle and none of the premises had both positive cattle and positive horses. Both VSV-NJ and VSV-IN were isolated from clinical cases.

In 1998 the index case of VS occurred in a horse in Tularosa, New Mexico; virus isolation was confirmed as VSV-IN on May 18. Overall, 6% of the 232 investigations conducted nationwide were positive for VS. Four states were affected, including Texas (1 positive premises), Colorado (102 positive premises), New Mexico (12 positive premises), and Arizona (15 positive premises). Once again, the highest number of premises positive for VS were premises housing equids (99%). Only one premises housed cattle positive for VS, and this occurred in only one cow.

Between 2004 and 2006, more than 750 premises housed affected animals in Arizona, Colorado, Idaho, Montana, Nebraska, New Mexico, Texas, Utah, and Wyoming.[9] In 2009 a total of five premises were affected, two premises in Texas and three in New Mexico. All five premises had only horses affected.[10] In 2010, four premises were reported: all in Arizona and all with only horses affected.[11]

Until recently, VS was considered endemic on Ossabaw Island, Georgia, where cattle, raccoons, white-tailed deer, horses, and feral swine were seropositive to VSV-NJ.[12-14] Recent serologic test results of white-tailed deer and feral swine and the failure to isolate VSV-NJ from sand flies on the island suggest the virus is no longer present.[15]

Vesicular stomatitis is a disease of the Western Hemisphere. Areas throughout South America, Central America, and Mexico are considered endemic for VS. There are reports of endemic VSV and other vesiculoviruses in Brazil,[16,17] Argentina,[18] Colombia,[19] and other South American countries.[16] Extensive research in Costa Rica has demonstrated the endemic nature of the virus and the disease.[20-23] Work conducted by the author in El Salvador also indicated that the virus and disease are endemic in that country. A review of VS in Mexico revealed that cases occurred in every year between 1981 and 1995, with both serotypes identified in most years. VS has a national distribution in Mexico, although most cases occur in the southern states of Chiapas, Veracruz, and Tabasco. Disease is considered endemic in the central area of Mexico, but at a lower level than in southern states; viral activity in the northern area of Mexico is sporadic.

Transmission

Vesicular stomatitis viruses are considered arboviruses because they use insect vectors as their primary means of transmission. Although experimental and epidemiologic evidence for the role of arthropods as biologic vectors in the transmission of VSV is convincing, the mechanisms of virus acquisition by arthropod hosts and potential amplification of disease and the identity of reservoir hosts remain unconfirmed. Propagation of VSV outbreaks may be enhanced by movement of infected horses and spread by direct contact between infected and uninfected mammalian hosts.

Arthropod Vector Transmission

Both the temporal and spatial characteristics of VS outbreaks suggest an association with arthropod abundance. Outbreaks of VS in the southwestern United States typically begin in late spring or early summer and continue through late fall, with northward progression of disease over this period. Index cases for outbreaks in the United States are usually identified in southern New Mexico, Texas, or Arizona. New cases occur as warmer weather induces insect hatches and cease when cold weather predominates, inhibiting vector hatches.

The evidence for arthropod transmission of VSV is most compelling for sandflies (Lutzomyia shannoni)[24-28] and black flies (Diptera: Simuliidae).[29] Other species of insects may also be competent biologic or mechanical vectors of VSV (Table 24-1). Black flies are competent experimental vectors for VSV-NJ, and this virus has been isolated from Simuliidae trapped in the wild during outbreaks of VS.[29,30] Simulium

vittatum (black fly) females intrathoracically infected with virus transmit infectious virus in their saliva after 10 days.[29] Efficient transmission of VSV-NJ occurs between infected and noninfected black flies co-feeding on nonviremic deer mice, suggesting that black flies could act as a transfer vector between nonviremic vertebrate hosts and domestic livestock.[31-33] Recent experiments with domestic cattle showed transmission from infected to noninfected black flies when feeding simultaneously and in close proximity on the same animal. Uninfected flies physically separated from infected flies by up to 11 cm were able to acquire virus.[34] These experiments suggest how VSV may be maintained and transmitted without a viremic reservoir host. The flight range of potential VSV insect vectors vary, but none would be adequate to explain the often large distances observed between either individual or clusters of infected premises. Analysis of backward wind trajectories during the VS outbreaks in 1982 and 1985 suggests the feasibility of infected insects being transported for long distances on wind currents and subsequently landing on noninfected premises many miles away.[35]

Other Forms of Transmission

During the VS outbreak in 1983, disease entered California through transport of infected cattle purchased in Idaho.[36] The only case of VSV infection identified in Texas during the 1995 outbreak was caused by movement of a horse from an area of VSV activity in New Mexico to Texas. This horse subsequently exhibited clinical signs of VSV infection after shipment.

Transmission of VSV by direct contact has been demonstrated between experimentally inoculated pigs.[37] Transmission occurred only when infected pigs had visible lesions. Resultant infections ranged from subclinical to clinical, with development of vesicular lesions. Seronegative pigs shed virus as early as 1 day after contact with infected pigs.

Arboviruses generally use vertebrate hosts as reservoirs for transmission by arthropods. A vertebrate reservoir is normally infective for hematophagous insects when viremic. However, viremia has not been detected in livestock species that exhibit clinical signs of VS. Many vertebrate species have serologic evidence of exposure to VSV and may serve as reservoirs of infection.

Bats (Myotis lucifugus lucifugus) subcutaneously inoculated with Cocal VSV were viremic for 10 days when housed at 22° C (71.6° F) and for 16 days when maintained in hibernation conditions.[38] These periods of viremia may be caused by active virus replication within the bats or may merely represent persistence of the original experimental inoculum. Virus is recoverable from spleen, liver, and brain homogenates for up to 8 months after experimental infection of immunocompetent Syrian hamsters with VSV-IN.[39] In deer mice (Peromyscus maniculatus), a potential reservoir species in the southwestern United States, VSV-NJ can be demonstrated by immunohistochemistry in central nervous system tissues and the heart for up to 5 days after inoculation.[40]

Risk Factors

The most important risk factors identified for VSV occurring on premises are related to animal management, insect population and control, and occurrence of positive animals on a premises. Management is a key risk factor identified in a case-control study of hoofstock conducted on 395 premises in Colorado, New Mexico, Utah, and Arizona.[41] Animals with access to a shelter or barn have a reduced risk of developing VS, and this is more pronounced for equine premises. Risk of developing disease is increased where animals have access to pasture. The protective effect of time in a sheltered environment was also supported in a more recent study.[9] On all premises where

Table 24-1 Insect Genera from which Vesicular Stomatitis Viruses Have Been Isolated

Genus	Common Name	Transmission
Tabanus	Horsefly	Yes
Chrysops	Deerfly	Yes
Aedes	Mosquito	Yes
Culex	Mosquito	Yes
Culicoides	Biting midge	Yes
Musca	Housefly	No
Hippelates	Eye gnats	No
Simulium	Black fly	Yes
Lutzomyia	Sandfly	Yes
Stomoxys	Stable fly	Yes

owners report increased insect populations and where animals are housed less than ¼ mile (0.4 km) from a source of running water, chances of developing VS are increased. A more recent case-control study supported these findings, suggesting that insect control and spending time in shelters decreased the odds for VS infection and that premises with grassland or pasture or that had a body of water were at higher risk.[9]

A retrospective case-control study of 52 premises with VS-positive animals, 33 with no VS-positive animals, and 8 nearby premises determined potential risk factors for VS in Colorado in 1995.[42] Premises-level and animal-level data, including management practices and ecologic variables, were collected. Premises with at least one seropositive animal in 1996 were significantly more likely to be case premises in 1995 than were control premises. For case premises, there was an association between serologic status of the animals in 1996 and clinical disease status in 1995. No significant premises-level or animal-level risk factors were identified in this study.

Pathogenesis

The molecular basis of VSV pathogenesis is typical of viral infections, with a series of events terminating in the release of progeny virions and cell death. Virus attaches to cell surface receptors through the G-protein spike. Penetration and uncoating of viral particles occur, and transcription and replication commence. Ultimately, new viral particles are assembled at the cellular plasma membrane. The matrix (M) protein plays a specific role in the attachment of condensed nucleocapsids to the plasma membrane and to subsequent budding of the new virions.[43] Inhibition of cellular RNA, deoxyribonucleic acid (DNA), and protein synthesis occurs before cellular rounding that results from M-protein–induced disruption in the cytoskeleton.[44]

Infection of epithelium with VSV induces intercellular edema in the Malpighian layer, and the epithelial cells become separated by vacuolar cavities.[45,46] Cellular necrosis occurs concomitant with edema; cells shrink in size but do not undergo lysis. The infiltration of inflammatory cells, including granulocytes and monocytes, eventually results in cellular lysis. Vesicles develop when the necrotic, edematous mucosa breaks free from underlying tissue, forming a cavity filled with cellular exudates. Separation occurs at the basal layer (stratum basale) of the epithelium. Intercellular fluid accumulation, cellular necrosis, and inflammatory cell infiltration result in vesicle formation within 48 hours of experimental inoculation. Vesicles rapidly disappear resulting from seepage of edema fluid.

A recent study examining lesion development and virus replication kinetics demonstrated that VSV replicated successfully and extensively in the keratinocytes in the coronary bands but not on the skin of the neck of cattle. Vesicular lesions developed only at the sites of inoculation with peak viral replication occurring between 24 and 48 hours postinoculation. Replicating virus was detected in the lymph nodes draining these sites only at 24 hours postinoculation. Interestingly, lesions were significantly more severe when black flies were used to inoculate virus, suggesting that components in the saliva enhance VSV infection and pathology.[47]

Clinical Findings

The clinical signs of VSV infection occur in cattle, horses, swine, and rarely, llamas (Figs. 24-1 through 24-4). Signs follow a typical viral incubation period of 3 to 7 days. An initial febrile

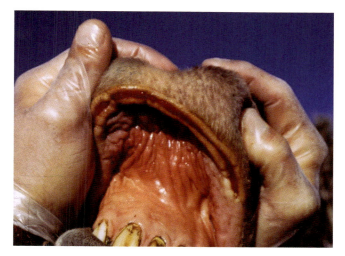

Figure 24-1 Ulceration of oral mucosa at mucocutaneous junction in horse caused by vesicular stomatitis virus (VSV) infection.

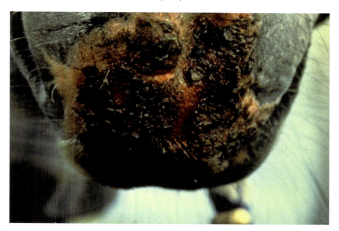

Figure 24-2 Crusting lesion of horse's muzzle caused by infection with vesicular stomatitis virus serotype New Jersey (VSV-NJ).

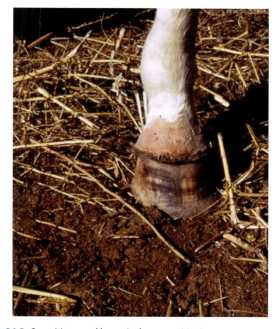

Figure 24-3 Coronitis caused by vesicular stomatitis virus serotype New Jersey (VSV-NJ) infection.

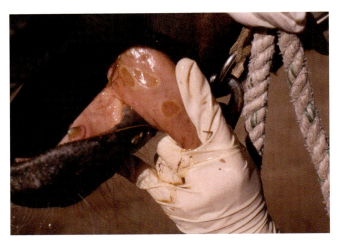

Figure 24-4 Lingual vesiculation and ulceration in horse caused by vesicular stomatitis virus (VSV) infection.

period is followed by ptyalism in cattle and horses.[48-50] Lesions of the oral mucosa present as raised, blanched, and rarely, fluid-filled vesicles. The dorsolingual surface is often affected, but the gingival surfaces, palate, and mucocutaneous junctions may also exhibit lesions.[49] Vesicles are very short lived and rupture, leaving ulcerations and erosions. Lesions often coalesce to form large, denuded areas of oral mucosa with epithelial tags. Vesicular and ulcerative lesions outside the oral mucosa occur on the snout of pigs; teats of cattle; and coronary bands of pigs, cattle, and horses. Teat lesions are not as common as oral lesions but may be associated with severe secondary cases of mastitis. Lesions of the feet typically manifest as coronitis, with edema and inflammation extending from the coronary band proximally up the lower leg. Foot lesions are much less common than oral lesions in outbreaks in the southwestern United States.

Crusting or scabbing lesions of the muzzle, ventral abdominal wall, prepuce, and udder may appear in affected horses. These lesions typically start as discrete, small (approximately 1-cm) erosions that quickly coalesce so that large, crusted, or scabbed areas are observed. These lesions are often located in areas of the body favored by hematophagous arthropods. Vesicular stomatitis viruses have been isolated from these crusting or scabbing lesions.

Subclinical infections are common in livestock during outbreaks of VS. One study reported disease prevalence of 44.7% in horses, with a seroprevalence of 61.0%. Only 4.5% of cattle on these premises had clinical signs, whereas 67.6% were seropositive to VSV-NJ.[51] In another study, disease prevalence ranged from 0% to 30%, with the seropositivity ranging from 14% to 100%.[52] Extensive herd testing conducted on an equine operation in 1995 confirmed the extensive nature of subclinical infections. In this study, 26% of horses examined were considered clinically affected with VS at 30 days. Of these horses tested, 67% were positive by the competitive enzyme-linked immunosorbent assay (cELISA), and 77% were positive by the virus neutralization test (VNT). An additional 12% of first test-negative horses were positive by the VNT at 60 days. The retested animals, combined with the original horses tested, provided an overall seroprevalence of 81% by the VNT, demonstrating substantial subclinical virus activity.

Stomatitis and other ulcerative, erosive, or vesicular diseases not caused by VS also occur in horses.[53] Trauma of the oral and nasal cavities and coronary bands from any cause is the primary differential diagnosis for VS in horses. Sunburn is also often confused with VS. Very few infectious agents, other than VSV and other vesiculoviruses, have been definitively associated with vesicle formation in horses. In some cases, infections with equine arteritis virus, Jamestown Canyon virus, caliciviruses, and equine herpesviruses may result in oral ulcers and erosions. Wood shavings of the *Simaroubaceae* family (containing the compounds quassin or neoquassin) used as bedding material can cause apparent "outbreaks" of ulcerative stomatitis in groups of horses, as can physical trauma induced by coarse forage or plant awns, including triticale hay.

Cantharidin is the toxin contained in blister beetles (*Epicauta* spp.), which may be present in baled alfalfa hay. Ingestion of the beetles can cause vesicular or ulcerative lesions, as well as severe systemic signs. Adverse reactions to the administration of pharmaceuticals or over-the-counter medications, including nonsteroidal antiinflammatory drugs (NSAIDs), may cause ulceration or erosion of the oral mucosa, generally in combination with systemic manifestations.

Pemphigus foliaceus, equine exfoliative eosinophilic dermatitis and stomatitis, squamous cell carcinoma, and melanoma can mimic the clinical picture of vesicular stomatitis. Recently, several apparent outbreaks of ulcerative stomatitis were reported in horses in the United States and New Zealand. Extensive investigations failed to determine any infectious or other cause for these outbreaks. The most significant differential diagnosis for VS in nonequine species is foot-and-mouth disease, which does not occur in horses.

Diagnosis

Three approaches to diagnosis of VSV infection are available: (1) antibody detection through a variety of serologic tests, (2) virus detection through isolation methods, and (3) detection of viral genetic material by molecular techniques.

Detection of antibodies to VSV is accomplished by VNT, complement fixation test (CFT), or ELISA. The VNT is considered the standard serologic test for VSV antibodies. The World Animal Health Organization (OIE) recognizes the VNT as a prescribed test for international trade.[54] Samples with detectable antibody at greater than a 1:40 dilution are considered positive for international trade purposes. The CFT is also recognized as a prescribed test for international trade purposes, and samples with titers greater than 1:5 dilution are considered positive.[54]

Numerous ELISAs have been developed for detection and quantitation of VS antibodies,[55-57] but most recently the cELISA has become the serologic test of choice for screening purposes during outbreaks of VS in the United States. The cELISA is considered a prescribed test for international trade by the OIE. A sample is considered positive if the absorbance is greater than or equal to 50% of the absorbance of the diluent control.

An ELISA capable of detecting the immunoglobulin M (IgM) class of antibody to VSV (MAC-ELISA) was developed after the 1982 outbreak of VS in the southwestern United States.[58] It facilitates detection of recent exposure to VSV. This assay is not a prescribed test for international trade as determined by the OIE.

A comparison of the most common diagnostic tests for VSV (VNT, CFT, cELISA, MAC-ELISA) by examination of experimentally inoculated animals indicates that the cELISA performs comparably to the VNT. The relative sensitivity and specificity of the cELISA compared with the VNT is 88% and 99%, respectively.[59] Positive MAC-ELISA and cELISA responses consistently appear 1 to 2 days before CFT seroconversion, but all animals revert to MAC-ELISA–negative status by 49 days after exposure. In a recent report, comparison of the VNT and cELISA on 1106 samples collected from cattle on sentinel farms in Costa Rica indicates very good agreement between the two tests.[60] The current serologic diagnostic testing scheme employed during outbreaks of VS in the United States is to screen samples with the cELISA and CFT and, if necessary, confirm by the VNT.

For virus isolation, vesicle fluid, epithelial tags, or swabs from fresh lesions are the ideal diagnostic sample. Vesicular stomatitis viruses are easily propagated in cell culture and induce cytopathic effects (CPEs) on an assortment of cell types, including Vero, BHK-1, and IB-RS-2 cells.[53] Fluorescent antibody (FA) staining using conjugates specific for VSV-NJ and VSV-IN may be employed for serotype differentiation.[61]

The detection of genomic sequences of VSV may be used to identify the presence of virus in tissue or swab samples. Many polymerase chain reaction (PCR) assays to detect various genomic sequences of VSV have been developed but are used primarily at this time for research purposes.[62-67]

The report of a potential foreign animal disease (FAD) by a practitioner initiates standardized investigation procedures by animal health officials (see Chapter 63). The private veterinary practitioner is of paramount importance in this diagnostic scheme, and practitioners trigger the process by calling an animal health official. One of three different officials may be contacted: the nearest FAD diagnostician (FADD), a specially trained animal health official, if the practitioner knows these officials; the state veterinarian's office; or the Animal and Plant Health Inspection Service, Veterinary Services (APHIS-VS), area veterinarian in charge (AVIC) office.

Early and frequent discussions between practitioners and animal health officials are encouraged. Animal health officials depend on practitioners to report suspicious findings, and in most states, practitioners are obligated to do so. Animal health officials expect practitioners to report suspect FAD as soon as possible. Delays in reporting may have catastrophic effects on disease control, so "erring on the side of caution" is a reasonable response and will be supported by animal health officials. A practitioner's first call to the local FADD or AVIC may be merely to discuss their observations before formally reporting suspicious lesions or signs. The AVIC ultimately determines if an FAD investigation will be initiated.

Reasonable approaches to quarantine are generally the rule during the initial phases of an investigation. The continued medical care of the affected animal remains the responsibility of the practitioner and owner, and the practitioner should employ biosecurity and biocontainment measures to prevent the spread of disease. All investigative procedures conducted by the FADD are done at no charge to the owner or practitioner. Blood, tissue, and other samples are collected by the FADD and submitted to laboratories specializing in the diagnosis of FADs, either the National Veterinary Services Laboratories (NVSL) in Ames, Iowa, or Plum Island, New York. State and university diagnostic laboratories are not routinely used for diagnostic testing. Samples collected by practitioners may be submitted by the FADD, but in most situations, new samples are collected. In rare instances, private practitioners submit biologic samples directly to the laboratories.

Results for all samples are sent by telephone or e-mail to the AVIC and the FADD. It is generally the responsibility of the FADD to provide results to the owner and referring veterinarian immediately after receiving results. If test results are negative for an FAD, quarantines and hold orders are released, and further diagnostic procedures and testing are the responsibility of the owner and veterinary practitioner.

Therapy

Vesicular stomatitis is typically short-lived and self-limiting. No specific treatment is indicated, and most horses recover in 7 to 14 days. Even in severe cases, supportive care is adequate. Strict biosecurity practices, including wearing disposable protective gloves and washing hands frequently, should be instituted to prevent the spread of disease among horses and to human handlers (see Chapter 62).

Frequent rinsing of lesions with mild antiseptic solutions or application of topical antibiotics may help prevent secondary bacterial infections. Softening of grain or pellets with water may ease mastication when oral lesions are present and help prevent weight loss. Dehydration of sufficient severity to require intravenous fluid support is rare.

Prevention

The concept of using a virulent live VSV as a vaccine was first proposed in the 1920s.[68] Cattle inoculated intramuscularly with VSV did not develop lesions and when challenged with virus locally were resistant.

A special license was obtained from the U.S. Department of Agriculture (USDA) in 1967 to produce and sell a live VSV-NJ lyophilized vaccine. Sale of this vaccine in the United States was discontinued in 1972.[69] The same vaccine was used in Guatemala for many years with reported success.

A commercially available, killed–VSV-NJ vaccine was used in Colorado during the 1985 outbreak, but serologic data regarding its immunogenicity and efficacy are not available.[70] Two doses of this formalin-killed cell culture–derived vaccine were administered intramuscularly 30 days apart to lactating and nonlactating adult cattle. Geometric mean titers peaked 21 days after the second vaccination at 1:530 and declined to a geometric mean titer of 1:65 by 175 days after vaccination. During the 1995 VSV outbreak, three commercial dairies approved to use a killed autogenous vaccine produced from a 1995 isolate of virus were enlisted in a field trial.[71] All vaccinated cattle generated serum neutralizing antibodies to VSV-NJ, but immunity waned quickly to low levels by 250 days after vaccination. There was no indication that wild-type virus infected livestock on these operations or on nearby operations, so vaccine efficacy could not be determined in either of these studies.

A DNA vaccine that expresses the glycoprotein gene of VSV-NJ elicits neutralizing antibody responses in mice, calves, and horses.[72] Manipulation of the VSV genome may ultimately lead to novel attenuated live-VSV vaccines that are safe and efficacious. One such strategy currently under investigation is the translocation of the N gene, which reduces mortality in mice without reduction in the ability to generate a protective immune response.[73]

Public Health Considerations

Three laboratory workers infected with VSV through exposure to experimentally infected animals[74] complained of fever, general malaise, and muscle pain. Two of the individuals handled experimentally infected cattle, and the third was splashed with virus-containing material while harvesting infected allantoic fluids. Mild stomatitis was observed in two of the three individuals. Recovery was complete and rapid without specific therapy. Although no virus was isolated from any of these individuals, high neutralizing antibody titers to VSV-NJ were detected.

In the 1950s, laboratory workers at the Agricultural Research Laboratory in Beltsville, Maryland, were routinely tested for VSV complement-fixing antibodies.[75] A summary of this work indicated that VS in humans appears as an acute, self-limiting infection with signs similar to influenza. Overall, 96% of laboratory workers and animal handlers had positive titers to VSV, although only 57% of those with positive titers could recall having clinical signs.

An investigation of owners and handlers of infected cattle was conducted during an outbreak of VS in 1965.[76] Forty-one persons were interviewed, and specimens were collected for virus isolation and serologic testing. Eight persons who lived or worked on ranches where cattle were confirmed to have been infected with VSV-IN had serologic evidence of exposure to VSV. Fever, general malaise, myalgia, nausea, and pharyngitis were observed. Vesicular lesions of the gums occurred in two people.

A study of veterinarians, research workers, and regulatory personnel exposed to VSV during an outbreak in Colorado in 1982 revealed that the prevalence of neutralizing antibody was higher in exposed persons with clinical signs than in those without a history of clinical illness.[77] Higher risk of seropositivity was observed for individuals who examined the oral cavity of infected animals, who had open wounds on hands or arms, and who examined horses rather than cattle. Overall, infection rates among exposed humans were low.

The complete reference list is available online at www.expertconsult.com.

Papillomavirus Infections

25

Kelly P. Sears and Debra C. Sellon

Equine papillomavirus types 1, 2, and 3 have been isolated from acquired papillomas (warts), genital papillomas, and aural plaques in horses. A large number of studies have implicated bovine papillomavirus types 1 and 2 in the pathogenesis of equine sarcoid, a form of nonmetastatic cutaneous fibrosarcoma, but a causal link has not been confirmed by fulfilling Koch's postulates. Each of these disorders is discussed separately in this chapter.

Equine Warts

Etiology

Papillomaviruses are small, nonenveloped viruses with icosahedral symmetry, 72 capsomers, and a double-stranded, circular DNA genome. They are classified on the basis of their species of origin and the degree of homology with other papillomaviruses isolated from the same species.[1] Most papillomaviruses infect epithelial cells, causing proliferative lesions described as true papillomas; however, some types infect both the epithelium and underlying fibroblasts with resultant fibropapillomas.[2] Lesions induced by papillomaviruses are usually benign and self-limiting. Some papillomaviruses are oncogenic; in particular, human papillomavirus (HPV) types 16 and 18 are associated with cervical carcinoma.[3] All the open reading frames (potential coding regions) of the viral genome are located on a single strand of viral DNA. The early region of the genome encodes proteins necessary for cell transformation (E5, E6, and E7) and replication and transcription regulatory proteins E1 and E2. The late region codes for structural capsid proteins (L1 and L2). The early and late gene regions are separated by a regulatory region containing the origin of replication and many of the control elements for viral transcription and replication.[1]

Cutaneous papillomas (warts) of the horse are proliferative skin lesions caused by infection with *Equus caballus* papillomavirus type 1 (EcPV-1). Lesions are most often observed on the muzzle and lips of young horses (Fig. 25-1) but may also appear on ears, eyelids, genitalia, or distal limbs.[4] *Equus caballus* papillomavirus type 1 has been isolated, characterized, and cloned

from equine warts.[5] Two additional equine papillomaviruses have been identified.[6] *Equus caballus* papillomavirus type 2, a mucosotropic equine papillomavirus, has been isolated from papillomas and squamous cell carcinomas (SCC) affecting the genital area of horses.[7,8] *Equus caballus* papillomavirus type 2 was also recently isolated from an atypical, nongenital SCC with bovine papillomavirus type 1 (BPV-1) also being isolated from these lesions.[9] A third equine papillomavirus was recently isolated from an ear papilloma and is suspected to be the cause of aural plaques.[6] The three viruses vary in their open reading frames (ORFs) for the early genes E6 and E7.

Congenital equine papillomatosis is much less common than acquired disease.[10-16] Congenital lesions do not spontaneously regress, but surgery is usually curative.[16] Although in utero infection by a latent papillomavirus has been suggested as an etiology of these lesions, there has been no genetic or antigenic evidence to support this.[13,17]

Epidemiology

Most horses with cutaneous papillomatosis (warts) are less than 3 years of age. There are no breed or gender predilections. Disease can be spread by fomites or by close contact with affected horses. Spread is common when young horses are brought together in large groups for show, sale, or breeding.[4]

Pathogenesis

In 1951, Cook and Olson[18] demonstrated that intradermal or subcutaneous injection of filtrates of equine papillomas results in growth of typical papilloma lesions within 60 to 70 days. Inoculation by skin scarification produces similar results. Lesions regressed spontaneously within 50 to 100 days. Similar injections into calves, lambs, dogs, rabbits, and guinea pigs did not result in lesions.[18] Natural infections are thought to require contact of virus with damaged skin (environmental trauma, ectoparasites, ultraviolet light damage).[16] The incubation period is estimated at approximately 60 days and may be influenced by the dose of virus, route of exposure, and immunity of the host.[16,19]

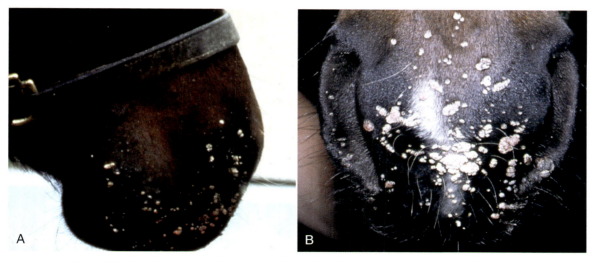

Figure 25-1 Typical appearance of warts on muzzle and lips of young horse. *(Courtesy Dr. Melissa Hines.)*

Histopathologic studies of naturally occurring equine warts suggest that lesions are initiated by basal cell hyperplasia without viral antigen production. As lesions develop, there is prominent acanthosis with cellular swelling and fusion, as well as marked hyperkeratosis and parakeratosis.[20] Hypomelanosis of lesions may be related to a disturbance in melanin synthesis.[21] Regression of papillomas is associated with an increase in the number of hyperfunctional Langerhans' cells at the dermoepidermal junction and infiltration of T lymphocytes.[22] Natural immunity is strong, and, in most horses, warts disappear spontaneously 1 to 6 months after they initially appear.[16] Investigators in one report documented persistent penile papillomas in a gelding and the lesions remained static for 24 months.[8]

Clinical Findings

Horses with equine cutaneous papillomatosis usually have multiple lesions, most frequently on the muzzle and lips but occasionally occurring on the distal limbs, genitalia, ears (Fig. 25-2), and eyelids.[4,16] Equine warts vary in size from 0.1 to 2 cm in diameter. When they first appear, warts are often slightly raised, flat, smooth, and flesh colored. As they proliferate in number and size, they become verrucous, gray, and hyperkeratotic with development of fronds, resulting in a cauliflower-like appearance.[4] Single or multiple lesions may be oval or irregular in outline, dry, gray or red in color, and with rough, wrinkled, or smooth surfaces. Depigmentation may occur as warts slough. Genital lesions are suspected to have the potential to progress to SCC[8,23]; genital papillomas should be considered potential premalignant lesions.[24]

Diagnosis

A diagnosis of equine warts is usually obvious based on history, clinical signs, and age of the affected horse. Additional diagnostic testing is rarely performed. If needed, cutaneous biopsy would provide a definitive diagnosis. Verrucous sarcoids resemble warts in their gross appearance and predilection for the face. Proliferative lesions in older horses should be considered sarcoids until proved otherwise.

Pathologic Findings

Biopsy of papilloma lesions may reveal histologic changes characteristic of one of the three phases, including growth,

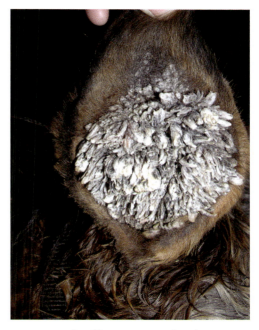

Figure 25-2 Severe, frondlike warts in ear of yearling Quarter Horse.

development, and regression. In the initial growth phase, basal cell hyperplasia with few viral inclusions, prominent acanthosis, and moderate orthokeratotic and parakeratotic hyperkeratosis are seen.[24] Papillated epidermal hyperplasia, koilocytosis, hypomelanosis, and increased quantity of irregular keratohyalin granules are typically seen in the development phase. Intranuclear inclusion bodies are also seen in some lesions. In the final phase, regression of papillomas is associated with an increase in the number of hyperfunctional Langerhans' cells at the dermoepidermal junction and infiltration of lymphocytes, as well as increased proliferation of fibroblasts.[4,16,20,25]

Therapy

A variety of therapies have been proposed for equine warts. However, most lesions resolve spontaneously within a few months of appearance, making it difficult to ascertain the true efficacy of any therapeutic intervention. If lesions persist beyond

6 to 9 months, an underlying immune deficiency should be suspected.

Most horses with warts do not require treatment. If removal is necessary for immediate esthetic enhancement, cryosurgery with a two-cycle, freeze-thaw-freeze technique is a valid treatment. Chemical cautery with trifluoroacetic acid is also considered safe and effective. A solution of 25 g anhydrous trifluoroacetic acid, 3 g water, and 20 g glacial acetic acid is applied to affected tissues only. Adjacent tissues should be protected with petroleum jelly. Applications are repeated on the fourth and seventh days after initial treatment.[4] Topical treatment with podophyllin (50% podophyllin, 20% podophyllin in 95% ethyl alcohol, 2% podophyllin in 25% salicylic acid) and undiluted medical grade dimethylsulfoxide (DMSO) may be used once daily until remission occurs. There is no scientific evidence to support the theory that surgical excision of some lesions enhances or hastens regression of remaining lesions. Recurrence after surgical excision has been reported.[4,16] A variety of immunomodulatory drugs, including mycobacterial cell wall extracts and *Propionibacterium* extracts, have also been recommended for treatment of equine warts, but there are no efficacy studies published to date. Autogenous vaccines for treatment of equine warts are controversial, and to the authors' knowledge, there are no scientific reports documenting their efficacy. Bovine wart vaccines are not effective in horses.

Prevention

Affected horses should be isolated from uninfected animals. Skin trauma from the environment or ectoparasites should be minimized. Disinfection of premises and equipment with formaldehyde or lye has been recommended after exposure to a horse with warts but is not practicle or environmentally safe.[4,16]

Public Health Considerations

There are no reports of human disease secondary to equine papillomavirus infection.

Aural Plaques

Etiology and Pathogenesis

Aural plaques (papillary acanthoma, hyperplastic dermatitis of the ear) are raised, depigmented lesions on the inner surface of the pinnae of the ear.[16,26-28] Papillomavirus has been demonstrated in these lesions by electron microscopy (EM) and immunohistochemistry (IHC).[29] The pathogenesis of aural plaques in horses is unclear. Lesions often appear worse in the summer and fall, possibly because of fly irritation.

Clinical Findings

There are no age, breed, or gender predilections for occurrence of aural plaques in horses.[11] Lesions are often bilateral and progress from small, smooth, depigmented papules and plaques to larger, often coalescent, hyperkeratotic plaques (Fig. 25-3). Aural plaques do not spontaneously regress, and they may be more active in the summer, possibly in association with black fly bites. Plaques are not sensitive, pruritic, or painful but may be considered esthetically displeasing by owners. Similar lesions may occur around the anus and vulva.[16,30]

Diagnosis

The diagnosis of aural plaques is usually made on the basis of clinical signs. Biopsy is usually not indicated, but if performed,

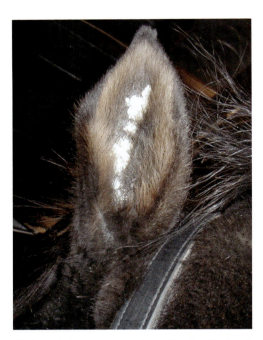

Figure 25-3 Aural plaques in ear of horse. *(Courtesy Dr. Erin Groover.)*

lesions appear histologically identical to verruca plana, a wartlike disease of humans, with epithelial proliferation and epidermal hypomelanosis.[30]

Treatment and Prevention

Aural plaques are not considered to spontaneously regress. Torres et al[31] performed a pilot study validating the efficacy of topical imiquimod, a synthetic imidazoquinoline amine immunomodulator. Lesions were treated with a 5% imiquimod cream (Aldara, 3M Pharmaceuticals, St Paul, MN). The plaques were treated 2 or 3 times per week, every other week, until resolution (1.5 to 8 months), however, there were no untreated controls in this study to compare regression time or to verify lack of spontaneous regression. The most common side effect was local inflammation at the site of application. Lesions did recur in 2 of the 16 cases during the follow-up period. Use of fly repellents is recommended to minimize secondary irritation or infection of lesions.[30]

Sarcoids

Sarcoids are locally aggressive but nonmetastatic, fibroblastic skin tumors of equids. They are the most common neoplasm of horses, donkeys, and mules. They may occur on any part of the body but have a predilection for the head, ventral abdomen, and legs. These tumors are seldom life threatening but may cause esthetic and performance-limiting problems, depending on their location, size, and rate of growth. A variety of therapies have been proposed, with minimal to moderate success. Recurrence of tumor after treatment is a significant problem regardless of the type of treatment attempted.

Etiology

A viral etiology for equine sarcoids was postulated as early as 1936 by Jackson.[32] In 1948, Olson demonstrated that intradermal inoculation of horses with cell-free extracts from bovine skin tumors containing BPV caused lesions resembling equine sarcoids.[33,34] Ragland et al[35] described an epizootic of equine sarcoid in 1966 and confirmed the ability to induce sarcoidlike lesions in horses by inoculation with BPV in 1969.[36,37] Lesions regressed spontaneously, and inoculated horses developed a humoral immune response to BPV. Subsequent studies by a variety of investigators have demonstrated the presence of deoxyribonucleic acid (DNA) and ribonucleic acid (RNA) from BPV-1 and -2, or closely related viruses, and expression of the BPV-1 and -2 major transforming protein, E5, in equine sarcoids.[38-54] Bovine papillomavirus DNA can be detected from normal skin of horses and peripheral blood mononuclear cells of horses affected with equine sarcoid and, to a lesser extent, in the skin of unaffected horses, suggesting the possibility of viral latency.[41,43,49,55,56]

Bovine papillomaviruses are the causative agents of bovine warts with at least 10 distinct bovine viruses associated with either fibropapillomas or papillomas.[2] Two of the bovine fibro-papilloma viruses (BPV-1 and -2) are recognized as the likely causative agents of equine sarcoids.[57-59] Sequence analysis of BPV DNA from equine sarcoids suggests the possibility of equine sarcoid-specific variants of BPV.[52,53]

Despite the lack of evidence of a productive infection or detectable antibodies to BPV, viral DNA exists episomally in equine cells. This genetic material, however, does not integrate in the host cell genome.[47,60] An increasing volume of evidence suggests that BPV-1 proteins play a crucial role in the transformation of fibroblasts into the highly invasive cells characteristic of sarcoids.[57,61] Yuan et al showed that expression of the BPV-1 genome enhances cell proliferation, induces invasiveness, and contributes to anchorage-independent growth to equine fibroblasts.[57,61,62] This evidence supports the conclusion that BPV is the causative agent of equine sarcoids.[57]

Like all papillomaviruses, BPV is very resistant to physical and chemical inactivation.[32] It remains viable after 30 minutes at 67°C (152.5°F), is stable at a pH between 4 and 8, is stable in ether, and survives in 50% glycerol when frozen or lyophilized.[63] These properties suggest that BPV may be able to survive for a long time in the environment, providing a source for exposure long after cattle are removed[41]; however, extensive environmental surveys have not been performed. One study was unable to identify BPV DNA in the environment of affected and healthy horses, except for the environment of one horse living in contact with a cow with warts.[41]

Suggestions that other viruses may be causally related to equine sarcoid are unsubstantiated. A retrovirus identified in a cell line originating from an equine sarcoid was determined to be an endogenous virus that was unrelated to the sarcoid.[64,65] Equine cutaneous papillomaviruses, the etiologic agent of equine warts, are not causally related to equine sarcoids.[5]

Epidemiology

Equine sarcoids are the most common dermatologic neoplasm in horses, donkeys, and mules worldwide, accounting for an estimated 20% of all equine tumors[66] and as many as 90% of all skin tumors.[67] The incidence of sarcoid tumors in the general population of horses is not known. Sarcoids accounted for 0.7% of all equine cases presented to the Cornell University Veterinary Hospital between 1975 and 1987 and to the Ohio State University between 1976 and 1985.[68]

Sarcoid tumors most frequently develop in horses less than 8 years of age, but lesions may occasionally be observed in yearlings.[25,68] Equine sarcoids appear less likely to develop in horses after 7 years of age.[69-72] Young male equids are at increased risk of disease.[53,71,73,74]

In cool northern climates, sarcoids are most often observed on the head and abdomen of horses; in warmer climates the limbs are more frequently affected.[68] It remains uncertain whether contact with cattle is a risk factor for equine sarcoids.[32,74] No evidence indicates that castration increases the risk of paragenital sarcoids in donkeys.[73] However, a donkey living in close contact with affected donkeys is more likely to develop sarcoid tumors than the average donkey.[75]

Evidence for genetic predisposition for development of sarcoid tumors includes varying disease prevalence in specific breeds[74,76,77] and increased incidence of lesions in some equine families.[35,78,79] Additionally, the presence of specific equine leukocyte antigen (ELA) alleles (A1, A3, A5, B1, W3, and W13) are associated with increased risk of sarcoid development in multiple breeds.[3,25,77,80-84] Sarcoids may occur in any breed of horse, but they are seen more frequently in Quarter Horses and less frequently in Standardbred horses than in the general equine population.[74,76,77] Several studies have shown that the frequency of the ELA W13 allele in horses with sarcoids is high regardless of breed. However, the majority of horses with the W13 allele never develop a sarcoid tumor, suggesting that environmental factors (most likely BPV) and other genetic factors are also important for disease development.

Pathogenesis

The manner by which BPV induces equine sarcoid lesions is uncertain. Hypotheses include transmission of virus by direct or indirect contact with infected horses and cattle and transmission by insects.[3,75,85] Finlay confirmed that multiple species of flies harbor BPV-1 DNA that is commonly found in equine sarcoids further supporting the possibility of an insect vector.[86] Genetic sequences specific for BPV have been identified from skin of normal horses with no sarcoid lesions and from normal skin of horses with sarcoid tumors, suggesting the possibility of viral latency.[41,43,49,56] Nucleic acid from BPV cannot be demonstrated in lymphocytes, liver, spleen, or lymph nodes of affected horses.[54,87,88]

Regardless of the manner of initial contact with BPV, it is clear that BPV alone is insufficient to induce sarcoid lesions in horses. The immunologic status of the horse, genetic background, and skin trauma may play a role in initiation of disease.[41]

Sarcoid lesions may arise spontaneously or may occur at the site of a prior wound. Rubbing or biting at truncal or limb lesions may precede appearance of lesions on lips and eyelids. Indirect transmission by tack is also possible. Metastasis to internal organs has not been reported. Recurrence after surgical resection, cryotherapy, immunotherapy, or chemotherapy is common.

Clinical Findings

Although sarcoid tumors may occur on any part of the body, either singly or in clusters, the most common sites are the head, ventral abdomen, groin, axillae, and limbs.[67,69,89] Approximately 14% to 84% of affected horses have multiple lesions.[16,80,90,91] Lesions are usually firm on palpation because of fibroblastic proliferation. The overlying epidermis may be thick, rough, and hyperkeratotic or ulcerated. Sarcoid tumors may occur in the subcutaneous tissues as firm, movable masses with an intact covering of grossly normal skin.[69,92]

The gross appearance of sarcoids may vary, but lesions are generally classified as one of six types consisting of verrucous, nodular, fibroblastic, malevolent, mixed, or occult.[25,81,90,93,94] Lesions may be pedunculated or sessile.

Nodular, subcutaneous sarcoids are most likely to occur in the groin, sheath, or eyelid region (Fig. 25-4). These lesions may progress to typical ulcerated fibroblastic sarcoids with time or traumatic insult.

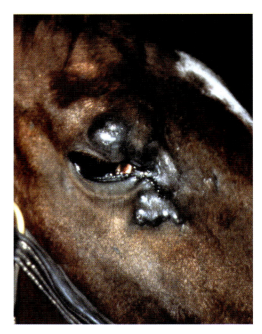

Figure 25-4 Nodular, subcutaneous sarcoid of eyelid of horse. *(Courtesy Dr. Melissa Hines.)*

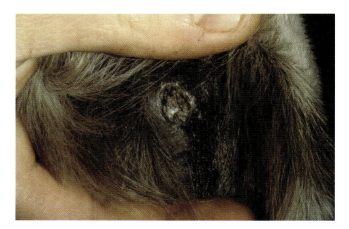

Figure 25-5 Verrucous sarcoid on ear of horse. *(Courtesy Dr. Wendy Duckett.)*

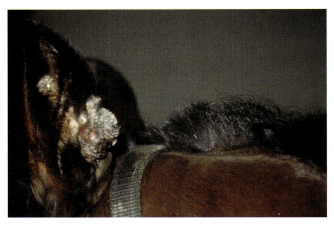

Figure 25-6 Fibroblastic sarcoid on ear of horse.

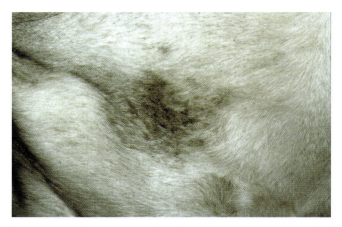

Figure 25-7 Occult sarcoid on shoulder of horse. *(Courtesy Dr. Wendy Duckett.)*

Verrucous sarcoids resemble equine warts, with a dry, horny, cauliflower-like surface that is partially or totally hairless[95] (Fig. 25-5). These sarcoids are usually small to medium in size, measuring less than 6 cm in diameter. They can remain static in size and shape for years but may undergo transformation and become fibroblastic if traumatized.[95] Verrucous sarcoids appear more frequently around the face, neck, axilla, groin, sheath areas, and coronary band.[69]

Fibroblastic sarcoids are raised and ulcerated, resembling "proud flesh" and may become quite large (>20 cm diameter; Fig. 25-6). Differential diagnoses include granulation tissue, squamous cell carcinoma, cutaneous habronemiasis, and pythiosis.

Malevolent sarcoids exhibit behavior typical of malignant neoplasms being both aggressive and invasive. Multiple ulcerated lesions may be seen, and lymphatic involvement is common. These nodules are often found on the face, jaw, axilla, elbow, and medial thigh. Mixed sarcoids have characteristics of both verrucous and fibroblastic types.[25]

Occult sarcoids are slow-growing tumors that are flat with slightly thickened skin and a mildly roughened surface[95] (Fig. 25-7). This presentation is partially or totally devoid of hair and seems to favor areas of the body with sparse hair growth, including the skin around the mouth, eyes, neck, and medial aspects of the forearm and thigh. These lesions may progress to verrucous sarcoids.[25] Trauma to occult sarcoids, surgical or otherwise, can stimulate fibroblastic proliferation of the tumor and should be avoided if possible. Differential diagnoses for occult sarcoids include dermatophytosis, dermatophilosis, demodicosis, staphylococcal folliculitis, onchocerciasis, and alopecia areata.[65,67]

Diagnosis

Diagnosis of sarcoid tumors in horses is usually suspected on the basis of characteristic clinical signs. Because lesions may grossly resemble papillomas, granulation tissue, fungal or bacterial granuloma, habronemiasis, solar keratosis, squamous cell carcinoma, neurofibroma, melanoma, and fibrosarcoma, histologic examination of biopsy specimens is required for a definitive diagnosis. Biopsy of static verrucous and occult sarcoids is usually not indicated because intervention may prompt transformation into an aggressive, fibroblastic type of lesion.[96] Partial removal of a sarcoid tumor may stimulate aggressive regrowth of tissue. If possible, wide excision of the entire mass should be performed at biopsy to decrease the likelihood of recurrence.

Because autotransplantation of an equine sarcoid tumor may occur, surgical instruments that contact the tumor should not be used on healthy adjacent skin.[95]

Samples should be submitted to an appropriate diagnostic laboratory in 10% neutral buffered formalin. Small tumors may be submitted intact; representative samples should be cut from the excised tumor and submitted if lesions are large; however, it is always best to try to submit samples that confirm clear margins of removal. Biopsy samples should be examined by an experienced veterinary pathologist to facilitate an accurate diagnosis. The most common incorrect diagnoses are fibroma, fibrosarcoma, neurofibroma, and granulation tissue—the subsequent treatment of which may lead to inappropriate therapy.[67]

Pathologic Findings

Histologically, equine sarcoids are characterized by fibroblastic and epidermal proliferation with associated epidermal hyperplasia and dermoepidermal activity.[16,35,78] The dermis contains collagen fibers and fibroblasts in a classic whorled, tangled, or herringbone pattern, and mitotic figures may be numerous (Fig. 25-8). Tumor cells are spindle or fusiform to stellate shaped. Fibroblasts at the dermoepidermal junction frequently orient perpendicularly to the basement membrane in a picket-fence pattern.[16] If present, the overlying epidermis is hyperplastic and hyperkeratotic. Occult sarcoids may exhibit only focal epidermal hyperplasia and hyperkeratosis, with underlying junctional fibroblastic proliferation.[16] The junction between tumor and normal tissue is not always clear, making it difficult to assess surgical margins histopathologically.[95]

Therapy

A wide variety of therapeutic strategies have been proposed for treatment of equine sarcoid tumors. The specific treatment selected should be determined after consideration of the tumor site, size, type, and aggressiveness; clinical experience of the attending veterinarian; and the availability of services, equipment, and facilities.[69,97] Static verrucous and occult sarcoids are usually not treated because intervention may prompt transformation to an aggressive, fibroblastic type of sarcoid.

Determining the comparative efficacy of treatment for equine sarcoid tumors is difficult because of the large variation in tumor size, location, and treatment methods. Almost all reports of treatment efficacy originate from large veterinary referral hospitals, where horses treated for sarcoid tumors are likely to have large, multiple, recurrent, and highly aggressive

tumors. Success rates for therapy in this population may be expected to be less than success rates in private practice, where horses tend to have solitary, less aggressive lesions.

Surgical Resection

Surgical resection, even with wide margins of normal tissue, is not generally recommended as a sole therapy for equine sarcoids because of a recurrence rate estimated at 50% to 64%, usually within 6 months.[98] Testing of the surgical margins for BPV DNA may aid in determining the likelihood of recurrence and necessity of other therapeutics.[81] However, surgical resection (including normal tissue margins of 0.5-1.0 cm) is often used to debulk tumors and improve the effectiveness of adjunctive therapies (e.g., cryotherapy, laser surgical excision, hyperthermia, irradiation, photodynamic therapy, immunotherapy, chemotherapy). Split-thickness skin grafts may facilitate epithelial covering of the wound with faster healing, less granulation tissue, and a better cosmetic result.[69,97,98]

Cryotherapy

Cryotherapy with liquid nitrogen is a common adjunctive therapy for equine sarcoids after surgical debulking of lesions. One-year cure rates for cryotherapy are estimated at 70% to 100%.[67,99-107] Horses are sedated or anesthetized to facilitate restraint during the procedure. Lesions are frozen two or three times to $-20^{\circ}C$ to $-30^{\circ}C$, with complete thawing to room temperature between each freeze. Monitoring tissue temperature with cryoprobes diminishes the likelihood of inadvertent freezing of sensitive normal tissues in the area and ensures complete freezing of the tumor. Thermocouple needles are placed in the subcutaneous tissues beneath the tumor and along the periphery of the lesion. Treated tissues undergo necrosis, with local swelling and inflammation. Healing occurs by secondary intention or delayed closure, which may result in scarring or regrowth of white hair from damage to hair follicles.[98] The average time to complete healing is 2.4 months (range: 1.0-3.5 months).[108]

Adverse consequences of cryotherapy are usually related to damage to adjacent normal tissues and facial nerve paralysis; septic arthritis, loss of the upper eyelid, and evisceration of the globe have been described.[102,106] There are limited reports of spontaneous regression of multiple sarcoids after cryotherapy of one or two lesions, suggesting that cryotherapy may enhance the immune response of the horse.[106] Because spontaneous regression occurs, however, no scientific data support intervention solely to induce remission.

Carbon Dioxide Laser Therapy

Carbon dioxide (CO_2) laser therapy has been advocated for treatment of equine sarcoid tumors, with a success rate (no recurrence at the same site for 6 or 12 months) of 62% to 81%.[109,110] Animals presenting with multiple sarcoids were more likely to experience tumor recurrence, which was significantly lower in donkeys than in horses.[110] Approximately 58% of equids in one study developed new sarcoid lesions elsewhere on the body after laser therapy.[110] Swelling is minimal after laser resection, and the horse exhibits minimal pain to palpation of the surgical wound. If sufficient normal skin is available, primary closure of the surgical site can be performed.[67] Treatment with CO_2 laser requires specialized equipment and training, limiting its use to veterinary specialty hospitals.

Hyperthermia

Radio-frequency current–induced hyperthermia resulted in sarcoid tumor regression, with no recurrence at 7 to 12 months in three horses.[111] There have been no additional reports of its use since 1983, however, making it difficult to assess the efficacy of this modality for sarcoid therapy.

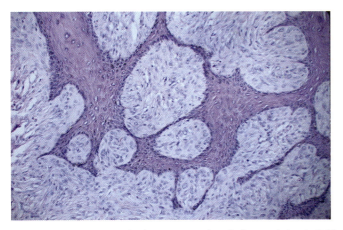

Figure 25-8 Photomicrograph of equine sarcoid, with characteristic spindloid cells and elongate rete pegs of adjacent epidermis.

Irradiation

Brachytherapy of sarcoid tumors provides continuous delivery of a high radiation dose directly to the tumor while sparing adjacent healthy tissue. Isotopes used for interstitial brachytherapy of equine sarcoids include permanently implantable seeds of radon-222 or gold-198; removable needles of radium-226, cobalt-60, or iridium-192; and iridium-192 seeds. Response rates range from 50% to 100%.[67] Brachytherapy has been particularly useful for treatment of small periorbital sarcoids, with success rates of up to 100%.[67,112-114] In a study of 155 horses treated with iridium-192 interstitial brachytherapy for periocular tumors, adverse effects included palpebral fibrosis (10.4%), cataract (7.8%), keratitis and corneal ulceration (6.9%), permanent hair loss (21.7%), and hair dyspigmentation (78.3%).[114]

The use of brachytherapy is severely limited by the need to maintain a horse in a radiation safety–approved area and the need to comply with all state and federal radiation safety laws. Hyperthermia may be combined with brachytherapy for synergistic tumor killing.[115]

Photodynamic Therapy

Photodynamic therapy involves the administration of a photosensitizer to a patient. The drug accumulates in tumor tissue and is activated by visible light to a higher energy state from which free radicals and reactive oxygen are formed. Intratumoral injections of the photodynamic agent hypericin into three sarcoid tumors on a donkey resulted in an 81% reduction in tumor volume at the end of therapy (25 days) and a 90% reduction after 2 months.[116] Further evaluation of this type of therapy is needed before it can be recommended for general use.

Immunotherapy

Immunotherapy with an attenuated strain of *Mycobacterium bovis* (bacille Calmette-Guérin [BCG]), mycobacterial cell wall preparations in oil, and mycobacterial cell wall skeleton–trehalose dimycolate combinations have been widely used for treatment of equine sarcoids, especially periocular lesions.[16,67,117,118] Treatments are administered by intralesional injection every 2 to 3 weeks for an average of four treatments.[16] Debulking before initiating intralesional therapy is recommended. Inflammatory reactions with ulceration and necrosis are common within minutes to days of injection. Some patients experience fever, increased white blood cell count, and general malaise.[119] Occasional reports of anaphylactic reactions after repeated use of BCG have led to recommendations that horses be medicated with flunixin meglumine and corticosteroids before BCG injection.[16,120] Intralesional BCG injections have also been associated with lymphangitis[119] and septic arthritis.[121] Reported response rates for treatment of periorbital sarcoids with BCG range from 69% to 100%, with best results for treatment of fibroblastic and nodular lesions.[108,118,121] Remission rate with BCG therapy of sarcoid lesions elsewhere on the body is approximately 48%, with the poorest response reported for lesions on the legs and in the axillary region.[108] Complete resolution of lesions may require 6 weeks to 1 year or more.[108,119,120,122]

Controlled studies of immunotherapy for equine sarcoids using agents other than BCG are lacking. Systemic immunomodulator therapy with nonviable *Propionibacterium acnes* (EqStim, Neogen Corp, Lansing, MI) has been advocated for treatment of equine sarcoid.[69] Protocols include intralesional or intravenous injections once weekly for 6 to 8 weeks, with eventual necrosis and sloughing of the lesion.

Autogenous vaccines have been proposed as immunotherapeutic agents for equine sarcoid tumors.[72,123-125] In 1999, Kinnunen et al[123] reported the use of an autogenous vaccine in 21 horses. All horses had surgical debulking of tumor, and resected tissue was used to prepare vaccine. Only 1 of 12 horses with a primary tumor had a recurrence of tumor after therapy.

In contrast, four of nine horses with recurrent tumors before this study had recurrences after treatment with autogenous vaccine. However, disease-free intervals for both groups of horses were significantly longer than for horses treated with conventional surgery alone.[123] A recent vaccination trial with a papillomavirus-like particle (VLP) vaccine showed promising results for the development of protective immunity.[126] Sarcoid regression has been reported in several horses with refractory sarcoid after transplantation of tissue from one horse into another horse.[69] However, the transfer of tumor tissue and tumor extracts carries a risk of tumor production rather than tumor regression, as well as risk of transmission of other infectious diseases. Because other types of therapy work well for many horses without these risks, this type of therapy is not recommended.[69]

Chemotherapy

A variety of topical and intralesional chemotherapy protocols have been described for treatment of horses with sarcoids. These therapies are usually applied after surgical debulking of a lesion but may be efficacious as a sole therapy for small tumors. Administration of chemotherapeutic agents should be undertaken with caution to avoid human contact with potentially toxic agents. Gloves and appropriate protective eyewear should be worn for topical application and intralesional injection of most agents.

Daily topical application of 5-fluorouracil, a fluorinated pyrimidine antimetabolite that interferes with DNA biosynthesis, or podophyllin, an irritant cathartic, has been used successfully to treat some sarcoid lesions.[69,92,98] Treatment may be continued for up to 90 days. Topical 5-fluorouracil cream applied daily to occult and verrucose periorbital lesions (not directly on margin of eyelid) was successful in eliminating lesions in six of nine horses.[118] The other three horses improved, but lesions recurred in a fibroblastic form over the next 3 to 36 months.

Multiple other topical agents have been used with reported anecdotal success. A bloodroot extract containing *Sanguinaria canadensis*, puccoon, gromwell, distilled water, and trace minerals (Animex, NIES, Las Vegas, NV) has been used to treat a variety of skin lesions, including equine sarcoids.[69] It preferentially kills tumor cells, and the lesion sloughs in 7 to 10 days. Another bloodroot plant extract product (XXTERRA, Larson Laboratories, Fort Collins, CO) is marketed for treatment of equine sarcoids, with claims of changing the antigenicity of the sarcoid cells so that the immune system recognizes them as foreign with resultant tissue rejection.[69,92,98] Product literature instructs that the paste be applied topically to the lesion and covered with a bandage for 4 to 5 days. Application of the product with bandaging should be repeated until the lesion sloughs. In a small pilot study, imiquimod (Aldara, 3M Pharmaceuticals) was applied topically 3 times per week for up to 8 months. Eighty percent of the treated lesions showed at least 75% reduction in size with complete resolution in 60%. No recurrence was seen during the follow-up period (4-60 months).[127]

An experimental topical ointment containing a variety of heavy metals and the antimitotic compounds 5-fluorouracil and thiouracil (AW-3-LUDES) was described by Knottenbelt and Kelly[118] but is not widely available. The ointment is applied daily or every other day for three to five treatments. A response is anticipated in 5 to 10 weeks, with necrosis and sloughing of sarcoid tissue. Caution must be exercised if this compound or other chemotherapeutic agents are used for treatment of periorbital sarcoid. Inadvertent contact between these agents and sensitive ocular tissues can result in serious adverse effects.

A recent study also assessed the efficacy of topical acyclovir in treating sarcoids. Acyclovir is an antiviral typically used to treat herpesvirus lesions, utilizing viral and cellular thymidine kinases (TKs) to activate it.[128,129] Papillomaviruses, however, lack TKs and are unable to convert aciclovir to its active form.[129,130] Despite BPV itself being unable to activate the drug, topical application of a 5% cream has shown some success. Forty-seven sarcoids were treated on 22 horses with daily topical application of the 5% cream for 2 months. Complete regression was observed in 68% of the lesions with no recurrence during the follow-up period (6-18 months) or documented adverse effects.[129]

Intralesional injections or implants of chemotherapeutic agents result in a high local drug concentration for extended periods. Implants may consist of a high-molecular-weight collagen matrix that contains a chemotherapeutic agent (cisplatin or 5-fluorouracil) and a vasoactive modifier such as epinephrine.[69,98] Alternatively, sterilized sesame oil may be used to slow drug release and increase tumor/plasma drug concentration ratio. Intratumoral treatment of 19 horses with cisplatin (Platinol, Bristol Myers Squibb, Princeton, NJ) resulted in a 1-year disease-free period for 87% of horses.[131] Theon et al[132] also reported a 92% and 77% relapse-free survival rate at 1 and 4 years, respectively, after surgical debulking combined with perisurgical wound injection of cisplatin and sesame oil injections. Intratumoral injection of 5-fluorouracil has also been asssessed. Thirteen horse were treated every 2 weeks by intratumoral injection for a period of 14 weeks with complete resolution in 61.5% of cases (3-year follow-up period). In this study, lesions greater than 13.5 cm in diameter and those refractory to previous therapies were less likely to resolve.[133]

Perioperative cisplatin in sesame oil injections are recommended when surgical debulking results in a site that cannot be surgically closed and an open wound that is less than 5 cm in largest diameter. The first treatment is administered at surgery. Instructions for preparation of the drug from powder are available.[134] Tumor dosage is planned as 1 mg of cisplatin per cubic centimeter of tissue to be injected. All visible tumor and a margin of normal tissue of 1 to 2 cm should be injected.

The target volume is injected through multiple sites using a parallel-row or field-block technique. Rows of injections should be 0.6 to 0.8 cm apart. Number and frequency of treatments vary with differing protocols. A standard therapy may include 4 intratumoral treatment sessions at 2-week intervals.[134] In a retrospective study of 573 equidae treated with intratumoral cisplatin, 96% of the treated sarcoid lesions resolved after a course of 4 treatments, and the overall cure rate (local control after 4 years) was 93.3%.[135] All treatment effects from intralesional cisplatin in sesame oil are local. Acute inflammatory reactions may occur but usually resolve quickly. Phenylbutazone or flunixin meglumine may be administered if necessary to minimize discomfort.

Cisplatin is mutagenic and carcinogenic, and the reader is referred to other sources for a detailed discussion of appropriate chemotherapy precautions to protect the health of the owner and the veterinarian.[134]

Other recent studies have assessed the efficacy of Ting point acupuncture and subcutaneous injection of *Viscum album* subsp. *austriacus* (mistletoe) extract. Both resulted in size reduction of the lesions, with complete regression in a small percentage treated with mistletoe.[136,137]

Prevention

To the author's knowledge, there are no management strategies or treatment techniques to prevent development of sarcoid tumors in horses.

Public Health Considerations

There is no evidence that BPV is infectious for humans, and sarcoid tumors of horses are not considered a zoonotic disease.

The complete reference list is available online at www.expertconsult.com.

CHAPTER

26 Miscellaneous Viral Diseases

Kenneth William Hinchcliff

Miscellaneous Orbivirus Infections

The genus *Orbivirus* within the *Reoviridae* family includes 22 distinct species, each of which has multiple serotypes. The orbivirus that is most commonly associated with horses is African horse sickness (see Chapter 16). Because these viruses are transmitted by many diverse insect vectors and have a wide host range, there are likely some equine pathogens as yet to be described. Most of the miscellaneous orbiviruses currently described are geographically distinct, but future analyses will elucidate their genetic relationships and provide evidence of their evolution.

Equine Encephalosis

Etiology and Epidemiology

Equine encephalosis virus (EEV) is an insect-borne orbivirus transmitted by a variety of *Culicoides* spp.[1] and is closely related to bluetongue and epizootic hemorrhagic disease viruses.[2] It has characteristics in cell culture similar to African horse sickness[3] (see Chapter 16). There are multiple serotypes of EEV that infect equids of southern, eastern, and western Africa, with serologic evidence of infection or virus isolation from equids in Kenya, Botswana, Namibia, South Africa, Ghana, The Gambia, and Ethiopia but not Morocco.[4,5] Seven serotypes have been identified as circulating among equids in South Africa,[4] with additional phylogenetically distinct isolates from horses in Israel.[6] The virus was detected in horses in Israel in 2008 when it caused a mild febrile illness in large numbers of horses.[7] The virus isolated from horses in Israel was phylogenetically distant to those serotypes circulating in South Africa and similar to an isolate obtained from horses in Ghana.[5] Horses, donkeys, and zebras in southern, western, and eastern Africa frequently have antibodies to the virus, indicating widespread infection of these equids. Antibodies to EEV were found in 77% of 1144 horses, 57% of 518 horses, 49% of 4875 donkeys, and up to 88% of zebras in South Africa.[1,4,8,9] All of 144 equids (horses and donkeys) sampled in The Gambia, 129 of 159 (81%) in Ghana, and 206 of 220 (94%) in Ethiopia had serologic evidence of infection by EEV.[5] None of 120 horses sampled in Morocco had serologic evidence of infection.[5] Zebra foals develop antibodies to the virus within months of losing their maternally acquired passive immunity.[10] Elephants seldom have antibodies to EEV.[4]

Seroprevalence in Thoroughbred yearlings has varied in South Africa markedly from year to year. In a study conducted between 1999 and 2004, seroprevalence ranged between 17.5% and 34.7% (of approximately 500 sampled each year) in most years but was as low as 3.6%.[11] In this study, serotypes 1 and 6 were the predominant serotypes identified and in a small percentage of horses, there was indication of infection with multiple serotypes.[11]

Equine encephalosis virus replicates in midges, although the rate of replication differs, depending on species of midge and strain of the virus. The genetic and phenotypic stability of strains of the virus are unknown, and there exists the potential for emergence of new strains or recognition of currently undetected strains, as demonstrated by the recent isolation of a phylogenetically distinct form of the virus from horses in Israel and Ghana. Variations in pathogenicity are not recognized but might exist. There is independent persistence of virus serotypes in a maintenance cycle based on observation of increased rates of seasonal seroconversion to a specific serotype with ongoing low level of infection by other serotypes.[4,11] For example, infection by serotype 1 is most common (60%), whereas infection by serotype 2 is uncommon (0.7%), despite the latter having been first documented as infecting horses in 1967.[11]

Clinical Findings

The clinical importance of EEV is uncertain, but three syndromes described are asymptomatic infection, clinical disease, and on less evidence, encephalitis. Seroconversion without evidence of clinical disease in closely managed horses suggests that in most instances infection by the virus is asymptomatic. Most infections are subclinical based on the high seroprevalence rate and lack of reports of disease outbreaks. Clinical signs commonly attributed to EEV infection include fever, lassitude, edema of the lips, and congested mucous membranes as reported in horses in Israel in 2008 and 2009.[7] The virus was originally isolated from a horse with signs of neurologic disease, hence the name. However, the disease associated with infection by EEV is poorly documented and given the high prevalence of infection, EEV might be falsely incriminated as the cause of more severe neurologic disease in some situations. Acute neurologic disease, abortion, and enteritis are anecdotally reported. In an outbreak report in late 2008 in Israel, the morbidity rate on 60 premises varied from 2% to 100%. No horses died of the disease during that outbreak.[7] Disease associated with EEV has not been recorded in donkeys or zebras.[1]

Diagnosis

Characteristic abnormalities in serum biochemistry or hematology are not reported. Antibodies to the virus are detected by serum neutralization assays (which are serotype specific) and enzyme-linked immunosorbent assay (ELISA), which is not serotype specific. Complement fixation and agar gel immunodiffusion tests have been used to detect group-specific antibodies. A group-specific, indirect sandwich ELISA detects EEV antigen and does not crossreact with African horse sickness virus, bluetongue virus, or epizootic hemorrhagic disease virus.[12] A competitive ELISA suitable for use with serum from horses, donkeys, or zebras detects antibodies to all seven EEV serotypes while not detecting antibodies to other orbiviruses (such as African horse sickness or bluetongue virus).[13]

Pathologic Findings

Necropsy examination reveals cerebral edema, localized enteritis, degeneration of cardiac myofibers, and myocardial fibrosis, but whether these abnormalities are attributable to EEV is unclear.[3] Definitive diagnosis of individual animals is difficult at the current time because of the high prevalence of seropositive animals and the ill-defined clinical and necropsy characteristics of the disease. Detection of seroconversion and/or virus isolation associated with clinical signs consistent with the disease in groups of horses permits detection of outbreaks of the disease such as occurred in Israel.[7] There are no recognized measures for treatment, control, or prevention. There is no vaccine.

Public Health Considerations

The virus does not appear to cause disease in humans.

Peruvian Horse Sickness Virus

Peruvian horse sickness virus (PHSV) is an orbivirus described as causing neurologic disease in horses in Peru.[14] The outbreak in Peru in 1997 caused the death of 104 horses, which is a mortality rate of approximately 1.25% and a case fatality rate of 78%. A genetically identical virus has been isolated from horses dying of neurologic disease in northern Australia.[14] Serologic surveillance in that area demonstrates antibody to PHSV in 11% of horses. The disease is described as causing motor incoordination, sagging jaw, tooth grinding, and stiff neck, with death in 8 to 11 days.

Miscellaneous Alphavirus Infections

Getah Virus

Etiology and Epidemiology

Getah virus is an alphavirus within the Semliki Forest complex of togaviruses.[15] These are small, enveloped viruses with a single-stranded, positive sense ribonucleic acid (RNA) genome. Getah virus causes disease in horses and pigs. Getah virus is reported from Japan, Hong Kong, China, southeast Asia, Korea, and India.[15,16] Reports from the 1960s document antibodies to Getah virus in animals in Australia, but the presence of this virus in Australia has not been confirmed with modern techniques that are able to differentiate antibodies to Getah virus from those of the related Ross River virus and other viruses in this complex. There are no reports of disease caused by Getah virus in Australia. There is considerable sequence homology between Getah and Ross River virus genomes.[17] There is temporal but not geographic variability among isolates of Getah virus from southeast Asia and Japan.[18,19]

Getah virus is arthropod borne, and infection is through the bite of an infected mosquito. The life cycle of Getah virus has not been completely determined. The virus is maintained in the mosquito-vertebrate-mosquito host cycle typical of arboviruses. The definitive, amplifying vertebrate host for Getah virus is unknown, although a number of vertebrates, including horses, cattle, and pigs, can be infected by the virus. Antibodies to the virus have been detected in humans.[15] Horses and pigs become viremic and presumably can infect mosquitoes, although this does not appear to have been confirmed experimentally. The virus is assumed to be maintained in a mosquito-pig-mosquito cycle in those areas in which there is mosquito activity year round.[20] Persistence of the virus in areas in which mosquito activity is seasonal has not been explained, and whether transovarial or transtadial transmission occurs within the mosquito population is not reported.[20]

There is suspicion that during outbreaks of disease Getah virus is spread by horse-to-horse contact, based on the rapidity of spread among horses, the short duration of the outbreak, and the lack of mosquito activity at the time that some horses developed the disease.[21,22] However, experimental evidence suggests that this route of spread is likely of limited importance in propagation of epidemics because of the low concentration of virus in nasal and oral secretions of infected horses and the large inoculum required to cause disease in horses by the intranasal route.[23]

The prevalence of serologic evidence of infection of horses by Getah virus in Japan ranges from 8% to 93%, depending on the region of the country in which the samples were collected and the disease history of the band or stable of horses.[21,24] Seroprevalence was 17% in India and 25% in Hong Kong.[23,25] These results confirm the widespread incidence of subclinical infection of horses by Getah virus in endemic areas.

Clinical Findings

Disease associated with Getah virus infection is characterized by pyrexia, edema of the limbs, and an abnormal gait, often described as "stiffness."[21,22] Eruptions of the skin, urticaria, and submandibular lymphadenopathy are reported in some horses with the disease in Japan but not in India.[21,22] The clinical disease persists for 7 to 10 days. Abortion is not a feature of the disease and foals born of mares that have had the disease during gestation are normal.[21] Subclinical infection is very common in endemic areas. Getah virus has been isolated from aborted swine fetuses and transplacental transmission occurs.[26]

Hematologic abnormalities induced by Getah virus infection in horses include lymphopenia.[21] Increases in serum activity of muscle-derived enzymes, such as creatine kinase, are not characteristic of the disease. Affected horses can have mild to moderate hyperbilirubinemia secondary to inappetance.[21]

Diagnosis

Diagnosis of disease caused by Getah virus is achieved by detection of clinical signs consistent with the disease, isolation of the virus from blood of affected horses, and seroconversion to the virus.[19] Interpretation of serologic data from horses in Japan is hindered by the widespread use of a vaccine against Getah disease that induces detectable antibodies to Getah virus in serum.[24,27]

Pathologic Findings

Reports of postmortem examination of horses with disease caused by Getah virus are limited to experimental studies because the disease is typically not fatal. Horses with disease induced by inoculation with pathogenic Getah virus typically have mild changes, including atrophy of splenic and lymphoid tissue with destruction of lymphocytes, and perivascular and diffuse infiltration of focal skin lesions by lymphocytes, histiocytes, and eosinophils. Lesions in the central nervous system are equivocal and limited to mild perivascular cuffing in the cerebrum and small hemorrhagic foci in the spinal cord.[28]

Treatment of affected horse is supportive. Affected horses might benefit from administration of analgesics and antipyretics

such as phenylbutazone. Administration of antimicrobials is not indicated in uncomplicated cases.

Prevention

An inactivated virus vaccine is available in Japan for immunization of horses against disease caused by Getah virus.[24] The vaccine, which is combined with that for Japanese encephalitis (JE), is considered effective. Minimizing the exposure of horses to infected mosquitoes is prudent, although the efficacy of this technique in preventing infection is unknown. During outbreaks of disease caused by Getah virus, it is also prudent to isolate affected horses, given the potential for horse-to-horse spread of the virus.

Public Health Considerations

Disease in humans caused by Getah virus has not been documented.

Ross River Virus

Etiology and Epidemiology

Ross river virus is an alphavirus within the Semliki Forest complex of togaviruses. These are small, enveloped viruses with a single-stranded, positive sense RNA genome. There is considerable sequence homology between Getah and Ross River virus genomes.[10] Ross River virus causes disease in both humans and horses.[29-31]

Ross River virus is found in most areas of continental Australia, Tasmania, West Papua and Papua New Guinea, New Caledonia, Fiji, Samoa, and the Cook Islands.[16] There is geographic genetic variability among isolates of Ross River virus.[18,19]

The virus is arthropod borne, and infection is through the bite of an infected mosquito. The virus is maintained in the mosquito-vertebrate-mosquito host cycle typical of arboviruses. The vertebrate hosts of Ross River virus include a large number of eutherian, marsupial, and monotreme mammals and birds.[16] Macropod species, including kangaroos and wallabies, are assumed to be the most important amplifying hosts, although this is debated.[16]

There is a high incidence of Ross River virus infection of horses in endemic regions of Australia, and the prevalence is increased with year-round mosquito activity. In a 1998 study, the number of seropositive horses in Queensland, an area with year-round mosquito activity, was approximately 80%, whereas the number of seropositive horses around the Gippsland Lakes in southern Australia, a region with seasonal mosquito activity, was 50%.[27] Outbreaks of clinical disease attributed to Ross River virus infection of horses occurred in southeastern Australia in late 2010 and early 2011[29] and were also associated with serologic and virologic evidence of infection by Murray Valley encephalitis virus and Kunjin virus, which is a lineage of West Nile virus (Fig. 26-1). During the outbreak that was associated with unusually wet summer conditions in an area characterized by hot, dry summers, 392 horses on 271 premises were suspected or confirmed to have been infected by one or more of these arboviruses.

Clinical Findings

The disease associated with Ross River virus infection of horses is typified by pyrexia; petechial hemorrhages; submandibular lymphadenopathy; lameness, including "stiffness," swollen joints, or distal limbs; inappetence; reluctance to move; and mild colic.[29-31] Horses are often described as being ataxic,[31] although the neurologic basis of this sign is unclear. Any previous skepticism regarding the pathogenicity of Ross River virus in horses was addressed by the outbreak of disease caused by Ross River virus during 2010 and 2011 in southeastern Australia.[31] Disease associated with confirmed Ross River virus infection was

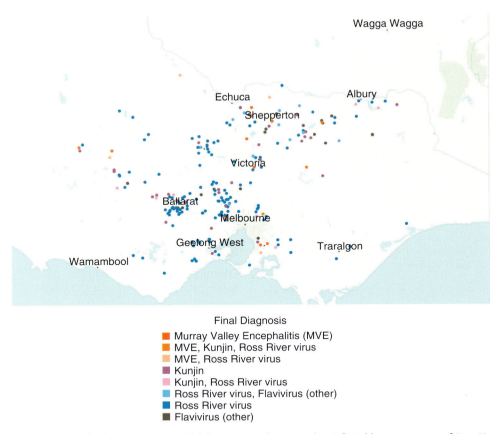

Figure 26-1 Map of southeastern Australia depicting sites at which horses were documented as infected by one or more of Ross River virus, Murray Valley encephalitis virus, Kunjin virus (a lineage of West Nile virus), and unidentified flaviviruses. *(Figure provided by Dr. Roger Paskin, Department of Primary Industries, Victoria, Australia.)*

characterized by ataxia, stiff gait, depression, edema, listlessness, pyrexia, and reluctance to walk. Horses infected experimentally with Ross River virus have minimal clinical signs of disease.[33] The duration of disease caused by Ross River virus in horses is uncertain, and some veterinarians consider that the disease can persist for weeks to months or recur in horses.

There are insufficient reports of disease to determine if characteristic or diagnostic abnormalities in serum biochemistry or hematology occur in affected horses. An elevated concentration of fibrinogen in plasma is reported in all of three horses with the presumptive disease that were tested.[30]

Diagnosis

Diagnosis of infection by Ross River virus is confirmed by virus isolation from serum or heparinized blood samples collected during the acute phase of the disease or detection in serum of antibodies to the virus.[29] Detection of immunoglobulin M (IgM) antibodies to Ross River virus is indicative of recent infection, whereas detection of IgG or neutralizing antibodies is indicative of more distant infection.[29,30] Seroconversion confirms exposure and presumably infection by the virus. Isolation of Ross River virus has been achieved from horses with IgM antibody to the virus but not with IgG antibody, likely because of the temporal pattern of antibody appearance in blood of infected horses.[29] In addition to culture of the virus in mice or tissue culture, Ross River virus can be detected in blood and synovial fluid using a reverse transcriptase–polymerase chain reaction (RT-PCR).[30] It is important to remember that subclinical infection of horses in endemic regions is very common and that this high rate of subclinical infection increases the risk of incorrect clinical diagnosis of disease as being attributable to

infection by the virus. It is possible that clinical abnormalities in a horse with Ross River viremia or serum antibodies to the virus are actually not attributable to infection by Ross River virus. This is important in that there are no reports of postmortem examination of horses with disease confirmed to be caused by Ross River virus. Thus case definition in terms of postmortem confirmatory diagnostics has not been established.

Therapy

Treatment of affected horse is supportive. Affected horses might benefit from administration of analgesics and antipyretics such as phenylbutazone. Administration of antimicrobials is not indicated in uncomplicated cases.

Prevention

Control measures have not been evaluated, but minimizing the exposure of horses to infected mosquitoes is prudent, although the efficacy of this technique in preventing infection is unknown. There is no vaccine to prevent infection or disease of horses by Ross River virus.

Public Health Considerations

Disease associated with Ross River virus infection is common in humans in Australia, with an estimated 4800 cases per year and much larger numbers during epidemics of the disease.[34] The horse is believed to be an amplifying host of the virus because experimentally infected horses can infect mosquitoes.[35] Direct transmission from the horse to humans, which has not been demonstrated, but would be most likely to occur in humans with occupational exposure. The disease in humans is characterized by mild pyrexia and constitutional signs initially, with subsequent development of a rash on the skin and oral lesions. Arthritis or arthralgia is common and affects primarily the wrists, knees, ankles, and small joints of the extremities. These signs and symptoms can persist for 2 to 3 months, and the disease can relapse.

Miscellaneous Flaviviruses

Powassan Virus

The Powassan virus, a flavivirus, occurs in Ontario and the eastern United States and produces a nonsuppurative, focal necrotizing meningoencephalitis in horses.[36] Approximately 13% of horses sampled in Ontario in 1983 were serologically positive to the virus. Experimental intracerebral inoculation of the Powassan virus into horses resulted in a neurologic syndrome within 8 days.[37] Clinical findings include a "tucked-up" abdomen, tremors of the head and neck, slobbering and chewing movements resulting in foamy saliva, stiff gait, staggering, and recumbency. Pathologically, there is a nonsuppurative encephalomyelitis, neuronal necrosis, and focal parenchymal necrosis. The virus has not been isolated from the brain.

Murray Valley Encephalitis Virus

Etiology and Epidemiology

Murray Valley encephalitis (MVE) virus is a type of arbovirus (flavivirus) spread by mosquitoes and causes outbreaks of encephalitis in humans in Australia[38] and a nonsuppurative polioencephalomyelitis in horses.[39,40] Transmission involves the bite of infected mosquitoes and the primary vector during epidemics is the mosquito *Culex annulirostris*, although other mosquito species may be involved in other aspects of MVE virus ecology. The primary hosts in Victoria of MVE virus during years of high virus activity are believed to be wild water birds.[38]

Antibodies against MVE virus have been detected in a wide range of animals, including horses, pigs, marsupials, poultry, and wild birds, but there is no definitive evidence that MVE virus causes disease in most of these species. During late 2010 and early 2011, an outbreak of disease in horses associated with infection by MVE virus occurred in southeastern Australia.[31] The disease caused by MVE virus was part of a complex of arboviral diseases afflicting horses during the period. Horses were infected, and some had clinical signs associated with infection by MVE, Ross River virus, Kunjin virus (a lineage of West Nile virus [WNV]),[41] a variant of WNV distinct from Kunjin virus (WNV$_{NSW2011}$), and an unidentified flavivirus[31,42] (see Fig. 26-1). Some horses had serologic or virologic evidence of simultaneous infection by more than one arbovirus.[31] The outbreak occurred during an unusually wet summer season, in an area characterized by hot and dry summers, and after 7 years of severe drought. There was markedly higher vegetation cover, usually high numbers of mosquitoes, and an increase in populations of wild water birds during the period of the outbreak.

Clinical Findings

Clinical signs associated with infection by MVE virus are predominantly neurologic and include ataxia, depression, hyperesthesia, hypermetria, and prolonged recumbency.[31,39,43] The onset of clinical signs can be acute, and signs can mimic those of colic.[39] However, neurologic disease in horses characterized by depression, changes in temperament, and incoordination in conjunction with high levels of MVE antibodies has been observed sporadically in areas where MVE virus is known to have been active.[31,38,39,40] The case fatality rate in horses infected with one or more arboviruses was approximately 10%,[31]

although the proportion of deaths attributable to MVE is uncertain.

Therapy and Prevention

There is no specific treatment for this flavivirus.

There is no vaccine, and prevention is based on minimizing exposure of susceptible horses to mosquitoes.

Miscellaneous Bunyaviridae

There are a number of viruses in the *Bunyaviridae* family that cause disease in horses in the Western Hemisphere.[44] Neuroinvasive disease is primarily reported in humans, and cases are most commonly reported along the eastern-half of the United States with focal areas of higher incidence along the Appalachian mountain range and the upper Mississippi basin. The viruses are maintained in a mosquito-vertebrate host-mosquito or midge-vertebrate host-midge cycle; occasionally, horses are infected and develop signs of neurologic disease.

California Group

The California serogroup of viruses are mosquito-transmitted viruses of the family *Bunyaviridae* that can cause acute encephalitis in horses.[45,46] There are 12 serotypes isolated in Africa, Europe, Asia, and North and South America. La Crosse virus, snowshoe hare virus, and Jamestown Canyon virus are three serotypes that have been isolated in Canada and California and that have the potential to cause disease in humans. The snowshoe hare virus is the most widely occurring arbovirus in Canada and is maintained in an amplification cycle involving small mammals, such as snowshoe hares, and mosquitoes, primarily of the *Aedes* genus.[46] In one reported case, an affected horse recovered completely within 1 week, and there was seroconversion to the snowshoe hare serotype of the California serogroup of viruses.[47] Approximately 15% of horses in southern California have antibodies to Jamestown Canyon virus in horses.[48] The virus has been isolated from vesicular lesions in a horse.[49]

Cache Valley virus has been isolated from a clinically normal horse, and the high seroprevalence of specific antibody suggests enzootic transmission.

Main Drain virus has been isolated from a horse with severe encephalitis in California.[45] Clinical findings included incoordination, ataxia, stiffness of the neck, head pressing, inability to swallow, fever, and tachycardia. The virus is transmitted by rabbits and rodents and by its natural vector, *Culicoides variipennis*.

Paramyxoviridae

Nipah virus is a member of the *Paramyxoviridae* family of the order Mononegavirales and is a cause of encephalitis in humans and pigs in southeast Asia.[50] The virus is a member of the *Henipavirus* genus (which includes the Hendra virus; see Chapter 17) that is transmitted from frugivorous bats (*Pteropus* spp.) to pigs, among which it spreads horizontally to other pigs and humans. Horses can be exposed and develop antibodies to the virus, and there is one anecdotal report of dilated meningeal vessels in a horse from which Nipah virus was isolated.[50]

Salem virus, a paramyxovirus, has been isolated from horses, but disease associated with this virus is questionable.[51] The virus was implicated as a cause of an outbreak that started in the northeastern United States on a racetrack in Salem, New Hampshire, in the early 1990s. Once the virus was isolated, subsequent studies demonstrated widespread seropositivity in healthy horses. Subsequent spontaneous outbreaks similar to this first outbreak failed to demonstrate seroconversion in the face of disease. In an experimental infection of one horse, only transient increase in rectal temperature and mild lymphopenia was observed.

Other Viruses

Nigerian equine encephalitis, a disease with low morbidity but high mortality, is characterized by fever, generalized muscle spasms, ataxia, and lateral recumbency of 3 to 5 days' duration. The virus has not been identified, but the only report describes the lesions as consistent with an alphavirus. Lagos bat virus, a pathogenic *Lyssavirus*, is highly endemic in this area.[52]

An orthopoxvirus was associated with an outbreak of severe cutaneous disease in horses in southern Brazil.[53] The disease was characterized by papules and vesicles progressing to proliferative and exudative lesions on the muzzle, external nares, and external and internal lips. The vesicles eroded, and the proliferative lesions eventually bled and progressed to moist crusts and scars. None of the 14 affected animals died, and signs lasted approximately 6 to 12 days.

Australian bat lyssavirus (ABLV), a member of the Rhabdoviridae family, causes fever, lethargy and ataxia progressing to seizures and death in some infected horses in Australia. This is the only member of the lyssavirus genus (which includes rabies virus) known to be present in Australia. There is some evidence that rabies vaccine may provide cross protection against ABLV infection. There have been several reported cases of a rabies-like illness in humans after being bitten or scratched by an animal.

The complete reference list is available online at www.expertconsult.com.

27 Laboratory Diagnosis of Bacterial Infections

Barbara A. Byrne

This chapter is written to aid the veterinary clinician in collecting samples for bacterial culture, understanding the methods used to detect bacteria, interpreting results, and ensuring that optimal results are received from the microbiology laboratory.

Direct Microscopic Examination

The direct microscopic examination of samples taken from sites of suspected bacterial infection is an essential component for detection and interpretation of microbial isolation and identification results. A variety of staining methodologies can be used to examine clinical specimens. The most common methods include the Gram stain and Wright's stain. Less frequently used stains include acid-fast, periodic acid–Schiff, and silver stains.

Samples should be examined for the presence and type of inflammation. A Wright's stain is preferred for this evaluation because most cells are poorly recognized with Gram stain. The smear should be evaluated for inflammatory cells, such as neutrophils and macrophages, and the morphologic condition of the cells. Degenerate cells, characterized by swollen nuclei, loss of cytoplasmic detail, and nuclear destruction, are highly suggestive of a septic process and an indication that a culture should be performed on the sample. A Wright-Giemsa stain will also detect bacteria, although the Gram-staining characteristics will not be apparent. The presence of both intracellular and extracellular bacteria is consistent with an infection rather than mere contamination. Bacteria are frequently observed when samples are obtained from normally colonized sites such as mucous membranes; however, they should not be accompanied by significant inflammation if only normal flora is present.

If fixed tissue sections are the only sample available for evaluation, several staining techniques can be used. With the standard hematoxylin and eosin (H&E) stain, bacteria will appear blue in color. Several silver-based staining methods are available to better visualize bacteria. These stains may be particularly helpful to observe leptospiral organisms in tissues. Available tissue Gram-staining techniques include the Brown and Brenn method, which can be used to identify the gram reaction of organisms in fixed tissues.

Every sample submitted for bacterial culture should receive a Gram stain to facilitate detection of bacteria. This methodology is rapid and simple to perform and can give vital information regarding the potential pathogens present. Examination of the Gram-stained specimen can indicate the relative number of bacteria present. The gram reaction, either gram positive or gram negative, and bacterial morphology can be used to develop a list of possible etiologies that can be used for empiric antimicrobial drug selection (Table 27-1). Certain morphologies and staining characteristics can be consistent with the presence of anaerobic bacteria and indicate that the sample should also be

Table 27-1 Gram Stain Reaction and Morphology of Common Bacterial Pathogens of Horses

Pathogen	Morphology
Gram-Positive Organisms	
Streptococcus equi subsp. *equi*	Cocci, often in long chains
Streptococcus equi subsp. *zooepidemicus*	Cocci, often in short chains
Rhodococcus equi	Pleomorphic coccobacilli
Corynebacterium pseudotuberculosis	Pleomorphic coccobacilli, diphtheroid
Dermatophilus congolensis	Cocci, "railroad track"
Actinomyces spp.	Rods, coccobacilli to filamentous and branching
Staphylococcus aureus	Cocci
Clostridium spp.	Rods, sometimes with spores
Gram-Negative Organisms	
Escherichia coli	Rod
Klebsiella spp.	Rod
Actinobacillus spp.	Rod
Pasteurella spp.	Rod
Salmonella spp.	Rod
Pseudomonas spp.	Rod
Leptospira spp.	Curved rods
Bacteroides spp.	Rod
Fusobacterium necrophorum	Rods, tapered ends

incubated anaerobically (Fig. 27-1). For example, observation of large, gram-positive rods (with or without spores) or long, tapered gram-negative rods suggests *Clostridium* spp. or *Fusobacterium* spp. infection, respectively. Failure to observe bacteria on a Gram stain does not rule out an infection because bacteria need to be present in fairly high numbers, 10^4 to 10^6/mL, to be detected.

Some artifacts appear similar to bacteria in a Gram stain. As noted, the Gram stain is not particularly useful for identifying inflammatory cells because they usually stain pink with poor detail. Portions of cells, particularly the nucleus, can stain purple and may even look similar to dense clumps of gram-positive cocci in thick preparations. Therefore it is best to look for bacteria in areas of the smear that are less dense. Equine respiratory secretions contain abundant mucus that stains pink. Occasionally, these strands can appear as long, pink, rodlike structures. They can be differentiated from true bacteria by their variation in size and length and irregular thickness.

Acid-fast (Ziehl-Neelsen) or modified acid-fast (Kinyoun) stains can be used to help identify members of the nocardioform-actinomycete group of bacteria, including *Mycobacterium* spp. (acid fast), *Rhodococcus equi* (weakly acid fast), and *Nocardia* spp. (weakly acid fast). Bacteria that are acid fast retain the stain carbolfuchsin and appear bright pink because of the waxy outer membrane containing mycolic acid (Fig. 27-2).

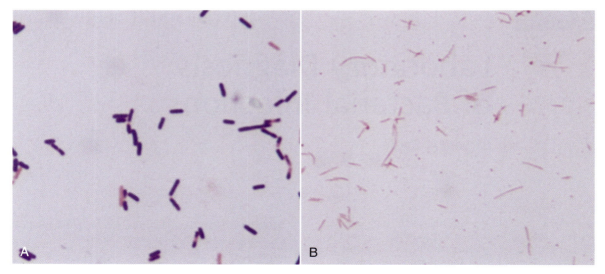

Figure 27-1 Gram stain of two anaerobic rods demonstrating characteristic morphology. **A,** *Clostridium perfringens.* **B,** *Fusobacterium necrophorum.*

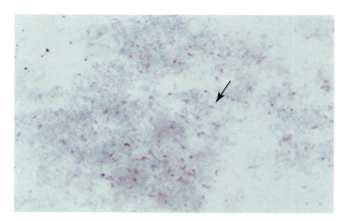

Figure 27-2 Kinyoun acid-fast stain of *Nocardia* spp. Acid-fast bacteria *(arrow)* appear bright pink or fuscia colored.

Direct detection of bacterial antigen in a sample can be accomplished using immunologic techniques such as direct immunofluorescence or immunohistochemistry. These techniques utilize antibody specific for the target organism and bind bacteria within the specimen. Bound antibody is subsequently visualized using fluorescent or light microscopy, respectively. Diseases for which these techniques are used include detection of *Leptospira* in urine and *Clostridium* in tissues such as liver or muscle. Fluorescent antibody testing can be a rapid means for diagnosis of certain infections, but it requires antibody specific for the organism and fresh or frozen specimens or tissues.

Sampling for Bacterial Culture

Indications

Clinical signs suggestive of but not pathognomonic for bacterial infections include fever, pain, and swelling. Clinicopathologic findings consistent with a bacterial infection include increased white blood cell (WBC) count with a neutrophilia and possibly a left shift, increased plasma fibrinogen and other acute-phase protein concentrations, and hyperglobulinemia. All of these findings are unlikely to be present, and their absence does not rule out the possibility of infectious disease. Cytologic examination of fluid or cells collected from the site of a suspected infection generally reveals neutrophilic inflammation and in some cases a granulomatous or pyogranulomatous response. Degenerate neutrophils are a strong indication that a septic process is present, and bacterial culture should always be performed.

Samples Most Appropriate for Culture

Ideally, specimens from sites that are normally sterile, such as joint fluid, peritoneal fluid, and blood, are the best samples to collect for culture because any bacteria isolated are likely causative. Culture of clinical samples obtained from sites that are colonized with bacterial flora, such as nasal or oral mucous membranes, will usually yield normal bacterial flora of that region (Box 27-1).[1] This may result in spending the client's money and expending the laboratory's efforts needlessly to identify many nonpathogenic bacteria and could result in inappropriate use of antimicrobial drugs. Because many of these bacteria can also be opportunistic pathogens, it is difficult to determine if they are causing the clinical condition. For example, collection of purulent discharge from the nasal passage of a horse will certainly yield bacteria that are potentially pathogenic, such as *Streptococcus equi* subsp. *zooepidemicus,* but their detection does not mean this bacterium is the cause of the discharge. It is preferable to identify the specific site of infection, such as sinus, guttural pouch, or lung, and collect the sample for culture from that location.

Several exceptions to this rule can be made. In general, if the clinician is trying to detect a pathogen not present in colonized sites in clinically normal animals, the laboratory can specifically target identification efforts toward that organism or use selective media to enhance pathogen detection. Detection of *Streptococcus equi* subsp. *equi* from a nasal or pharyngeal swab would be appropriate because the microbiology laboratory can focus on β-hemolytic streptococcal isolates for definitive identification. Box 27-2 provides a list of specimens to be collected for bacterial culture of different body systems.

Methods for Collection

Tissue (collected as an aspirate or biopsy) and fluids are the best samples to collect for bacterial isolation. In general, larger

---

Box 27-1 Common Normal Bacterial Flora of Horses for Selected Sites

Oral and Nasal Cavities and Pharynx
Streptococcus equi subsp. *zooepidemicus*
Streptococcus spp. (nonhemolytic or α-hemolytic)
Pasteurella
Escherichia coli
Actinomyces spp.
Enterobacter spp.
Actinobacillus spp.
Anaerobes, including *Peptostreptococcus anaerobius*, *Bacteroides fragilis*, *Bacteroides* spp., *Fusobacterium* spp.

Skin
Streptococcus
Staphylococcus aureus
Coagulase-negative staphylococci
Micrococcus
Corynebacterium spp.

Lower Genitourinary Tract
Streptococcus spp.
E. coli
Enterobacter spp.
Bacillus spp.
Staphylococcus spp.

Ocular Conjunctiva
Streptomyces spp.
Staphylococcus spp.
Bacillus spp.
Streptococcus spp. (α-hemolytic, β-hemolytic)
E. coli
Moraxella spp.
Acinetobacter spp.

Box 27-2 Samples and Tissues to Select for Common Conditions and Diseases of Major Organ Systems

- *Septicemia:* Blood culture.
- *Pneumonia:* Tracheal secretions, best collected by transtracheal aspiration.
- *Enteritis* or *colitis:* Feces more appropriate than swab of rectal contents to collect sufficient volume for enrichment to detect pathogens. At necropsy, select from the site closest to the lesion.
- *Genitourinary system* (including abortion): Multiple samples needed, and submission of entire selection for culture and microscopic examination is best to optimize identification of the etiology (abortion): fetal stomach contents, liver, lung, heart, fetal heart blood, spleen, placenta, dam serum (for serology). A guarded swab is optimal for culture of the uterus.
- *Nervous system:* Cerebrospinal fluid, or brain/spinal cord at necropsy.
- *Integumentary system:* Skin biopsy or aspiration of unruptured pustule/vesicle.
- *Musculoskeletal system:* Joint fluid, bone, affected muscle (e.g., necrotizing myositis).

---

samples increase the likelihood that a causative pathogen will be isolated because the sample can be centrifuged to concentrate any bacteria. Samples should be collected as aseptically as possible and placed in a sterile container. Submission of samples in a syringe is acceptable, but the needle should be removed and the syringe capped to avoid inadvertent injury and introduction of bacteria to personnel. Swabs are not the best choice for sampling because they hold only a small amount of material, and some swabs are made of substances that inhibit bacterial growth. Occasionally, however, a swab will be the only choice for sampling. Recently, the use of flocked swabs has been advocated as they can enhance specimen collection and release of

material for culture.[2] Swabs are often not appropriate for fecal or intestinal cultures because of their inadequate sample volume. It is best to submit multiple samples in individual containers to eliminate the possibility of cross-contamination.

Suspected Anaerobic Infection

The clinician should decide before submission whether anaerobic culture is necessary so that the sample can be handled appropriately (see Chapters 41 and 42). For example, when emphysema is detected within a tissue, such as in necrotizing myositis, anaerobic culture would be indicated. Likewise, anaerobic infections are common in abscesses, pneumonia, and pleuritis of horses. Anaerobic culture of tissues from an animal that has been dead for many hours may not be worthwhile because anaerobes will proliferate and disperse throughout the carcass. For example, observation of gram-positive rods typical of *Clostridium* spp. in muscle in a 24-hour-old carcass would not be clearly indicative of clostridial myonecrosis.

Many anaerobes are highly sensitive to oxygen and will die during transport if not protected appropriately. Therefore they should be stored and transported in an environment that minimizes their exposure to the atmosphere. Tissues or a generous volume of fluid (several milliliters) are the best samples for anaerobic culture. If a swab must be used for an anaerobic culture, it should be placed in a semisolid prereduced transport medium, such as anaerobic transport media (Anaerobe Systems, Morgan Hill, CA) or Port-a-Cul (BD Diagnostic Systems, Franklin Lakes, NJ), to minimize air exposure. Similarly, liquid or small tissue samples should be placed on top of the transport media and pushed down into the gel to preserve the anaerobic environment. Aerobic swabs are unacceptable for anaerobic culture. Even anaerobic swabs poorly support anaerobic organisms and should only be used for short-term (a few hours) transport to the laboratory.

Blood Culture

Neonatal foals are the equine patients at greatest risk for septicemia or bacteremia (see Chapter 6). However, blood culture may also be considered in older foals and adults when bacteremia or septicemia is suspected. Many systems are available for culturing blood, including conventional broth-based, biphasic broth-based, and lysis-concentration/filtration methodologies.

The conventional broth-based method uses bottled liquid-broth medium into which the patient's blood is inoculated. The amount of blood necessary varies with the volume of broth. Generally, a 1:10 blood/broth ratio is used. Most broth culture systems contain sodium polyanetholesulfonate (SPS) to inactivate bactericidal components of the blood inoculum and act as an anticoagulant. Some blood culture bottles contain resin for absorption or inactivation of antibiotics. Others utilize prereduced broth media to support growth of anaerobic bacteria. Inoculated broth is incubated at 35°C to 37°C (95°F-98.6°F) for 24 hours, then sampled for direct examination, Gram stain, and subculture onto solid media to isolate colonies. If no growth is detected, the broth is sampled again at 48 hours and 5 to 7 days after inoculation or when macroscopic changes, such as turbidity or gas bubbles, are observed. The broth culture medium allows proliferation of bacteria before subculture to solid agar and will help to detect bacteria present in low numbers. However, the broth method will require a minimum of 48 hours before colonies can be detected. Automated blood culture systems will detect carbon dioxide (CO_2) production within the bottle and can indicate a positive culture more quickly than routine daily subculturing and obviates the need for repeated routine subculture.

Broth cultures have the disadvantage that contaminating bacteria will proliferate and could easily outnumber the "true" pathogen, resulting in misidentification of the causative bacterium or a false-positive result. The biphasic broth-based method uses a broth medium for culture enrichment and a solid-agar medium that can be inoculated directly from the broth without entering the bottle, decreasing the likelihood of inadvertent contamination.

Lysis-centrifugation blood culture methodologies lyse phagocytes, and the sample is either centrifuged or filtered to concentrate the bacteria. The resulting pellet is plated to solid culture media. The lysis-centrifugation system allows detection of bacteria within 24 hours of collection, and the number of bacterial colony-forming units can be enumerated. Some studies have indicated it can be more sensitive than conventional broth methods.[3] However, in the author's experience, this technique is less sensitive than broth-based methods. The lysis-centrifugation technique has advantages for isolation of fungi and *Mycobacterium* spp.[3,4]

Although rare, anaerobic infections can be identified with either a broth or lysis method if a prereduced solid medium (e.g., *Brucella* blood agar) and incubation under anaerobic conditions are used for culture. Alternatively, a broth-based method specific for anaerobic culture can be used.

It is best to collect at least one culture before administration of antibiotics, but the horse owner or farm manager may have already given antimicrobial drugs before the veterinarian's arrival. If the animal has been treated before blood collection, testing is still possible because both methods (broth, lysis) will dilute the drug to subtherapeutic levels, and SPS will inactivate some aminoglycosides. Additionally, a resin-containing broth blood culture media can be obtained to absorb antibiotic drugs. An in vitro study demonstrated that when blood containing therapeutic levels of an aminoglycoside was inoculated with *Escherichia coli* and subsequently inoculated into broth blood culture medium, bacteria could be recovered more readily from the resin-containing blood culture broth than media without the resin.[5] However, these resins may not completely inactivate newer antimicrobial drugs such as ticarcillin, imipenem, and aztreonam.

Because bacteria may only be present in the blood intermittently, several samples should be obtained. Even in foals with septicemia, the number of organisms in each milliliter of blood may be quite low; therefore a larger volume of blood for culture, such as 10 mL, is preferred to a smaller volume such as 1 to 2 mL. If only these smaller volumes can be obtained, pediatric-sized blood culture bottles are available.

Many protocols can be followed for appropriate sampling for bacteremia; one is presented here. Up to four blood samples may be collected in a 24-hour period. After clipping and shaving the site for venipuncture, the area is thoroughly disinfected by repeated application of 10% povidone-iodine or other suitable skin antiseptic and allowed to dry. Although not ideal, an intravascular catheter can be used for collection of one sample, but the access port must also be thoroughly disinfected. The stopper on the blood culture bottle or lysis-centrifugation tube should be cleaned with alcohol and allowed to dry. Two samples should be taken from two different sites approximately 10 minutes apart. Antibiotic administration can then be started. The final two cultures can be taken any time within the next 24 hours. These last two samples should be collected immediately before the next antimicrobial drug administration, when the drug concentration is likely to be at its nadir. This timing will increase the likelihood of detecting bacteremia; sampling from different sites will help to distinguish contaminating bacteria from pathogenic bacteria. The causative organism should be cultured from more than one sample and is almost always present in a pure culture. The presence of multiple colony or bacterial types suggests contamination.

Joint Culture

Isolation of bacteria from joints can be difficult because bacterial numbers are frequently very low. Joint fluid is a sample that is relatively easy to collect, but false-negative culture results when enrichment is not performed are common.[6] A biopsy of synovial membrane might enhance bacterial isolation, but this recommendation is controversial, and the sample is difficult to obtain, often requiring general anesthesia and arthroscopy. Joint fluid can be inoculated into blood culture broth to allow proliferation of bacteria in very low numbers, increasing the likelihood for detection of the causative bacterium. Several papers have demonstrated the superiority of using either manual or automated blood culture systems over simple direct agar culture or use of enhancement broths.[7,8] Alternatively, joint fluid can be concentrated using a lysis-centrifugation blood-culture system. In humans, use of a lysis-centrifugation method is superior to broth inoculation. However, direct comparison of use of the lysis-centrifugation method with a blood culture system for detection of septic arthritis in horses demonstrated that use of blood culture medium was superior.[7,9]

Wounds

Sampling a fresh wound at the time of first treatment can be of doubtful utility because the results will demonstrate contaminating organisms that may or may not lead to infection. Culture of an established wound with signs of infection (e.g., heat, swelling, discharge) is clearly indicated. The superficial areas of the wound should be thoroughly cleaned and debrided before obtaining a sample; otherwise, superficial bacteria will be isolated. Culture of deep regions, including a biopsy of affected tissues, is most likely to lead to identification of the causative bacterium. Aspiration of fluid from deep tissues is an additional method that is useful for sample collection.

Sampling for Enteric Infections

The major bacterial pathogens cultured from horses with enteritis include *Salmonella* spp., *Clostridium perfringens*, and *Clostridium difficile* (see Chapters 35 and 41). Samples for culture of intestinal contents should be collected, whenever possible, from the site of the lesion rather than merely collecting fecal material. This is especially important for suspected clostridial enteritis. Selective enrichment broths are used to detect *Salmonella* spp. or *C. difficile* in intestinal and fecal samples. When submitting samples, be sure to indicate the likely pathogen(s) causing the clinical signs and include the age of the horse so that the appropriate media and culture conditions can be utilized.

Clostridial Enteritis

Anaerobic cultures from fecal material of horses are not routinely done at all microbiology laboratories. Therefore clinicians submitting samples from horses with suspected C. *perfringens* enteritis should specifically request culture for this agent. In cases of C. *perfringens* enteritis or enterotoxemia, intestine from the affected region is preferred over feces at necropsy. The intestine should be collected within 1 to 2 hours of death because clostridial organisms will rapidly proliferate throughout the intestine immediately after death, increasing the chance of isolation. Thus, in cases with a long postmortem interval, isolation of C. *perfringens* without concurrent detection of toxin can be of doubtful significance. Positive isolation should also be correlated with the presence of appropriate histologic lesions. Currently, only a few diagnostic laboratories offer detection of the C. *perfringens* toxins alpha, beta, iota, or epsilon for typing (other than the enterotoxin), making confirmation of a causative role of *C. perfringens* in enteritis difficult. An enzyme-linked immunosorbent assay (ELISA) is available to detect *C. perfringens* alpha, beta, and epsilon toxins in intestinal samples.[10] Many laboratories can perform genetic testing on isolates to identify toxin genes, although gene detection does not always indicate production of toxin in vivo or in vitro. Several commercial kits may be used to identify *C. perfringens* enterotoxin; however, this toxin is of unknown or doubtful significance in horses.

If *Clostridium difficile* enteritis is suspected, this should be indicated on the submission form because broth enrichment, specialized media, and toxin testing are optimal for diagnosis. *Clostridium difficile* toxin A and/or B and *C. difficile* antigen ELISA test kits are commercially available, and these tests can provide a means for rapid diagnosis of *C. difficile* enteritis. (For further discussion of diagnosis of clostridial enteritis in horses, see Chapter 41.)

Ocular Infections

The most common indication for culture of ocular tissues is the presence of a corneal ulcer, particularly those that are healing poorly or melting (see Chapter 10). A culturette may be used to sample the cornea, but gentle scraping to collect a small amount of tissue will more likely yield a causative organism. Although most bacteria typically associated with ocular infections are readily cultured in the laboratory, some infections are caused by streptococci that require additional nutrient supplementation (e.g., chocolate agar or *Staphylococcus* feeder streak) to be isolated successfully.[11] Equine corneal ulcer samples should also be cultured for fungal organisms as they frequently complicate these lesions (see Chapter 46).

Botulism and Tetanus

Not all laboratories have the capability to detect botulinum toxin or *Clostridium botulinum* (see Chapter 43). The best way to diagnose botulism is detection of toxin in blood or intestinal contents of the animal; however, many tests have inadequate sensitivity since low levels of toxin can cause clinical signs in horses. Sampling the suspected origin of the toxin (feed, water) for presence of toxin or *C. botulinum* culture is the best approach. These samples can be sent to the microbiology laboratory, then forwarded or submitted directly to the laboratory equipped to perform the assays to speed analysis.

Clostridium tetani is difficult to grow and frequently is not isolated from affected animals (see Chapter 44). The laboratory can perform a Gram stain on tissue smears to identify typical gram-positive bacilli with spores that enlarge the end of the bacterium and have a "tennis raquet" appearance typical of *C. tetani*. In most cases; however, tetanus is a clinical diagnosis.

Sample Transport

Samples should be kept cool and shipped to the appropriate laboratory as soon as possible after collection. Samples are best shipped on ice or frozen gel pack by overnight delivery to preserve bacterial viability. Some bacteria might survive freezing, but it will result in fewer numbers in the tissue and decrease the likelihood of isolation. In hot weather, samples will warm up quickly, so additional cold packs may be needed. If possible, avoid shipping over the weekend, when samples may sit in warm locations before delivery to the laboratory on Monday. If the sample has been inoculated into anaerobic transport media, the sample should be held and shipped at room

---

Box 27-3 Examples of Fastidious Organisms or Those Requiring Specialized Media or Culture Conditions

- *Mycobacterium* spp.: Other than atypical mycobacteria
- *Mycoplasma*
- Anaerobes
- *Clostridium*: Different media used for various species
- *Leptospira*
- *Listeria*: Cold enrichment for neural tissues
- *Salmonella*: Selection and enrichment
- Nutritionally variant *Streptococcus*

---

temperature. All samples should be contained within a sealed container (e.g., bag or tube), and a second sealed container should surround the specimen in case the primary container breaks or leaks. Absorbent material should also be placed in the package in case of leakage. Federal and state guidelines should be followed as appropriate.

Submission

To familiarize the clinician with isolation procedures in the bacteriology laboratory, it is important to explain how samples are handled for bacterial isolation. Not all samples are inoculated on all types of media to isolate every possible bacterial species, particularly from colonized sites such as the gastrointestinal tract. Some sites should be normally sterile, in which case all organisms present should be identified. Organisms that require special culture characteristics (e.g., anaerobes), fastidious growth, or enrichment procedures are handled in special ways to enhance or select for their isolation (Box 27-3). The type of media and conditions used to isolate and identify bacteria in the laboratory are determined by the horse's signalment, history, and clinical findings specified by the clinician, as well as the source of the sample. Thus it is important that the clinician provide a limited history, if possible, and any lesions or clinical signs detected. Likewise, if a particular bacterial species is suspected, it should be included. The laboratory can then use this information to establish any specialized culture conditions needed to detect suspected agents.

Notify the laboratory if your list of differential diagnoses includes a disease highly infectious for humans such as anthrax, coccidioidomycosis, histoplasmosis, blastomycosis, and mycobacterial infections. Even if the infection is not contagious to humans directly from the animal, some pathogens, such as the dimorphic systemic fungal infections, are highly infectious to laboratory workers when grown in culture. Warning the laboratory that these pathogens might be present will allow appropriate protective precautions to be implemented.

Interpretation of Isolation and Identification Results

Most laboratories will provide the clinician with results that include the Gram stain findings from the sample submitted, bacterial species identified, and their relative quantity. Results obtained from culture and isolation should be interpreted in the context of the organism(s) identified, Gram stain and cytology results, source of the sample, whether a mixed bacterial population was identified, quantity of bacteria, and clinical presentation.

Any bacterium isolated from a normally sterile site should be considered significant if the microscopic examination is consistent with a septic process and the organism matches the Gram stain. Isolation of some bacterial species will lead the clinician to suspect contamination such as *Bacillus* spp., α-hemolytic *Streptococcus*, and coagulase-negative *Staphylococcus*. These organisms, when found as part of a mixed bacterial population in the sample in low quantity, can be contaminants. Although any of these bacteria can cause infection given appropriate circumstances, the clinician should carefully evaluate all findings before concluding they are the primary cause of a disease process.

If the culture is collected from a site normally colonized with bacterial flora, it is expected that a variety of bacteria will be identified. If a bacterial species identified is not part of the normal flora for the site, it could be related to the disease condition. Bacteria present in very high numbers relative to other species could be directly related to the clinical signs; however, their proliferation could be in response to a condition, not the cause.

Results from urine cultures should always include quantification of bacterial numbers in colony-forming units per milliliter (CFU/mL). Because the lower genitourinary tract is colonized with bacteria, urine samples, whether collected by catheterization or free catch, will almost always have some contamination. Bacteria in concentrations greater than 40,000 CFU/mL from a midstream free catch or 1000 CFU/mL in a catheterization sample are considered significant; 20,000 to 40,000 CFU/mL by midstream catch and 500 to 1000 CFU/mL by catheterization are considered suspicious for infection.[12] Urinalysis and cytology results should also reflect an active sediment consistent with infection.

Molecular Methods for Detecting Bacterial Pathogens

Advances in genetic techniques have allowed development of several methods to detect and identify bacterial pathogens. Most use the basic concept that complementary single

strands of deoxyribonucleic acid (DNA) hybridize to one another. DNA polymerases, DNA restriction enzymes, hybridization, and gel electrophoresis are all tools utilized in these techniques.

Polymerase Chain Reaction

The most common technique used in molecular detection is the polymerase chain reaction (PCR). This method amplifies target DNA in vitro using a thermostable DNA polymerase. In short, the PCR reaction uses DNA oligonucleotides specific for the target that prime the polymerase reaction after binding; a DNA polymerase and nucleotides are used to synthesize a copy of the target DNA. Multiple cycles in which the DNA is melted to make single strands, annealing where the temperature is lowered to allow primer binding, and extension for DNA copying lead to many copies of the target DNA, which can then be more easily detected. The DNA product is visualized using agarose gel electrophoresis. Theoretically, 10^9 or more copies can be made from a single-target DNA molecule; but in practical use, most assays require the presence of 10 to 1000 targets (bacterial genomes).

A more recent variation of the PCR reaction is quantitative or real-time PCR. This technique uses the general PCR reaction, but as the DNA copies are synthesized, a fluorescent reaction is generated. A fluorescent molecule is intercalated in the target DNA and released as a copy is made, or a fluorescent-labeled probe specific for the target sequence is displaced by the growing DNA chain (TaqMan, Applied Biosystems, Carlsbad, CA; Fig. 27-3). An advantage of the quantitative PCR is that the reaction and detection can take place simultaneously, reducing the time for testing and results. Also, the test has increased sensitivity, and the probe displacement allows additional specificity.

The polymerase chain reaction is best used to detect bacteria that cannot be cultured in vitro, are difficult to cultivate, take

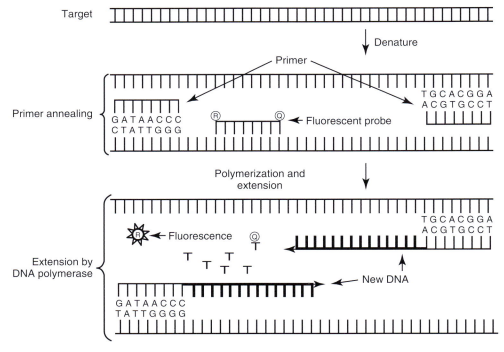

Figure 27-3 Real-time polymerase chain reaction (PCR) using the TaqMan technology. The PCR reaction amplifies target DNA with multiple cycles of denaturation, annealing, and elongation of new DNA strands. A probe complementary to the target sequence is labeled at the 5′ end with a fluorescent reporter molecule, R, and at the 3′ end with a quencher, Q, that dampens fluorescence. As DNA polymerization occurs, the Taq polymerase digests the probe, releasing the fluorescent molecule. The resulting fluorescence can be measured as repeated cycles release additional reporter fluorescence.

a prolonged time for isolation and identification, or are present in such low numbers that culture is inadequately sensitive. The technique is rapid and extremely sensitive. Bacteria for which PCR has been used to enhance detection include *Lawsonia intracellularis*, *Streptococcus equi* subsp. *equi*, *Anaplasma phagocytophilum*, and *Neorickettsia risticii*.[2,13-18]

Another application of PCR is for detection of bacteria within the joint, where cultures are frequently negative in adults despite a high suspicion of bacterial infection based on cytology. Bacteria are broadly targeted by using primers that recognize all eubacterial 16S ribosome genes (rDNA). One study demonstrated that PCR followed by reverse line blot hybridization (a method to determine species of bacteria amplified) was more sensitive for detecting joint sepsis (89%) than culture and isolation alone (38%) or culture following incubation in blood culture broth (78%).[19,20] One further advantage of PCR is that it can be performed on archival frozen or formalin-fixed tissues when the organism is no longer viable. Detection of bacterial messenger ribonucleic acid (mRNA) by reverse transcriptase PCR can also be conducted to verify that the organism was viable in the tissue.

Polymerase chain reaction detection of pathogens has several disadvantages. The technique is relatively expensive and requires some specialized equipment, depending on the methodology used. There must be adequate sample to allow extraction of DNA for the PCR reaction, and some samples will contain substances that interfere with the reaction, leading to false-negative results. Something must be known about the target organism so that appropriate oligonucleotide primers can be used. Even if broadly recognizing 16S rDNA primers are used, additional sequencing must be performed to identify the pathogen present. Thus it can be difficult or impossible to identify novel agents. Furthermore, PCR does not yield a bacterial isolate to use for antimicrobial sensitivity testing. Because no isolate is obtained, it also is difficult to compare isolates between patients to understand the molecular epidemiology and ecology of the infection. Although the sensitivity of PCR is very useful, contamination of the PCR reaction or sample can occur, leading to false-positive results. It is essential that the laboratory performing these tests have adequate positive and negative controls to interpret results.

Use of DNA probes is an older technique in which DNA isolated from a sample is hybridized with a labeled DNA probe specific for a particular pathogen. The probe technique is less sensitive than PCR because there is no amplification step and about 10^4 DNA copies/mL are required for most detection methods.[21] This technique has largely been replaced by more sensitive PCR assays; however, DNA probes can be useful to identify bacterial species in amplified DNA products or on bacterial isolates. Deoxyribonucleic acid hybridization can also be used in fluorescent in situ hybridization to detect bacterial species within a fresh tissue, but it is largely a research technique.

Toxin Gene Detection

Molecular methods may also be used to further characterize isolated bacteria. PCR and multiplex PCR, where multiple oligonucleotide primers are used in a single reaction to detect multiple targets, have been developed to detect toxin genes in *Clostridium perfringens* and *Escherichia coli*.[22] Polymerase chain reaction methods have been developed and are used by research and human bacteriology laboratories to detect antimicrobial resistance genes.[23,24] The use of microarrays to detect bacterial pathogens and antimicrobial resistance genes, although largely a research tool at this time, may eventually be important for resistance-gene characterization.[25-29]

Molecular Epidemiology

Identification of related isolates can be very useful for investigation of outbreaks and nosocomial infections. A variety of techniques, including pulsed-field gel electrophoresis (PFGE) or multilocus sequence typing (MLST), may be used to genotype isolates in order to determine the relatedness between isolates of the same species. These techniques can be used to explore whether bacteria have a similar source in a disease outbreak and to evaluate clonal spread of highly virulent bacteria.[30-33] In PFGE genotyping, genomic DNA is isolated from the bacterium and digested with an endonuclease that cuts infrequently, resulting in extremely large DNA fragments. These fragments are separated by PFGE, and a banding pattern results. The banding pattern can be compared for similarity between isolates. Bacteria with the same PFGE profile, or "fingerprint," are considered related.[34,35] In MLST, multiple genes are sequenced and the sequences are compared between isolates to determine the type.[36] Multilocus sequence typing is often considered a more descriminatory test in detecting strain differences. The advent of high-throughput whole-genome sequencing holds promise for detailed analyses of phylogenetic relationships between different bacterial strains.[37]

Antimicrobial Susceptibility Testing

Indications

Antimicrobial susceptibility testing should be considered when a bacterial pathogen is isolated. Some bacteria will have a predictable susceptibility pattern; accordingly, some laboratories elect not to perform this testing. These organisms include *Streptococcus*, *Corynebacterium*, and *Actinomyces* spp. Often, the susceptibility of a particular organism to antimicrobial drugs can be inferred from previous testing results from the practice population and can be used for empiric therapy. Susceptibility testing is always indicated for a number of pathogens, however, because their susceptibility to different drugs can vary and resistance can be acquired rapidly. These pathogens include *Pseudomonas* spp., *Staphylococcus* spp., and all enteric organisms such as *E. coli*, *Enterobacter*, *Serratia*, and *Klebsiella* spp. Failure to respond to appropriate antimicrobial therapy is another strong indication for sensitivity testing.

Methods

The two major methods for testing for antimicrobial drug susceptibility are agar diffusion, most frequently using the Kirby-Bauer method, and broth dilution, in which microdilution techniques are most common. All testing and interpretation should be performed in accordance with recommendations of the Clinical and Laboratory Standards Institute (CLSI) so that results are repeatable and able to be compared between laboratories (http://www.clsi.org). In the agar diffusion method, bacteria, at a single concentration, are spread over Mueller-Hinton agar to create a lawn, and discs impregnated with the drugs to be tested are placed on the lawn. The plates are incubated 18 to 24 hours, and the diameter of the zone of inhibition, or the area where bacteria do not grow, is measured. Zone size correlates with susceptibility (Fig. 27-4). The advantages of the Kirby-Bauer method are ease, little need for specialized equipment, and the different drugs used in testing can be changed readily. Disadvantages are that some bacteria grow poorly or not at all on the media, and the minimum inhibitory concentration (MIC) cannot be determined.

When broth microdilution methodology is used, a set concentration of bacteria is inoculated into each well of a 96-well plate containing an antimicrobial drug. A number of drugs can be tested on each plate at the discretion of the laboratory or plate manufacturer. Each drug is tested at several different concentrations; twofold dilutions are centered around the plasma levels expected in the patient when the drug is administered at recommended dosages. The plate is incubated 18 to 24 hours, and each well is examined for growth. Growth in a well indicates that the bacterium is not sensitive to the drug at that concentration. The lowest drug concentration at which there is no growth is considered the MIC (Fig. 27-5). The MIC will be unique for that particular isolate.

Interpretation

The CLSI establishes interpretation of antimicrobial sensitivity testing as sensitive, intermediate, or resistant, based on either the diameter of the zone of inhibition or the MIC. In the broth microdilution method, a "breakpoint," or the highest concentration of drug at which the bacterium would be considered susceptible, is used. The interpretations have been established using in vitro testing and in vivo clinical responses to the antimicrobial drug at corresponding concentrations. When an MIC is determined, a drug with an MIC greater than the breakpoint concentration is considered resistant and this drug is unlikely to be effective in vitro against the bacterium tested. The "sensitive" interpretation indicates that the drug is expected to be effective against the tested bacterium at label or recommended dosages. An "intermediate" interpretation suggests that for drugs that have flexibility in the dosage range, the drug could be effective at the higher recommended dosages and/or frequencies. The standards do not indicate the ability to penetrate to the site of infection or conditions found at the site. In several cases the predicted sensitivity in vitro does not correspond to clinical efficacy, particularly when the organism is intracellular or within a body compartment that is difficult to penetrate such as the central nervous system.

Serologic Diagnosis of Bacterial Diseases

Several bacterial (and fungal) infections can be diagnosed by detection of antibody specific to the pathogen. The presence of antibody indicates exposure to the bacterium or vaccination. Infection may have occurred in the past and been cleared or may be ongoing, depending on the organism and the test used. Serologic results must be interpreted in light of the clinical presentation, the prevalence of the organism in the geographic region, and the equine population at risk. Ideally, the serologic test will have little or no cross-reactivity with other bacteria, will be sensitive enough to detect low levels of antibody, and will be highly repeatable. The organism should not be part of the normal flora or one to which horses are regularly exposed; a positive result could merely indicate exposure, and many horses would have a positive result. Quantitative serologic tests (e.g., ELISA) can be helpful to follow the course of infection where rising antibody levels indicate recent exposure or infection.

Serologic testing is most useful to diagnose disease caused by bacteria that are difficult or impossible to isolate such as *Leptospira* spp. (see Chapter 32), *Lawsonia intracellularis* (see Chapter 34), *Anaplasma phagocytophilum* (see Chapter 39), *Neorickettsia risticii* (see Chapter 46), and *Borrelia burgdorferi* (see Chapter 33). Additional conditions that indicate use of serology include infections for which it is difficult or impossible

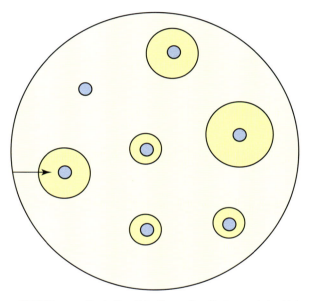

Figure 27-4 Diagram illustrating Kirby-Bauer disc dilution antimicrobial susceptibility testing. *Arrow* indicates zone of inhibition.

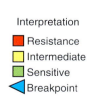

Interpretation

■ Resistance
■ Intermediate
■ Sensitive
◄ Breakpoint

Figure 27-5 Broth microdilution antimicrobial susceptibility testing. Drug concentrations of ampicillin are indicated in micrograms per milliliter (μg/mL). *Arrowhead* indicates the "breakpoint," or the highest concentration at which the bacterial minimum inhibitory concentration (MIC) is interpreted as sensitive. Growth in wells is seen as a dark pellet. Growth above the breakpoint would indicate resistance to the drug. Minimum inhibitory concentration for ampicillin for this bacterium would be 16 μg/mL and interpreted as "susceptible."

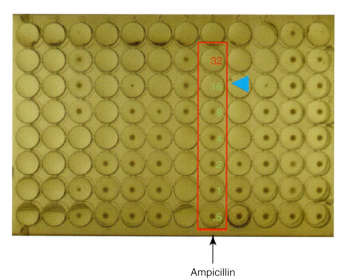

Ampicillin

to obtain a sample, as in horses with a suspected abdominal abscess.

Interpretation of a positive serologic test can be difficult because a positive test could mean that the horse was only exposed to the pathogen or vaccinated and does not have an active infection. A commercially available diagnostic ELISA detects immunoglobulin G (IgG) to the M protein of *Streptococcus equi* subsp. *equi* infection (see Chapter 28). Detection of IgM specific for the targeted organism aids interpretation because IgM is an immunoglobulin synthesized in the acute active stages of disease.

Blood should be collected in a serum (red-top) tube and allowed to clot fully. Subsequently, the sample should be centrifuged shortly after collection and the serum removed and transferred to a new sterile tube to avoid contamination with bacteria. Blood stored on the clot for prolonged periods may hemolyze, which can interfere with some serologic tests. If the sample will not be used within a few days, it should be stored frozen to preserve antibody integrity.

The complete reference list is available online at www.expertconsult.com.

CHAPTER

28

Streptococcal Infections

Andrew Stephen Waller, Debra C. Sellon,* Corinne R. Sweeney,*
Peter J. Timoney,* J. Richard Newton,* and Melissa T. Hines*

Overview

Debra C. Sellon

The streptococci are gram-positive, catalase-negative, facultative anaerobic, coccoid, or ovoid bacteria. The numerous species of streptococci may be described on the basis of the nature and extent of their hemolytic activity as alpha-hemolytic (α-hemolytic), beta-hemolytic (β-hemolytic), and nonhemolytic species (Fig. 28-1). Many of the most significant streptococcal pathogens in human and veterinary medicine are β-hemolytic, producing complete clearing of blood agar medium because of lysis of erythrocytes in the media. In α-hemolytic reactions, erythrocytes are not completely lysed, and growth is surrounded by greenish color of the agar resulting from streptococcal action on hemoglobin (see Chapter 27). Nonhemolytic streptococcal species have no effect on blood agar.[1]

In 1928 an American bacteriologist, Rebecca Lancefield, published a study of the chemical composition and antigenicity of hemolytic streptococci. In 1933 she described a classification of streptococci into groups according to their ability to induce production of antibodies that cause precipitation of streptococci from solution. These groups are now known as the *Lancefield groups*. The Lancefield group A streptococci, most notably *Streptococcus pyogenes*, are important streptococci in human medicine; in contrast, the group C streptococci *Streptococcus equi* subsp. *zooepidemicus* and *S. equi* subsp. *equi* assume greater importance in equine medicine. Although the Lancefield groupings remain phenotypically useful, it is now known that unrelated species of β-hemolytic streptococci may produce identical Lancefield antigens and that strains that are genetically related at the species level may have heterogenous Lancefield antigens.[1] Molecular analysis of streptococcal organisms have revealed that the bacteria formerly classified as group D streptococci, or enterococci, are better classified in the separate genus *Enterococcus* (see Chapter 45) and the group N streptococci, or lactococci, should be classified in the genus *Lactococcus*.

This chapter discusses individually the major streptococcal pathogens of horses, including *S. equi* subsp. *equi*, *S. equi* subsp. *zooepidemicus*, and *S. pneumoniae*. A variety of other streptococcal infections have been described in horses as nonspecific commensal organisms or sporadic etiologic agents of disease. Notable among these reports for the severity of associated disease, streptococcal toxic shock was reported in a horse in which *Streptococcus mitis* was cultured from the blood.[2]

Streptococcus equi Subsp. *equi*

*Corinne R. Sweeney, Peter J. Timoney, J. Richard Newton,
and Melissa T. Hines**

Disease caused by *S. equi* subsp. *equi* infection in horses, commonly referred to as "strangles," was described in early veterinary science literature and first reported by Jordanus Ruffus in 1251. Although its official name is *S. equi* subsp *equi*, there is compelling evidence that it is derived from an ancestral *S. zooepidemicus* as a "genovar" or "biovar" of the latter.[1-3] In particular, comparison of the completed *S. equi* strain 4047 and *S. zooepidemicus* strain H70 genomes highlight gene loss and gain events that shed light on the evolution of this host-restricted pathogen from an ancestral *S. equi* subsp. *zooepidemicus* strain.[1] However, the descriptive terms *S. equi* and *S. zooepidemicus* are still appropriate based on their ability to cause distinct infectious diseases and are used in this discussion.

Etiology

Streptococcus equi is a gram-positive coccoid bacterium that typically appears in pairs or chains. Colonies on blood agar plates are often (but not always) mucoid, honey colored, and surrounded by a wide zone of beta hemolysis. Its colony morphology can be identical to that of *S. zooepidemicus* (see later

*The authors acknowledge and appreciate the original contributions of these authors, whose work has been incorporated into this chapter.

*Modified from Sweeney CR, Timoney JF, Newton R, Hines MT: *Streptococcus equi* infections in horses: guidelines for treatment, control and prevention of strangles. J Vet Intern Med 19:123–124, 2005.

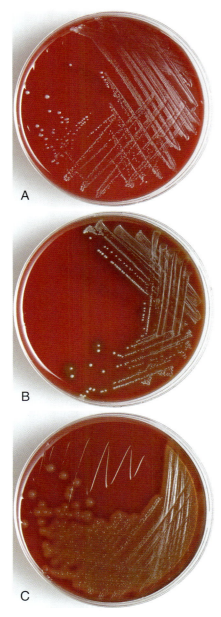

Figure 28-1 Cultures of streptococci on blood agar. **A,** Nonhemolytic streptococci; note the absence of a zone of hemolysis around the colonies. **B,** Alphahemolytic streptococci; note the greenish discoloration because of partial hemolysis. **C,** Beta-hemolytic streptococci; note the complete zone of hemolysis and clearing of agar around the bacterial colonies.

bacteria can be traced, at least hypothetically, to specific lesions within the DNA of *S. equi*, which serve to reduce its ancestral properties and increase its ability to cause rapid abscessation of lymph nodes.[1]

The *S. equi* genome encodes 29 known or putative cell surface proteins that are identified by the presence of a specific LPXTG motif, which is processed by sortase enzymes that attach the C-terminal end of the protein to the peptidoglycan cell wall.[1] *S. zooepidemicus* strains encode additional sortase-processed cell surface proteins; strain H70 encodes 39. These include the FimII, FimIII, and FimIV pilus loci.[1,8] Pili are hair-like projections from the bacterial surface, which are thought to play an important role in the adherence of streptococci to host tissues.[9,10] The reduced complement of pili and other sortase-processed proteins on the surface of *S. equi* may limit the variety of host tissues to which *S. equi* can attach, thus restricting the number of niches that it can occupy.

Surface proteins can also play an important role in immunoevasion. The sortase-processed M proteins of streptococci are antiphagocytic, acid-resistant fibrillar molecules that project from the cell wall surface in an arrangement whereby two identical molecules are coiled around each other.[11] The M protein of *S. equi* (SeM) is approximately 58 kilodaltons. The C-terminal two-thirds of SeM is predicted to have an alpha-helical coiled-coil structure and shares close sequence similarity with SzM of *S. zooepidemicus*,[12] whereas the N-terminal third is predicted to possess noncoiled-coil single strands and is unique to *S. equi*.[13] Its antiphagocytic action is a result of binding fibrinogen to the N-terminal half of the molecule and immunoglobulin G4 (IgG4) and IgG7 subclasses to the central region.[14-17] This interaction masks C3b-binding sites on the surface of the bacteria and inhibits the alternative C3 and classic C5 convertases.[18] The N-terminal portion of SeM is highly diverse,[12,19-22] with 114 different SeM types identified to date (http://pubmlst.org/perl/mlstdbnet/agdbnet.pl?file=sz_seM.xml [last accessed 24 January 2012]). The variable region may also be deleted in isolates recovered from the guttural pouches of persistently infected carriers,[23] although these strains remain virulent in horses (Chanter et al, unpublished data).

Differentiation of *S. equi* from *S. zooepidemicus* through its lack of fermentation of ribose, lactose, and sorbitol[4] may also have consequences on the properties of *S. equi*. Carbohydrate metabolism in streptococci plays an important role in colonization of mucosal surfaces.[24] Specialization of *S. equi* has probably rendered these pathways redundant, resulting in their loss.[1]

S. equi lacks a phage-resistance system encoded by a clustered regularly interspaced short palindromic repeat (CRISPR) locus.[1,25,26] In support of this increased vulnerability to phage attack, the SeP9 bacteriophage is lysogenic in *S. equi* but does not replicate in *S. zooepidemicus*.[27] Consequently, *S. equi* is thought to survive phage attack by incorporating phage DNA into its own genome, thereby becoming lysogenic. The *S. equi* strain 4047 genome contains four different prophage (φSeq1 to φSeq4), which may each contribute to the adaptation of *S. equi* to its unique pathogenic niche.[1]

The φSeq1 prophage does not encode any obvious virulence factor, but does lysogenize and has been proposed to kill susceptible bacteria, which may impede attachment of *S. equi* and its invasion of the lymphatic system. Such a mechanism is also seen in a lysogen of *Salmonella enterica* serovar Typhimurium, which releases low titers of phage that lysed competing nonlysogenic strains.[28] Alternatively, emerging genome data suggest that *S. equi* strains contain a diverse array of prophage at this genome location, raising the possibility that the uptake of phage DNA at this position may serve as a phage resistance mechanism and that these differences may partly explain differences in the virulence or behavior of individual *S. equi* strains (Harris et al, unpublished data).

discussion), and so it is often differentiated by its inability to ferment lactose and sorbitol.[4] However, it should be noted that some strains of *S. zooepidemicus* also fail to ferment these sugars,[1] thus deoxyribonucleic acid (DNA)-based tests that differentiate *S. equi* from *S. zooepidemicus* based on DNA restricted to *S. equi* can offer a more sensitive and potentially more robust means of diagnosis.[5]

S. zooepidemicus and *S. equi* usually infect horses by entering the nose or mouth. *S. zooepidemicus* then colonizes the mucosal surface and tonsillar tissues of the nasopharynx. In contrast, *S. equi* does not colonize the nasopharynx and is often not detected by nasopharyngeal swabs or washes taken 24 hours postinfection. Interestingly, unlike *S. zooepidemicus*, *S. equi* does not persist in the tonsil and only rarely infects other animals,[6] including humans.[7] The differences in the behavior of these

The φSeq2 prophage encodes a putative phospholipase A$_2$ with 98% predicted amino acid (aa) sequence identity with SlaA, of *S. pyogenes* M3 strain MGAS315. SlaA acquisition by *S. pyogenes* has been associated with increased morbidity and mortality in humans.[29] Deletion of *slaA* reduced colonization in an upper respiratory tract macaque model of pharyngitis and reduced virulence in a mouse intraperitoneal infection model.[30] The *slaA* gene is present in around a third of *S. zooepidemicus* strains, suggesting that this toxin may also be important to this opportunistic pathogen.[1] Furthermore, the gene encoding a second putative phospholipase A$_2$ toxin, SlaB, was present in all strains of *S. equi* and *S. zooepidemicus* examined.[1] However, the precise contribution of these toxins to both *S. equi* and *S. zooepidemicus* virulence remains unknown.

The φSeq3 and φSeq4 prophage encode four bacterial superantigens (SeeL and SeeM encoded on φSeq3 and SeeH and SeeI encoded on φSeq4), which share homology with the superantigens of *S. pyogenes* and may have even been exchanged between these two bacterial species.[1,31-34] Superantigens are potent immunostimulatory molecules that disrupt host immune responses through their ability to bypass the conventional mechanism of MHC-restricted antigen presentation.[35-37] SeeI, SeeL, and SeeM of *S. equi* have been shown to stimulate proliferation of equine peripheral blood mononucleated cells (PBMC) in vitro.[31,34,38] Furthermore, a febrile response in ponies was elicited by SeeI but not by SeeH.[31] The presence of three *S. zooepidemicus* superantigen-encoding genes (*szeF, szeN,* and *szeP*) was significantly higher in isolates from non-strangles lymph node abscesses,[39] suggesting that superantigens play an important role in the ability of these isolates to cause disease in lymph nodes. Interestingly, because superantigens exert their effects through binding to major histocompatibility complex (MHC) class II and T-cell receptors (TCR) molecules, differences in the amino acid sequences between individual horses may influence the magnitude of the resultant superantigen-effects and the subsequent severity of disease. Human leukocyte antigen (HLA) class II polymorphisms are known to influence the nature of T-cell responses to *S. pyogenes* superantigens[40] and the risk of severe streptococcal infection in humans.[41] The recently sequenced equine genome will provide the opportunity to identify equine MHC class II molecules recognized by *S. equi* sAgs and quantify the risks associated with the production of particular alleles thereof.[42]

In common with many other pathogenic bacteria, *S. equi* produces a hyaluronic acid capsule that mimics the molecule in vertebrate tissue and shields the bacterium from immune recognition.[43] It appears that strains producing different levels of capsule in vitro retain the same ability to infect horses,[44] either because the multitude of antiphagocytic mechanisms exploited by *S. equi* confer a level of redundancy or because other factors expressed by strains may compensate. *S. equi* encodes and produces a nonsecreted hyaluronate lyase on φSeq4 with low activity[45] but lacks a functional copy of the genome-encoded hyaluronate lyase,[1] whose orthologs have a broader substrate range and greater activity.[46] Reduced hyaluronic acid and chondroitin turnover may explain why *S. equi* infection rarely spreads beyond the lymphatic system and why the majority of horses recover from strangles despite possessing extremely high bacterial loads during the acute phase of disease.

S. equi also produces an array of additional virulence factors, including the β-hemolytic toxin streptolysin S,[47] those that bind factor H[48] and cleave immunoglobulin[49,50] or interleukin 8 (IL-8) and other CXC chemokines.[51,52] However, the acquisition of an iron-uptake system, the equibactin locus, has been proposed to represent the speciation event in the evolution of *S. equi* from an ancestral *S. zooepidemicus* strain.[1] The acquisition of iron is an essential process for all pathogenic bacteria.[53] The equibactin locus encoded on ICESe2 is absent from all *S.*

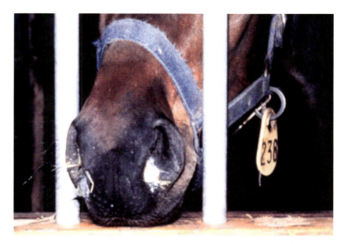

Figure 28-2 Purulent nasal discharge in horse with strangles.

zooepidemicus strains examined to date.[1] The locus encodes a nonribosomal peptide synthesis (NRPS) system resembling the yersiniabactin system of *Yersinia pestis*,[54] the causative agent of bubonic plague, typified by lymph node abscessation, in humans.[55]

Epidemiology

Transmission

Purulent discharges from horses with active and recovering strangles are an important and easily recognizable source of new *S. equi* infections among susceptible horses (Fig. 28-2). Transmission of infection occurs when there is either direct or indirect transfer of *S. equi* within these purulent discharges between affected and susceptible horses. Direct transmission refers to horse-to-horse contacts, particularly through normal equine social behavior involving mutual head contact. Indirect transmission occurs through the sharing of contaminated housing, water sources, feed or feeding utensils, twitches, tack, and other less obvious fomites, such as the clothing and equipment of handlers, caretakers, farriers, and veterinarians, unless appropriate barrier precautions are in place to prevent spread of *S. equi*.

Inapparent Carrier Horses

Transmission of *S. equi* that originates from outwardly healthy animals incubating the disease or that are inapparent persistently infected carriers of the organism plays a significant role in the establishment of new outbreaks.[56-59] Abscesses in the retropharyngeal lymph nodes rupture into the guttural pouches and drain via the nasal passages (Fig. 28-3). However, in a proportion of cases (approximately 10%), incomplete drainage leads to drying and hardening of purulent material, which forms chondroids that contain and maintain viable populations of *S. equi* (Fig. 28-4). Evidence indicates that some horses continue to harbor *S. equi* in chondroids within their guttural pouches, or within their sinuses for up to and possibly over 5 years after clinical signs have resolved. *S. equi* is shed intermittently from these reservoirs, draining via the nose into drinking water, feed troughs, and onto other fomites as described. In this situation the source of infection may not be readily apparent, and clinical signs may appear unexpectedly in animals with close contact to these carriers or in naïve new arrivals onto premises with endemic subclinical infection.[56-59] Introductions of persistently infected carriers into herds may be a source of new outbreaks, even in well-managed groups of horses. Adequate control for strangles cannot be achieved without recognition of this category of animal and implementation of appropriate methods for their detection and treatment.

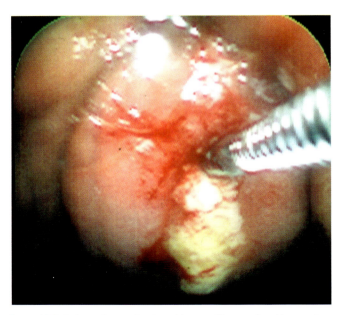

Figure 28-3 Endoscopic examination of horse with strangles. Abscessed retropharyngeal node has ruptured into the guttural pouch after being touched by the endoscopic biopsy instrument.

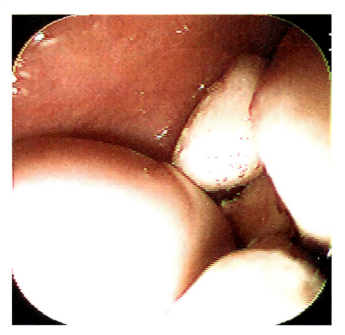

Figure 28-4 Endoscopic examination of guttural pouch of horse with chondroids.

Environmental Persistence of *S. equi*

S. equi does not persist for long in the environment, surviving for less than 1 to 3 days on wood, metal, or rubber surfaces and for only 1 or 2 days on these surfaces if the weather was sunny.[60] This lack of environmental persistence highlights the importance of acutely and persistently infected horses in the long-term persistence and transmission of *S. equi*.

Pathogenesis

S. equi enters through the mouth or nose and attaches to cells in the crypt of the lingual and palatine tonsils, as well as to the follicular-associated epithelium of the pharyngeal and tubal tonsils. A few hours after infection, the organism is difficult to detect on the mucosal surface but is visible within cells of the epithelium and subepithelial follicles. Translocation occurs in a few hours to the mandibular and suprapharyngeal lymph nodes that drain the pharyngeal and tonsil region.[61] Failure of neutrophils to phagocytose and kill the streptococci appears to be caused by a combination of the hyaluronic acid capsule, antiphagocytic SeM protein, and the many other antiphagocytic factors released by the organism.[62] This culminates in the accumulation of many extracellular streptococci in the form of long chains surrounded by large numbers of degenerating neutrophils. Bacterial enzymes, such as streptolysin and streptokinase, may contribute to abscess formation by damaging cell membranes and activating plasminogen. Superantigens and equibactin may also play an important role by misdirecting the immune response in a less potent direction and enhancing iron acquisition.

Although strangles predominantly involves the upper airways, including the guttural pouches and associated lymph nodes, metastasis to other locations occasionally occurs. Spread may be hematogenous or through lymphatic channels, which results in abscesses in lymph nodes and other organs of the thorax and abdomen. This form of the disease has been known as "bastard strangles." Bacteremia occurs on days 6 to 12 in horses inoculated intranasally with virulent *S. equi*.[63]

The first clinical sign of infection is a rapid increase in rectal temperature to 103° F (39.4° C) or higher, generally between 3 and 14 days after exposure. In addition, blood fibrinogen concentrations and white blood cell and neutrophil counts increase. Abscess development is rapid and often accompanied by lymph accumulation in afferent lymphatics. However, nasal shedding of *S. equi* usually begins after a latent period of 4 to 14 days and ceases between 3 and 7 weeks after resolution of the acute phase of disease,[5,64] providing an opportunity to separate recently infected from noninfected horses before they have the opportunity to transmit *S. equi*. Intermittent shedding persists beyond this period in some horses, and these persistently infected carriers may harbor *S. equi* in their guttural pouches or other areas of the upper respiratory tract for months or years.[56-59]

Approximately 75% of horses develop solid immunity to *S. equi* after recovery from infection.[65] The other 25% of infected horses are susceptible to reinfection within months, probably because of a failure to produce or maintain adequate concentrations of appropriate mucosal and systemic antibodies or through a natural increased susceptibility. Strong anti-*S. equi*-specific antibody responses occur after infection in most horses. Older horses with residual immunity have limited susceptibility to *S. equi* and often develop a mild form of strangles termed "*catarrhal strangles*."[5] However, despite the lack of classic clinical signs of strangles, these horses will shed virulent *S. equi* in nasal secretions in sufficient numbers to be a serious threat of transmission of disease to young or naïve horses.

Colostrum from mares that have recovered from strangles contains IgGb and IgA, with specificities similar to those found in the nasopharyngeal mucus of convalescent horses.[66] These antibodies recirculate to the nasopharyngeal mucosa after a foal ingests colostrum and provide resistance to infection until approximately the time of weaning.

Although it was widely believed that the SeM protein is a major protective antigen, it is clear that other antigens are also important. A recombinant protein-based vaccine that did not include SeM protected horses against subsequent experimental challenge with virulent bacteria.[67] Several aspects of *S. equi* pathogenesis are important to consider in the design and implementation of strangles control programs (Box 28-1).

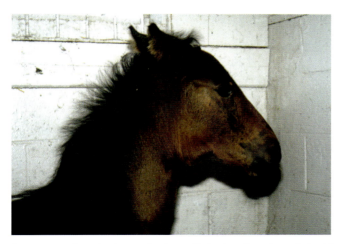

Figure 28-5 Enlarged, abscessed submandibular lymph node in foal with strangles.

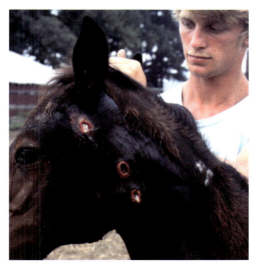

Figure 28-6 Multiple rupture sites of abscessed retropharyngeal and submandibular lymph nodes in foal with strangles.

Box 28-1 Aspects of Pathogenesis Important in Control and Prevention of Strangles

- Shedding does not begin until 1 or 2 days after onset of pyrexia. New cases can therefore be isolated before they transmit infection.
- Nasal shedding persists for 2 to 3 weeks in most animals. Persistent guttural pouch infection may result in intermittent shedding for years.
- Field and experimental data support the conclusion that disease severity depends on challenge load and duration.

Clinical Findings

Strangles is characterized by abrupt onset of fever followed by upper respiratory tract catarrh, as evidenced by mucopurulent nasal discharge (see Fig. 28-2) and acute swelling, with subsequent abscess formation in submandibular and retropharyngeal lymph nodes (Fig. 28-5). The term *strangles* was coined because affected horses sometimes were suffocated by enlarged lymph nodes that obstructed the airway. Severity of disease varies greatly depending on the immune status of the animal. Older horses often exhibit a milder form of the disease characterized by nasal discharge, small abscesses, and rapid resolution of disease, whereas younger horses are more likely to develop severe lymph node abscesses that subsequently open and drain (Fig. 28-6).

Fever is the first clinical sign and persists as lymphadenopathy develops and abscesses mature. Pharyngitis causes dysphagia, and affected animals may become anorexic or reluctant to eat and often stand with the neck extended. Attempts to swallow food and water may be followed by reflux of these substances from the nares. Depression and listlessness are common signs. Pharyngitis, laryngitis, and rhinitis may occur and contribute to bilateral nasal discharge, which is serous initially and rapidly becomes mucopurulent and then purulent, profuse, and tenacious. Accumulation of purulent exudates may cause a snuffling or rattling upper respiratory sound. Nasal and ocular mucosae may become hyperemic, and there may be purulent ocular discharge from which *S. equi* might be isolated.

Lymphadenopathy is a major clinical sign (see Figs. 28-5 and 28-6). The submandibular and retropharyngeal lymph nodes are involved with about equal frequency in *S. equi* infections and become swollen and painful about 1 week after infection. The first sign of lymphadenopathy is often hot, diffuse, painful edema. Serum may then ooze from the overlying skin for several days, as the lymph node abscesses mature before rupturing to drain tenacious creamy pus, which does not have a foul odor. Other lymph nodes of the rostral neck (parotid, cranial cervical, and retropharyngeal) are also frequently involved and may abscess. Retropharyngeal lymph nodes may drain into and cause empyema of the guttural pouch. Natural drainage of these deeper abscesses to the skin may take several days or weeks, and the swelling can exert pressure on the pharynx, larynx, trachea, and esophagus, causing severe dyspnea, stridor, and dysphagia. Retropharyngeal lymph node abscessation is not always associated with swelling that can be appreciated externally. Periorbital abscesses can cause marked swelling of the eyelids. Abscesses of the lymph nodes at the thoracic inlet can cause severe tracheal compression, asphyxia, and death. Coughing is not a significant feature in most cases, although some horses develop a soft, moist cough that becomes more productive and increasingly severe as the disease progresses. Squeezing the larynx will often cause marked pain, stridor, and gagging, followed by a retching cough and extended neck position when the neck is released. Expulsion of large quantities of pus from the nose or mouth with coughing usually indicates empyema of the guttural pouch.

Manifestations Associated with Severe Lymph Node Enlargement

Abscessation, particularly of the retropharyngeal lymph nodes, may result in obstruction of the upper respiratory tract. The enlarged lymph nodes may compress the pharynx, larynx, or trachea, necessitating a tracheostomy in severe cases (Fig. 28-7). Temporary laryngeal hemiplegia, resulting from damage to the recurrent laryngeal nerve from enlargement of either the retropharyngeal or the anterior cervical lymph nodes, may also contribute to dyspnea. Four of 15 horses with complicated strangles had upper respiratory tract obstruction requiring tracheostomy, and death was attributed to the obstruction in two of these horses.[68] Dysphagia may also occur as a result of lymph node enlargement or guttural pouch empyema.

Complications Associated with Metastatic Spread of Infection

Internal Infection

Approximately 20% of horses with strangles experience some type of complication, and the presence of complications greatly

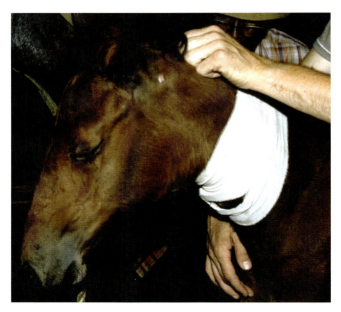

Figure 28-7 Temporary tracheostomy in midcervical region of foal with strangles. The tracheostomy alleviated the severe dyspnea associated with strangles in this foal. The tracheostomy tube and the site of insertion must be cleaned twice daily to keep the airway free of purulent debris.

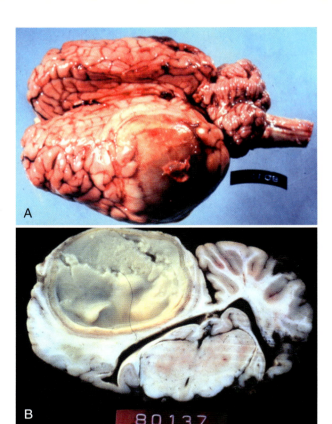

Figure 28-8 **A** and **B,** Cerebral abscess caused by S. *equi* infection in yearling Arabian colt.

increases the case-fatality rate.[68] Of 74 horses with strangles on a 235 horse farm, 15 (20.3%) had complications; case-fatality rate in horses with complications was 40% compared with an overall case-fatality rate of 8.1%.[68] Complications with strangles include spread of infection to parts of the body other than the head and neck, immune-mediated processes, and agalactia in mares.[5]

S. equi may potentially infect any anatomic site. The term *bastard strangles* is often used to describe metastatic abscessation. The organism may spread hematogenously, through lymphatic migration or close association with a septic focus, as when connecting structures (e.g., cranial nerves) allow transport of the organism or when there is direct aspiration of purulent material. Common sites of infection include the lung, mesentery, liver, spleen, kidneys, and brain. Respiratory distress may be caused by tracheal compression resulting from enlargement of the cranial mediastinal lymph nodes. Suppurative bronchopneumonia is an important sequela of strangles. Of 15 horses with complications associated with strangles, 5 had pneumonia or pleuropneumonia, and 3 of 5 deaths were attributed to pneumonia, making this the most common complication resulting in death.[68,69] Another important complication of strangles is extension of infection to the sinuses or guttural pouches.[57,59,68] In a general study of guttural pouch empyema, *S. equi* was isolated in 14 of 44 horses, and 5 of 74 horses with strangles had guttural pouch disease.[69] Infection of the guttural pouch is of particular importance because the guttural pouch is the most common site for prolonged carriage of the organism.[59,70] Horses with infection in the sinuses may also become carriers.

Other reported conditions associated with *S. equi* infection include myocarditis, endocarditis, panophthalmitis, periorbital abscesses, ulcerative keratitis, paravertebral abscesses, cerebral abscesses, septic arthritis, and tenosynovitis.

The prevalence of metastatic abscessation is generally low. However, in a recent study in which outbreaks of strangles on two farms were investigated, 7 of 25 (28%) developed metastatic abscessation.[5,71] Of these, euthanasia was performed in five horses, four of which had neurologic signs and confirmed

cerebral abscesses (Fig. 28-8). The reason for the high incidence of complications, particularly neurologic disease, on these farms is unclear, but possible theories include a high infectious dose, the virulence of the strains involved, differences in host susceptibility, and other, unidentified factors.

The diagnosis and treatment of metastatic *S. equi* infections may be more difficult than for uncomplicated strangles. The specific means of diagnosis vary depending on the site of infection and whether there are concurrent signs of classic strangles. For infections, such as bronchopneumonia, guttural pouch empyema, and sinusitis, appropriate samples can be collected for culture.

Diagnosis of internal abscesses is often difficult. A history of exposure to *S. equi* and laboratory results consistent with chronic infection, anemia, low-grade fever responsive to penicillin, hyperfibrinogenemia, and hyperglobulinemia are supportive of the diagnosis of metastatic abscessation. Treatment of *S. equi* infection that has spread requires long-term antimicrobial therapy and appropriate local treatment or drainage of abscesses, if possible.

It has been suggested that antimicrobial treatment after development of an abscess might contribute to metastasis, based on the theory that protein synthesis by the organism is altered by antimicrobial treatment. Further, a reduced immunogen level results in suboptimal immune response. Currently, no experimental infections or clinical data support the theory that antimicrobial treatment increases the prevalence of bastard strangles. In the study by Spoormakers et al,[71] antibiotics were not used in any of the cases before complications were identified, yet the incidence of significant complications was high, and it is known that metastatic infection has occurred in other outbreaks where antibiotics have not been used.

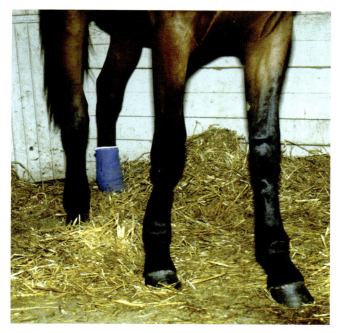

Figure 28-9 Marked edema of all four distal limbs in yearling Standardbred with purpura hemorrhagica secondary to recent *S. equi* infection.

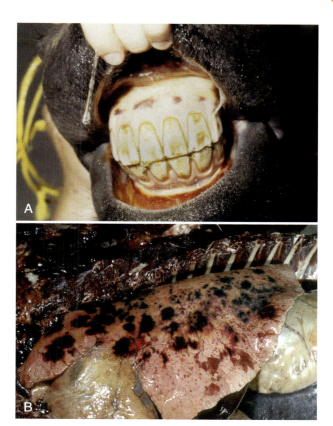

Figure 28-10 A, Petechial hemorrhages of oral mucous membranes in horse with purpura hemorrhagica. **B,** Hemorrhages on surface of lungs in horse with purpura hemorrhagica.

Immune-Mediated Complications

Purpura Hemorrhagica

Purpura hemorrhagica is an aseptic necrotizing vasculitis characterized primarily by subcutaneous edema, most frequently involving the head, limbs, and trunk (Fig. 28-9), and petechiation and ecchymoses of the mucous membranes (Fig. 28-10). Severe edema may result in oozing from the skin surfaces, and sloughing of the skin may occur (Fig. 28-11). In some horses the vasculitis may affect other sites, such as the gastrointestinal (GI) tract, lungs, and muscle, resulting in signs that include colic, respiratory difficulties, and muscle soreness. Leukocytoclastic vasculitis on histologic examination of skin is consistent with a diagnosis of purpura hemorrhagica. In those cases associated with *S. equi* infection, isolation of the organism and demonstration of elevated IgA and IgG titers to *S. equi* are also supportive.

Corticosteroids are the primary treatment for purpura. Generally, dexamethasone at 0.1 to 0.2 mg/kg, followed by a tapering-dose regimen, is used. In those cases in which purpura is associated with active bacterial infection or the horse is considered at high risk of developing infection, appropriate antibiotic therapy is also indicated. Nonsteroidal antiinflammatory drugs (NSAIDs) may be of some benefit in some cases of purpura. Supportive care, including intravenous (IV) fluids, hydrotherapy, and bandaging, may also be indicated.

Although the exact pathogenesis of purpura hemorrhagica is not fully understood, it appears to be a vasculitis caused by the deposition of immune complexes in blood vessel walls. Purpura is often associated with *S. equi* infection but may also occur in response to a number of different antigens. Of 53 horses with purpura, 17 were exposed to or infected with *S. equi*, and 5 were vaccinated with *S. equi* M protein; the remaining 31 cases either were associated with other organisms or had no known cause.[72] One of the four horses with purpura was euthanized because of the severity of the skin necrosis.[68] Similarly, 3 of 22 horses with purpura secondary to exposure to *S. equi* did not survive.[72]

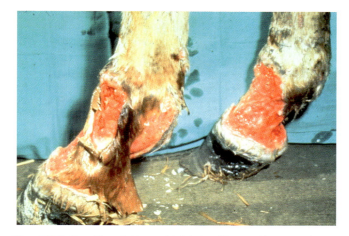

Figure 28-11 Sloughing of skin on distal limbs of horse with purpura hemorrhagica. *(Courtesy Dr. Warwick Bayly.)*

Myositis

Two types of myopathy—muscle infarction and rhabdomyolysis with progressive atrophy—have been documented in horses after exposure to *S. equi*.[73-75] These syndromes are presumed to be immune mediated, although through different mechanisms, and are most likely a manifestation of purpura hemorrhagica (Fig. 28-12). Many horses with purpura exhibit mild elevation in serum creatine kinase (CK) activity resulting from vasculitis within the muscle and mild muscle necrosis. Even with aggressive corticosteroid therapy and antibiotics, the prognosis is

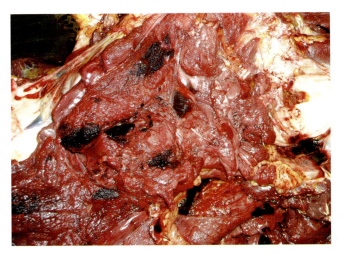

Figure 28-12 Infarcts in muscle of horse with *S. equi* myopathy. *(Courtesy Dr. Babetta Breuhaus.)*

Box 28-2 Nasal Wash Procedure for Diagnosis of *S. equi*

1. Prepare 50 mL of warm physiologic saline solution in a syringe.
2. Insert a 15-cm length of soft rubber tubing (5-6 mm in diameter) into the ventral nasal meatus to the level of the nasal canthus.
3. Inject the warm saline through the rubber tubing.
4. Collect the saline wash in a sterile specimen cup as it flows out of the nostril.
5. Submit the nasal washing as soon as possible to an appropriate diagnostic laboratory.

---

guarded. Affected horses should be treated with corticosteroids, and muscle mass may return to normal. If there are signs consistent with concurrent infection, antibiotics are also indicated.

Glomerulonephritis and Myocarditis

Streptococcal antigens have been suggested as a trigger for development of myocarditis and proliferative glomerulonephritis. In one horse with chronic renal failure, streptococcal antigens were documented in the diseased glomeruli, although this animal was infected with *S. zooepidemicus*.[76]

Agalactia

Agalactia has been reported in broodmares with strangles.[5] Infection of the mammary glands is possible, but the mammary glands are usually normal, and the agalactia is thought to be secondary to the fever, anorexia, and lethargy associated with infection. Although generally not life threatening, this complication may preclude mares from making adequate milk for their foals.

Diagnosis

Culture

Culture of nasal swabs, nasal washes, or pus aspirated from abscesses remains the "gold standard" for detection of *S. equi*. Specimens should be plated on Columbia colistin–nalidixic acid (CNA) agar with 5% sheep or horse blood added. The presence of other β-hemolytic streptococci, especially *S. zooepidemicus*, may confound interpretation of cultures. Unlike *S. equi*, most strains of *S. zooepidemicus* ferment sorbitol and lactose.

Nasal washes are more effective than swabs in detection of small numbers of *S. equi* because a greater surface area within the internal nares is sampled[77] (Box 28-2). However, culture

may be unsuccessful during the incubation and early clinical phases. *S. equi* is normally not present on the mucosa until 24 to 48 hours after the onset of fever; therefore horses monitored by daily rectal temperature measurements during an outbreak may be recognized early and isolated to limit transmission of *S. equi*.

Polymerase Chain Reaction

A polymerase chain reaction (PCR) assay is available to detect DNA specific to *S. equi* and offer an adjunct to culture.[77] The test can be completed in a few hours, so results may be available on the same day that samples are taken. However, PCR does not distinguish between dead and live organisms, thus care must be taken when sampling horses to note the order in which samples are taken because sterilized equipment may contain enough DNA to confound the results from subsequent horses. In addition, clinical samples that contain polymerase inhibitors or abundant *S. equi* may give negative PCR results, despite positive culture of *S. equi* from the same sample. PCR is approximately three times more sensitive than culture.[57,77]

PCR accompanying culture of a nasal swab or wash may be used in a control program to select animals for guttural pouch endoscopy.[57] In a clinical setting, especially with a farm facing endemic strangles or a sudden outbreak of strangles, PCR is useful to detect inapparent carrier horses, determine *S. equi* infection status before transport, determine *S. equi* infection status after transport before commingling, and determine the success of eliminating *S. equi* from the guttural pouch.

Serology

Fifteen or more surface exposed or secreted proteins of *S. equi* elicit strong serum antibody responses during infection and convalescence. The most reactive and best studied of these is SeM.[13] Proprietary enzyme-linked immunosorbent assays (ELISA) for measuring *S. equi*-specific antibody responses are commercially available (EBI, IDEXX, Lexington, KY and Animal Health Trust, Newmarket, UK[78]) and are useful for diagnosing recent (but not necessarily current) *S. equi* infection. The SeM assay used in the United States has also been used to determine the need for booster vaccination and to diagnose purpura hemorrhagica and metastatic abscesses (Table 28-1). However, these tests do not distinguish between responses to the available *S. equi* vaccines and natural infection. Comparison of titers obtained from sequential samples may provide an indication of exposure and infection status. Serum titers peak about 5 weeks after exposure and can remain high for over 6 months.

Clinicians should remember that considerable variation exists in the responses of individual horses when interpreting ELISA results. Horses at risk for development of purpura may be hyperresponders to SeM and make very strong antibody responses. Such animals, with SeM titers in excess of 1:3200, should never be vaccinated (J.F. Timoney, unpublished data).

Therapy

Appropriate treatment of horses with strangles usually depends on the stage and severity of the disease. Veterinary opinion on whether to use antibiotic treatment remains divided. However, most horses with strangles require no treatment other than proper rest and a dry, warm stall and provision of soft, moist, and palatable food of good quality while letting the disease run its course. Food and water should be easily accessible to the horse but not others.

Horses with Early Clinical Signs

During an outbreak, immediate antibiotic therapy of new cases in the early acute phase with fever and depression may be

Table 28-1 Interpretation of SeM-Specific ELISA

Result	Titer	Interpretation
Negative		No SeM-specific antibodies detected. This result may occur in a horse with no previous exposure to *S. equi* or vaccine or with recent exposure to *S. equi* (<7 days).
Weak positive	1:200-1:400	SeM-specific antibodies detected at a very low level. This is an equivocal result and may represent very recent or residual antibody from exposure to *S. equi* or vaccine in the remote past. Repeat testing is recommended in 7 to 14 days to confirm recent exposure.
Moderate positive	1:800-1:1600	SeM-specific antibodies detected at an intermediate level. This level may occur in a horse at 2 to 3 weeks after exposure or when the infection occurred 6 months to 2 years previously.
High positive	1:3200-1:6400	SeM-specific antibodies detected at a high level. High levels are found 4 to 12 weeks after infection or following vaccination: 1 to 2 weeks with injectable form or 2 to 4 weeks with intranasal form. Vaccination is contraindicated in horses with existing high levels of antibody (>1:1600).
Very high positive	>1:12,800	SeM-specific antibodies detected at a very high level. These levels are often found in horses with metastatic abscess or purpura hemorrhagica (immune-mediated vasculitis) after exposure to strangles vaccine or *S. equi*.

SeM, M protein of *S. equi*; *ELISA*, enzyme-linked immunosorbent assay.

curative and may prevent focal abscessation. Antibiotics should be given for 3 to 5 days. Experimental infected ponies treated with antibiotics at onset of fever usually do not develop lymph node abscessation because, at this early stage, the antibiotics have adequate access to the bacteria. Unfortunately, antibiotic treatment may inhibit synthesis of protective antigens and the development of protective immunity may not be stimulated.[79] Such horses remain susceptible to reinfection once treatment is discontinued if they are exposed to *S. equi*.

It has been argued on theoretic grounds that treatment of strangles with antibiotics is contraindicated because killing the organisms is indirectly affecting the development of immunity, thereby increasing the risk of bacteremia, septicemia, and metastatic abscessation. However, no experimental or clinical data exist to support such a phenomenon.

Horses with Lymph Node Abscessation

Once an external lymphadenopathy is detected in an otherwise alert and healthy horse, antibiotic therapy is probably contraindicated. Although it provides temporary clinical improvement in fever and lethargy, it only prolongs the inevitable enlargement and eventual rupture of lymph node abscesses. Antibiotics may suppress the bacteria within the lymph nodes sufficiently for a time, only to have a simmering infection flare and abscessation return when the antibiotics are discontinued.

Therapy should be directed toward enhancing maturation and drainage of the abscesses. Topical treatments such as ichthammol or a hot pack may be applied to promote maturation of the lymph node abscess, although objective controlled data supporting the use of these techniques are lacking. Surgical drainage of lymphadenopathies is sometimes indicated if abscesses do not rupture spontaneously; however, it is critical to wait until the abscess has matured and thinned out ventrally. Earlier surgical intervention may only result in minimal exudate drainage and continued lymph node swelling because the abscess has enough internal structure (honeycomb loculations) to block drainage through a single surgical incision. Daily flushing of the open abscess with a 3% to 5% povidone-iodine solution should be continued until the discharge ceases.

The use of NSAIDs, such as phenylbutazone or flunixin meglumine, may improve the horse's demeanor by reducing fever, pain, and inflammatory swelling at the site of the abscesses. This in turn may encourage eating and drinking. Consideration must be given to the complications seen after NSAID use in dehydrated and anorectic horses.

Even in the face of detectable lymphadenopathy, if the horse is febrile, depressed, anorexic, and especially manifesting dyspnea as a result of partial upper airway obstruction, antibiotic therapy is indicated to decrease abscess size and prevent complete airway obstruction. Rarely, affected horses may require intensive supportive therapy, including IV fluids, feeding by nasogastric tube, and tracheostomy (see Fig. 28-7). An animal requiring a tracheostomy should be given systemic antimicrobial drugs to prevent secondary bacterial infections of the lower respiratory tract.

Some clinicians believe that antibiotic therapy after abscesses have ruptured is indicated because it may hasten recovery, improve appetite, and reduce loss of body condition.

Horses with Complications

Horses that develop complications from strangles should receive appropriate symptomatic and supportive therapy, as previously discussed with the clinical findings associated with each type of complication.

Drugs of Choice for Therapy

Penicillin is generally considered the drug of choice for the treatment of nonpneumococcal streptococcal disease, with alternative drugs used depending on ease of administration or the site of infection. Other agents for therapy include cephalosporins and macrolides. Based on in vitro antimicrobial susceptibility testing, in which testing methods follow Clinical and Laboratory Standards Institute (CLSI) guidelines, the majority of *S. equi* isolates are susceptible to trimethoprim-sulfadiazine (TMS). However, this may or may not translate to in vivo efficacy.[80,81] *S. equi* is consistently sensitive to penicillin, which is thus considered the antibiotic of choice. Laboratories handling hundreds of *S. equi* strains have noted no emerging antibiotic resistance to penicillin by *S. equi* or *S. equi* subsp. *zooepidemicus*.[82] The incidence of resistance to most other drugs is low, with the exception of aminoglycoside resistance, including gentamicin, which is consistently observed.

Prevention

Vaccination

Most horses develop a solid immunity during recovery from strangles, which persists in more than 75% of animals for 5 years or longer.[83] This indicates that stimulation of a high level of immunity is biologically feasible given appropriate presentation of protective immunogen(s). The basis of acquired resistance to strangles is not understood but is believed to reside in part in antibodies to SeM and other immunogens unique to *S. equi* and may require both systemic and mucosal responses.

Earlier bacterin-type vaccines have been superseded (North America and Australia) by adjuvant extracts of *S. equi* prepared by hot acid or by mutanolysin plus detergent extraction. Hot acid cleaves and removes acid-resistant proteins, and carbohydrate mutanolysin (muramidase) hydrolyzes the bacterial cell wall, releasing intact surface proteins in the presence of detergent. Both types of vaccine contain the immunogenic SeM and are potent stimulators of an antibody response. However, the efficacy of extract vaccines has been disappointing, with little published data to support significant protection. One study suggested a reduction in the clinical attack rate of 50% in vaccinates a few weeks after the final booster.[84] Adverse reactions include soreness or abscesses at injection sites and occasional cases of purpura hemorrhagica.

An attenuated, nonencapsulated strain of *S. equi*, Pinnacle I.N. (Fort Dodge Animal Health, Fort Dodge, IA), with defects in carbohydrate utilization and designed to mimic the immunity provided through natural infection, stimulated a high level of immunity against experimental challenge.[77] This acapsular strain was derived following chemical mutagenesis to induce random mutations throughout the bacterial genome. Such nondefined point mutations are prone to back mutation and thus to reversion to full virulence and although this vaccine may protect up to 100% of horses,[85] it has not been licensed for sale in Europe due to safety concerns. These include nasal discharge, lymphadenitis, submandibular abscesses, and occasional purpura haemorrhagica following I.N. vaccination. Safety issues include residual virulence with formation of slowly developing mandibular abscesses in a small percentage of vaccinates, nasal discharge, and occasional cases of immune-mediated vasculitis (purpura). Because the vaccine contains live *S. equi*, accidental contamination of remote injection sites will result in abscess formation at these locations. Therefore, ideally, no other vaccinations are given concurrently or given before administration of the intranasal vaccine. Live vaccine should be administered only to healthy, nonfebrile animals free of nasal discharge and with no known contact with infected or exposed animals.

A live attenuated strain of *S. equi*, Equilis StrepE, has been approved for sale in Europe and marketed by Intervet. This strain was attenuated by the deletion of the *aroA* gene[12] and was 10^4-fold attenuated during intraperitoneal mouse challenge studies. Intramuscular vaccination of horses conferred 100% protection from subsequent *S. equi* challenge, but severe injection site reactions precluded the use of this route. However, submucosal vaccination with 10^9cfu into the inside of the upper lip was found to protect 50% to 100% of horses from the development of lymph node abscesses following intranasal *S. equi* challenge. Using this vaccination method, small pustules appeared at the site of injection from which the live vaccine strain could be isolated.[86] The presence of these pustules may be critical for the generation of an effective immune response since on dose reduction, reduced injection site reactions correlated with decreased protection.[86] The vaccine is limited by a short (3-month) duration of immunity, although boosting of horses vaccinated up to 6 months previously in the face of an outbreak has been shown to improve clinical outcome.

The administration of the Pinnacle I.N. or Equilis StrepE interferes with the culture, PCR, and ELISA diagnostic tests and may confound subsequent screening procedures. Furthermore, persistently infected carriers have a measurable anti-*S. equi* immune response and it is unlikely that vaccination will resolve their *S. equi* infection. Therefore horses vaccinated with live vaccines should always be treated as if they are potentially infectious to naïve animals.

Vaccination of mice with recombinant SeM was protective,[87] but these promising results were not repeated on vaccination and challenge of horses.[88] However, exploitation of the emerging *S. equi* genome sequence data identified several more *S. equi* proteins that conferred protection in a mouse infection model.[89,90] This work led to the identification of a combination of seven *S. equi* antigens that proved to be highly protective in

Welsh mountain ponies.[67] Such recombinant protein vaccines do not contain live *S. equi* and thus offer a reduced risk of adverse reactions and the ability to use normal screening (culture, PCR, and ELISA) strategies. These vaccines are not yet commercially available.

Quarantine and Bacteriologic Screening

Prevention of strangles through quarantining and screening is difficult to achieve without specific measures to reduce the risk of inadvertent introduction of *S. equi* infection through subclinical carriers. The owner, farm manager, or trainer should always be questioned as to the possible exposure of the animal to strangles. Prevention through quarantining and screening is further complicated where frequent moving and mixing of horses occur during the breeding season and at racetracks and where strangles outbreaks have not been appropriately investigated and controlled.

Wherever possible, animals being introduced to a new population of horses should be isolated for 3 weeks and screened for *S. equi* by repeated nasopharyngeal swabs or lavages (three samples taken at weekly intervals) or a single guttural pouch endoscopy and lavage. Samples should be tested for *S. equi* by both culture and PCR; animals testing positive should be kept in isolation for further investigation and treatment.

High standards of hygiene should also always be maintained to avoid indirect transmission between quarantined and resident horses. The use of specific quarantine equipment is recommended, and if dedicated staff are not available, quarantined horses should always be handled after the existing herd.

Control of Outbreaks

Outbreak Investigations

Investigation of strangles outbreaks should begin with an interview of horse owners to obtain a detailed history and to evaluate the potential extent of the disease problem. The review should identify affected groups of horses and allow the geography of the premises and the management practices to be assessed for further risks and future opportunities for disease control.

A practical disease control strategy should then be agreed on and implemented (Table 28-2). This strategy may need to be adapted to the individual circumstances of specific premises and outbreaks and can be summarized as follows:

- All movements of horses on and off the affected premises should be stopped and segregation and hygiene measures implemented immediately.
- Cases of strangles should be maintained in well-demarcated "dirty" or "red" (i.e., *S. equi*–positive) quarantine areas. Note that separation of cases from in-contacts is recommended to minimize the infectious dose received by these horses and the severity of any ensuing disease.
- Horses that have been in contact with cases should also be maintained in a separate well-demarcated "amber" area.
- Remaining unexposed horses to be managed by separate personnel in "green" areas.
- Rectal temperatures of all horses (always moving from "green" to "amber" to "red") should be taken at least once daily during an outbreak to detect, promptly segregate, and possibly treat new cases.
- The aim of the control strategy, after resolution of clinical signs and bacteriologic screening, is to move horses from the "red" to "green" areas where nonaffected and noninfectious horses are kept.
- Every precaution should be taken to ensure high hygiene standards throughout the premises for the duration of the outbreak. Regular disinfection of water troughs or buckets will minimize the infectious dose received by in-contacts.

Table 28-2 Goals and Associated Measures Used to Control Transmission of *S. equi* on Affected Premises

Goal	Measures
1. To prevent the spread of *S. equi* infection to horses on other premises and to new arrivals on the affected premises.	Stop all movement of horses on and off the affected premises immediately and until further notice. Horses with strangles and their contacts should be maintained in well-demarcated "dirty," "red," or "amber" (i.e., *S. equi*–positive) quarantine areas. Clustering of cases in groups should allow parts of the premises to be easily allocated as "dirty" and "clean" ("green") areas.
2. To establish whether convalescing horses are infectious 3 weeks after clinical recovery.	At least three nasopharyngeal swabs or lavages are taken at approximately weekly intervals from all recovered cases and their contacts and tested for *S. equi* by culture and polymerase chain reaction (PCR). Horses that are consistently negative are returned to the "clean" area.
3. Investigate all outwardly healthy horses in which *S. equi* is detected either by culture or PCR.	Endoscopy of the upper respiratory tract and guttural pouches.
4. To eliminate *S. equi* infection from the guttural pouches.	Healing of lesions through a combination of flushing and aspiration with saline and removal of chondroids using endoscopically guided instruments. Topical and systemic administration of antimicrobials to eliminate *S. equi* infection.
5. To prevent indirect cross-infection by *S. equi* from horses in the "dirty" area to those in the "clean" area of the premises.	Personnel should use dedicated protective clothing when dealing with infectious animals and should not deal simultaneously with susceptible animals. If this is unavoidable, infectious horses should be dealt with after susceptible animals ("green" to "amber" to "red"). Strict hygiene measures are introduced, including provision of dedicated clothing and equipment for each area, disinfection facilities for personnel, and thorough stable cleaning and disinfection methods. After removal of organic material from stables, all surfaces should be thoroughly soaked in an appropriate liquid disinfectant or steam-treated and allowed to dry. This should be repeated if possible. Manure and waste feed from infectious animals should be composted (inactivation of bacteria by heat) in an isolated location. Pastures used to hold infectious animals should be rested for 4 weeks. Care should be taken to disinfect water troughs at least once daily during an outbreak. Horse vans should be hosed clean and disinfected after each use.

- Screening of all incontact "amber" and unexposed "green" horses by ELISA is recommended to identify those horses that may have had subclinical infection or be persistently infected carriers that may predate the outbreak.
- Screening of all convalescing cases after clinical recovery and ELISA-positive healthy horses should be conducted using three consecutive swabs or lavages of the nasopharynx taken at weekly intervals, with special care taken to maintain good hygiene and avoid inadvertent transmission between horses during sampling.
- Swabs or lavage fluid should be tested for *S. equi* by conventional culture and PCR.
- Endoscopy of the upper respiratory tract and guttural pouches should be performed in all outwardly healthy horses in which *S. equi* is detected, either by culture or PCR. Lavage samples from guttural pouches should then be tested for *S. equi* by culture and PCR.
- Sites such as the cranial nasal sinuses or tonsils should be considered in horses that continue to harbor *S. equi* in the absence of pathology or infection of the guttural pouches.

Carriers with *S. equi* Infection of Guttural Pouches

Detection

Diagnosis of *S. equi* infection associated with guttural pouch empyema with or without chondroids following strangles is best achieved by direct visual assessment of both pouches using endoscopy. Cytologic assessment and culture and PCR for detection of *S. equi* in lavage samples collected by a sterile disposable catheter passed through the biopsy channel of the endoscope are recommended to accompany visual examination because infection and inflammation may be present in the absence of obvious and visible pathology. Diagnosis of guttural pouch empyema with or without chondroids may also be made by radiography of the guttural pouch area, although changes may not be visible in all cases.

Box 28-3 Gelatin-Penicillin to Treat *S. equi* Infection of Guttural Pouches

To make 50 mL of gelatin-penicillin solution:

1. Weigh out 2 g of gelatin (Sigma G-6650 or household grade), and add 40 mL of sterile water.
2. Heat or microwave to dissolve the gelatin.
3. Cool gelatin to 45° C to 50° C.
4. Add 10 mL of sterile water to 10 million units (10 megaunits) of sodium benzylpenicillin G.
5. Mix penicillin solution with the cooled gelatin to make a total volume of 50 mL.
6. Dispense into syringes, and leave overnight at 4° C to set.

S. equi may be cultured from lavages collected by direct percutaneous sampling of the pouch, although this is not recommended because of the high risk of injury to important anatomic structures in the region.

Treatment

Appropriate methods of treatment of guttural pouch empyema in individual horses depend on the consistency and volume of the material within the pouches. Repeated lavages of pus-filled pouches by rigid or indwelling catheters using isotonic saline or polyionic fluid, with subsequent lowering of the head to allow drainage or use of a suction pump attached to the endoscope, assist in the elimination of empyema. Sedation aids in implementation of the endoscopy and facilitates drainage of flush material from the guttural pouches by lowering the horse's head.

Administration of both topical and systemic benzylpenicillin appears to improve treatment success rate. Verheyen et al[70] have reported on the method of delivering a gelatin-penicillin mix (Box 28-3). The gelatin-penicillin mix is more effective at remaining in the pouches than a straight aqueous solution and is a useful way of delivering a large dose of penicillin where it is needed. Instillation is easiest through a catheter inserted up the nose and endoscopically guided into the pouch opening. The catheter works best with the last 1 inch bent at an angle to aid entry under the pouch flap. Recommendations include elevating the horse's head after infusion.

Topical instillation of 20% (w/v) acetylcysteine solution has also been used to aid the treatment of empyema. Acetylcysteine has a denaturing and solubilizing activity by disrupting disulfide bonds in mucoprotein molecules, thus reducing mucus viscosity and theoretically facilitating natural drainage. Erythema of the mucus membranes lining the guttural pouch has been observed after instillation of 20% (w/v) acetylcysteine solution. More long-standing cases, in which there is inspissation of the purulent material that does not readily drain into the pharynx, are more difficult to treat topically because they can be refractory to large-volume irrigation. Use of a memoryhelical polyp retrieval basket through the biopsy channel of the endoscope allows nonsurgical removal of chondroids, even when present in large numbers and in conjunction with empyema (J.R. Newton, unpublished data). When combined with topical and systemic antimicrobial treatment, this is usually sufficient to cure severe guttural pouch lesions. Surgical hyovertebrotomy and ventral drainage through Viborg's triangle carry inherent risks of general anesthesia and surgical dissection around major blood vessels and nerves, as well as *S. equi* contamination of the hospital environment (see Chapter 1). Scarring of the pharyngeal openings of the guttural pouch may preclude both natural drainage of purulent material and endoscopic access to the guttural pouches. Such animals may require conventional surgical or endoscopically guided laser treatments to break down scar tissue and allow access to the pouches.

Hygiene Measures

Particular care should be taken with hygiene measures during strangles outbreaks to prevent indirect transfer of *S. equi* from infectious horses (including potential subclinical carriers) to susceptible animals (see Chapter 62). Personnel should use dedicated protective clothing when dealing with infectious animals and should not deal simultaneously with susceptible animals. If this is unavoidable, infectious horses should be dealt with after susceptible animals. Only dedicated equipment should be used for infectious horses and thoroughly disinfected between animals. In disinfecting stables used by infectious horses, care should be taken to ensure thorough cleaning to remove all organic material. Particular care must be taken with feed and water troughs, as well as wooden fencing or other wooden surfaces. Manure and waste feed from infectious animals should be composted in an isolated location. Personnel dealing with susceptible animals should avoid contact with waste from infectious horses.

After removal of organic material from stables, all surfaces should be thoroughly soaked in an appropriate liquid disinfectant or steam-treated and allowed to dry; this should be repeated if possible. After thorough cleaning and soaking in liquid disinfectant, wooden surfaces should be treated with a suitable preservative or sealed with epoxy paint. Pastures used to hold infectious animals should be rested for 4 weeks; no evidence exists for prolonged survival of *S. equi* on pastures. Care should be taken to disinfect water troughs at least once daily during an outbreak. Horse vans should be hosed clean and disinfected after each use.

S. equi does not present any additional problems with disinfection of equipment than do any other bacterial species. Normal commonsense approaches should be adopted at all times, such as ensuring physical removal of visible organic material and using an appropriate disinfectant with proven action against *S. equi* and following the manufacturer's guidelines on dilution.

The Horserace Betting Levy Board in the United Kingdom has established guidelines on strangles in its Codes of Practice, which can be viewed at the following Web address: http://codes.hblb.org.uk/. The British Horse Society has also produced a series of guidelines for the prevention and resolution of strangles outbreaks, which can be viewed at: http://www.bhsscotland.org.uk/uploads/5/4/5/3/5453271/001_steps__web_pdf.pdf.

Public Health Considerations

Cases of *S. equi* infection in debilitated humans have been reported.[7,91] Animal handlers, caretakers, veterinary practitioners, pathologists, and equine postmortem attendants should take particular care to avoid unnecessary contamination from infectious horses, especially avoiding respiratory and oral contamination by purulent material. *S. equi* is highly host adapted, however, and infections of humans have rarely been confirmed.

Streptococcus equi Subsp. *zooepidemicus*

Debra C. Sellon and Andrew S. Waller

Etiology, Epidemiology, and Pathogenesis

Streptococcus equi subsp. *zooepidemicus* (*S. zooepidemicus*) is a Lancefield group C β-hemolytic streptococcus that is considered a part-mucosal commensal of the oral cavity, pharynx, and respiratory tract of horses. It causes disease as an opportunistic pathogen of the respiratory tract (rhinitis, bronchitis, pneumonia) and reproductive tract (endometritis) of horses after virus infection, heat stress, or tissue injury.[2,64,92-96] This organism is the most frequently isolated pathogen from equine joints, lymph nodes, nasal cavities, and lungs.[64]

S. zooepidemicus shares 98% DNA homology with *S. equi* but can be differentiated microbiologically by its ability to ferment lactose and sorbitol but not trehalose. The population of *S. zooepidemicus* strains is extremely diverse as highlighted by multilocus sequence typing.[2] This scheme currently differentiates 279 different strains of *S. zooepidemicus*, including two types of *S. equi*, which falls within this genetic typing scheme (http://pubmlst.org/perl/mlstdbnet/mlstdbnet.pl?file=sz_profiles.xml).

The SzM protein of *S. zooepidemicus* lacks the N-terminal variable domain of the SeM protein of *S. equi*,[12] the equibactin iron-uptake system, some other surface exposed or secreted proteins and the pyrogenic exotoxins SeeH and SeeI.[1] However, some *S. zooepidemicus* strains produce superantigens, including homologs of SeeL and SeeM and the novel superantigens SzeF, SzeN, and SzeP.[1,39] The presence of superantigen-encoding genes was significantly associated with isolation from non-strangles lymph node abscesses,[39] suggesting that *S. zooepidemicus* strains differ in their potential to cause disease. Some genetically related groups of *S. zooepidemicus* were also significantly more likely to have been isolated from the respiratory tract and others from cases of endometritis and abortion.[2]

Isolates from the tonsils and pharynx of horses usually show less encapsulation than *S. equi*. This may be as a result of decreased hyaluronate lyase activity by *S. equi*.[1,45] Hyaluronate lyase activity may enhance tissue dissemination of some *S. zooepidemicus* strains.[45]

Serum antibodies to the sortase-processed SzP protein of *S. zooepidemicus* are opsonic and protective in mice and may contribute to protection in horses, at least when the homologous strain is used.[97-99] Specific IgA and IgG antibodies in nasopharyngeal secretions may play a role in protection.[64] However, the prolonged and frequent upper airway infections of young foals suggest that effective immunity is not acquired until later in life,[93,100] probably at a point when individual horses have been infected with and developed immunity toward a variety of different *S. zooepidemicus* strains.

Clinical Findings

S. zooepidemicus is associated with several clinical syndromes in horses. It causes endometritis in "susceptible mares" (see Chapter 8) and is one of the most frequent causes of infectious abortion and placentitis,[95,96] resulting in significant annual losses to the industry. *S. zooepidemicus* is the most common bacterial isolate from horses with pneumonia[82,102,103] and shipping fever (see Chapter 1).[92] There is growing evidence of close involvement with repeated respiratory tract infections in young animals up to 3 or 4 years old and lower airway inflammation in foals and Thoroughbred horses in training.[93,100]

Therapy

Most β-hemolytic streptococci from horses are susceptible to β-lactam antibiotics, including penicillin, ampicillin, and ceftiofur.[82] Many isolates are also susceptible to trimethoprim-sulfonamide combinations and oxytetracycline. Specific therapy will depend on the site and severity of disease. (See Chapters 1 and 8 for treatment of respiratory tract and reproductive tract infections, respectively.)

Prevention

Prevention of equine disease caused by *S. zooepidemicus* is difficult because of the opportunistic nature of the infection. Control is best achieved by decreasing stress and treating predisposing medical conditions or stressors (e.g., viral infection, transport, uterine fluid accumulation) appropriately and promptly. Immunization of mares with bacterial extracts provides some resistance to endometritis caused by this organism.[103] However, development of vaccines for prevention of infection will be complex due to diversity of common strains, opportunistic nature of infection, and the concern of glomerulonephritis associated with immune complex formation.[2,76]

Public Health Considerations

There are numerous reports of *S. zooepidemicus* infection of people.[104-107] Outbreaks of glomerulonephritis have been linked to consumption of unpasteurized milk and cheese products contaminated with *S. zooepidemicus*.[104] Also, the many reports of *S. zooepidemicus* bacteremia, meningitis, and arthritis in people have frequently been traced to animal contact.[107-113] Despite these reports of human disease caused by *S. zooepidemicus* infection, this is considered a rare zoonosis, especially when the frequency of human exposure to the organism is considered.

Streptococcus pneumoniae

Debra C. Sellon

Etiology

Streptococcus pneumoniae is an α-hemolytic streptococcus occasionally isolated from healthy horses and those with respiratory tract disease.[93,100,114,116] It is a facultative anaerobe, and its growth in culture can be enhanced by a carbon dioxide–enriched environment. *S. pneumoniae* is an important cause of community-acquired pneumonia (pneumococcal pneumonia), meningitis, and septicemia in people, although oropharyngeal carriage in healthy humans is common. This organism may also cause pneumonia in a variety of other animals, but isolates from guinea pigs and horses appear to be distinct from those that infect other animals, including humans.[116]

Pathogenesis

Only *S. pneumoniae* capsule type 3 has been isolated from horses.[117] Although more than 80 different capsule types have been isolated from people, capsule type 3 is recognized as a particularly pathogenic strain and is associated with a higher mortality than other types of pneumococci.[118] However, equine isolates lack both the hemolytic cytotoxin pneumolysin and the major autolysin gene *lytA*, which are considered important virulence factors,[119] providing one possible explanation to the usually subclinical disease produced in horses.

Clinical Findings and Therapy

S. pneumoniae has been isolated from the respiratory tract of healthy horses and on several occasions from the lungs of pneumonic foals.[114,120] As in humans, the incidence of inapparent carrier status seems to be higher in young horses.[120] *S. pneumoniae* is associated with lower airway disease in training Thoroughbreds, although with a lower prevalence than *S. zooepidemicus*.[93,100] Experimental infection of ponies produced lobar pneumonia, with inflammation in the trachea typical of the disease seen in training horses.[115]

Horses with *S. pneumoniae* respiratory tract disease should be treated with appropriate antimicrobial therapy based on antimicrobial sensitivity testing. Most isolates are expected to be susceptible to β-lactam antibiotics. Additional symptomatic and supportive care should be provided if indicated.

Public Health Considerations

The isolation of *S. pneumoniae* from the respiratory tract of horses suggests the possibility of zoonotic infection; however, equine strains of *S. pneumoniae* differ from their human counterparts[116] and zoonotic transmission has not been demonstrated to date.

The complete reference list is available online at www.expertconsult.com.

Staphylococcal Infections

J. Scott Weese

Etiology

The *Staphylococcus* genus consists of a diverse group of over 50 different species and subspecies of gram-positive cocci. They are common commensals of various body sites in different animal species, and although many are of limited clinical relevance, a small number of staphylococci are among the most important opportunistic pathogens in horses.

Staphylococcal species are typically divided into two groups based on the ability to produce coagulase (Box 29-1). Coagulase-positive species are the main pathogenic staphylococci in horses, and among those, *Staphylococcus aureus* accounts for the vast majority of infections. Although typically associated with infections in dogs and cats, *Staphylococcus pseudintermedius* infections have been reported in horses,[1,2] and anecdotal information suggests *S. pseudintermedius* infections, especially methicillin-resistant *S. pseudintermedius* (MRSP), may be an emerging issue in equine medicine. Another coagulase-positive species, *Staphylococcus delphini*, can also be encountered in equine infections,[3] yet its overall role in disease is probably limited. Misidentification of (or inadequate attempts by laboratories to differentiate) coagulase-positive staphylococci may hamper our understanding of the relative roles of these different species.

There is a wide range of coagulase-negative staphylococci (CoNS; see Box 29-1),[1,4-7] and they are typically considered of limited virulence, although there may be variability in the pathogenicity of different CoNS species. Most often, CoNS only cause infections in hospitalized or otherwise compromised hosts. Difficulties in differentiating different CoNS and minimal effort by diagnostic laboratories to speciate CoNS has hampered proper understanding of the relative role of different CoNS in disease, and it is possible that some CoNS are more pathogenic than others.

Many staphylococcal species can be found in healthy and diseased horses as part of the normal microflora, particularly in the nasal passages, intestinal tract, skin, and conjunctiva. Staphylococci can be found in or on the vast majority of horses,[4] and it is reasonable to suspect that staphylococci could be found somewhere in virtually all horses, with even a moderate degree of effort. A diverse collection of CoNS tends to predominate as commensals, but even the more pathogenic coagulase-positive staphylococci are common.[4,8]

Antimicrobial Resistance

Staphylococci, particularly *S. aureus*, have been notable in their tendency to acquire resistance to antimicrobials, and introduction of new drugs (often to treat resistant *S. aureus*) has typically lead to further development of resistance. Certain patterns of antimicrobial resistance among staphylococci have been recognized for years and are not unexpected. In particular, resistance to penicillin is widespread[9-11] because of acquisition of β-lactamase genes by *S. aureus*. Other patterns of resistance are more recent and continue to evolve, with the most notable being methicillin resistance. Methicillin-resistant *S. aureus* (MRSA) is of tremendous concern in human medicine[12] because it is associated with considerable morbidity and mortality, along with other health care challenges such as high economic cost and increased duration of hospitalization. Methicillin resistance is mediated by the gene *mecA*. This gene encodes production of an altered penicillin-binding protein 2a (PBP2a) that possesses low affinity for β-lactam antimicrobials, rendering methicillin-resistant staphylococci resistant to virtually all β-lactams (penicillins, cephalosporins, carbapenems). Often, methicillin-resistant staphylococci are also resistant to various other antimicrobials, and treatment options may be limited.

Although typically considered a human hospital-associated pathogen, MRSA was identified in horses in the 1990s[13,14] and is now widely disseminated in the horse population internationally. Initial reports of MRSA infections in horses described soft tissue infections typically linked to known or suspected contact with infected or colonized people. Subsequently, larger numbers of MRSA infections were identified in horses in equine hospitals and on horse farms, along with recognition of a pool of colonized clinically normal carriers, transmission of MRSA between horses, and transmission between humans and horses (in both directions).[15-17] Identification of MRSA colonization in horses indicated that a silent pool of infectious horses could be present, complicating control of this pathogen and facilitating widespread dissemination. Methicillin-resistant *S. aureus* colonization rates vary between studies and regions (Table 29-1) but indicate a small but still concerning prevalence of MRSA

Box 29-1 Examples of *Staphylococcus* Species Based on Coagulase Production

Coagulase Positive
S. aureus
S. pseudintermedius
S. intermedius
S. delphini
S. schleiferi subsp. coagulans
S. hyicus*

Coagulase Negative
S. epidermidis
S. xylosus
S. equorum
S. schleiferi subsp. schleiferi
S. lentus
S. sciuri
S. capitis
S. haemolyticus
S. hominis
S. vitulinus
S. warneri

*Variable coagulase reaction.

Table 29-1 Methicillin-Resistant *Staphylococcus aureus* (MRSA) Colonization of Horses

Country	Group	Prevalence	Reference
Belgium	Hospitalized horses	12/30 (40%)	62
United Kingdom	Healthy horses on farms	4/678 (0.6%)	33
Australia	Hospital admissions	8/216 (3.7%)	80
United Kingdom	Healthy horses on farms	0/296	81
	Horses being examined by a veterinarian	3/152 (3%)	
Ireland	Healthy horses on farms	4/236 (1.7%)	82
	Horses presented to private veterinary practices	5/64 (7.8%)	
	Horses presented to academic hospital	15/319 (4.7%)	
Italy	Healthy horses	1/159 (0.6%)	1
Canada	Various	6/458 (1.3%)	28
The Netherlands	Hospital admissions	24/259 (9.3%)	21
Canada	Healthy horses on farms	0/497	83
Belgium	Hospital admissions	12/110 (11%)	26
Canada	Hospital admissions	69/3372 (2.0%)	20
United States	Healthy horses on farms	2/293 (0.7%)	84
Slovenia	Healthy horses on farms	0/300	85
Canada	Hospital admissions	61/2283 (2.7%)	61
Canada and the United States	Healthy horses on farms	46/972 (4.7%)	17
United Kingdom	Horses on farms	0/40	86
	Horses at equine hospital	8/67 (12%)	

carriage in most areas. Recognition of MRSA colonization in horses in various regions continues to rise, but it is unclear whether this is because of continued emergence of the bacterium or increased surveillance. True regional variation does seem to exist for unknown reasons.

Risk factors for MRSA colonization have only been superficially explored. Farm size (regular contact with >20 horses) was the only risk factor identified in a study of colonization of horses on farms.[18] Treatment with ceftiofur or an aminoglycoside was associated with nosocomial MRSA colonization,[19] whereas previous identification of MRSA on the farm, previous colonization of the horse, antimicrobial administration within 30 days, and admission to the neonatal intensive care unit (ICU) were risk factors for colonization at the time of equine hospital admission.[20] Methicillin-resistant *S. aureus* colonization at the time of equine hospital admission has been identified as a risk factor for development of MRSA infection during hospitalization.[19]

Evaluation of the types (strains) of MRSA that are found in horses can provide interesting insights into this pathogen. One clone, a sequence type (ST) 8 clone referred to as USA500 or CMRSA-5 in the United States and Canada, respectively, has been found as a predominant strain in horses internationally.[18,19,21-24] This is a recognized human epidemic clone that is uncommon in humans, and the high prevalence in some horse populations suggests that is adapted for survival in horses compared to most other MRSA strains. Other human epidemic clones can be found in horses, albeit less commonly. More recently, a different strain of MRSA has been found in horses, particularly in northern Europe, and this may represent an emerging problem. This strain, a livestock-associated strain

referred to as ST398 (or clonal complex 398) has been increasingly identified in horses in both equine hospitals and the general horse population,[21,25-27] with one study at a Belgian referral hospital reporting colonization of 11% of horses at the time of admission.[26] This strain has been found in a Canadian horse,[28] and it is unclear whether it is a rare issue outside of northern Europe or an emerging pathogen.

Although MRSA attracts the most attention, other methicillin-resistant staphylococci can also be problematic. Recent evidence suggests that MRSP may also be an emerging issue in horses. Currently, MSRP is uncommon or at least uncommonly diagnosed; however, MRSP is of concern because of the high level of drug resistance that is typically present. For unexplained reasons, MRSP tend to be resistant to many more antimicrobials than MRSA,[29] and there may be few to no viable treatment options with some MRSP infections. Methicillin-resistant *Staphylococcus pseudintermedius* is an important pathogen in dogs, and the prevalence can be quite high in dogs in some areas,[29,30] but it is unknown whether MRSP in horses originates in dogs. Rare infections with methicillin-resistant *S. delphini* have also been encountered.

Methicillin resistance is common among CoNS,[7,31,32] although methicillin-resistant CoNS are not as important clinically as methicillin-resistant coagulase-positive staphylococci because CoNS are much less likely to cause disease. Methicillin-resistant CoNS colonization rates can be high (e.g., 30%-40%),[32,33] and although they certainly can cause infections, this colonization rate appears to be uncommon. Methicillin-resistant strains are not inherently more virulent than their susceptible counterparts, they are just harder to treat if an infection develops, and the presence of methicillin-resistance in CoNS should not necessarily raise concern. Indeed, it is reasonable to suspect that methicillin-resistant CoNS could be found in a majority of healthy horses.

Pathogenesis

Staphylococci can possess an impressive array of virulence factors that enable them to colonize and cause disease. Most virulence factors have been identified in *S. aureus*, but some may also be found in other staphylococci. Exozymes, including coagulase, protease, hemolysins, hyaluronidase, collagenase, lipase, and nuclease, facilitate colonization and growth in vivo. Staphylococcal enterotoxins (SEs), also classified as "pyrogenic staphylococcal superantigens," are produced by various coagulase-positive staphylococci and are primarily associated with food poisoning in humans. Because this disease is not recognized in horses, SEs are probably of limited concern in equine isolates, although they have been found in *S. aureus* and *S. pseudintermedius* of equine origin.[34,35] Biofilm formation may be important both as a mechanism to colonize body sites and in the development of infections. Bacterial biofilms have only been minimally investigated in horses, yet biofilm production has been identified in staphylococci, such as *S. aureus*, *S. pseudintermedius*, and *S. epidermidis* from other species,[36-39] and it is likely to occur in equine isolates. Biofilm formation facilitates persistence of infection, evasion of the host immune response, and resistance to the effects of antimicrobials and may be particularly important in surgical site infections, especially those involving surgical implants.

Toxic shock syndrome toxin 1 (TSST-1) is another pyrogenic staphylococcal superantigen and is associated with staphylococcal TSS in humans. Toxic shock syndrome toxin 1 is unique in its ability to cross intact mucosal surfaces, and systemic disease can result from localized infections. Toxic shock syndrome associated with TSST-1 has been reported in a horse,[40] but this disease appears to be very rare. Exfoliative toxin (ETs) is responsible for skin exfoliation in staphylococcal scalded-skin syndrome in humans and has been associated with skin infection in a horse.[35,41] A similar toxin, *S. intermedius* exfoliative toxin, is commonly found in *S. pseudintermedius*,[42] but its relevance in horses is completely unclear. The Panton-Valentine leukocidin (PVL) is predominantly found in human MRSA, particularly community MRSA,[43] and is of unclear relevance in horses.

The mere presence of staphylococci in or on a host does not mean that disease is occurring or will occur. Staphylococci are opportunists, and one or more risk factors typically must be present before disease can occur. Risk factors for development of clinical infection in humans include surgery, trauma, concurrent infection, skin lesions, and immunocompromise, although there is an increasing incidence of community-associated MRSA infection in people without traditionally accepted risk factors.

Risk factors for development of staphylococcal disease in horses have not been adequately evaluated but are likely similar to those reported in humans. Risk factors for MRSA infection are not known but may relate to colonization risk factors as described.

Clinical Findings

Staphylococci can be involved in infections of virtually any body system, although skin and soft tissue infections (including surgical site infections) and joint infections are most common.[14,21,23,25,44-46] Clinical signs depend on the location of infection, virulence of the involved strain, and host factors. Severity of disease can range from mild local infection to septicemia and toxemia. The clinical presentation of staphylococcal infection can be quite variable, and clinical signs cannot differentiate staphylococcal infection from infection caused by another opportunistic pathogen.

Most clinical reports of *S. aureus* infections (Fig. 29-1) describe infections of wounds and incisions, subcutaneous tissues (cellulitis), bones and joints, and skin as being most common, although a wide range of infections have been reported, including pyelonephritis, tracheitis, metritis, lymphangitis, fistulous withers, pleuritis, meningitis, and sinusitis.[9,44,45,47,48] *Staphylococcus aureus* is a leading cause of septic arthritis, especially postinjection septic arthritis.[44,49-52]

There are limited reports of *S. pseudintermedius* infection in horses, although it can presumably cause disease similar to that caused by *S. aureus*, with a predominance of skin and soft tissue infection and less frequently septic arthritis, tenosynovitis, and osteomyelitis.[1-3,7]

Less information is available for other staphylococci. *Staphylococcus hyicus* has been implicated as a cause of pastern dermatitis ("greasy heel"), postarticular injection septic arthritis, and fistulous withers,[45,47] although the incidence of disease is probably quite low. Coagulase-negative staphylococci, particularly *S. epidermidis*, have also been identified in septic arthritis, tenosynovitis, osteomyelitis, and other musculoskeletal infections,[7,45,53,54] yet the relatively limited virulence of CoNS means that infections in otherwise healthy horses are rare. More often, CoNS are associated with nosocomial infections, particularly infections of invasive devices such as IV catheters.[46]

Methicillin-Resistant Staphylococci

Methicillin-resistant staphylococci do not cause different types of infections than methicillin-susceptible staphylococci. Wounds and postoperative infections predominate in reports of MRSA

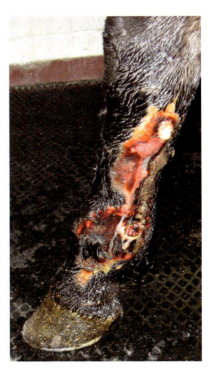

Figure 29-1 Severe skin and soft tissue infection caused by methicillin-susceptible *Staphylococcus aureus*.

infections, although catheter site infections, pneumonia, osteomyelitis, septic arthritis, and bacteremia have also been identified.* A difference in severity between susceptible and resistant infections does not necessarily exist. MRSA can cause disease ranging from very mild to rapidly fatal, just like methicillin-susceptible *S. aureus*, because *mecA* and other resistance genes just confer drug resistance not virulence properties. However, antimicrobial resistance can have an impact on outcome if inappropriate antimicrobial therapy is used, either in the absence of culture or while awaiting culture results. Poor outcomes from multidrug-resistant staphylococci are mainly the result of the failure to promptly identify the resistant pathogen (as opposed to increased inherent virulence), thus prompt identification of antimicrobial resistance is critical.

Diagnosis

Cytologic evaluation of aspirates, biopsies, or swabs can provide a suspicion of staphylococcal infection by identification of gram-positive cocci, ideally with concurrent cytologic or histologic evidence of disease. This does not confirm staphylococcal infection because staphylococci cannot be distinguished from other gram-positive cocci (e.g., streptococci, enterococci), but a strong suspicion can sometimes be made in infections where staphylococci are commonly involved and where streptococci and enterococci are rare (e.g., skin infection).

Isolation of staphylococci in appropriate clinical specimens is the standard for diagnosis. Staphylococci are rather hardy organisms that are easy to isolate using standard culture methods. Therefore diagnosis can be achieved in most cases through submission of an appropriately collected sample for bacterial culture. Joints are a notable exception; it is often difficult to

*References 9, 13, 14, 23, 25, 55-57.

isolate infectious agents from septic joints, and negative synovial fluid cultures do not rule out staphylococcal infection.

Laboratories must identify coagulase-positive staphylococci to the species level or at a minimum differentiate *S. aureus* from *S. intermedius* group (the group that includes *S. pseudintermedius*) because there are different antimicrobial susceptibility testing breakpoints[58] and because of greater zoonotic disease concerns with MRSA. Susceptibility results for generically identified "coagulase-positive staphylococci" should not be considered valid, and proper speciation must be obtained. Failure to differentiate CoNS is probably of little concern because it is unlikely that knowing the species would impact subsequent laboratory testing or case management.

Traditionally, oxacillin has been used as the indicator of methicillin resistance, but oxacillin is a poor inducer of resistance in some *S. aureus* strains (and methicillin-resistance may be missed), so cefoxitin is now used as the indicator of MRSA. However, cefoxitin is poorly effective for detection of MRSP,[59] and oxacillin testing is required for this species. Staphylococci that are oxacillin or cefoxitin resistant are considered methicillin-resistant, and inherently resistant to all β-lactams. Confirmation of methicillin resistance can be performed with PBP2a latex agglutination test or *mecA* polymerase chain reaction (PCR), yet this is uncommonly performed by diagnostic laboratories.

It is important to consider the ecology of *Staphylococcus* spp. when interpreting culture results. Because staphylococci may be found on many body sites in normal animals, isolation does not necessarily indicate a role in disease. In particular, isolation of *Staphylococcus* spp. from the oral cavity, nasal cavity, pharynx, vagina, or skin (or from samples potentially contaminated by bacteria from those sites) may simply be identification of the normal microflora. This is of particular concern with CoNS because they are commonly found but uncommonly cause disease. Factors, such as the disease process, typical pathogens, the expected resident microflora, sample site, sampling technique, and amount of bacterial growth, can help differentiate relevant isolation from contamination. For example, a deep culture of a postoperative infection through aseptically prepared skin is likely more relevant than a quick, superficial swab of an infected site or body surface. The high prevalence of staphylococcal colonization of humans can further complicate interpretation of results because contamination of the diagnostic sample by hand contact could result in a false-positive result. Isolation of CoNS should be interpreted with caution, particularly when there may have been contamination with commensal staphylococci. If CoNS are isolated in combination with another pathogenic microorganism (e.g., *Escherichia coli*, *S. aureus*, *Streptococcus zooepidemicus*), the CoNS is often disregarded. However, the potential for CoNS infection should not be completely dismissed, particularly in hospitalized animals.

Other Diagnostic Methods

Molecular diagnostic testing, particularly PCR, is increasingly available from commercial diagnostic laboratories. Polymerase chain reaction has the advantage of being fast and potentially highly sensitive, resulting in shorter turnaround times. Polymerase chain reaction also has inherent disadvantages of being able to detect dead microorganisms and not being able to provide antimicrobial susceptibility results. Additionally, increased sensitivity may not be desirable for pathogens like staphylococci that are easy to grow and may be present at low levels as contaminants in many situations. Advantages and limitations of PCR testing must be considered prior to its use, and there is unfortunately almost no information available regarding sensitivity, specificity, and predictive values of commercial assays. Therefore their role in clinical testing is completely unclear at this time.

Methicillin-Resistant *Staphylococcus aureus* Screening

In many human hospitals, MRSA screening is an important infection control measure, allowing for prompt identification of potentially infectious patients. It can also identify patients that might be at greater risk of MRSA infection, which may result in more prompt anti-MRSA treatment if infection develops or proactive MRSA decolonization in some situations. However, although MRSA screening has clearly been shown to be both medically and economically beneficial in humans,[60] the role of screening in horses is not well understood. Methicillin-resistant *Staphylococcus aureus* screening could be considered as part of the evaluation of hospital or farm infection control programs, with factors such as the incidence of disease, prevalence of colonization, risk of exposure to positive horses, nature of the horse population (e.g., foals or hospitalized horses versus healthy adults on farms) and cost used to determine whether it is useful and appropriate. Screening has been used as part of MRSA eradication attempts on farms[16] and as routine infection control surveillance in areas that have a reasonably high prevalence of MRSA in the referral population.[20,61] Nasal swabs are most commonly used for MRSA screening, but the addition of skin swabs has been shown to increase sensitivity.[62] Enrichment culture of nasal swabs also increases the sensitivity of testing.[23]

In human medicine, PCR screening for MRSA is becoming increasingly popular because of its sensitivity in detecting colonized individuals and the rapid turnaround time, which facilitates prompt use of infection control measures.[63] High quality and validated assays are available for use in humans, but effectiveness in humans does not necessarily mean effectiveness in equine specimens, as was demonstrated with one human assay.[55] Despite the fact that *mecA* PCR has been marketed as an MRSA test for horses, it is ineffective because *mecA* is present in other methicillin-resistant staphylococci.

Treatment

Treatment of staphylococcal infections will depend on the location and severity of infection and the antimicrobial susceptibility of the isolate. Culture and susceptibility (C&S) testing is essential to guide treatment. In certain situations, staphylococcal infection should be considered likely and empiric treatment chosen according to typical staphylococcal susceptibility patterns. In particular, iatrogenic septic arthritis should be treated as penicillinase-producing staphylococcal infection until proved otherwise.[49] Empiric treatment to cover MRSA is rarely indicated but may be considered in situations in which there is a high likelihood of MRSA infection and when the implications of initial treatment failure are high (e.g., a neonatal foal known to be colonized with MRSA that develops septic arthritis).

In most situations, systemic antimicrobial therapy is required for treatment of staphylococcal infections. Drug choices should be based on in vitro antimicrobial susceptibility in combination with other patient and drug factors (e.g., penetration, concentration, activity at site of infection, drug interactions). "Antibiogram" information is very important because of the variability in antimicrobial susceptibility, the paucity of published data regarding susceptibility patterns, and the questionable ability to extrapolate susceptibility data from referral facilities in limited geographic regions. Knowledge of staphylococcal susceptibility trends on the farm, in the hospital, or in the region can provide more useful information.

Because most staphylococci are resistant to penicillin, a β-lactamase resistant β-lactam or other drug class should be used initially if staphylococcal infection is suspected. β-lactamase inhibitors, such as clavulanic acid or sulbactam, are widely used in combination with penicillins in humans and other animal species, but their use is rather limited in horses because of an inability to safety administer oral preparations and lack of availability of parenteral formulations in many regions. Accordingly, cephalosporins are most commonly used.

The emergence of methicillin-resistant staphylococci has created significant challenges. In addition to being resistant to all β-lactams, including cephalosporins and carbapenems (e.g., imipenem), methicillin-resistant staphylococci are often resistant to a variety of other antimicrobials. Although β-lactam antimicrobials will be ineffective, it is important to remember that not all MRSA isolates are highly drug resistant and some may only be resistant to β-lactams. Therefore identification of an MRSA infection does not mean that "big-gun" antimicrobials are required, particularly in non–life-threatening infections. However, high-level resistance to multiple antimicrobial classes does occur, and some MRSA isolates will be resistant to most antimicrobials present on typical veterinary antimicrobial panels. An expanded antimicrobial susceptibility panel should be requested when good antimicrobial options are not present on the initial report. Typically, MRSA is susceptible to one or more of chloramphenicol, doxycycline, or amikacin, and these may all be reasonable options, depending on the case. In vitro susceptibility to fluoroquinolones is often reported; however, there are concerns about using fluoroquinolones for MRSA or MRSP infections because of the potential for rapid development of resistance during treatment and the often unpredictable clinical response despite in vitro susceptibility.

Topical therapy may be effective in uncomplicated superficial (e.g., wound, incision) infections. Silver sulfadiazine, a combination of 1% silver sulfadiazine and 0.2% chlorhexidine digluconate, fusidic acid, 1% hydrogen peroxide cream, honey, or mupirocin may be useful.[64-68] A variety of essential oils (e.g., tea tree oil) and other compounds, such as allicin (garlic extract), have in vitro antistaphylococcal activity[69-72]; however, clinical efficacy is unclear. Some essential oils, such as tea tree oil, have been shown to have cytopathic effects on host cells[73,74] and therefore may be contraindicated. It is preferable to use topical compounds with proven safety and efficacy, ideally in horses but alternatively in other mammalian species.

Local or regional therapy using intraarticular administration, regional limb perfusion, intraosseous infusion, injection of antimicrobial-containing gel matrices, or implantation of antimicrobial impregnated materials (e.g., polymethylmethacrylate [PMMA] beads) can be very useful in some types of infections, providing high antimicrobial levels at the site of infection. A limited study of regional limb perfusion with gentamicin (1 g) was successful in the treatment of experimentally induced *S. aureus* septic arthritis.[75] Intraosseous infusion of gentamicin with the horse standing might also be useful for treatment of orthopedic infections.[76] These approaches are usually combined with appropriate systemic antimicrobial therapy.

Prognosis

Prognosis for staphylococcal infections is highly variable and depends on the location and severity of infection. Infections can range from mild and easily treated to difficult-to-treat or rapidly fatal. Antimicrobial resistance can potentially worsen the prognosis if appropriate therapy is not started or is delayed, but the presence of an MRSA (or other MR-staphylococcal) infection does not inherently carry a poor prognosis. A multicenter retrospective study of MRSA infections reported an 84% survival rate.[44]

Prevention

Staphylococci are common opportunists, so measures to reduce staphylococcal infections largely involve reducing the risk of development of any opportunistic infection. Good general management, prompt treatment of illnesses, proper wound care, judicious antimicrobial therapy, judicious use of invasive devices, proper disinfection of surgical equipment, and the use of appropriate aseptic practices for surgery and intraarticular injection may all play a role in prevention of staphylococcal disease.

In equine hospitals, more specific efforts are directed at MRSA prevention because of the potential difficulties in treatment and zoonotic disease concerns and the potential for outbreaks. Horses that are infected or colonized with MRSA should be considered infectious. Ideally, they should be isolated and handled with barrier precautions, including gloves, gowns (or dedicated coveralls or laboratory coats), and overboots (or dedicated boots). The entire stall environment can be contaminated, as can medical or handling items,[77] so barrier precautions should be used whenever the stall is entered or potentially contaminated items are handled. Any items that have been in contact with the horse or the environment should be disinfected or discarded after use. Staphylococci are susceptible to all common disinfectants, provided that concentration and contact time are adequate and organic debris does not inhibit disinfection.

Aggressive infection control practices are more practical in equine hospitals as compared to farms, based on personnel training, facility infrastructure, and the generally short duration of hospitalization. Isolation of horses may be more difficult on farms, and isolation may be of limited use on a farm where MRSA is endemic in horses and/or horse personnel. The main effort should be directed at implementation of a good general infection control program to limit entry and dissemination of MRSA. This includes aspects such as cohorting risk groups, minimizing contact with new or transient horses, isolation of new arrivals, reduction of direct contact between large groups of horses, ensuring cultures are submitted when infections develop, and good personal hygiene practices (especially hand hygiene). Enhanced practices should be used when a horse is known to be infected or colonized with MRSA, but the intensity of precautions may vary with the ability of the farm to implement infection control measures and whether MRSA may already be present on the farm. Ideally, colonized horses should be housed so that they cannot come into direct contact with other horses and contact with humans is minimized. In situations where the farm is able to implement infection control measures and/or when there is no evidence that MRSA is already present on the farm, short-term use of an aggressive infection control intervention is justifiable. Methicillin-resistant *Staphylococcus aureus* control in horses is facilitated by the observation that MRSA carriage in horses tends to be transient, with most horses eliminating MRSA naturally within a few weeks.[24] Therefore short-term use of enhanced precautions may allow for elimination of MRSA from an infected or colonized horse and prevent dissemination of MRSA on the farm. Active measures, such as systemic, intranasal, or nebulized antimicrobials, to eliminate MRSA colonization have not been shown to be effective and are not currently recommended.

Public Health Considerations

The main public health concerns involve MRSA because it is a significant human pathogen and the strains of MRSA that are found in horses are almost always strains that are found in

Table 29-2 Methicillin-Resistant *Staphylococcus aureus* (MRSA) Colonization in Equine Veterinary Personnel and Horse Owners

Country	Group	Prevalence	Reference
Australia	Equine veterinarians	19/89 (21%)	87
The Netherlands	Equine hospital personnel	16/170 (9.4%)	21
International	Equine veterinarians	26/257 (10%)	88
International	Large animal veterinary personnel	11/96 (16%)	89
Canada and the United States	Horse owners and veterinarians	14/107 (13%)	17

humans. Transmission of MRSA between horses and humans is increasingly recognized and is of concern in the horse industry and the veterinary profession. High rates of MRSA colonization have been reported in horse owners and equine veterinarians (Table 29-2); it is clear that MRSA can move between horses and humans, in both directions. Although there are few published reports, MRSA skin and soft tissue infections of equine origin have been identified.[23,27,78] The risk of zoonotic transmission is probably highest on breeding farms and in equine hospitals because of the frequency and nature of contact. Limited information is available regarding optimal measures to reduce zoonotic MRSA transmission. General infection control and hygiene practices are probably critical, and in a study of equine veterinarians, good hand hygiene practices were associated with significantly lower MRSA colonization rates.[79]

There is limited concern about zoonotic transmission of other staphylococci. Methicillin-resistant *Staphylococcus pseudintermedius* is a very rare cause of human infection, despite rather common exposure from dogs, so it appears to be poorly adapted to humans. However, infections can occur so basic infection control measures are indicated when handling infected horses. CoNS are common and of limited clinical concern in people in the general population.

The complete reference list is available online at www.expertconsult.com.

CHAPTER

30 Dermatophilosis

Rosanna Marsella

Dermatophilosis is a common pustular and crusting skin disease of horses caused by *Dermatophilus congolensis*.[1] Various names have been used to describe this disease in horses, including streptothricosis, cutaneous actinomycosis, rain rot, mud fever, and dew poisoning.

Etiology and Epidemiology

Dermatophilus congolensis is a gram-positive, non–acid-fast, facultative anaerobic, branching actinomyces.[2] Genotypic and phenotypic variation between isolates has been demonstrated.[3-5] *Dermatophilus congolensis* has a distinct life cycle and exists in two morphologic forms, hyphae and zoospores.[6,7] Hyphae are composed of filaments that break into coccoid cells. These cells mature into flagellated zoospores, which represent the infective stage.[8]

The natural habitat of *D. congolensis* is unknown.[1,9] Many attempts to isolate the organism from the soil have failed,[10] even when soil samples were collected from the immediate environment of diseased animals.[11] In one study, however, *Dermatophilus* was isolated from the soil, and its survival appeared to depend on the type of soil and the water content.[12] Organic matter has a protective effect on the microorganism. Because the pathogenicity of *Dermatophilus congolensis* was preserved in soil, it is hypothesized that soil could act as a temporary reservoir for the organism. *Dermatophilus* can also survive in the skin of animals that are clinically normal, potentially acting as source of infection once favorable conditions are present.[13,14] Crusts from affected animals represent an important source of contagion for spreading lesions on the same animal and possibly the infection of other animals in the same herd.[15]

Pathogenesis

Establishment of infection with *D. congolensis* appears to depend on a variety of factors, including the virulence of the strain, the general health of the animal, skin trauma, and moisture.[16] Zoospores germinate, producing hyphae under favorable conditions. Hyphae penetrate the epidermis and spread from the initial area, triggering an inflammatory response.[17,18] Coccal cells are released from crusts to establish new sites of infection.

Virulence of the Strain

Strain differences in virulence affect the ability of *D. congolensis* to establish infection in the host.[19-22] Randomly amplified polymorphic DNA and pulsed-field gel electrophoresis techniques have been successfully used for molecular typing of *Dermatophilus congolensis*. Isolates from the same animal species or from the same geographic location are not always closely related genetically.[23] More specifically, variability may be observed in hemolytic activity on blood agar,[24] phospholipases,[25] proteases and lipases,[4,26] mucoid nature of colonies, motility, flagella density and polarity, capsule width, restriction enzyme profiles of bacterial deoxyribonucleic acid (DNA), protein electropherotype, and carbohydrate content. Hemolytic activity and enzyme activity of proteins and lipids appear to be important determinants of infectivity.[5] *Dermatophilus* also produces ceramidases,[27] which are thought to play a role in the pathogenesis of the disease through their protective and cell regulatory functions in the epidermis.

The extracellular products of *Dermatophilus* have proteolytic activities,[28] including the ability to digest keratin, which could play an important role in the establishment of the infection.[29,30] Zoospores are the most likely source of extracellular proteases, and their ability to function at a wide pH range enables the bacterium to adjust to the pH variations of inflamed skin.[30] Because the stratum corneum is filled with lipids and proteins,[31] it is reasonable to speculate that *D. congolensis* may use lipases and proteases to penetrate this barrier. Proteases may have a role in acquisition of nutrients and may initiate or inactivate host inflammatory protease cascades or cytokines.

Skin Trauma and Insects

Dermatophilus is unable to infect intact skin but can readily infect traumatized skin.[32] Various insects and ticks play a role as vectors for the transmission of *Dermatophilus* and as causes of trauma, which makes the skin more susceptible to the infection.[33,34] The inflammatory response triggered by biting flies provides a suitable growth medium for *Dermatophilus*.

Climatic Conditions and Host Factors

Moisture causes the release of infective zoospores of *D. congolensis*,[1] resulting in an increased incidence of this disease during wet seasons and heavy rainfall.[9,32,35,36] Rainfall contributes to the infection in several ways such as increasing the population of hematophagous flies, which cause skin damage and initiate inflammation at feeding sites, and contributing to maceration, which decreases the barrier function of skin. Increased temperature and humidity have been hypothesized to play a role as well. Zoospores are attracted by low concentrations of carbon dioxide and repelled by high concentrations.[37]

Host factors that influence susceptibility to infection include poor body condition, malnutrition,[38-40] stressful conditions, and glucocorticoids.[41] Any disruption in the skin barrier due to trauma (e.g., insect bites, pruritus due to other conditions) can facilitate the establishment of the infection. Resistance in some animals may have a genetic component and appears to be associated with major histocompatibility complex (MHC) haplotypes and variation in serine composition.[37,42]

Immune Responses to *Dermatophilus*

Both humoral and cell-mediated responses are triggered by infection with *D. congolensis*.[43-47] Resistance to infection may be related to antibody production,[48] T-cell activation,[49] and nonspecific immune mechanisms such as epidermal hyperproliferation and neutrophil chemotaxis.[50-52] Several reports, however, indicate that no correlation exists between serum antibodies and resistance.[53,54] Therefore it is likely that location of antibodies may be more important than serum titers.

As the hyphae of *D. congolensis* spread in the epidermis, antigens are released that are captured by Langerhans' cells and presented to T cells at the site of infection. Dense accumulations of mononuclear cells are found in infected skin. Chronic lesions contain both CD4+ and CD8+ T lymphocytes in equal proportions, whereas acute lesions on their way to resolution contain primarily CD4+ T cells.[55] The epidermal proliferation found in this disease could be the result of cytokines secreted by T cells, as well as secondary self-trauma.

Clinical Findings

The clinical features of dermatophilosis are fairly characteristic.[56] The primary lesions are papules, which mature into pustules. Because pustules are transient, only epidermal collarettes and areas of focal alopecia are often seen (Fig. 30-1). Lesions easily become exudative, and hairs are matted together to form thick crusts in which the hairs are embedded (Fig. 30-2).[57] When crusts are removed, the underlying skin is often eroded, painful, and prone to bleeding (Fig. 30-3). Purulent exudate may be observed in active lesions, whereas chronic lesions tend to have dry crusts with more diffuse scaling and alopecia (Figs. 30-4 and 30-5). Frequently, these lesions are misdiagnosed as a fungal infection. It is important to remember that bacterial infections are much more common in horses than fungal infections.

The distribution of lesions is characteristic of *Dermatophilus*.[58] The rump, dorsal thorax, and face are usually affected when lesions are triggered by heavy rainfall (Figs. 30-6 and 30-7). The saddle area may be most affected in horses, where

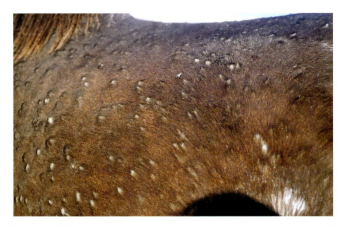

Figure 30-1 Focal areas of alopecia on dorsal area of horse with dermatophilosis.

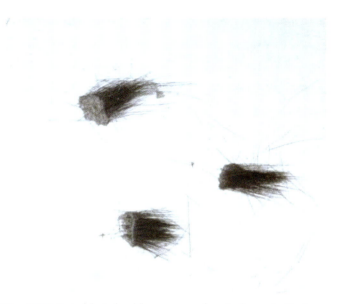

Figure 30-2 Typical "paintbrush" appearance of crusts observed with dermatophilosis. The hairs are matted and become embedded in the crust.

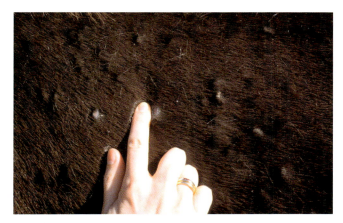

Figure 30-3 Area underneath the crusts is often eroded and sensitive to the touch.

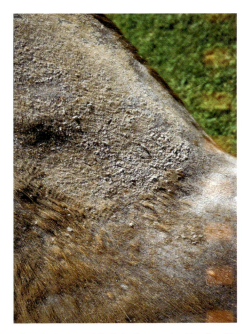

Figure 30-4 Chronic dermatophilosis is characterized by dry skin and diffuse scaling.

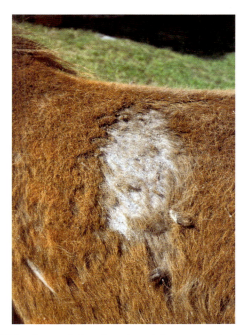

Figure 30-5 Focal areas of alopecia coalesce to form more extensive alopecia and scaling in a horse with dermatophilosis.

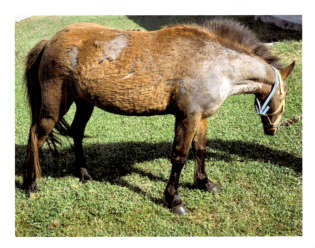

Figure 30-6 The dorsum is often affected in horses that develop dermatophilosis after heavy rainfall.

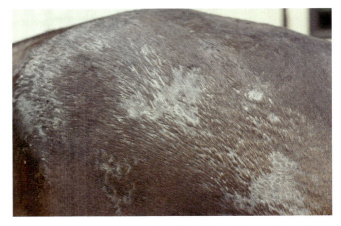

Figure 30-7 The rump area may be affected by scaling and alopecia in a chronic case of dermatophilosis caused by excessive exposure to rain.

trauma and moisture result from riding. *Dermatophilus* lesions are frequently aggravated by *Staphylococcus* spp. infections. In some horses, lesions are primarily found on the distal limbs (e.g., pasterns, coronets, heels). In these horses, lameness and edema may be present. Horses with white areas may develop severe erythema at these sites (Fig. 30-8); photosensitization has been hypothesized to be involved in the pathogenesis of these lesions. Alternatively, it may be that sunburn due to lack of pigment lowers the local immunity and facilitates the establishment of *D. congolensis*.

Diagnosis

Diagnosis of dermatophilosis is based on suggestive history, typical clinical signs, and supportive cytology and histopathology, if necessary.[59] In horses with generalized distribution, bacterial folliculitis caused by *Staphylococcus*, dermatophytosis,

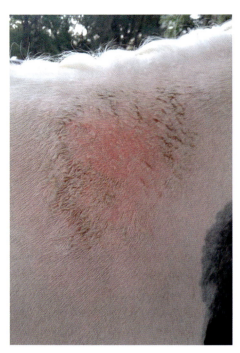

Figure 30-8 Lesion of dermatophilosis in horse with actinic damage due to the lack of pigmentation.

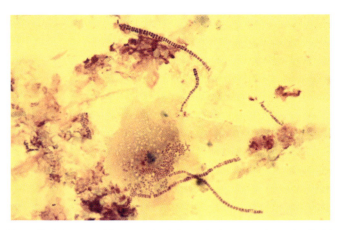

Figure 30-9 *Dermatophilus congolensis* in cytologic preparation stained with Diff-Quik. Note the typical "railroad tracks" appearance of this bacterium.

demodicosis, pemphigus foliaceus, and generalized granulomatous disease should be considered as differential diagnoses.[60] Dermatophilosis involving distal limbs must be differentiated from contact dermatitis, contact photosensitization, atypical dermatophytosis, pastern folliculitis, and pastern leukocytoclastic vasculitis.

Cytology

For a definitive diagnosis, a portion of a crust should be minced and mixed with a few drops of water on a glass slide, air-dried, heat-fixed, gram-stained, and examined microscopically. Touch preparations of the soaked undersurface of a new crust may also be useful to identify the organism. Romanowski stain (Diff-Quik) can be used as a rapid staining technique to identify the organism. When present, *D. congolensis* is observed under oil immersion as branching organisms. It is common to identify *Staphylococcus* spp. on cytology from affected horses. The filaments can usually be seen dividing both transversely and longitudinally into thick bundles of coccoid forms (Fig. 30-9). In chronic cases, cytology may be negative, and it may be necessary to culture the organism.

Culture

Dermatophilus congolensis grows easily on blood agar when incubated at 37°C (98.6°F) with increased carbon dioxide. If severe secondary infection is present, other organisms may overgrow the plate, and special isolation techniques may be necessary.

Pathology

Crusted lesions should be selected for biopsies, and care should be taken that crusts are sectioned and embedded, even when they lift off the biopsy, because the most characteristic microscopic feature is a stratified or layered crust. Crusts are made of alternating layers of parakeratotic and orthokeratotic keratin and accumulations of degenerating neutrophils.[61] Large numbers of organisms are usually present within the crust in acute cases. Severe epidermal hyperplasia, suppurative luminal folliculitis, intracellular edema, and perivascular infiltration of the dermis with neutrophils (especially in acute lesions), mononuclear cells, and plasma cells (especially in chronic lesions) are also often observed. Organisms are best visualized using Giemsa or Brown and Brenn stains.

Therapy

One of the most important components of clinical management for horses with dermatophilosis is to keep animals dry. Most horses recover spontaneously within a month of being moved to a dry environment. Topical therapy is also important. Various products have been used for treatment of equine dermatophilosis. Benzoyl peroxide shampoos are antibacterial[62] and keratolytic, helping with the removal of crusts. Topical therapy should be applied at least once weekly. Shampoo should be allowed to contact the skin for 10 to 15 minutes. Excessive scrubbing should be discouraged because it leads to trauma in the hair follicles and increases the risk of furunculosis. It is important not to share grooming tools between affected and nonaffected horses to minimize spread of the organism. For localized lesions, topical mupirocin (Bactoderm; Pfizer Inc, Pfizer Animal Health, NY), a drug with excellent antibacterial properties and skin penetration, may be used.[63,64] Other topical options include stannous fluoride 0.4% applied daily and oxychlorine spray to be used several times daily. Both products are rapidly bactericidal and constitute a valid alternative to labor intensive shampoo therapy.

Systemic antimicrobial therapy may be necessary for treatment of horses with severe or generalized dermatophilosis. *Dermatophilus congolensis* is usually sensitive to a variety of antibiotics,[65] including erythromycin, penicillin, sulfonamides, and gentamicin. Most often, penicillin G (22,000 IU/kg) is used for short-term treatment, and trimethoprim-potentiated sulfonamides (15-20 mg/kg twice daily) are used for longer treatment periods (minimum treatment period of 3 weeks). Treatment should be extended 7 to 10 days past the clinical resolution of lesions to minimize the likelihood of a relapse. Horses should be monitored for development of colitis and bone marrow suppression. Unfortunately, previously infected animals may not develop immunity and may relapse when favorable conditions are present.

Prevention

The most effective method for prevention of equine dermatophilosis is to minimize exposure to excessive moisture and insects. Insect repellents (e.g., 2% permethrin, FlyPel) should be applied at least once daily in tropical climates where high humidity and rainfall are present. Topical antibacterial therapy with antibacterial shampoos (e.g., benzoyl peroxide) is also helpful to decrease the bacterial load on the skin.

Public Health Considerations

Dermatophilosis is a rare zoonosis. In humans it can cause pitted keratolysis, painful or pruritic folliculitis, or subcutaneous nodules.[66-68] Immunosuppressed individuals may be more susceptible to disease.[69]

The complete reference list is available online at www.expertconsult.com.

CHAPTER

31 *Rhodococcus equi*

Melissa T. Hines

Rhodococcus equi infection was first described in horses in 1923.[1] It is now recognized worldwide as a major cause of disease in foals 3 weeks to 6 months of age. The most common clinical manifestation is pyogranulomatous pneumonia, although a number of other clinical problems may be identified. The disease has the potential to cause significant losses, especially on farms where it is endemic. Infrequently, *R. equi* causes infection in adult horses, generally thought to be associated with immunosuppression. *R. equi* has been isolated from a wide variety of species, including cats, dogs, goats, cattle, camelids, pigs, crocodiles, and other indigenous animals. Clinical disease is uncommon in these species, and infection is often localized. *R. equi* is now considered an important pathogen in immunocompromised human patients, particularly those infected with human immunodeficiency virus (HIV).

Etiology

Rhodococcus equi, previously known as *Corynebacterium equi* and *Mycobacterium equi*, is a facultative intracellular bacterium that resides within macrophages.[2,3] A proposal to reclassify this organism as *Prescottia equi*, a new genus within the *Corynebacteriales* order, is under consideration but this chapter will use the currently accepted classification within the genus *Rhodococcus*.[3a] Rhodococci belong to the family Nocardiaceae, order Actinomycetales. *R. equi* is a pleomorphic, gram-positive organism with a rod-coccus life cycle.[2,4] Depending on growth conditions and the phase of the life cycle, it may appear either coccoid or as long rods or short filaments with rudimentary branching. The organism is aerobic, nonmotile, asporogenous, and partially acid-fast. In vitro, optimal growth occurs at 30° C (86° F) and at a pH between 7.0 and 7.5.[3,5]

Rhodococcus equi is a member of a unique phylogenetic group within the Actinomycetales, known as the *mycolata*.[2,6] This group contains a number of pathogenic genera in addition to *Rhodococcus*, including *Mycobacterium*, *Corynebacterium*, and *Nocardia*. The distinguishing feature of the mycolata is their distinct, lipid-rich cell envelope that contains mycolic acids, a large proportion of which are linked to the peptidoglycan-arabinogalactan cell wall polysaccharide and glycolipids. This characteristic cell envelope forms a permeability barrier to hydrophilic compounds, making a permeability pathway, such as those provided by porins, necessary.[7] The unique mycolic acid-containing cell envelope of *R. equi* is clinically significant because it is thought to play a role in survival of the bacteria under harsh conditions, such as within macrophages, and may also influence antibiotic susceptibility patterns.[6-8]

There are numerous strains of *R. equi* that include both virulent and avirulent variants. Strains may be identified by a variety of characteristics, including the degree of virulence, serotyping, and restriction endonuclease digestion of genomic and plasmid deoxyribonucleic acid (DNA).[9-16] In one study, 44 strains were identified among 209 isolates, with 5 strains accounting for more than half of the isolates.[17] It appears that a small number of strains account for clinical disease, and that in some cases, disease may be caused by simultaneous infection with multiple strains.[17,18]

Virulent strains of *R. equi* are characterized by their ability to survive and replicate within macrophages (Fig. 31-1). This ability is associated with the presence of a large virulence

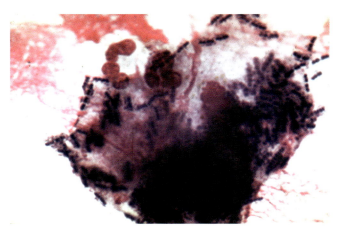

Figure 31-1 *Rhodococcus equi* in equine macrophage. Virulence is associated with the ability of *R. equi* to survive and replicate within macrophages.

plasmid of approximately 80 to 90 kilobases (kb), which was initially identified in isolates from diseased foals.[12-14,19] A number of different strains carry the virulence plasmid, and these strains appear to be geographically widespread.[17] Based on analysis of DNA from the virulence plasmids of various isolates, at least 10 distinct but closely related plasmids have been identified.[20-27] The virulence plasmid has been sequenced and contains 73 coding sequences that can be grouped into four regions based on open reading frame amino acid sequence similarity and predicted protein function.[28,29] Three of these regions contain genes that encode proteins involved in functions such as conjugation, replication, stability, and segregation. The presence of genes resembling those required for conjugation suggests that the virulence plasmid may be transferred from virulent to avirulent strains, although this has not been demonstrated. The fourth region of the virulence plasmid is an approximately 27.5-kb pathogenicity island (PAI) that is crucial for the virulence of *R. equi* in foals. This PAI was most likely acquired through horizontal gene transfer from an uncertain bacterial source in the soil. It encodes 6 full-length virulence-associated protein (Vap) genes (A, C, D, E, G, and H) and 3 truncated Vap pseudogenes (VapF, I and X). The first Vap to be identified was VapA, a highly immunogenic surface lipoprotein of 15 to 17 kilodaltons.[12,13,19,30] Vaps C, D, and E are secreted, but unlike VapA, are not anchored to the cell wall.[31] The Vap genes show little homology with known genes in other species, suggesting that *R. equi* employs novel virulence mechanisms. Of the Vap genes, only VapA has been shown to play a role in virulence, although its precise function is unknown.[14,15,32-35] VapA is necessary for the replication of *R. equi* within macrophages, increases the cytotoxicity of *R. equi* for murine macrophages, and is required for pathogenicity in foals.[6,14,15,32-34,36] However, although VapA is required for virulence, it is not sufficient. Some additional virulence determinants that have been identified within the PAI are genes for two regulatory proteins, virR and orf8.[35,37,38] The loss of either regulator results in decreased transcription of VapA. The vcgB gene *(orf 10)* also has a potential role in virulence.[39] In addition, genes on the virulence plasmid appear to influence chromosomal gene expression patterns, which may affect intracellular survival.[40]

Multiple other factors, such as additional regulatory systems, characteristics of the mycolic acid-containing cell envelope, and interactions with iron, influence virulence.[8,15,41-45] Strains of *R. equi* with longer mycolic acid carbon chains in the cell envelope are more lethal in mice and cause greater granuloma formation than those with shorter mycolic acid carbon chains.[8,46] The polysaccharide capsule has been suspected to be a virulence factor, but a mutant strain lacking a capsule was shown to multiply in isolated macrophages and was virulent in mice.[47] Virulence is linked to resistance to β-lactam antibiotics in a study of nonplasmid-containing *R. equi* strains isolated from humans, but a similar association has not been recognized in foals.[48-50]

Gene expression by bacteria is often regulated by complex networks that respond to environmental signals. At least five environmental signals, including temperature, pH, oxidative stress, magnesium, and iron, contribute to the regulation of gene expression within the PAI of *R. equi*.[6,31,51-55] Because the conditions that upregulate expression generally tend to be present when there is bacterial interaction with the host, the pattern of gene expression is consistent with the role of these genes in virulence. Maximal expression of VapA occurs at high temperature (37°C [98.6°F]) and low pH (6.5).[51,52]

Almost all clinical isolates of *R. equi* from horses contain the virulence plasmid and express VapA, but this is not true of isolates from other species.[6,15,25,56-59] A second plasmid, 79 to 100 kb in size, has been identified that expresses VapB but not VapA.[6,15,60,61] Although this plasmid has not been associated

with naturally occurring disease in foals, it can cause disease after experimental inoculation and appears to be of intermediate virulence.[62] In isolates from swine, 60% are positive for VapB, whereas other isolates lack a plasmid.[63] In human patients affected with *R. equi*, strains may contain VapA or VapB or may lack a virulence plasmid.[60,64] It is unclear if the severely immunocompromised status of the majority of human patients with *R. equi* allows relatively avirulent organisms to produce disease or if there are distinct, species-specific virulence determinants.

Epidemiology

R. equi is widespread in soil and in the feces of herbivores, especially horses.[65-75] Because *R. equi* is present on virtually all horse farms, exposure of horses is common worldwide. In soil samples the greatest numbers of organisms are found in surface soil, with almost no bacteria found at a depth of 30 cm (1 foot) or more.[74] *R. equi* can be isolated from the feces of adult horses, reaching numbers of 10^2 to 10^3/g of feces.[68,72-74] This generally represents acquisition from contaminated soil and passive intestinal carriage in adult horses, rather than actual colonization of the intestine. In foals, *R. equi* can be first isolated from the feces at about 1 to 2 weeks of age, with most foals becoming positive by 4 weeks of age.[72,76] Up to the age of about 3 months, *R. equi* can actively multiply in the intestine of foals, reaching concentrations of 10^4 to 10^5/g of feces or higher and then declining to adult concentrations. Foals with rhodococcal pneumonia often swallow sputum infected with large numbers of virulent organisms, which may then multiply in the intestine, resulting in high numbers in the feces and significant environmental contamination.

Under suitable conditions, *R. equi* can multiply further in the environment. *R. equi* grows substantially better in soil enriched with feces than in soil alone, and it is hypothesized that the organic acids in manure, such as acetate and propionate, support growth.[5] The organism tends to replicate better at a relatively warm temperature and in a neutral soil (pH 7.3) compared with an acidic soil (pH < 5.5).[5] In addition, decreased soil moisture and decreased pasture cover have been associated with high numbers of environmental *R. equi*.[77] In some cases, a single gram of soil may contain millions of virulent *R. equi*.[68,72-74,78]

Inhalation of dust particles containing virulent *R. equi* is the major route of infection in foals. Experimentally, aerosolized bacteria and intratracheal or intrabronchial inoculation of bacteria in foals can produce pulmonary lesions similar to those of natural infection.[79-81] *R. equi* has been isolated from the air on farms, with the number of organisms in the air increasing on dry, windy days.[73,82-85] Although ingestion is a common route of exposure, in most cases it does not result in clinical disease.[68,72,86,87] Rarely, *R. equi* infection is acquired through contamination of a wound.[88,89] Once infection is established, *R. equi* may disseminate to distant sites by hematogenous spread. Foals are generally exposed to *R. equi* early in life, but the time when foals actually become infected has not been well established. Following experimental intrabronchial challenge the incubation period varies from approximately 3 days to 4 weeks, depending on the severity of the challenge.[14,81,87,90] Under field conditions the incubation period is uncertain and probably varies, depending on several factors such as the number of virulent bacteria, the age of the foal, and individual host defense mechanisms. It has been theorized that the age of onset of clinical disease is associated with the waning of maternal antibody.[68,72,91] However, a statistical study, as well as epidemiologic evidence, suggests that at least on endemic farms foals may become infected earlier, possibly during the first several days of life.[92-94] The median age at diagnosis on most endemic farms is 35 to 50 days. Also, while foals remain susceptible to infection over a wide age range, younger foals appear to be more susceptible than older foals.[62,79-81,95]

Exposure of foals to *R. equi* is common because the organism is present on most horse farms, but the prevalence of clinical disease varies widely between farms and years, ranging from 0% to 100%.[68,89,96-100] On many farms the disease is unrecognized, whereas on others it is either sporadic or endemic. Many endemic farms have prevalence rates of 13% to 25%. The mortality rate is also highly variable, with death or euthanasia occurring in 0% to approximately 30% of cases.[93,96,100-102]

Numerous studies have attempted to explain the difference in prevalence between farms and to identify risk factors for the development of rhodococcal disease. These studies have evaluated variables such as soil and airborne concentrations of *R. equi*, soil geochemistry, breeding-farm characteristics, management and preventive health practices, and foal-related factors.[89,103-106] It was initially proposed that the prevalence of rhodococcal pneumonia correlated with the number of *R. equi* bacteria in soil, but this was not supported by soil cultures.[67,107-110] Subsequently, it was hypothesized that farms with endemic disease were more heavily infected with virulent strains of *R. equi* than those farms where disease was not present, but the evidence has not uniformly supported this theory.[24,48,75,111] Martens et al[48] compared 33 farms with *R. equi* and 33 farms without a history of *R. equi* and found no significant associations between disease status and isolation of *R. equi* from soil or detection of VapA in soil isolates. Thus it appears that the risk of foals on a given farm for developing rhodococcal disease cannot be determined by soil culture and VapA results. One study evaluated soil samples from affected and unaffected farms for multiple factors, including pH, salinity, and nitrate, and found no association between any soil factor and the *R. equi* disease status of the farms.[97] A study of 171 mare-foal pairs in Kentucky indicated that dams of foals with *R. equi* pneumonia did not shed more *R. equi* in their feces than dams of unaffected foals.[112] Rhodococcal pneumonia has been associated in some studies with high airborne concentrations of *R. equi* and dry, dusty conditions.[73,82,85,96] In a study of Thoroughbred breeding farms in Australia, airborne concentrations of *R. equi* were correlated with disease incidence, and high concentrations were found in association with holding pens/lanes, warmer ambient temperatures, low soil moisture, reduced grass height, and later dates in the foaling season.[82] In a study in Kentucky, airborne concentrations of virulent *R. equi* were increased by the presence of horses at the sampling site and were lower between midnight and 6 AM than at other times, suggesting that an increased density and activity of horses at sites will increase airborne concentrations.[85]

Some associations between rhodococcal disease and environmental management have been identified, although individual study results have varied significantly. In general, most studies have supported an association between high foal density and disease, as well as between high mare and foal numbers and disease.[100,104,105,111] Also, farms with large acreage and a population of transient mares and foals tended to be at a high risk for foals developing rhodococcal pneumonia.[104-106] There has been no evidence that poor farm management or lack of attention to preventive health practices contributes to the probability of rhodococcal pneumonia.[104,106] The role of housing has been evaluated, but the results have been conflicting. Depending on the study, both concrete and dirt floors in foaling stalls have been associated with an increased risk of developing rhodococcal disease, whereas some studies have indicated that foaling at pasture may decrease the risk of disease.[104,106]

Limited studies have attempted to identify host factors of foals that influence the outcome of exposure to *R. equi*.

Chaffin et al[113] evaluated hematologic and immunophenotypic parameters in foals on endemic farms before the onset of clinical disease.[113] Foals with a lower number of segmented neutrophils or a CD4:CD8 ratio of less than 3.0 appeared to have a higher risk of developing rhodococcal pneumonia. However, the data were confounded by farm-related differences and there was considerable overlap between values for affected and unaffected foals, making the significance of these findings unclear. Flaminio et al[114] found that absolute and proportional B-cell concentrations were greater in foals with active *R. equi* pneumonia than in healthy foals of the same age. It has also been suggested that genetic factors may play a role in susceptibility to *R. equi*, in part because limited data suggest an association between foal death caused by *R. equi* and the type of transferrin, an iron-binding protein with differing genotypes and variable bacteriostatic properties.[115] Another hypothesis is that infection of foals with equine herpesvirus type 2 (EHV-2) is a predisposing factor for invasion of the respiratory tract by *R. equi*.[116,117] At this time, host factors that influence susceptibility to *R. equi* in foals are poorly understood.

Pathogenesis

Mechanisms of Disease

The infectivity of *R. equi* is limited to cells of the monocyte/macrophage lineage, and the basis of this organism's pathogenicity is its ability to replicate in and eventually destroy macrophages.[6,15,34,118] Although the function of the virulence plasmid is not fully understood, it is essential for full virulence and *R. equi* strains cured of the virulence plasmid are unable to survive and replicate in macrophages and are avirulent for foals and mice.[12,13,15,32,81] Defining the mechanisms by which rhodococci survive and replicate within macrophages and the role of the virulence plasmid are key to understanding the pathogenesis of the disease. The presence of the virulence plasmid does not appear to influence the uptake of *R. equi* by macrophages as both virulent and avirulent strains are phagocytosed to a similar extent.[33,119] *R. equi* can enter the macrophage via several mechanisms, and the specific mechanism used affects the ability of the organism to survive within the cell. A primary means of entry is through activation of the alternate complement pathway with fixation of complement and binding to the macrophage complement receptor type 3 (CR3), also known as Mac-l (CD11b/CD18).[120-123] In general, complement receptor-mediated phagocytosis is not associated with a high level of production of reactive oxygen intermediates and proinflammatory mediators, possibly allowing the organism to avoid classic macrophage-killing pathways.[122] Brumbaugh et al[123] reported that phagocytosis of *R. equi* by equine macrophages was not associated with a functional respiratory burst. In addition, *R. equi* can enter the cell through the Fc receptor after opsonization with specific antibody.[6,124-126] This route is associated with increased activation of phagocytes and possibly enhanced killing of *R. equi* in comparison to complement receptor-mediated phagocytosis. Another possible means of entry into the cell is via interaction with the macrophage mannose receptor, which may be associated with delayed phagosome-lysosome fusion.[127,128]

Virulent strains of *R. equi* continue to multiply once within the membrane-enclosed vacuoles of the macrophage, whereas avirulent strains multiply at low levels initially and cease to grow after approximately 6 hours.[8,34] The means by which virulent *R. equi* avoids the killing mechanisms of macrophages are not fully understood, although it appears there is a complex alteration of the normal phagocyte maturation process, which is at least in part regulated by the virulence plasmid.[119,124,125,130] In studies with murine macrophages, phagosome-lysosome fusion occurred with both virulent and avirulent *R. equi*. However, with virulent *R. equi*, the phagolysosomes did not acidify normally and maturation of the phagolysosome was ultimately blocked.[119,129] Also, virulent *R. equi* have developed several means to enhance intracellular survival. Among these are the ability to effectively acquire essential nutrients, such as iron; the modulation of cytokine production; and the presence of antioxidant defense mechanisms, such as catalase, that protect the organism from reactive oxygen metabolites.[54,55,124,129-131]

The replication of *R. equi* within macrophages ultimately results in the death of the host cell. In vitro, macrophage degeneration is apparent approximately 8 hours after infection and is marked by 24 hours.[124,125] Cell death occurs by necrosis rather than apoptosis. The cytotoxicity requires viable bacteria and is linked to virulence, although the exact mechanisms are unclear. Based on studies in murine macrophages, the cytotoxicity of *R. equi* is strongly upregulated by the presence of VapA-expressing plasmids.[33] Isolates with a VapB-expressing plasmid are less virulent and have a lower cytotoxic potential, whereas isogenic strains without a plasmid are avirulent with a very low cytotoxic potential.

Large numbers of cells migrate to the site in response to infection with *R. equi*, ultimately resulting in granuloma formation. The precise signals that influence granuloma formation are largely unknown, but it is clear that a complex network of cytokines and chemokines is involved. Although granulomas may help contain and control infection, they may also contribute to the pathology of disease because they are associated with the secretion of several inflammatory mediators and may allow proliferation of organisms and cause the loss of pulmonary function.[133]

Immunity to *Rhodococcus equi*

The mechanism of protective immunity to *R. equi* has important implications for the control of disease. Although the outcome of exposure to *R. equi* is clearly affected by the dose and virulence of the organism, the host immune response is also critical. Virtually all foals are exposed to *R. equi* early in life, but most do not develop disease. Adult horses are essentially resistant to infection because of the acquisition of protective immunity. Thus it appears that most foals are capable of developing effective immune responses, which subsequently protect them for life. The mechanisms of this protective immunity are not fully understood, and although much emphasis has been placed on the role of cellular immunity, it appears that all aspects of the immune system are involved.[134,135]

Role of Innate Immunity

Innate immune responses play an important role in the control of *R. equi* and strongly influence adaptive immune responses.[134-137] This includes the responses of macrophages and dendritic cells. Although the replication of *R. equi* in nonactivated macrophages is critical to the pathogenesis of disease, at the same time the killing of *R. equi* by activated macrophages is important in the control of infection. Mice with macrophages that are deficient in either of two radical-generating pathways have an increased susceptibility to infection with *R. equi*.[138] Macrophage activation by *R. equi* in mice involves toll-like receptor 2 (TLR-2).[136,139,140] Because human neonates have diminished TLR-induced responses compared with adults, it has been hypothesized that inefficient TLR-2 signaling could contribute to the enhanced susceptibility of neonatal foals to *R. equi*.

Neutrophils may also be important in controlling *R. equi* early in the course of infection.[132,138] The induction of a neutrophil deficiency in mice during the first week after experimental rhodococcal infection resulted in more severe disease

Box 31-1 Commercial Sources of *R. equi* Hyperimmune Plasma

Lake Immunogenics, Inc. (USDA licensed: Pneumomune-Re)
348 Berg Road
Ontario, NY 14519
585-265-1973 or 800-648-9990
lakeimmunogenics.com

Plasvacc USA, Inc. (USDA licensed: Equiplas R, Equiplas REA)
1535 Templeton Road
Templeton, CA 93465
805-434-0321 or 800-654-9743
plasvaccusa.com

MgBiologics (USDA licensed: ReSolution *R. equi* antibody)
2366 270th St.
Ames, IA 50014
515-769-2340 or 877-769-2340
mgbiologics.com

Veterinary Immunogenics, Ltd. (European licensure: Hypermune-RE)
Carleton Hill
Penrith
Cumbria
CA11 8TZ
United Kingdom
+44 (0) 1768 863881
veterinaryimmunogenics.com

PRO-SER S.A.
Av. Leandro N. Alem 1698
(2752) Capitan Sarmiento; Buenos Aires, Argentina
(02478) 482373, from abroad +54 2478 482373
labproser.com.ar

USDA, United States Department of Agriculture.

and significantly increased tissue concentrations of *R. equi*.[141] It has been hypothesized that a defect in neutrophil function contributes to disease in foals, but in general, neutrophils from foals are fully bactericidal.[121,124,142-146]

Role of Antibody

Antibody also plays a significant role in immunity to *R. equi*. It appears to be most important in the initial stages of infection and does not afford complete protection. Some mechanisms by which antibody may contribute to immunity include blocking the initial stages of cellular infection, altering the route by which bacteria enter the macrophage, and decreasing the bacteria's ability to arrest maturation of the phagosome.[134,135]

Several lines of evidence support a role for antibody in protection against *R. equi*. The age of onset of clinical disease in foals often coincides with the waning of maternal antibody, although other factors undoubtedly contribute to the age-related susceptibility of *R. equi* as well. Antibodies to *R. equi*, including antibodies to VapA, are widespread in horses and are found in the majority of foals within the first 3 months of age.[13,147-150] An inverse correlation may exist between antibody concentrations and disease severity and prevalence.[120,148,149,151] After challenge of immune adult horses with virulent *R. equi*, the antibody response is characterized predominantly by increases in concentrations of IgGa and IgGb, which are important isotypes in opsonization and complement fixation.[152] In experiments in vitro, opsonization with *R. equi*-specific antibody increased phagosome-lysosome fusion and significantly enhanced the killing of *R. equi* by alveolar macrophages from foals.[124]

Additional evidence supporting a role for humoral immunity in protection against *R. equi* comes from studies of passive immunization through the administration of hyperimmune plasma (HIP) (Box 31-1). Several studies investigating the protective effect of HIP have been performed in both mice and foals with varied results.[24,93,98,99,153-160] Specifically in foals, although the administration of HIP does not always have a significant protective effect, it can prevent or reduce the severity of pneumonia in foals that are either experimentally or naturally infected with *R. equi*.[93,98,99,155-159] Hyperimmune plasma does not alleviate clinical signs or alter the course of the disease when administered to foals 7 days after experimental challenge with *R. equi*, suggesting that HIP is primarily effective in the prevention of infection rather than treatment.[156]

It is uncertain which specific components of HIP are responsible for enhancing protection against *R. equi*. In addition to immunoglobulin, HIP contains a number of substances, including fibronectin, complement factors, interferon, and other cytokines. In a study by Hooper-McGrevy et al,[161] the same degree of protection was provided by purified immunoglobulin specific for VapA and VapC as by HIP, suggesting that this immunoglobulin was the primary component of HIP that conferred protection. In contrast, in an experimental model in colostrum-deprived foals, Perkins et al[157] found no difference in the incidence and severity of disease after administration of normal equine plasma as compared to HIP. Because the survival rate for foals in both groups was approximately 70% without antibiotic therapy, both normal and HIP were thought to provide some protective effect, although there was no untreated control group. It was therefore concluded that either only a small amount of antibody was sufficient to enhance protection or that factors in the plasma other than immunoglobulin were responsible for the protective effect.

Several studies have evaluated the protection provided by the ingestion of colostrum from mares immunized against *Rhodococcus*. Martens et al[162] found that the passive immunization of foals by ingestion of colostrum from mares immunized with live *R. equi* did not provide protection against experimental challenge. Similarly, in field studies by Madigan et al,[98] in which pregnant mares were immunized with a *R. equi* bacterin, and by Prescott et al,[158] in which pregnant mares were immunized with a VapA extract, foals were not protected from natural infection with *R. equi*. In contrast, in a field study by Cauchard et al,[163] in which pregnant mares were immunized with either VapA protein or whole killed *R. equi*, vaccination did appear to provide protection. In general, the protection provided by colostrum has not been as consistent as that with HIP.

Role of Cellular Immunity

Cell-mediated immunity should play a major role in the control of *R. equi* because it is an intracellular pathogen, and considerable evidence supports this. Much of this evidence comes from a mouse model of rhodococcal disease, although there are some data in horses. Clearance of intracellular pathogens by T cells generally involves secretion of cytokines and direct cytotoxicity. In mice, both CD4+ and CD8+ T lymphocytes contribute to immune clearance of *R. equi* from the lung.[164-166] Mice with CD4+ T cells but no CD8+ T cells are able to clear pulmonary infection completely, whereas mice with CD8+ T cells but no CD4+ T cells are able to decrease bacterial numbers but not completely clear infection. Thus CD4+ T lymphocytes appear to be both necessary and sufficient for clearance of *R. equi*.[164-166] CD4+ T lymphocytes are further characterized as T helper 1 (Th1) or T helper 2 (Th2) cells, depending on their cytokine secretion patterns.[167] CD4+ Th1 cells secrete primarily interferon gamma (IFN-γ), a potent activator of macrophage microbicidal activity, whereas CD4+ Th2 lymphocytes secrete predominantly the interleukins IL-4, IL-5, and IL-13, which potentiate the humoral immune response. In mice, secretion of IFN-γ by CD4+ Th1 lymphocytes appears to be absolutely required for clearance of *R. equi*.[165] Adoptive transfer of an *R. equi*-specific CD4+ Th1 cell line mediates clearance in immunodeficient nude mice that normally are unable to control pulmonary bacteria.[166] In contrast, nude mice that receive an *R. equi*-specific CD4+ Th2 cell line are unable to clear bacteria and develop prototypic pulmonary lesions. Also, Th17 cells are

now recognized as an important T helper subset in protection against intracellular pathogens especially at mucosal sites, and these cells may play a role in the control of *R. equi*.[168-170] Even though CD4+ cells are critical in the control of rhodococcal infection, CD8+ T lymphocytes also contribute. Like CD4+ Th1 cells, they can produce IFN-γ. Another possible important effector function of CD8+ cells is the recognition and lysis of *R. equi*-infected cells, as demonstrated for the related pathogen, *Mycobacterium tuberculosis*.[171,172]

Limited data in horses support the observations in mice that protective immunity to *R. equi* involves both CD4+ and CD8+ T lymphocytes. Adult horses challenged intrabronchially with virulent *R. equi* do not develop clinical disease and effectively clear bacteria from the lung in association with increased numbers of CD4+ and CD8+ lymphocytes at the site of infection.[173] T lymphocytes from bronchoalveolar lavage (BAL) fluid of challenged horses proliferate when stimulated with *R. equi* antigen, and both CD4+ and CD8+ T lymphocytes from the site express IFN-γ. In addition, T lymphocytes from the blood and BAL fluid of adult immune horses have *R. equi*-specific cytolytic activity.[174] These cytotoxic T lymphocytes (CTLs) appear to be primarily CD8+ and have the ability to kill in a major histocompatibility complex (MHC) class I unrestricted fashion. They appear to recognize unique bacterial lipids from the cell wall.[175]

Immunity to *Rhodococcus equi* in Neonatal Foals

The immune responses of neonates differ both quantitatively and qualitatively from those of adults.[176-180] Not only are neonates immunologically naïve, but they also have several immunologic functions that are diminished as compared to adults, some of which have been documented in foals. For example, antigen-presenting cells from foals have lower expression of CD1 and MHC class II as compared to cells from adult horses.[181,182] In addition, *R. equi*-specific CTL activity is relatively low in 3-week-old foals, with activity increasing to adult horse levels by 8 weeks of age.[183] Oral inoculation of foals with *R. equi* can accelerate the development of *R. equi*-specific CTL.[184] The ability of monocytes, lymphocytes, and neutrophils to produce and regulate cytokines is also influenced by age.[145,179,180,185-187] In general, neonates are thought to have a Th2 bias and a diminished ability to generate the type 1 responses necessary for clearance of intracellular pathogens.[179,185] However, a diminished ability to produce both IFN-γ and IL-4 has been demonstrated in foals, suggesting there is not a clear polarization toward a Th2 response in foals.[188-190] Foal monocyte-derived dendritic cells are able to respond to *R. equi* and express the Th1-inducing cytokine IL-12.[181] Also, experimental infection of young foals with virulent *R. equi* results in IFN-γ production and antibody responses similar to those seen in adult horses.[191,192] Sturgill et al[193] did not find any significant association between IFN-γ or IL-4 secretion early in life and subsequent development of pneumonia.

The age-related differences in the immune responses of neonates as compared to adults have been hypothesized to account for the unique age-associated susceptibility of foals to rhodococcal pneumonia. However, despite these differences, the majority of foals are able to mount a successful immune response and do not develop significant clinical disease following exposure. Currently, the basis of the age-related susceptibility is not clear but is most likely multifactorial.

Clinical Findings

Clinical disease caused by *R. equi* is most common in foals 3 weeks to 6 months of age, with signs most often developing before 4 months of age.[93,100,101,107,194] Respiratory tract disease occurs most frequently, although other systems may be affected as well, either independently or in conjunction with pulmonary involvement. General clinical signs often associated with rhodococcal disease, regardless of the site of infection, include fever, lethargy, and decreased appetite.

Rhodococcal infection may remain subclinical. When clinical disease does develop, it is often insidious in nature. Because of the foal's ability to compensate and the slow spread of infection, early clinical signs are often subtle, making the disease difficult to detect. Although infection is generally chronic, clinical signs often appear acutely when the disease becomes severe, leading to the description of an "acute on chronic" disease. Occasionally, foals may be found dead or in acute, severe respiratory distress with high fever.

Pulmonary Disease

The most common manifestation of *R. equi* infection in foals is chronic pyogranulomatous bronchopneumonia with abscessation and associated suppurative lymphadenitis.[100,107,108,194] Of 131 cases with *R. equi* infection, suppurative pneumonia was confirmed in 115.[194] In a review of 40 cases of equine lung abscesses, 32 cases were identified in foals 6 months of age or younger, with *Streptococcus equi* subsp. *zooepidemicus* cultured from 20 of 34 and *R. equi* cultured from 13 of 34 cases.[195] Occasionally, *R. equi* is cultured with other pathogens, including *Pneumocystis carinii*.[196] *R. equi* has rarely been cultured from foals with the syndrome of bronchointerstitial pneumonia and respiratory distress, but it is not believed to be the primary cause of this condition.[197]

It is important to minimize stress during the physical examination of foals with suspected rhodococcal pneumonia so as not to exacerbate respiratory distress. In a study of 161 foals with *R. equi* pneumonia, the most common clinical signs were cough (71%), fever (68%), lethargy (53%), and increased respiratory effort (43%).[94] Tachypnea and tachycardia are also common. In severe cases, mucous membranes may be cyanotic. Nasal discharge is an inconsistent finding. Although many affected foals are in good body condition, weight loss or failure to grow may occur, especially in chronic cases. Findings on auscultation of the lung are variable and often do not correlate with the severity of pneumonia. If the foal can tolerate it, the sensitivity of auscultation may be enhanced by inducing the foal to breathe deeply using a rebreathing bag or cupping a hand over the nostrils for a few seconds. Inspiratory and expiratory crackles and wheezes may be audible and are often most prominent cranioventrally. In some cases, only large airway sounds are present, suggesting consolidation. With severe consolidation or extensive peripheral abscess formation, lung sounds may be decreased. This may also indicate pleural effusion, although effusion is only occasionally seen in association with rhodococcal pneumonia.[198] In one case, respiratory distress was identified in association with a focal mediastinal abscess without concurrent pulmonary involvement.[199] Thoracic percussion, as well as ancillary diagnostic aids such as radiography and ultrasonography, can help detect areas of consolidation, abscessation, or pleural fluid.

Extrapulmonary Disorders

Numerous extrapulmonary disorders (EPDs), including extrapulmonary sites of infection and immune-mediated disorders, have been associated with *R. equi* infection.[194,200,201] Retrospective studies from referral centers have found the prevalence of EPDs to be 66% to 74%, although this is higher than what some clinicians recognize.[200,201] EPDs may occur either with or without pneumonia and can be subclinical and difficult to

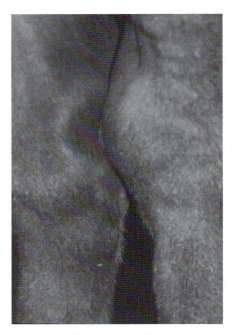

Figure 31-2 An immune-mediated polysynovitis may be recognized in association with *R. equi* infection. Although any joint may be affected, the tibiotarsal and stifle joints appear to be most often involved. Typically, joint effusion occurs with minimal or no lameness.

recognize antemortem. One study of 150 foals identified 39 separate EPDs, with multiple EPDs occurring concurrently in some foals.[201] In this study, survival was lower in foals with EPDs as compared to those without (43%: 48/111 versus 82%: 32/39).

Abdominal Disease

Enterocolitis, typhlitis, abdominal abscesses, peritonitis, and adhesions have been reported in association with *R. equi*.[100,194,198,202,203] In the review of 131 foals with *R. equi* by Zink et al,[194] approximately 50% of foals with bronchopneumonia on necropsy also had intestinal lesions, and an additional 4% of foals had intestinal lesions without pneumonia. Of the foals with intestinal lesions, only 38% had any history or clinical signs related to intestinal disease. Colic and diarrhea are the predominant signs in those foals with intestinal involvement that do manifest clinical signs. In chronic or severe cases, there may be a loss of body condition. Some foals develop significant ascites, which is typically associated with extensive granulomatous inflammation of the colonic mucosa and submucosa. *R. equi* has been identified in association with *Lawsonia intracellularis* in a 26-month-old colt with chronic diarrhea.[204]

Nonseptic Polysynovitis

Nonseptic polysynovitis has been documented in approximately one third of *R. equi* cases, and can be an early manifestation of disease.[101,200,201] There is variable effusion of one or more synovial structures, but in contrast to septic arthritis, there is generally no or minimal lameness (Fig. 31-2). Multiple joints are typically involved, with the tibiotarsal, stifle, carpal, and fetlock joints being frequently affected.[101,201] Evaluation of synovial fluid reveals a nonseptic, mononuclear pleocytosis with no bacterial growth and histologic examination reveals a lymphoplasmacytic synovitis.[101,205,206] The effusion generally resolves as the rhodococcal infection clears.

The pathogenesis of this nonseptic polysynovitis has been hypothesized to be immune-mediated.[205,206] This theory has been supported by the presence of immunoglobulin within the synovial membrane of three affected foals.[206] Additionally, rheumatoid factor activity, which results from antibodies directed against the Fc portion of immunoglobulin, has been identified in the synovial fluid of a foal with *R. equi* pneumonia and reactive arthritis.[205] However, heavy intrabronchial challenge with virulent *R. equi* has also been shown to result in a polysynovitis without lameness in which *R. equi* can be initially cultured from the synovial effusion.[14] Thus an alternative hypothesis for the polysynovitis in some cases is that bacteremia leads to a short-lived septic polysynovitis, which is followed by ongoing nonseptic inflammation after clearance of the organism.

Bone and Joint Disease

Septic arthritis and osteomyelitis may be observed either alone or with other signs of rhodococcal disease.[100,194,207-210] These conditions can be distinguished from nonseptic polysynovitis by the degree of lameness along with cytologic evaluation and culture or PCR of joint fluid or aspirates. Some foals have an associated cellulitis. Several cases of *R. equi* vertebral osteomyelitis have been reported.[211,212] In general, early signs of vertebral osteomyelitis may include a stiff gait, reluctance to move, and pain on palpation. However, the diagnosis is usually not made until the infection extends to the epidural space, causing signs of spinal cord or nerve root compression such as paresis, ataxia, paralysis, or cauda equina syndrome. The specific signs vary, depending on the severity and site of the lesion. Although radiography may be useful in the diagnosis, in four of six cases, radiographs were normal despite the presence of extensive lesions on necropsy.[212-214] Therefore nuclear scintigraphy, computed tomography (CT), or magnetic resonance imaging (MRI) may be indicated. The prognosis is generally poor, although a foal that presented for urinary incontinence associated with diskospondylitis involving the sacral vertebrae responded to debridement and long-term antimicrobial treatment.[212]

Diseases of Other Body Systems

A variety of other conditions have been sporadically recognized in association with *R. equi*. Abscesses have been seen in almost every tissue, including the brain.[87,89,100,200,215] In addition, other problems have been documented such as dermatitis, ulcerative lymphangitis, and cellulitis, which has been reported secondary to wounds or skin damage by the larvae of *Strongyloides westeri*.[214,216] Pericarditis, endocarditis, nephritis, hepatitis, cholangitis, and hepatoencephalopathy have also been reported, as have uveitis, panophthalmitis, and hypopyon (Fig. 31-3).[100,194,200,217,218] Immune-mediated hemolytic anemia, immune-mediated thrombocytopenia, and telogen effluvium have been described.[201,219]

R. equi has rarely been isolated from aborted equine fetuses and infertile mares.[194,220-227] The significance of isolating the organism has been unclear in some cases, but *R. equi* has been confirmed as a cause of placentitis and abortion with fetal pneumonia.[223,224,227] A case of fetal infection and abortion has been seen in association with an avirulent strain.[228]

Infection in Adult Horses

Rhodococcal disease is uncommon in adult horses as most adults are immune to infection, but sporadic cases have been reported.[190,229-235] As in foals, the most common clinical signs are related to suppurative bronchopneumonia (Fig. 31-4). Occasionally, pleuritis may be recognized. Other reported signs include intestinal disease, lymphadenitis, wound infections,

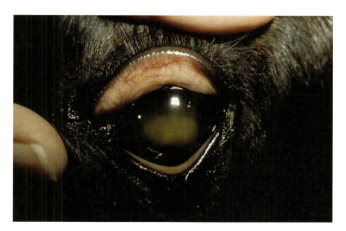

Figure 31-3 Hypopyon associated with *R. equi* in a foal.

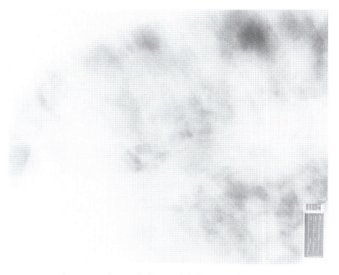

Figure 31-4 Thoracic radiograph from adult horse with *R. equi* pneumonia. There is a severe, multifocal, coalescing alveolar pattern. Rhodococcal disease is uncommon in adult horses and is generally thought to be associated with immunosuppression. Clinically, the most common manifestation in adults has been suppurative bronchopneumonia, similar to that recognized in foals,

and osteomyelitis. In both cases in which the organism isolated from adult horses was assessed, the virulence plasmid was present.[231,232] It is thought that adult horses with *R. equi* infection are immunocompromised, and although the immune status has not been assessed in every case, immunodeficiency was reported in two cases.[230,234]

Diagnosis

The ability to make a rapid, accurate diagnosis of rhodococcal disease is important because early recognition and treatment can improve the prognosis. Based on clinical signs alone, it is difficult to distinguish pneumonia caused by *R. equi* from that caused by other pathogens. The American College of Veterinary Internal Medicine (ACVIM) consensus statement has reviewed evidence related to the diagnosis, treatment, control, and prevention of *R. equi* infection and has made recommendations based on the strength of the evidence.[236] For

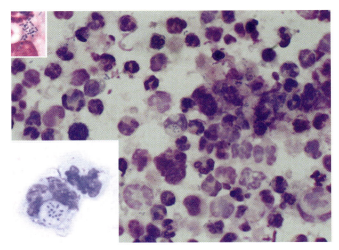

Figure 31-5 Cytology of tracheobronchial fluid from foal with rhodococcal pneumonia. There is increased cellularity, characterized primarily by macrophages and neutrophils. Intracellular organisms are often identified in macrophages *(top inset)* and may also be found within neutrophils *(bottom inset)*. *R. equi* may appear coccoid or as rods or short filaments with rudimentary branching. It is often described as "coccobacillary." *(Courtesy Dr. Andrea Bohn.)*

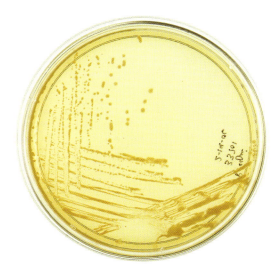

Figure 31-6 *R. equi* in culture. Colonies are typically irregularly round, smooth, semitransparent, and mucoid. After several days in culture, colonies often develop a characteristic salmon-pink color.

bronchopneumonia, the consensus statement recommends that diagnosis be based on bacteriologic culture or amplification of the VapA gene using polymerase chain reaction (PCR) from a tracheobronchial aspirate (TBA) from a foal with one or more of the following: (1) clinical signs of lower respiratory tract disease, (2) cytologic evidence of septic airway inflammation, or (3) radiographic or ultrasonographic evidence of bronchopneumonia.[236] For extrapulmonary infections, it is recommended that diagnosis be based on culture or PCR amplification of VapA from samples from the site of infection. In cases in which *R. equi* may not be detected at the site, such as polysynovitis or uveitis, diagnosis should be based on identification of *R. equi* from a TBA or other primary site of infection. Amplification of VapA by PCR should not be used alone because it does not allow for either identification of other bacterial pathogens or in vitro antimicrobial susceptibility testing of *R. equi* isolates. The evidence supporting these recommendations was felt to be strong. A number of additional tests have been evaluated for the diagnosis or *R. equi*, some of which may be supportive.

Cytology

The presence of intracellular gram-positive pleomorphic rods on cytologic evaluation of fluid specimens supports a diagnosis of rhodococcal infection (Fig. 31-5). Immunostaining procedures have also been used to aid in the detection of organisms.[237,238] The organisms may be present in low numbers and difficult to detect. Sweeney et al[101] reported that organisms consistent with *R. equi* were seen on cytology of tracheobronchial fluid in 61% of 48 culture-positive foals. Similarly, using an indirect fluorescent antibody technique, 62.3% of tracheal aspirates from 53 foals with experimentally induced rhodococcal pneumonia were positive.[237]

Culture

Culture and subsequent phenotypic analysis of the isolate by classic morphologic and biochemical tests has been the "gold standard" for the diagnosis of *R. equi*. Typically, the organism is cultured from a TBA, which may be obtained by a variety of techniques.[237,239] When collecting the sample, stress to the

patient must be considered as some foals are in severe respiratory distress. Other samples, such as joint fluid or peritoneal fluid, can be cultured as appropriate based on the case. Blood culture appears to be a sensitive means of diagnosis in human patients with *R. equi*, and although blood cultures are not routinely performed in foals with suspected *R. equi* infection, intermittent or persistent bacteremia might be more common than previously recocognized.[100,240-242] In a study by Reuss et al,[201] 11 of 19 foals had positive blood cultures and these foals were less likely to survive than foals that were blood culture negative.

Colonies of *R. equi* usually appear on solid media within 48 hours of aerobic culture, although longer incubation may be necessary, especially for samples collected from foals that have been treated with antibiotics.[3,100,237,243,244] Occasionally, the organism may be isolated only under anaerobic conditions after antimicrobial therapy.[243] Colonies of *R. equi* generally appear irregularly round, smooth, semitransparent, and mucoid (Fig. 31-6). They typically have a characteristic salmon-pink color, which may not develop until 4 to 7 days in culture. Other pathogens may be isolated concurrently with *R. equi*.[101,196,245] It is generally assumed without further testing that the isolates of *R. equi* from clinically ill foals are virulent strains. However, isolates can be analyzed for the presence of virulence plasmids and virulence-associated antigens.[56,239,246,247]

The reliability of culture of TBAs in the diagnosis of rhodococcal pneumonia has varied among studies.* In some studies, essentially all foals in which *R. equi* was isolated from the lung parenchyma at necropsy had positive antemortem cultures from tracheobronchial fluid, but in other studies the results have not been as consistent. When combining the results of three studies, Giguere et al[249] reported an overall sensitivity of 86%.

Nucleic Acid Amplification and Polymerase Chain Reaction

A number of PCR techniques have been developed to amplify either chromosomal or plasmid DNA of *R. equi* in a variety of samples.[250-259] These techniques have generally been shown to be rapid and reliable, detecting small numbers of organisms.

---

*References 86, 100, 102, 195, 240, 248.

Using primers for VapA, virulent strains of *R. equi* can be identified in less than 24 hours. PCR assays based on genes other than VapA may be useful in identifying strains from environmental samples or from species other than horses, particularly human patients; however, amplification of VapA is recommended for use in foals with clinical disease.[236]

The results of studies assessing the accuracy of PCR have varied widely depending on several factors such as the specific assay and the "gold standard" for comparison. Sensitivities have ranged from approximately 10% to 100% and specificities from 78% to 91%.[237,240,252,260] However, most but not all studies have found PCR to be more sensitive than bacterial culture.

Cytology, culture, and PCR may all identify *R. equi* from the trachea of foals with subclinical disease or with simple contamination of the airways from inhaling *R. equi* from the environment. In one study on a farm with endemic rhodococcal pneumonia, 77 of 216 foals with no signs of respiratory disease (35%) had positive cultures of tracheobronchial fluid.[261] Therefore it is important to interpret culture and PCR results in the context of the entire case, including the physical examination findings, laboratory evaluation, and diagnostic imaging. Detection of *R. equi* from a foal without any evidence of disease is most likely incidental.[236] Similarly, identification of *R. equi* in nasal swabs or feces cannot be taken as evidence of rhodococcal disease.[239,240,262-264] *R. equi* may be present in nasal swabs as a result of contamination of the upper airways from inhalation of dust. Also, *R. equi* can be present in the feces of many normal horses.[66,76,262,263] At the same time, negative fecal cultures do not rule out infection. Despite the fact that infected foals often swallow contaminated sputum, in one study only 5 of 30 foals (17%) with confirmed *R. equi* pneumonia had positive fecal cultures.[261] Thus a single fecal sample from a foal has no diagnostic value. One study has advocated weekly quantitative fecal cultures as an aid in the early diagnosis of *R. equi* enteritis because the bacterial count per gram of feces increased at the onset of clinical signs.[263]

Serologic Tests

Serologic assays developed to detect *R. equi*-specific antibodies include several enzyme-linked immunosorbent assays (ELISAs), an agar-gel immunodiffusion (AGID) test, and synergistic hemolysis inhibition assays.[148,237,265-278] The presence of antibody could indicate maternal transfer of antibody, exposure, or infection associated with either subclinical or clinical disease. Assays to detect antibody have been used in research to measure the humoral immune response to *R. equi*. Although they have also been used in the clinical diagnosis of rhodococcal infection, independent studies evaluating their performance have demonstrated either low sensitivity, low specificity, or both. In general, the studies confirmed that antibodies, including those specific for VapA, were present in many foals regardless of their disease status. Some antibody could be maternally derived, but titers increased significantly over time in all assays, suggesting that foals are routinely exposed to *R. equi*, including virulent strains. One study evaluated the testing of paired sera, but this failed to improve the diagnostic accuracy.[276] It has been suggested that serologic tests may be of more value as a diagnostic test if used on nonendemic farms, but this has not been assessed.[275,276] The ACVIM consensus statement recommends that serology not be used as a diagnostic test for *R. equi* pneumonia.[236]

Ancillary Diagnostic Tests

Clinical Pathology

A complete blood count (CBC), fibrinogen, and serum biochemistry profile can provide useful information in the evaluation of patients with suspected rhodococcal infection.[100]

However, the abnormalities are nonspecific, reflecting the presence of inflammation. Hyperfibrinogenemia is the most consistent laboratory finding, although rare cases may have normal fibrinogen concentrations. Neutrophilic leukocytosis with or without monocytosis is also common. One study demonstrated that a white blood cell (WBC) count >20,000 cells/uL, fibrinogen concentration >700 mg/dL and evidence of pulmonary abscessation on imaging were more likely to be found in foals with pneumonia caused by *R. equi* than in foals with pneumonia caused by another pathogen.[279] However, there is significant variation in fibrinogen concentrations and WBC counts both within foals known to be infected with *R. equi* and compared to foals infected with another pathogen, limiting the value of these tests as specific diagnostic tests or prognostic indicators.* Thrombocytosis, which is often associated with acute or chronic inflammation, has also been reported in conjunction with *R. equi* infection, but this finding is variable.[100,241] Hyperglobulinemia may be seen in some foals.

Serum amyloid A (SAA) is an acute-phase protein that has been proposed as a useful inflammatory marker in infectious disease. In one limited study, foals with *R. equi* had increased concentrations of SAA.[280] Concentrations of SAA decreased in recovered foals before fibrinogen concentration increased and neutrophil count decreased, suggesting that SAA concentrations could be useful in monitoring treatment response. A study that evaluated SAA concentrations in foals before and during clinical rhodococcal pneumonia found that concentrations of SAA were variable and could not be used reliably either as an ancillary diagnostic tool or as a screen for early detection of disease.[281]

Diagnostic Imaging

Thoracic radiography is frequently used to evaluate foals with suspected *R. equi* pneumonia.[100,101,237,245,278,282] Typically, there is a prominent alveolar pattern with regional consolidation. Often, discrete nodular and cavitary lesions consistent with pulmonary abscessation are seen, and in some cases, gas is detectable within the abscesses (Fig. 31-7). Evidence of tracheobronchial lymphadenopathy may be present, characterized by nodular densities displacing the trachea dorsally. In foals with severe respiratory distress and a marked bronchointerstitial pattern, the syndrome of sporadic bronchointerstitial pneumonia should be considered. The cause of this syndrome is unclear, and although occasional cases have cultured *R. equi*, its role in the pathogenesis is unclear.[197] A miliary pattern characterized by distinct reticulonodular lesions was described in three of five foals concurrently infected with *R. equi* and *Pneumocystis carinii*.[196] Ultrasonography (US) of the thorax and abdomen can yield valuable information in the evaluation of cases with suspected rhodococcal disease.[100,283-285] With respect to the thorax, US does not image lesions with overlying aerated lung, and thus the technique is primarily useful in identifying peripheral lung involvement and may not evaluate the full extent of the lesions. In most affected foals, however, peripheral lesions are present.[283,284] When thoracic US was compared with radiography in 17 foals with confirmed *R. equi* pneumonia, the findings were essentially in agreement in 15 of 17 foals.[283] Lesions were identified by US in the remaining two foals but were less severe than those identified by radiography.

Radiographic or ultrasonographic detection of pulmonary abscesses can be useful in raising the index of suspicion of rhodococcal pneumonia but is not recommended as a definitive diagnostic test.[195,236] Other pathogens, such as *Streptococcus zooepidemicus*, can also cause abscessation and should be considered, especially in foals over 3 months of age.[195] In addition, evidence of abscessation may be absent in some cases of

*References 101, 195, 236, 245, 249, 279.

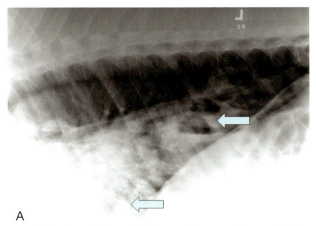

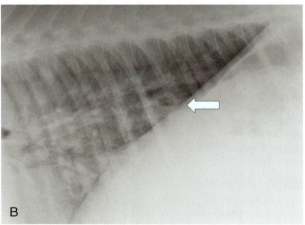

Figure 31-7 Thoracic radiographs from two foals with rhodococcal pneumonia. **A,** Severe, structured interstitial pattern with multiple, large, cavitating masses *(arrows)* typical of *R. equi.* **B,** Mild to moderate, diffuse, structured interstitial pattern, with numerous small nodules and masses and at least two moderate-sized cavitary lesions *(arrow)*. *(Courtesy Dr. Greg Roberts.)*

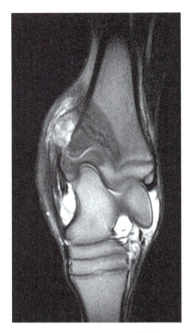

Figure 31-8 Magnetic resonance imaging (MRI) of left tarsus of foal with septic physitis, metaphysitis, and epiphysitis caused by *R. equi* (coronal proton-density image). There is a decrease in signal from the medial aspect of the tarsus and extending beyond the midline. Fluid in the soft tissue on the medial aspect most likely represents purulent material. The lesion in the tarsus demonstrated by MRI was much more extensive than that visualized radiographically. *(Courtesy Drs. Kelly Farnsworth and Pat Gavin.)*

rhodococcal pneumonia, and only a mild to severe bronchointerstitial pattern may be recognized.

Advanced imaging techniques, such as CT, MRI, and scintigraphic imaging, may be indicated in some foals with *R. equi* infection, especially when there is extrapulmonary involvement. High-resolution CT has been used to define lesions in human patients with *R. equi* pneumonia.[286] CT was used to diagnose a mediastinal abscess causing severe respiratory distress in a foal with an atypical clinical presentation of *R. equi*.[199] MRI and CT have been used to diagnose septic physitis in foals (Fig. 31-8). Scintigraphic perfusion imaging was used to demonstrate pulmonary perfusion defects in affected areas of the lung in four foals with experimental rhodococcal pneumonia.[155] The findings correlated well with radiographic and necropsy lesions.

Pathologic Findings

The gross lesions characteristic of *R. equi* pneumonia are multiple firm nodules separated by congested and partly atelectatic lung (Fig. 31-9).* The nodules vary in size, with some foci

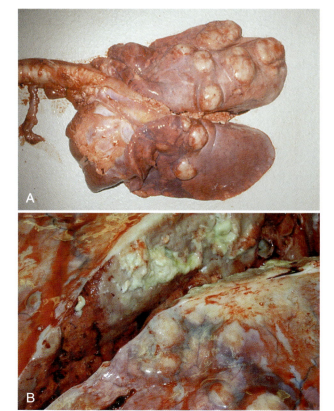

Figure 31-9 A, Multiple pulmonary abscesses characteristic of *R. equi* pneumonia. **B,** Caseous exudates on cut section of rhodococcal abscess. *(Courtesy Dr. Seth Harris.)*

---

*References 79, 80, 86, 194, 261, 287.

coalescing to form large lesions. Occasionally, multiple miliary pyogranulomatous foci are present. Although the distribution of lesions may vary, lesions are typically bilateral and are most severe in the cranioventral regions. Occasionally, lesions are widely distributed throughout the lung. The lesions are often described as abscesses when circumscribed and as suppurative bronchopneumonia when less well defined. They consist of areas of caseous necrosis, and in most cases, there is no distinct fibrous capsule around the necrotic tissue. The presence of pleural fluid is uncommon. Grossly, the bronchial lymph nodes are often enlarged and edematous, and caseonecrotic foci may be present. Emphysematous lymphadenitis has been described in a foal with rhodococcal pneumonia.[288]

Histologically, the lesions are predominantly pyogranulomatous. Early lung lesions are characterized by a cellular influx into the alveolar spaces, consisting largely of macrophages and multinucleate giant cells with fewer neutrophils. Intact bacteria are typically observed within macrophages and giant cells. Lymphocytes and plasma cells are present in moderate numbers, primarily in the alveolar septa and other interstitial zones. As the disease progresses, necrosis involves the alveolar septa and spreads to affect large areas of the pulmonary parenchyma, producing the caseous necrotic foci observed macroscopically. Numerous degenerate bacteria-laden macrophages are present. Frequently, a pyogranulomatous lymphadenitis is also present histologically.

The most common sites involved in *R. equi* infection other than the lung are the intestinal tract and mesenteric lymph nodes. There may be a multifocal enterocolitis and typhlitis, associated primarily with Peyer's patches in the ileum and areas of lymphoid tissue in the cecum and colon. Similar to the bronchial lymph nodes, mesenteric and colonic lymph nodes may be enlarged and have caseonecrotic foci. Occasionally, a large abdominal abscess will form, most often in a mesenteric lymph node. Peritonitis and adhesions may be present. Histologically, the intestinal lesions consist of pyogranulomatous inflammation of lymphoid tissue with fibrinonecrotic ulceration of the overlying epithelium.

The lesions of *R. equi* infection can be more widespread, suggesting hematogenous dissemination of the organism. Some of the lesions identified include septic arthritis, vertebral osteomyelitis, hypopyon (see Fig. 31-3), and ulcerative lymphangitis. Abscesses may develop at almost any site. Lesions of placentitis and fetal pneumonia in an aborted fetus have been reported in association with *R. equi* infection.[232]

R. equi can be isolated from tissues at necropsy in most cases. In addition, immunohistochemistry on impression smears and formalin-fixed tissue specimens can be used as a diagnostic aid and can be as sensitive as bacterial culture.[289-292] To identify virulent *R. equi* specifically in tissues, monoclonal antibodies directed against the 15- to 17-kDa antigens associated with virulence have been used.[290,291]

Therapy

Antimicrobial Therapy

The ACVIM consensus statement recommends the use of a macrolide (erythromycin, azithromycin, or clarithromycin) in combination with rifampin for treatment of infection caused by *R. equi* in foals (Table 31-1).[236] This recommendation is based on pharmacokinetic studies, in vitro data, and retrospective studies, but because there are no randomized controlled studies, the level of evidence for this recommendation is considered moderate. No specific recommendation is made for treatment of foals infected with isolates that are resistant to macrolides and rifampin.

Table 31-1 Antibiotics Frequently Used to Treat *Rhodococcus equi* in Horses

Drug	Dosage
Erythromycin (estolate, stearate, phosphate ethylsuccinate, lactobionate)	25 mg/kg orally (PO) every 6 to 8 hours (q6-8h)
Azithromycin	10 mg/kg PO q24h for 5 days, then q48h thereafter
Clarithromycin	7.5 mg/kg PO q12h
Rifampin	5-10 mg/kg PO q12h or 10 mg/kg q24h

In most cases, erythromycin, azithromycin, or clarithromycin is given in combination with rifampin. In one retrospective study, clarithromycin-rifampin was found to be the most effective therapy.[92]

R. equi is an intracellular pathogen that causes pyogranulomatous inflammation, and therefore effective antimicrobials must have good tissue and macrophage penetration and function in a relatively acid environment. Although *R. equi* is sensitive to a wide variety of antimicrobials in vitro, this often does not correlate with in vivo efficacy.[100,101,293,294] For example, aminoglycosides appear to be highly active against *R. equi* in vitro. However, in one case series, none of the 17 foals treated with gentamicin and penicillin survived despite all isolates being susceptible to gentamicin in vitro, whereas 13 foals treated with erythromycin and rifampin survived.[101]

Treatment of foals with the macrolide antibiotic erythromycin in combination with rifampin began in the late 1980s. The use of this combination significantly improved the success of treatment from a survival rate of approximately 20% to 30% to 60% to 90%.[100-102,295-297] Two newer generation macrolides, azithromycin, an azalide, and clarithromycin, a semisynthetic macrolide, have been demonstrated to be useful alternatives to erythromycin. Rifampin and the macrolides are lipid-soluble antibiotics capable of intracellular penetration and are concentrated in granulocytes and macrophages. The drugs are usually bacteriostatic but may be bactericidal at high concentrations. The use of a macrolide in combination with rifampin has been recommended both because the drugs are synergistic against *R. equi* and because the development of resistance to either drug is decreased when used in combination.[100,293,298,299] Interestingly, some recent studies have demonstrated that concurrent treatment with rifampin significantly decreases concentrations of clarithromycin and potentially other macrolides in plasma, pulmonary epithelial lining fluid (PELF) and bronchoalveolar cells.[300,301] Still, there are no clinical studies comparing the efficacy of the combination of a macrolide with rifampin to a macrolide alone, and further studies are needed before changing treatment recommendations.[236]

The pharmacokinetics and in vitro susceptibility of *R. equi* to macrolides and rifampin have been investigated.[294,302-307] In the case of macrolides, plasma concentrations tend to generally be poor predictors of in vivo efficacy against respiratory pathogens as compared to concentrations at the site of infection such as in PELF and bronchoalveolar cells.[308] It appears that, despite differences in bioavailability and elimination, azithromycin, clarithromycin, and the various formulations of erythromycin are all capable of reaching therapeutic concentrations at the site of infection. Compared with erythromycin, azithromycin and clarithromycin are more chemically stable; have a greater bioavailability after oral administration, especially in the absence of fasting; and achieve higher concentrations in tissues and phagocytic cells. These properties tend to allow for lower dosages and longer dosing intervals when using the newer macrolides. Concentrations of clarithromycin in PELF and bronchoalveolar cells of foals have been shown to be higher than concentrations of either azithromycin or erythromycin.[302,307,309] However, azithromycin was released more slowly from the cells resulting in more sustained tissue concentrations.

Randomized prospective studies comparing the efficacy of the various macrolides in foals with pneumonia are lacking. In a retrospective study of foals admitted to a referral hospital, the efficacy of azithromycin (n = 20), clarithromycin (n = 18), and erythromycin (n = 24) was compared.[96] All foals except one in the azithromycin group were treated concurrently with rifampin. The results indicated that clarithromycin-rifampin was superior to erythromycin-rifampin or azithromycin-rifampin, especially in foals with severe radiographic lesions. There was no advantage of azithromycin-rifampin over traditional therapy with erythromycin-rifampin except for the convenience of once-daily dosing. These results may not necessarily apply when foals are screened and treatment is started early before the establishment of severe lung lesions. In one study of foals with experimental *R. equi* pneumonia, the addition of streptolysin O to clarithromycin/rifampin therapy resulted in lower bacterial counts in the lungs and longer survival times.[310]

Horses with rhodococcal infection often require prolonged antibiotic therapy regardless of the treatment protocol. Treatment is frequently continued for 3 to 12 weeks, although a shorter duration of therapy may be sufficient if the disease is recognized early.[100,101,236,311] Criteria often used for the cessation of therapy include resolution of clinical signs, normalization of plasma fibrinogen concentrations, and radiographic or ultrasonographic resolution of lung lesions. In some affected foals, such as those with well-established abscesses or osteomyelitis, a longer than average treatment period may be indicated. In contrast, some foals with subclinical ultrasonographic lesions can clear the infection without treatment, but there are currently no validated means to distinguish these foals from those that will progress to clinical disease.[312]

The use of a macrolide in combination with rifampin is generally well tolerated in foals, but several adverse effects have been reported, including diarrhea, hyperthermia, and respiratory distress.[313-315] Many of the reports involve erythromycin, although this may be due to its extended period of use in comparison to the newer macrolides. In a study of 143 pneumonic foals, the risk of adverse effects was greater in foals treated with erythromycin than in foals treated with trimethoprim-sulfamethoxazole or penicillin.[313] Of the 73 foals treated with erythromycin, either alone or in combination with rifampin or gentamicin, 26 (36%) developed diarrhea, 18 (25%) developed hyperthermia, and 11 (15%) developed respiratory distress. Colitis has been observed in mares of foals being treated orally with erythromycin-rifampin, and in one study, *Clostridium difficile* was cultured from 5 of 11 (45%) of such mares with diarrhea.[315-317] Although many cases of antibiotic-associated colitis are self-limiting in both foals and mares, occasional cases are severe and fatal. In the study comparing macrolides in foals, diarrhea was observed in 17% of foals treated with erythromycin, 5% of foals treated with azithromycin, and 28% of foals treated with clarithromycin.[96] No difference was found between the groups in the proportion of foals that developed severe diarrhea requiring fluid therapy. The incidence of hyperthermia and respiratory distress resulting from antimicrobial therapy was not critically evaluated because both are common clinical signs in foals affected with *R. equi*. However, anecdotal reports suggest that these reactions do occur with the newer macrolides.[236]

The identification of a long-acting antimicrobial effective against *R. equi* could result in less frequent administration and improved compliance. Tulathromycin, a semisynthetic macrolide, appears to have poor in vitro activity against *R. equi*, and although it concentrates in bronchoalveolar lavage cells, it was not as effective as azithromycin-rifampin when investigated in foals.[318-320] Tilmicosin, another long-acting macrolide, is also poorly active against *R. equi* and can result in significant swelling at the injection site in foals.[309] As a result of these studies, tulathromycin and tilmicosin are currently not recommended for use in foals with rhodococcal pneumonia.[236] In comparison, another long-acting macrolide, gamithromycin, is active against *R. equi* in vitro, and intramuscular administration at a dosage of 6 mg/kg maintains bronchoalveolar cell concentrations above the MIC$_{90}$ for approximately 7 days.[321] Further investigations into the safety and clinical efficacy of gamithromycin are needed.

The majority of *R. equi* isolates are sensitive to erythromycin, clarithromycin, azithromycin, and rifampin, but resistant strains have been encountered.[205,293,294,322-330] In a 2010 study, the overall prevalence of resistant isolates in Texas and Florida over a 10-year period was 4% and the odds of death were 7 times higher in foals infected with resistant isolates.[330] This study also demonstrated that isolates were sometimes misclassified as resistant so that retesting may be required for validation of resistance. Resistance to erythromycin and especially rifampin can develop rapidly, particularly when these drugs are used as monotherapy. *R. equi* isolates from foals have been documented to develop resistance to rifampin after monotherapy and to both erythromycin and rifampin during therapy.[205,324] Anecdotally, the development of resistance to clarithromycin and azithromycin in treated foals has also been observed. Resistance to rifampin develops as a result of mutations in the RNA polymerase beta subunit encoded by the *rpoB* gene.[326,327] The molecular mechanisms of resistance to the macrolides have not been determined, but there is significant cross-resistance between the macrolides.[331] The susceptibility pattern of macrolide or rifampin resistant isolates to alternative antibiotics is variable.[320,330]

It is occasionally necessary to consider alternative antimicrobials to the macrolide-rifampin therapy because of resistance, diarrhea, or financial concerns. Currently, there are no data to make specific recommendations for the treatment of horses when the macrolide-rifampin combination cannot be used, and selection is based on susceptibility of the isolate and anecdotal information. A trimethoprim-sulfonamide combination (15-30 mg/kg q8-12h) can be effective, especially when treating mild disease or when continuing treatment in a foal that has made a good initial response to macrolide-rifampin therapy.[332] Using trimethoprim-sulfonamide with rifampin has been suggested, but pharmacokinetic and efficacy data are not available. Oral doxycycline in combination with rifampin has been used with anecdotal success to treat foals with rhodococcal pneumonia, and pharmacokinetic studies support that doxycycline concentrations in serum, PELF, and BAL cells are above the MIC$_{90}$.[333] Also, the doxycycline-rifampin combination has been shown to be synergistic in vitro.[299] Enrofloxacin (5 mg/kg orally q 24h) alone or in combination with other antibiotics (ceftiofur or rifampin) has been used successfully to treat a limited number of foals with culture-confirmed *R. equi* pneumonia.[100] However, enrofloxacin may result in lameness, joint effusion, and cartilage lesions in foals.[100,334-336] Chloramphenicol achieves high concentrations in phagocytic cells in other species, but only approximately 70% of *R. equi* isolates are susceptible. Telithromycin, a semisynthetic ketolide with activity against many macrolide-resistant gram-positive bacterial isolates, has been investigated in foals.[337] The intragastric administration of 15 mg/kg q 24h resulted in adequate concentrations to treat macrolide-susceptible *R. equi* isolates, but administration of the same dose q 12h yielded concentrations only adequate for the treatment of approximately 50% of the macrolide-resistant *R. equi* isolates. An in vitro study suggests that equine antimicrobial peptides may be promising alternative candidates for the control of resistant *R. equi* infections.[338] In foals in which significant diarrhea develops, intravenous erythromycin lactobionate (5 mg/kg diluted in saline and administered as a slow infusion q6h) has been recommended.[100] The use of an aminoglycoside in combination with either macrolides or rifampin is controversial; it was demonstrated in vitro that activity against *R. equi* can be diminished when these drugs were used in combination.[100,293,298,299] In a clinical study of 72 foals, however, the survival rate and ability to race as 3-year-olds were similar for foals treated with gentamicin and rifampin as for those treated with erythromycin and rifampin.[339]

Additional Therapy

Additional therapy may be beneficial depending on the specifics of the case. If another pathogen is isolated with *R. equi*, an additional antimicrobial may be indicated depending on the susceptibility of the organism. Supportive care is important, including maintaining adequate nutrition and hydration, as well as maintaining foals in a cool, well-ventilated environment. Arterial blood gas assessment will help determine if oxygen therapy is indicated. Oxygen may be delivered by pharyngeal insufflation or by percutaneous transtracheal oxygenation in severely hypoxic foals. Bronchodilators, such as aminophylline, theophylline, clenbuterol, and albuterol, are rarely helpful clinically.[100] In addition, concurrent administration of erythromycin and to a lesser extent clarithromycin with either aminophylline or theophylline may result in increased plasma concentrations of these bronchodilators, potentiating their toxicity. Nebulization with saline, antimicrobials, or bronchodilators have been advocated, but there are no data regarding their efficacy. Nonsteroidal antiinflammatory drugs (NSAIDs) should be used judiciously to reduce fever and improve attitude and appetite. Recently, an in vitro study demonstrated that polyunsaturated fatty acid-enriched macrophages have improved phagocytic and microbicidal activity against *R. equi*, suggesting that fatty acid supplementation might be beneficial.[340] Although data are limited, based on an experimental model of *R. equi* pneumonia in foals, specific hyperimmune plasma was ineffective in treating disease once infection was established.[156] In cases with infection at a site other than the lungs, such as septic arthritis or osteomyelitis, local therapy may be indicated in addition to systemic antibiotics. Regional limb perfusion with erythromycin has been used in the management of septic physitis associated with *R. equi*.[341] In foals with abdominal abscesses, drainage, surgical removal or marsupialization may be considered, although abdominal adhesions often complicate surgery. Immune-mediated extrapulmonary disorders generally improve as the infection resolves.

Prognosis

The survival rate for foals with *R. equi* pneumonia varies from approximately 60% to 90% with current antimicrobial therapies.[93,96,101,102,295] At farms using screening programs to identify disease early, survival may approach 100%, whereas at referral centers where the disease is probably more severe, survival rates range between 59% to 72%. Clinical and hematologic variables associated with survival from rhodococcal pneumonia have varied widely between studies. In a retrospective study of 115 cases from 6 veterinary medical teaching hospitals, the overall survival rate was 72%.[296] Extreme tachycardia (heart rate >100), respiratory distress, and severe thoracic radiographic abnormalities were more likely in nonsurviving foals than in surviving foals. Clinicopathologic abnormalities were not associated with survival. The proportion of foals that survived was significantly higher in Standardbreds (80%) than in Thoroughbreds (61%). In a study of 81 foals, overall survival was 69%.[96] Radiographic scores, heart rate, and fibrinogen concentrations were significantly higher in nonsurvivors, whereas arterial oxygen and platelet counts were significantly higher in survivors. Only fibrinogen concentration was retained in the logistic regression model. There was no significant difference in survival among breeds in this study. In another study of 39 foals, respiratory rate, temperature, WBC count, and fibrinogen concentration were higher in nonsurvivors.[245] The results of studies correlating the severity of radiographic lesions and prognosis have varied, but in one study the severity of alveolar pattern and number of cavitary lesions was associated with a poor outcome in foals with *R. equi*.[98,100,245,342] However, caution should be used when using radiographic findings as a prognostic indicator because many individual surviving foals have had severe lesions.[98,100,245]

The prognosis has generally been poor in cases of abdominal abscesses and osteomyelitis, although some horses respond to aggressive treatment.[212,233] Similarly, while some adult horses have been successfully treated, the prognosis in adults tends to be poor, possibly because of delayed identification of the problem and underlying immunosuppression.[233,235]

Several studies have attempted to evaluate the long-term effects of *R. equi* pneumonia on pulmonary function and athletic performance. In a study by Ainsworth et al,[343] five horses that had recovered from rhodococcal pneumonia and five healthy controls were evaluated by endoscopy, radiography, hematologic and BAL analyses, and pulmonary function testing. There were no significant differences in these parameters between groups, suggesting that horses that recover from *R. equi* pneumonia do not have detectable evidence of residual lung damage. The pulmonary function of seven Standardbreds that had recovered from *R. equi* pneumonia was evaluated during intense treadmill exercise, and gas exchange was not compromised compared with reference values for normal Standardbreds.[344]

A number of studies have evaluated racing performance. In a study of 11 horses previously affected with *R. equi* pneumonia, 7 eventually raced, and 4 of the 7 won races.[345] In another study, 54% of foals (45/83) surviving *R. equi* infection eventually raced at least once, compared with 65% of foals in the general population.[296] No physical examination, laboratory results, or radiographic findings were identified that were predictive of whether foals went on to race. The racing performance of foals that went on to race was not significantly different from that of the general U.S. population of racing horses. Thus, although *R. equi* infection was associated with a decreased chance of racing as an adult, the performance of those foals that did go on to race was not impaired. Similarly, in a study by Bernard et al,[346] *R. equi* in foals did not have a negative influence on racing performance as evaluated by 2- and 3-year-old race earnings. In general, the prognosis for performance after successful treatment of uncomplicated *R. equi* pneumonia should be regarded as excellent.

Prevention

Potential strategies for the prevention and control of *R. equi* include decreasing the size of the infective challenge, early detection of disease, chemoprophylaxis/immunostimulants, and either passive or active immunization.

Decreasing the Size of Infective Challenge

The outcome of exposure to *R. equi* is partially determined by the size of the infective challenge, as with most infectious diseases. Therefore practices targeted at decreasing the number of organisms in the environment could potentially decrease the incidence of disease, but data supporting their efficacy are limited. Many studies have been based on historical controls and have multiple compounding factors. As a result, the ACVIM consensus statement concludes that although management changes could be beneficial in the control or prevention of rhodococcal disease, there is currently inadequate evidence to support specific environmental interventions and further research is needed.[236]

It is generally felt that the risk of rhodococcal disease increases with the number and density of mares and foals on a farm, although studies evaluating this association have had varying results.[100,104,111] In one report, decreasing the number of mares at a farm reduced the cumulative incidence of *R. equi* relative to preceding years, and there are similar anecdotal reports.[248] This information is difficult to interpret given the normal year-to-year variation that can occur within farms, although it is reasonable that reducing density be considered as an approach for decreasing the incidence of *R. equi*.[101,236]

Another strategy considered for decreasing exposure to *R. equi* is to decrease the number of soil bacteria by manure management, even though neither the presence nor the concentration of virulent *R. equi* in soil at breeding farms has been correlated with either increased odds or increased cumulative incidence of *R. equi* pneumonia.[48,82,111] Horse manure is believed to contribute to environmental contamination with *R. equi* both because it often contains bacteria and because it contains volatile fatty acids that enhance the growth of *R. equi* once in the environment.[5,72] Therefore, in addition to simply decreasing the number of animals to decrease the amount of manure, it has been recommended to remove horse manure frequently from stalls, paddocks, and pastures and to either not spread manure on pastures as fertilizer or to compost the manure before spreading.[78,100,347] In epidemiologic studies, however, manure removal or avoiding spreading manure on pastures, regardless of whether it was composted or not, did not significantly alter the risk for development of *R. equi* pneumonia.[104,106] These management practices may still be potentially beneficial in controlling parasitic or other infectious diseases.

R. equi infection has been linked to raising foals in a dusty environment, but it has been difficult to document this objectively. Still, it has been theorized that efforts to reduce dust in the environment, such as reseeding and irrigating to promote growth of grass, as well as using water sprinklers in paddocks, may reduce aerosolization of dust particles that may contain *R. equi* and thus help decrease the incidence of rhodococcal infection. Airborne concentrations of *R. equi* were correlated with disease incidence at Thoroughbred breeding farms in Australia; irrigation of holding pens at a farm with rhodococcal pneumonia reduced the frequency of recovery of virulent *R. equi* in air samples from the pens, although there was no reduction in the cumulative incidence of *R. equi* pneumonia at the farm.[82,83]

One study demonstrated that foals from farms with endemic *R. equi* were significantly less likely to have foaled in a pasture than in a stall or small paddock.[104] Stall confinement may expose foals to high concentrations of organisms and poor ventilation, contributing to the development of disease. However, one study of three farms in Ireland demonstrated lower airborne concentrations of virulent *R. equi* in barns than in paddocks.[83]

It has been discussed whether isolation of foals with *R. equi* pneumonia is warranted, but there is currently no evidence that *R. equi* is contagious between foals.[118,236,348] As compared to either adult horses or uninfected foals, infected foals generally shed higher concentrations of *R. equi* in their feces, probably because these foals swallow sputum with large numbers of virulent organisms which may then multiply within the intestine.[72,73,75,76] Also, airborne concentrations of virulent *R. equi* were higher in samples from the breathing zone of pneumonic foals than in samples from lanes and pens at their farm, but there was no difference in samples from the breathing zones of pneumonic foals and healthy controls, suggesting that diseased foals do not represent a greater risk than other foals for aerosol transmission.[348] Thus, although infected foals are certainly a source of environmental contamination, exposure is so widespread in the environment that the ACVIM consensus statement concluded that there is no evidence to indicate that affected foals should be isolated from other foals.[236]

Early Detection of Disease

The early recognition of *R. equi* pneumonia may reduce losses and limit the duration and thus the costs of therapy. Therefore the ACVIM consensus statement recommends that some form of screening for early identification of disease be used at farms with endemic *R. equi*, even though the level of evidence to support this recommendation was considered weak because of the lack of controlled studies.[236] Implementing screening at farms with only sporadic *R. equi* pneumonia may not be warranted.

A number of approaches have been recommended for early diagnosis of rhodococcal disease. As thorough comparisons between the various screening tests have not been made, it is difficult to recommend a specific test. The preferred approach may vary with the incidence of disease and the resources available.[236] Higuchi et al[273] suggested that physical examination of foals at 30 and 45 days of age was useful for early diagnosis of *R. equi* infection on endemic farms. Similarly, Prescott et al[349] found that twice-weekly complete physical examinations with careful auscultation of the thorax was successful in the early diagnosis of infection and in preventing mortality. Serologic surveillance has also been recommended, but it is unreliable.[100,276,350]

Other strategies for early detection of *R. equi* pneumonia include serial monitoring of WBC count and fibrinogen concentration and thoracic US. A prospective study of 162 foals from a farm with endemic *R. equi* infection evaluated the efficacy of WBC count, fibrinogen concentration, and the AGID test for early identification of *R. equi*-infected foals.[249] Although both WBC count and fibrinogen concentration were useful in detecting early *R. equi* infection, the WBC count was more sensitive and specific. It was recommended that WBC counts of foals should be evaluated monthly on farms with endemic *R. equi* infection. Foals with WBC concentrations of 13,000 cells/μL or greater should receive a careful physical examination, and foals with WBC concentrations of 14,000/μL or higher should be considered candidates for additional diagnostic testing such as thoracic radiography or US. Serologic testing using the AGID was not accurate in predicting disease. Thoracic US of foals starting at 30 days of age and repeated at 2-week intervals until 16 to 20 weeks of age may be effective in reducing subclinical and clinical disease associated with *R. equi*.[284] Some advantages of US are that it can be sensitive and performed relatively quickly with immediately available results.[283,284] Culture of air samples from the breathing zone of young foals was not useful in predicting subsequent rhodococcal pneumonia.[351]

A consequence of any screening program is that greater numbers of foals will be treated for presumptive *R. equi* pneumonia, including some foals with subclinical disease or with another disease. Treatment of all subclinically affected foals may not be necessary as some may recover without treatment.[312] However, because it remains unknown which foals might recover spontaneously and because the disease can be so severe, it is common to treat all foals with positive screening tests. Thus, not only are screening programs associated with financial costs, they may also be associated with an increased risk of adverse events related to treatment and the further development of drug resistance.

Chemoprophylaxis and Immunostimulants

Prophylactic use of macrolides or other classes of antimicrobial drugs to prevent rhodococcal disease is not recommended because of conflicting evidence of efficacy and concerns about the selection of antibiotic-resistant bacteria. Two controlled studies with different designs have evaluated the use of azithromycin for chemoprophylaxis.[352,353] In a randomized, controlled trial of 338 foals at 10 farms, treatment reduced the cumulative incidence of *R. equi* pneumonia.[352] In contrast, in a study of 70 foals at one farm in Germany, treatment did not change the incidence of disease, although the age at onset of pneumonia was delayed in treated foals.[353] Regardless, antibiotic use is not considered an acceptable approach for chemoprophylaxis because of the pressure for emergence of antibiotic resistance among bacteria.[333]

Gallium is a metal-based compound with antimicrobial properties that has been demonstrated to reduce replication of *R. equi* in culture and within macrophages and to reduce tissue concentrations of *R. equi* in mice after experimental infection.[354,355] It appears to be bioavailable and safe in foals.[356-360] Unfortunately, chemoprophylaxis with gallium maltolate failed to reduce the incidence of *R. equi* in a placebo-controlled trial of 438 foals on 12 breeding farms.[94] Also, although treatment of mares with oral gallium nitrate significantly reduced their fecal concentrations of virulent *R. equi* over time, there was no change in airborne concentrations of *R. equi* shortly after foaling.[361]

Immunostimulants, such as inactivated *Parapoxvirus ovis*, *Propionibacterium acnes*, and unmethylated CpGs, have been investigated in foals for their potential to enhance the host defense mechanisms during the period of high susceptibility to *R. equi*.[146,193,362-364] These immunostimulants can improve ex vivo or in vitro phagocytic cell function and cytokine induction in foals. However, in a trial of foals on a farm with endemic *R. equi*, treatment with inactivated *Parapoxvirus ovis* did not affect the proportion of foals that developed clinical or ultrasonographic evidence of pneumonia.[193]

Passive Immunization

Intravenous administration of licensed hyperimmune plasma (HIP) containing antibody against *R. equi* may aid in the prevention of *R. equi* pneumonia on endemic farms. The ACVIM consensus statement feels the level of evidence for this recommendation is moderate.[234] In some studies, this practice has been effective in significantly reducing the incidence of rhodococcal pneumonia after experimental or natural challenge.[98,99,155,158] However, other studies have failed to document a statistically significant protective effect.[93,157,159] For example, in a randomized clinical trial of 165 Thoroughbred foals on a farm with endemic *Rhodococcus*, there was no statistically significant difference in the incidence of *R. equi* pneumonia in foals receiving HIP (19.1%) as compared with untreated foals (30%).[93] Despite the somewhat varying results, the potential beneficial effects and relative safety of administering HIP have made its use relatively common. In a survey of 65 endemic farms, 36 (56%) administered HIP.[104] It is recommended to use a commercially available licensed plasma product from hyperimmunized horses to ensure some standard of potency, purity, and safety.[236] There appears to be no advantage to using plasma produced by immunizing horses with farm-specific isolates.

The optimal protocol for the administration of HIP has not been determined, and differences in the age at administration, dose, and product may account for some of the variability between studies. Since no benefit was seen when HIP was administered after experimental challenge, plasma should optimally be given before exposure to *R. equi*.[156] The exact time of exposure of most foals is unclear but likely occurs early in life, especially on endemic farms.[92,95] However, early administration of HIP may result in a waning of passively transferred antibodies to nonprotective concentrations when some foals are still susceptible. Most studies have administered approximately 1 liter of plasma between 1 and 60 days of age.[93,98,99,159] In the study of 165 foals on an endemic farm, 950 mL of plasma was administered at 1 to 10 days of age and again at 30 to 50 days of age.[93] Because the majority of treated foals that developed pneumonia did so before the administration of the second dose, it was postulated that administration of the second dose at an earlier age may have been more beneficial. The ideal time for HIP administration may vary from farm to farm. Further research is needed to determine the ideal age and minimum effective dose. As transfusion of HIP is not completely protective, its use does not eliminate the need for careful monitoring of foals at risk.

Active Immunization

The development of an effective vaccine for *R. equi* would clearly be beneficial and has been an area of active research. Most foals exposed to virulent *R. equi* mount a protective immune response and remain immune as adults, which suggests that the induction of protective immunity by active immunization should be possible. However, the development of an efficacious vaccine has proven difficult despite the use of multiple strategies for active immunization of mares and foals.

There are several challenges to developing an effective vaccine in a neonatal foal. Because of inherent characteristics of the neonatal immune system, it may be difficult to stimulate the correct type of immune response (i.e., the protective phenotype). In addition, because of immunologic naïveté, foals may not be able to mount an immune response of the required magnitude rapidly enough to prevent infection.[176-180] Another possible challenge is overcoming potential interference by maternal antibody. However, this may be less important with *R. equi* than with some other pathogens because the T-lymphocyte responses that play a significant role in immunity to *R. equi* may be less affected by maternal antibody than humoral responses.[365,366]

Several candidate vaccines have been investigated, but as yet none has been developed for widespread use. The administration of killed virulent *R. equi* does not elicit protective immunity in mice or protect foals from experimental infection.[367,368] Immunization of foals with two exoenzymes produced by *R. equi*, cholesterol oxidase, and phospholipase C did not prevent the development of disease after experimental challenge, although severe clinical signs did not develop in either vaccinated or control foals in this study.[369] A number of vaccines have been evaluated for the prevention of *R. equi* under field conditions, including an inactivated *R. equi* vaccine with and without EHV-2, a preparation of soluble antigens of *R. equi* that include VapA and "equi factor" exoenzymes, and an EHV-2 subunit vaccine.[116,370,371] Although studies have suggested that these vaccines could provide some protection against *R. equi*, data are limited.

Infection with avirulent *R. equi* does not result in protection, suggesting that the virulence plasmid encodes antigens critical to protective immunity.[367,372] Several studies have focused specifically on the potential of VapA as an immunogen. Vaccination with VapA results in the production of VapA-specific antibodies in both horses and mice.[30,152,158,159,373-376] A study in mice demonstrated that immunization with VapA significantly enhanced clearance of organisms from the liver and spleen after experimental challenge.[30] Other studies, however, have suggested that VapA vaccines are unable to prevent bacterial replication despite their immunogenicity.[373,374] In a study by Prescott et al[158] on an enzootic farm, vaccination of mares and their foals with a VapA extract did not protect foals from natural infection with *R. equi* despite the presence of opsonizing antibody. Limited data from a study in pregnant mares suggest that the use of a VapA candidate vaccine could result in passive antibody-mediated protection of foals and warrants further investigation.[163]

Exposure to live virulent *R. equi* elicits protective immunity in both foals and mice. Specifically in foals, oral immunization with live virulent *R. equi* protected foals against experimental challenge, confirming that young foals can mount a highly effective protective immune response.[377,378] Foals that were orally immunized developed high concentrations of antibody specific to VapA and VapC but not to other Vap proteins, indicating that VapA and VapC are highly immunogenic.[378] Although oral immunization with live virulent bacteria is protective, it is not considered a practical means of widespread vaccination because of the risks of developing disease in some individuals and disseminating large numbers of organisms into the environment. Efforts to develop a safe, effective vaccine for *R. equi* are ongoing. An effective vaccine will most likely induce both humoral and cellular immunity and will direct the immune response to the protective phenotype. Several strategies for vaccination are under investigation, including DNA vaccination, the use of salmonella expressing VapA, co-immunization with recombinant lactococci secreting VapA and leptin, and the use of a recombinant bacille Calmette-Guerin (BCG) vaccine expressing VapA antigen.[379-386] Also, the use of attenuated strains of *R. equi*, including strains with mutations in genes involved in steroid metabolism, is being investigated.[379,381,387,388]

Public Health Considerations

R. equi is an emerging pathogen in human medicine and is most often recognized as an opportunistic infection in immunocompromised patients.[64,389-391] The first case of *R. equi* infection in a human patient was not reported until 1967, and only about 12 additional cases were reported during the next 15 years. However, coincident with the emergence of HIV infection and advances in organ transplantation and cancer treatment, the incidence of *R. equi* in humans has greatly increased since the early 1980s. Improvements in laboratory diagnosis and enhanced awareness of the disease have also contributed to the increase in reported cases. In the past 15 years, at least 100 cases of *R. equi* infection in humans have been reported in the medical literature.[64,390,391] Approximately 85% to 90% of human patients with *R. equi* are immunocompromised, with these patients being divided between those with human immunodeficiency virus (HIV) infection and those who are otherwise immunocompromised as a result of disease, immunosuppressive medications, or both. These immunocompromised patients often have concurrent infections with other opportunistic pathogens. Only about 10% to 15% of *R. equi* infections occur in seemingly immunocompetent hosts.

R. equi infection in human patients is thought to be acquired by inhalation, inoculation into a wound or mucous membrane, or ingestion. The soil is believed to be the most common source of infectious organisms. The possible role of other routes of *R. equi* acquisition, including human colonization and person-to-person transmission, is poorly understood.[64,392,393] Unlike in foals, in which essentially all isolates from clinical cases express VapA, only 20% to 25% of isolates recovered from human patients express VapA.[64]

The clinical manifestations of *R. equi* infection in human patients are varied, and the organism has been isolated from almost every site in the body. As in foals, pulmonary infection, often resulting in pyogranulomatous pneumonia, is common, being recognized in approximately 84% of immunocompromised patients and approximately 42% of immunocompetent patients.[64,389] Localized infections, often associated with wounds, represent about 50% of reported cases in immunocompetent hosts.[389] Combination antibiotic therapy is the mainstay of treatment, and empiric two-drug regimens typically include erythromycin, rifampin, and/or ciprofloxacin.[64,389] Numerous other antimicrobial agents have also been recommended, including vancomycin, imipenem, and aminoglycosides. Surgical drainage of abscesses in sites of poor antibiotic penetration is probably beneficial. The mortality rate among immunocompetent patients is approximately 11%, compared with rates of 50% to 55% among HIV-infected patients and 20% to 25% among non–HIV-infected immunocompromised patients.

Exposure to domesticated animals, especially horses and pigs, may play a role in some cases of *R. equi* infection in humans, although only one-third of all patients have a history of exposure to horses or pigs.[64] However, it is recommended that immunocompromised patients with significant exposure to domesticated animals be cautioned regarding the possible risk of *R. equi* infection.

The complete reference list is available online at www.expertconsult.com.

CHAPTER

Leptospirosis

32

Melissa T. Hines

Leptospirosis is a bacterial disease of worldwide distribution caused by spirochetes of the genus *Leptospira*. The disease affects humans, domestic animals, and wildlife, including reptiles and amphibians. The first formal report of leptospirosis was in human patients by Adolf Weil over 100 years ago, leading to the name Weil's disease.[1,2] Subsequently, leptospirosis was identified in dogs and livestock. The first report of naturally occurring leptospirosis in horses was in 1947 in Russia.[3] In horses the disease has most often been associated with abortion and equine recurrent uveitis; however, sporadic cases of renal and hepatic disease have also been reported.

Etiology

The order Spirochaetales includes two families of spiral bacteria, *Spirochaetaceae* and *Leptospiraceae*, which share unique morphologic and functional features[4,5] (Fig. 32-1). The genus *Leptospira* is within the family *Leptospiraceae* and includes a large number of both pathogenic and nonpathogenic bacteria. Morphologically, all the leptospires are indistinguishable and are flexible, tightly coiled, unicellular bacteria. At least one end is hook shaped, leading Stimson[6] in 1907 to initially name the organism *Spirochaeta interrogans* because of the resemblance to a question mark. The organisms are slender, with a diameter of approximately 0.1 to 3.0 μm and a length of 6 to 20 μm. The helical coil amplitude is 0.1 to 0.15 μm.

Structurally, the leptospires have a helical protoplasmic cylinder consisting of nuclear material, cytoplasm, and the cytoplasmic membrane and peptidoglycan cell wall[4,7] (Fig. 32-2). There are two axial flagella, or axial filaments, each attaching

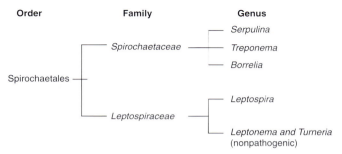

Order	Family	Genus
		Serpulina
	Spirochaetaceae	Treponema
		Borrelia
Spirochaetales		Leptospira
	Leptospiraceae	Leptonema and Turneria (nonpathogenic)

Figure 32-1 Classification of major spirochetes of veterinary importance.

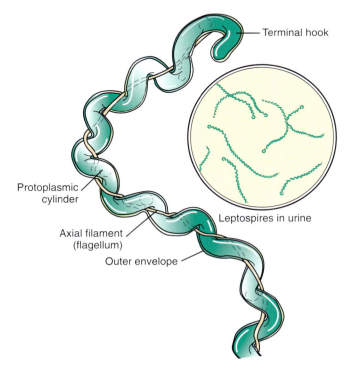

Terminal hook

Protoplasmic cylinder

Axial filament (flagellum)

Outer envelope

Leptospires in urine

Figure 32-2 Ultrastructure of pathogenic leptospires. *(From Greene CE, editor: Infectious diseases of the dog and cat, ed 3, St Louis, 2006, Saunders; courtesy University of Georgia, Athens.)*

at opposing ends of the organism by platelike insertion discs. The distal end of each flagellum is not attached and extends toward the center of the cell, sometimes overlapping the flagellum from the opposite end. These flagella facilitate motility. As with other spirochetes, the leptospires have a double-membrane structure in which the cytoplasmic membrane and peptidoglycan cell wall are closely associated and are overlaid by an outer membrane that surrounds the protoplasmic cylinder and periplasmic flagella. This outer membrane is rich in lipopolysaccharide (LPS), the composition of which is similar to that of other gram-negative bacteria, but with less potent endotoxic activity.[8,9] Despite the gram-negative characteristics of leptospires, they do not stain well with conventional bacteriologic dyes. Therefore other techniques, such as darkfield microscopy, silver impregnation, and immunologic staining, have been developed for identification of leptospires.

Leptospires are obligate aerobes with an optimum growth temperature of 28° C to 30° C (82.4° F-86° F).[4] Although slow growing, they can be isolated on artificial media, a characteristic that is unique among spirochetes. They require either long-chain fatty acids or long-chain alcohols as a primary energy source.

The leptospiral genome is approximately 5000 kilobases (kb) in size and consists of two sections, a 4330-kb chromosome and a smaller 359-kb chromosome.[10-12] No other plasmids have been identified. Evidence suggests horizontal transfer of genetic material within the genus. The genome has been sequenced, and a number of leptospiral genes have been cloned.

Classification of organisms within the genus *Leptospira* is complex and has been undergoing revision. Currently, two separate systems of classification are used: (1) the traditional phenotypic classification system based on serotyping and (2) a genotypic classification system based on deoxyribonucleic acid (DNA) homology.

In the traditional serologic classification system, the leptospires are grouped into two species, the pathogenic species *Leptospira interrogans* and the nonpathogenic, saprophytic species *Leptospira biflexa*.[4,5,12] Within each species, the "serovars" are organized into "serogroups" based on shared antigenicity. In this system, *L. interrogans* contains at least 218 serovars organized into 23 serogroups, and *L. biflexa* contains at least 60 serovars organized into 28 serogroups.

Analysis of leptospiral DNA by DNA hybridization revealed significant genetic heterogeneity within the two phenotypic species, *L. interrogans* and *L. biflexa*, resulting in the reclassification of species based on DNA homology.[13-15] Currently, 17 "genomospecies" of *Leptospira* have been defined, and further taxonomic revisions are likely.[14,16-19] Serologic testing is used within the genomospecies to identify serovars (Table 32-1). The name *L. interrogans* is used to identify species in both the phenotypic and the genotypic classification systems, causing some

Table 32-1 Genomospecies Identified with Selected Serovars of *Leptospira*

Serovar	Genomospecies
Australis	*interrogans*
Autumnalis	*interrogans*
Bratislava	*interrogans*
Canicola	*interrogans*
Grippotyphosa	*interrogans, kirschneri*
Hardjo	*interrogans, borgpetersenii, meyeri*
Icterohaemorrhagiae	*interrogans, inadai*
Pomona	*interrogans, noguchii*
Sejroe	*borgpetersenii*

confusion. Therefore *L. interrogans* sensu stricto, meaning "in the strict sense," is sometimes used to denote the specific genomospecies, whereas *L. interrogans* sensu lato, meaning "in the broad sense," is used when referring to the more general phenotypic species. For the purposes of this chapter, *L. interrogans* and its associated serovars in capital letters will be used.

The two systems of classification do not correspond. The genomospecies of a strain cannot be predicted by the serogroup or serovar, and serologically similar leptospires may belong to different genomospecies. In addition, both pathogenic and nonpathogenic serovars may occur within the same genomospecies. Within some serovars, there is sufficient genetic heterogeneity that the same serovar may be found in multiple genomospecies.

The genotypic classification system is taxonomically correct, but in part because of the lack of simple molecular identification methods, many diagnostic laboratories retain the serologic classification of leptospires. Also, in most veterinary literature published to date, leptospires are identified by the classic serologic system. Therefore most descriptions in this chapter refer to organisms classified by serotyping.

Epidemiology

Leptospirosis is maintained in nature by subclinically infected maintenance hosts, also known as *reservoir hosts* or *definitive hosts*.[4,5,12] These maintenance hosts, which include numerous wild and domestic animal species, serve as a source of infection for incidental or accidental hosts, including humans (Table 32-2). Specific serovars of *Leptospira* are generally found in particular maintenance host species, and epidemiologic studies suggest that these host preferences may vary both with geographic regions and over time. In the maintenance hosts the organism is considered to be host adapted, and infection is endemic. Although the host is highly susceptible to infection, the organism is usually of low pathogenicity, and disease is usually subclinical or mild. There is generally prolonged excretion of leptospires in the urine, making these maintenance hosts the primary source of environmental contamination and transmission to other species.

In contrast, incidental hosts typically have a low susceptibility to infection but are more likely to develop acute, severe disease when they do become infected. Incidental hosts generally shed organisms for relatively short periods, making them inefficient transmitters of disease. For most serovars of *Leptospira*, horses are incidental hosts. However, recent evidence suggests that as with cattle and pigs, horses may be a maintenance host for *L. interrogans* serovar Bratislava.[20-25]

The primary source of exposure to *Leptospira* is infected urine. Maintenance hosts may shed organisms in the urine for prolonged periods because of chronic infection of the renal tubules.[12,26-28] The organism can also be spread through aborted fetuses, placental tissues, uterine discharges, and milk. Contact with the organism may occur either directly or indirectly through contaminated soil, bedding, feed, or drinking water. Once in the environment, leptospires may survive for several weeks under favorable conditions, which is generally a warm, moist environment such as stagnant or slow-moving warm water. Survival is favored by a neutral or slightly alkaline pH and inhibited by a pH of less than 6 or greater than 8. Therefore organisms can survive only transiently in undiluted acidic urine. Ambient temperatures of 10° C to 25° C (50° F-77° F) favor survival, and temperatures lower than 7° C to 10° C (44.6° F-50° F) or higher than 34° C to 36° C (93.2° F-96.8° F) are detrimental. The organism is susceptible to freezing and drying. Some evidence indicates that leptospires may survive in insects or other invertebrate hosts, but the significance of this is unknown.[29,30]

Although contact with infected fluids is the most common means of direct transmission of leptospirosis, venereal and transplacental transfer have been documented in some species.[12,26,28] Leptospiral organisms have been found in the semen of infected bulls, and transmission by natural breeding or artificial insemination can occur but is uncommon. In humans, transmission through sexual intercourse during convalescence has been reported.[31] Data in horses are limited, but there are currently no reports of leptospiral transmission through semen or embryo transfer.[32] Fetal infection has been documented in foals after localization in the pregnant uterus, resulting in resorption, abortion, stillbirth, or weak neonatal foals.[20,21,33-38]

Seroprevalence

Serologic surveys to assess the prevalence of antibody to leptospiral organisms have been performed in multiple species, including horses. These studies confirm that there is widespread exposure to *Leptospira* worldwide and that exposure is significantly more common than clinical disease. Specifically, in horses, seroprevalence has varied from 1% to 95%, depending on the geographic location and the serovars assessed.[20,22,23,39-66]

In some studies, horses were more likely to be seropositive than other domestic animal species.[42,47,49,50,64] Titers to a wide variety of serovars have been reported in horses, and although there is variation between studies, in general, titers to *Leptospira interrogans* serovars Icterohaemorrhagiae, Bratislava, Pomona, Ballum, and Grippotyphosa tend to be most common. Various serovars of leptospires have also been isolated from bacteriologic surveys of horses at necropsy.[34,51,59] Studies in The Netherlands, Northern Ireland, Canada, and Kentucky suggest that at least in these regions, horses may be a maintenance host for serovar Bratislava because of the prevalence of this serovar.[20-25] One study suggested that the Sejroe

Species: Selected Serovars	Known Primary Reservoir Hosts	Domesticated Animal Hosts	People	Wildlife
L. interrogans Sensu Stricto				
Bratislava	Rat, pig, cow, hedgehog, horse?	Horse, dog, cow	+	+
Pomona	Cow, pig, skunk, opossum	Horse, dog, cat, sheep, goat, rabbit, cavy	+	+
Icterohaemorrhagiae	Rat	Horse, dog, cat, cow, pig, cavy	+	+
Hardjo	Cow, occasionally sheep	Horse, dog, pig, sheep	+	+
Canicola	Dog	Horse, dog, cat, cow, pig	+	+
L. kirschneri				
Grippotyphosa	Vole, raccoon, skunk, opossum	Horse, dog, cat, cow, pig, sheep, goat, rabbit, gerbil, cavy	+	+

Table 32-2 Selected Serovars of *Leptospira* Identified in Horses and Their Hosts

serovar may be maintained in the racing horse population in Korea.[65]

Risk Factors

Several studies have assessed risk factors for exposure to leptospirosis in horses. An early study in Australia did not find any correlation between increased moisture in the environment and seroprevalence.[60] In a Canadian study of 1923 horses in which the seroprevalence ranged from 0.8% to 94.6% depending on the serovar, age was significantly associated with the presence of titers, with the chance of being seropositive increasing by approximately 10% with each year of life.[48] In addition, horses managed individually, such as horses at a track, were about half as likely to be seropositive as those managed in groups, such as rodeo horses. Some other studies, but not all, have shown an increase in prevalence with increasing age.* Barwick et al[67,68] evaluated sera from 2551 horses on 572 farms in the state of New York and used a multidimensional indexing system to identify risk factors associated with seropositivity to various serovars. Although findings varied, depending on the specific serovar assessed, age was again identified as a risk factor, as were certain management practices. The density of horses turned out together, as well as exposure to rodents, wildlife, and potentially contaminated soil and water, could be associated with increased risk of seropositivity to some serovars. Additionally, some studies have demonstrated a seasonal association depending on the serovar.[61,65]

Abortion, Stillbirths, and Neonatal Deaths

Well established as a cause of abortion in cattle and swine, leptospirosis has been sporadically reported as a cause of abortion in horses since the 1950s, but problems in making an accurate diagnosis have made determination of the true prevalence difficult.[36,69,70] Even so, leptospirosis has been confirmed as a significant cause of abortion, stillbirth, and perinatal death in horses in locations worldwide.[34-37,71-80] In a study reviewing the pathology case records of 3527 cases of abortion, stillbirth, and perinatal death in horses, fetoplacental infection caused by bacteria was diagnosed in 628 cases, of which leptospirosis was identified in 78.[75] In comparison, equine herpesvirus was diagnosed in 143 cases. Related studies in Kentucky have found leptospirosis in 2.5% to 4.4% of submissions of equine fetuses, stillborn foals, and placentas.[71-73] Multiple serovars of *Leptospira* have been associated with abortion, with serovar Pomona type kennewicki being among the most common.[34-37,72,73,79] Mixed infections with multiple serovars have also been documented.[77]

Several studies have evaluated the risk of urinary shedding by mares on farms with leptospiral abortions. Leptospiruria was documented in at least some mares that had aborted and also other seropositive horses on the farms.[21,25,73,77] For example, Donahue et al[73] identified leptospires in the urine of 14 of 67 mares within 10 days of leptospiral abortion (20.9%). However, a study of three central Kentucky horse farms with a history of leptospiral abortions found no evidence of long-term urinary shedding of *Leptospira* by horses with high leptospiral antibody titers.[25]

Equine Recurrent Uveitis

Uveitis is a disease with multiple etiologies; leptospirosis is identified as one of the causes in both human and equine patients. In horses, several serovars of *Leptospira* have been associated specifically with equine recurrent uveitis (ERU), with Pomona being frequently incriminated.[81-83]

As with equine abortions, it has been difficult to establish an accurate prevalence of leptospiral uveitis, in part the result of difficulties in making a definitive diagnosis. However, it appears that there are geographic differences in prevalence, with *Leptospira* spp. having only a minor role in ERU in the United Kingdom.[81,83]

Pathogenesis

The usual portal of entry for leptospires is by penetration of mucous membranes and abraded or soft, moist skin. Occasionally, organisms may enter by inhalation, ingestion, or animal bites. As with most infectious diseases, the outcome of exposure to leptospires depends on the dose, virulence, and host susceptibility. After entry into the lymphatics and bloodstream, the organisms multiply and are carried to multiple organs. Bacteremia typically occurs 4 to 10 days after initial exposure. There is no apparent tissue tropism, and leptospires replicate in many tissues, including the kidneys, liver, spleen, central nervous system (CNS), eye, mammary gland, and genital tract. The action of the axial flagella and the release of hyaluronidases may facilitate invasion, especially into the CNS and eye. Fetal infection can occur following localization in the pregnant uterus. The organism may persist, most often in renal tubular epithelial cells.

The exact mechanisms by which leptospires cause disease are not completely understood. One feature of the disease is systemic vasculitis. Studies in mice suggest that the endothelial cell membrane of small vessels is disrupted by the intercalation of a glycolipoprotein toxin that displaces host long-chain fatty acids required to maintain vascular cell wall integrity.[84] The damage to the vascular endothelium allows for further migration of spirochetes into the tissues, as well as capillary leakage and hemorrhage, with disruption of tissue architecture, ischemia, and necrosis. There is a broad spectrum of clinical signs depending on the specific tissues affected and the severity of the infection.

Clear differences exist in the virulence of different isolates of *Leptospira*, but information relative to specific virulence factors and their role in pathogenesis is limited. Several outer membrane proteins, including LPS, may contribute to virulence. Highly immunogenic, LPS is responsible for the serovar specificity of leptospires.[12,85] Although leptospiral LPS exhibits endotoxic activity in biologic assays, it is of low potency.[8,9,86-88] Outer membrane components may play a role in the pathogenesis of interstitial nephritis, and the outer envelope may have an antiphagocytic function.[8,89-91]

Factors in addition to the outer membrane proteins most likely contribute to the virulence of leptospires. Toxins other than LPS are produced by some pathogenic strains. Several serovars, including Pomona and Hardjo, produce hemolysins.[92,93] Protein and glycolipoprotein cytotoxins have also been identified.[12] Virulent leptospires can induce apoptosis in vitro and in vivo, and increased concentrations of inflammatory cytokines, such as tumor necrosis factor alpha (TNF-α), are found in patients with leptospirosis.[94] A study in horses with leptospirosis examining the activity of the antiinflammatory/antioxidative enzymes platelet-activating factor acetylhydrolase and paraoxonase-1 suggested that subclinical infection may be associated with a low grade systemic inflammatory response and oxidative stress.[95]

Immune-mediated mechanisms may also play a role in the pathogenesis of leptospirosis in several species. This is supported in part by the observation that significant clinical disease

*References 25, 41, 61, 65, 67, 68.

may be present even after apparent clearance of the majority of organisms.[12] In human patients, levels of circulating immune complexes correlate with disease severity, and in surviving patients, circulating immune complex concentrations decrease concurrently with clinical improvement.[96] A number of auto-antibodies, including antiplatelet antibody, have been detected in clinical leptospirosis, but their role in pathogenicity is uncertain.[12] In horses, evidence indicates that immune mechanisms may be important in some cases of ERU.[97-101]

The humoral immune response appears to be primarily responsible for the control of infection and immunity to leptospires.[12,102,103] Antibodies, which are predominantly directed against outer envelope epitopes, are generally produced within a few days of infection. Immunity usually is specific to the inciting serovar and closely related serovars, although some broadly reactive antigens have also been described. After opsonization by antibodies, organisms are cleared by the reticuloendothelial system. However, when there is infection by a host-adapted serovar in a maintenance host, concentrations of antibody may remain low, allowing organisms to persist, primarily in the kidney. Fetal infection, especially in the third trimester, may result in a specific antibody response that can be protective. Passive immunity can be transferred by antibodies alone, and although cell-mediated immune responses to leptospires do occur, they are currently thought to have a minimal role in protection.[12] The duration of immunity to leptospirosis is uncertain.

The pathogenesis of leptospiral-induced inflammation in ERU has not been fully elucidated despite considerable research, with evidence supporting a role for both persistent infection and autoimmune mechanisms. The presence of *Leptospira* within the eye may cause direct damage, initiate a local immune response to the bacteria, or incite an autoimmune reaction through molecular mimicry. Actual continued infection may not be necessary to induce immune-mediated ocular inflammation because any release of inflammatory cytokines could reactivate memory T cells that react with ocular antigens.[97,104] Some studies have documented persistent leptospiral infection in horses with ERU, although the findings have not been consistent.[105-113] In a U.S. study by Faber et al,[105] 21 of 30 horses (70%) with ERU had leptospiral DNA in the aqueous humor detectable by polymerase chain reaction (PCR), compared with 1 of 16 control horses (6.25%).[105] Vitreous humor samples were cultured in several European studies of ERU, and *Leptospira* was isolated in 9% to 50% of vitreous humor samples from eyes with uveitis, with the most common serogroup being Grippotyphosa.[106-110] The prevalence of the serogroup Grippotyphosa led to the hypothesis that although many pathogenic serovars may penetrate the eyes, only a few are able to persist.[110] However, in a study of horses in the southeastern United States, leptospiral DNA was not detected in the aqueous humor or vitreous of horses with ERU or clinically normal horses.[82] It was concluded that although leptospiral organisms may have helped initiate ERU in some cases, the continued presence of the organisms did not play a direct role in the pathogenesis of the disease.

There is considerable evidence supporting a role for immune mechanisms in the pathogenesis of leptospiral ERU. In particular, a delayed-type hypersensitivity response has been suggested.[97,114] Horses exposed to *L. interrogans* can produce cross-reactive antibodies that bind to cornea, lens, ciliary body, and/or retina in addition to *Leptospira*.[98-101,104,115-118] After inoculation with killed leptospiral organisms, antibodies reacting with cornea have been found in tears, aqueous humor, and serum of horses.[99] In addition, horses inoculated with either killed *Leptospira* or equine cornea develop cross-reacting antibody and corneal opacity.[98] Specifically, a 90-kilodalton (kDa) leptospiral protein has been identified that shares antigenicity with a 66-kDa equine corneal protein.[116] This protein appears to be present in several serovars of *L. interrogans* sensu stricto, but it is not present in the nonpathogenic *L. biflexa* sensu stricto or in *L. borgpetersenii* serovar Tarassovi strain Perepelicin, which is pathogenic but has not been associated with ERU.[117] Additional leptospiral proteins that may contribute to the immunopathogenesis of ERU include LruA, LruB, and LruC.[118-120]

Clinical Findings

Clinical leptospirosis in horses has been primarily associated with abortion and ERU, although sporadic cases of systemic disease have also been reported. After experimental induction of leptospirosis in horses, fever was the most consistent clinical sign, with anorexia, listlessness, and icterus observed in some cases.[121-124] The majority of experimentally infected horses exhibited leukocytosis and neutrophilia during acute infection, and hyperbilirubinemia was occasionally seen. Although not a consistent finding, some horses developed uveitis, generally several months after exposure.

Abortion, Stillbirth, and Neonatal Disease

Leptospiremia may lead to infection of the reproductive organs, and in pregnant animals, this may result in fetal resorption, hydrallantois, abortion, stillbirth, and premature or weak neonates.[35,71-76,79,80,125] In an outbreak of leptospirosis associated with flooding on a farm with 70 broodmares, there were 8 abortions, a stillbirth, 3 neonatal deaths, and a case of neonatal illness in a 6-week period.[77] Abortion has also been associated with mixed *Leptospira* and equine herpesvirus type 1 (EHV-1) infection.[73,126] Leptospiral abortions most often occur in middle to late gestation. Although affected placentas may appear grossly normal, they more frequently are diffusely thick, edematous, and hemorrhagic. The chorioallantoic membrane may appear mucoid and discolored. In some cases, inflammation of the umbilical cord or funisitis may be present as well, generally appearing as diffuse discoloration of the umbilical cord.[127] In a study of 80 clinically normal embryo donor mares, there was no correlation between the seroreactivity of the mare to *Leptospira* and the embryo recovery rate.[128]

Equine Recurrent Uveitis

Uveitis in horses has been described after natural and acquired infection with leptospires.[82,105,113,121-123,129-133] Although the condition generally occurs months to years after infection, some cases may be more acute. Signs are typically recurrent or persistent. In a study by Wollanke et al,[109] 38% of the 120 horses from which *L. interrogans* was isolated from the vitreous had been clinically affected for longer than 1 year. Despite the association between ERU and leptospirosis, it is important to remember that most exposure to leptospires does not result in uveitis and that uveitis may have many other causes.[81,83,131,134,135]

The signs of ERU include miosis, blepharospasm, photophobia, aqueous flare, iritis, ciliary injection, and occasionally keratitis (Fig. 32-3). Chronically, there may be synechia, cataract formation, atrophy of the corpora nigra, chorioretinitis, altered iris color, and ultimately blindness. These clinical signs are nonspecific and do not distinguish cases of leptospiral uveitis from those with other causes. Interestingly, a study of 112 horses with ERU by Dwyer et al[134] suggested that leptospiral uveitis may be more severe than ERU from other causes because horses with uveitis that were seropositive to leptospires were 4.4 times

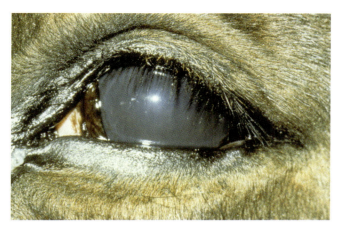

Figure 32-3 Uveitis in equine eye characterized by miosis, aqueous flare, and corneal edema. Leptospirosis is one cause of equine recurrent uveitis (ERU); however, making a definitive diagnosis can be difficult. (*Courtesy Dr. Brian Gilger.*)

more likely to lose vision than were seronegative horses with uveitis.

Systemic Disease in Adults and Foals

Although exposure to leptospires is common in the equine population, systemic disease appears to occur infrequently. However, clinical leptospirosis has been sporadically reported in horses of all ages. In several reports of leptospirosis in neonatal and premature foals, infection was most likely acquired in utero.[33,35,70,77,136] Signs included weakness and icterus, and in one foal, hematuria and dysuria were present. Leptospirosis has also been diagnosed in slightly older foals. Leptospires were isolated from the urine of a 5-week-old foal with signs of dullness and poor body condition on a farm on which multiple foals had died by 14 weeks of age.[137] Also, leptospirosis was thought to be involved in the deaths of 12 foals 4 to 12 weeks of age on one farm over a 3-year period.[24] These foals had severe respiratory distress with lethargy and pyrexia. Other signs included jaundice in one foal, an unsteady gait in one foal, and diarrhea in two foals. The disease was rapidly fatal, and hemorrhagic pneumonia was found in all foals on necropsy. *Leptospira interrogans* serovar Lora was isolated from the blood of one foal, two foals had high microscopic agglutination test (MAT) titers in single sera, and two others had marked increases in the MAT titers in paired sera.

Reports of clinical leptospirosis in adult horses have described fever, anorexia, and lethargy.[135,138,139] Icterus and hepatic dysfunction have also been reported.[45,129,132] Acute renal failure associated with leptospirosis has been documented in a 7-year-old stallion, a 3-month-old filly, and a 7-month-old filly.[140-142] Common signs in these cases included anorexia and lethargy, and two of the three horses were febrile. Laboratory evaluation revealed leukocytosis with hyperfibrinogenemia, azotemia, and isosthenuria. Ultrasound revealed enlarged kidneys in two of the three cases. A renal biopsy was only performed in the 3-month-old foal and confirmed tubulointerstitial nephritis.[141] All affected horses responded to antimicrobial therapy. In a 2-year-old filly with a nonulcerative keratouveitis resulting in blindness, leptospiral organisms were identified in the kidney, suggesting the ocular disease was associated with a systemic infection with *Leptospira*.[133] One study of 119 racing Thoroughbreds in Brazil suggested that subclinical leptospirosis may impair performance.[143]

Diagnosis

Leptospirosis should be considered as a differential diagnosis in patients with compatible clinical signs such as abortion, uveitis, and renal or hepatic disease, especially when the history suggests exposure to contaminated urine. However, making an accurate diagnosis of leptospirosis can be problematic because of the difficulty in identifying the organism and the high seroprevalence in the equine population. Therefore a number of methods for diagnosing leptospirosis have been developed, and studies are ongoing to develop simpler, more reliable methods.

Direct Detection Methods

Leptospires are difficult to visualize by standard light microscopy as they stain weakly or not at all with traditional stains. Therefore darkfield microscopy is the most common means of microscopic identification.[4] The organisms appear as slender, silver rods with hooked end(s) and are motile if viable. The helical coils may give the organism a "beaded" appearance. Although darkfield microscopy can provide a presumptive diagnosis of leptospirosis, the technique is not highly sensitive or specific. Approximately 10^4 to 10^5 leptospires/mL are necessary for one organism to be visible per field. Other motile bacteria and filamentous cellular extrusions or fibrin strands can be mistaken for leptospires.

Several samples, such as blood, urine, cerebrospinal fluid (CSF), milk, and macerated tissue, can be examined by darkfield microscopy. Usually, however, the organism is identified in urine because relatively large numbers of leptospires can be shed in the urine of infected animals. Diuresis with furosemide appears to dislodge leptospires from the kidney, and if the patient is well hydrated, it is recommended to administer furosemide and collect midstream urine from the second urination to facilitate recovery.[144] Urine should generally be examined within 20 minutes because the organism can deteriorate rapidly, especially in highly alkaline or acidic urine. If the urine cannot be examined promptly, it is recommended to neutralize the pH or to add formalin, in which case the leptospires will be killed and nonmotile, but morphology will be maintained. Leptospires may also be demonstrated in blood during the bacteremic phase of acute illness. Usually, too few organisms are present in the CSF for detection by darkfield microscopy, but occasionally organisms will be seen. When low numbers are present, centrifugation of the sample may help to concentrate the organisms. Transmission-electron microscopy has been used for the detection of leptospira in the vitreous body of horses.[112]

Immunofluorescence and immunoperoxidase staining have been used to increase the sensitivity of direct microscopic examination.[4,5] In particular, the fluorescent antibody test (FAT) has improved the ability to identify leptospires in fluids and tissues or tissue impression smears. Although the characteristic morphology of leptospires may be less evident when using FAT compared with darkfield microscopy, FAT is more sensitive, can detect degenerated organisms, and can be serovar specific. Several other methods to detect leptospiral antigens in clinical samples have been evaluated but are not currently in widespread clinical use. These include a radioimmunoassay (RIA), an enzyme-linked immunosorbent assay (ELISA), a double-sandwich ELISA, and an immunomagnetic antigen capture assay.[12,145]

A variety of histopathologic stains have been applied to the detection of leptospires in tissues.[4,5,146] Leptospires were first visualized using silver staining, and the Warthin-Starry stain, a modified silver stain, is widely used for histologic examination. Dieterle's and Steiner's are other modified silver stains that have also been used. In some cases, leptospires can be seen by light

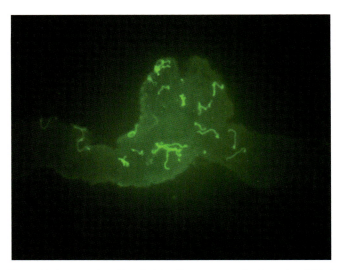

Figure 32-4 Leptospires identified by fluorescent antibody testing (100×). *(Courtesy Dr. Lindsay Oaks.)*

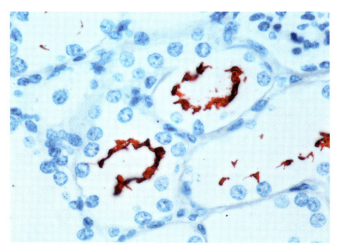

Figure 32-5 Immunohistochemical staining demonstrating spirochetes in renal tubules aggregating along luminal borders of tubular epithelial cells. *(Courtesy Dr. Tim Baszler.)*

microscopy in tissue sections or on air-dried smears with Giemsa stain. Both immunofluorescent (Fig. 32-4) and immunohistochemical (Fig. 32-5) methods have been useful in detecting leptospiral antigens and intact leptospires in tissue specimens.

Culture

Culture has been considered the "gold standard" for the diagnosis of leptospirosis, but the sensitivity is considered to be low.[4,5] Leptospires are fastidious, slow-growing organisms, and some serovars may require incubation for 4 to 6 months. Organisms are cultured in special media, most often Ellinghausen, McCullough, Johnson, and Harris medium (EMJH), at 28° C to 30° C (82° F-86° F). Leptospires are readily overgrown by contaminants, and adding antibiotics or 5-fluorouracil may improve recovery. After culture, isolates can be identified using DNA profiles and serology. Occasionally, leptospires have been cultured from fluids and tissues of healthy dogs, therefore culture may not always be diagnostic of clinical illness.[29]

Proper timing and handling of samples for culture are essential to the recovery of leptospires because of the fastidious nature of these organisms. Although leptospires may be isolated from a variety of specimens, culture of blood and urine is most common. Culturing multiple samples of both blood and urine, ideally prior to the initiation of antibiotic therapy, may improve the recovery rate. As with direct detection of organisms, it has been recommended to use furosemide to dislodge leptospires from the kidney before collecting urine midstream from the second urination.[144] Urine shedding typically begins within 2 weeks of infection and may continue intermittently for prolonged periods, especially in chronic cases. Blood cultures are generally obtained during the first 4 to 10 days of infection, when infected animals are most likely to be leptospiremic. If indicated, CSF samples can be collected for culture in this same time frame. Leptospires may also be cultured from tissue samples collected by biopsy or at necropsy.

Optimally, samples should be inoculated into culture media immediately. However, this is often not possible, in which case samples should be either diluted 1:10 with 1% bovine serum albumin, buffered saline, or culture media or inoculated into transport media. If not diluted immediately, blood should be anticoagulated with sodium oxalate, preservative-free heparin, or sodium polyethylene sulfonate; citrate anticoagulants should be avoided because they inhibit the growth of leptospires. Urine pH should be adjusted to neutral if necessary. When shipped, tissue and fluid samples should be kept in transport media or on ice but not frozen.

DNA Methodology

A number of molecular techniques, including dot blotting, DNA hybridization, genomic probes, and PCR, have been applied to the identification of leptospires in various species.[78,147-150] Currently, PCR is the most frequently used of these assays in veterinary medicine. PCR has been used in urine and semen of cattle, and some, but not all, studies have shown PCR to be more sensitive than FAT or culture for the detection of organisms.[147,151-154] In a study of horses with ERU, 21 of 30 horses (70%) with ERU had leptospiral DNA in the aqueous humor detectable by PCR, compared with 1 of 16 control horses (6.25%).[105] Only 6 of 27 horses with uveitis (22.2%) in this study were culture positive in the aqueous humor, all of which were positive by PCR, leading to the conclusion that PCR was more reliable than culture for detecting leptospires in the aqueous humor. Additionally, PCR has been used to detect *Leptospira* in placental tissues and premature or aborted foals, as well as in the investigation of wildlife reservoirs.[38,78-80,149]

Animal Inoculation

The intraperitoneal inoculation of urine, blood, tissue suspensions, and environmental samples into weaning gerbils, hamsters, or guinea pigs has been used in the diagnosis of leptospirosis.[4] Blood samples from the inoculated animals are used to inoculate media and to assess the serologic response.

Serology

Diagnosis of leptospirosis has often been based on serology because of the difficulties in direct identification and culture of the organism. Antibodies are usually present in blood about 5 to 7 days after the onset of signs, and concentrations may remain elevated for years after exposure. Antibodies have also been detected in a variety of clinical samples in addition to blood; the most important in horses being aqueous humor.

The reference method for serologic diagnosis of leptospirosis is the MAT, in which sera are reacted with live antigen suspensions of various leptospiral serovars.[4,12,155] The MAT detects both immunoglobulin M (IgM) and immunoglobulin G (IgG) antibodies. Results are read by darkfield microscopy, with the end-point being the highest dilution of serum at which 50% of the leptospires are agglutinated. It is a serogroup-specific assay, although cross-reaction may occur between some serogroups, especially in acute-phase samples. In general, the MAT has high specificity, but sensitivity may be low. In particular, infections by host-adapted strains in reservoir hosts may not be identified because antibody concentrations are often low. The MAT can be a challenging assay to implement and interpret, and there have been several modifications. In addition, a macroscopic agglutination test and agglutination assays that utilize formalinized antigens have been used.

Serologic tests must be interpreted with caution because of the widespread exposure of horses to leptospires. The MAT has been employed in most epidemiologic surveys of seroprevalence, with titers of 100 or higher being considered positive. In the diagnosis of clinical disease, serology is most useful in diagnosis of acute infections in incidental hosts, in which antibody responses tend to be greater than in reservoir hosts or chronic infections. A single elevated titer, generally 800 or greater, detected in association with clinical signs is suggestive of acute infection. Detection of a fourfold change in antibody titer in paired sera obtained 2 weeks apart is considered to be stronger evidence for a diagnosis of leptospirosis. However, especially in cases of abortion or uveitis, acute infection may have occurred earlier, and there may be no change in titer. Although vaccination of horses for leptospirosis is not common, vaccination will cause a detectable antibody response that cannot be differentiated from natural exposure.

A number of additional techniques for the detection of leptospiral antibodies have been developed, including complement fixation, ELISA, indirect hemagglutination assay, and intradermal skin testing.[12,26,155-157] The most widely used of these assays in veterinary species is the ELISA, which is specific and has greater sensitivity than the MAT.[155] Either IgM or IgG can be detected by ELISA. Because IgM is the initial antibody produced, a positive IgM-specific ELISA suggests infection within the previous month.

Diagnosis of Abortion, Stillbirth, and Neonatal Deaths

Several *Leptospira* serovars have been associated with abortion, stillbirth, and neonatal deaths. High leptospiral titers in aborting mares, as well as positive fetal antibody titers, are considered supportive of a diagnosis of leptospirosis. The level of titers observed in aborting mares varies widely, with most titers ranging from 1:100 to 1:1600, and titers of 1:204,800 and higher occasionally seen.[25,71-73,76,77] Aborting mares often have titers to multiple leptospiral serovars, and these titers do not necessarily correspond with the cause of abortion.[25,37,76,77] Also, in an investigation of three Kentucky horse farms, no correlation was found between the serovar that caused abortion in the previous year and the prevalence of positive titers to that serovar in horses tested on that farm the following year.[25]

Numerous diagnostic techniques have been used to confirm leptospirosis as the specific cause of abortion or stillbirths, including isolation of the organism, demonstration of spirochetes on histopathology, a positive FAT for the organism, and PCR. It is important to evaluate both fetal tissues and placenta. In 74 cases of leptospiral abortion in Kentucky, organisms were cultured in 60.8% of cases (45/74).[73] The diagnosis was supported by FAT and MAT in the remaining cases. In a similar study of 71 cases (51 aborted fetuses and 16 stillborn foals), spirochetes were identified in the allantochorion and/or kidney with the Warthin-Starry stain in 69 of 71 cases, 56 of 60 cases were positive using the direct FAT, and leptospires were isolated

from fetal tissues in 20 of 42 cases.[76] PCR has been used in cases of abortion and premature birth and appears to be a relatively rapid and reliable diagnostic tool.[78-80,149]

Diagnosis of Equine Recurrent Uveitis

Confirming leptospirosis as the definitive etiology in cases of ERU can be difficult. The significance of serum antibody is unclear because of the relatively high seroprevalence in the equine population and conflicting results from studies of ERU. Several studies have demonstrated a positive relationship between ERU and leptospiral seroreactivity.[45,134, 58-160] For example, in the Dwyer et al[134] study of 372 horses, seropositive horses were 13.2 times more likely to have uveitis than seronegative horses. However, other studies have failed to confirm a significant association between ERU and serum antibody concentrations.[105,106,135,161] A study of 30 horses with ERU and 16 control horses found no correlation between serologic results and the presence of leptospiral DNA or organisms in the aqueous humor.[105] In another study, 4 of 41 horses with ERU and positive *Leptospira* cultures in the vitreous were seronegative.[106]

Such studies have caused many investigators to conclude that serologic testing is of low sensitivity and specificity in the diagnosis of leptospiral-related uveitis.[105,106,135,161] Some suggest that the presence of antibodies to *Leptospira* in the aqueous or vitreous humor is more accurate than serology in establishing a diagnosis of leptospiral uveitis, especially with evidence of local production of antibody, as suggested by intraocular titers that exceed serum titers, or comparison with total IgG concentrations or albumin.[106-108,135,139,162] However, Wollanke et al[109] concluded from a study of 242 horses with ERU and 39 control horses that even vitreous antibody titers that are 4 times higher than serum titers may not be a sensitive test for the diagnosis of ERU associated with *L. interrogans* infection. Also, in a study of 52 horses with ERU, 17 horses with ocular inflammation not related to ERU, and 24 normal horses, there was no significant difference in titers of anti-*Leptospira* antibodies in either serum or aqueous humor between the 3 groups.[82] Intraocular production of antibodies against *Leptospira* organisms was only demonstrated in two horses, one with ERU and one with non-ERU inflammation.

Demonstration of leptospiral organisms or DNA within the eye may be useful in the diagnosis of leptospiral uveitis, as some cases may have persistent infection.[105-112] Both aqueous and vitreous humor can be sampled and assessed by culture, PCR, or examination by electron microscopy. In addition, ocular tissues can be evaluated should enucleation be indicated.

Pathologic Findings

Leptospirosis is characterized by vasculitis with endothelial damage and inflammatory infiltrates composed of monocytic cells, plasma cells, histiocytes, and neutrophils.[12] Lesions can be found in multiple tissues because the organism can replicate in many sites. In horses with systemic leptospirosis, icterus, pulmonary hemorrhage, glomerulonephritis renal interstitial edema, and tubulointerstitial nephritis have been reported.[24,129,141]

Gross and histologic lesions have been identified in the placenta and fetus in many cases of leptospiral abortion.[34,37,76,146,163] In a study of 71 cases (51 aborted fetuses and 16 stillborn foals), gross lesions were found in 80.3% of fetuses, stillborn foals, and placentas, whereas microscopic lesions were observed in 96%.[132] The lesions, which were consistent with those identified in other studies, included gross placental lesions of edema, cystic allantoic nodules, and necrosis of the chorion with necrotic mucoid exudates. Histologic placental lesions included thrombosis, vasculitis, mixed inflammatory cell infiltration of the stroma and villi, hyperplasia of allantoic epithelium, and villous necrosis and calcification. In the fetus or stillborn foal, gross abnormalities were most common in the liver, being identified in 23 cases, whereas abnormalities were identified in the kidneys of 7 cases. The liver was enlarged, mottled, and pale to yellow. Histologically, there was hepatocellular dissociation, mixed leukocytic infiltration of the portal triads, and giant cell hepatopathy. The kidneys were swollen and edematous with white radiating streaks in the cortex and medulla. Microscopically, there was suppurative and nonsuppurative nephritis. Additional lesions included pulmonary hemorrhages, pneumonia, and myocarditis. Gross and microscopic evidence of funisitis has also been reported in association with leptospiral abortion.[127]

Therapy

Appropriate treatment for leptospirosis varies, depending on the severity and duration of clinical signs, as well as the site of infection. Some cases may resolve spontaneously or with only supportive therapy. However, specific antimicrobial therapy may be indicated in some patients.

Well-controlled studies related to the efficacy of antibiotic treatment for leptospirosis in any species are limited. Results between in vitro and in vivo studies of antibiotic susceptibility have been conflicting. Also, antibiotic efficacy may vary when treating patients with acute versus chronic disease. Some antibiotics to which leptospires tend to be susceptible include penicillin, ampicillin, amoxicillin, cefotaxime, ceftiofur, erythromycin, and ciprofloxacin.[164-170] Resistance to some antibiotics, including sulfonamides, chloramphenicol, and cephalothin, has been documented for some isolates. Whereas in vitro susceptibility to streptomycin and tetracyclines was intermediate in some studies, these drugs have been clinically effective in the treatment of leptospires.[171-173] Currently, penicillin and doxycycline are most often recommended for treatment of leptospirosis in human patients.[12,174-178] Although the effects of antibiotic therapy on outcome and duration of clinical illness have been variable, a consistent finding in human studies has been the prevention of leptospiruria or a significant reduction in its duration.[174,175,177,178] Similarly, dihydrostreptomycin, tetracycline, and erythromycin have been shown to prevent urinary shedding in laboratory animals.[179-182] Reports on the efficacy of dihydrostreptomycin in eliminating the carrier state in cattle and swine have been variable.[173,182-184]

No specific studies have addressed antibiotic therapy for leptospirosis in horses. Some recommended antibiotics include penicillin, oxytetracycline, streptomycin, dihydrostreptomycin, and erythromycin.[20,168] In one limited study, tetracycline, penicillin, and dihydrostreptomycin did not eliminate shedding in horses, although the dosages and duration of treatment may not have been adequate.[21] Penicillin has been administered to pregnant mares with rising leptospiral titers in late gestation, with the delivery of clinically normal foals, although the significance of this is uncertain.[21] In the reported cases of acute renal failure in horses, two horses were treated with penicillin and the third with ticarcillin–clavulanic acid, all with a positive outcome.[140-142] A premature foal with hematuria and leptospiruria was successfully treated with penicillin and amikacin sulfate.[33] In all cases, appropriate adjunctive therapy, such as intravenous fluids and furosemide, was given. Because horses with clinical leptospirosis may be azotemic, it is important to consider the potential for nephrotoxicity when selecting a specific antibiotic.

Equine Recurrent Uveitis

Treatment for ERU typically consists of a combination of anti-inflammatory agents and mydriatics. Recently, implantation of a sustained-release delivery system for the immunosuppressant drug cyclosporine has shown some efficacy.[185] Some treatments have been targeted specifically for *Leptospira*-associated uveitis. Vitrectomy and replacement of vitreous with a saline solution of gentamicin has been recommended for treatment of ERU. In a study of 38 horses with follow-up of at least 6 months, owners reported no further uveitis episodes in 42 of 43 eyes.[106] Some vision was maintained in 31 of 43 eyes (72%), whereas 12 of 43 (28%) were blind. It was thought that improvement was primarily caused by removal of persistent intraocular bacteria, as well as inflammatory mediators and cells that contribute to the progression of intraocular inflammation.

In view of the evidence of persistent infection with *Leptospira* in some horses with ERU, more aggressive antibiotic therapy may be indicated, but to date, no controlled studies have assessed therapeutic efficacy.[105-110] Administration of doxycycline via nasogastric tube at 10 mg/kg every 12 hours did not result in appreciable concentrations of the drug in the aqueous and vitreous in normal eyes and a higher dosage may be needed.[186,187] Enrofloxacin administered at 7.5 mg/kg intravenous (IV) every 24 hours resulted in concentrations above the reported MIC for *Leptospira interrogans* serovar Pomona in the aqueous humor following disruption of the blood-aqueous barrier.[188] However, the value of systemic or local antibiotics in the treatment of suspected leptospiral-induced ERU remains unclear and further study is indicated.

Anecdotally, it has been suggested that vaccination of horses with leptospiral vaccines may either decrease subsequent episodes of uveitis or potentially worsen the disease by stimulating the autoimmune response. In one study, 41 horses with ERU were vaccinated with either a vaccine containing 6 serovars of *Leptospira* (20 horses) or a placebo (21 horses).[104] Although the vaccine appeared to increase the days to recurrence of uveitis, it failed to slow the progression of the disease. These data do not support the use of vaccination against leptospirosis as adjunctive therapy for horses with ERU. However, there was no exacerbation of ocular disease, with only one horse developing a local injection site reaction.

Prevention

Limiting exposure to stagnant water and to potential carriers, such as cattle, swine, rodents, and wildlife, may help to control leptospirosis.[20,26] On one farm with leptospiral abortions, abortions ceased when horses were no longer fed by spreading feed on the ground.[73] Numerous wildlife of various species had been observed in the area during feeding. Infected animals should be isolated and contaminated areas cleaned and disinfected. For people in high-risk environments, doxycycline once weekly is effective for short-term prophylaxis.[189,190] This practice is controversial because of concerns about developing antibiotic resistance, and it has not been recommended for prevention of disease in horses.

Vaccination against leptospirosis is common in some species. Although currently no vaccines are approved for use in horses, limited studies have assessed the response of horses to vaccination with leptospiral bacterins.[104,191-194] It appears that horses mount an antibody response after vaccination. To date, the only adverse effect documented has been infrequent local injection site reactions. Anecdotally, vaccination has been used on farms with leptospiral abortions and uveitis, but no controlled data support its efficacy. In a study by Rohrbach et al,[104] vaccination was used in horses with preexisting ERU in an attempt to modulate the disease, but not to prevent initial infection with leptospires. For a vaccine to be effective, it would be important for the appropriate serovars to be included. There are ongoing studies to develop new vaccines for *Leptospira* such as a DNA vaccine expressing the hemolysin-associated protein 1.[195] Potentially, some of these vaccines may be cross-protective.

Public Health Considerations

Leptospirosis is perhaps the most widespread zoonosis in the world. Recently the prevalence has been increasing, resulting in the description of leptospirosis as a reemerging disease.[12,196-198] The incidence is greatest in geographic regions with warm climates, and within the United States, the highest incidence is found in Hawaii. The spectrum of signs in human patients is broad. In most cases the disease is subclinical or mild; however, 5% to 10% of patients may develop severe icteric leptospirosis with multisystemic involvement.[12,198] The mortality in these patients typically ranges between 5% and 15%.

The source of human infection is usually either direct or indirect contact with the urine of an infected animal. Occupation has been established as a significant risk factor for humans, with farmers, especially dairy farmers, veterinarians, and abattoir workers, among those at increased risk.[12,199] Certain recreational activities, such as water sports and hunting, have also been shown to increase the risk of exposure.[12] It has been suggested that horses could play a role in the transmission of leptospirosis in urban tropical areas based on the finding of leptospires by PCR in the urine of Thoroughbreds in Rio de Janeiro, Brazil.[200]

Personnel should be careful when dealing with infected animals to limit exposure. Latex gloves should be worn when handling urine or urine-contaminated materials. Areas contaminated with urine should be washed with detergent and treated with disinfectants such as iodophors. Prophylactic antibiotic therapy may be indicated if exposure to urine or tissues from an infected animal has occurred. In the case of the weanling with acute renal disease caused by *L. interrogans*, personnel closely involved in the treatment of the horse were treated with doxycycline for 1 week.[142]

The complete reference list is available online at www.expertconsult.com.

---

33 Lyme Disease

Thomas J. Divers

Etiology

Lyme disease is caused by at least three strains of the spirochete *Borrelia burgdorferi* sensu lato complex,[1,2] which includes several worldwide species and multiple variants of each species. The North American strain is *B. burgdorferi* sensu stricto,[3] which may have several strain variations.[4] In Europe, *B. afzelii* and *B. garinii* are responsible for most cases of Lyme disease.[5] In Asia, *B. garinii* is most common. *Borrelia burgdorferi* organisms are helical-shaped, gram-negative, unicellular spirochetes with flagellar projections.[6] *Borrelia burgdorferi* bacteria are not free-living organisms and quickly die outside a host. They are maintained in a 2-year enzootic life cycle that involves ixodid ticks (*Ixodes scapularis* in the eastern United States and *I. pacificus* on the west coast of North America) and mammals.[6] The white-footed mouse, which provides a continual source of the spirochete, and deer, which maintain the tick vector, are the most common mammals involved in maintaining the life cycle of this spirochete (Fig. 33-1).

Epidemiology

The seroprevalence of *B. burgdorferi* in horses in the United States is not known but is likely much higher than in humans but with similar geographic distribution (Fig. 33-2). The mid-Atlantic and northeastern states have a high seroprevalence, as do areas of Minnesota and Wisconsin extending into southern Canada. Seropositive horses are rare in the Rocky Mountain states, the Dakotas, Nebraska, and some other areas of the United States. In one New England survey, 45% of horses had *Borrelia* antibodies.[7] In a Wisconsin study, 118 of 190 horses were serologically positive.[8] In central Europe, there is a high level of antibody positive horses.[9-11] Lyme disease in humans seems to be more common in the northern hemisphere but does occur in the southern hemisphere, including Brazil and Australia.

Infection in horses is caused by attachment and prolonged (>24 hours) feeding of infected adult *Ixodes* spp. ticks. Female ticks are likely the competent vector for horses and can be identified by the complete arch over the anus (see Fig. 33-1). Adult males rarely feed. Nymphs are responsible for a high percentage of infections in humans because they are small and often escape visual inspection.[5] It is not known if the immature stages transmit the spirochete to horses. *Ixodes scapularis* adults are most active in the fall and throughout winter when temperatures are above freezing. Once feeding begins, the organism begins its complicated up-and-down regulation of genes to enhance survival in the host. Exact pathogenesis of *Borrelia* in the horse is not known. After experimental infection of ponies, the organism appears to reside mostly in skin near the tick bite, as well as in connective tissue and muscle and around nerves and blood vessels near synovial membranes.[13] A lymphocytic

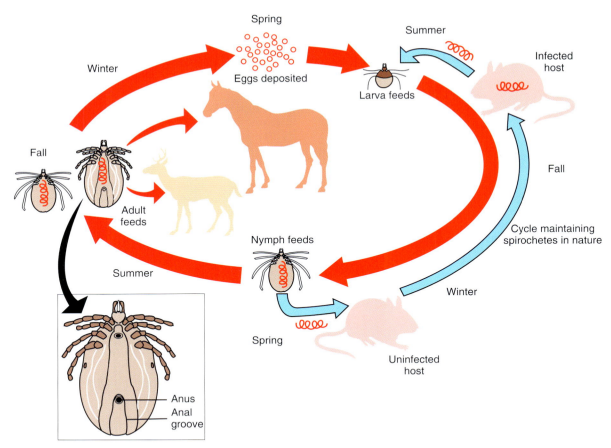

Figure 33-1 Two-year enzootic cycle of *Borrelia burgdorferi* and distinguishing features of *Ixodes* species ticks. *Inset,* Female ventral abdomen.

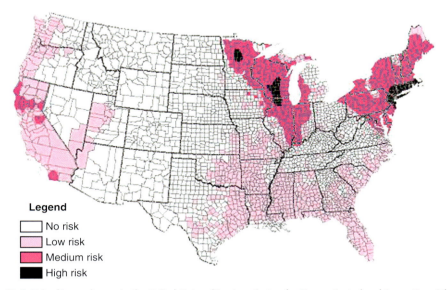

Figure 33-2 Risk of Lyme disease in the United States. *(Courtesy Centers for Disease Control and Prevention, Atlanta.)*

plasmacytic reaction may occur within these tissues, and in experimentally infected ponies, this reaction was associated with the highest concentration of the *Borrelia* organism.[13,14]

The species of *Borrelia* may have predilection for causing disease in certain body sites. In human borreliosis, *Borrelia afzelii* may be mostly associated with skin disease, whereas *B. garinii* is more neurotropic and *B. burgdorferi* is the species to most commonly cause joint disease.

The organism lives in the tick gut and is transferred to animals during blood meals. Generally, 24 to 48 hours of attachment is required to transfer the organism successfully from the tick to the mammalian host.[12] This time may be needed for the organism to downregulate an outer membrane protein (OspA), which may be important to maintain survival in the mammalian host.[15] Conversely, other surface proteins (e.g., OspC, OspE, OspF) that are in low concentration in the tick gut are upregulated, particularly OspC in the tick salivary gland, to enhance complement resistance and other methods of immune evasion in the mammalian host.[16] The changes in expression of surface proteins may be triggered by the blood meal. Other proteins, such as the C6 peptide found in a dominant invariable region of the variable major protein like gene VisE, permit antigenic variation, ensuring survival in the host.[17] Many other components of the agent may be important for infection but these are not entirely understood.[18] *Borrelia burgdorferi* may also survive in the host by residing in collagen and connective tissue likely related to low-molecular-weight decorin-binding proteins, having no requirement for iron and by possibly forming resistant cysts within the host.[19-21] Persistent infection, especially following antibiotic treatments, has been very controversial in humans, and most studies do not support any such syndrome of chronic infection/chronic Lyme disease following appropriate antibiotic therapy.[22,23] Conversely, a recent article provided evidence that both a cyst (round bodies) and biofilm-like colonies exist which have some potential to cause chronic disease.[24]

Clinical Findings

A wide variety of clinical signs have been attributed to *Borrelia* infection in horses, but demonstration of cause and effect has been difficult to document in most cases. Clinical signs most often attributed to equine Lyme disease include stiffness and lameness in more than one limb, muscle tenderness, hyperesthesia, lethargy, and behavioral changes.[25-30] Unlike human Lyme disease, joint effusion has been minimal in most Lyme-suspect horses. Muscle wasting and pain over the thoracolumbar area have been present in a few horses with high serum titers (Fig. 33-3).

There have been several cases of confirmed or suspected neuroborreliosis. In one report, two horses were diagnosed with Lyme neuroborreliosis and both had chronic, necrosuppurative-to-nonsuppurative, perivascular-to-diffuse meningoradiculo-neuritis on necropsy examination.[32] Hyperesthesia, lumbar pain, and muscle wasting were the initial clinical findings followed by ataxia of all four limbs, facial nerve paralysis, and finally, head tremors with depression in one horse. The second horse had a 3-year history of asymmetric muscle wasting and facial paralysis that had not responded to equine protozoal myeloencephalitis (EPM) treatment and was eventually diagnosed as a peripheral neuropathy that responded to dexamethasone, but, after discontinuing the treatment, the horse relapsed

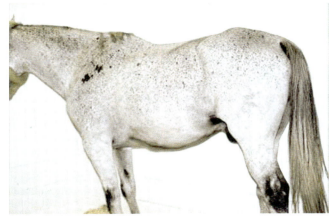

Figure 33-3 Muscle wasting and pain over the thoracolumbar area in horse with high serum titer.

with marked muscle wasting, ataxia, and depression. No cerebrospinal fluid (CSF) was evaluated, but, on necropsy, spirochetes were identified by Steiner silver impregnation in both cases, predominantly in the affected dura mater of brain and spinal cord. No spirochetes were identified by Silver stain within the neural parenchyma or within neurogenic atrophied muscle. *Borrelia burgdorferi* sensu stricto was identified by polymerase chain reaction (PCR) with highest spirochetal burdens in tissues with inflammation, including spinal cord, muscle, and joint capsule. In another report, a horse with severe neck stiffness that progressed to ataxia had lymphohistiocytic meningitis and *B. burgdorferi* deoxyribonucleic acid (DNA) in the CSF.[31] That horse had originally responded to doxycycline treatment but relapsed after discontinuing the treatment. Another case in a Thoroughbred hunter that presented for lameness and ataxia had lymphocytic pleocytosis and *Borrelia* PCR-positive CSF. The horse responded well to doxycycline but had some deterioration when treatment was discontinued.[33]

Two other suspect horses the author examined had ataxia and severe lymphocytic infiltration of the meninges. There are other published reports of neurologic dysfunction in a horse attributed to Lyme disease.[25,26] From these accumulated reports, it would appear that ataxia and lumbar muscle wasting caused by lymphohistiocytic meningitis and radiculoneuritis with occasional fasciculations and neck stiffness are characteristic of neuroborreliosis in the horse. Cerebrospinal fluid (CSF) would likely have a lymphocytic pleocytosis and might be PCR positive for *Borrelia burgdorferi*. In another case report, panuveitis and arthritis was reported in a pony.[34] Recently, bilateral uveitis in two horses was found to be the result of *Borrelia* infection of the eye.[35] *Borrelia* was found on cytologic examination and confirmed by PCR in the vitreous in both horses. No organisms were observed in the aqueous, although one aqueous sample was PCR positive. *Borrelia* was also observed with silver stain in the inflamed uveal tissue. In addition to the uveitis, one of the horses had a history of hyperesthesia and the other had muscle wasting over the topline. A chronic multifocal lymphohistiocytic ganglioradiculitis and neuritis with presumptive neuronal degeneration in the spinal nerves was found in the second horse along with inflammatory lesions in multiple organ systems, including the heart, lung, liver, spleen, kidney, skin, skeletal muscle, and nervous tissue. Inflammatory cells were predominantly lymphocytes though often accompanied by plasma cells, histiocytes, and/or neutrophils. The distribution of the infiltrates was often within connective tissues or centered on blood vessels. Another report describes a horse with multiple lymphohistiocytic cutaneous nodules over the masseter muscle 3 months following removal of a tick (Fig. 33-4); this horse was confirmed as having Lyme pseudolymphoma. The horse responded completely to doxycycline treatment as might be expected for a cutaneous form of borreliosis.[36]

The high fever and limb edema typically reported in association with *Borrelia* seroconversion are most often the result of *Anaplasma phagocytophila* infection because many ticks are concomitantly infected with both *Borrelia* and *A. phagocytophila*.[37]

Experimental infection of ponies caused consistent lesions in the skin and inconsistent lesions in muscle, fascia, nerves, and perisynovial tissues, but clinical signs were not observed. Except for the lymphocytic/histiocytic dermatitis, the pathology has been mild in most of the experimentally infected ponies. Until clinical signs can be experimentally reproduced, the association between *B. burgdorferi* infection and clinical disease in many horses will remain speculative and no doubt somewhat controversial.

The diagnosis of Lyme disease is most common in sport horses, but this might be because subtle clinical signs of stiffness and hyperesthesia are most easily recognized in sport horses and may not be related to any genetic predisposition for disease.

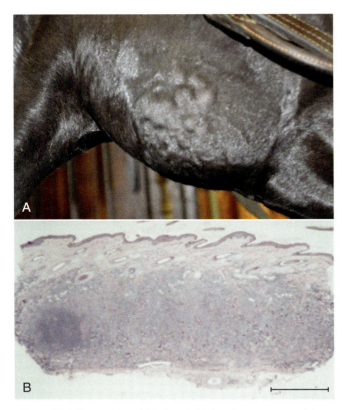

Figure 33-4 Horse with multiple lymphohistiocytic cutaneous nodules.

Diagnosis

The diagnosis of exposure to *Borrelia* can usually be determined by serology but to definitively diagnose that a horse is currently infected is more difficult and to determine whether clinical disease is associated with *Borrelia* is extremely difficult. Enzyme-linked immunosorbent assay (ELISA) or immunofluorescent antibody (IFA) testing have been the preferred screening tests for detection of antibodies indicating exposure. If the ELISA value is not greater than the laboratory control, it suggests no exposure, distant exposure but no current infection, or recent infection (within 1-2 months).[13] A repeat sample taken in 2 months that remains negative would help rule out recent infection.[13] Experimentally infected ponies successfully treated with antibiotics (no organisms found at euthanasia) had titers that decreased to preinfection ELISA units 4 months after treatment was initiated.[38] Antibiotic-treated ponies that remained infected at euthanasia had some decrease in titer during antibiotic treatment, but never as low as preinfection, and had a rebound increase in titer after discontinuing antibiotic therapy.[17] In field-infected and treated cases, this same magnitude of decline in ELISA antibody level is rarely seen. The value of the C6 SNAP test (IDEXX Laboratories, Westbrook, ME), based on antibody to a peptide that reproduces the sequence of the invariable region 6 (an immunodominant, conserved region), has good correlation with the ELISA in horses; specificity is better than sensitivity.[39] Vaccination should not cause the C6 to be positive. In humans the C6 antibody cannot always be used to assess treatment outcome or the presence of active infection but has comparable sensitivity to Western blot for diagnosing Lyme disease.[40,41]

The principal value of the Western blot assay is both in separating horses that are ELISA positive because of natural infection from horses that are ELISA positive because of

vaccination or from cross-reacting flagellar antigen exposure. In experimentally infected ponies, the Western blot assay was positive at 8 to 10 weeks after infection, versus 6 to 8 weeks for the ELISA.[13] Recently, a multiplex antibody bead test for OspA, OspC, and OspF quantitative antibody detection has been used in the serodiagnosis of equine Lyme disease.[42] The concept is that high levels of OspA would suggest vaccination, OspC would indicate recent infection (antibody against this antigen typically increases with early infection and then declines after 3-4 months), and OspF would suggest either chronic infection or more long-lasting antibodies. OspA antibodies have been found in a higher percentage of nonvaccinated horses with the multiplex assay than were detected by Western blot (WB) testing. The clinical significance of this finding and clinical practice value of the multiplex assay in determining time of infection, active versus past infection, and response to treatment could be significant but may require further investigations with a large number of field cases or ideally with experimentally infected and treated horses.

Clinical signs were not obvious in ponies experimentally infected with *Borrelia*, and a large number of apparently asymptomatic horses are seropositive; therefore clinical diagnosis is difficult and should be based on clinical probability of Lyme disease (knowledge of most common anatomic location of the organism in the horse, reported clinical syndromes), ruling out other diseases, and laboratory testing. Polymerase chain reaction and/or histopathology (usually a lymphoplasmacytic or histiocytic inflammation) on CSF or tissues can be helpful. To complicate the relationship between infection and clinical signs further, the most common drugs (oxytetracycline, doxycycline, and now minocycline) used to treat *Borrelia* in the horse have antiinflammatory properties that may alleviate musculoskeletal pain in horses, thus preventing response to therapy from being used as a diagnostic test.[43]

Pathologic Findings

Lesions in experimentally infected horses are mostly limited to a lymphohistiocytic reaction in the skin surrounding the site of the tick attachment and lymphoid hyperplasia of regional lymph nodes.[13,14,38] One experimental pony had a mononuclear cell reaction in cutaneous muscle and the panniculus, especially surrounding small arteries and nerves. Perivascular, perineural mononuclear inflammation is reported in human patients with Lyme disease.[44] One pony had a nonsuppurative synovitis with mononuclear subsynovial perivascular infiltration. Perivascular mononuclear cell aggregates also formed around small arteries adjacent to the perineurium of peripheral nerves, including the ulnar, facial, sciatic, labial, and fibular nerves and the dorsal spinal nerve roots. A perivascular mononuclear inflammation was also present in skeletal muscle in multiple areas.[44] All these changes have been reported in human patients with Lyme disease, and the association of these lesions with Lyme disease in experimental ponies is strengthened by the observation that all lesions in the one pony were most severe on the side of the body where the ticks were attached.[44] Pathologic findings in case reports include lymphohistiocytic inflammation of synovial membranes, meninges, nerve roots, and uveal tissue; in many cases, this inflammation is around blood vessels or nerves.

Therapy

The three most frequently used drugs for treatment of Lyme disease in horses are intravenous (IV) tetracycline and oral (PO) doxycycline or minocycline. In experimental ponies, IV tetracycline was more effective than PO doxycycline for eradicating *Borrelia*.[38] Intravenous tetracycline obtains much higher tissue concentrations than PO doxycycline, which has low bioavailability after per os administration in the horse.[45] If blood concentrations were equal, one would expect doxycycline to be the preferred drug because of better volume of distribution. Doxycycline cannot be administered by the IV route to horses because of potential adverse effects.[46] Tetracycline should not be given orally to horses because of low bioavailability and risk of active drug reaching the colon and causing diarrhea (unlike PO doxycycline, where much of the unabsorbed drug is inactive in the colon).[47] Minocycline has better oral bioavailability than doxycycline in the horse, and because it is less protein bound, it attains higher concentration in CSF and aqueous fluids than does doxycycline in the horse.[48] In humans, doxycycline treatment for only a few days for cutaneous Lyme disease or for 2 months for lameness or neuroborreliosis is still considered by many the gold standard for therapy; most reports suggest this treatment eliminates the infection.[5] Because of the low bioavailability of doxycycline in the horse and possibility of more long-term infection in horses than humans prior to treatment, this protocol may not be as successful in the horse. Group III cephalosporins are sometimes used for neuroborreliosis in humans but may not be better than doxycycline treatments.[5] Penicillin and amoxicillin are sometimes used for cutaneous Lyme diseases but are probably inferior to doxycycline.[5] In the one report on a cystic form of *Borrelia*, doxycycline was not effective against this form in vitro but metronidazole was moderately effective.[24] In that same report, the biofilm colonies were resistant to both doxycycline and metronidazole.[24] In both humans and horses the organism is resistant to fluroquinolones.[49]

The exact dose and the frequency and duration of therapy with tetracycline and doxycycline in the treatment of *Borrelia* infection are not known. A common intensive treatment scenario in clinical practice has been to give IV tetracycline 6.6 mg/kg every 24 hours (q12h) for 7 to 10 days, followed by PO doxycycline 10 mg/kg q12h or PO minocycline 4mg/kg q12 for 1 to 2 months. Although IV tetracycline (5 mg/kg q24h for 28 days) was 100% effective in eradicating *Borrelia* from experimentally infected ponies (treatment initiated 4 months after infection) and causing ELISA titer to return to baseline,[38] this same protocol has not been as effective in causing a decline in ELISA antibody in horses with naturally occurring infections.[50] It is unknown if this discrepancy is the result of treatment failure caused by prolonged field infections prior to treatment, reinfection, and/or molecular mimicry maintaining a persistently high serum antibody concentration. Even with aggressive antibiotic treatment protocol, ELISA titers may not decline remarkably before treatment is discontinued and may remain high for many months. Sensitivity of the WB, C6 SNAP test, and the Luminex assay in determining successful treatment have not been documented but all would be better than the ELISA. The C6 SNAP test is not quantitative in the horse, which makes changes more subjective. It is possible that cyst forms may be present in some chronically infected human or horse cases, and these are not killed by tetracyclines. Metronidazole may be effective against the cyst forms but is not effective against free-living *Borrelia*.[51] In refractory cases, it may be reasonable (but with unproven efficacy) to treat with both a tetracycline family drug and metronidazole. In humans, a chronic immune synovitis occurs in approximately 20% of chronic infections even after successfully treating the infection.

Other classes of drugs used to treat *Borrelia* in humans have no practical advantages over tetracyclines (e.g., ampicillin), are toxic when given orally to adult horses (e.g., macrolides), or were not as effective in the experimental pony study (e.g., ceftiofur [Naxcel, Pharmacia & Upjohn, Kalamazoo, MI]).[38] If IV tetracycline is administered as treatment, renal function should be monitored since tetracycline-induced acute renal failure can develop in horses. Use of a tetracycline class drug in pregnancy could result in abnormal fetal development.

Prevention

The means for prevention of Lyme disease in endemic areas may include (1) the prevention of tick exposure or prolonged (>24 hours) attachment, (2) the provision of early antimicrobial treatment after known *Ixodes* exposure, or (3) vaccination. Various insecticidal sprays can be used to prevent tick infection, but most are not approved for use in horses and efficacy in the horse is unproven. Currently, no adverse effects are known to result from use of the more common canine tick sprays (e.g., fipronil [Frontline, Merial, Duluth, GA]; Advantix [Bayer, Shawnee Mission, KS]) in the horse. Permethrin-based insecticides are approved for use in horses, but efficacy against ticks is not well documented. Any use of insecticides approved for dogs and close observation for ticks should be performed most diligently in late summer, fall, and early winter (after fly season) because this is the most common time for adults to attach. If ticks are found on a horse, they can be examined to determine if they are *Ixodes* spp. (see Fig. 33-1), the only genus of North American tick known to transmit *B. burgdorferi*.

Ponies were completely protected against experimental infection by vaccination with a recombinant OspA antigen vaccine when infected ticks were attached 92 days after the third vaccination.[14] Duration of protection in the horse, adverse effects, and efficacy of the currently available canine vaccines are unknown. Differentiation of natural exposure antibody from an OspA vaccine antibody response can often be made by either immunoblot testing, multiplex PCR, or C6 SNAP test. Several canine-approved Lyme vaccines are available and are commonly used in horses. All could result in production of protective antibodies, and the author is not aware of adverse effects being reported. The proper dose and frequency of administration are undetermined, but in the experimental vaccine study, neutralizing antibodies declined significantly within 5 months after the last vaccine inoculation. The decision to vaccinate is complicated because of the belief of many that the incidence of clinical disease in exposed horses is low. Clinical disease in high level sport horses appears to be more common, and vaccination has therefore been used frequently in that population of horse. Although vaccination following prior infection is more questionable, it is possible that horses can become reinfected if they do not develop or maintain protective antibody (i.e., antibody against OspA).

Public Health Considerations

There are minimal public health considerations associated with equine Lyme disease. A significant number of Lyme-infested horses with clinical signs of lameness or behavioral changes are positive for spirochetemia or spirocheturia (53% and 20%, respectively, in one study[28]), but it is considered unlikely that adult ticks feeding on horses would move to humans. Seroprevalence in horses in an area might be an important sentinel for risk of human Lyme disease in the same area.

The complete reference list is available online at www.expertconsult.com.

Lawsonia intracellularis

Nicola Pusterla, Connie J. Gebhart, Jean-Pierre Lavoie,* and Richard Drolet*

Etiology

Lawsonia intracellularis is the etiologic agent of the recently recognized and emerging intestinal disease in horses called *equine proliferative enteropathy* (EPE). *Lawsonia intracellularis* is an obligate intracellular, curved, gram-negative bacterium that resides freely within the apical cytoplasm of infected intestinal enterocytes.[1] It causes proliferation of the affected enterocytes, resulting in a thickened small and sometimes large intestine. *Lawsonia intracellularis* can only be grown in vitro in cell culture and requires a specific atmosphere for growth. Besides horses, *L. intracellularis* infects many species of domestic and wild animals, including pigs, hamsters, rabbits, foxes, deer, ferrets, ostriches, and nonhuman primates. Equine proliferative enteropathy was first reported in horses in 1982 by Duhamel and Wheeldon.[2] Since 1996, several reports of sporadic cases and outbreaks on breeding farms have been described.[3-20] In the last few years, reported cases of EPE have been increasing, occurring primarily in postweaning foals and occasionally in adult horses. The disease has almost reached a worldwide occurrence and has been reported in the United States, Canada, Europe, South Africa, Australia, Brazil, and Japan.

Molecular investigations of *L. intracellularis* isolates from proliferative enteropathy lesions of a variety of animal species, including horses and hamsters, showed 98% homology of the 16S-ribosomal deoxyribonucleic acid (rDNA) gene to pig isolates.[21] Moreover, phenotypic characterization of outer membrane proteins and immunoblots of different *L. intracellularis* isolates using several antibodies and more sensitive molecular characterizations of the *L. intracellularis* genome demonstrated only minor differences among isolates. None of these differences appears to be antigenically relevant. Recently, the whole genome of a porcine *L. intracellularis* isolate was sequenced and analyzed for the presence of variable number tandem repeat (VNTR) sequences.[22] Variable number tandem repeat sequences in the genomes of prokaryotes are often associated with a high level of polymorphism and enable bacterial strain differentiation with substantial discriminatory power. Use of these *L. intracellularis* VNTR sequences provides a sensitive method for analysis of the genetic relatedness of *L. intracellularis* bacteria or DNA obtained from various temporal and geographic locations and from various animal species. This provided insight into the phylogenetic relatedness of these isolates. Molecular VNTR sequence profiles of *L. intracellularis* isolates from various documented outbreaks of proliferative enteropathy occurring in pigs, horses, ostriches, spider monkeys, ferrets, and hamsters were analyzed. The patterns that emerged provide some insight into the sources and phylogenetic relatedness of *L. intracellularis* isolates from different species. Variable number tandem repeat sequence types obtained from pigs were very different from those obtained from horses or other nonpig

species. Little or no genetic variation was found between isolates from within outbreaks for any animal species or in multiple temporal samples taken from the same outbreak site. Slight variations between isolates obtained from outbreaks at different geographic locations were found, but these differences were minor. Marked variation in VNTR types were found, however, between isolates from pig sources and those obtained from non-pig sources including horses (Fig. 34-1).

Epidemiology

In pig populations, intestinal adenomatosis is maintained by chronic carriers, allowing transmission of *L. intracellularis* from one pig generation to the next.[23] Mice and rats are important reservoirs of *L. intracellularis* on piggeries with the percentage of polymerase chain reaction (PCR)-positive animals varying substantially between farms (4% to 83%).[24-26] Rodents appear to be suitable reservoir hosts because of their susceptibility to *L. intracellularis*, their close contact to domestic animals, and their high reproductive rate, which maintains *L. intracellularis* across generations. The source of infection has not been determined for horses. Exposure to pig feces has been suggested as a potential source of infection for horses since the first reported cases of EPE. However, in most cases of EPE, no history or evidence of direct or indirect exposure to pigs or pig feces has been reported. Further, multilocus VNTR profile of pig and equine isolates differ greatly.[22] A recent experimental study has

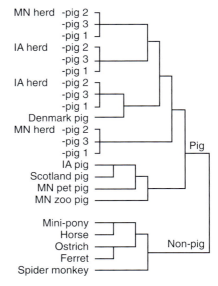

Figure 34-1 Dendrogram showing representative variable number tandem repeat (VNTR) sequence relationships between *Lawsonia intracellularis* isolates from various animal species and geographic sources. *MN,* Minnesota; *IA,* Iowa.

*The authors acknowledge and appreciate the original contributions of these authors, whose work has been incorporated into this chapter.

shown host specificity for *L. intracellularis* isolates cultured from pig or horse intestines.[27] The study showed that clinical signs, longer periods of shedding, and stronger serologic immune responses were observed in animals infected with species-specific isolates. Previous studies have shown that a variety of wild and domestic animals, including dogs, cats, rabbits, opossums, skunks, mice, and coyotes, can shed *L. intracellularis* on farms with diagnosed EPE cases.[28-29] On a recently identified farm in California endemic for EPE, 7.5% of fecal samples and 27% of serum samples from cottontail rabbits tested PCR positive and seropositive for *L. intracellularis*, respectively.[29] Of interest was that on this farm, a large population of cottontail rabbits lived in the hay barn and had direct access to the hay fed to the horses. An epidemiologic investigation on this farm showed rabbit feces on top of hay bales but also in the feeders of the weanling foals, suggesting that the foals developing EPE were likely exposed to *L. intracellularis* via the oral ingestion of infected rabbit feces. Similar to rodents, lagomorphs may represent an effective reservoir/amplifier host because of their large population, their close contact to horses, and their short reproductive cycle. It still remains to be determined how *L. intracellularis* became endemic in the rabbit population on this farm.

Feco-oral transmission of *L. intracellularis* has been documented in naïve foals housed with clinically infected foals experimentally challenged with an equine isolate of *L. intracellularis*.[30] A recent study demonstrated that feces from rabbits experimentally infected with an equine isolate of *L. intracellularis* served as infectious material to weanling foals.[31] Although infected rabbits and foals remained asymptomatic, infection was supported by fecal shedding of *L. intracellularis* and detection of specific antibodies to *L. intracellularis*. Although the natural infectious dose for foals has not been determined, pigs receiving as low as 10^5 *L. intracellularis* have been shown to develop infection.[32] Recent work suggested that 1 g of infectious feces would suffice to deliver this challenge dose.[25] Likely, the initial transmission of *L. intracellularis* occurs via the accidental ingestion of infectious feces from one of the described or as yet undetermined amplifiers/hosts. Amplification of *L. intracellularis* and environmental contamination leading to exposure rates of up to 100% of resident foals are likely to occur secondary to the shedding of large quantities of *L. intracellularis* from either clinically or subclinically infected foals.

In piglets, large group size, weaning, transportation, diet change, and mixing have been associated with clinical disease.[1] Predisposing factors, such as the stress of weaning, overcrowding, decline in *L. intracellularis*-specific colostral antibodies, endoparasitism, and introduction of new animals, have been suggested in the development of EPE in foals.[7] In pigs, infection and fecal shedding of *L. intracellularis* may persist for as long as 12 weeks.[33] In contrast, the horse may have a shorter duration of infectivity; experimentally infected foals showed an onset and duration of fecal shedding between 10 and 14 days and 17 and 27 days, respectively.[30,34] *Lawsonia intracellularis* can survive in environmental conditions for 1 to 2 weeks at 5°C to 15°C.[35]

Pathogenesis

The pathogenesis of EPE has remained poorly investigated, and most of the information available has been extrapolated from experimentally infected hamsters, pigs, and rabbits. Comprehensive studies of lesion development and evolution have been conducted in pigs[36] and hamsters.[37] Morphologic studies of early lesions in experimentally infected animals indicate that enterocyte hyperplasia is directly preceded by the presence of the intracellular organism.[36,37] In vivo, the onset of hyperplasia

associated with proliferative enteropathy follows an increase in numbers of intracellular *L. intracellularis* in enterocytes. Likewise, resolution of the lesions is closely related to disappearance of the intracellular organisms, indicating a correlation between the two events.[1] The means by which *L. intracellularis* produces hyperplasia is unknown. No other cytopathologic effects on infected enterocytes are seen in vivo or in vitro. Inflammation becomes evident in later-stage lesions and is not characteristic of the primary lesion.

Convalescent pigs have a degree of immunity to reinfection.[32] Animals challenged a second time, after cessation of fecal shedding, were evaluated clinically and their feces were tested by PCR to detect shedding. Animals previously infected did not shed detectable numbers of *L. intracellularis* and had no clinical signs. The cell-mediated immune response may be an important feature in protecting animals from reinfection with *L. intracellularis*. Descriptive immunocytologic studies of intestinal tissue sections of pigs affected by proliferative enteropathy reveal a mild infiltration of cytotoxic T cells, macrophages, and B lymphocytes carrying major histocompatibility complex (MHC) class II structure at the beginning of the cell-mediated immune response.[38]

Immunohistochemical studies of intestinal sections of naturally infected pigs also demonstrated a large accumulation of immunoglobulin A (IgA) in the apical cytoplasm of proliferating enterocytes.[38] Further, interferon gamma (IFN-γ) is produced by peripheral blood mononuclear cells (PBMCs) of both pigs and horses following specific stimulation,[33,39,40] and IgA is detected in intestinal lavages of challenged pigs.[32] Similarly, IFN-γ played a role in limiting intracellular infection and increased cellular proliferation in experimentally infected mice.[41]

Clinical Findings

There are characteristic signalment, seasonality, clinical signs, and blood work abnormalities associated with EPE. The disease is generally manifested in foals less than 1 year of age, and in North America, EPE is often seen between August and January.[16] Although the disease is commonly seen in weanling foals 4 to 7 months of age, cases of EPE have been seen in young adults (Pusterla, personal communication). Lethargy, anorexia, fever (>38.5°C [101.3°F]), peripheral edema (ventrum, sheath, throatlatch, and distal limbs; Figs. 34-2 and 34-3), weight loss

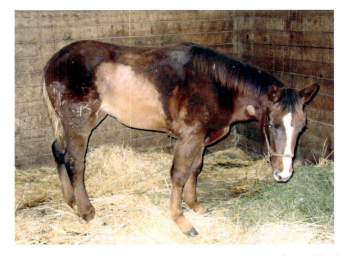

Figure 34-2 Ventral and distal limb edema in a 7-month-old Thoroughbred filly with equine proliferative enteropathy (EPE).

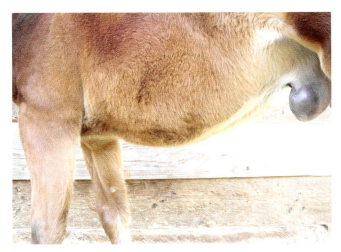

Figure 34-3 Ventral and sheath edema in an 8-month-old Quarter Horse colt with equine proliferative enteropathy (EPE).

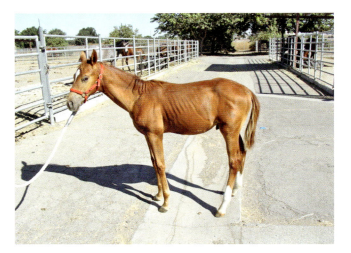

Figure 34-4 Severe weight loss in a 5-month-old Quarter Horse colt with equine proliferative enteropathy (EPE).

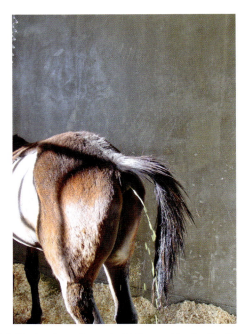

Figure 34-5 Diarrhea in an 8-month-old Thoroughbred colt with equine proliferative enteropathy (EPE).

(Fig. 34-4), colic, and diarrhea (Fig. 34-5) are among the most common clinical findings in affected foals. Early clinical signs are generally nonspecific and include mild depression, partial anorexia, and fever. Although diarrhea is commonly seen in affected foals and can vary from cow pie to watery, some affected foals may have normal fecal character. Foals with EPE may also have concurrent disorders such as respiratory tract infections, gastric ulcerations, and intestinal parasitism. Signs of EPE may resemble those of more common gastrointestinal disorders such as parasitism; bacterial infections (*Clostridium* spp., *Salmonella* spp., *Rhodococcus equi*, *Neorickettsia risticii*); rotavirus, coronavirus; ulcerations; sand accumulation; intestinal obstruction; and intoxication with plants, chemicals, and pharmacologic agents such as nonsteroidal antiinflammatory drugs (NSAIDs) or antimicrobials. Similar to pigs, the disease can be subclinical in foals. Subclinical disease is characterized by a self-limiting and transient decrease of total serum protein concentration coupled with decreased daily weight gain when compared to unaffected foals.[30,34] It will remain to be determined if growth retardation or unthriftiness are associated with subclinical infection.

The most consistent laboratory finding of clinical EPE is hypoproteinemia caused by hypoalbuminemia. Total protein is generally less than 5.0 g/dL, and albumin is usually less than 2.0 g/dL. In a recent case report,[16] hypoalbuminemia was the only consistent clinicopathologic abnormality of 57 affected foals, with albumin concentrations ranging from 0.9 to 3.3 g/dL (normal reference range 2.7 to 4.2 g/dL). The exact mechanisms by which hypoalbuminemia develops in affected foals has not been investigated. It appears that a combination of decreased feed intake, coupled with malabsorption and protein-losing enteropathy as a result of the proliferative nature of the disease may represent likely mechanisms by which low albumin occurs.[42] Affected foals may also demonstrate nonspecific blood abnormalities such as anemia or hemoconcentration, leukocytosis or neutropenia, hyperfibrinogenemia, increased activity of muscle enzymes, and electrolyte abnormalities (hypocalcemia, hypochloremia, and hyponatremia). Urine analysis to rule out protein-losing nephropathy and cytologic evaluation of abdominal fluid to rule out protein lost to a third space are generally unremarkable.

Diagnosis

A presumptive diagnosis of EPE is generally made based on the age of the affected animal, clinical signs, hypoproteinemia/hypoalbuminemia, presence of thickened small intestinal loops on ultrasonographic evaluation, and ruling out other causes of enteropathy and protein losses. Abdominal ultrasonography, although not very sensitive, may show segments of thickened small intestine (Fig. 34-6) and excessive abdominal fluid. In these cases, abdominocentesis will yield a noninflammatory transudate. An antemortem diagnosis is generally confirmed via PCR detection of *L. intracellularis* in feces or rectal swab and/or serology.

It is essential to combine both molecular and serologic diagnostic testing because these modalities have high analytical specificity but variable sensitivity, depending on the situation. Negative PCR results can be expected if the fecal samples are collected from foals with prior antimicrobial treatment or during advanced disease stage when *L. intracellularis* organisms are no longer expected in the feces. Negative serologic results can be expected in the early stage of the disease when humoral immune responses are not yet strong enough to be detectable by serology. Further, differences in sensitivity among different PCR and serologic assays can lead to divergent results. Among PCR assays, the use of real-time platform has been shown to yield the best sensitivity and to reduce the likelihood of cross- or carry-over contamination (i.e., false-positive results).[43-45] Several serologic assays, including indirect fluorescent antibody test (IFAT), enzyme-linked immunosorbent assay (ELISA), and immunoperoxidase monolayer assay (IPMA), have all been validated and established for pigs.[46-49] However, a preliminary comparative study using equine serum samples has shown that IPMA is the most accurate of all serologic tests to determine the presence of specific anti-*Lawsonia intracellularis* antibodies in foals with EPE (Gebhart, personal communication).

Based on clinical observations, it appears that the exposure rate to *L. intracellularis* is higher than the clinical attack rate; however, assuming that index cases are only the apex tip of the pyramid, it is always advisable to test herdmates to determine their exposure and clinical status. This is best achieved by collecting blood to determine the level of anti-*Lawsonia intracellularis* antibodies by serology and to measure total protein concentration by refractometry. Another more expensive alternative is to measure total protein and/or albumin concentrations by chemical analysis. Polymerase chain reaction testing of feces from healthy herdmates is not advised in this situation because of the expense of testing and low rate of positivity. Also, the results from previous epidemiologic studies show that healthy herdmates rarely shed detectable *L. intracellularis*.[50,51] Daily syndromic surveillance of all herdmates is also recommended in order to recognize early stages of disease. This is best achieved via daily physical examination, including rectal temperature and the regular assessment of weight, allowing the calculation of daily weight gain. A positive titer by IPMA ($\geq$60) in a healthy herdmate with no hypoproteinemia should be viewed as past exposure with no apparent disease or possibly early, not yet clinically apparent EPE. Seropositive or seronegative clinically healthy herdmates with hypoproteinemia (<5.0 g/dL) or hypoalbuminemia (<3.0 g/dL) should undergo further diagnostic testing (white blood cell count, abdominal ultrasound examination, fecal PCR) to determine if *L. intracel-*

lularis infection is the cause of the hypoproteinemia. Treating foals with suspected EPE based only on clinical findings and hypoproteinemia/hypoalbuminemia is not recommended because of the risk associated with the use of antimicrobials. Healthy seronegative herdmates with no hypoproteinemia should continue to be monitored daily for clinical signs and monthly or bimonthly for hypoproteinemia and/or hypoalbuminemia and detectable antibodies to *L. intracellularis*. Any foal developing clinical signs of EPE should undergo a thorough diagnostic workup. Further, clinically affected foals or foals with suspected clinical EPE should be separated from the rest of the healthy herdmates to decrease environmental contamination until their shedding status has been determined by PCR. It has been previously shown that experimentally infected foals start shedding *L. intracellularis* 5 to 17 days prior to developing hypoproteinemia and clinical signs.[30] It is this prodromal stage of subclinically infected foals that is likely responsible for the environmental contamination and exposure of susceptible foals.

Pathologic Findings

Lesions are most commonly seen in the ileum, near the ileal-cecal junction, and appear as a thickening of the mucosa. Gross lesions are not evident in all cases of EPE and may often be overlooked. Intestines show an irregular, patchy subserosal edema. The ileal mucosa is thickened with deep folds and chronically affected animals may have patches of pseudomembrane covering the mucosa (Fig. 34-7). Hypertrophy and thickening of the muscularis mucosa may occur in chronically affected or recovering animals (Fig. 34-8). Histologically,

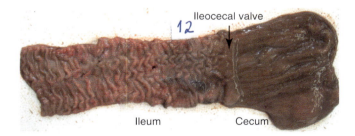

Figure 34-7 Gross lesions of equine proliferative enteropathy (EPE). Ileal-cecal junction of an affected 5-month-old foal showing thickened ileal mucosa with a corrugated appearance.

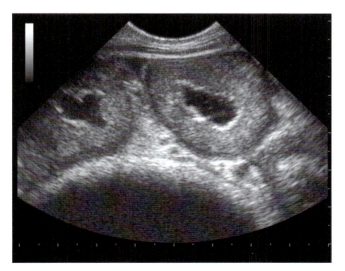

Figure 34-6 Ultrasound image showing thickened section of small intestinal wall in a 5-month-old Quarter Horse filly with equine proliferative enteropathy (EPE). The wall thickness measured 4.3 mm (normal wall thickness $\leq$3 mm).

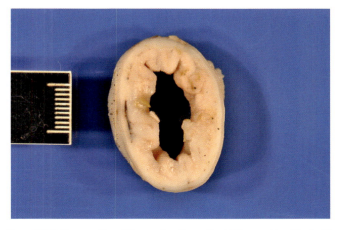

Figure 34-8 Cross-section of ileum of an 8-month-old Thoroughbred foal with equine proliferative enteropathy (EPE) showing diffusely thickened intestinal wall.

adenomatous proliferation occurs among the epithelial cells in the crypts of the small intestine, in association with the presence of curved, intracellular bacteria in the apical cytoplasm of these enterocytes.[2,3,7] Severe EPE is diagnosed by the demonstration of hyperplasia of the crypt glands with an increased number of mitotic figures and marked reduction or absence of goblet cells in routine hematoxylin and eosin preparations (Fig. 34-9); however, for visualization of the bacteria in the cytoplasm of enterocytes, special stains are necessary. The histologic lesions of PE are unique and inflammation is not normally a hallmark of disease. Warthin-Starry silver stain allows the detection of the bacteria in histologic sections, improving the diagnostic sensitivity, but the technique has limitations when applied to autolyzed and necrotic samples.[1] Immunohistochemistry procedures, using postmortem tissue or biopsy material with an antibody specific for *L. intracellularis*, have been used successfully to diagnose EPE (Fig. 34-10).

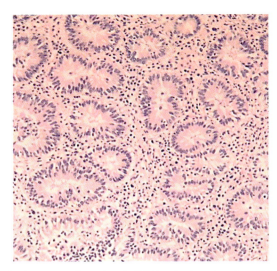

Figure 34-9 Hematoxylin and eosin (H&E)-stained section of small intestine from an 8-month-old foal with equine proliferative enteropathy (EPE) showing marked hyperplasia of crypt glands with lack of goblet cells.

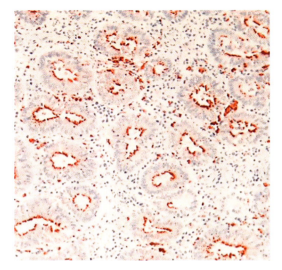

Figure 34-10 Immunohistochemical stained section of small intestine from an 8-month-old foal with equine proliferative enteropathy (EPE). *Lawsonia intracellularis*–specific antibody stains the bacteria lining the apical cytoplasm of the affected crypts *(red areas)*.

Therapy

It is important to treat affected animals early, before lesions become advanced and result in marked weight loss and critically low serum protein values. Treatment of EPE in horses involves the use of antimicrobials such as macrolides, alone or in combination with rifampin, chloramphenicol, oxytetracycline, or doxycycline administered for 2 to 3 weeks. The choice of antimicrobial in the treatment of EPE should take into account the risk of inducing disturbance of the gastrointestinal flora and renal toxicity. This is especially a concern when treating older foals with severe hypoalbuminemia. In addition, supportive care, such as intravenous (IV) fluids, plasma transfusion, parenteral nutrients, and antiulcer drugs are commonly used to treat affected foals. Concurrent medical conditions should also be addressed. Rapid clinical improvement following treatment is to be expected; however, it may take weeks for the hypoproteinemia to resolve. Spontaneous recovery of clinically affected foals has not been documented, and treated foals usually survive the disease. Long-term sequelae have not been reported; however, clinically affected and successfully treated foals sell for an average of 68% of the average price of unaffected foals by the same stallion.[16]

Prevention

The monitoring of a herd with endemic status follows guidelines similar to those for herds with diagnosed index cases. This includes the regular physical evaluation of resident foals and the monthly or bimonthly assessment of total protein concentration and monthly serologic status. Monitoring for exposure to *L. intracellularis* and hypoproteinemia/hypoalbuminemia should begin at least 4 weeks prior to the historic first detection of clinical cases. Monthly data, including concentration of total solids or albumin and weight gains, should be evaluated for each foal and compared to the previous month's data to determine decreasing trends potentially associated with early disease. Recent work performed in central Kentucky has shown a seasonality to EPE cases, with peak cases recorded in November and December.[16] Year-to-year variations, depending on climatic conditions, can be expected; however, most of the EPE cases are seen between August and January in the northern hemisphere, which relates to the age of the foals. Considering the cost of treating a foal with clinical EPE, this monitoring program is cost-effective, especially if concentration of total serum solids can be assessed by farm personnel. The lack of epidemiologic data regarding potential natural reservoir hosts, as well as the lack of information pertaining to the biology of *L. intracellularis*, precludes the institution of any management changes on endemic farms. Early recognition of clinical cases and separating them from the rest of the susceptible foals until full recovery or cessation of fecal shedding appear to be logical biosecurity measures to prevent spread and environmental contamination. Further, maintaining good pest control and preventing nonequine domestic and wild animals access to feed and feeding areas may potentially minimize the risk of disease spread.

Prevention strategies have been best described in pigs using in-feed antimicrobials and a commercially available *L. intracellularis* vaccine.[33,52-54] Recent work has shown that detectable humoral and cellular responses can be measured in foals administered an avirulent live *L. intracellularis* vaccine.[34,55-57] The recently established vaccine protocol has shown that the intrarectal administration of 30 mL of either the lyophilized or the frozen-thawed formulation of the avirulent *L. intracellularis* vaccine given twice, 30 days apart, yielded the strongest immunologic responses.[55] The *L. intracellularis* vaccine is safe, and the administration well tolerated by foals. Further, the avirulent *L. intracellularis* vaccine has not been associated with the induction of clinical disease in pigs or foals. Fecal shedding for up to 12 days has been documented following intrarectal vaccine administration in foals.[55] Using the previously mentioned protocols, vaccine efficacy has been evaluated in the field and, more recently, under experimental conditions. A field efficacy trial performed on EPE endemic farms in central Kentucky in 2008 showed that vaccinated foals maintained higher daily weight gains and higher total protein concentrations when compared to a nonvaccinated, naturally seroconverted group.[58] Because of the low incidence of disease reported on the study farms, no difference in attack rate between vaccinated and nonvaccinated foals could be determined. The overall decreased disease prevalence in the study population may have been associated with the ongoing vaccine trial on these farms because disease prevalence in central Kentucky did not change in 2009 compared to 2008. Potential explanation of the decreased number of clinical cases was the elimination of so called "super shedders" and possible exposure of nonvaccinated foals to *L. intracellularis* vaccine organism shed in the feces of recently

vaccinated foals. Under experimental conditions, weanling foals vaccinated intrarectally with an avirulent live vaccine against *L. intracellularis* were protected against clinical and subclinical EPE following challenge exposure with a virulent *L. intracellularis* isolate of equine origin.[34] This was determined by lack of clinical disease, absence of hypoproteinemia and sonographic abnormalities compatible with EPE, and a significant reduction in *L. intracellularis* fecal shedding in vaccinated foals compared to nonvaccinated foals. Further, average daily weight gains from the vaccinated foals over the entire study period were similar to the control foals and significantly higher when compared to the nonvaccinated foals, highlighting the benefit of the vaccine in the prevention of subclinical disease. The extralabel use of the *L. intracellularis* vaccine should be considered on naïve and endemic farms in an attempt to reduce or prevent EPE. Timing of vaccine administration should again be synchronized with historic disease occurrence. Further, routine monitoring for clinical signs and hypoproteinemia/hypoalbuminemia is still recommended, even when vaccine prophylaxis is used.

The complete reference list is available online at www.expertconsult.com.

The complete reference list is available online at www. expertconsult.com.

CHAPTER

35 Salmonellosis

Jorge A. Hernandez, Maureen T. Long, Josie L. Traub-Dargatz,* and Thomas E. Besser*

Etiology

Salmonellosis is disease caused by an enteric or systemic infection with a bacterium of the genus *Salmonella*. Salmonellae are gram-negative, facultative, rod-shaped bacteria that belong to the family Enterobacteriaceae. The *Salmonella* genus contains two species, *Salmonella enterica* and *Salmonella bongori* of which *S. enterica* is the type species. *S. enterica* has six subspecies designated I (subsp. *enterica*), II (subsp. *salamae*), IIIa (subsp. *arizonae*), IIIb (subsp. *diarizonae*), IV (subsp. *houtenae*), and VI (subsp. *indica*) with more than 2400 serovars.[1-5]

All species and subspecies are considered pathogens, but the virulence of many is undefined. The vast majority of clinical cases are associated with a single subspecies, *S. enterica* I (commonly designated *S. enterica* subsp. *enterica*) with approximately 1450 serovars that account for about 99.5% of mammalian infections.[4] Basic multilocus enzymatic electrophoretic studies confirmed greater than 85% sharing of genetic information based on serovar associations.[3,6-11] Molecular epidemiologic studies and high-throughput genomic technologies (*Salmonella* genus project: http://www.sanger.ac.uk/Projects/Salmonella/) are redefining the classification and evolutionary relatedness of these microbes that have been previously grouped based only on antigenic relationships.

Current nomenclature for the *Salmonella* species requires that the species designation *(Salmonella)* be followed by the subspecies designated as a roman numeral.[1] The serotype follows and is capitalized (not italicized). The Centers for Disease Control and Prevention (CDC) and World Health Organization (WHO) require that a serotype designation be preceded by "ser" or "serotype" the first time it is designated within a report. Afterward, the name may be shortened and written as the genus name followed directly by the serotype name (e.g., *Salmonella* Anatum or *Salmonella* Dublin). Historically, the serotype name derived from the geographic area in which the serotype was first identified, but more modern serotypes are designated by an antigenic formula that includes designation of the subspecies, the somatic (O) antigen, and the flagellar (H) antigen. To make it more confusing, serotypes of the I and II subspecies are still designated in the literature by the location of first isolation. Because most of the mammalian and thus horse isolates are *S. enterica* I, the *genus* (ser.) location nomenclature will be used in this text.

In horses, the most frequently occurring serovars isolated from clinical cases vary somewhat from year to year, but the top four or five serovars are consistently among the most frequently identified serovars in equine salmonellosis cases in the United States.[12-18] The relative ranking of these common serovars undergoes periodic shifts as epidemic or epizootic strains emerge and disappear. Because only 700 to 1000 isolates are officially serotyped each year, the reporting may vary from year to year because testing related to small outbreaks may bias the data. From 2000 through 2004, *S.* Newport increased in

*The authors acknowledge and appreciate the original contributions of these authors, whose work has been incorporated into this chapter.

relative frequency, with the emergence of the North American cmy-2 cephalosporinase-producing strains becoming second to the common food-borne pathogen *S*. Typhimurium (Table 35-1). *S*. Newport has remained a common isolate through the decade as of 2009.[19-22] *Salmonella* Agona, Anatum, and Javiana have been either third or fourth most common over the last 10 years. In the last 5 years, a serovar with the new designation I 4,[5],12:i:- has increased to frequency similar to *Salmonella* Agona and Braenderup; the latter was responsible for outbreaks in wildlife and domestic animals worldwide.

Some *S. enterica* subtypes and serovars produce distinct clinical syndromes that result in their classification as "host-adapted"

or "non–host-adapted."[23] In general, host-adapted serovars produce systemic infections characterized by bacteremia, fever, and systemic signs. In host-adapted salmonellosis, diarrhea is not observed or, if present, is a relatively minor component.[23] The equine host-adapted serovar, *S*. Abortusequi, causes a disease with bacteremia and infectious abortion as its principal manifestations. In contrast, non–host-adapted serovars typically produce localized infections of the intestine and colon with enterocolitis and diarrhea as the predominant components.[23]

Epidemiology

Nonhospitalized Horses

Source of Infection

The source of infection in individual horses and in outbreaks of salmonellosis in groups of horses is often not definitively identified. Unless surveillance for infection is ongoing, the source of infection may be difficult to determine retrospectively. The primary route of exposure is likely oral intake of the organism, and the multiple potential sources of infection for equids (Fig. 35-1) include consumption of contaminated water or feed and oral contact with the feces of infected animals, contaminated environmental surfaces, or animal care worker's contaminated hands or equipment. Aerosol exposure to the agent has been proposed in other animal species.[24,25] Although evidence

Table 35-1 Frequently Occurring Equine Salmonellosis Serotypes

	1999-2004			2005-2009	
Serovar	Number	% of Total	Serovar	Number	% of Total
Typhimurium	1435	29%	Typhimurium	846	25%
Newport	729	15%	Newport	373	11%
Agona	679	14%	Javiana	312	9%
Anatum	290	6%	Anatum	217	6%
All others	1918	38%	All others	1652	49%
Total	4982		Total	3400	

Data derived from U.S. Animal Health Association *Salmonella* Committee, National Veterinary Service Laboratories, 1998 to 2004; and CDC Surveillance 2005 to 2009.

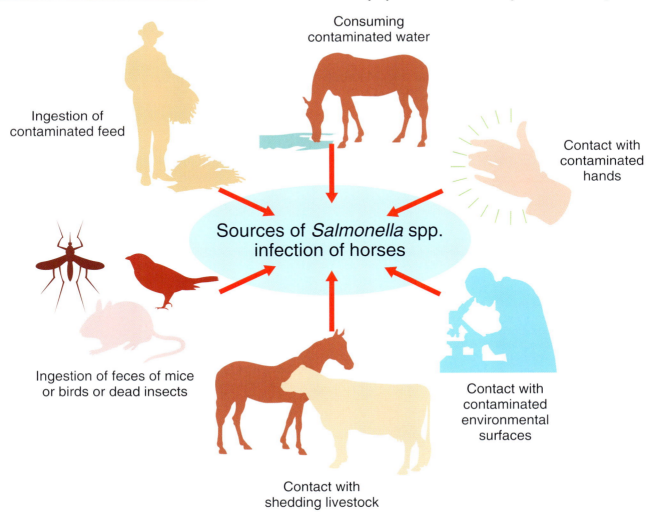

Figure 35-1 Examples of the multiple potential sources of *Salmonella* exposure to equids.

of this route of exposure in horses is lacking, it theoretically could occur.

Clinically normal horses shedding *S. enterica* in their feces potentially pose a risk to animals with which they have direct contact and can contaminate the environment, which serves as a source of the organism for susceptible animals.[26] A larger percentage of horses appears to shed the organism in summer than in winter months.[27-30] Other livestock could also be a source of transmission to horses. Through surveillance of all large animal hospital patients, cattle (specifically dairy cattle) have been found to shed *S. enterica* more than equids or other large animal patients.[31]

Salmonellae can persist in the environment in fecal matter for months to years depending on the serotype, moisture content, and temperature conditions.[32,33] In one study, *S.* Dublin persisted in dried bovine feces for up to 5 years.[34] In another study, *S.* Cholerasuis was more persistent when feces were in the dried (13 months) versus wet form (3 months).[32]

Feed is a potential source of *S. enterica* for horses. Most commercial equine feeds are manufactured using good manufacturing procedures (GMP), but none are certified to be *Salmonella* free. Pelleting likely decreases the number of salmonellae in contaminated feed, depending on the temperature used in the processing procedure.[35] However, livestock feed can be contaminated with *S. enterica* as established by a survey by the Food and Drug Administration (FDA) of processors of either animal or vegetable protein products used in animals.[36] *Salmonella* spp. were detected in 56.4% of animal protein and 36% of vegetable protein products sampled (4350 total). In another FDA report, 34% of animal protein–derived feed samples were positive for *Salmonella* in 2002 and represented 27 serotypes.[37] *S.* Anatum persisted for 429 days in ground feed and 299 days in meat and bone meal, *S.* Infantis was present at 723 days in feed and at 588 days in meal, and *S.* Enteritidis survived approximately the same amount of time in feed and meal (728 days in feed and 750 days in meal).[38] It was speculated that these non–host-adapted strains survived longer than host-adapted types evaluated, such as *S.* Typhisuis and *S.* Cholerasuis.[38] The National Animal Health Monitoring System (NAHMS) survey estimated that 0.4% of grain or concentrate that was the primary feed source for horses was positive for *S. enterica*, but the serotypes detected were not those typically associated with clinical disease in horses.[29] Contaminated feed has been identified definitively as a source of infection in an outbreak of salmonellosis due to *S.* Ohio among neonatal foals in California.[39] One other report identified maize silage as containing *S.* Typhimurium that resulted in fatal diarrhea and colic in horses to which it was fed.[40]

Equine feed sources, such as hay, grain, and other concentrate sources, could become contaminated after arrival at the equine premises from the feces of rodents and birds or bodies of insects. Rodents have been proposed as a reservoir for *Salmonella* spp.[35,41] and carried the same strain as affected horses in one equine salmonellosis outbreak.[42] Insects, such as flies, can become contaminated with *Salmonella* spp.[35,43] Pastures could become contaminated with *Salmonella* spp. from infected animals and wildlife, organic fertilizers, bone meal, contaminated runoff, and contaminated water supply. Soils have been reported to remain positive for *Salmonella* spp. for a variable period from 120 to 280 days.[43]

The role that contaminated water sources play in equine salmonellosis is unknown, but *Salmonella* survives in pond water for 115 days.[43] In a national study of equine health and management, 10% to 33% of equine operations used surface water as the primary water source for equids.[29] This likely varies with the serotype of *Salmonella* and environmental temperature, as well as other characteristics of the water (e.g., pH, salinity). Freezing reduces the total number of organisms, but survivors may remain viable and infective for months.[43]

Prevalence

The wide range in the reported prevalence of salmonellosis in equids depends on the study design from which these data are drawn. Salmonellosis is defined as infection with the organism and the occurrence of detectable signs of disease secondary to infection, although some reports of equine salmonellosis include animals shedding the organism without signs of disease.[27,44,45] This is likely in part a result of the transition from early investigations focusing only on animals with clinical disease to the current interest in surveillance of the general population or overall hospital population for shedding of the organism. All of these factors need to be considered when describing *Salmonella* infection or shedding by equids.

For the purposes of this discussion, three types of *Salmonella*-infected horses may exist: asymptomatic horses with or without fecal shedding; horses shedding organisms with concurrent diarrhea; and horses with other gastrointestinal (GI) clinical signs (nondiarrheic) and shedding organism.[27,46,47] In describing prevalence, the first distinction to make is whether the prevalence being reported is for a population of ill equids, the entire equine hospital population, or the general equine population on their home premises. If one assumes that salmonellosis equates to some clinical disease associated with the infection, it is thus distinct from the prevalence of equids shedding the organism in their feces. Therefore the horses with clinical disease or salmonellosis would be a subset of the total number of horses that shed the organism in their feces. It stands to reason that the prevalence of clinical salmonellosis in the general equine population is unknown because in many cases only the number of cases is reported without provision of the number of animals at risk in the whole population. Essentially, the only study that examined true prevalence of fecal shedding in the equine population whether normal or associated with disease was a national study of the general horse population sampled while on their home premises and based on a single sample per animal; this result was 0.8%.[48] The prevalence of fecal shedding by horses in this study was higher in the summer months (1.1%) than in the winter months (0.2%) and in the southern region (1.4%) than in the northern region (0.2%) of the United States.[48] A total of 16 different serotypes were identified, with the most common serotype being Muenchen, followed by Newport, Schwartzengrund, and Typhimurium.

Risk Factors

Infection with *S. enterica* and the subsequent development of clinical disease depends on multiple factors in horses (Fig. 35-2). Age may be a risk factor for development of clinical illness, with foals more likely to develop disease than adults.[30,49,50] Stress may be a predisposing factor for initiating equine salmonellosis, and horses may be carriers of *Salmonella* spp. and may not shed the organism in their feces until stressed. Stress is difficult to define, and what may predispose one animal to disease if infected may not predispose the next. Various factors have been associated with increased prevalence of salmonellosis or shedding of the organism in feces by equine populations including transportation or shipping,[51-55] surgery,[52,56] feed withdrawal,[52] change in feed,[29] antimicrobial treatment,[51,57-59] deworming,[60] colic,[61] and diarrhea.[53] Some of these factors may be an outcome of the infection rather than predisposing factors such as the association with diarrhea.

Possession of normal intestinal flora and motility likely make horses more resistant to colonization with *Salmonella* spp.[62] Challenge studies that vary the doses of *Salmonella* organisms ingested by horses subjected to feed change or restriction or to different antimicrobial regimens that may alter GI flora have

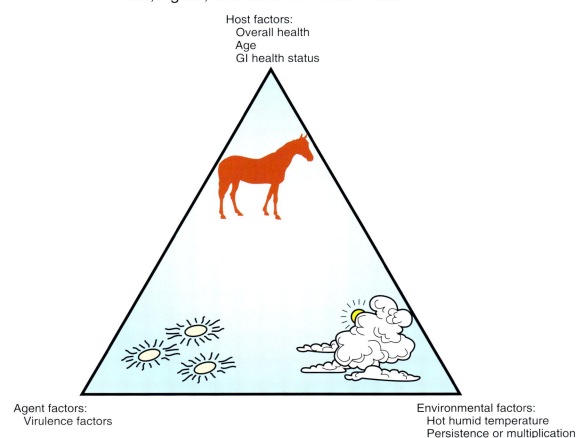

Figure 35-2 Triad of disease factors resulting in *Salmonella* infection. Disease results when multiple risk factors come together, including those associated with the *host* (e.g., age, antimicrobial treatment), the *agent* (e.g., virulence, infective dose), and the *environment*.

not been reported. Fasting and diet change could alter the normal bacterial flora. Both stress and antimicrobial treatment may alter the normal flora in horses and thus predispose to colonization and eventually to disease associated with *Salmonella* infection.[63] The barrier effect of the indigenous intestinal flora that prevents establishment and multiplication of potentially pathogenic bacteria is called *colonization resistance*.[64] Although little is known about the complexity of interactions among indigenous microflora of the intestine in the horse, disturbances of the normal flora may predispose to colonization and multiplication of pathogenic bacteria.[65] A syndrome of antibiotic-associated diarrhea is often associated with proliferation of different enteric pathogens, such as *Salmonella* spp., *Clostridium difficile,* and *Clostridium perfringens.*[66]

In one of the few experimental studies of the impact of various stressors on experimentally infected equids, Owen et al[52] reported that transportation of experimentally infected ponies resulted in reactivation of the *Salmonella* infection. Details regarding the duration and method of transportation are lacking in this report, and during transport the ponies also had feed deprivation as an additional stressor. The authors noted that treatment with oxytetracycline resulted in prolonged fecal shedding of *Salmonella* spp. in treated ponies. However, in human infection, prolonged fecal shedding has been observed with many antibiotics.

Hospitalized Horses

Source of Infection

Environmental contamination can be an important source of nosocomial *Salmonella* infections (or spread of infections) in hospitalized horses.[30,42,50,67-71] In one study, persistence of S. Typhimurium in the environment was identified as the source of nosocomial infection for several horses.[68] In that study, S. Typhimurium was isolated from hospital personnel, shared equipment, and stalls. A hospitalized foal was identified as the point-source of infection. In another study, environmental contamination was suggested to be the source of infection for other horses during an outbreak of salmonellosis due to S. Typhimurium in a university hospital.[70] The point source of environmental contamination was a horse that presented with colic. S. Typhimurium was isolated from stall drains, surgery pads, forklift tires, and the ambulatory garage floor. In a different study, environmental contamination contributed to the widespread nature of infection during an outbreak of S. Infantis in horses and food animals.[42] S. Infantis was isolated from hospital workers' hands, rectal thermometers, mice trapped in the hospital facility, and mats in stalls and recovery rooms; the original source of S. Infantis was not determined.

Hospital environments can serve as reservoirs, leading to the persistence of *Salmonella* in hospitals over protracted periods.

In a study that followed an outbreak of salmonellosis due to *S.* Infantis, isolates obtained from patients or the hospital environment over a period of 9 years were compared.[31] Results of the genetic analysis in combination with clear epidemiologic links indicated that environmental contamination arising from the outbreak persisted across years despite rigorous hygiene and biosecurity precautions and may have led to subsequent nosocomial infections. In another study in Australia, 28 isolates of multidrug-resistant (MDR) *S.* Heidelberg obtained from horses over a period of 6 years were compared[69] and indicated that the MDR isolates from the veterinary hospital originated from a common source.

Several studies have reported different levels of environmental contamination in hospitals that had been forced to close because of outbreaks of nosocomial *Salmonella* infections in horses. In the study of nosocomial *S.* Infantis, a total of 148 environmental samples were collected for bacterial culture after disinfection during the first 7 weeks of the outbreak; this outbreak strain was isolated from six samples (4%).[42] In another study involving hospital closure and disinfection, the outbreak strain, an MDR *S.* Typhimurium was isolated from 3 of 241 environmental samples[68]; in contrast, 28 of 237 samples (12%) tested positive by polymerase chain reaction (PCR). In another study involving a third veterinary school hospital in the United States, during the hospital's closure (10 weeks), 1110 environmental samples were collected and tested, and 12 samples (1%) tested positive for *Salmonella* by culture; 8 of 12 samples were collected from stall drains and the remaining samples were collected from surgery pads, a stall wall, forklift tires, and the ambulatory garage floor.[70] In another study,[161] environmental samples were collected 2 weeks, 1 month, and 2 months before the hospital was closed (because of an outbreak of nosocomial *S.* Newport infections in horses) and 36/120 or 30%, 8/25 or 32%, and 15/171 or 9% samples tested positive for *Salmonella*, respectively. The results in that study show evidence of extensive and repeated environmental contamination in the hospital caused most likely by ineffective cleaning and disinfection procedures.

Routine environmental sampling procedures for detection of *Salmonella* contamination in hospital facilities is important to establish a baseline and a threshold level that justifies enhanced surveillance and infection control measures. In one study,[71] an active surveillance program that included periodic sampling and testing of horses and the hospital environment on admission and during hospitalization allowed early detection of nosocomial *Salmonella* transmission and hospital contamination. During the summer months in 2006, 8 of 145 or 6% of large animals were classified as infected with an outbreak strain of *S.* Newport. In addition, the outbreak strain was recovered from 42 of 295 or 14% of environmental samples, which was an indication that widespread environmental contamination had occurred. Clear differences in the frequency of *S.* Newport recovery before and during the epidemic period triggered enhanced surveillance and infection control measures to mitigate the risk of disease transmission in hospitalized horses and hospital contamination. This is a recent example of a successful surveillance program that allowed early detection and mitigation of new cases of nosocomial *Salmonella* infections in hospitalized horses without resorting to hospital closure.

Prevalence

One of the first studies of the prevalence of fecal shedding among the general hospitalized equine population was conducted as a surveillance program at a university teaching hospital in the late 1970s. A total of 1451 horses were sampled, with a reported 3.2% prevalence of fecal shedding of *Salmonella*.[72] The serotypes identified included Typhimurium,

Typhimurium var. Copenhagen, Infantis, Montevideo, Meleagridis, and Drypool, as well as untypable isolates. Seasonal variability was marked in detection of fecal shedding, with the highest incidence in the late summer and early fall and the lowest in the spring. Of the 46 horses shedding *Salmonella* in this study, 18 had diarrhea and 7 deaths were attributed to salmonellosis. Since this early report, many more reports on the prevalence of shedding *Salmonella* by hospitalized equids have been published. In a study of the general equine hospitalized population (anticipated hospital stay ≥3 days, 246 horses), the prevalence of fecal shedding was 7%, with serotypes identified including Oranienburg, Newport, and Arizona, in descending order of frequency, followed by Newington, Drypool, Anatum, Thompson, and Meleagridis, each represented by single isolates.[29,55] Only 3 of the 18 culture-positive horses in this study were admitted for diarrhea.

The prevalence of *Salmonella* infection as a cause of disease among hospitalized horses with diarrhea has been evaluated in a Dutch study.[73] During 1990 and 1991, 380 fecal samples were collected from horses that were referred for treatment of diarrhea. Most horses had a single fecal sample collected from the rectum, or if they died soon after arrival, samples were collected at necropsy. Of these samples, 18% (69/380) were positive for *Salmonella* spp. with the most common serotype being *S.* Typhimurium (43/69).

Some reports on the prevalence of fecal shedding of *Salmonella* spp. were based on a subset of the hospital population, for example, patients admitted for colic or needing intensive care. The prevalence of fecal shedding among colic patients (246 horses, with an average of three samples per horse) at a veterinary teaching hospital was 9%.[53,56] The serotypes were Typhimurium, Infantis, Muenchen, and Anatum, in descending order of frequency, followed by a similar number with Oranienburg, Montevideo, and Thompson, all with the same frequency. In a second study of colic patients (based on culture of feces or rectal swab samples) the prevalence was 13% (100 horses, with an attempt to collect five samples per horse, unless it died before day 5), and the most common serotype identified was Senftenberg, followed by Typhimurium, then London and Agona.[57] Senftenberg was the most frequently isolated serotype from horses "without colic" in this report. In a survey of equids admitted to a veterinary teaching hospital intensive care unit over a 4-year period (1583 horses, with daily collection of fecal samples for culture), the overall prevalence of shedding was 5.5%, and the most common serotypes identified were Typhimurium and Krefeld; other types identified included Anatum, Agona, Enteritidis, Heidelberg, Muenster, Newington, Oranienburg, Poona, and Tennessee.[74]

Risk Factors

Risk factors associated with nosocomial *Salmonella* infections in hospitalized hoses ware investigated in an attempt to identify exposure factors that may influence health policy to prevent disease transmission. During an outbreak investigation of *S.* Saintpaul in hospitalized horses, the odds of nosocomial *Salmonella* infection were higher in horses with a presenting complaint of colic, in horses receiving parental antibiotics, and in horses intubated with nasogastric tubes.[75] In that study, because bacteriologic culturing of nasogastric tubes had not been performed, it was not possible to determine whether the association between *Salmonella* isolation and nasogastric intubation meant that *Salmonella* was transmitted by the tube itself or by associated materials and procedures. In another study, the odds of nosocomial *Salmonella* infection were higher in hospitalized horses with large colon impactions, longer duration of treatment with potassium penicillin, and mean ambient temperature ≥80° F.[19]

Several studies have indicated that abdominal surgery may be a predisposing factor for nosocomial *Salmonella* infections in hospitalized horses, but more research is needed to establish abdominal surgery as a risk factor. In one study, abdominal surgery was suspected to increase the risk of nosocomial *Salmonella* infection in hospitalized horses.[19] However, the odds of nosocomial infection associated with surgery were not different between case and control horses. In another study, 18 of 33 equine inpatients infected with a nosocomial strain of S. Typhimurium had surgery.[70] In that study, however, the frequency and type of surgery in noninfected horses was not reported. Finally, a more recent study identified abdominal surgery as a predisposing factor associated with nosocomial *Salmonella* infections in hospitalized horses. In that study, the odds of nosocomial *Salmonella* infection were 8 times higher in horses that underwent abdominal surgery compared to horses that did not undergo abdominal surgery.[50] In many hospitals, horses that undergo abdominal surgery are treated with antimicrobials, which may cause disturbances in the ecologic balance between the host and its normal microflora. Antimicrobial drugs eliminate intestinal flora that are antagonistic to *Salmonella* organisms, which is an environment that can make equine inpatients that undergo abdominal surgery more susceptible to nosocomial *Salmonella* infections. Ekiri et al hypothesized that surgical stress may cause severe alterations of host-defense mechanisms in horses that undergo abdominal surgery.[50]

High caseload in hospitals has been suspected to be a risk factor for nosocomial *Salmonella* outbreaks; however, published studies have failed to establish high caseload as a risk factor. One hypothesis is that cleaning procedures may not be as stringent as in periods of low caseload, and the staff itself may play a role in disease transmission.[75] During the outbreak investigation of nosocomial S. Saintpaul infections in hospitalized horses, limitations in data collection affected the ability to adequately examine caseload as a predisposing factor for nosocomial *Salmonella* infections. In another study, high caseload was not identified as a risk factor for nosocomial *Salmonella* infections in hospitalized horses.[50] In that study, the number of horses shedding *Salmonella* during hospitalization was not different between time periods of low and high caseload. Thus it is logical to propose that for high caseload to be a predisposing factor for nosocomial *Salmonella* outbreaks two factors must be present: (1) a high frequency of horses shedding *Salmonella* and (2) low quality standards of cleaning and disinfection.

Carrier Horses

The prevalence of carrier horses that are not shedding *Salmonella* in their feces as detectable by culture is difficult to determine. There are few studies of long-term, repeated fecal culture and sampling of mesenteric lymph nodes and other sites where *Salmonella* spp. may reside. In one study in England of 85 equids undergoing necropsy for various causes other than salmonellosis, 20% had *Salmonella* spp. isolated from one or more sites, with the mucosa of the cecum and large colon being the most common sites harboring the organism. No details on culture or sampling method were included in this report.[76] A culture survey at one equine slaughter plant showed a 70% prevalence of carrier horses.[77] In a second slaughter plant study, the prevalence of isolation was 27%.[78] In a study of 102 horses that underwent necropsy between April and December 1994 at a veterinary teaching hospital, only two foals had *Salmonella* spp., which was recovered from the mesenteric lymph nodes.[79] These authors concluded that the results of cross-sectional studies using culture to identify *Salmonella* infection should be interpreted with caution because the results of prevalence from a single facility may not reflect the prevalence of infection in the general population. In one of the slaughter plant surveys, the authors speculated that the horses were becoming infected while at the slaughter plant because the serotype of *Salmonella* identified was similar to that obtained from birds

sampled from corrals where the horses were housed before slaughter.[80]

Pathogenesis

Salmonella bacteria are transmitted by the fecal-oral route. In experimental studies, most animals require oral administration of very high numbers ($\geq 10^8$) of *Salmonella* organisms to cause disease, although work with horses indicate that smaller inoculums may result in asymptomatic disease with prolonged shedding.[81] Before establishing colonization of the ileum and colon, ingested *Salmonella* must survive a series of host-derived obstacles, such as salivary bactericidal enzymes, stomach acid, intestinal proteases, lysozymes, antimicrobial peptides and bile salts, complement, and phagocytes, as well as interference by the gut microbiome, including nutrient competition and bacteriocins.[23] Anything that interferes with the activity of these nonspecific responses is likely to decrease greatly the infectious dose of *Salmonella* required to cause disease, a process termed *facilitation*. For example, oral antacid preparations or administration of drugs that decrease gastric acid secretion increases the risk of salmonellosis, presumably from increased passage of viable bacterial cells into the intestinal tract.[52,82] Similarly, antimicrobial treatment that disrupts the normal microbiome increases the risk of salmonellosis, along with several other causes of infectious enteritis.[52] Many of the stress factors that predispose to salmonellosis, including transportation, sudden feed changes, spoiled feedstuffs, and other illnesses, probably act at least in part by affecting the innate resistance of the horse through the mechanisms previously described, for example, by disrupting the natural GI bacterial flora, reducing GI motility, or reducing the stomach acid or other natural barriers to colonization.

Most of the factors that determine success for *Salmonella* have been derived from S. Typhimurium and distinctive virulence factors for mediating disease include the type III secretion system (T3SS 1 and 2), fibrae, flagellin, and bacterial deoxyribonucleic acid (DNA). As a facultative cellular bacteria, *Salmonella* attaches and invades many cells, from intestinal epithelium to phagocytes of the immune system. Fimbriae are now recognized as pattern-recognition receptors that activate signalling pathways in macrophages by binding either on the cell surface or within the phagosome.[83-85]

The two secretion systems of *Salmonella* and fimbriae consisting of 13 loci are required for biofilm formation, attachment, and colonization of the gut without invasion. The fimbriae and flagellin can induce uptake of *Salmonella* independent of the T3SS system. In the gut, *Salmonella* invades enterocytes, M cells, and dendritic cells. Invasion frequently goes beyond the gut even with the nontyphoidal subspecies, resulting in the invasion of lymph nodes and spleen[86] (Fig. 35-3). *Salmonella* spp. invasion of the intestinal epithelium involves a rearrangement of the epithelial cell cytoskeleton in an exquisitely regulated event of T3SS effector proteins of which there are 7 to 9 proteins (Sip A, SipC, SopB/SigD, SodC-1, SopE2, and SptP).[87] Additional proteins are injected into the cytosol that disrupt immune signalling such as mitogen-activated protein (MAP) kinases and nuclear factor-kappa B (NF-κB) ligases limiting tissue macrophage cytotoxicity.

The pathologic events of salmonellosis result in neutrophil recruitment, intestinal inflammation, and increased fluid secretion into the intestinal lumen.[88] During attachment and invasion, *Salmonella* T3SS effectors induce a massive recruitment of neutrophils through effectors such as eicosanoid hepoxilin A3. An important mediator of this process is the cytokine interleukin-8 (IL-8; now also termed *CXCL8*), secreted by epithelial cells in response to *Salmonella* infection. The specific

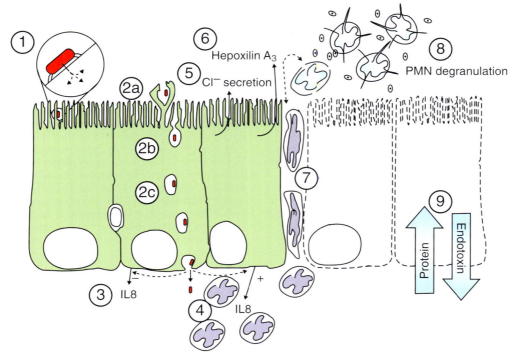

Figure 35-3 Schematic of events in pathogenesis of *Salmonella* enterocolitis. *1, Salmonella* bacteria penetrate the intestinal mucous layer and bind to epithelial cells with one or more fimbrial adhesions. The type 3 secretion system, *Salmonella* pathogenicity island 1 (SPI1), is activated, and effectors are injected into the epithelial cells. *2, Salmonella* SPI1 effectors trigger actin rearrangements, resulting in bacteria-mediated endocytosis *(2a)*, internalization *(2b)*, and eventually transcytosis *(2c)* of *Salmonella* bacteria. *3, Salmonella* SPI1 effectors trigger transcytosis of bacterial flagellin, which interacts with toll-like receptor 5 *(TLR5)* at the basolateral cell surfaces, triggering a cascade of cellular signals and resulting in release of interleukin-8 *(IL-8)* and other chemotactic molecules. *4,* IL-8 and other chemotaxins attract large numbers of polymorphonuclear *(PMN)* leukocytes to the epithelial basolateral cell surface. *5, Salmonella* SPI1 effectors trigger increased chloride *(Cl⁻)* secretion from the epithelial cells, probably mediated through increased inositol polyphosphate concentrations within the epithelial cells. *6, Salmonella* SPI1 effectors trigger release of hepoxilin A₃ at the apical surface. *7,* Hepoxilin A₃ acts as a chemoattractant, drawing PMNs through the intercellular spaces and through the tight junctions to reach the intestinal lumen. *8,* PMN degranulation is triggered at the epithelial cell apical surfaces, releasing inflammatory mediators and causing necrosis of the epithelial cells. *9,* Loss of the epithelial barrier functions results in increased leakage of protein-rich fluid into the intestinal lumen and increased absorption of bacterial endotoxin.

trigger for IL-8 secretion is thought to result from an interaction of *Salmonella* flagellin with the toll-like receptor (TLR) 5 at the epithelial basolateral cell surface.[89] The proinflammatory effects of flagellin are also caused by its interaction with the T3SS-SPI1 effector SopE2.[90]

Release of inflammatory mediators by large numbers of activated neutrophils has long been considered central to the inflammation associated with salmonellosis.[53,89,91] This inflammation results in massive epithelial damage, including sloughing of large areas of the epithelium with subsequent pseudomembrane formation. Inflammation and epithelial necrosis result in loss of serum protein into the lumen, with resultant hypoproteinemia typical of severe salmonellosis. Damage to the intestinal epithelium and the presence of invading salmonellae in the submucosa also result in release of endotoxin into the circulation, with septic and endotoxin circulatory shock. (see Chapter 11). In addition to their roles in epithelial invasion and neutrophil chemotaxis, T3SS effectors such as SopB in the cytosol lead to protein kinase B (AkT) activation, which triggers increased fluid secretion at the site of infection. Downstream of AkT activation, inositol phosphates are increased, which mediate increased chloride ion secretion followed by movement of water into the intestinal lumen.[92,93]

The bacterium provoke the host immune response nonspecifically through the many pathogen- and danger-associated molecular pathogen patterns that include lipopolysaccharide (LPS), flagella, and bacterial DNA, both extracellularly and intracellularly through TLR4, TLR5, and TLR9. These in turn produce Pro-IL-1B and Pro-IL-18, apoptotic proteins, and many inflammatory mediators.

The hallmarks of host-adapted *Salmonella* serovar pathogenesis, including that of *Salmonella* Abortusequi, are invasion, bacteremia, and disseminated disease, primarily without enteritis. On reaching the submucosa, these strains are internalized in macrophages and disseminate through lymphatic and blood circulations, resulting in bacteremia and colonization of the target organs (e.g., placenta, testicle) typical of this agent.

Clinical Findings

Horses infected with *S. enterica* may show a range of clinical signs, from inapparent shedding of the organism to peracute death.[45-47,94] Based on the classic papers by Smith et al[44] in 1979, Owen et al[46] in 1979, and Roberts and O'Boyle[47] in 1982, four syndromes were consistently reproduced experimentally using *S.* Typhimurium in the first two studies and *S.* Anatum in the third. The clinical syndromes were remarkably consistent, including: (1) asymptomatic disease, (2) mild febrile disease without significant change in fecal consistency, (3) toxic enterocolitis, and (4) sepsis. Within these syndromes, variation in GI signs, including severe ileus and gastric reflux, large colon impaction, small colon impaction, and small intestinal obstruction were observed. *S. enterica* is not usually cultured from horses with chronic diarrhea, although persistent, watery feces is a sequelae of severe enterocolitis in *Salmonella* spp.–positive horses that experience long-term hypoproteinemia. Other syndromes in adult horses can include abortion and infectious cholangiohepatitis.

Inapparent *Salmonella* infections are most likely to be experimentally induced with a lower dose infectious inoculum. In challenge experiments, asymptomatic horses shed *Salmonella* for 7 to 31 days.

In a cross-sectional study of horses on 972 premises in 28 states, the overall prevalence of *Salmonella* spp. detected by culture in feces was 0.8% of resident horses and varied from 1% to 17% of horses associated with equine hospital environments. In APHIS/CDC data, submissions are scant compared to species tested for food-borne surveillance.[12-15] The Salmonella serovars isolated from asymptomatic horses generally reflect the literature reported outbreaks of new serovars such as with S. *oranienburg* in California in 2013.[95] Otherwise, only 10 to 20 isolates per annum are reported from nondiarrheic horses; these usually include S. Anatum and S. Newport.

The relative risk these asymptomatic horses pose to a healthy, nonhospitalized adult population is not known; however, in a study of horses that tested positive to *S. enterica*, there was limited risk to stablemates after discharge.[96] However, higher risk was attributed to stablemates if comingled with horses that received oral antibiotics. The risks of *Salmonella* spp. to hospitalized horses have been previously discussed in this chapter.

Mild GI disease characterized by delayed onset of disease but rapid fecal shedding characterizes the second form of the disease.[45-47,94] In experimental infection, horses generally start shedding *Salmonella* spp. within the first few days. Increased rectal temperature, depression, and anorexia usually occurred within the first week followed by diarrhea of a short duration (1-3 days). Change in fecal consistency was mild in this group, generally consisting of soft, ill-formed feces. Horses that demonstrate limited evidence of impending circulatory collapse often recover spontaneously, and there is limited mortality associated with these clinical signs.

The third form of salmonellosis that has been reproduced experimentally is "toxic" enterocolitis characterized by a fulminant, often pipe stream diarrhea within 2 to 3 days of inoculation. Most affected horses start shedding within 1 to 3 days after inoculation and continue shedding for several days if they survive.[45-47,94] Feces appear voluminous because of the frequency and high water content. Before this change in fecal consistency, horses are often febrile, extremely depressed, and anorexic. GI pain, increased heart rate, increased respiration, and injected mucous membranes are common. Horses will have decreased borborygmi and possibly tympany on abdominal auscultation. These horses may become bacteremic during this syndrome. Without intensive supportive care, horses will succumb to circulatory failure likely from both sepsis and dehydration; horses can present recumbent and nonresponsive. Laminitis is a common sequelae.

As with most vertebrates, peracute sepsis can occur in adult horses.[45-47,94] In experimentally infected adult horses, this is characterized by profound depression, increased rectal temperature, and anorexia without significant diarrhea and often no fecal output. It is these horses in which severe ileus and gastric dilation can be most common.[97] Horses can be extremely tachycardic with heart rates often between 80 and 90 beats per minute because of profound circulatory collapse. This syndrome is usually fatal despite aggressive circulatory support; on necropsy, *S. enterica* can be isolated from liver, mesenteric lymph nodes, and kidneys.

Foals, depending on age, may present with neonatal septicemia with or without diarrhea, diarrhea, and osteomyelitis.[98-107] Clinical signs of enterocolitis can manifest as any of the syndromes in adults; osteomyelitis, arthritis, and omphalophlebitis, however, are the most common concurrent conditions and sequelae. Foals are significantly more likely to be blood culture positive and irrespective of syndrome are fecal positive. In foals that do not survive, the organism can be isolated from multiple organs, including lungs. As in calves, affected foals may have evidence of interstitial pneumonia.

Equine salmonellosis caused by *S. Abortus equi*, a host-adapted serovar, is called *equine paratyphoid*.[108-110] Although originally described in the United States, Asia, and Europe, this agent has not been identified in the United States and Europe for several decades but has caused outbreaks in locally endemic foci in Japan. This strain causes abortion at 7 to 8 months of gestation in mares. The organism has also been associated with fistulous withers and orchitis. In foals, septicemia and osteomyelitis/arthritis occur in neonates and 1- to 3-month-old foals. This organism is transmitted mainly by the fecal-oral route, but stallions can transmit the organisms through semen. The organism is maintained in the population by subclinical carriers.

Diagnosis

Clinical Pathology

Clinicopathological changes of *Salmonella* infection can vary from mild shifts in electrolytes to profound evidence of endotoxemia and plasma volume shifts.[63] In both experimentally and clinically infected asymptomatic horses, there may be limited hematologic and serum biochemical changes. In symptomatic horses, hematologic changes may include neutropenia with or without left shift. Neutropenia usually precedes the onset of clinical signs, and the severity of neutropenia is associated with the severity of disease. Neutrophil counts often rebound with mature leukocytosis common later in the course of the disease. Thrombocytopenia may accompany the neutropenia. Consistent with fluid volume shifts, horses can have increased packed cell volume (PCV) with severely affected horses displaying increases to over 50%. Consistent with increased PCV, there can be relatively increased blood urea nitrogen (BUN), total solids, total protein, and albumin. In some horses with severe disease, total solids, protein, and albumin concentrations may be normal in the face of dehydration, indicating the need for intravenous (IV) oncotic support in addition to crystalloid replacement therapy. Common electrolyte and acid-base disorders include hyponatremia, hypochloremia, hyperkalemia, and metabolic acidosis. Blood lactate can also be high.[63]

Detection of the Organism

The CDC/Pan American Health Organization (CDC/PAHO) defines human salmonellosis as patients with appropriate clinical findings, including asymptomatic infections, and concurrent laboratory confirmation of *Salmonella* from a clinical specimen. The same definition can be applied to horses with clinical signs of diarrhea, abdominal pain, and inappetence of variable severity. Both asymptomatic and extra-intestinal manifestations of salmonellosis may occur. Laboratory confirmation of this diagnosis currently requires the isolation of *Salmonella* from a clinical specimen obtained from the suspected case. The CDC further defines a probable case as that which has clinical symptoms and is linked epidemiologically to a confirmed case (http://wwwn.cdc.gov/NNDSS).

Bacterial isolation is the most definitive means of confirming the presence of *Salmonella* organisms. With the use of selective enrichment and multiple selective plating agars, bacterial isolation is a highly sensitive diagnostic method.[111] Nevertheless, false-negative cultures are thought to occur frequently because of low concentration of the organism in the feces at particular stages of the disease. Multiple serial bacterial cultures are frequently recommended to increase the sensitivity of culture,[45,61,112] despite the increased likelihood of false-positive results caused by detection of passive shedding of the organism. Because of the number of enrichment steps required, detection in culture of *Salmonella* when the organism is shed at low concentrations may take a week or more from the onset of culture.[111,113]

Bacterial isolation is required for determining the serotype and the antimicrobial resistance of the infecting *Salmonella* spp. and thus aids establishing appropriate treatment and an accurate prognosis. In addition, comparative phenotypic or genetic analyses of *Salmonella* isolates, critically important in the epidemiologic investigation of potential outbreaks of disease, require the availability of viable bacterial isolates.

Fecal specimens (at least 1 g) are most often used for bacteriologic culture of *Salmonella*. Although enrichment cultures of larger volumes of fecal specimens tend to increase the likelihood of isolating *Salmonella*, practical limits are imposed by the volumes of media required, and multiple small samples may be a more rewarding approach. Culture of rectal mucosal biopsies has also been recommended for diagnosis and in at least some situations may be more sensitive for diagnosis than fecal culture.[114] Unlike the situation with host-adapted serovars, horses with enteric salmonellosis inconsistently experience bacteremia and blood cultures are often unrewarding except in neonatal foals. Bacteremia is thought to occur most frequently in salmonellosis, affecting young animals (1-6 months) or foals with failure of passive transfer, and blood culture would be warranted in these patients.

Postmortem specimens for bacteriologic culture should include cecal and colonic contents, mesenteric lymph nodes, liver, and spleen, as well as any other sites where clinical history or gross lesions indicate localization of the infection. Cultures of these necropsy specimens may be positive even when repeated fecal cultures are negative, and whether antimicrobial therapy has or has not been administered.

Once isolated, isolates should be sent to National Veterinary Services Laboratory to identify the serovar. In addition, strain-specific identification of *Salmonella* isolates within serovars is useful to identify potential nosocomial and other common-source outbreak strains and for the purposes of reporting. *Salmonella* strain typing can be accomplished by different methods, including phenotypic procedures such as phage typing and antimicrobial resistance typing.[8,9] Phage typing is a highly reproducible and discriminatory method, but this procedure is not widely available.[9] More recently, genetic typing with pulsed-field gel electrophoresis (PFGE) has been increasingly used as a means of identifying strain types of *Salmonella* infection.[10,11] Both phage typing and PFGE typing may be insufficiently discriminatory to identify subtypes within disseminated clonal types of *Salmonella* spp. Whole genome sequencing of bacterial isolates, including *Salmonella* spp., is becoming more economical, and several projects for serovar Typhi and others are underway. Finally, bacterial arrays have been used as a reliable, robust method to identify broad phylogenetic relationships that can illuminate bacterial evolution and explain trends in host adaption and virulence.

In investigating and implementing infection control measures with a known or suspected outbreak of salmonellosis, it is often useful to assess the degree and nature of environmental contamination. More information about approaches to identifying environmental *Salmonella* contamination is available elsewhere.[16,42,115,116]

A limitation of using bacteriologic culture is the time required to obtain laboratory results (3 to 5 days). As a result, several studies have assessed the diagnostic performance of PCR-based tests for detecting *Salmonella* in fecal samples in horses.[117-121] One advantage of using PCR tests is that results can be obtained in 2 days, thus allowing an earlier implementation of appropriate infection control measures. However, despite the availability of rapid PCR tests for detection of *Salmonella*, its acceptance as a diagnostic and surveillance tool for detection of *Salmonella* shedding in horses has been limited. One concern has been the potential misclassification (false positives) of horses classified as negative to *Salmonella* shedding after testing negative on one to seven fecal samples by using bacteriologic culture methods. For example, in one study[122] among 152 horses without clinical signs of salmonellosis that tested negative on one fecal sample by bacteriologic culture, 26 (17%) tested positive by PCR. In another study,[119] among 105 hospitalized horses without clinical signs of salmonellosis that tested negative on ≥5 consecutive fecal samples collected at 24-hour intervals, 76 (72%) tested positive by PCR. In both studies[119,122] the PCR protocol targeted the *Salmonella* histidine transport operon gene.

Four additional studies have assessed the diagnostic performance of real-time PCR tests for detecting *Salmonella* spp.[121] in fecal specimens in horses.[113,118,120] In these studies, the reported sensitivity (true positives) of the PCR tests evaluated ranged from 80% to 100%, when bacteriologic culture was used as the gold standard. The reported specificity (true negatives) ranged from 85% to 98%. Real-time PCR tests that produced the highest combined sensitivity and specificity targeted the SpaQ gene[118] or the InvA gene of *Salmonella*.[120,121]

Although the use of PCR protocols for early detection of *Salmonella* shedding in horses is promising, a PCR-based surveillance system has some limitations. A positive PCR result indicates the presence of genetic material from *Salmonella*, but it does not allow other phenotype or genotype characterization that is required to confirm nosocomial *Salmonella* infections in hospitalized horses or contamination of hospital facilities caused by the widespread outbreak of a *Salmonella* strain. A PCR test with high sensitivity and high specificity, relative to culture, is desired for early detection of *Salmonella* shedding in hospitalized horses.

Serologic Testing

Serologic testing for exposure to *Salmonella* antigens is possible but is not widely available. Seropositive animals are not necessarily actively infected, and actively infected animals may be seronegative early in the infection. Antigenic differences between some infecting strains and some serologic tests may also result in false-negative results.

Pathologic Findings

The gross pathologic findings in horses with salmonellosis are typically those of enteritis or enterocolitis. The predominant necropsy lesion is that of diffuse fibrinous or hemorrhagic inflammation of the cecum and colon. The mucosa may show superficial necrosis, and grayish pseudomembranes may adhere to the mucosa. Circumscribed focal mucosal ulcers underlain by edematous submucosa may develop in more chronic cases. The mesenteric lymph nodes are enlarged and may exhibit hemorrhage and edema.

Elsewhere in the GI tract, the stomach may be hyperemic with edema and focal hemorrhages. Small intestinal changes may vary from simple congestion to a mucoid or hemorrhagic exudate. Histologically, the most severe lesions are typically found in the cecum and colon. Hemorrhage and superficial coagulative necrosis with a predominantly mononuclear cell infiltrate are the principal findings. Fibrinocellular exudates may be attached to the necrotic epithelium. The capillaries of the lamina propria are frequently occluded by fibrin thrombi. "Para-typhoid nodules," small foci of hepatic necrosis that may be associated with aggregations of inflammatory cells, are not always present but are suggestive of salmonellosis when observed.

Therapy

Antimicrobial Treatment

The use of antimicrobials for treatment of adult horses with salmonellosis is controversial.[63] Generally, antibiotic treatment of adult horses with salmonellosis is avoided, although some cases may warrant such treatment.[62] In adult human infections, treatment with antibiotics did not alter the length of illness.

Treatment of inapparent *Salmonella* infections with antimicrobial drugs has not proved to be an effective means of eliminating the carrier state. Because there is a paucity of information on the benefits versus disadvantages of antimicrobial treatment of equine salmonellosis, it is difficult to make definitive recommendations on the use of antimicrobials to treat adult horses with enterocolitis caused by *Salmonella* infection.[26] Antimicrobial therapy should be discontinued in horses that develop diarrhea while receiving antimicrobial drug(s).[123]

It has been suggested that antimicrobial treatment of adult horses with enterocolitis caused by *Salmonella* infection does not alter the course of the enterocolitis[63] or duration of shedding of the organism in feces.[45,63] Use of antimicrobials may be justified in some patients because of the risk for septicemia from severe neutropenia or persistent fever, the translocation of bacteria across the injured epithelium of the bowel, the presence of an indwelling IV catheter, or the presence of widespread endothelial damage.[26,123] Most clinicians decide on a case-by-case basis whether to institute antimicrobial treatment in adult horses with enterocolitis suspected or confirmed to be caused by salmonellosis. The choice of antimicrobials should be individualized based on the antimicrobial susceptibility pattern of the isolate from the patient or from past experience with isolates from that farm, hospital, or geographic region. A lipid-soluble drug would be optimal because *Salmonella* spp. can be intracellular. Combinations of gentamicin and a beta-lactam drug are often administered to horses with colitis of undetermined origin and to horses with confirmed salmonellosis, but this regimen has the disadvantage of poor intracellular penetration and the risk of renal toxicity (gentamicin).[45]

Papich[62] has suggested that, if antimicrobials are used, the drug of choice for treatment of salmonellosis in horses is a fluoroquinolone. This drug was selected because it has an injectable form (enrofloxacin 5-10 mg/kg IV every 24 hours [q24h]), favorable pharmacologic features (intracellular penetration), bactericidal activity, and minimal effect on the anaerobic intestinal flora. Fluoroquinolones should not be administered to young foals because of concerns about their adverse effect on cartilage. For foals with salmonellosis, Papich[62] suggests a beta-lactam drug such as an extended-spectrum cephalosporin or ampicillin-sulbactam alone or in combination with an aminoglycoside (gentamicin or amikacin). Oral ciprofloxacin was associated with colitis in four Standardbred horses in part because of poor absorption after oral administration, and Weese et al[124] suggest that because this drug does not reach therapeutic levels after oral administration and may cause colitis, the oral route should be avoided in horses.

Because some isolates of *Salmonella* from horses, especially those with clinical illness, can be MDR, the choice of an antimicrobial before the availability of an antibiogram on the isolate is even more challenging. In addition, the use of some antimicrobials may apply selection pressure toward enhanced ability of MDR *Salmonella* spp. to colonize equine patients.[125]

In neonatal foals, bacteremia is more likely, so antimicrobial therapy is indicated, especially if there is an associated bone or joint infection.[123] Choice of antimicrobial should be based on antibiogram of the isolate if possible. Joint lavage and limb perfusion may also be considered in patients with bone or joint infection.[126-128]

Merritt et al[97] proposed using enrofloxacin and an immunostimulant in the treatment of horses with chronic diarrhea that are shedding *Salmonella* in the feces, implying a favorable outcome to treatment.

Fluid and Colloidal Therapy

Initial assessment should include determination of hydration status, plasma electrolyte concentration (sodium, potassium, chloride, calcium, magnesium), acid-base status (venous blood gas or total carbon dioxide [CO_2]), serum glucose, and osmolality.[129] Generally, large volumes of polyionic IV fluids are required for treatment of adult horses with severe enterocolitis caused by salmonellosis. Goals of fluid therapy include replacement of fluid and electrolyte losses and maintenance of fluid, electrolyte, and acid-base balance after replacement has occurred. Frequent measurement of serum electrolytes, assessment of acid-base status, and PCV/total protein (TP) monitoring are indicated because a wide variety of abnormalities may occur in horses with salmonellosis.[45] Systemic inflammatory response syndrome (SIRS), such as occurs with endotoxemia and sepsis, often results in increased vascular permeability, reduced vascular responsiveness, and myocardial depression (see Chapter 11). Hypoalbuminemia is common and results in decreased oncotic pressure.[130] These factors predispose to reduced circulating volume and inadequate perfusion. The need to augment replacement or maintenance fluids is based on repeated evaluation of serum electrolytes.[129]

In patients with complications, such as hypovolemic shock, significant ongoing fluid losses, and hypoalbuminemia, IV administration of colloidal solutions may be indicated. Small-volume colloidal administration may be accomplished over a short time to expand the intravascular volume by osmotic redistribution from the extracellular fluid. Several commercially available colloids are available, including plasma and hydroxyethyl starch (HES). Experimental studies have shown HES to be superior to plasma for treatment of endotoxic shock in attenuation of endotoxin-induced vascular permeability. Hypertonic saline (HYS) may be indicated as an adjunct to intravascular resuscitation. In hypovolemic shock, HYS may be important in stabilization of the cardiovascular system. It is important that isotonic replacement fluids be given with HYS. HYS is contraindicated in patients with renal failure, cardiac dysrhythmias, hypernatremia, hypokalemia, thrombocytopenia, or coagulopathies.[129]

Clinicians should pay careful attention to catheter selection, placement, and maintenance in horses with enterocolitis and endotoxemia because such patients are at increased risk of venous thrombosis. More expensive, polyurethane catheters may prove to be more economical because they can be left in place longer than catheters made of alternative materials and may reduce the risk of thrombosis in horses with severe GI disease.[129] Any signs of heat, pain, swelling, or thickening of the vein should prompt immediate catheter removal, and if sepsis is suspected, the catheter should be submitted for bacterial culture.

For further information on fluid treatment of diarrheic equine patients, the reader is referred to in-depth reviews on the subject.[129,130]

Treatment of Endotoxemia and Inflammation

There are five principal goals of treatment for endotoxemia: (1) prevention of movement of endotoxin into the circulation; (2) neutralization of endotoxin before it interacts with inflammatory cells; (3) prevention of synthesis, release, or action of inflammatory mediators; (4) prevention of endotoxin-induced cellular activation; and (5) general supportive care with IV fluids or colloids and inotropic agents (as previously addressed).[131]

Prevention of movement of endotoxin into the circulation needs to be addressed at the bowel level. Di-tri-octahedral (DTO) smectite (Biosponge; Platinum Performance, Buellton, CA) is a natural, hydrated aluminomagnesium silicate containing chelated macrominerals and microminerals available for use in horses.[131,132] Although the mechanism remains speculative, DTO reduced the duration of diarrhea and the frequency of defecation in horses with experimentally induced colitis.[133] Further controlled studies to determine the in vivo efficacy of DTO in horses with salmonellosis are needed.

Neutralization of toxin before activation of inflammatory cells can be attempted in two ways: administration of antiendotoxin antibodies or administration of polymyxin B, which forms a stable complex with lipid A. The conclusions of various studies of serum or plasma products enriched with antiendotoxin antibodies have been variable. Additional controlled studies need to be performed using strict entrance criteria and in which antiendotoxin antibodies or nonspecific immunoglobulins are administered early in the course of the disease.[131] With the recent report of fatal serum hepatitis associated with commercial plasma transfusion in horses, the benefit of this treatment must be weighed against the risk of this potential, although rare, complication.[134] Polymyxin B has been evaluated in several experimental studies and is currently used in clinical cases for the treatment of endotoxemia in horses.[135,136] It is optimal to initiate polymyxin treatment (1000-6000 units/kg q8-12h) as early in the course of endotoxemia as possible.[136] Use of polymyxin B should be avoided in horses with renal compromise.

Preventing or reducing the synthesis, release, or effect of inflammatory mediators secondary to endotoxemia includes treatment of horses with nonsteroidal antiinflammatory drugs (NSAIDs) such as flunixin meglumine. The NSAIDs have been the main means of treatment of horses with endotoxemia for decades. These drugs inhibit cyclooxygenase and thus the formation of arachidonic acid metabolites. Another class of drug used for treatment of horses with endotoxemia is pentoxifylline (8 mg PO q8h).[131] During in vitro experimental studies, this drug reduced production of cytokines, thromboxanes, and expression of tissue factor while increasing plasma concentration of prostaglandin I_2. However, during in vivo experiments in horses, pentoxifylline had limited benefit.[137] Other drugs are being explored for the treatment of endotoxemia through inhibition of the production, release, or effect of inflammatory mediators, but most of these are not available for clinical use. Corticosteroids are likely contraindicated in treatment of salmonellosis because of their immunosuppressive effect.[63,131]

New treatments are being developed and tested for their ability to interfere with endotoxin-induced cellular activation.[131] These new treatments seek to modulate proinflammatory and antiinflammatory mediators in response to endotoxin (see Chapter 11).

Colonic Flora Modulation

The prevalence of fecal shedding of *Salmonella* in the postoperative period of equine colic patients was not reduced with the use of two commercially prepared probiotic products.[53,138] Possible reasons for failure of these products include lack of viable organisms in the product, failure of the organisms to remain viable in the GI tract, and inappropriate quantities of organisms to provide an intestinal flora barrier to colonization with *Salmonella* spp.[132] A recent study demonstrated the potential benefit of *Lactobacillus pentosus* WE7. This organism is acid and bile tolerant and moderately inhibitory to growth of *Salmonella* spp. in vitro.[139] A randomized masked placebo study of the efficacy of this organism on the shedding of *Salmonella* in high-risk equine patients is warranted.

Other Treatment Considerations

All horses with diarrhea should be isolated from other animals, and barrier precautions should be used to minimize the exposure of other animals and human handlers to the feces of diarrheic horses during treatment (see Chapter 62). These horses should be housed in an area where insect, rodent, and bird control is optimal.

Horses with severe disease should be kept as comfortable as possible. An effort should be made to keep the horse's coat and skin clean of feces; surfaces such as the perineum may require frequent cleaning, and topical application of skin protection products is warranted. Affected horses should be protected from extremely cold or hot and humid environmental conditions. These horses should be housed with plenty of bedding in case they want to lie down. The stall should be kept reasonably clean by frequent removal of soiled bedding and replacement with fresh bedding. A cushioned stall floor is ideal because these horses are prone to laminitis. If cushioning of the stall with mats is not an option, then application of hoof support with padding using various materials cut to fit over the sole of the hoof and attached with tape is indicated.

All horses with diarrhea should have access to fresh water unless gastric dilation and ileus are a part of the disease process. Some horses will consume electrolyte solutions orally, which may reduce the amount of IV supplementation required; therefore offering an electrolyte bucket along with access to plain fresh water is indicated.

Special attention to diet is warranted for horses with diarrhea. Efforts should be made to provide clean feed (not contaminated with diarrheic feces) in small amounts several times a day to encourage consumption and to adequately monitor feed intake. The horse should be offered several options of types of feed to enhance feed consumption if appetite is reduced. Feeds that are low bulk and low in soluble carbohydrate are ideal such as complete pelleted rations, good-quality grass hay, or judicious amounts of alfalfa hay. Small amounts of fresh grass may stimulate anorectic horses to eat, but large amounts of lush pasture should be avoided. If the horse is hypoproteinemic, provision of a complete pelleted ration or alfalfa hay will provide a source of protein in the diet. If the horse is unwilling or unable to eat for an extended time, addressing protein and calorie malnutrition is warranted through parenteral nutrition. Equine patients prone to hyperlipemia or those that are underweight require nutritional support more quickly than horses in optimal body condition. A detailed description of parenteral nutrition is beyond the scope of this chapter, and the reader is directed to other sources of information on this topic.[138,140]

It is important in any horse with diarrhea to monitor vital signs and select laboratory tests frequently to determine the need for and most appropriate change in therapy. Monitoring horses with enterocolitis for early signs of laminitis is very important so that treatment for laminitis can be promptly implemented. For more information on the pathogenesis, treatment, and prevention of laminitis, the reader is referred to reviews on this topic.[141,142]

If the horse is showing signs of abdominal pain that is refractory to management with NSAIDs such as flunixin meglumine, consideration should be given to administration of more potent analgesics on an as-needed basis. Options for pain management would include administration of butorphanol, potentially in combination with xylazine or detomidine. In some horses with enterocolitis, a constant-rate IV infusion of butorphanol may be necessary. Other sources of information on management of abdominal pain in horses are available.[143,144]

Prevention

Options for prevention of salmonellosis in equids can be separated into two broad categories: (1) prevent or minimize exposure and (2) optimize host resistance if exposed.[145] *Salmonella* spp. are ubiquitous enough that avoiding all exposure is likely not feasible; however, means are available to minimize both frequency and dose of exposure.

Reducing Exposure to *Salmonella* Species

Exposure of horses to *Salmonella* spp. can be minimized by reducing chances of oral exposure to the organism. This can be accomplished by using biosecurity and biocontainment strategies on the farm and in veterinary hospitals (see Chapter 62). The following overview of options for reducing risk of exposure to *Salmonella* provides selected examples to illustrate the preventive measures.

New arrivals to the farm or resident horses returning to the farm from high-risk situations, such as from veterinary hospitals, should be isolated from the resident equine population for 14 to 21 days to reduce the chances of exposing the resident horse population to the organism. Housing horses in veterinary hospitals based on risk level may reduce cross-contamination between patients. For example, colic patients could be kept stalled separately from elective orthopedic cases.

Providing horses on farms with access to pastures that are well maintained can reduce the bacterial load. Avoiding overcrowding and overgrazing will decrease the fecal load on pastures, as well as keep grasses longer and allow horses to avoid grazing where other horses have defecated. Avoiding common-use turnout areas for hospitalized horses will minimize exposure. If grazing of hospitalized horses is desirable, providing grass in raised beds or hydroponically produced grass should be considered.

Using feeds that are manufactured with good manufacturing procedures and that do not contain animal protein sources may reduce the likelihood of feed-related exposure to *Salmonella* spp. Pelleted feeds may be less likely to contain live bacteria because of the heating process. Horse feeds should be stored so that rodent and bird fecal contamination is minimized by using rodent-proof containers and keeping lids closed.

Although challenging, control of insect, rodent, and bird access to equine housing areas should be considered, especially in the areas where horses are fed. Block open rafters in barns using wire mesh nailed to the rafters to reduce bird roosting above horse stalls and feed storage areas. Keeping the quantity of available feed to a minimum will reduce rodent and bird populations. Insect control can be accomplished by removing livestock fecal material from stalls and disposing of feces away from horse housing areas. Utilize professional vermin control personnel to provide control plans.

Water sources for horses should be tested for quality, including coliform counts, and can be tested for specific pathogens. Run-off from fecal disposal areas should be regulated, and if horses have access to irrigation ditches, creeks, or ponds, these water sources should be tested.

Regular removal of livestock feces from stalls and pastures reduces the load of enteric bacteria in the horse's environment.

Disposal sites for feces should be distant from the equine housing area and pastures. Serious consideration should be given to drainage systems used in horse barns so that the materials going down the drains do not run off onto horse pastures, paddocks, or feeding sites. For example, in an outbreak of salmonellosis in neonatal foals, the mares were suspected to be shedding *S.* Ohio in their feces at the time of foaling. Control measures included cleaning and disinfection of the surfaces in the foaling barn, thorough bathing of mares immediately after foaling, frequent removal of mare's feces from the stall, and giving the newborn foal colostrum from a bottle before suckling from the udder. These measures appeared to prevent further cases.[143,146] Actual monitoring of fecal shedding by horses and the environmental contamination in high-risk areas (e.g., veterinary hospitals) can allow for rapid intervention to control spread of *Salmonella* spp.[144,147]

Cleaning and disinfection of equipment used on equine patients between uses or use of dedicated equipment for high-risk patients is important in controlling spread of *Salmonella* between hospitalized patients. These include all medical and nonmedical implements that come into contact with *Salmonella*-infected or at-risk horses. Use of dedicated thermometers also reduces the risk of fecal-oral spread of bacteria.

Environmental control measures for prevention of salmonellosis include designing farm and hospital facilities to allow for thorough cleaning and disinfection and keeping equine housing areas cooled during hot and humid weather conditions to reduce the risk of *Salmonella* overgrowth in the environment and reduce susceptibility of ill horses to severe salmonellosis if exposed.[148] *Salmonella* spp. can persist and perhaps even multiply in the environment and this is enhanced through the continued presence of the organism in fecal and any organic debris. Thus proper disinfection is one of the most important means to control certain infectious equine diseases, especially the enteric pathogens such as *Salmonella*.[149] The stall and surrounding areas for any known *Salmonella*-positive animal should be considered contaminated and appropriate barrier precautions taken. Once the horse has left the facility, cleaning and disinfection should be implemented and the effectiveness of these procedures monitored.

It is important to emphasize cleaning the environmental surfaces as part of the process. Physically removing these materials by cleaning is an important first step. Basic concepts include cleaning from top to bottom and farthest from a drain toward the drain and cleaning from the least toward the most contaminated areas.

Personal protection is a hallmark of personal safety and reducing the spread of infectious diseases. Use of footbaths or mats with disinfectant is a common measure to control trafficking of pathogenic microorganisms in livestock operations and veterinary hospitals.[31,38] Alternative approaches include use of dedicated footwear in a particular facility or area in the hospital (e.g., isolation facility, colic aisle way). Often a combination of these methods is used. An important part of optimal patient care includes the regular use of effective hand hygiene when handling all horses whether a patient or not. The product type to be used should be considered, as well as the regular implementation of the methods by hospital personnel. Several veterinary hospitals are now using not only handwashing but also disinfectant hand gels as part of their infection control strategies.[150]

Optimizing Resistance

Vaccination to stimulate specific immunity is one option often undertaken in control of infectious diseases.[145] However, no commercial vaccine is currently available for prevention of salmonellosis in horses.

Recently, a conditionally licensed *S.* Newport bacterial extract vaccine for use in cattle has become available, but no such product exists for horses. Other options for improving resistance of horses to salmonellosis include reducing stress when possible (see earlier discussion on host resistance). Feasible options for reducing stress and maintaining normal GI flora that may act as a barrier to colonization by *Salmonella* include judicious use of antimicrobials and gastric ulcer medications, minimizing dietary changes, and keeping the environmental temperature cool during hot and humid weather conditions.

Supplementation with probiotics in the limited number of studies conducted to date have not reduced the fecal shedding of *Salmonella* by hospitalized equine colic patients.[151]

Public Health Considerations

Salmonellosis is an important zoonotic disease estimated to cause more than 1 million cases of diarrheal disease, 15,000 hospitalizations, and 400 human deaths annually in the United States.[152] The economic costs of salmonellosis are considered the largest single contributor to the overall burden of human acute bacterial enteric disease, which was estimated at almost $8 billion in 1989.[153]

Although it is generally assumed that most cases of human salmonellosis result from food-borne exposure, other important routes of infection exist. The prevalence of contamination of horsemeat with *Salmonella* at slaughter plants is of concern from a public health perspective because horsemeat is exported from the United States to some countries for human consumption. Contamination of horsemeat and food-borne transmission of *Salmonella* by horsemeat have been reported.[68,69,154,155] In some countries, horsemeat is consumed raw as steak tartare. A link between contaminated horsemeat and an outbreak of human illness in France caused by MDR *S.* Newport has been reported.[155] Because horsemeat consumption is rare in the United States, a more significant route of infection is transmission by direct or indirect contact with infected animals. Direct contact with infected horses is a significant risk factor for zoonotic transmission of *Salmonella* spp.[70,71,156,157] This risk is presumably greater for contact with clinically ill animals with salmonellosis. Indirect animal contact may also result in significant exposure to *Salmonella*; household environmental contamination of workers exposed to a veterinary *Salmonella* outbreak is quite common.[158] Although direct contact transmission from horses to humans does occur, such reports appear to be infrequent[148,159] (JL Traub-Dargatz, Colorado State University, personal communication).

More recently, North America has seen the emergence of a new epidemic, MDR serovar, *Salmonella* Newport.[160] This new epidemic *Salmonella* is of particular concern from a public health viewpoint because of its cmy-2–encoded decreased susceptibility to extended-spectrum cephalosporin drugs, including ceftriaxone and ceftazidime and the veterinary drug ceftiofur. These cephalosporin drugs are considered the drugs of choice for childhood *Salmonella* infections that require antimicrobial therapy when fluoroquinolone drugs are contraindicated. This *S.* Newport strain has been reported as the cause of significant problems with equine nosocomial infection and raises concerns about direct-contact transmission to veterinary hospital staff and clients.[160,161]

The complete reference list is available online at www.expertconsult.com.

36 Glanders

Anthony N.B. Kettle and Paul L. Nicoletti*

Glanders is one of the oldest recorded diseases of equids with zoonotic potential known since ancient times. Disease symptoms were recorded by Hippocrates in 425 BC and was given the name "melis" by Aristotle in 350 BC.[1,2] The common etiology of these diseases was first demonstrated by Viborg at the end of the eighteenth century.[2] The etiologic agent, now known as *Burkholderia mallei*, was isolated in 1882 by Loeffler and Schütz from the liver and spleen of an infected horse.[1,3] The mallein test for diagnosis of glanders was developed in 1890.[4]

By the second half of the nineteenth century, glanders was widespread in horses in North America, and a major epidemic of disease occurred in association with movement of horses during and after the Civil War.[1,4,5] *Burkholderia mallei* was reportedly used as a biologic warfare agent in World Wars I and II and the Russian invasion of Afghanistan.[6] *Burkholderia mallei* is now regarded as a select agent (category B, U.S. Centers for Disease Control and Prevention) and all experimental work must be carried out in a Level 3 Biosafety facility.[7,8] Disease caused by *B. mallei* must be reported to the World Organization for Animal Health (formerly the Office International des Epizooties [OIE]) in Paris.

Etiology

Burkholderia mallei (formerly *Pseudomonas, Bacillus, Pfeifferella, Loefflerella, Malleomyces, Actinobacillus, Corynebacterium,* and *Mycobacterium*) is a short, rod-shaped, gram-negative, aerobic, facultative intracellular, nonmotile, and non–spore-forming bacterium. The organism survives outside the host for varying periods of time, depending on many factors. Virulence factors of *B. mallei* include capsular polysaccharide, lipopolysaccharide,

*The authors acknowledge and appreciate the original contributions of these authors, whose work has been incorporated into this chapter.

and type III and VI secretion pathways.[9-12] Capsular polysaccharide is essential for virulence in hamsters and mice.[12] An acapsular mutant of *B. mallei* failed to induce disease in experimentally infected horses.[13] In addition, a complex quorum-sensing network and a two-component transcriptional regulatory system are required for maximal virulence in hamsters.[14]

Epidemiology and Pathogenesis

Although occasional cases of glanders occur in cats, dogs, goats, and sheep, the principal hosts are horses, donkeys, and mules. Recently, natural infection has been reported in camels as well.[15] Carnivores, such as lions, may be infected from ingestion of contaminated meat as occurred in the Tehran Zoo in 2010. Mice and guinea pigs can be experimentally infected. Both acute and chronic forms of the disease are found; horses typically are chronically infected, whereas donkeys and mules are more likely to develop the acute form. Chronically infected equids are the only known reservoir for *B. mallei*. Human infections can occur by aerosol transmission from infected animals and are frequently fatal if untreated.

Glanders is restricted geographically to Eastern Europe, Asia, North Africa, South America, and the Middle East. It is considered endemic in Iraq, Turkey, Pakistan, India, Mongolia, and China,[16-23] where reported outbreaks appear to be increasing in the last 10 to 20 years. Reports of recent outbreaks in Brazil, Bahrain, Lebanon, and Kuwait have appeared in the veterinary literature[22,23] and on the OIE Website. Glanders has been eradicated from Europe, Australia, and North America by a rigorous policy of culling animals that are positive by complement fixation test (CFT), serum agglutination test, or the mallein test. An accidental human infection occurred in a laboratory worker in 2000,[24] but there have been no naturally occurring cases of glanders in North America for more than 60 years. The last case in animals in the United States was in 1942.

Burkholderia mallei is a niche-specific derivative of *Burkholderia pseudomallei*.[25,26] The primary route of infection in horses is through the ingestion of feed or water contaminated by the nasal secretions of infected horses.[1] The disease can be spread by subclinically infected horses. Poor sanitation, crowding, and immunosuppression from parasitism are considered risk factors. The incubation period varies from a few days to many months. The disease has been the target of eradication efforts for many decades because of its clinical effects in equids and its public health implications. The increasing number of outbreaks in recent years led to the classification of glanders as a reemerging disease.

Clinical Findings

Historically, glanders is described as either acute or chronic, but clinically it may be difficult to distinguish between the two forms. It is perhaps better to regard chronic glanders as a progressive disease comprised of acute episodes occasionally interspersed with periods of latency. The host factors determining the course of the infection are unknown. Donkeys are most likely to die from acute disease within 7 to 10 days, whereas horses may either die rapidly or live for several years with chronic abscessation.

Acute glanders is characterized by bronchopneumonia and septicemia with a moderate to high fever, depression, and rapid weight loss. Frequently, highly infectious mucopurulent to hemorrhagic nasal discharge forms crusts on the external nares. Submaxillary lymph nodes are frequently swollen, painless, and seldom rupture.

Chronic glanders is typically described as one of three forms: cutaneous (farcy), nasal, or pulmonary, although in practice there is much overlap between the three forms.

In the cutaneous form, nodules develop into crater-shaped ulcers discharging a thick yellow exudate (Fig. 36-1, *A*) and generally track the lymphatic vessels to regional lymph nodes. The lymph vessels become swollen and corded with nodules appearing at intervals en route (Fig. 36-1, *B*). The cutaneous lesions may appear anywhere on the body, but typically the limbs and especially the hindlimb are more frequently affected.

The nasal form is characterized by frequent snorts to clear the nasal passages as nodules form on the nasal septum and erupt to discharge a thick tenacious yellow exudate (Fig. 36-2).

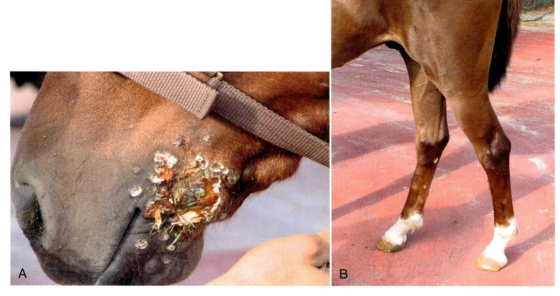

Figure 36-1 **A,** Crater-shaped ulcers with exudate. **B,** Swollen cutaneous lymphatics with nodules. *(Courtesy Dr. U. Wernery, Central Veterinary Research Laboratory, Dubai, UAE.)*

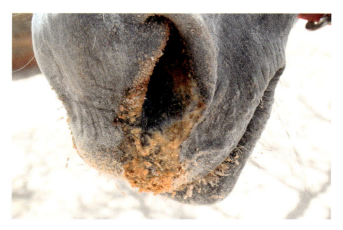

Figure 36-2 Nasal exudate in horse with glanders. *(Courtesy Dr U. Wernery, Central Veterinary Research Laboratory, Dubai, UAE.)*

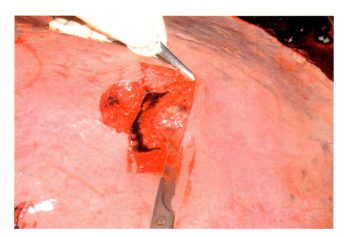

Figure 36-4 Pulmonary granulomas in lungs of horse with glanders. *(Courtesy Dr U. Wernery, Central Veterinary Research Laboratory, Dubai, UAE.)*

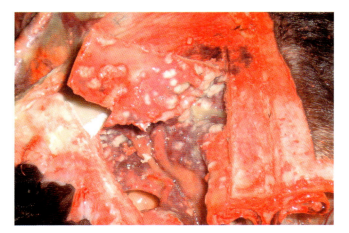

Figure 36-3 Granulomas and ulcers (stellate scar) in nasal septum of horse with glanders. *(Courtesy Dr U. Wernery, Central Veterinary Research Laboratory, Dubai, UAE.)*

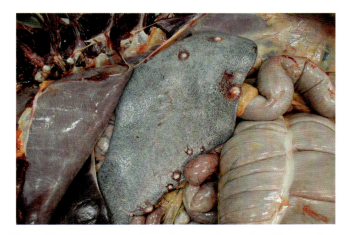

Figure 36-5 Abscesses on spleen of horse with glanders. *(Courtesy Dr U. Wernery, Central Veterinary Research Laboratory, Dubai, UAE.)*

The nasal discharge may become hemorrhagic as nodules rupture, leaving large ulcers that heal forming stellate scars (Fig. 36-3). There is a regional lymphadenopathy, and the glottis may become swollen, which leads to dyspnea.

The pulmonary form is an extension of the nasal form to the lower respiratory tract with the formation of round, grayish, firm nodules within the lungs (Fig. 36-4). Similar abscesses may be found on the liver and spleen (Fig. 36-5), and occasionally, orchitis may occur in stallions (Fig. 36-6).[1,16,27]

Diagnosis

Glanders must be differentiated from other chronic infections of the upper respiratory tract, including strangles *(Streptococcus equi* subsp. *equi)*, ulcerative lymphangitis *(Corynebacterium pseudotuberculosis)*, pseudotuberculosis *(Yersinia pseudotuberculosis)*, and sporotrichosis *(Sporotrichum* spp.), and from epizootic lymphangitis *(Histoplasma farciminosum)*. In humans, glanders also needs to be differentiated from melioidosis *(Burkholderia pseudomallei)*.[28]

The test for glanders listed in the OIE Terrestrial Manual in 2012 for international trade is the CFT. Historically, the mallein test (Fig. 36-7) was used to eradicate glanders from North

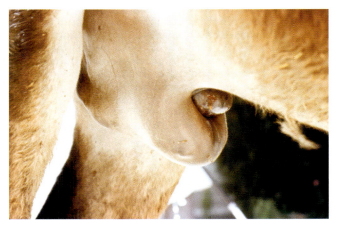

Figure 36-6 Swollen sheath in horse with orchitis caused by glanders.

America and Britain at the turn of the twentieth century since the CFT was not available for glanders until 1913. Early reports indicated the CFT was less sensitive than the mallein test.

Mallein is a heat-treated solution of water-soluble proteins, primarily lipopolysaccharide (LPS), extracted from *B. mallei*.[29] The intradermal-palpebral application of the test is acknowledged as the most sensitive, reliable, and specific of the mallein

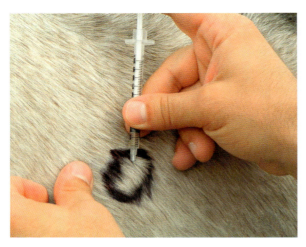

Figure 36-7 Performing the intradermal mallein test. *(Courtesy Dr U. Wernery, Central Veterinary Research Laboratory, Dubai, UAE.)*

tests for glanders. The immunologic basis for the test is primarily a stimulation of memory T cells. Anergy may result in a false-negative reaction. False-positive reactions may also occur. In negative horses, mallein may induce antibodies that are detectable for up to 19 weeks after injection.[30]

The CFT is currently the test used for international trade, but a number of nonspecific false-positive results occur.[30] These false positives are thought to derive at least in part from the use of crude cell-antigen preparations and also from cross-reactions with other bacteria.

Recently, a Western immunoblot technique has been proposed (but has yet to be validated) for resolving the false positives found in the CFT for use in areas with low glanders prevalence.[31] Several other serologic tests and diagnostic techniques are now available for glanders diagnosis, including polymerase chain reaction (PCR), agglutination, indirect hemagglutination, enzyme-linked immunosorbent assay (ELISA), counter immunoelectrophoresis, Rose-Bengal staining, and competitive ELISA (cELISA).[32] Culture and immunohistochemical staining for bacterial antigen may be used. Although rarely used, guinea pigs are highly susceptible, and an acute purulent orchitis occurs in a few days after inoculation of material (Strauss test). A lack of sensitivity of this procedure and culture has been reported.[17] Recent advances in our understanding of *B. mallei* and the increasing availability of molecular diagnostic tools may soon result in a new generation of more sensitive and specific diagnostic tests for glanders in horses.[32]

Therapy

Euthanasia and slaughter of equids with glanders are strongly recommended and may be mandatory in some countries. Although there are relatively few studies of antimicrobial susceptibility patterns of *B. mallei*, it appears that this organism is resistant to many antimicrobial drugs, including β-lactam antibiotics.[33-36] A recent study examined the antimicrobial susceptibility patterns of 15 isolates of *B. mallei* to 35 antimicrobial agents.[36] The most effective drugs in vitro included imipenem, ceftazidime, ciprofloxacin, piperacillin, doxycycline, and aminoglycosides. There were no obvious differences in susceptibility patterns among human, animal, and environmental isolates. Recently, experimental work has been done with granulysin and silver carbine compounds.[37] The availability of several *B. mallei* genome sequences has greatly facilitated the development of new therapeutics; however, much work remains to be done to determine a suitable treatment regimen for horses. The difficulty with treatment in horses is in determining whether the infection has been eliminated.

Prevention

Glanders has been successfully eliminated from most countries through rigorous slaughter of animals with a positive mallein test. Quarantine of in-contact animals and pretesting of horses for movement are necessary components of disease control. A wide variety of national and international regulations exist, and glanders is a reportable disease for the OIE and many countries.

There is no vaccine for prevention of glanders in animals. Research efforts currently are focused on development of a vaccine for people in case the organism becomes an instrument of bioterrorism. A recent report highlights promising results for a vaccine using T-helper epitopes,[38] and a series of protective antigens have been identified by genome analysis that may also be useful in the development of a vaccine.[39]

Public Health Considerations

Glanders is a rare but serious zoonotic disease. Most human cases are ultimately traced to direct contact with *B. mallei* through exposure to infected animals or laboratory exposure to the organism.[24,27,41] The organism often enters via cutaneous exposure through the hands or arms. The incubation period is estimated to be a few days to several weeks but can be much longer. Local suppuration and regional lymphadenopathy with fever and lethargy are often the first symptoms.[24] Dissemination of infection occurs 1 to 4 weeks after lymph node involvement becomes apparent. Systemic effects may include abscesses in the liver, spleen, lungs, pleura, subcutis, and muscles.[24,27,40,41] Mortality in acutely affected people with untreated disease approaches 95% within 3 weeks. As previously mentioned, several antibiotics have reliable activity against *B. mallei*[24,33-36] and are usually used in combination against *B. mallei* infections. In a recent report of glanders in a laboratory worker, treatment with imipenem and doxycycline for 2 weeks, followed by azithromycin and doxycycline for 6 months, was successful (in vitro susceptibility testing did not support the use of azithromycin).[24,27] Glanders in human patients may be difficult to diagnose because of a lack of awareness and rarity of human disease.[27]

The complete reference list is available online at www.expertconsult.com.

37 Brucellosis

Debra C. Sellon and Paul L. Nicoletti*

In 1897, Bang[1] described *Bacillus abortus*, the agent of infectious abortion of cattle. In 1920, Meyer and Shaw[2] placed the organism in the genus *Brucella*, and *Brucella abortus* was first associated with fistulous withers of horses in 1929. Brucellosis may have been the disease responsible for the "plague of Athens" described by Thucydides in the fifth century BC and the historical context for Sophocles' tragic play, *Oedipus Rex*.[3] Today, brucellosis remains the most prevalent bacterial zoonosis worldwide with more than 500,000 new cases reported in humans annually.[4]

Chromosomal deoxyribonucleic acid (DNA) analysis supports the use of the natural host species as a valid phenotypic characteristic for species classification of the genus *Brucella*.[5,6] Infections in horses usually involve the cattle pathogen *B. abortus*, although infections with *Brucella suis* have also been reported. Equine infection with *B. abortus* is associated with septic supraspinous bursitis ("fistulous withers"),[7-9] atlantal bursitis ("poll evil"),[9] other bursal infections,[10] septic arthritis,[11] vertebral osteomyelitis,[12] and abortion.[13,14] *Brucella suis* has been isolated from horses with septic bursitis, aborted equine fetuses, and the internal organs of a mare with no external signs of disease.[15,16] Because infection of horses with *B. abortus*, although rare, is more common than infection with *B. suis*, this chapter focuses on brucellosis caused by *B. abortus* unless otherwise indicated.

Etiology and Epidemiology

Brucellosis in horses is caused by infection with species of the genus *Brucella*, especially *B. abortus* and *B. suis*. There are no reports of successful natural or experimental infection of horses with *B. melitensis* or *B. canis*.[17] *Brucella* spp. are nonmotile, aerobic, intracellular gram-negative cocci or short rods that are usually arranged singly or less frequently in pairs, short chains, or small groups.[5] They require complex media for growth in culture, and many strains require supplementary carbon dioxide (CO_2) for optimal growth on primary isolation. On clear media, colonies are transparent, raised, and convex with a smooth, shiny surface. They appear as a pale honey color by transmitted light.[5] The optimum temperature for growth is 37°C (98.6°F), but growth occurs between 20°F and 40°C (68°F and 104°F).[5]

Brucella abortus infections have been reported worldwide but have been effectively eradicated from several European countries, Japan, and Israel. Cattle are the most common natural hosts for *B. abortus*, but the organism has also been isolated from horses, American bison, buffalo, and yaks.[3] Most horses with brucellosis have a history of contact with cattle.[9,10,14] In 1937, Duff[18] examined 85 horses with fistulous withers; *B. abortus* was isolated from 80% of these horses. Of the horses with brucellosis, 92% had reported contact with cattle, and 56 horses were from farms where cattle had brucellosis.[18] *Brucella suis* most often infects swine but may also infect horses and cattle.

Brucella spp. may be transmitted by ingestion, inhalation, or direct contact through skin abrasions or mucous membranes. It is presumed that most horses acquire infection from cattle. *Brucella abortus* has been isolated from equine feces and urine and from aborted equine fetuses, suggesting that horses are a potential source of infection to cattle.[14,19,20] However, experimental infections indicate that horses do not excrete the organism in sufficient numbers to infect susceptible cattle in close contact.[20,21]

There is no apparent age, gender, or breed susceptibility to the organism in horses, although most cases have been reported in horses older than 3 years.[8] Brucellosis is considered a zoonotic disease (see section on Public Health Considerations).

Pathogenesis and Clinical Findings

There is almost no available information on the pathogenesis of brucellosis in horses. It is difficult to induce clinical signs of brucellosis experimentally in horses; the typical route of experimental infection is by intraconjunctival inoculation.[20,21] In this model, infected horses developed mild fever, and *B. abortus* was isolated from blood and internal organs of some horses weeks after inoculation, but no obvious clinical signs were observed.

Infection of people with *Brucella* spp. is thought to occur by food-borne ingestion but may also occur through the respiratory system or by exposure of mucosa or skin abrasions to organisms present in contaminated body fluids, tissues, or carcasses. The organism infects host macrophages, dendritic cells, and trophoblasts. As with most intracellular organisms, expression of gamma-interferon appears to be critical for limiting *Brucella* infection. The organism elicits only a moderate inflammatory response, which is likely a strategy for immune evasion. Molecular mechanisms that lead to intracellular persistence are being investigated. Excellent recent reviews of the pathogenesis and immune response to *Brucella* spp. are available.[22,23]

Many horses that are seropositive for *B. abortus*, which suggests exposure or infection with the organism, exhibit no recognizable clinical signs. In horses that develop clinical disease, *B. abortus* appears to have a predilection for infection of the tendons, muscles, bones, and joints. It is often associated with septic bursitis of the supraspinous bursa over the second and third dorsal vertebral spinous processes (fistulous withers) or supraatlantal bursa over the first and second cervical vertebra (poll evil). However, *B. abortus* is not the only potential etiologic agent in horses with fistulous withers. In geographic areas with a low prevalence of infection in cattle, *B. abortus* is rarely isolated from horses with fistulous withers.[8,24]

Fistulous withers secondary to *B. abortus* infection is characterized by a profuse serofibrinous exudate with varying degrees

*The authors acknowledge and appreciate the original contributions of these authors, whose work has been incorporated into this chapter.

of necrosis and formation of distended fistulous tracts of varying size (Figs. 37-1 and 37-2). The onset of clinical signs may be abrupt or insidious. Early clinical signs may include localized pain, heat, and swelling of the bursa without obvious external fistulation or exudate. Lethargy and general stiffness may be present.[7] The bursa ruptures, and purulent exudate drains from the fistula. There may be apparent healing, fibrosis, and refistulation. The exudate often contains multiple bacteria, including *Streptococcus* spp., *Staphylococcus aureus*, and *Actinomyces bovis*. Horses with fistulous withers that are seropositive to *B. abortus* are significantly more likely than seronegative horses with fistulous withers to have radiographic evidence of osteomyelitis of underlying dorsal spinous processes.[8]

There are reports of brucellosis as a cause of abortion in mares and isolation of *B. abortus* from equine fetuses.[13,14,25,26] This appears to be rare, however, and brucellosis cannot be considered an important cause of abortions in horses. Bursitis, tenosynovitis, arthritis, and osteomyelitis have been reported in other areas of the body.[9-12,27]

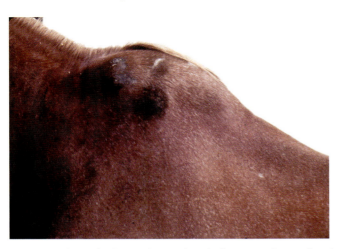

Figure 37-1 Chronic fistulous withers with multiple tracts in horse infected with *Brucella abortus*.

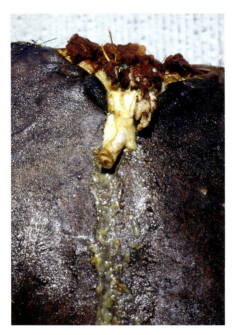

Figure 37-2 Severe postsurgical lesions and exudation in horse with fistulous withers.

Diagnosis

Brucella spp. should be considered as a cause of fistulous withers or poll evil, especially in horses that have commingled with cattle in endemic areas. Bacterial confirmation may be difficult because other bacteria are frequently found in exudates and may overgrow *B. abortus*, making the organism difficult to isolate. However, culture of aspirates from lesions or from affected tissues collected at surgery or necropsy is indicated to attempt confirmation of the diagnosis.

Because of the difficulty that may be encountered in attempts to culture *B. abortus* from horses with fistulous withers, concomitant serologic testing for detection of specific antibodies is recommended. A wide variety of serologic tests for brucellosis are available but few of them have been validated for horses and there is little or no comparative information on which to determine a preferred test for this species. The card test, a test widely used for screening of *B. abortus* in cattle, has poor specificity with frequent false-positive results.[28] The plate agglutination test is more sensitive and specific for diagnosis of brucellosis in cattle.[28,29] A titer of 50 or higher is considered positive.[9,24] A low number of false-positive results may be observed with these tests, and there are reports of *B. abortus* isolation from seronegative horses.[9] Other serologic tests that can be performed include tube agglutination, complement fixation, Coombs' (antiglobulin), mercaptoethanol, enzyme-linked immunosorbent assay (ELISA), brilliant green/crystal violet IgM test (rivanol), and agar gel diffusion. An increase in titer is considered diagnostic but may not occur in horses with long-standing infections. In these horses, a single high titer in combination with appropriate clinical signs should be considered diagnostic.

Therapy

Many therapies and combinations of therapies have been described for treatment of horses with brucellosis, including systemic antimicrobials, lavage, surgical resection of lesions, and administration of strain 19 vaccine. The preferred treatment in uncomplicated human brucellosis is doxycycline-aminoglycoside combination.[30,31] Although *Brucella* spp. are generally sensitive to tetracyclines, chloramphenicol, streptomycin, and selected sulfonamides, apparently there is insufficient diffusion into all affected sites, and treatment of horses solely with antimicrobials is rarely effective. Lavage of draining tracts with antiseptic or antimicrobial solutions has been recommended and may provide analgesic, antiseptic, and antifibroblastic effects.[8] Aggressive surgery has been recommended for some affected horses.[8] Removal of all diseased tissue is necessary and may be difficult. Postsurgical healing is often slow and may not be complete (see Fig. 37-2).

Administration of *Brucella* vaccine is reported to be an effective extralabel treatment for horses with *B. abortus* infection.[8,9,32-34] A survey of Florida veterinarians was conducted to ascertain perceived successes of various treatment regimens in horses with fistulous withers.[34] Treatment with strain 19 vaccine and antibiotics was considered successful in 37 of 46 horses (80.4%). Treatment with strain 19 vaccine alone was considered successful in 22 of 29 horses (75.8%). Treatment regimens have varied from a single dose (2-5 mL) of strain 19 vaccine administered subcutaneously to a series of three doses (5-8 mL) administered at 10-day intervals.[9,32,33] Subcutaneous administration of the vaccine has been associated with severe local and systemic reactions, including increased temperature, increased respiratory rates, inappetence, local inflammatory responses, and local abscessation.[9,32,33] In one report, three of four horses that received intravenous strain 19 vaccine died; the remaining horse recovered completely within 4 weeks.[8]

Prevention and Public Health Considerations

Horses should not be housed or pastured with *B. abortus*–seropositive cattle. Properly fitted saddles and harnesses may help to minimize trauma to the withers and reduce the incidence of disease. Effective parasite control programs to eliminate infestation with *Onchocerca* spp. and to control fly populations may also be beneficial.[7]

Brucellosis is a zoonotic disease. In the United States, human brucellosis is seen most frequently in slaughterhouse workers, farmers, dairymen, veterinarians, travelers to endemic areas, and laboratory workers.[35] Largely as a result of effective measures to control disease in animals, the number of human cases of brucellosis in the United States has decreased dramatically, from more than 6000 cases in 1947 to fewer than 200 per year since 1980.[35] Despite the low incidence in the United States and most industrialized countries, brucellosis remains one of the most common zoonotic diseases worldwide, with an especially high prevalence in the Mediterranean Basin and Arabian Peninsula, Central Asia, the Middle East, India, Mexico, and some areas of South America.[30,31] Most human patients are thought to be infected after exposure to livestock, consumption of raw milk and dairy products, or through occupational exposure (e.g., veterinarians, butchers, laboratory technicians).[30]

Infection in humans may result in subclinical disease (no apparent symptoms), acute disease, localized disease, relapsing infection, or chronic disease. Acute disease is characterized by malaise, chills, sweats, fatigue, and weakness. Some patients may also complain of myalgia, weight loss, arthralgias, or cough. Fever is common and may have an undulating or intermittent pattern.[35] Localized infection with *B. abortus* may occur in almost any organ, and clinical signs are related to the specific site of infection. As many as 10% of patients with brucellosis will relapse after apparent successful antimicrobial treatment. Relapse may occur as long as 2 years after initial treatment. Chronic infection longer than 1 year is characterized by persistent fatigue, malaise, and depression resembling chronic fatigue syndrome.[35]

Reports of brucellosis in humans in contact with infected horses are rare. However, there are reports of accidental infection of veterinarians with *B. abortus* from strain 19 vaccine.[36,37] The poor survival of *Brucella* in purulent exudate is probably one explanation for the limited reports. *Brucella abortus* infection is a reportable disease in the United States. Regulatory authorities may require that seropositive horses be quarantined or euthanized.[7]

The complete reference list is available online at www.expertconsult.com.

38 Contagious Equine Metritis

Michaela Kristula

Etiology

Contagious equine metritis (CEM) is a transmissible bacterial venereal disease of horses caused by *Taylorella equigenitalis*, a gram-negative coccobacillus.

Epidemiology

Taylorella equigenitalis is transmitted by either carrier stallions or mares directly during mating or by indirect genital contact with contaminated fomites (vaginal speculums, artificial vagina, or wash buckets).[1] There is evidence that transmission of *T. equigenitalis* through the use of fresh cooled or extended semen (with antibiotics) from an infected stallion is possible[2] but most likely infrequent.[1] The risk of transmission of *T. equigenitalis* through frozen semen has not been established.[1]

Contagious equine metritis was first reported in 1977 in Newmarket, England,[3] and the disease spread rapidly among horses in Europe. Two carrier Thoroughbred stallions imported from France were thought to have introduced the disease into the United States in 1978,[4] causing significant economic losses. Recently, pulsed-field gel electrophoresis (PFGE) confirmed that the 1978 CEM outbreak was caused by the two imported carrier thoroughbred stallions, each carrying a different strain of *T. equigenitalis*.[5] Further small-scale outbreaks of CEM were reported in 1979 in Trakehners in Missouri, in 1982 in thoroughbreds in Kentucky, and in 2006 in Lipizzaners in Wisconsin.[1] These outbreaks had minor economic consequences and were linked to imported carrier animals.[1] In 2008, a U.S.-origin stallion undergoing routine testing for semen export cultured positive for CEM. An epidemiologic investigation by the U. S. Department of Agriculture Animal Plant Health Inspection Service (USDA-APHIS) identified 23 stallions and 5 mares as infected with CEM in the United States.[6] Genetic profiles generated by PFGE identified a single common strain in all the infected horses,[5] and the suspected source of the outbreak was a stallion imported from Denmark in late 2000.[5,6] A significant finding of the 2008 domestic CEM outbreak was that most of the carrier stallions identified were exposed to *T. equigenitalis* through contaminated fomites at semen collection centers in the United States. An Arabian stallion in California tested positive for *T. equigenitalis* in 2010, with a PFGE strain not previously seen in this country.[5] The positive stallion was from Belgium but had been imported to the United States from the United Arab Emirates, a country not known to be affected by CEM.[2,7] In July 2011, the USDA National Veterinary Services Laboratories confirmed that an Arabian stallion born in Arizona tested positive for *T. equigenitalis* with a strain not previously identified in the United States, and an investigation for its source is ongoing.[7]

Taylorella asinigenitalis, a new species of *Taylorella*, was isolated from donkey jacks in the United States in 1997 and 1998.[8,9] In 1997, *T. asinigenitalis* (California strain) was isolated from a donkey jack in California.[8,9] In 1998, *T. asinigenitalis* (Kentucky strain) was isolated from two donkey jacks, a stallion, and seven nurse mares bred to them in Kentucky.[8-10] Experimental infection of mares was only possible with the Kentucky jack isolate of *T. asinigenitalis* not the California strain. Exposure to the Kentucky strain resulted in a clinical response and seroconversion consistent with CEM,[8] although mares naturally exposed to the Kentucky strain during the outbreak were not reported as developing any clinical signs.[10] Further evidence of *T. asinigenitalis* was not found in the United States until 2011, when a strain of *T. asinigenitalis* was isolated from a miniature donkey undergoing export quarantine (P. Timoney, personal communication). *Taylorella asinigenitalis* was isolated from a stallion in Sweden in 2004[11]; a stallion, mare, and 22 male donkeys between 1995 and 2008 in France[12]; and from 2 donkey jacks in Italy in 2008.[13] The origin and prevalence of *T. asinigenitalis* in horses and donkeys is not known, but risk factors for transmission are likely similar to *T. equigenitalis*.[10] More field studies are needed to establish the epidemiologic relationships between *T. asinigenitalis* in donkeys and horses.

Contagious equine metritis remains a clinically and economically important disease of horses.[14] Although national and international control procedures have reduced the incidence of CEM,[15,16] the disease has been detected in many countries, including Japan, Australia, most European countries, Iran, Turkey, and Brazil.[17] Contagious equine metritis has the potential to cause widespread outbreaks of short-term infertility in mares because of the increased international movement of stallions that occurs.[14,17]

Pathogenesis

In the mare, *T. equigenitalis* typically causes an intense neutrophilic endometritis (Fig. 38-1) that subsequently resolves with a subacute neutrophilic mononuclear endometrial response.[8] Stallions are inapparent carriers of *T. equigenitalis* on their external genitalia.[18] The bacteria may persist for an extended period

and are most frequently isolated from the fossa glandis and urethral sinus. The organism can also be isolated from the distal end of the urethra, the prepuce, and surface of the penis.[19] Schluter et al[20] isolated *T. equigenitalis* from the urethra, testis, epididymis, and seminal vesicles of an infected stallion at postmortem, suggesting *T. equigenitalis* can be transmitted through seminal fluid.

Clinical Findings

Infected stallions do not show clinical signs. Clinical signs in infected mares range from copious purulent vaginal discharge (Fig. 38-2) for up to 14 days after mating to shortened diestrous intervals unaccompanied by other clinical signs.[18] *Taylorella equigenitalis* typically causes temporary infertility in the mare. The acutely infected mare does not usually conceive. If pregnancy is successful, mares may still abort or produce foals at term that are also carriers. The variation in clinical disease in exposed mares is due to variation among strains of *T. equigenitalis*.[1] Bleumink-Pluym et al[21] demonstrated biologic differences between strains of *Taylorella*, and proposed strains differed in pathogenicity. Some mares recover spontaneously, whereas a smaller percentage of mares become chronic carriers, with the bacteria localizing most often in the clitoral sinuses and fossa and occasionally in the uterus.[1]

Diagnosis

The bacteriologic culture method for identification of *T. equigenitalis* is the "gold standard" method for preexport and preimport certification and detection of the carrier state. Cultures must be placed in Amies transport media with charcoal (BBL CultureSwab Plus Amies, Becton, Dickinson and Company, Sparks, MD) and refrigerated (4° C-6° C) during transit to a

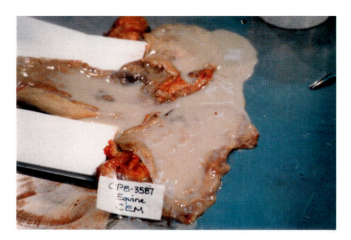

Figure 38-1 Purulent discharge and endometritis caused by *T. equigenitalis* in the uterus of a mare at postmortem. *(Courtesy the Maryland Department of Agriculture.)*

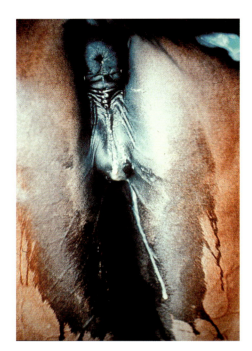

Figure 38-2 Purulent discharge caused by *T. equigenitalis* in a mare. *(Courtesy Dr. Don Simpson.)*

National Veterinary Services (NVSL)-approved laboratory[22] within 48 hours, then inoculated onto Eugon agar (with 10% chocolated horse blood) and CEM-selective agar. The plates are incubated at 37° C (98.6° F) for at least 7 days in an atmosphere of 5% to 10% carbon dioxide. Bacteria from suspicious colonies that are gram-negative, react positive to oxidase and phosphatase tests, and do not grow aerobically on blood agar are identified as presumptive CEM bacteria by agglutination with rabbit serum. Confirmatory testing is performed at NVSL by the polyclonal fluorescent antibody test.[22] Even with improved bacteriologic techniques, false negatives are common, particularly in imported stallions.[23-25] False-negative diagnoses are common because *T. equigenitalis* is fastidious and slow growing, and other bacteria that live in the genital tract of the horses overgrow *T. equigenitalis* despite inhibitors in the media.[24]

No serologic test is reliable for the diagnosis and control of CEM.[26] The complement fixation test (CFT) for CEM is of value for detecting infections in acutely infected mares[26,27] but is not reliable for identifying chronically infected mares.[26,28] The CFT is of no value for identifying infected stallions because stallions do not develop a demonstrable serum antibody response after exposure.[26,27] To date, no serologic differences have been observed between different strains of *T. equigenitalis*.[16]

Various polymerase chain reaction (PCR) tests have been developed to detect *T. equigenitalis*.[23,29,30] Real-time PCR testing for the detection of *T. equigenitalis* shows great promise to improve the specificity, sensitivity, and speed of identification of *T. equigenitalis* compared to culture.[30-32] Real-time PCR testing directly from genital swabs[32] can discriminate *T. equigenitalis* from *T. asinigenitalis*. Recent and future developments in molecular technology should enable epidemiologic analysis of different strains of *T. equigenitalis* and explain the pathophysiology and differences in virulence of different *T. equigenitalis* strains.[16]

Import Requirements

Contagious equine metritis was classified as a reportable disease in the United States following the outbreak of CEM in 1978 in Kentucky. After a second outbreak of CEM in Missouri in 1979, the disease was eradicated from the United States by rigorous testing, treatment, quarantine, and surveillance of infected and exposed horses. Mandatory testing of imported mares and stallions for *T. equigenitalis* was implemented to prevent reintroduction of CEM. Approximately 2500 horses are imported from CEM-affected countries annually and tested for CEM in U.S. quarantine stations.[6]

Currently, horses may be imported into the United States from CEM-infected countries after meeting preimport requirements and testing negative for dourine, glanders, equine piroplasmosis, and equine infectious anemia at the U.S. port of entry. Additionally, mares and stallions over 731 days of age are required to undergo further test procedures for CEM at a state-approved CEM quarantine facility.[33] These tests are carried out by an accredited veterinarian under supervision by either state or federal officials.

At the CEM quarantine facility, swabs are taken from both the mare's clitoral fossa (Fig. 38-3) and sinuses (Fig. 38-4) on three occasions, 3 days apart, for bacterial culture of *T. equigenitalis*. On the third culture, the clitoral sinuses are flushed with a ceruminolytic agent (Cerumene, Evsco Pharmaceuticals, Buena, NJ) and 0.2% nitrofuracin solution (Equi-Phar Nitrofurazone, Squire Laboratories, Revere, MA) and packed with 0.2% nitrofuracin ointment. The area is subsequently scrubbed with 4% chlorhexidine gluconate (Betasept, Purdue Frederick,

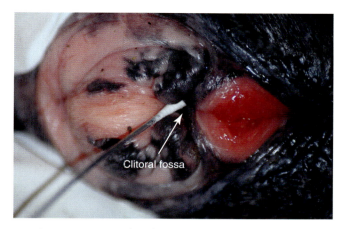

Figure 38-3 Location for culture of the clitoral fossa in the mare.

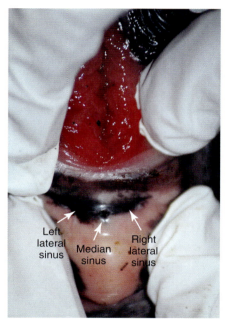

Figure 38-4 Location of the clitoral sinuses for culture in the mare. Stretching of the clitoral fossa enabled the orifice of the median sinus to be visualized in the photograph.

Norwalk, CT) and packed with 0.2% nitrofurazone ointment for 4 more days. Mares testing positive for CEM have the option of being returned to the country of origin or being treated.

For stallions, three separate swabs are obtained from the prepuce and surface of the penis (Fig. 38-5), the fossa glandis (Fig. 38-6), and the urethral sinus (Fig. 38-7). If the stallion is negative for *T. equigenitalis*, it is subsequently mated to two test mares and the stallion's external genitalia are scrubbed for 5 days with 4% chlorhexidine gluconate and packed with 0.2% nitrofurazone ointment. Three sets of cultures are taken from the stallion's test mare's clitoral sinuses and fossa at 3, 6, and 9 days after mating. A CFT for CEM is performed on each test mare at 15 days after mating. Stallions testing positive for CEM have the option of either being treated, castrated, or returned to their country of origin.

In the 2008 domestic CEM outbreak, carrier mares and stallions were identified using the existing import regulations previously described and augmented by additional testing requirements.[2] Most of the domestic carrier stallions (20 of 23) were identified on prebreeding cultures,[1,2] although only 18 out of 23 were identified on the first culture. Three of the 23 carrier stallions were found positive by test breeding susceptible mares followed by bacteriologic culture and serology of the test mares.[2] This contrasts with data on imported carrier stallions from U.S. quarantine stations, where a smaller percentage were identified on prebreeding cultures.[1,25] However, in both U.S. quarantine stations and the 2008 domestic CEM outbreak, the test breeding of stallions to test mares has been critical for the detection of carrier stallions negative on bacterial culture for *T. equigenitalis*.[2,25] More research is needed to determine the value of validating a PCR test and incorporating the PCR test into the current regulatory requirements.[2]

In 2010, the USDA tested 292 stallions for CEM.[2] The stallions were either actively breeding or previously imported into the United States.[2] None of the 292 stallions tested positive for *T. equigenitalis*.[2] Based on the resolution of the 2008 domestic CEM outbreak and the negative testing results of the 292

stallions, the USDA declared the United States free of *T. equigenitalis* in December 2010.[2] The United States could not maintain the 12-month CEM-free status because in 2011 the USDA reported the Arabian stallion from Arizona as positive for CEM. Because of the domestic outbreaks of CEM, many countries no longer recognize the United States as CEM-free and have placed restrictions on U.S. equine imports.[6]

Despite requiring preimport testing for CEM in CEM-affected countries of origin, at least 28 CEM positive horses have been identified during quarantine in the United States during the past 10 years.[6] As a result of the domestic CEM incidents in 2006 and 2008, APHIS is in the process of strengthening the CEM regulations by amending the regulations regarding the importation of horses from countries affected with CEM. This includes incorporating additional certification requirements for imported horses 731 days of age (2 years of age) or less and adding new testing protocols for horses over 731 days of age.[6] Additionally, the rules will be strengthened for importing Spanish Purebred horses,

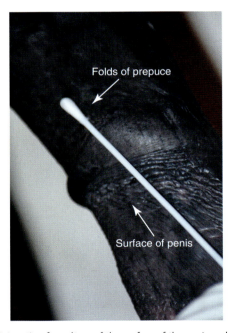

Figure 38-5 Location for culture of the surface of the penis and folds of the prepuce in the stallion.

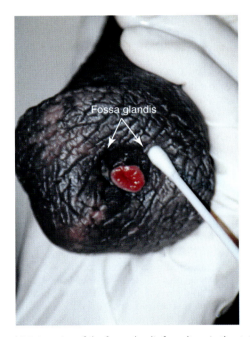

Figure 38-6 Location of the fossa glandis for culture in the stallion.

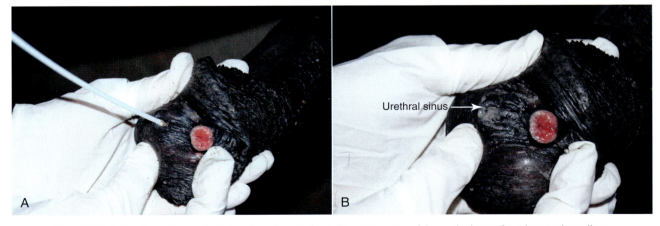

Figure 38-7 **A,** Location of the urethral sinus for culture in the stallion. **B,** Location of the urethral sinus for culture in the stallion.

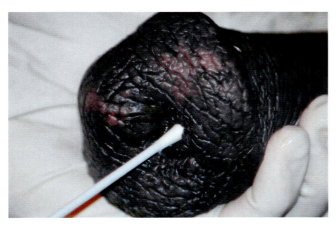

Figure 38-8 Location of the terminal urethra—proposed new culture site for the stallion.

Thoroughbred horses, and temporarily imported competition and entertainment horses.[6]

To increase the likelihood of detecting CEM in imported mares, the following amendments to the regulations are likely to be adopted[6]: (1) an additional culture sample from either the distal cervix or the endometrium will be required on the third set of samples and (2) a CFT will be required on arrival at a state's CEM quarantine facility. In addition, the time frame to complete sampling will be extended to a 12-day period with no less than 72 hours between each set of samples.

To increase the likelihood of detecting CEM in imported stallions, the following amendments to the regulations are likely to be adopted[6]: (1) an additional culture site from the stallion's distal urethra will be required (Fig. 38-8), (2) an additional culture sample from either the distal cervix or the endometrium will be required on the third set of samples from each test mare, (3) the CFT on the test mares will be required on day 21 instead of day 15 after breeding. In addition, the allowable time frame to complete all three culture sets on the test mares will be extended to a 12-day period, with specimens collected anytime between the third and fourteenth day after breeding and a minimum of 72 hours between each set.

Therapy

Although isolates of *T. equigenitalis* are distinguished by their variable sensitivity to streptomycin, the bacteria is sensitive to most common antibiotics such as penicillin, ampicillin, tetracycline, and trimethoprin-sulfamethoxazole.[34,35] The USDA guidelines for treatment of CEM-infected mares and stallions are the same as the prophylactic treatment schedule outlined for routine testing for CEM. For an infected mare, the clitoral

sinuses are flushed with a ceruminolytic agent and 0.2% nitrofuracin solution and packed with 0.2% nitrofurazone ointment. The clitoral sinuses and fossa are subsequently scrubbed for 4 more days with 4% chlorhexidine gluconate and packed with 0.2% nitrofurazone ointment. The external genitalia of the infected stallion are scrubbed for 5 days with 4% chlorhexidine and packed with 0.2% nitrofurazone ointment. Both treated stallions and mares are retested for CEM no less than 21 days after completion of treatment as previously described.

The USDA treatment protocols are not always effective, and a more aggressive combination of both topical and systemic antibiotics is required to treat some CEM-positive stallions and mares.[20,25,36,37] A treatment regimen with either oral trimethoprim-sulfamethoxazole 30 mg/kg twice daily (Mutual Pharmaceutical, Philadelphia) or an antibiotic choice based on sensitivity, along with cleaning of external genitalia (as previously described) and packing with 1% silver sulfadiazine cream (Thermazene, Kendall, Mansfield, MA), is recommended.[25] The addition of local antibiotics to the uterus of an infected mare may also be beneficial.

During the 2008 domestic CEM outbreak, 3 of 23 carrier stallions and 1 of 5 carrier mares remained culture positive after initial treatment following the USDA treatment protocol.[2] The treatment was switched to topical 1% silver sulfadiazine, and all horses were confirmed culture negative.[2]

Prevention and Control

Stringent control methods and regulations for horse movement continue to be necessary to minimize and control the spread of CEM. Control measures are based on taking bacterial swabs prior to breeding to establish freedom of disease and using strict hygiene measures during breeding activities. Specifically, disposable gloves should be worn and changed between horses, equipment should be either disposable or sterilized between horses, and clean water should be used for each horse. Although there is an increasing awareness of CEM in the United States, prebreeding cultures for CEM are not routinely requested except by organizations engaged in the collection of stallions for artificial insemination.

With the estimated annual market of export of U.S. horses valued at $300 million,[14] the United States seeks to regain its CEM-free status to both facilitate international trade in horses and protect the U.S. domestic equine population and industry.

Public Health Considerations

There is no evidence that *T. equigenitalis* affects humans.[38]

The complete reference list is available online at www.expertconsult.com.

Anaplasma phagocytophilum Infection

Nicola Pusterla and John E. Madigan*

Etiology

Anaplasma phagocytophilum (formerly *Ehrlichia equi*) is the etiologic agent of equine granulocytic anaplasmosis (EGA; formerly equine granulocytic ehrlichiosis). *Anaplasma phagocytophilum* has recently been classified based on genetic analysis in the genera *Anaplasma*, with *Anaplasma marginale*, which causes infectious anemia in cattle by infecting erythrocytes, and *Anaplasma platys*, which causes canine cyclic thrombocytopenia by infecting platelets.[1]

Because 16S ribosomal ribonucleic acid (rRNA) gene sequences differ only up to three bases (99.1% homology) among former *E. equi*, *E. phagocytophila* (cause of tick-borne fever in Europe), and the recently discovered human granulocytic ehrlichiosis (HGE) agent, these organisms are now all considered strains of *A. phagocytophilum*. *Ehrlichia equi*, *E. phagocytophila*, and the HGE agent are also closely related on the basis of morphology, host cell tropism, and antigen analysis by indirect fluorescent antibody tests.[2] The deoxyribonucleic acid (DNA) sequences of the 16S rRNA gene from the peripheral blood of naturally infected horses in Connecticut and California are identical with those of the HGE agent.[3] Moreover, infective human blood from HGE patients injected into horses causes typical EGA, can be transmitted to other horses, and induces protection in horses to subsequent challenge with *E. equi*.[4,5] These data suggest that the agent of EGA and HGE are conspecific. *Anaplasma phagocytophilum* has been cultured in vitro using the tick-embryo cell line IDE8[6] and a human promyelocytic leukemia cell line HL60.[7]

Anaplasma phagocytophilum is found in membrane-lined vacuoles within the cytoplasm of infected eukaryotic host cells, primarily neutrophilic and eosinophilic granulocytes. These inclusion bodies consist of one or more coccoid or coccobacillary organisms approximately 0.2 µm in diameter, as well as large granular aggregates called *morulae*, which are approximately 5 µm in diameter. Organisms are visible under high, dry, or oil-immersion objective with light microscopy. They stain deep blue to pale blue-gray with Giemsa or Wright-Leishman stains. Electron microscopy reveals loosely packed, ovoid to round *A. phagocytophilum* organisms in several membrane-lined vacuoles of equine granulocytes. The size of vacuoles ranges from 1.5 to 5 µm in diameter.

Epidemiology

Equine granulocytic anaplasmosis occurs during late fall, winter, and spring. The horse represents an aberrant host, and it seems unlikely that infected horses could serve as effective reservoirs of *A. phagocytophilum* because the presence of the organism in an affected animal is generally limited to the acute phase of the disease. Horses of any age are susceptible, but the clinical manifestations are less severe in horses younger than 4 years.[8] Horses from endemic areas have a higher seroprevalence of antibody to *A. phagocytophilum* than horses from nonendemic areas, suggesting the occurrence of subclinical infection in some animals.[9] Further, horses introduced into an endemic area are more likely to develop EGA than native horses.

Persistence of *A. phagocytophilum* has not been demonstrated in naturally infected horses. However, infection with *A. phagocytophilum* can persist in experimentally infected horses for at least 129 days, but the continued presence of the organism is not associated with detectable clinical or pathologic abnormalities.[10] The disease is not contagious by direct transmission, but infection can be transferred readily to susceptible horses with transfusion of as little as 20 mL of blood from horses with active infection. Most often, one infected horse is observed in a group of horses in the same pasture. The disease, first reported in the late 1960s in the foothills of northern California, has since been reported in horses in Washington, Oregon, New Jersey, New York, Colorado, Illinois, Minnesota, Connecticut, Florida, Wisconsin, and outside the United States, in Canada, Brazil, and Europe.

In recent years, EGA has been experimentally transmitted by the western black-legged tick *(Ixodes pacificus)*[11] and the deer tick *(Ixodes scapularis)*.[12] Further, an epidemiologic study in California showed that the spatial and temporal pattern of EGA cases closely paralleled the well-characterized life history and distribution of *I. pacificus*, but not other ticks typically associated with horses.[13] In the eastern and midwestern United States, *I. scapularis* is the vector of granulocytic anaplasmosis, and small rodents, such as white-footed mice, chipmunks, and voles, as well as the white-tailed deer, are potentially important reservoirs.[14] In California, white-footed mice, dusky-footed wood rats, cervids, lizards, and birds have been proposed as reservoirs.[15,16] In Europe, where granulocytic anaplasmosis is transmitted by the sheep tick *(Ixodes ricinus)*, the reported reservoir hosts are wild rodents, deer, and sheep.[17]

Pathogenesis

The pathogenesis of EGA is poorly understood. After entering the dermis by tick-bite inoculation and spread, presumably through lymphatics or blood, ehrlichiae invade target cells of the hematopoietic and lymphoreticular systems. Ehrlichiae replicate within vacuoles of professional phagocytes. Whether or how these granulocytic ehrlichiae directly injure cells is not known, despite evidence of cytolytic activity in vitro.[7] Granulocytic ehrlichiae are suspected to initiate a cascade of

*The authors acknowledge and appreciate the original contributions of these authors, whose work has been incorporated into this chapter.

localized pathologic inflammatory events after invading organs such as spleen, liver, and lungs. Subsequent tissue injury is thought to be mediated locally by accumulating inflammatory cells and systemically by induction of proinflammatory responses.[18] The mechanism by which sufficient cells are removed to cause pancytopenia is unknown. However, the presence of normal cellularity or diffuse hyperplasia of bone marrow, combined with hemophagocytosis in spleen and lymph nodes, and the presence of infected granulocytes in spleen and lung support peripheral sequestration, consumption, and destruction of normal blood elements as the major mechanisms for ehrlichia-induced pancytopenia.[18]

Granulocytic anaplasmosis caused by *A. phagocytophilum* triggers dysfunction or suppression of host defenses, and an early paper describes that horses infected with *A. phagocytophilum* are predisposed, as are humans and sheep, to develop opportunistic infections and secondary infections with bacteria, fungi, and viruses.[19] During infection, animals develop defects in both humoral and T-cell–mediated immunity and abnormalities in normal neutrophil phagocytic and migratory functions.[20]

Immunologic studies with *A. phagocytophilum* indicate both a cell-mediated and a humoral immune response to clinical infection. Horses that recover from experimental infections develop antibody responses by 21 days after infection.[21] In naturally infected horses, antibody titers peak 19 to 81 days after the onset of clinical signs. Humoral immunity persists for at least 2 years and does not appear to depend on latent infection or carrier status.[22,23]

Clinical Findings

The incubation period after experimental exposure of horses to infected ticks is 8 to 12 days and after needle inoculation of infectious blood, 3 to 10 days. The incubation period for natural infection is believed to be less than 14 days. This estimate is based on the time of onset of clinical signs in horses that had presumptive exposure to ticks while on a trail ride before returning to a nonendemic area for EGA.

The severity of clinical signs of EGA varies with the age of the horse and the duration of the illness.[8] This can make clinical recognition of EGA difficult at the first examination. Adult horses over 4 years of age generally develop characteristic progressive signs of fever, depression, partial anorexia, limb edema, petechiation, icterus, ataxia, and reluctance to move. Clinically and experimentally, it appears that horses less than 4 years of age tend to develop milder signs, including moderate fever, depression, moderate limb edema, and ataxia. In horses less than 1 year of age, clinical signs may be difficult to recognize, with only a fever present. During the first 1 to 2 days of infection, fever is generally high, fluctuating from 39.4° C to 41.3° C (102.9° F-106.3° F). Initial clinical signs are reluctance to move, ataxia, depression, icterus (Fig. 39-1), and petechiation of nasal septum mucosa (Fig. 39-2). Weakness and ataxia can be severe, to the point that horses will sustain fractures after falling. Staggering is often seen, and the tendency to assume a base-wide stance suggests proprioceptive deficits. Partial anorexia develops in most affected horses. Limb edema (Fig. 39-3) and more severe signs of disease develop by days 3 to 5, with fever and illness lasting 10 to 14 days in untreated horses. Heart rate is often modestly high (50-60 beats/min). Rarely, there is cardiac involvement with development of cardiac dysrhythmias. Ventricular tachycardia and premature ventricular contractions have been observed with the usual clinical signs. The clinical course of the disease ranges from 3 to 16 days. The disease is normally self-limiting in untreated horses; fatalities can result

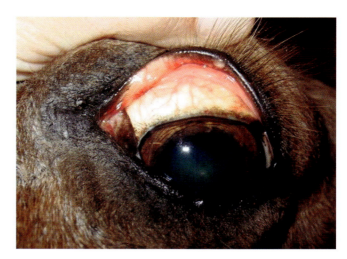

Figure 39-1 Horse infected with *Anaplasma phagocytophilum* showing icteric sclera.

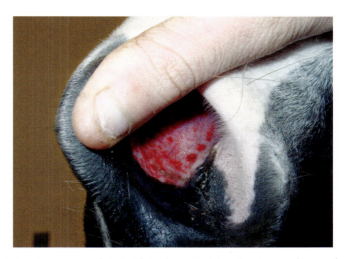

Figure 39-2 Horse infected with *A. phagocytophilum* showing petechiation of nasal septum mucosa.

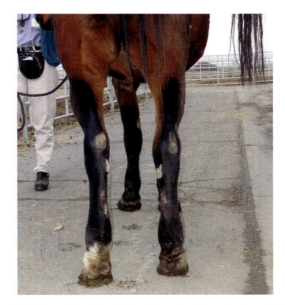

Figure 39-3 Horse infected with *A. phagocytophilum* showing distal limb edema.

from secondary infection and from injury secondary to trauma caused by incoordination. Abortion has not been observed in pregnant mares, and laminitis has not been reported as part of the clinical syndrome.

The initial stage of the disease is characterized by the development of a fever and may be mistaken for a viral infection. The differential diagnoses for EGA include purpura hemorrhagica, liver disease, equine infectious anemia, equine viral arteritis, and encephalitis.

Laboratory abnormalities in horses affected with EGA may include leukopenia, thrombocytopenia, anemia, icterus, and characteristic inclusion bodies (morulae) in neutrophils and eosinophils. The morulae are pleomorphic, blue-gray to dark blue in color, and often have a spoke-wheeled appearance.

Diagnosis

Diagnosis is based on awareness of geographic area for infection, typical clinical signs, abnormal laboratory findings, and visualizing characteristic morulae in the cytoplasm of neutrophils and eosinophils in a peripheral blood smear stained with Giemsa or Wright's stain (Fig. 39-4). Because affected horses are leukopenic, a greater percentage of neutrophils can be examined by use of the buffy coat preparation and subsequent staining. The number of cells containing morulae varies from less than 1% of

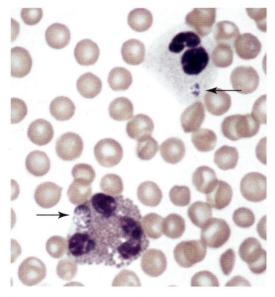

Figure 39-4 *Anaplasma phagocytophilum* inclusions *(arrows)* in neutrophilic and eosinophilic granulocytes of horse with equine granulocytic anaplasmosis (buffy coat smear, Giemsa stain, 1000×).

cells initially to between 20% and 50% of neutrophils by days 3 to 5 of infection. However, more than three ehrlichial inclusion bodies need to be seen on a blood smear to consider the diagnosis definitive.

Culture is rarely attempted for horses infected with *A. phagocytophilum.* Alternatively, an indirect fluorescent antibody test is available, and paired-titer testing with a significant (fourfold or greater) rise in antibody titer to *A. phagocytophilum* can be performed to confirm recent exposure retrospectively.[9] However, because inclusion bodies are always visible during the midstage of the febrile period, antibody testing is not usually required to make a definitive diagnosis.

Recently, several polymerase chain reaction (PCR) assays have been developed for members of the *A. phagocytophilum* genogroup and are considered to be highly sensitive and specific.[24-26] Polymerase chain reaction analysis is useful for the diagnosis of EGA, particularly during early and late stages, when the number of organisms may be too small for diagnosis by microscopy (Fig. 39-5).

Pathologic Findings

The characteristic gross lesions observed in experimentally infected horses are hemorrhages, usually petechiae and ecchymoses, and edema. Edema is observed in the legs, ventral abdominal wall, and prepuce. Hemorrhages are most common in the subcutaneous tissues, fascia, and epimysium of the distal limbs. Histologically, there is inflammation of the small arteries and veins, primarily those in the subcutis, fascia, and nerves of the legs, as well as in the ovaries, testes, and pampiniform plexus.[19] Vascular lesions may be proliferative and necrotizing, with swelling of the endothelial and smooth muscle cells, cellular thromboses, and perivascular accumulations, primarily of monocytes and lymphocytes but also, to a lesser extent, neutrophils and eosinophils. Mild inflammatory vascular or interstitial lesions have also been reported in the kidneys, heart, brain, and lungs of animals necropsied during the course of the disease.[18] The ventricular tachycardia and premature ventricular contractions occasionally observed in affected horses are thought to be associated with myocardial vasculitis. Further, horses with a chronic bacterial infection may develop an exacerbation of the preexisting lesion (bronchopneumonia, arthritis, pericarditis, lymphadenitis, cellulitis).[19]

Therapy

The intravenous administration of oxytetracycline at 7 mg/kg body weight once daily for 5 to 7 days has been an effective treatment for EGA.[8] Prompt improvement in clinical appearance and appetite and decrease in fever are noticed within

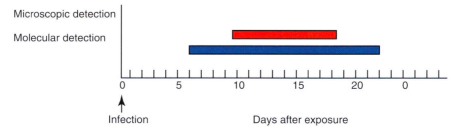

Figure 39-5 Microscopic and molecular detection time of *A. phagocytophilum* in blood of horse experimentally infected with *Ixodes scapularis.*

12 hours of treatment. Failure of defervescence within 24 hours strongly indicates another cause for illness. On rare occasions, horses treated for less than 7 days relapse within the following 30 days. When untreated, the disease can be self-limiting in 2 to 3 weeks if no concurrent infection is present, but weight loss, edema, and ataxia are increased in severity and duration. In treated horses, ataxia will persist for 2 to 3 days, and limb edema may persist for several days. Inclusion bodies generally are difficult to find after the first day of treatment and are no longer present within 48 to 72 hours. Supportive measures are recommended in severe cases, including fluid and electrolyte therapy, supportive limb wraps, and stall confinement of severely ataxic horses to prevent secondary injury. The prognosis in EGA is considered excellent in uncomplicated cases, in sharp contrast to some of the differential diagnoses.

Prevention

At present, no vaccine is available against EGA, and prevention is limited to the practice of tick control measures such as the use of permethrin repellent products.[27]

The complete reference list is available online at www.expertconsult.com.

40 Neorickettsia risticii

Nicola Pusterla and John E. Madigan*

Etiology

Neorickettsia risticii (formerly *Ehrlichia risticii*) is the etiologic agent of equine neorickettsiosis (EN), also called Potomac horse fever, *equine monocytic ehrlichiosis* or *equine ehrlichial colitis*. *Neorickettsia risticii* has recently been classified based on genetic analysis in the genera *Neorickettsia* among three other species: *Neorickettsia sennetsu* (human agent of Sennetsu fever), *Neorickettsia helminthoeca* (agent of salmon poisoning in the dog), and an ehrlichia-like bacterium present in the metacercarial stage of the fluke *Stellantchasmus falcatus* (SF agent).[1] Based on sequence analysis of the 16S ribosomal ribonucleic acid (rRNA) gene, *N. risticii* shares 98.9% homology with *N. sennetsu*, 94.8% with *N. helminthoeca*, and 99.1% with the SF agent. Strain variance has been determined among 11 *N. risticii* strains, with a maximum divergence of 0.7%.

Neorickettsia risticii is a gram-negative coccus and stains dark blue to purple with Giemsa stain and Romanowsky's stain, red with Macchiavello stain, and pale blue with hematoxylin and eosin (H&E). The organism tends to occupy one side of the cytoplasm rather than being symmetric and is generally round. *Neorickettsia risticii* divides by binary fission and is found in membrane-lined vacuoles within the cytoplasm of primarily macrophages and glandular epithelial cells in the intestine of the horse. The organism is rarely observed in peripheral blood monocytes. In cell culture or host cells, *N. risticii* occurs in two different forms, either singly or in groups (morulae), the former being 0.8- to 1.5-µm electron-lucent and the latter 0.2- to 0.4-µm electron-dense bodies. *Neorickettsia risticii* has been successfully cultured in human histiocytic lymphoma cells and in canine, equine, and murine monocytes.

Epidemiology

Equine neorickettsiosis was recognized originally in 1979 along the Potomac River in the state of Maryland.[2] Equine neorickettsiosis is known to occur in 44 of the United States, three Canadian provinces (Nova Scotia, Ontario, Alberta), South America (Uruguay, Brazil), Europe (The Netherlands, France), and India. Isolation or detection of the causative agent from clinical cases of the disease using conventional cell culture or molecular detection by polymerase chain reaction (PCR) has only been reported from 14 states (California, Illinois, Indiana, Florida, Kentucky, Maryland, Michigan, New York, New Jersey, Ohio, Oregon, Pennsylvania, Tennessee, Texas, Virginia, and Washington), Nova Scotia, Uruguay, and Brazil.

The epidemiology of *N. risticii* has been the subject of intensive research efforts for more than 20 years. The disease typically occurs near freshwater streams and rivers and on irrigated pastures, mainly during middle to late summer (May to November). The seasonal incidence of the disease, the geographic distribution of EN, and the experimental transmission by the intradermal route implied the involvement of a blood-sucking arthropod as a vector. The historic connection between other ehrlichial agents and tick vectors prompted many to regard ticks as prime candidates for the transmission of *N. risticii*. Therefore many studies focused on identifying an arthropod vector for EN. Despite intensive investigation, however, no evidence was found for spread of the disease by arthropod vectors such as ticks.[3]

The causative organism is present in the feces of experimentally infected horses and can be experimentally transmitted by the oral route using feces from infected horses. These findings, together with the close serologic and molecular relationship between *N. risticii* and *N. helminthoeca* isolated from flukes, suggest that the vector of *N. risticii* may not be an arthropod but instead a helminth closely associated with aquatic habitats. Barlough et al[4] provided strong evidence that trematodes, which

*The authors acknowledge and appreciate the original contributions of these authors, whose work has been incorporated into this chapter.

use operculate freshwater snails as intermediate hosts, may be involved in the life cycle of *N. risticii*. This theory was confirmed when deoxyribonucleic acid (DNA) of *N. risticii* was detected by nested PCR in operculate snails (*Pleuroceridae: Juga* spp.) collected from stream waters in a northern California pasture where EN is endemic. The results of sequencing PCR-amplified DNA from a suite of genes (16S rRNA, groESL heat shock operon, and 51-kDa major antigen genes) indicated that the source organism was clearly related to the type strain of *N. risticii*. The PCR-amplified product is associated with the presence of virgulate cercariae in the snail secretions[5] (Fig. 40-1). The number of snails harboring the trematode stages varied from 3.3% to 93.3%, and the number of PCR-positive snails (3.3%-20%) appears to depend on the size of the snails, the month of collection, and geographic origin.

In northern California, the species of snail incriminated in the life cycle of *N. risticii* is *Juga yrekaensis*, a common pleurocerid snail, which inhabits fresh or brackish stream water in the northwestern United States (Fig. 40-2). Additionally, DNA from *N. risticii* has been detected in virgulate cercariae in lymnaeid snails (*Stagnicola* spp.) from northern California, in virgulate xiphidiocercariae isolated from pleurocerid snails *(Elimia livescens)* in central Ohio, and from pleurocerid snails *(Elimia virginica)* in central Pennsylvania, suggesting that other types of snails may also harbor infected trematodes.[5-7] This type of trematode is known to become encysted in the second intermediate

host. *Neorickettsia risticii* DNA has been detected by PCR in mesocercariae and metacercariae in various aquatic larval, nymphal, and adult insects such as caddisflies, mayflies, damselflies, and dragonflies in northern California and in central Pennsylvania[7,8] (Fig. 40-3). Polymerase chain reaction investigations suggest that the prevalence of aquatic insects harboring *N. risticii* varies from 10% to 80%.

Recently, two potential helminth vectors, *Acanthatrium* spp. and *Lecithodendrium* spp., both infected with *N. risticii*, were found in the intestine of bats and birds collected in northern California and Pennsylvania[9,10] (Fig. 40-4). Further, transstadial

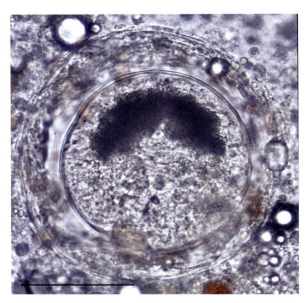

Figure 40-3 Photomicrograph of metacercaria collected from caddisfly larva (bar = 0.2 mm). *(From Madigan JE, Pusterla N: Vet Clin North Am Equine Pract 16:487, 2000.)*

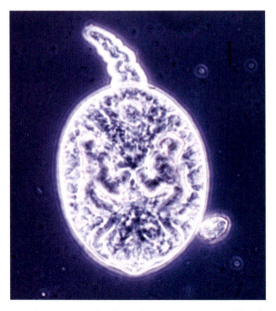

Figure 40-1 Photomicrograph of virgulate cercaria released by pleurocerid snails of genus Juga (bar = 0.01 mm).

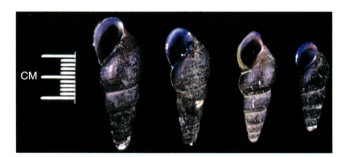

Figure 40-2 Juga yrekaensis pleurocerid snails collected from equine neorickettsiosis endemic region in northern California (bar = 1 cm).

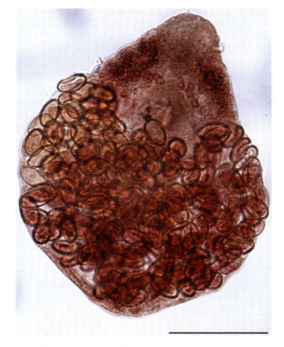

Figure 40-4 Photomicrograph of adult Acanthatrium trematode collected from intestine of Myotis yumanensis bat (bar = 0.5 mm). *(From Madigan JE, Pusterla N: Vet Clin North Am Equine Pract 16:487, 2000.)*

transmission of *N. risticii* in the vector *Acanthatrium oregonense* was recently documented by molecular characterization.[11]

These trematodes belong to the *Lecithodendriidae* family, common parasites of bats, birds, and amphibians in North America, which use pleurocerid freshwater snails as first intermediate hosts and aquatic insects as second intermediate hosts. Additional trematodes, members of the *Lecithodendriidae* or other families, may also act as vectors of *N. risticii* in other endemic regions of the United States.

Since *N. risticii* was first identified, no definitive reservoir host of the organism has been proposed. Seroepidemiologic studies have revealed the presence of antibody titers specific to *N. risticii* in domestic and wild animals, such as dogs, cats, coyotes, pigs, and goats, from regions in which EN is endemic.[12] A variety of nonequine mammalian species, such as mice, dogs, cats, and cattle, are susceptible to *N. risticii*.[13-15] Based on vertical transmission of *N. risticii* in the trematode *Acanthatrium oregonense* and detection of *N. risticii* DNA in the blood, liver, or spleen of bats and swallows, it is speculated that these insectivores act as both definitive host of the helminth vector and natural reservoir of *N. risticii*.

The biologic activity of *N. risticii* in infected vectors has been recently investigated by the inoculation of PCR-positive trematode stages into horses and mice. Horses injected subcutaneously with *N. risticii* PCR-positive trematode stages (virgulate cercariae and sporocysts) collected from *J. yrekaensis* snails developed clinical signs and hematologic changes consistent with EN.[16] Furthermore, *N. risticii* was transmitted to mice using PCR-positive metacercariae isolated from caddisfly larvae (*Dicosmoecus* spp.).[8] These data confirm that *N. risticii* is associated with a helminth vector and illustrate the value of PCR technology as a screening method for epidemiologic studies.

Pathogenesis

The mode of transmission of *N. risticii* has remained one of the greatest mysteries of EN. *N. risticii* has been successfully transmitted by the intravenous, intramuscular, subcutaneous, intradermal, and oral routes using whole blood from naturally infected horses or with infected cell culture material.[17-21] In light of recent epidemiologic discoveries concerning the vector

of *N. risticii* and its helminth hosts, horses could conceivably be exposed to *N. risticii* through skin penetration by infected cercariae or by consuming infected cercariae in water or metacercariae in a second intermediate host such as an aquatic insect. One horse fed adult caddisflies (*Dicosmoecus gilvipes*) in northern California[22] and two horses fed adult caddisflies (*Cheumatopsyche campyla*, *Hydropsyche hageni*) or a mixture of adult caddisflies and mayflies (*Leucrocuta minerva*) in central Pennsylvania developed EN.[7] These studies attempted to mimic the natural route of infection with *N. risticii* and showed that oral transmission using infected aquatic insects was not only possible, but also that the clinical disease produced was similar to that seen in naturally infected horses. Aquatic insects, such as caddisflies and mayflies, represent a likely source of infection because of their abundance in the natural environment, their high infection rate with *N. risticii* as determined by PCR, and the mass hatches regularly observed during summer and fall. Under natural conditions, horses grazing near rivers or creeks will ingest adult insects along with grass (adult insects live near water and are likely to die there) or consume adult insects trapped on the water surface. Horses also may consume insects that are attracted by stable lights and subsequently accumulate in feed and water (Fig. 40-5). A serosurvey performed at two Ohio racetracks in 1986 reported that cases of PHF were associated with certain barns, as well as specific stalls in those barns.[23] Aquatic insects might have been present in larger numbers in those locations, perhaps attracted by specific lighting, and were accidentally ingested by the horses in their food. A recent outbreak of EN in Minnesota and Iowa was the first one to incriminate mayflies as significant vectors for horses.[24] The use of night lighting was determined to be a consistent risk factor during that outbreak.

After natural or experimental transmission in horses, *N. risticii* infects blood monocytes. Although the pathogen is readily phagocytized by monocytes, it appears to elude the host's defense mechanisms by inhibiting lysosomal fusion with phagosomes.[25] *Neorickettsia risticii* can be isolated by cell culture from the peripheral blood monocytes of infected horses as early as 6 days after ingestion of adult aquatic insects harboring the organism, and bacteremia can persist up to 2 weeks after spontaneous resolution of clinical signs.[7] *Neorickettsia risticii* also has a predilection for the intestinal wall, especially that of the large colon. Colonic epithelial cells, mast cells, and tissue

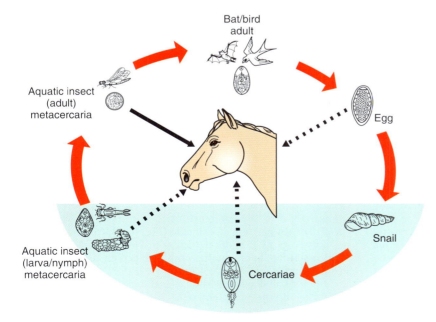

Figure 40-5 Life cycle of helminthic vector of Neorickettsia risticii and natural route of transmission. Solid black arrow represents demonstrated route of transmission with adult aquatic insects. Dashed black arrows represent possible routes of infection with trematode eggs, free cercariae, or larval/nymphal aquatic insect stages.

macrophages are the targets of infection. Lesions are confined to the gastrointestinal tract. The resultant diarrhea is thought to be caused by loss of epithelial cell microvilli, reduction in electrolyte transport, and increase in intracellular cyclic adenosine monophosphate (cAMP) in infected intestinal cells. All these mechanisms contribute to the reduced luminal absorption of electrolytes (sodium and chloride) and increased water losses in the large and small colon.[26]

Neorickettsia risticii causes significant immune depression in mice and detectable alterations of the immune system in horses. Whether a clinically significant immune depression occurs in horses is unclear. Recovered horses are resistant to development of clinical disease by rechallenge for a least 20 months. Humoral and cell-mediated immune responses appear to have significant roles in conferring protection against *N. risticii*. Antibodies can be protective when they block the pathogen's attachment to or penetration of host cells. This occurs by several mechanisms such as blocking ehrlichial binding to its specific receptor, by inhibiting ehrlichial metabolism, or by conferring antibody-dependent cell-mediated cytotoxicity. However, the presence of antibodies does not always correlate with clearance of ehrlichial organisms and presence of protective immunity. This has been shown with horses that have been vaccinated with a killed *N. risticii* vaccine and subsequently developed clinical disease after natural exposure.[27] Antibodies induced by a killed vaccine may not be effective because protective antigens may only be expressed during cell invasion or replication. Cell-mediated immunity likely plays a dominant role in protecting the host from *N. risticii* infection, as shown for other rickettsial infections.

Clinical Findings

The incubation period for *N. risticii* infection in horses is approximately 1 to 3 weeks. In two recent studies, horses fed aquatic insects harboring *N. risticii*–infected metacercariae developed clinical signs 9 to 15 days after oral challenge.[7,22] The clinical features of EN have been extensively reported over the years. Naturally occurring cases of EN are typified initially by an acute onset of mild depression and anorexia, followed by a biphasic increase in body temperature ranging from $38.9°C$ to $41.7°C$ ($102°F$ to $107°F$). At this stage, decreased intestinal sounds can be auscultated.

Within 24 to 48 hours, moderate to severe diarrhea ranging from "cow pie" to watery consistency develops in approximately 60% of affected horses. The onset of diarrhea is often accompanied by mild abdominal discomfort. Some horses develop severe toxemia and dehydration, which result in cardiovascular compromise characterized by increased heart rate and respiratory rate and congested mucous membranes. Subcutaneous edema along the ventral abdomen has also been observed in horses with EN. Laminitis can supervene as a severe complication of EN in as many as 40% of affected horses. Laminitis may progress, despite resolution of other clinical signs. Interestingly, laminitis has only been reported in naturally infected horses and probably reflects as-yet undetermined pathophysiologic mechanisms related to the natural route of transmission. It should be emphasized that a horse with EN may present with all or any combination of these clinical signs.

Case-fatality rates vary from 5% to 30% and depend mostly on the strain involved. Fatalities are associated with toxemia and severe laminitis. Long-term problems appear to be related to sequelae such as laminitis. To date, no evidence exists that *N. risticii* infection results in chronic disease. Attempts to isolate *N. risticii* by culture or PCR after clinical signs have abated have been unsuccessful.

Transplacental transmission of *N. risticii* has been reported in natural and experimental infections, and the organism may induce abortion or resorption of the fetus or produce weak foals, which require extensive neonatal care. Pregnant mares, which exhibit clinical signs of EN, can subsequently abort around 7 months of gestation, regardless of the severity of infection.[28,29] In mares experimentally infected at 90 to 120 days of gestation, abortion occurred at 65 to 111 days after inoculation.[30] Abortions are spontaneous with a fetus in fresh condition. Gross findings of the fetuses include meconium staining and petechiation of external surfaces.

Hematologic findings vary in the early stage of EN from a transient leukopenia (white blood cell count <5000/μL), characterized by a neutropenia and a lymphopenia, to a normal hemogram, despite evidence of systemic toxicity.[31] A common finding in cases of EN is a marked leukocytosis (>14,000/μL), usually observed within a few days of disease onset. Increases in both packed cell volume and plasma protein concentration secondary to dehydration and hemoconcentration can occur. A transient nonregenerative anemia and thrombocytopenia may develop and can be profound in some horses. Horses often present with evidence of a hypercoagulable state, characterized by significant changes in plasma fibrinogen, fibronectin, factor VIII, and plasminogen. In contrast to the tick-borne *Anaplasma phagocytophilum* (see Chapter 39) infection, visual observation of *N. risticii* in peripheral blood monocytes is rarely successful.

Diagnosis

A provisional diagnosis of EN is often based on the presence of typical clinical signs and the seasonal and geographic occurrence of the disease. A definitive diagnosis of EN, however, should be based on the isolation or detection of *N. risticii* from the blood or the feces of infected horses. Serologic testing using indirect fluorescent antibody or enzyme-linked immunosorbent assay (ELISA) test formats is of limited value as a diagnostic tool because antibody levels to *N. risticii* may not be detectable for some time after infection. Paired serum titers must be evaluated; single titers are useless for confirmatory testing of EN. The reliability of the indirect immunofluorescence technique for antibody detection has been questioned because the test yields a high percentage of false-positive results.[32]

Isolation of the agent in cell culture from the peripheral blood of affected patients, although possible, can take from several days to weeks of culture before detection is successful and is not routinely available in many diagnostic laboratories. The recent development of *N. risticii*–specific PCR assays has greatly facilitated and hastened the diagnosis of EN.[33,34] In experimentally and naturally infected animals, PCR performed on feces and peripheral blood was more sensitive than culture.[35] Conventional PCR assays, however, are time-consuming and prone to contamination. Real-time PCR platforms associated with automated nucleic acid extraction allow the detection of *N. risticii* DNA within the same day of sample receipt, making this technology a much more practical assay for routine diagnostic testing.[36] To enhance the chances of detection of *N. risticii*, the assay should be performed on blood, as well as fecal samples, because the presence of the organism in blood and feces may not necessarily coincide (Fig. 40-6). Another routine application of PCR is the detection of *N. risticii* DNA in fresh or formalin-fixed and paraffin-embedded colon tissue, allowing postmortem diagnosis.

Differential diagnoses should include peritonitis and any clinical syndrome of enterocolitis such as salmonellosis, clostridial diarrhea, or intestinal ileus secondary to displacement or

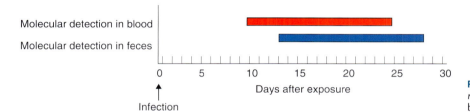

Figure 40-6 Molecular detection time of *Neorickettsia risticii* by real-time polymerase chain reaction (PCR) in blood and feces of horses with Potomac horse fever.

obstruction. Diagnostic tests specific to ruling out these diseases should be concurrently pursued.

Pathologic Findings

Gross necropsy findings in the acute stage of EN disease include distended large colon and cecum filled with watery contents. Mucosal hyperemia and ulceration and areas of necrosis and hyperplasia of lymphoid follicles and lymph nodes may also be observed. Microscopic changes include areas of moderate to severe lymphohistiocytic infiltration of the submucosa and lamina propria of the cecum and large colon.[26] Lack of severe lesions and absence of neutrophil infiltration are important in the differential diagnosis of EN. Both silver stain and immunoperoxidase procedure using a specific antibody to *N. risticii* can demonstrate rickettsial organisms in intestinal epithelial cells and macrophages in paraffin-embedded tissue specimens. Although not routinely done, electron microscopy can be used to detect *N. risticii* infection during disease.

Changes in fetuses aborted because of *N. risticii* infection are consistent, unique, and diagnostic of this abortion syndrome. Fetuses have increased volume of feces within the small and large intestine and liver discoloration. Microscopic findings include lymphohistiocytic enterocolitis, periportal hepatitis, lymphohistiocytic myocarditis, and severe splenic inflammation characterized by both intense lymphohistiocytic infiltration and lymphoid necrosis.[28-30] *N. risticii* can be recovered by cell culture from bone marrow, spleen, lymph node, colon, and liver of aborted fetuses.

Therapy

Horses with EN can be treated successfully by the intravenous (IV) administration of oxytetracycline at 6.6 mg/kg twice a day, when given early in the clinical course of the disease. A response to treatment is usually seen within 12 to 24 hours, associated with a decrease in rectal temperature followed by an improvement in demeanor, appetite, and borborygmal sounds.[37] The disease does not progress after initiation of treatment. If therapy is begun early in the course of EN, clinical signs frequently resolve by the third day of treatment. No more than 5 days of antimicrobial therapy are usually needed. Whether treatment of clinically affected broodmares during the diarrheal stage of disease prevents subsequent abortion remains unknown. In horses exhibiting signs of enterocolitis, IV administration of polyionic fluids is extremely important to prevent hypovolemia and shock. Addition of calcium, magnesium, and potassium to fluids may be necessary in horses with prolonged anorexia and

fluid losses. Concurrent use of nonsteroidal antiinflammatory drugs (NSAIDs), such as flunixin meglumine (0.25 mg/kg IV or orally [PO] every 8 hours [q8h]) or phenylbutazone (2.2-4.4 mg/kg IV or PO q12h) is indicated. Horses developing severe protein-losing enteropathy associated with decreased albumin concentrations may benefit from plasma transfusion. Preventive measures for laminitis, the most common potentially lethal sequela of EN, should be implemented as well. Although no specific therapy is universally recognized to prevent laminitis, the authors recommend stall confinement of affected horses, use of foot support (deep bedding, padded support), ice for the feet, and administration of NSAIDs as previously described.

Prevention

Several inactivated, whole-cell vaccines based on the same strain of *N. risticii* are commercially available and have been used in endemic areas for several years to protect horses from EN. Vaccination has been reported to prevent all clinical signs except fever in 78% of experimentally infected ponies.[38] Protection conferred by this vaccine appears to be much shorter in duration than protection after natural infection, which can last up to 2 years. For unexposed horses, considering the time required to develop immunity after vaccination, the short-lasting humoral immunity, and the existence of antigenic variations in the field, it is questionable how much benefit the vaccine will provide under field conditions. Vaccine failure has been reported and attributed to antigenic and genomic heterogeneity among *N. risticii* isolates.[27] Vaccine failure may also be caused by lack of protection at the site of exposure because the natural route of transmission seems to be the oral route. An improved vaccine for EN is strongly desired in the future.

If vaccination of horses is performed using inactivated vaccines, the primary series should include two vaccines given 4 weeks apart. A third dose should be given if the patient is a foal that received the first dose at less than 5 months of age. Thereafter, boosters should be administered at 4- to 6-month intervals. *Neorickettsia risticii*–induced abortion is not prevented by vaccination.

The ingestion of aquatic insects carrying infected trematodes is probably the only means of transmission of *N. risticii* under natural circumstances. In endemic regions, control measures should limit access of susceptible horses to freshwater streams, ponds, and irrigated pastures during peak incidence, as well as reducing night lights on horse facilities to minimize the attraction of water insects during mass hatches.

The complete reference list is available online at www.expertconsult.com.

Enteric Clostridial Infections

J. Scott Weese

Etiology

The genus *Clostridium* comprises a diverse group of gram-positive, anaerobic, spore-forming bacteria, most of which are nonpathogenic and important components of the intestinal microflora (Figs. 41-1 and 41-2). Only a small number of the more than 300 recognized *Clostridium* species are enteropathogens (Box 41-1), and the common consideration of clostridia as "bad" bacteria has led to oversimplification of the role of this

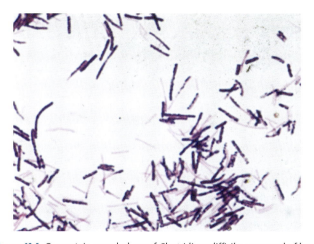

Figure 41-1 Gram stain morphology of *Clostridium difficile* composed of long, thin rods. The variable staining appearance *(pink to purple)* may be encountered in cultures after 48 hours or longer.

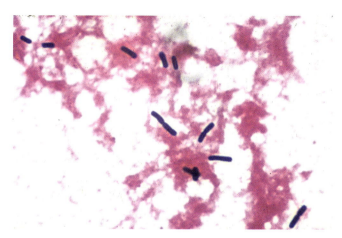

Figure 41-2 Gram stain appearance of *Clostridium perfringens*, demonstrating the characteristic appearance of short, thick, gram-positive *(purple)* rods.

genus in disease and excessive broad assumptions about the relationship between clostridial abundance and gut health. In reality, it appears that clostridia are important components of the intestinal microflora, and disruptions of the healthy intestinal ecosystem are actually associated with a loss of clostridial abundance and diversity.[1] However, although many clostridial species are probably important for health and only a small percentage of species are potential enteropathogens, a small group of clostridia account for considerable morbidity and mortality in horses. In particular, *Clostridium difficile* and *Clostridium perfringens* are important enteropathogens and in some areas are the most frequently identified causes of colitis.[2]

Epidemiology and Pathogenesis

Clostridium difficile

Clostridium difficile is a fastidious anaerobe that can be found in the intestinal tract of horses and numerous other species, as well as in the environment (see Fig. 41-1). As a spore-forming bacterium, it exists in two states; vegetative cells and spores. The vegetative form is the active growing form that causes disease in the intestinal tract. It is highly susceptible to oxygen and dies quickly outside the body.[3] The spore form, in contrast, is highly tolerant of oxygen, disinfectants, and a variety of other stressors and can persist outside of the body for years. As a result, the vegetative form is responsible for disease, whereas the spore form is the infectious form that is acquired through fecal-oral exposure. Presumably, *C. difficile* spores are most often ingested directly from feces and contaminated farm environments, but exposure through food and water cannot be discounted.

The epidemiology and pathophysiology of *C. difficile* infection (CDI) in horses are incompletely understood. Although an important cause of colitis, *C. difficile* can also be found in healthy individuals, particularly in young foals and horses treated with antimicrobials (Table 41-1). The point prevalence of *C. difficile* shedding in healthy adult horses is low, but *C. difficile* exposure may be quite common and shedding transient.[4] This was highlighted by one study that reported a 5.5% point prevalence but a 40% cumulative prevalence when horses were tested monthly for a year.[4] Therefore it is possible that horses very regularly ingest *C. difficile*, yet eliminate the organism in a short period of time, only to be reexposed in the future, typically with no evidence of disease. This is important to consider when evaluating the pathophysiology of disease because simple exposure to *C. difficile* is rarely enough to induce disease.

Development of CDI involves proliferation of *C. difficile* in the intestinal tract and production of *C. difficile* toxins. Most *C. difficile* strains possess genes that encode production of toxin A, an enterotoxin, and toxin B, a cytotoxin. A minority of strains produce only toxin B, and these are able to cause disease.[5] Additionally, some strains may produce a binary toxin (CDT),

Box 41-1 *Clostridium* Species that can be Found in the Intestinal Tract of Horses*

Species that are Associated With Enteric Disease in Horses	Species that have not Been Associated With Enteric Disease in Horses
C. difficile	C. aceticum
C. perfringens	C. aldrichii
C. septicum	C. aminobutyricum
C. sordellii	C. aminophilum
	C. aminovalericum
	C. asparagiforme
	C. baratii
	C. bartlettii
	C. bifermentans
	C. bolteae
	C. botulinum
	C. butyricum
	C. cadaveris
	C. carnis
	C. cellobioparum
	C. chauvoei
	C. clostridioforme
	C. cochlearium
	C. cylindrosporum
	C. diolis
	C. disporicum
	C. estertheticum
	C. formicaceticum
	C. glycolicum
	C. haemolyticum
	C. hathewayi
	C. hiranonis
	C. hylemonae
	C. indolis
	C. josui
	C. kluyveri
	C. leptum
	C. litorale
	C. lituseburense
	C. longisporum
	C. methylpentosum
	C. novyi
	C. pasteurianum
	C. phytofermentans
	C. polysaccharolyticum
	C. propionicum
	C. saccharobutyricum
	C. sardiniense
	C. scindens
	C. sphenoides
	C. sporogenes
	C. sticklandii
	C. subterminale
	C. symbiosum
	C. tertium
	C. tetani
	C. tetanomorphum
	C. thermocellum
	C. ultunense
	C. xylanolyticum

*Unpublished data from M Costa and JS Weese.

Table 41-1 Prevalence of *Clostridium difficile* Shedding by Nondiarrheic Horses

Country	Population	N	Prevalence	Reference
Sweden	Adults	140	0%	108
Sweden	Adults	273	0%	109
	Adults with colic	65	0%	
	Foals <14 days of age	56	29%	
	Foals treated with erythromycin and rifampin	16	44%	
Canada	Adults	255	0.4%	2
	Foals	47	0%	
Canada	Race horses	540	7.6%	21
	Broodmares	120	5.8%	
	Adults admitted to a teaching hospital	82	4.9%	
Italy	Adults	42	33%	110
United States	4H club horses	25	8%	111
Australia	Adults	112	0%	24
Slovenia	Adults and foals	20	5%	112

strain can be found in horses and concern has been expressed that it might be an emerging problem in horses in some regions.[4,19,21] There has been inadequate investigation of the role of strain in disease in equine CDI, and it is unclear whether hypervirulent strains are an issue. In general, the strains that are found in horses are the same that are found in humans,[21-24] raising concern about the potential for interspecies transmission.

Since healthy horses appear to be frequently exposed to *C. difficile*, certain factors must account for why some individuals develop disease while others remain healthy. In humans, antimicrobial therapy and hospitalization are the main risk factors for development of CDI. Penicillins, cephalosporins, and clindamycin have typically been considered the highest-risk antimicrobials in humans, although attention has recently shifted toward humans treated with fluoroquinolones as a particularly high-risk group.[25-27] Other risk factors in humans include nasogastric intubation, immunosuppressive therapy, organ transplantation, presence of a gastrostomy or jejunostomy tube, and use of stool softeners.[28-30] The role of proton pump inhibitors (PPIs) in CDI in humans has been controversial, with conflicting data.[31-36] In basic terms, a wide range of factors that either increase the risk of *C. difficile* exposure, disrupt the protective gastrointestinal microflora, or suppress the immune system can be associated with CDI. Yet, there is increasing recognition of CDI in the absence of any known risk factors.[37-39]

There has been limited study of risk factors in horses. Antimicrobial therapy is presumably an important risk factor for development of CDI in horses and is often implicated in equine CDI, although CDI certainly can occur in horses in the absence of antimicrobial exposure and it does not appear that antimicrobial exposure creates a higher risk of CDI versus colitis of other etiologies.[40] The risk of antimicrobial-associated CDI and relative risk of different antimicrobials may vary geographically. This is perhaps best illustrated by Swedish reports of CDI in mares whose foals were being treated with erythromycin.[41] It was presumed that mares were being exposed to low levels of erythromycin during treatment of their foal, and CDI was experimentally reproduced with low-dose erythromycin administration.[42] There is essentially no information regarding other risk factors in horses. Potential risk associated with PPI use in horses has not been reported, although it cannot be discounted.

While most of the focus is on colitis, *C. difficile* has also been implicated as a cause of duodenitis/proximal jejunitis, although

the role of which is currently unclear.[6-9] Some strains lack toxin genes and are therefore clinically irrelevant.

Various strains of *C. difficile* can be encountered in horses. In humans, it is clear that certain strains are hypervirulent.[10-13] The greatest concern is the ribotype 027/NAP1 strain, which can be found in humans internationally and which has been identified in a horse.[14] There is also concern about ribotype 078, a strain that is increasingly identified in humans with community-onset CDI[15-18] and which is common in food animals.[16,18-20] This

Table 41-2 Prevalence of *Clostridium perfringens* in Healthy Adult Horses and Foals

Country	Population	N	Prevalence	Reference
United Kingdom	Adults	60	0%	113
United Kingdom	Foals	124	19%	114
Switzerland	Adults	58	1.7%	53
United States	Broodmares before foaling	124	19%	56
	Broodmares after foaling	116	30%	
	Foals 8-12 hours old	124	64%	
	Foals 3 days old	124	90%	
	Foals 1-2 months old	115	33%	
Japan	Foals	29	18%	115
Canada	Adults	135	0.7%	4

Table 41-3 Classification of *Clostridium perfringens* Isolates Based on Production of Toxins

	Toxins					
Type	Alpha	Beta	Epsilon	Iota	Beta-2	Enterotoxin
A	×				±	±
B	×	×	×		±	±
C	×	×			±	±
D	×		×		±	±
E	×			×	±	±

evidence is only available from a single study in one region, so the strength of this association is unclear.[43]

Clostridium perfringens

Clostridium perfringens is a rather ubiquitous bacterium that can be found in a wide range of animals and in the environment (see Figure 41-2). It has been described as being the most widely occurring pathogenic bacterium and is a recognized cause of enteric disease in horses of all ages[2,44-50]; however, a true understanding of its role in disease has proved somewhat elusive because of challenges with diagnostic testing.

This bacterium is well adapted for survival in the intestinal tract and in the environment, but the prevalence of fecal shedding varies greatly between different animal species. *Clostridium perfringens* actually appears to be uncommon (or at least uncommonly detected) in healthy adult horses but relatively common in foals and broodmares (Table 41-2). Although *C. perfringens* appears to be uncommonly present or present at sub-detectable levels in healthy adult horses, it probably colonizes and proliferates quickly in response to intestinal microflora disruptions, as can occur with stress, diet changes, antimicrobial therapy, and other enteric diseases.[51] This ability to proliferate in response to events complicates diagnosis, by clouding cause versus effect.

Although there may be diagnostic challenges as discussed later, there is little doubt that *C. perfringens* is an enteropathogen in horses, causing disease ranging from mild diarrhea to rapidly fatal colitis. As with *C. difficile*, the pathogenesis of disease is not well understood, and the reason that some horses develop disease while others are simply colonized likely involves a combination of host and bacterial factors. The study of risk factors in horses has been limited. One study evaluating foal management practices associated with *C. perfringens* diarrhea identified housing in a stall or drylot for the first 3 days of life; the presence of other livestock on the premises; delivery on dirt, sand, or gravel; and feeding of small amounts of hay and grain to the mare postpartum as risk factors for development of *C. perfringens* enteritis in foals.[47] Antimicrobial treatment is likely a risk factor as well in adult horses and foals, along with any factor that modifies the protective intestinal microflora.

The type of *C. perfringens* is also a very important determinant of disease. *Clostridium perfringens* isolates can produce a range of toxins, many of which are poorly understood. Isolates are classified into different types based on production of four major toxins: alpha, beta, epsilon, and iota (Table 41-3). In addition, a variety of other toxins may be produced, most notably beta-2 toxin and enterotoxin. Although beta-2 toxin and enterotoxin (*C. perfringens* enterotoxin [CPE]) are not classified as "major" toxins, they may be the most important toxins clinically and both have been associated with diarrhea in adult horses and foals.[2,45,46,52-55]

Type A is the predominant type in normal and diarrheic horses.[56,57] All type A strains produce alpha toxin in varying amounts, although the role of alpha toxin alone in production of disease is questionable. Type A strains have been associated with disease in horses, although this may be based on production of beta-2 toxin or enterotoxin by some strains not because of inherent pathogenicity of all type A strains. Currently, it is unclear whether type A strains that do not produce another toxin are clinically relevant in horses. Although less common, type C strains have been associated with enterocolitis in horses, with particularly severe disease in foals.[48,50,58-60] There are limited reports of disease caused by type B and D strains.[57] Most recent attention has been paid to CPE and beta-2. A correlation between the presence of beta-2 toxin and fatal enterocolitis has been reported,[53] but limited study has been performed and the true role of this toxin in disease is rather unclear. More information is available for CPE and an association between the presence of CPE or strains possessing the *cpe* gene and diarrhea has been reported in horses.[2,46] Conclusive evidence is still lacking, although there is perhaps more information indicating a role of this toxin in equine disease compared to any other *C. perfringens* toxin.

Other Clostridia

An etiologic agent is not identified in a large percentage of horses with colitis, and it is possible (or probable) that other clostridia may play a role in some of these cases for which a definitive etiology is never identified. Determining a role for other clostridia is complicated by our poor understanding of the range of clostridia that may be present in the intestinal tract, our limited understanding of the intestinal microflora, difficulties isolating many clostridia, and problems differentiating overgrowth of species in response to disease from disease caused by overgrowth. Accordingly, there is limited information about other clostridial enteropathogens. *Clostridium sordellii* and *Clostridium septicum* have attracted some attention,[61] however, minimal information is currently available.

Clinical Findings

The "classic" presentation of clostridial enteric disease is acute and often severe colitis, but the clinical presentation will vary, depending on a variety of factors, including the area of the gastrointestinal tract that is affected. Horses of any age can be affected, including foals less than 24 hours of age. Clostridial enteritis can range from mild self-limiting disease to rapidly fatal necrohemorrhagic enterocolitis. It is impossible to differentiate CDI from *C. perfringens*–associated diarrhea or disease caused by other clostridia. It is similarly impossible to differentiate clostridial enteritis from types of enteritis, such as salmonellosis, based on clinical signs.

Diarrhea is the most readily apparent clinical presentation of enterocolitis and is indicative of large colon disease. Varying degrees of depression, dehydration, toxemia, colic, anorexia, and pyrexia are typically present, although some horses may simply have mild diarrhea in the absence of any signs of systemic inflammation. In other cases, horses have an acute onset of severe disease, with significant diarrhea, abdominal pain, and systemic inflammatory response.[62] In particularly severe cases, profound disease may be present before the onset of diarrhea. It may be difficult to differentiate peracute colitis from intestinal accident, such as large colon volvulus, based solely on clinical presentation, and death may occur before diarrhea is observed.

Small intestinal involvement can occur concurrently with large colon disease; however, the small intestinal component is not usually readily identifiable. If only the small intestine and cecum are affected, diarrhea may not be observed because of the tremendous absorptive capacity of the large colon. In these horses, colic, depression, pyrexia, hypoproteinemia, toxemia, and leukopenia may be present. If the proximal small intestine is involved, gastric reflux may develop. Although not proved, it is possible clostridial disease localized to the small intestine may present with nonspecific clinical signs, including pyrexia, protein loss, and mild colic.

Mortality rates secondary to clostridial enterocolitis are highly variable. With acute CDI, mortality rates of up to 42% have been reported, with adult horses more likely to die than foals.[2] Conflicting data are available regarding mortality rates of CDI versus colitis of other etiologies,[40,62] and care must be taken when interpreting published mortality rates because they are biased toward severe cases presented to referral hospitals. Mortality data are limited for *C. perfringens*–associated diarrhea, but fatal disease certainly can occur and there have been anecdotal associations of *C. perfringens* with severe disease.

Complications, such as laminitis and thrombophlebitis, frequently develop in horses with colitis of any etiology, presumably from toxemia and systemic inflammatory response. Bacterial translocation has not been adequately studied in horses with colitis. It is logical to assume that loss of integrity of the intestinal mucosa would lead to translocation of intestinal microorganisms, yet extraintestinal infections, such as meningitis, endocarditis, arthritis, or pneumonia, are rarely identified in adult horses. Extraintestinal infection is a greater concern in foals. In some patients, thrombosis of major intestinal vessels, presumably because of disseminated intravascular coagulation (DIC) (Fig. 41-3), will result in rapid deterioration, with ischemic necrosis, severe pain, abdominal distention, and death.

Diagnosis

Clostridium difficile

The "gold standard" for diagnosis of CDI is detection of toxin B in feces using the cell cytotoxicity assay, but this test is time-consuming, expensive, and not readily available commercially. Clinically, diagnosis is usually based on identification of *C. difficile* toxin A or B or both in fecal samples. A variety of immunoassays are available and are widely used; however, only one (*Clostridium difficile* TOX A/B II ELISA, Techlab, Blacksburg, VA) has been specifically validated in horses.[63] This test, which detects both toxins A and B, was reported to have a sensitivity and specificity of 84% and 96%, respectively, compared to the

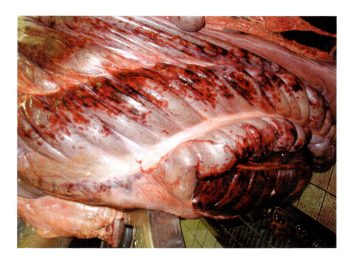

Figure 41-3 Disseminated intravascular coagulation (DIC) in a horse that died of severe *Clostridium difficile* infection. Note the widespread petechial and ecchymotic hemorrhages.

gold standard. A variety of other assays are available, yet preference should be given to tests that have been validated with equine feces because some human tests can perform poorly in samples from animals.[64]

The target of available immunoassays should be considered. Some commercial assays only detect toxin A, which will not detect disease caused by toxin A negative/B positive strains.[6] Immunoassays are also available for glutamate dehydrogenase (GDH), sometimes referred to as "*common antigen*," which is present in toxigenic and nontoxigenic strains. These tests can be rapid, cost-effective, and highly sensitive, at least in humans,[65] but suffer from limitations in specificity because they detect both toxigenic and nontoxigenic strains and the presence of the organism in the absence of toxin production. Because of the high sensitivity, low cost, and quick turnaround time, combination testing could be considered. With this approach, GDH immunoassay is used as a rapid screening test, with negative results having a high negative predictive value, and positive samples tested further by enzyme-linked immunosorbent assay (ELISA). The main advantage of this is the ability to quickly and confidently rule out CDI; however, it also depends on the same sensitivity in equine specimens as compared to humans, something that has not yet been proved.

A limitation of ELISA-based approaches is sensitivity. Although commercial ELISAs may have relatively high sensitivities when compared to the gold standard, it is accepted that the gold standard actually only has moderate sensitivity, so false negative results are common. In humans, concerns about false negative tests, because of the major impact of CDI in hospitalized patients and the potential for hospital-associated transmission, have led to increasing interest in rapidly and highly sensitive screening methods. Enrichment culture is a very sensitive method,[66] if done by a laboratory with adequate facilities and experience, yet the long turnaround time (5 to 10 days) precludes its use in a clinical setting. Real-time polymerase chain reaction (PCR) can be highly sensitive[67-69] and is increasingly being used in human healthcare settings because of the high sensitivity and short (<1 day) turnaround time. An additional advantage is that PCR can target toxin genes (typically *tcdB*, the gene encoding toxin B), thereby preventing false positives from nontoxigenic strains. However, the usefulness of real-time PCR (or any other test that detects the organism) decreases as the background prevalence of *C. difficile* colonization increases. In humans, it is assumed that *C. difficile* colonization is uncommon, so positive results most likely indicate infection. Additionally, a moderate false positive rate is considered acceptable because of the desire to identify as many infected patients as possible, to ensure prompt treatment and isolation. However, because colonization rates can be high in horses, real-time PCR may have limited clinical specificity. As the pretest likelihood of colonization increases (e.g., with young horses and horses treated with antimicrobials), the positive predictive value will decrease. Accordingly, the role of PCR and culture in diagnosis of CDI in horses is currently unclear. Because PCR could be highly sensitive, an adequately validated assay could be a useful screening tool and would confidently rule out CDI; however, PCR-positive/toxin-negative results would be expected, and interpretation of these is difficult. Culture is typically of limited availability and reserved for epidemiological or outbreak investigations. Typing of C. *difficile* isolates is rarely indicated clinically and most relevant for outbreaks or situations with atypical clinical presentations.

Clostridium perfringens

Diagnosis of C. *perfringens* enteritis is complicated. Identification of clostridial spores in fecal smears has been used by some clinicians, but spores are present in diseased and nondiseased animals. Fecal smears are not specific because of the abundance of commensal clostridia that cannot be differentiated visually from C. *perfringens*. *Clostridium perfringens* is relatively easy to isolate from feces, but positive culture results do not necessarily indicate disease, particularly in young horses, where colonization rates may be high. Additionally, the tendency of C. *perfringens* to overgrow in response to disruptions of the intestinal microflora limit the usefulness of culture, hampering differentiation of cause versus effect. Quantitative culture of C. *perfringens* provides no additional information, since there is no evidence that the number of C. *perfringens* shed relates to the presence or absence of disease. Negative culture results from a properly collected and tested sample may be useful to rule out C. *perfringens*–associated diarrhea; however, it is not known whether a single negative sample is adequate. Isolation of C. *perfringens* from a diarrheic horse is therefore, at best, slightly suggestive that C. *perfringens* might be involved.

Toxigenic culture, whereby C. *perfringens* isolates are tested by PCR to determine which toxin genes they contain, may provide additional information. Genotyping is likely most useful when strains are identified that are uncommon in normal horses and more commonly associated with severe disease such as that seen in neonatal hemorrhagic colitis caused by type C. Detection of strains containing enterotoxin or beta-2 toxin genes might also be useful; however, these strains can still be found in healthy horses,[52,56] so the possibility of false-positive results still remains. Toxigenic culture therefore provides some additional information but is only suggestive and is perhaps best suited as an adjunctive test such as to provide added confidence to positive ELISA results for CPE.

The detection of specific C. *perfringens* toxins directly in feces is preferable to detection of toxin genes because this indicates the elaboration of the toxin protein in situ. Two types of enterotoxin assays are currently commercially available, including the ELISA and reverse passive latex agglutination (RPLA) test.[2,54] The RPLA is thought to be less specific, and ELISA is more often used; however, it has not been validated in horses.

Polymerase chain reaction can be used to detect specific C. *perfringens* toxin genes in feces. Adequately developed and validated assays could have a high sensitivity and short turn-around time, which are distinct clinical advantages. However, issues of specificity remain because toxigenic C. *perfringens* can be found in the absence of disease. Polymerase chain reaction

is probably most useful when targeting toxin genes that are more likely clinically relevant, such as beta-2 and CPE, whereas testing directed only at alpha toxin is probably of limited usefulness. The combination of a positive ELISA with positive CPE gene PCR is probably the strongest evidence of C. *perfringens*–associated disease. Confident diagnosis of other disease caused by other strains and toxins remains difficult because of a lack of toxin-detection tests.

Other Clostridia

Diagnosis of other clostridia as causes of enteric disease is difficult. General anaerobic culture could be performed, but many clostridia are not readily isolated using standard methods. Further, it is difficult to impossible to ascribe disease to a certain bacterial species that is present in a fecal sample in the absence of organized research studies because of the relatively poor overall knowledge of the equine clostridial microflora. Presence of a specific *Clostridium* at high numbers in a diarrheic fecal sample might raise suspicion, but it can certainly not indicate infection. This was highlighted by a report of experimental lincomycin-induced colitis, in which *Clostridium cadaveris* was initially implicated as the cause[70] but subsequently refuted.[71] Introduction of molecular testing that can detect a range of clostridia will, if anything, cloud the picture further without concurrent clinical and epidemiologic studies to determine the relevance of results. Although PCR assays that detect various clostridia are commercially available, there does not appear to be any clinical utility at this time.

Treatment

Supportive care is the most important component of a treatment plan for clostridial enteritis of any presentation or etiology. Fluid therapy, oncotic support, and good nursing care are the hallmarks of treatment of colitis. If antimicrobial-associated diarrhea is present, cessation of antimicrobials is ideal, if possible. Often, if antimicrobials are required to treat an underlying condition, clinicians will change antimicrobials if diarrhea occurs; however, there is no evidence to indicate whether this is useful, of little effect, or likely to cause further intestinal microflora disruption.

Antimicrobial Therapy

Although sometimes used, there is little evidence to support broad-spectrum systemic antimicrobial therapy in adult horses with colitis. The goal of systemic antimicrobial therapy in horses with colitis is the prevention or treatment of clinically significant bacterial translocation because there is no evidence that systemic antimicrobials are effective against enteric clostridial overgrowth. Scant evidence exists to suggest that bacterial translocation is a significant clinical problem in adult horses, and antimicrobial therapy could further disrupt the already perturbed intestinal microflora. However, the real risks and benefits have not been adequately evaluated, and some clinicians choose to treat certain horses with systemic antimicrobials. In adult horses, systemic antimicrobial therapy is sometimes used in those with severe neutropenia, marked toxic changes in white blood cells, hemorrhagic diarrhea, or persistent or intermittent pyrexia; however, other clinicians do not use antimicrobials in those situations, with no readily apparent difference in outcome. Broad-spectrum antimicrobial therapy is probably indicated in all neonatal foals with colitis. Although there is also little published information about bacterial translocation in foals with clostridial colitis, the naïve immune system of neonatal foals probably increases the likelihood of extraintestinal infection and anecdotal experiences suggest that severe extraintestinal infections do occur in this population.

Specific antimicrobial therapy directed against enteric clostridia may be useful and is widely used clinically, although objective data are limited and it is likely that many cases would respond to supportive therapy alone. Antimicrobial susceptibility testing of enteric clostridia is rarely performed by diagnostic laboratories, and with acute colitis, the time delay involved with culture and susceptibility testing of anaerobes would be problematic. Therefore empiric treatment choices are usually made. Fortunately, development of resistance is less common in clostridia compared to common aerobic bacteria, so reasonable susceptibility assumptions can be made.

Metronidazole is widely used for the treatment of colitis in horses and has been reported to be effective in the treatment of idiopathic colitis.[72] Studies evaluating the efficacy of metronidazole in clostridial colitis in horses have not been reported. Metronidazole is commonly used for the treatment of CDI in humans and is widely used in horses with anecdotal success. Recently, concern has been expressed about the use of metronidazole in severe CDI in humans because of apparent decreasing efficacy.[73-75] Vancomycin is more often being used as first-line therapy in severe cases,[76] with recent approval of fidaxomicin providing another option.[77] However, metronidazole is still widely recommended as a first-line treatment in patients without severe disease.[78] The reason for decreasing response to metronidazole in humans is unclear and is not clearly associated with metronidazole resistance. Metronidazole resistance has been identified in *C. difficile* from humans[79-82] but appears to be quite rare. It is unclear whether the human experiences can or should be extrapolated to horses. There is no indication that metronidazole is becoming less effective in horses, but the variability in clinical presentation and outcome and sporadic nature of disease might complicate identification of decreasing efficacy. Metronidazole resistance has been reported among equine *C. difficile* isolates,[83] but this has only been from one region and has not been confirmed. Vancomycin has been used in horses with anecdotal success; however, no objective data are present and there are concerns about the use of this critically important human drug in horses. Fidaxomicin has not been studied in horses.

In the absence of objective data, use of metronidazole continues to be a reasonable first-line approach for CDI in horses. The author currently uses an empiric dosing regimen of 15 mg/kg orally (PO) every 8 hours (q8h) for horses of all ages. Metronidazole pharmacokinetics have been evaluated in healthy horses,[84] but neither intestinal lumen levels nor study of diarrheic horses has been reported. In humans, metronidazole levels in the intestinal lumen are quite high when diarrhea is present, allowing for treatment of colitis with lower doses than are used for systemic infections.[85] These may drop as diarrhea subsides, perhaps facilitating relapse as *C. difficile* spores (which are resistant to antimicrobials) could germinate and grow in the presence of an altered intestinal microflora and subtherapeutic drug levels. Whether this indicates the need for increased dosing as diarrhea resolves is unclear.

Almost no information is available for treatment of *C. perfringens*–associated diarrhea. Based on limited studies of antimicrobial susceptibility, metronidazole appears to be an appropriate choice. Zinc bacitracin has been evaluated as a treatment of colitis in horses.[86] This antimicrobial is effective against *C. perfringens* in vitro, but almost universal resistance among *C. difficile* isolates has been reported.[83,87] Zinc bacitracin is perhaps best used as a second-line therapy in cases in which CDI has been ruled out and when there has been poor response to metronidazole or when metronidazole is contraindicated (e.g., pregnant mares).

Toxin Adsorption

Although having no effect on clostridial organisms, adsorption of clostridial toxins in the intestinal tract might be a useful means of decreasing the severity of disease. Further, adsorption of endotoxin that is normally present in the intestinal tract could reduce clinical signs of endotoxemia that result when endotoxin is absorbed across a compromised mucosal barrier. Di-tri-octahedral smectite (Bio-Sponge, Platinum Performance, Buellton, CA) adsorbs *C. difficile* toxins A and B, *C. perfringens* enterotoxin, and endotoxin in vitro.[88,89] It is widely used for the treatment of colitis with anecdotal success, but clinical data are limited. Postoperative administration of di-tri-octahedral smectite was able to significantly reduce the incidence of diarrhea in horses that underwent colic surgery,[90] but there was no apparent effect on outcome. There are no known contraindications, including no impact on the effect of metronidazole in vitro.[89]

Probiotics

Probiotics are widely used in horses for prevention or treatment of diarrhea, with little evidence of efficacy. In humans, variable results have been obtained. A somewhat controversial meta-analysis reported evidence for efficacy of *Saccharomyces boulardii* for prevention of antimicrobial-associated diarrhea in humans,[91] but only weak evidence for efficacy in the treatment of CDI or other types of colitis. Overall, it has been stated that probiotics do not have a role in treatment or prevention of human CDI.[92]

Information is even more limited in horses. *Saccharomyces boulardii* has been evaluated as a treatment of undifferentiated colitis in horses, and although some encouraging differences were identified in a very small clinical trial, there was no impact on outcome.[93] Lactic acid bacteria (e.g., *Lactobacillus* spp., *Bifidobacterium* spp., *Enterococcus* spp.) are widely available in commercial probiotics, but no efficacy data are available. One area of concern with commercial probiotics is quality control because veterinary products rarely contain their stated ingredients.[94,95] There is probably no contraindication to the use of probiotics, except perhaps in very young foals.[96]

Fecal Transplantation (Fecal Microbiota Transplantation, Fecal Bacteriotherapy, Transfaunation)

The concept of transfaunation is certainly not new in veterinary medicine, although it is being investigated intensively in human medicine as a "novel" approach to the treatment of recurrent CDI, as well as other intestinal conditions. The logical premise is that disease is largely perpetuated by a markedly perturbed intestinal microflora and that restoration of this complex microbial population is required for disease resolution. Studies of fecal bacteriotherapy, which is infusion of feces from a healthy donor by enema or colonoscopy, have reported astoundingly high cure rates, often with a single treatment,[97-101] despite the procedure typically being reserved for patients with severe disease and poor response to conventional therapy.

There are anecdotal reports of fecal bacteriotherapy being used in horses, typically administration of fecal slurries by nasogastric tube, yet safety and efficacy data are lacking. This approach is worth considering in horses because it has been recently shown that the intestinal microflora is profoundly altered in horses with acute colitis,[1] and methods to restore the microbial balance may be critical for resolution of disease. Aspects of fecal bacteriotherapy, such as volume, dose, and frequency; whether to pretreat with a proton pump inhibitor (to reduce bacterial killing by gastric acid); and screening of donor samples, require study, but this approach may be appealing, particularly in cases that are poorly responsive to initial treatment.

Prevention

Prevention of Sporadic Clostridial Colitis

Essentially no objective information is available regarding prevention of clostridial colitis. However, certain factors are known or suspected to be risk factors for development of clostridial colitis, and modification of those is a reasonable approach to try to reduce the risk of disease. Since a major predisposing factor is thought to be disruption of the normal protective intestinal microflora, ways to prevent disruption of this complex microbial population should be considered. Prudent use of antimicrobials is likely one of the most important aspects. Antimicrobials should only be used when necessary, and drugs associated (even anecdotally) with a higher risk of colitis should be avoided unless other options are not available. Antimicrobials that have not been properly evaluated in horses should not be administered. Other factors that might increase the risk of disease, such as diet changes, high concentrate diets, transportation, and various stressors, should be limited as much as possible, with the understanding that many potentially high-risk practices are inherent in the horse industry and cannot be completely avoided.

Prevention of Transmision to Other Horses

Although *C. difficile* and *C. perfringens* can be found in healthy horses and in the farm environment, isolation of horses with active infection is recommended because of the large numbers of clostridia that they may be shedding while diarrheic. Ideally, strict isolation should be performed throughout the diarrheic phase and likely for a period after. This duration is not known as there is little information about shedding patterns of infected horses, but isolation for 3 to 7 days after clinical resolution is probably reasonable. Beyond strict physical separation from other horses, isolation of horses with colitis should include the use of barrier precautions (overboots or dedicated boots, specific barrier gown or other item to protect underlying clothing and skin, and gloves). Good hand hygiene is important. Since clostridial spores are resistant to alcohol, handwashing should be performed rather than application of alcohol-based hand sanitizers if clostridial contamination is a concern. Hands should be washed after any contact with the horse or its environment, even if gloves were worn.

Clostridial spores can persist for prolonged periods of time (years) in the environment. Spores are resistant to ultraviolet (UV) light, temperature changes, and desiccation, that effectively eliminate most vegetative bacteria. Additionally, spores are resistant to most disinfectants, complicating cleaning and disinfection of contaminated areas. Elimination of all clostridia from the environment is neither reasonable nor practical; however, measures should be taken to reduce high-level environmental contamination by affected horses and the overall environmental clostridial burden. All items that have been in contact with infected horses or their environment (e.g., medical instruments, buckets, shovels, wheelbarrow, feed bins, hay nets) should be disinfected or discarded. The stall and pasture environments are virtually impossible to disinfect. In these situations the goal should be to reduce the environmental burden. Careful cleaning to remove any remnants of feces is an important step. Sporicidal disinfectants can then be applied to some surfaces; however, disinfection of surfaces with heavy organic contamination (e.g., dirt floors, pasture) is futile. Bleach and accelerated hydrogen peroxide are the most common and practical sporicidal disinfectants.[102-105]

Outbreak Control

Although CDI is an important cause of outbreaks in human hospitals, outbreaks appear to be rare in equine hospitals. There is only one report of an outbreak in an equine facility,[106] although underreporting is certainly possible, and most cases of CDI encountered in equine hospitals are in horses that are presented with diarrhea. The reason hospital-associated transmission seems to be uncommon in horses is not clear. Transmission of *C. perfringens* seems to be of very limited concern in equine hospitals, with no outbreaks reported.

For reasons that are not understood, while these clostridia do not appear to be important causes of hospital-associated disease, outbreaks do occur on farms, although most of the available information is anecdotal. Outbreaks seem to be largely restricted to foals on breeding farms. If an outbreak is identified in adult horses, prompt investigation of potential antimicrobial contamination of feed is indicated. Lack of published information should not be taken as an indication of lack of impact because outbreaks in foals, particularly involving CDI, can be hard to control and highly problematic. In the author's experience, a typical pattern is identification of occasional cases of clostridial diarrhea in neonatal (1 to 7 days of age) foals at the start of the foaling season, with steady progression so that virtually all foals develop diarrhea as the foal season advances.

Outbreak control measures on farms have not been adequately investigated, and little additional guidance is available from anecdotal reports. Often, various interventions are attempted, including improved hygiene, changing of foaling areas, restriction of antimicrobial use, or prophylactic administration of metronidazole, di-tri-octahedral smectite, or probiotics. Fecal transplantation is a potential option for prevention of disease during outbreaks, particularly among foals, although safety and efficacy data are needed.

Vaccines are available for prevention of *C. perfringens*–associated disease in other species. These vaccines are designed to protect against types C and D, not enterotoxin or beta-2 toxin. Although there are anecdotal reports of the use of these vaccines in horses, particularly vaccination of mares during outbreaks in foals on breeding farms, vaccination with ruminant vaccines is not recommended because of the anecdotally high incidence of adverse effects (muscle irritation, abscess formation), lack of relevant strains, and lack of evidence of efficacy. A bacterin-toxoid vaccine targeting an equine-origin *C. perfringens* containing beta-2 toxin and CPE was shown to be safe and generate an immune response to phospholipase and beta-2 toxin in pregnant mares.[107] Antibodies against phospholipase C and beta-2 toxin were also produced in colostrum, and foals born to vaccinated mares had significantly higher serum antibody levels than control, suggesting the potential for efficacy. However, clinical efficacy has not been reported.

Probiotics are widely available commercially, and some are marketed for the prevention of diarrhea, particularly during antimicrobial therapy. There is currently no evidence that commercial probiotics are effective at prevention of clostridial enteritis in horses. It has been generally accepted that probiotics are, at worse, harmless; however, probiotic-induced diarrhea has been reported in neonatal foals,[96] likely from overgrowth of the probiotic in the poorly developed intestinal microflora with mild diarrhea from excessive organic acid production.

Public Health Considerations

Both *C. difficile* and *C. perfringens* are enteropathogens in humans, but public health risks associated with equine clostridial infections have not been adequately explored. The main concern involves *C. difficile* because it is a very important human pathogen and strains found in horses are generally indistinguishable from those found in humans.[4,6,21] However, transmission of *C. difficile* between horses and humans has not been confirmed and the true risk is unknown.

Regardless of the public health risks associated with clostridial infection, all horses with enteritis should be treated as infectious because of the possibility of salmonellosis. This is true even if clostridial disease is diagnosed because co-infection with *Salmonella* can occur. General infection control measures should be equally effective at reducing the risk of zoonotic transmission of clostridia or *Salmonella* spp. As fecal-oral pathogens, particular emphasis should be placed on avoiding contact with feces and good hand hygiene practices. Additionally, humans who may be at higher risk for contracting a zoonotic bacterial enteric disease, such as very young or very old persons, immunosuppressed individuals, and possibly those being treated with antimicrobials, should be restricted from contact with affected horses, with their environment, and with potentially contaminated items.

The complete reference list is available online at www.expertconsult.com.

42 Systemic Clostridial Infections

Debra C. Sellon and Simon F. Peek*

Clostridial Myonecrosis

Simon F. Peek

Etiology

Clostridial myonecrosis in horses is most often caused by infection with *Clostridium perfringens*,[1,2] although sporadic cases have been described in association with other *Clostridium* spp., including *C. septicum*,[1,3,4] *C. chauvoei*,[1,2,5] *C. novyi*,[1,6] *C. ramosum*, *C. sporogenes*,[1] and *C. fallax*.[7] The majority of cases in the literature have been single-species infections, but mixed infections have been reported.[1,3] These highly pathogenic clostridial organisms are gram-positive, spore-forming, anaerobic bacilli that can elaborate numerous potent exotoxins. Vegetative growth of these clostridial species is accompanied by production of dermonecrotizing and vasoactive toxins that lead to gas production, extensive tissue damage, and necrosis, as well as rapidly developing, life-threatening systemic toxemia.

Epidemiology

The prevalence of clostridial myonecrosis is low, and although the disease is sporadic, more cases appear to occur in certain regions. Many cases reported in the literature are from the northeastern[1,2,4] and midwestern[1,5,8] areas of the United States, but the disease may occur anywhere in the United States,[3] Canada,[9] Europe,[10] and the Southern Hemisphere.[7,11] Although species such as *C. perfringens* can frequently be cultured from the environment and soil wherever livestock are found, the means by which spores or vegetative organisms gain access to areas of affected soft tissue is not fully understood. Some of the species involved, including the most frequently isolated species, *C. perfringens*, can also be found within the gastrointestinal tract, in both the vegetative and the spore form, and some strains may be regarded as commensals. Spores of some clostridia (e.g., *C. sporogenes*, *C. histolyticum*) can be found in healthy equine muscle tissue, which suggests that after creation of appropriate anaerobic conditions, these spores may vegetate and begin exponential growth.[12] However, spores of species typically isolated from clinical cases of equine myonecrosis have not, as yet, been identified dormant within muscle tissue.

Most cases of equine myonecrosis temporally occur soon after parenteral injection of pharmacologic or biologic agents (≤48 hours) in the affected area of the body.[1,2,9] The condition is more common in the cervical musculature,[1-4,8,9] but occasional cases involving the gluteal muscles[1,8,9] and rarely the caudal thigh musculature[1] have been reported. Cervical and throatlatch lesions are sometimes encountered secondary to inadvertent perivascular leakage of pharmacologics intended for intravenous (IV) administration.[1] Traumatic wounds have rarely been associated with the condition.[1,9] A wide array of pharmacologic and biologic preparations have been incriminated as inciting causes of clostridial myonecrosis, including nonsteroidal antiinflammatories,[1,2,4,8,9] antihistamines,[1,2,9] multivitamins,[1,2,9] antipyretics,[1,7,13] dewormers,[2,9,14] vaccines, diuretics,[1] and synthetic prostaglandins.[13] The most frequently reported pharmacologic agent associated with the development of clostridial myonecrosis is flunixin meglumine, with the most cases occurring in the cervical region.[1-11,13,14]

Pathogenesis

Most information regarding the pathogenesis of clostridial myonecrosis comes from rodent models of infection. Because identical species of clostridia, specifically *C. perfringens* and *C. septicum*, are the most commonly recognized causes of human clostridial myonecrosis, it is reasonable to assume that etiologic-specific pathogenic factors are comparable. During vegetative growth of *C. perfringens*, the primary toxin implicated in the disease process is alpha (α) toxin, a dermonecrotic toxin with both phospholipase C and sphingomyelinase activity.[15] The definitive role that α-toxin plays during myonecrosis has been well established using controlled vaccine protection studies in which mice immunized against the C-terminal domain of the α-toxin were protected against lethal intramuscular (IM) doses of the organism, whereas unvaccinated controls were not.[16] Deletional mutants of *C. perfringens* in which the

*The authors acknowledge and appreciate the original contributions of these authors, whose work has been incorporated into this chapter.

structural α-toxin gene has been removed are nonpathogenic, and virulence is restored by recombination with a plasmid expressing the wild-type gene.[17] Other toxins that can be produced during vegetative growth by *C. perfringens* and other clostridial species include theta toxin (perfringolysin), kappa toxin (collagenase), and mu toxin (hyaluronidase).[15,18] Although other exotoxins elaborated by *C. perfringens* (and also other species) have highly potent and pathogenic effects extracellularly, no compelling evidence exists that they are required for lethal disease, as is the alpha toxin.

Many of the signs of systemic toxemia, cardiovascular collapse, and multiorgan dysfunction observed clinically in horses with clostridial myonecrosis can similarly be explained by observations made in rodent and rabbit models of gas gangrene. Alpha toxin directly suppresses myocardial contractility in vivo,[19] whereas theta toxin is a potent reducer of systemic vascular resistance.[20] Theta toxin has demonstrable ability to dysregulate polymorphonuclear/endothelial cell interactions, promoting leukostasis and interfering with normal cellular host responses to tissue injury at the active site of infection.[21]

Clinical Findings

Horses with clostridial myonecrosis demonstrate rapid soft tissue swelling, subcutaneous and deeper soft tissue emphysema, and rapid toxemia that may progress to circulatory collapse and multiorgan failure over just a few hours.[1-3] Clinicopathologic data from horses that have died acutely corroborate multiorgan failure and diffuse intravascular coagulation as two major pathologic processes that occur in terminally ill horses with clostridial myonecrosis.[1,2,8] Some horses that develop clostridial myonecrosis have a recent history of colic, resulting in the administration of IM analgesics, with subsequent myonecrosis in the region of the injection.[1,2,8,9] Some authors have postulated that colic may truly be a prodromal sign of equine clostridial myonecrosis,[4] drawing comparisons with the nausea and abdominal pain that are early symptoms of clostridial myonecrosis in human patients.[22,23]

Occasionally, horses with clostridial myonecrosis will develop hemolytic anemia/crisis after several days to 1 or 2 weeks of therapy.[1,24] This appears to be a distinct entity to the life-ending, diffuse intravascular coagulation that other horses develop in the early stages of the disease. It is not certain whether hemolytic events are a direct effect of the clostridial infection. Some clostridia (e.g., *C. septicum*) can elaborate one or more exotoxins with in vivo hemolytic activity.[22,23] Alternatively, hemolysis may be a potential immunologic complication of penicillin or other drug therapy.

Diagnosis

Clostridial myonecrosis may be presumptively diagnosed in any horse that develops acute-onset, rapidly progressive soft tissue swelling accompanied by emphysema in the area of a recent parenteral injection. Clostridial myonecrosis associated with penetrating traumatic wounds appears to represent a rare subset of cases.[1,9] Acute-onset cellulitis without emphysema should be viewed as suspicious for the disease, but confirmed by cytologic evaluation and Gram stain before aggressive fasciotomy or debridement is performed (Fig. 42-1). Ultrasonography of areas of postinjection cellulitis should be performed to identify areas of deeper emphysema and gas production that may not yet be palpable in the immediate subcutis. Definitive etiologic confirmation can be achieved by Gram stain and anaerobic culture of fluid aspirates from an affected soft tissue area. Numerous, characteristic gram-positive rods, sometimes with endospores present, can be easily visualized on air-dried smears, particularly from the periphery of an area of soft tissue emphysema.

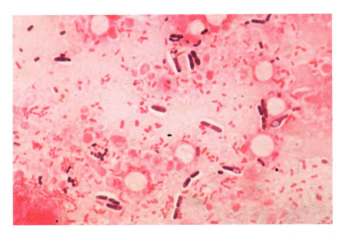

Figure 42-1 Gram stain of aspirate from subcutaneous tissues of horse with acute clostridial myonecrosis. Notice the numerous, large, gram-positive rods.

Speciation after anaerobic culture by genetic or fluorescent antibody techniques provides definitive confirmation and may guide prognosis.[1,25]

Real-time polymerase chain reaction (PCR) assays have been described for detection and differentiation of *C. chauvoei* and *C. septicum*.[26,27] These rapid techniques may be used for antemortem diagnoses in large animals, which has largely been unrewarding in the past because bioassay techniques and direct florescent antibody techniques are restricted to postmortem samples. Early identification of anaerobic versus aerobic infection may allow earlier intervention of appropriate antimicrobial therapy.

Therapy

Higher survival rates are associated with aggressive combinations of medical and surgical treatment.[1,2,4] Barotherapy has become a component of the approach to treatment of human cases of clostridial myonecrosis, but hyperbaric oxygen chambers are only beginning to become available for use in large animal veterinary medicine. Rapid therapeutic intervention with high doses of IV crystalline penicillins should be considered as soon as a presumptive diagnosis is made. Potassium penicillin at doses as high as 88,000 IU/kg every 2 hours (q2h) have been used, and conventional doses of 22,000 IU/kg q6h should be viewed as the minimum required dose, expense permitting.[25] Oral metronidazole (25 mg/kg q6h) is often included in therapy but is unlikely to reach the high tissue levels that may be achieved with IV penicillin.

Intensive fluid, electrolyte, and cardiovascular support is indicated in the acute stages of clinical disease because dehydration and systemic toxemia can be life threatening at this time.[1-3,25] Many affected horses become hypotensive, with diminished cardiac output and renal function, complicated by substantial myoglobin release and the potential for pigment nephropathy. Fenestration of affected soft tissues appears to be an important part of therapy, and clinicians are advised to be aggressive in incising areas of subcutaneous emphysema, extending the incisions into deeper tissues and adjoining areas of healthy tissue (Fig. 42-2). Because of the obtunded mentation of many affected horses and the rapid progression of tissue necrosis in affected areas, these procedures can usually be performed under sedation without the need for local anesthesia.[25] Frequent reevaluation of the horse for signs of spreading emphysematous cellulitis, necessitating repeated incisions and debridement, is advised. Local infusion of penicillin into tissue at the margins of debrided muscle may have some benefit in limiting the spread of the infection.

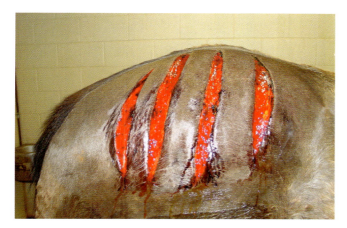

Figure 42-2 Fasciotomy/myotomy incisions in gluteal region of 2-year-old Quarter Horse filly that developed clostridial myonecrosis secondary to vaccination at the site. *(Courtesy Dr. Susan Semrad.)*

For horses that survive the acute stages of disease, prognosis will improve significantly. However, veterinarians should warn owners of the significant soft tissue and skin sloughing that will likely ensue over coming days to weeks (Fig. 42-3). Long-term wound care will often be needed, with many cases taking weeks to months before granulation and second-intention skin healing are complete. Cosmetically, some horses may heal with pigmentation changes and significant cicatrix formation (Fig. 42-4), but the visual appearance of healed wounds is often normal.[25]

Prognosis appears to vary according to the species of *Clostridium* involved. A much better prognosis is afforded to horses with soft tissue lesions associated with *C. perfringens* than to those with *C. septicum* or *C. chauvoei* infections.[1] The largest retrospective study published to date reported an overall survival rate of 73% for horses with clostridial necrosis when they were treated with a combination of aggressive medical and surgical therapy in a referral hospital setting. Horses with *C. perfringens* infection had a survival rate of 81%.[1] There was no gender predilection observed in that study, but the disease did appear disproportionately to affect Quarter Horses. Previous studies have demonstrated much higher case-fatality rates,[2,8,9] and therefore clinicians and owners should be mindful of the need for prompt, aggressive, and potentially expensive therapy if horses are to have the best chance of survival. The majority of horses that die will succumb within the first few days.

Prevention

Although bacterin-toxoids should be in common use for prevention of disease caused by *Clostridium tetani* in all horses (see Chapter 44) and *Clostridium botulinum* in susceptible and at-risk foal populations (see Chapter 43), there is no standard vaccination practice for the prevention of clostridial myonecrosis in horses. Current preventive methods focus on appropriate injection technique, particularly with respect to the location of IM administration of pharmacologic and biologic preparations. No protective effect appears to be gained from skin disinfection, hair clipping, or disinfection of the top of multidose vials before IM injection in preventing clostridial myonecrosis.[26] When administering IM injections, however, particularly in the neck, where the disease most often occurs, it is prudent to ensure appropriate needle placement. When administering potentially irritant substances, particularly if lay people are responsible for injecting flunixin meglumine, it may be prudent to encourage use of the larger, better-vascularized, caudal thigh musculature.

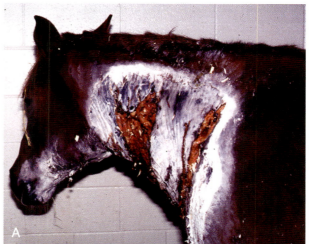

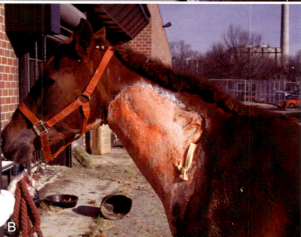

Figure 42-3 A, Mature Quarter Horse gelding showing skin and muscle sloughing 2 weeks after surgical fenestration of an area of clostridial myonecrosis in the cervical region. **B,** The same horse approximately 30 days after surgical fenestration showing near-complete granulation bed in prior area of clostridial myonecrosis.

Tyzzer's Disease

Debra C. Sellon

In 1917, Ernest Edward Tyzzer[28] described an infectious syndrome of gastrointestinal and hepatic disease in Japanese Waltzing mice that came to be known as Tyzzer's disease. He isolated and characterized the etiologic agent and reproduced the disease experimentally in mice. The etiologic agent was originally named *Bacillus piliformis*. However, in 1994, Duncan et al[29,30] demonstrated that the organism was more closely related to clostridial bacteria than to the *Bacillus* genus, and it was renamed *Clostridium piliformis*. In 1973, Swerczek et al[31] described focal bacterial hepatitis in foals in Kentucky attributable to infection with *Clostridium (Bacillus) piliformis*.

Etiology

C. piliformis (also *C. piliforme*) is a motile, pleomorphic, gram-negative, spore-forming, obligate intracellular bacterium. It is classified as an organism that is "extremely oxygen sensitive" (EOS) and is gram positive only if fixation and staining are performed under strictly anaerobic conditions.[31,32] *C. piliformis*

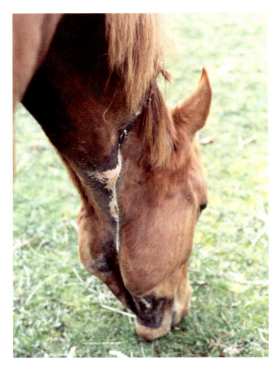

Figure 42-4 Scarring and skin depigmentation in a healed area of clostridial cellulitis and myonecrosis in throatlatch region associated with perivascular injection. *(Courtesy Dr. Susan Semrad.)*

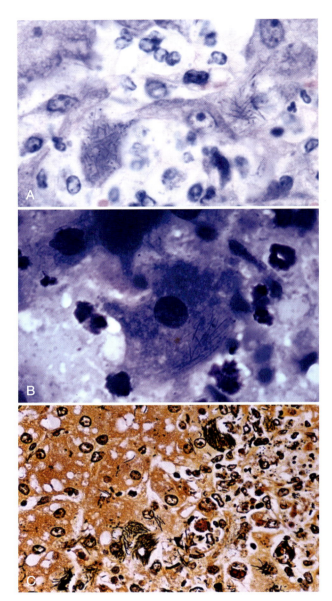

Figure 42-5 Photomicrographs of the liver of foals with Tyzzer's disease. Note the thin, filamentous bacilli visible within hepatocytes. **A,** Giemsa stain, 400×. **B,** Diff-Quik stain, 400×; imprint from liver of affected foal. **C,** Warthin-Starry (silver) stain, 160×. *(Courtesy Dr. Charles Leathers.)*

does not grow in cell-free media but can be propagated in the yolk sac of chick embryos or some types of cell culture. *C. piliformis* stains poorly with routine hematoxylin and eosin stains of formalin-fixed tissue samples. Silver impregnation or Giemsa stains facilitate visualization of the organism (Fig. 42-5). The large vegetative form of *C. piliformis* ranges from 8 to 40 mm in length. This vegetative phase is quite labile; in contrast, spores may survive for up to 1 year in soiled bedding at room temperature or for 1 hour at 56° C (133° F).

Epidemiology and Pathogenesis

Infection with *C. piliformis* has been reported in a variety of laboratory, wild, and domesticated mammalian species, including the horse,[30,33-49] cow,[50,51] dog,[52-55] cat,[56] rat,[57-63] mouse,[58,59,64-69] hamster,[69-71] gerbil,[72-74] guinea pig,[75-79] rabbit,[80-82] muskrat,[83-85] wombat,[86] red panda,[87] coyote,[88] snow leopard,[89] gray fox,[90] raccoon,[91] and serval.[92] Among laboratory animals, clinical disease is most common in rabbits, gerbils, hamsters, and guinea pigs. Infections of mice and rats are more likely to be subclinical.[62] There is one report of infection in a severely immunocompromised person.[93] There have been a few reports of infection in avian species.[94,95] Disease has been reported in horses in many parts of the world, including North America, Australia, Europe, and Africa.

The natural route of infection of horses with *C. piliformis* is unknown, but the most likely route of exposure is by ingestion of spores from the environment. This theory is supported by the distribution of lesions in affected animals[30,35,96] and experimental reproduction of disease in foals by oral transmission. Experimental infection of adult horses results in fecal shedding of the organism, and coprophagia may contribute to the likelihood of infection in foals.[46] The sporadic nature of the disease in foals suggests that direct transmission is unlikely.[50,97,98] However, clusters of disease may be observed on specific horse premises.[30,37,46,47]

Serologic studies suggest that there is widespread exposure of horses to *C. piliformis*.[98] Approximately 23% of horses tested had antibodies to the flagellar antigens of an equine *C. piliformis* isolate, 14% had antibody to epitopes of a rat isolate, and 5% had antibody to epitopes of a hamster isolate. This variability in seropositive rates between isolates suggests the possibility of multiple strains of bacteria that cause disease in horses.[99,100] However, shared epitopes among strains have also been identified,[99] making it difficult to determine whether only certain strains may cause disease in animals or whether individual strains may be restricted to specific host species.

In a study of affected and unaffected Thoroughbred foals on a farm in California, several risk factors for Tyzzer's disease were identified.[37] Data from nine affected foals from a population of 322 foals were examined. In the final multivariable logistic regression analysis, foals born between March 13 and April 13 were 7.2 times as likely to develop Tyzzer's disease as those born at other times; foals of nonresident (visiting) mares were 3.4 times more likely to be infected than resident foals; and foals of mares less than 6 years of age were 2.9 times as likely to develop disease as foals born to older mares. Seasonal risk may reflect management, environmental, or climatic factors that influenced disease incidence. The increased risk observed for foals born to nonresident mares and foals born to younger mares suggests that colostrum may be important for passive immunity in foals.[37] Hook et al[99] have demonstrated colostral transfer of antibodies to C. piliformis.

Very little is known about the pathogenesis of infection with C. piliformis in horses or other animals. Murine susceptibility to Tyzzer's disease varies with host strain, age, and immune status. Depletion of neutrophils or natural killer cells in experimentally infected mice increases the severity of disease, but macrophage depletion does not alter the course of disease.[101] In rodents and lagomorphs, outbreaks of disease are characterized by fatal diarrhea, with pathology predominantly observed in the gastrointestinal tract.[102]

Clinical Findings

Tyzzer's disease affects foals between 7 and 42 days of age.[37,43,47,48,98] Clinical signs include severe depression, fever, icterus, diarrhea, dehydration, and seizures. Some foals are found dead with no recognizable premonitory clinical signs. Almost all affected foals die; the overall course of disease is usually less than 48 hours from onset of clinical signs until death. Clinicopathologic abnormalities frequently include hemoconcentration, metabolic acidosis, hypoglycemia, hyperbilirubinemia, and increased hepatic enzyme activities.[37,43] Ultrasonographic examination of the abdomen of affected foals may reveal hepatomegaly with an increased vascular pattern.[43]

Diagnosis

Tyzzer's disease should be considered as a differential diagnosis for foals between 7 and 42 days of age with compatible clinical signs and laboratory evidence of hepatitis. The likelihood of this diagnosis is increased if previous cases of C. piliformis infection have been confirmed on the premises. Currently, no reliable antemortem laboratory tests are available to confirm a diagnosis of Tyzzer's disease in foals. Diagnosis is confirmed on postmortem examination by observation of typical gross and histopathologic lesions and observation of intracellular bacteria at the periphery of lesions when liver sections are stained appropriately (see Fig. 42-5).

Pathologic Findings

At postmortem examination, affected foals have a grossly enlarged liver with multifocal, light-colored areas in the liver capsule and parenchyma.[97] These light-colored areas correspond with areas of severe, random, diffuse acute to subacute hepatic necrosis.[45] Intracellular filamentous bacilli can be observed in parallel or random arrangements in hepatocytes at the periphery of these lesions if sections are silver-stained (Warthin-Starry stain). Occasionally, lesions consistent with enterocolitis or myocardial infection may be observed.[39,41,103]

Therapy

The prognosis for foals with Tyzzer's disease is poor. Three foals with presumptive C. piliformis infection did survive.[37,43] These foals received appropriate supportive care and antimicrobial therapy rapidly after they developed clinical signs. Because of difficulties cultivating C. piliformis in vitro, there is relatively little information regarding antimicrobial susceptibility patterns for this organism. The only available data are based on in vitro studies using embryonated eggs in which penicillin, tetracycline, erythromycin, and streptomycin were considered effective. Treatment of laboratory animals with either sulfonamides or corticosteroids can induce active Tyzzer's disease in carrier animals.[104] A 10-day-old foal that survived presumptive Tyzzer's disease was treated with sodium penicillin and trimethoprim-sulfadiazine.[43] In addition, the foal received intensive IV fluid therapy with dextrose, sodium bicarbonate, and potassium chloride solutions. Seizure activity was controlled with IM xylazine. Nutritional needs were met with IV parenteral nutrition. Additional supportive therapy included IV dimethyl sulfoxide and antiulcer prophylaxis. Clinical improvement was observed within 24 hours of initiation of therapy. Antimicrobial and antiulcer therapy was continued for approximately 3 weeks.

Prevention

No vaccines are available for prevention of Tyzzer's disease in foals. Because C. piliformis is most likely transmitted by a fecal-oral route, good farm hygiene may be beneficial for decreasing the likelihood of disease. Maintaining foals in well-grassed paddocks has been proposed as a preventive measure to decrease exposure to contaminated soil.[45] It is also recommended that all foals receive adequate passive transfer of immune globulins soon after birth. High-risk foals[37] should be closely monitored for the earliest signs of disease and treated aggressively as soon as these are recognized. Spores are reported to be sensitive to disinfection with 0.3% sodium hypochlorite[105]; however, this disinfectant is readily inactivated in the presence of organic matter and may not be an effective disinfectant for use in barns.

Public Health Considerations

There is a single report of human infection with C. piliformis in a severely immunocompromised patient.[93]

The complete reference list is available online at www.expertconsult.com.

Botulism

Pamela A. Wilkins

Botulism is a neuromuscular disorder of horses and other mammals caused by neurotoxins of *Clostridium botulinum;* similar disease has been described resulting from toxins produced by a few strains of *Clostridium baratii* and *Clostridium butyricum.* The first published reports of botulism in horses appeared in the early 1950s.[1] Disease characterized by flaccid paralysis may occur in adult horses or in foals—this has been termed *shaker foal syndrome.*[2-4]

Botulinum toxin is considered to be one of the most potent toxins known.[5] Although it has medicinal uses in the treatment of specific disorders,[5,6] clinical botulism is a serious, frequently fatal disease. The exotoxin causes paresis and paralysis by interfering with acetylcholine release at the neuromuscular junction.[6,7] Death is usually attributed to respiratory failure. Because of the pathogenicity of botulinum toxin, especially for humans, it has been placed on the list of select agents to facilitate control of dangerous biologic agents and toxins. Botulism can result from the ingestion of preformed botulinum toxin or the growth of *C. botulinum* in anaerobic tissues, with subsequent in vivo elaboration of toxin. Outbreaks of botulism resulting from consumption of contaminated feed can be devastating, with high morbidity and mortality.

Etiology

Clostridium botulinum is a gram-positive, saprophytic, spore-forming, anaerobic rod-shaped bacterium. Eight neurotoxins isolated from *C. botulinum* (A, B, Ca, Cb, D, E, F, and G) are distinguished by neutralization of biologic activity with type-specific serologic reagents and are classified in seven serogroups designated A through G. Bacterial strains are usually identified on the basis of the type of toxin produced (Table 43-1). Although all types of botulinum toxin produce an identical clinical disease, determination of the toxin type is important if antitoxin is used for treatment. Clinical botulism in horses has been attributed to *C. botulinum* types A, B, C, and D.

Clostridium botulinum spores are highly resistant to heat, light, and drying. Germination occurs under anaerobic conditions at temperatures of 15°C to 45°C (59°F-113°F). Toxin

Table 43-1 Mammalian Species Affected by Each Type of Botulinum Toxin

Botulinum Toxin	Mammalian Species Affected
A	Horse, human, cattle, ferret, mink
B	Horse, human, cattle
C	Horse, cattle, sheep, dog, cat, mink, ferret
D	Horse, cattle, sheep, dog
E	Human, mink, ferret
F	Human
G	—

may be released from vegetative cells by cell lysis or by diffusion through the cell wall within several days of germination. After release, the single-chain toxins are inactive until cleaved by bacterial or tissue proteases to the active dichain neurotoxin. All serotypes of botulinum toxin are composed of a heavy chain with a molecular weight of approximately 100 kDa and a light chain of 50 kDa connected by a single disulfide bond.

Epidemiology

Equine botulism is most frequently observed in Kentucky and the Mid-Atlantic region of the eastern United States, although the disease had been reported worldwide.[3,8] In the United States, horses are most often affected with type B or C botulism, although type A botulism has been confirmed in adult horses and foals and is predominant in the Western United States.[9]

Type B *C. botulinum* spores can be isolated from the soil of most geographic regions of the United States, but they are most common in the soil of the northeastern and Appalachian regions. In contrast, *C. botulinum* type A spores are more common in the soil in the western United States. The frequency of occurrence of types A and B food-borne botulism in humans parallels the distribution of these types in the soil.[10] A similar correlation between frequency of environmental isolation of a specific serotype of *C. botulinum* and the frequency of disease caused by that serotype is observed in horses in North America. Type B botulism is most often seen in the Mid-Atlantic states and Kentucky, type C occurs mainly in Florida, and type A has been observed predominantly in the western United States.

Pathogenesis

Equine botulism may occur after ingestion of preformed botulinum toxin in contaminated feed (forage poisoning),[11-15] ingestion of spores with elaboration of toxin within the gastrointestinal (GI) tract (toxicoinfectious botulism),[16] or contamination of wounds with *C. botulinum* and subsequent in vivo toxin production (wound botulism).[17] Ingestion of preformed botulinum toxin in decaying vegetable matter (grass, hay, grain, spoiled silage) or carcasses is the most common type of botulism observed in adult horses.[3,8] An outbreak of botulism type C was associated with bird droppings and a horse burial site.[18] Toxicoinfectious botulism is most common in foals 1 to 3 months of age, although it has been observed in foals as young as 7 days of age. Toxicoinfectious botulism may also be the cause of "grass sickness" in horses in Europe.[19-21]

Clostridial toxins are dichain structures with a molecular weight of approximately 150 kDa that are synthesized as single chains and posttranslationally cleaved into heavy (H) and light (L) chains. They are metalloproteinases that are structurally similar to tetanus toxin and that prevent the spontaneous or action potential–induced presynaptic release of acetylcholine at the neuromuscular junction.

Botulinum neurotoxin (BoNT) consists of a light chain that functions as a zinc-dependent endopeptidase and a heavy chain with two functional domains of approximately the same size. The N-terminal section of the H chain is the translocation domain that forms ion channels spanning endosomal membranes to facilitate translocation and activation of light chains. The C-terminal section of the H chain is the ganglioside-binding domain to facilitate binding and internalization of the toxin at the cholinergic neuron.[22]

Botulism intoxication occurs by a multistep process, involving each of the functional domains of the toxin, and can be summarized as the outcome of three distinct stages: (1) binding to the target cell and internalization, (2) translocation, and (3) inhibition of neurotransmitter release.

Binding to cholinergic nerve terminals is thought to require gangliosides and a protein receptor, possibly synaptotagmin for BoNT types A, B, and E.[23,24] Once bound to the cell surface, BoNT is internalized into an acidic compartment by endocytosis that is temperature and energy dependent. After internalization, the toxin cannot be neutralized by antitoxin.

Translocation is thought to involve a pH-dependent structural rearrangement of BoNT inside an acidic compartment within the cell, possibly synaptic vesicles or the endosomal compartment.[25,26] The active light chain is translocated to the cytosol, where it interacts with and eventually cleaves SNARE proteins (soluble N-ethylmaleimide-sensitive factor attachment protein [SNAP] receptor). SNARE proteins are a group of proteins that are critical for membrane fusion and exocytosis of neurotransmitters from the cell and include synaptobrevin (vesicle-associated membrane protein family [VAMP]), syntaxin, and SNAP-25.[22] The specific SNARE protein cleaved and the site of cleavage vary with the specific serotype of botulinum toxin. Botulinum neurotoxin types B, D, F, and G cleave members of the VAMP family of SNARE-complex proteins, whereas types A, C, and E cleave SNAP-25. Botulinum neurotoxin type C also has the capacity to cleave syntaxin.

Botulinum neurotoxin prevents exocytosis of acetylcholine at the neuromuscular synapse by the cleavage of SNARE proteins involved in the fusion of synaptic vesicles with the plasma membrane. Cleavage of SNARE proteins creates a nonfunctional complex in which coupling between calcium ion (Ca^{++}) influx and synaptic vesicle fusion is disrupted.[27] The cleavage of the SNARE proteins allows docking of the synaptic vesicle but prevents exocytosis. Increasing intracellular Ca can partially overcome the effects of BoNT type A.[22,28]

The extended duration of activity of BoNT at the neuromuscular junction is the root of the clinical problem and the reason for its recent application as a therapeutic tool in human medicine. Specific BoNT serotypes vary in their duration of action. For example, BoNT type A induces long-term inhibition (months) of neurotransmission, whereas BoNT type E induces a comparatively short-term inhibition (weeks).[29,30] The reasons for these differences have not been fully elucidated but may relate to the half-life of the light chain in the cytosol and to persistence of SNAP-25 fragments in the SNARE complex.

Clinical Findings

Clinical signs in horses with botulism are related to inhibition of acetylcholine release at the neuromuscular junction and resultant generalized lower motor neuron and parasympathetic dysfunction.[8,31] This includes dysphagia; flaccid paralysis; diminished pupillary reactivity; decreased eyelid, tongue, and tail

tone; and progressive flaccid tetraparesis and tetraplegia.[3,8,32] The time to onset of clinical signs after exposure to toxin varies from 12 hours to several days. Sudden, unexplained death of one or more horses may be the initial signal of the onset of an outbreak. Decreased eyelid, tongue, and tail tone may be observed early in disease. Horses that walk may have a stilted, short-strided gait without ataxia. Muscle trembling and weakness may be apparent, particularly in foals. Pupillary dilation with sluggish pupillary light reflexes is common. There is normal cutaneous sensation with depressed spinal reflexes. Pharyngeal paralysis is frequently observed in adult horses with botulism and may be confirmed by endoscopic examination of the upper airway.

Clinical signs may rapidly progress to recumbency. Tachycardia may occur, particularly in foals. Foals may appear or become constipated and dysuric. Signs of colic may be associated with diminished GI motility. Dyspnea and cyanosis may be present initially or terminally. Death is generally attributed to respiratory failure secondary to respiratory muscle paralysis.

Diagnosis

Diagnosis of botulism is primarily made on the basis of history and clinical signs after exclusion of other diagnostic possibilities.[3,8,32] Differential diagnoses include but are not limited to severe electrolyte imbalance (hyponatremia), tick paralysis, and postanesthetic myasthenic syndrome. Routine laboratory work, including complete blood count, serum biochemical profile, and urinalysis, is generally unremarkable unless secondary problems (e.g., infection, dehydration) have developed. Although characteristic electromyographic changes have been described in association with infant botulism and toxicoinfectious botulism in foals, electromyography (EMG) is not uniformly available, and most veterinarians are not trained to interpret this test properly.[33] One recent study suggests that rapid nerve stimulation of the peroneal nerve in horses with botulism produces characteristic changes that include decreased baseline M-wave amplitudes with incremental responses at high rates.[34]

Definitive diagnosis is usually based on detection of toxin in serum, feces, GI contents, or feed. A variety of tests, including enzyme-linked immunosorbent assay (ELISA), radioimmunoassay (RIA), passive hemagglutination, and polymerase chain reaction (PCR), have been described for identification of botulinum toxin; however, the diagnostic test of choice remains mouse inoculation. Serum or an extract of feed, feces, or GI contents is injected into the peritoneal cavity of mice, which are observed for classic clinical signs of botulism. The specific serotype of botulinum toxin present in a sample is determined by co-injection of mice with suspect samples and specific antisera. If appropriate antiserum is present, clinical signs will not occur. Although serum samples are occasionally positive for botulinum toxin by mouse inoculation assay, the quantity of circulating toxin is usually too small for detection.[3] Isolation of C. botulinum or its toxin from feedstuffs, feces, or GI contents or from lesions or wounds in the patient is strong circumstantial evidence of infection.[3,8]

Pathologic Findings

No pathologic findings are directly attributable to the effects of botulinum toxin. Pressure sores and regions of self-trauma may be seen in recumbent horses, and all patients, old or young, may have aspiration pneumonia secondary to dysphagia (Fig. 43-1). Gastric ulceration reported at postmortem examination in foals

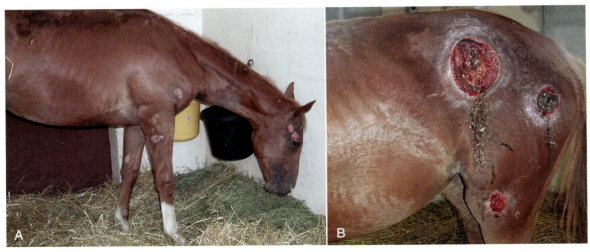

Figure 43-1 A, Mild pressure sores associated with recumbency in horse, caused by neurologic disease other than botulism. **B,** The same horse with severe pressure sores. *(Courtesy Dr. Amy Bentz, Chadds Ford, PA.)*

in the past may have been a reflection of the severity and progression of the disease rather than an inciting event. Gastric ulceration has been reported in association with severe illness in foals, but as intensive care techniques have improved, the incidence of gastric ulceration in nonsurviving patients at necropsy has decreased.[35]

In human infants, the large intestine is thought to be the site of colonization with *C. botulinum* and toxin-induced infection.[36]

"Grass sickness" (equine dysautonomia) appears to be a form of toxicoinfectious intestinal botulism in adult horses with fairly specific lesions, including degenerating neurons in peripheral autonomic ganglia, as well as in intramural intestinal ganglia, that stain positive for synaptophysin, a SNARE protein.[21,37,38]

Therapy

The efficacy of early administration of antitoxin in improving survival and decreasing length of hospital stay has been clearly demonstrated for humans and horses and is the mainstay of therapy.[3,8,32,39-44] Before the use of botulinum antitoxin in affected foals, the disease was almost uniformly fatal within 12 to 72 hours of the onset of clinical signs, except in very mildly affected horses.[32] Currently, equine-origin polyvalent (anti-B and anti-C) botulinum antitoxin (Botulism Laboratory, New Bolton Center, Kennett Square, PA) and monovalent (anti-B) botulinum antitoxin (Veterinary Dynamics, Templeton, CA) are commercially available.

Respiratory failure is almost uniformly the proximate cause of death in both adults and foals with botulism. Adults and foals with mild respiratory failure (normal pH and mild to moderate increase in arterial carbon dioxide tension [Pa_{CO_2}]) can frequently be treated with intranasal oxygen insufflation, positioning in sternal recumbency, and repeated arterial blood gas (ABG) monitoring to detect worsening respiratory failure. Close ABG monitoring is required for the first 24 to 48 hours of treatment because administration of botulinum antitoxin does not remove toxin already bound to receptors within the terminal neuromuscular junction of the axon, and the equine patient may deteriorate further during this period. Arterial blood gas analysis should also be performed if the patient's condition appears to change; these horses may suddenly alter their respiratory rate and pattern as respiratory failure worsens.

Increased nostril flare, decreased chest excursion, and restlessness may be physical indicators of worsening respiratory failure.

Foals with botulism and respiratory failure can be mechanically ventilated successfully.[44] Mechanical ventilation can ameliorate ABG abnormalities and allow time for the patient to recover cholinergic neuromuscular control. Volume-cycled ventilators tend to be better tolerated by foals. In synchronized intermittent mandatory ventilation (SIMV) mode, a minimum breath rate is set, along with a predetermined tidal volume and inspiratory flow rate, resulting in flow-controlled, volume-cycled mandatory breaths.[45] The sensitivity, related to the inspiratory effort the patient must generate to trigger a breath, should be set low in these horses. This is in recognition of their primary problem, botulism, and the muscular weakness associated with the disease.

Antimicrobial administration, although not required for treatment unless wound botulism is suspected, is frequently employed in an effort to prevent or reduce some of the complications of the disease such as aspiration pneumonia caused by dysphagia. Antimicrobial choice in botulism is influenced by the disease process being treated. Antimicrobial drugs that might potentiate neuromuscular blockage (e.g., procaine penicillin, aminoglycosides, tetracyclines) should be avoided.[46-48]

Nutritional management must be considered in horses with botulism and can generally be achieved in foals by feeding milk or milk replacer via indwelling nasogastric or nasoesophageal tubes* as small, frequent meals (every 2 hours). In adult horses, periodic nasogastric intubation of slurry meals can be provided. In prolonged cases, it may be beneficial to consider commercially available liquid diets. Parenteral nutrition is generally not necessary. Intravenous fluid support may be required until patients are able to drink water safely.

Nursing care is an important part of treatment, and equine patients should be protected as much as possible from development of decubital ulcers, corneal ulcers, and inadvertent aspiration. Frequent turning and slinging of adult horses are arduous tasks and require skill and persistence (Fig. 43-2). Ocular examination should be performed at least daily, and ocular lubricant ointments should be used to prevent exposure keratitis. Care should be taken to ensure the "down" eye is protected.

Survival rate for botulinum neurointoxication in appropriately treated foals less than 6 months of age is greater than 90%.

*Kangaroo, 12-French, 43-inch enteral feeding tube, Sherwood Medical, St. Louis, MO 63103.

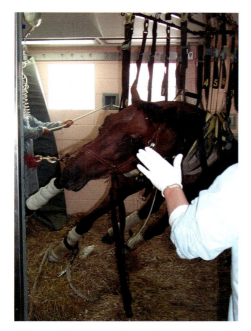

Figure 43-2 "Slinging" a horse. The sling used here is the Anderson sling; the horse is not yet upright. Slings can be used to support horses in a standing position or can be used as an aid to change position of recumbency in "down" horses. This horse has neurologic disease, not botulism, but botulism cases would be similarly handled. *(Courtesy Dr. Amy Bentz, Chadds Ford, PA.)*

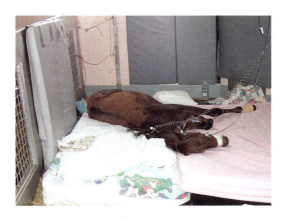

Figure 43-3 Weanling with botulism maintained in lateral recumbency on mattresses. Note intravenous line (coil) for fluid support and oxygen line providing intranasal oxygen insufflation. Two twin mattresses were required for this foal, and synthetic sheepskin was used to protect the body from pressure sores and skin maceration associated with prolonged recumbency. This weanling also received antitoxin and survived. *(Courtesy Dr. Amy Bentz, Chadds Ford, PA.)*

Approximately 50% of affected foals will require some form of ventilatory support, ranging from intranasal oxygen insufflation to mechanical ventilation, and all affected foals should have repeated ABG analysis performed during the first 48 hours of treatment (Fig. 43-3). Mechanical ventilation can ameliorate ABG abnormalities and allow time for the patient to recover

Box 43-1 Botulism Vaccination Protocol

Adult Horses
Broodmare: Initial three-dose series at 30-day intervals, with last dose 4 to 6 weeks before anticipated parturition date. Annually thereafter, 4 to 6 weeks prepartum.
Other adult horses: Should consider vaccination, particularly if in endemic regions. Initial three-dose series, then annual booster.

Foals
From vaccinated mares: Three-dose series of toxoid at 1-month intervals, starting at 2 to 3 months of age.
From unvaccinated mares: Foal may benefit from (1) toxoid at 2, 4, and 8 weeks of age; (2) transfusion of plasma from vaccinated horse; or (3) antitoxin (efficacy needs further study).

cholinergic neuromuscular control. Foals recovering from botulism are not protected after specific immunoglobulin G (IgG) from antitoxin is depleted, and they should be vaccinated.

Adult horses with botulism that remain standing have a good prognosis for recovery; however, it may require several weeks to months before affected horses regain sufficient strength to return to work. Horses that become recumbent have a poorer prognosis even with antitoxin administration and excellent nursing care. This is related in part to their size and the secondary effects of prolonged recumbency. The degree of respiratory compromise can be severe, and long-term (days) mechanical ventilation of adult horses is a difficult undertaking.

Prevention

Appropriate vaccination (*Clostridium botulinum* type B toxoid, Neogen, Tampa, FL) is thought to be almost 100% protective in adult horses[3,8] (Box 43-1). However, foals born to vaccinated dams can present with botulism, suggesting that reliance on passive transfer of immunity for protection of foals may be inadequate in endemic areas.[32] Failure of transfer of specific immunity to botulinum toxin can originate from failure of passive transfer of immunity. However, foals less than 2 weeks of age with adequate blood concentration of IgG (>800 mg/dL) have also been diagnosed with botulism. In these cases, the dose of toxin may have overwhelmed the available antitoxin, or the dam may not have produced sufficient specific antibody in response to the vaccination to provide adequate protection to the foal through colostrum. Older foals from vaccinated dams may have lost specific passive immunity by the time of their exposure to the toxin and before their own vaccination. In humans, plasmapheresis of patients no longer responding to botulinum toxin administered for medicinal purposes can return them to responder status, most likely by decreasing available specific IgG.[49]

Public Health Considerations

There is no zoonotic potential with equine botulism.

The complete reference list is available online at www.expertconsult.com.

Tetanus

Robert J. MacKay

Tetanus was first described in Egypt more than 3000 years ago and was familiar throughout the ancient world.[1,2] In 1890, von Behring and Kitasato demonstrated that rabbits produced neutralizing antibodies in response to the administration of small doses of tetanus toxoid.[3] Two years later, von Behring immunized sheep and horses against tetanus toxin to produce commercial quantities of antitoxin, and equine antitoxin was used extensively in injured soldiers during the first world war. In 1927, Ramon and Zoeller[4] developed a vaccine from tetanus toxoid; a similar vaccine for horses was first used in the 1940s.

Etiology

Tetanus is caused by exotoxins produced by *Clostridium tetani*, a motile anaerobic gram-positive bacillus. *Clostridium tetani* is a ubiquitous soil inhabitant and can be isolated from feces of domestic animals, including horses.[5,6] Endospores are formed that give the sporulating organism a drumstick appearance.[1] They are not completely destroyed by boiling but can be eliminated by autoclaving at 115° C (239° F) for 20 minutes.[7] Toxin may account for 5% of the mass of the organism during proliferative growth.[8] It has been estimated that the lethal dose for humans is 500 pg/kg.[9] Among animals, the horse is considered most sensitive to tetanus toxin.[10]

The most common route of infection is inoculation of wounds with *C. tetani* spores. Puncture wounds contaminated by manure, soil, or rusty metal are especially likely to cause tetanus. In 18 horses with tetanus after known wounding, 9 had lesions of the lower limb, 6 had punctures in the solar surface of the hoof, and 2 had wounds on the face.[11] Contaminated surgical sites, the postpartum uterus, injection abscesses, and infected umbilical structures are also potential sites for *C. tetani* infection. Injuries around the pastern associated with hobbling were prevalent sites of *C. tetani* infection in working horses, donkeys, and mules in Morroco.[12] Causative wounds were not found or reported in 55/107 (51%) equids with tetanus[11-13] and reportedly are not found in 15% to 30% of human cases.[14]

Epidemiology

Tetanus occurs in all parts of the world but is most likely found in closely settled areas that are intensively farmed. The climate and soil pH in the tropics may contribute to the increased prevalence of *C. tetani* and its availability to contaminate wounds.[15] Although the disease is rare in developed countries, tetanus is still important worldwide. In 1992, there were more than a million human deaths caused by tetanus,[16] and neonatal tetanus still causes an estimated 200,000 to 500,000 deaths annually in developing countries.[15] Tetanus was diagnosed in

0.07% of 97,000 working equids presented to Society for the Protection of Animals Abroad (SPANA) clinics in Morocco.[12] Young horses are overrepresented in some equine case series. Average ages were 4.3[13] and 3.4[11] years in European and North American reports, respectively.

Pathogenesis

The clinical signs of tetanus are caused by exotoxins encoded on a 75-kB plasmid.[17] Two toxins are produced: tetanolysin and tetanospasmin.[18] Tetanolysin damages viable tissue, thereby lowering the redox potential and creating favorable conditions for expansion of the anaerobic infection.[6] Tetanospasmin is produced as a single inactive 150-kD polypeptide comprising 3 linked domains: L, H_N, and H_C. The peptide is cleaved by tissue proteases into active heavy (H) and light (L) chains connected by a single disulfide bond. After its production by proliferating organisms, tetanus neurotoxin (TeNT; active tetanospasmin) diffuses locally and circulates in the bloodstream to neuromuscular junctions throughout the body. Tetanus neurotoxin does not enter the central nervous system (CNS) directly, except at the fourth ventricle. At motor nerve terminals, the lectin-like H_C domain is captured by "antennae" on the membrane polysialoganglioside GD_{1b} and routed to specific membrane protein receptors. The toxin is then internalized via clathrin-coated pits and transported retrograde in axons at 75 to 250 mm/day.[19] After 1 to 14 days the toxin enters the CNS, reaches the neuronal cell body, traverses the synaptic cleft, and binds irreversibly to presynaptic inhibitory interneurons.[2] Following H_C-mediated binding to membranes, the entire toxin is internalized through a process requiring H_N.[20] Within the endosome, the disulfide link is reduced and the L chain is released into the cytosol. The L chain is a zinc metalloproteinase that cleaves synaptobrevin, which is a component of the SNARE protein complex that is necessary for membrane fusion and exocytosis of neurotransmitter vesicles.[18,21] In inhibitory interneurons, the light chain thus prevents release of the inhibitory neurotransmitters glycine and gamma-aminobutyric acid (GABA).[22] This results in the sustained excitatory discharge of alpha motor neurons evident clinically as muscle rigidity and muscle spasms.[6]

Preganglionic autonomic neurons in the lateral column of the gray matter and parasympathetic centers in the brainstem are affected by a similar mechanism but with delayed kinetics compared to somatic motor neurons.[23] Autonomic dysfunction therefore occurs days after spasms begin, probably because of relatively slow transport of toxin in the autonomic nerves.[2] There is both a basal increase in sympathetic activity and episodes of intense hyperactivity ("autonomic storms") involving both α-adrenergic and β-adrenergic receptors. During autonomic storms there is up to a tenfold increase in the concentration of circulating epinephrine. The resulting sympathetic hyperactivity causes hemodynamic instability and is an important cause of death in ventilated tetanus patients.[24]

The toxin also acts at the neuromuscular junction to cause muscle paralysis.[25] This botulinum toxin-like effect causes the facial paralysis characteristic of the rare cephalic form of tetanus; however, any paralysis usually is overridden by spasmogenic effects at the inhibitory interneuron. Tetanus neurotoxin also has been shown in experimental animal studies to have a cortical convulsant effect.[26] Whether this contributes to tetanic spasms in horses is unknown.

Neuronal binding of toxin is thought to be irreversible.[27] Recovery requires sprouting and growth of new nerve terminals, a process that is completed in several weeks to months.

Clinical Signs

The time from wound inoculation by *C. tetani* to development of first clinical signs can be from 1 to more than 60 days, but usually is 7 to 21 days. In a series of 18 horses with tetanus, signs were first seen 2 to 21 days after wounding, with an average incubation period of 9 days.[11] In another report of 16 equids with tetanus and associated wounds, the incubation period ranged from 2 to 60 days, with a mean of 15 days.[13] The period of onset (time from first sign to first spasm) has not been reported for equine cases but probably is similar to the 1 to 7 days reported for humans.[1]

Generalized, localized, and cephalic forms of tetanus are described in humans.[1,6] By far, the most commonly recognized form in horses is generalized tetanus. Neonatal tetanus is always of this type. Probably because cranial somatic nerves are shorter then nerves to the limbs, the first signs of tetanus are associated with rigidity of muscles around the head and neck. Increased tonus of the masticatory muscles (trismus), rigidity of facial expression (risus sardonicus), and neck stiffness are typical presenting signs.[11,32-37] Prolapse of the membrana nictitans begins during this phase (Fig. 44-1).[10] The head and neck are held in an extended position, and the face has a fixed anxious expression. The ears and commissures of the lips are retracted caudally, and the upper eyelids are elevated. Often, the mouth is clamped shut and the jaws cannot be pried apart manually (lockjaw). Hyperthermia (usually >102.5° F) occurs in some horses during the early stages and rectal temperature may

rise further after tetanic convulsions. For example, 2 of 31 horses had temperatures of at least 38.5°C (101.3°F) at admission.[10,13]

In mildly affected horses, signs may be restricted to the head and neck (Box 44-1). In moderately affected horses that were injected with culture filtrate containing tetanus toxin, pelvic limb stiffness occurred about 30 hours after trismus.[38] Horses with moderate tetanus also exhibit signs of dysphagia because of pharyngeal involvement and rigidity extends to the muscles of the limbs, trunk, and tail. These horses also adopt a "saw-horse" posture with rigid extension of the neck, back, and limbs and elevation of the tailhead.[11,35,36] The gait appears stiff and stilted. In severe tetanus, affected animals are recumbent and respiratory muscles are affected. Spasm of intercostal muscles causes intermittent apnea.

In all cases of generalized tetanus, tonic spasms develop within days of the onset of rigidity. These can be initiated by external tactile, visual, emotional, or auditory stimuli or by voluntary movements such as posturing for urination or defecation. The dramatic responses to even minor stimuli can make a horse with tetanus appear hyperresponsive or hyperesthetic. When the face is touched, there is reflex retraction of the eye and prolapse of the nictitans.[10] Attempts to chew or suckle set off rounds of masseter contraction that are easily visible under the skin (Fig. 44-2). Reflex spasms may prevent an affected horse from reaching to the ground for food or water. Even if the horse is able to move ingesta to the pharynx, reflex pharyngeal and laryngeal spasms result in nasal regurgitation and stridor.

Because there is no reflex inhibitory control of movement, antagonistic flexor and extensor muscles contract simultaneously and with full power. The force of these contractions may cause rhabdomyolysis, intramuscular hemorrhage, tendon avulsion, and fracture of long bones or vertebrae. Extensors are generally more powerful than flexors, so the neck, torso, limbs, and tail are dramatically extended during spasms (Fig. 44-3). In foals, the head may even arch back over the torso. Efforts to stand may provoke cycles of violent muscle contraction of the limbs and trunk that pitch the horse back into recumbency. Even during apparent convalescence, muscle spasms can be disabling enough to cast an adult horse onto the floor of a stall.[34,39] Once down it is difficult for an adult horse with tetanus to regain its feet.[10]

Tetanus presents in a local form in approximately 2% of human cases.[2] Local tetanus, evident as muscle spasms at the

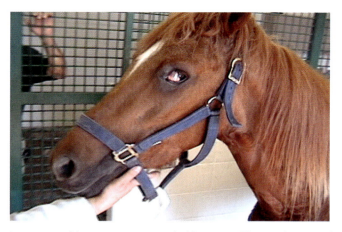

Figure 44-1 Mild tetanus in an 18-month-old Paso Fino filly recently imported from Puerto Rico with unknown vaccination history. This filly, shown in a frame from a video, had a 2-week history of bilateral "flashing" of the nictitans inducible with any kind of stimulation. The only other abnormal clinical sign was profuse sweating of the head and neck. The filly recovered uneventfully without treatment over the next 4 weeks.

Box 44-1 Classification of Clinical Severity

Mild
Anxious expression
Prolapsed nictitans
Trismus
Extended head

Moderate
As for *mild, plus*
Dysphagia
Hyperresponsiveness
Muscle spasms
Tail-head extension
"Saw-horse" stance
Stiff gait

Severe
As for *moderate, plus*
Lateral recumbency
Frequent severe spasms
Respiratory difficulties
Cardiovascular instability

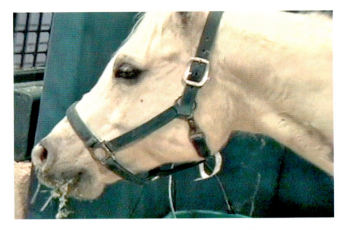

Figure 44-2 Moderate tetanus in a 16-year-old Thoroughbred gelding shown in a frame from a video. Note the contraction lines over the masseter fanning out ventrally and caudally from the front of the facial crest. This is characteristic of the spasms seen in horses with trismus. Also evident is the dilated left nostril, elevated dorsal eyelid and piece of hay clamped between the incisors. This gelding recovered over 6 weeks with nursing care and repeated sedation with acepromazine.

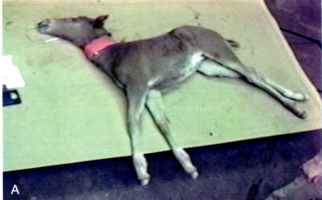

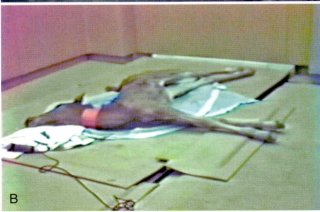

Figure 44-3 Severe generalized tetanus in a 2-week old Quarter Horse foal shown in frames from a video. Between spasms, this foal maintained a rigid extended posture **(A)** but when stimulated (e.g., by sound), the foal suffered generalized tetanic spasms **(B)**. This foal was euthanized soon after these images were taken. *(Frames from video courtesy Dr. Eleanor Green, Texas A&M University.)*

site of a tetanus toxin injection in the neck, was described in a single experimental horse.[38] The local form probably also occurs in naturally affected horses, although it has not been documented in the literature. Local tetanus is associated with low toxin load and/or partial humoral immunity. Rigidity and

spasms are restricted to muscles adjacent to the inciting wound. Cephalic tetanus usually begins with asymmetric facial paralysis, although any cranial nerve can be affected. Signs may progress to generalized tetanus with high mortality.

Disturbances of autonomic function occur after several days of muscle spasms.[24] There may be increased or fluctuant heart rate, increased or fluctuant blood pressure (up to 300 mm Hg systolic pressure[6]), and profuse sweating. Sweating and tachycardia are common in horses presenting with generalized tetanus. Mean heart rates at presentation of 61[11] and 57[12] beats per minute were reported for horses with tetanus at the time of presentation to referral clinics. It is not clear whether these signs represent TeNT-induced sympathetic overactivity or are physiologic responses to the pain and anxiety caused by muscle rigidity and spasms. Signs of sympathetic overactivity are usually overlooked until after muscle spasms have been controlled. It is reported that hypersalivation, increased respiratory secretion, and late-onset hypotension occur because of parasympathetic overactivity.[40]

Death usually occurs because of euthanasia of recumbent horses with uncontrollable paroxysmal muscle contractions or because of associated musculoskeletal injuries. Spontaneous deaths usually are attributed to compromised respiration. This may be because of laryngeal spasm and asphyxia; contractions of the chest wall, diaphragm, and abdomen; accumulation of excessive respiratory secretions; and aspiration pneumonia. Long bone or vertebral fractures may occur during muscle spasms or because of accidental falls. In humans and possibly horses, sudden death may occur because of cardiac or other effects of autonomic dysfunction.

Reduced intestinal borborygmi, infrequent defecation, colic, and dehydration are frequent nonneurologic signs of tetanus.

Diagnosis

This diagnosis is presumptive and based on clinical signs in the context of a history of poor, absent, or unknown vaccination against tetanus. An early and sensitive diagnostic test in the horse is transient prolapse of the membrana nictitans provoked by stimulation around the head. Typically, this response is elicited by lightly tapping the skin beneath the eye. Differential diagnoses to consider include myopathy, meningitis, colic, pleuritis, hyperkalemic periodic paralysis, trauma, epilepsy, and laminitis.

Gram stain of wounds reveal the characteristic drumstick-shaped gram-positive bacilli in about 30% of human tetanus patients,[28] but Gram stain and culture are seldom attempted in horses with tetanus. The clinically relevant dose of TeNT in equids is probably less than the 0.5 ng/kg estimate for humans, whereas the minimal lethal dose in 6-week-old National Institutes of Health (NIH) strain test mice is about 20 ng.[29] Therefore it is very unlikely that toxin could be detected in the blood of an affected horse by mouse bioassay. The mouse challenge test can be used for assay of tissue fluids from the presumptive site of inoculation. With the development of a real-time polymerase chain reaction (PCR) assay for the TeNT gene,[30] confirmation of C. tetani in culture without bioassay is now possible.

Necropsy findings of horses with tetanus are nonspecific, with secondary signs of musculoskeletal trauma and pulmonary congestion, atelectasis, and edema most common.[11,13] The diagnosis has been confirmed definitively postmortem in one human case by detection of TeNT in spinal cord ventral horn cells by immunohistochemical staining with an antibody directed against tetanus toxin fragment C.[31]

Therapy

Therapy for tetanus should have the following objectives: (1) provision of a safe quiet environment; (2) elimination of *C tetani* and unbound toxin; (3) sedation, muscle relaxation, and relief of pain (Table 44-1); and (4) general support.

Horses should be moved carefully to a large well-bedded stall. All possible external stimuli, including light and noise, should be minimized. Feed and water should be hung so that the horse does not need to lower its head.[41] Horses in danger of falling may be maintained in a body sling,[41] tackle and girdle,[42] stocks, or walking frame.[43]

If a recent wound or other infection can be identified, it must be opened, cleaned, debrided, and flushed. Tetanus antitoxin (TAT) can be infiltrated into the tissues around the lesion, although this procedure is not now recommended in protocols for treatment of human tetanus.[6] Penicillin traditionally has been given to kill remaining *C. tetani* organisms; however, the drug has been found to have potential anti-GABA and proconvulsant activities.[44] Metronidazole now is considered the antimicrobial of choice[1] and has outperformed penicillin in two clinical trials of human patients.[45,46] It can be given at 20 to 30 mg/kg orally (PO) every 12 hours (q12h) for 3 to 5 days. If the horse's condition precludes oral medication, give 40 to 60 mg/kg per rectum, or 10 to 20 mg/kg intravenously (IV) every 6 to 8 hours (neonates).

Although some evidence suggests that massive parenteral doses of TAT reduce mortality in experimental tetanus in mice, active toxin that is already bound is not accessible to serotherapy. By the time a horse shows clinical signs, circulating toxin is not detectable.[11] No effect of TAT dose has been found in retrospective studies of equine tetanus patients, although the numbers are small. Notwithstanding the lack of evidence for large TAT doses, it is prudent to ensure neutralization of any

residual unbound toxin by administration of at least 10,000 IU IV, intramuscularly (IM), or subcutaneously (SC) and repeat daily for 3 to 5 days. Because TAT does not cross the blood-brain barrier, large doses have been given intrathecally to patients with tetanus. The results of intrathecal therapy as reported in small case series in horses have been inconclusive[11,13,42,47]; however, metaanalysis of the major human studies performed up until 1991 did not reveal any survival advantage for this route of TAT administration.[48] Notwithstanding the general lack of historical evidence, intrathecal TAT continued to be given over the last 2 decades, especially by physicians in the Indian subcontinent, and a new metaanalysis of 12 studies of both neonatal and adult cases detected a statistical survival advantage for intrathecal versus IM TAT.[49] Administration of TAT has been associated with acute hepatic necrosis in horses.[50,51] The first clinical sign of this potentially fatal adverse reaction may appear 4 to 10 weeks after administration of TAT and has been reported in horses that received TAT for treatment of clinical tetanus.[52]

Sedatives and muscle relaxers are used to control muscle spasms and rigidity. The traditional approach in humans has been the combination of a phenothiazine-based ataractic sedative such as chlorpromazine with a GABAergic agent such as diazepam or phenobarbital.[2] In horses, chlorpromazine[11,32,41,53] is the most common such treatment, although acepromazine,[34,35] promazine,[35] and propionyl promazine[40] have also been used. In moderately affected horses, obvious muscle relaxation occurs within minutes of treatment and lasts for hours. Chlorpromazine additionally has α-adrenergic antagonist and anticholinergic actions that may help suppress autonomic overactivity.[1] Pentobarbital sodium is sometimes recommended for additional muscle relaxation in horses but must be titrated very carefully to avoid recumbency.[11,41] Phenobarbital, at a dose of 10 mg/kg IV and then by nasogastric (NG) tube q8h, provided effective muscle relaxation for a neonatal foal with tetanus that had not to that point been controlled by high and frequent doses of diazepam.[43] Large doses of diazepam are very effective for short-term control of muscle rigidity in humans, and the drug (in combination with xylazine) appeared effective for treatment of severe signs in two horses.[11] Diazepam may be given IV to horses and repeated as necessary to control muscle spasms. In light of potential cumulation of diazepam and respiratory or CNS depression, however, diazepam may be inappropriate for long-term treatment.[54] Midazolam has a relatively short half-life and can be used as a constant infusion but is usually too expensive for use in adults. Additional strategies under study to increase GABA in patients with tetanus include pyridoxine (vitamin B6),[55] intrathecal baclofen,[56] and sodium valproate.[57]

Methocarbamol,[37] glycerol guaiacolate,[35] mephenesin, and d-tubocurarine[58] have all been used for muscle relaxation in horses with tetanus but have not found wide application. The direct muscle relaxant dantrolene is used in horses for prevention of myopathy[59] and might have application to the treatment of tetanus. This drug has been used successfully in human tetanus.[60]

Magnesium, which was first used more than 100 years ago to treat tetanus,[61] has multiple potentially useful actions against spasms and autonomic dysfunction and is inexpensive. It blocks neuromuscular transmission, interferes with catecholamine release from nerves and the adrenal medulla, reduces receptor responsiveness to released catecholamines, antagonizes the actions of calcium, and is an anticonvulsant and vasodilator.[2,62,63] Interestingly, electromyography (EMG) studies show that magnesium tends to spare the respiratory muscles, which is a marked advantage. In a randomized controlled trial comparing magnesium sulfate (MgSO₄) infusion with placebo in patients with severe tetanus, magnesium was significantly associated with reduced requirements for other drugs to control muscle

Table 44-1 Drugs for Sedation or Muscle Relaxation in Horses with Tetanus

Drug	Action(s)	Dose (mg/kg)	Interval (hr)	Route
Acepromazine	S, MR, AA	0.02-0.1	6-12	IV, IM
Butorphanol/ xylazine*	S, AA, AN	0.1/0, then 0.018/0.39 per hr	CRI	IV
Chloral hydrate	S	5-10 mg/kg	PRN	IV
Chlorpromazine	S, MR, AA	0.4-1.0	6-12	IV, IM
Dantrolene sodium	MR	2-8	24	PO
Diazepam	S, MR, AA	0.1-0.2	PRN	IV
Glyceryl guaiacolate†	MR	To effect	PRN	IV
Methocarbamol	MR	10-55	6-12	IV, PO
Magnesium sulfate (MgSO₄)‡	MR, AA	50, then 5-20 per hr	CRI	IV
Midazolam	S, MR	0.1-0.2 per hr	CRI	IV
Morphine	S, AA, AN	0.1-1	PRN	IV, IM
Pentobarbital sodium†	S, MR	1-3	6-12	IV
Phenobarbital sodium	S, MR	10-20, then 2-10	8-24	IV, PO
Promazine	S, MR, AA	0.4-1	6-12	IV, IM
Xylazine	S	0.25-1	PRN	IV, IM

S, Sedative; *MR*, muscle relaxant; *AA*, antiadrenergic; *AN*, analgesic; *PRN*, *pro re nata* (as needed); *CRI*, constant-rate infusion; *IV*, intravenous; *IM*, intramuscular; *PO*, oral.

*Do not give loading dose of xylazine.

†Serious risk of recumbency during treatment.

‡Infusion rate can be increased by 5 mg/kg/hr every 6 hours (q6h) until control achieved. Serum concentrations and electrocardiogram (ECG) should be monitored frequently as described in text.

spasms and tetanus-associated cardiovascular instability.[62,63] Parenteral $MgSO_4$ is used widely and safely in horses for treatment of cardiac arrhythmia[64] and is recommended for neonatal encephalopathy[65]; however, signs of toxicity have been reported in horses given large amounts of enteral $MgSO_4$, so treatment needs to be monitored closely.[66] In human patients, it is recommended that serum/plasma magnesium concentration is kept between 2 and 4 mM (4.9 to 9.8 mg/dL) and that an electrocardiogram (ECG) is recorded and monitored continuously. Infusion is discontinued if the width of the QRS complex increases by more than 25%.

In addition to magnesium infusion, a variety of approaches have been used for treatment of autonomic overactivity in human patients with tetanus.[1] These have included reserpine, clonidine, angiotensin-converting enzyme (ACE) inhibitors, adenosine, α-adrenergic blockers (chlorpromazine, phentolamine), β-blockers (propranolol, esmolol, labetalol), atropine, verapamil, and intrathecal bupivicaine.[6,63,67] Treatment has not been particularly successful and, with the exception of chlorpromazine, has little obvious application in the horse. Morphine sulfate infusion is now used to suppress extreme sympathetic hyperactivity in human patients, as well as to induce sedation.[28] It acts centrally by reducing sympathetic tone in the cardiovascular system and controls cardiac instability without cardiac compromise. Repeated dosing of morphine at analgesic doses has been associated with behavioral and gastrointestinal side effects in horses.[68] Continuous infusions of the opioid agonist-antagonist butorphanol in combination with xylazine[69] (see Table 44-1) or other $α_2$-adrenergic agonists may provide the desired combination of autonomic suppression and sedation in horses with tachycardia, systemic hypertension, excessive sweating, hyperthermia, or other signs of autonomic dysfunction.

Intensive supportive therapy during at least the initial few days of signs is essential. In horses that cannot eat or drink, IV fluids and nutrition can be provided.[33] Enteral nutrition may be given via an indwelling NG or esophagostomy tube. If there is stridor, a tracheotomy should be performed and tracheotomy tube placed. Because muscle rigidity and spasms reportedly are extremely painful in humans with tetanus, analgesia should be provided in well-hydrated horses with a nonsteroidal antiinflammatory drug (NSAID) such as flunixin meglumine or equivalent or an opioid such as butorphanol or methadone. Full paralysis and mechanical ventilation of a severely affected foal is theoretically possible. Except for the need for paralysis with a drug, such as pancuronium, management would be akin to that used for botulism of foals[70] and likely would require 1 to 3 weeks of ventilation.

Prognosis

The fatality rate is at least 50% in most reports[12,13,39] and was 75% and 68% in the most recent North American and European series, respectively.[11,13] All horses that subsequently died were recumbent by 24 to 48 hours after admission. In surviving horses, there usually is stabilization of signs in 2 to 7 days, with gradual recovery over the next several weeks.* However, one

horse reportedly remained stiff at 6 months but was normal at 9 months after onset of signs.

On the basis of various prognostic scoring systems used for human tetanus[1] and the few small equine series published, negative prognostic indicators are incubation period less than 7 days, period of onset (time from first sign to first spasm) less than 2 days, umbilical or uterine entry site, no vaccination within the previous year, and presence of comorbid disease. Severe signs at presentation, recumbency, or initial rapid progression of clinical signs all are predictive of poor outcome.

Prevention

Tetanus has long been preventable by vaccination with inexpensive toxoid preparations. Nonvaccinated adult horses should be given an initial 2-dose series of tetanus toxoid administered 3 to 6 weeks apart. Protective responses are usually attained within 2 weeks after the second dose. Current recommendations are to give booster doses annually thereafter or additionally at the time of injury or surgical procedure.[71,72] Broodmares should be revaccinated 4 to 6 weeks before foaling to provide for colostral transfer of immunity to their foals. Passively transferred antibody suppresses the immunoglobulin G (IgG) response of foals to toxoid vaccination at 3 months but not 6 months of age.[73] Therefore it is recommended that foals from vaccinated mares be given a three-dose initial series beginning at 4 to 6 months of age, with a second dose 4 to 6 weeks later and the third dose at 11 to 12 months.[71,72] Foals from nonvaccinated mares are vaccinated 3 times at 4-week intervals beginning at 1 to 4 months of age.[72] The magnitude of serologic responses to vaccination with tetanus toxoid depend on the particular product used, with the type of adjuvant likely the most important variable. Vaccination with North American products adjuvanted with carbopol resulted in several-fold higher IgGb and IgG(T) titers than did those adjuvanted with squalene adjuvant.[74] Horses vaccinated with a European product that uses ISCOM-Matrix adjuvant had serum titers 24 months beyond a booster vaccination that were well above the 0.02 IU/mL serum tetanus toxin-binding enzyme-linked immunosorbent assay (ELISA) titer considered protective.[75] Despite the wide range of serologic responses mounted by vaccinated horses, tetanus has only been reported in unvaccinated horses or in horses improperly vaccinated.

Tetanus antitoxin is produced by hyperimmunization of donor horses with tetanus toxoid. Administration of one vial of antitoxin (1500 IU) to a nonvaccinated horse provides immediate protection that lasts for 2 to 3 weeks. Antitoxin is indicated in foals from nonvaccinated mares and in any wounded horse that has not been vaccinated within the previous year. In these cases, antitoxin and toxoid should be administered concurrently, with separate syringes at separate sites. Because the use of antitoxin is associated with hepatic necrosis (serum hepatitis) in a small number of horses, antitoxin should not be given in horses that are adequately covered by toxoid vaccination.[50]

The complete reference list is available online at www. expertconsult.com.

---

*References 11, 13, 32, 34, 36, 39.

Miscellaneous Bacterial Infections

Debra C. Sellon, Sharon J. Spier, Mary Beth Whitcomb, Marta Gonzalez Arguedas,*
Maureen T. Long,* J. Lindsay Oaks,* and Melissa T. Hines*

Corynebacterium pseudotuberculosis

Sharon J. Spier and Mary Beth Whitcomb

Etiology

Corynebacterium pseudotuberculosis is a gram-positive, pleomorphic, rod-shaped, intracellular, facultative anaerobe with worldwide distribution. It is the etiologic agent of ulcerative lymphangitis, external subcutaneous abscesses, and internal infection in horses. In North America, disease is most prevalent in the southwestern United States, but cases of *C. pseudotuberculosis* infection have been reported throughout the United States. Infection has been reported in sheep, goats, cattle, buffalo, camelids, equids, and humans.

C. pseudotuberculosis grows well at 36° C (96.8° F) on blood agar in 24 to 48 hours, and it forms small, pinpoint-diameter, whitish, opaque colonies surrounded by a weak zone of hemolysis. Because of the high content of lipids in the bacterial cell wall, particularly corynomycolic acid, the colonies spatter in a flame and can be pushed across the agar surface.[1] The high content of lipids may facilitate survival of the organism in macrophages.[2]

Two species-specific biotypes of *C. pseudotuberculosis* have been identified based on differences in nitrate reduction,[3] and deoxyribonucleic acid (DNA) fingerprinting techniques have revealed multiple strains.[4-7] Biotypes isolated from small ruminants are nitrate negative, whereas those from horses are nitrate positive. From the result of DNA studies, the terms "biovar equi" for nitrate-positive and "biovar ovis" for nitrate-negative strains were proposed.[3] Natural cross-species transmission does not seem to occur between sheep and horses; however, cattle can have infection from either biotype.[3]

The whole genome sequence of several equid strains of *C. pseudotuberculosis* has been reported.[8-11] Genetic sequencing of multiple isolates from sheep, goats, and horses from Chile demonstrates the presence of bacterial rpoB gene polymorphisms that segregate by host species.[12]

Epidemiology

Three forms of *C. pseudotuberculosis* infection have been described in horses: ulcerative lymphangitis or limb infection, external abscesses (Fig. 45-1), and internal infection. Ulcerative lymphangitis presents as severe cellulitis, with involvement of lymphatic vessels in one or more limbs and multiple draining ulcerative lesions. In a retrospective study of *C. pseudotuberculosis* infection in horses from California, horses with ulcerative lymphangitis comprised only 1% of the cases, whereas external abscesses occurred in 91% and internal abscesses in 8% of the

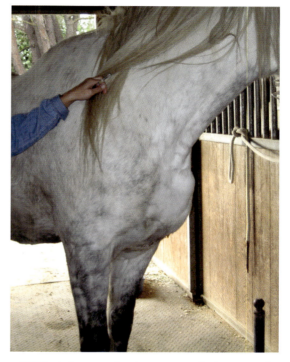

Figure 45-1 Typical pectoral abscess caused by *Corynebacterium pseudotuberculosis.*

cases.[13] Horses of all breeds and gender may develop any of the three forms of disease, although mares may be overrepresented and Thoroughbreds underrepresented in studies by Doherr.[14] In one recent study of internal infection, mares seemed to be overrepresented.[15]

The biologic reservoir for *Corynebacterium pseudotuberculosis* is soil. The equine biovar is able to survive and multiple in different types of soil under a wide range of environmental conditions. The addition of manure to soil appears to favor survival, presumably by providing essential fatty acids and micronutrients that enhance bacterial growth and multiplication.[16]

The portal of entry of this soil-borne organism is thought to be through abrasions or wounds in the skin or mucous membranes. Many insects have been incriminated as vectors for the transmission of the disease to horses, and recent studies have shown that *Haematobia irritans, Musca domestica,* and *Stomoxys calcitrans* can act as vectors for this disease[17] (Figs. 45-2 and 45-3). The regional location of abscesses suggests that ventral midline dermatitis predisposes the animal to introduction of the organism. Because of the variable incubation period, ventral midline dermatitis may not be present during maturation of the abscesses.

*The authors acknowledge and appreciate the original contributions of these authors, whose work has been incorporated into this chapter.

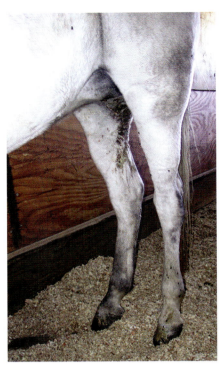

Figure 45-2 Houseflies (*Musca domestica*) feeding on exudate draining from abscess. Flies are vectors for *C. pseudotuberculosis*.

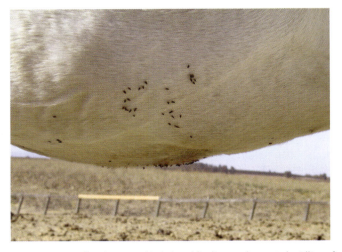

Figure 45-3 Horn flies (*Haematobia irritans*) feeding on the ventral midline of horse. Ventral midline dermatitis is a predisposing factor for *C. pseudotuberculosis* disease in horses, and the bacteria can be found in this species of fly.

Temporal and spatial analysis suggests that the disease can be transmitted through horse-to-horse contact or from infected to susceptible horses by insects, other vectors, or contaminated soil; the incubation period is 3 to 4 weeks.[18] The organism survives for up to 2 months in hay and shavings and more than 8 months in soil samples at environmental temperatures.[16,19,20]

The incidence of disease fluctuates considerably from year to year, presumably because of herd immunity and environmental factors such as rainfall and temperature. To date, the definitive environmental factors supporting the spread of infection have not been determined.[14] Disease incidence is seasonal, with highest number of cases occurring during the dry months of the year, which is late summer and fall in the southwestern United States, although cases may be seen all year. Horses with internal infection are more frequently seen 1 to 2 months after the peak number of cases with external abscesses.[21]

Horses of all ages may be affected, although the low incidence of disease in foals less than 6 months of age suggests that passive transfer of immunoglobulins offers protection in foals born in endemic areas. A case-control study in an endemic area revealed young adults (<5 years) and horses in contact with other horses on summer pasture had increased risk of infection. Horses housed outside or with access to an outside paddock appeared to be at higher risk than stabled horses.[22]

Pathogenesis

The pathogenesis of *C. pseudotuberculosis* infection in horses is poorly understood. The incubation period appears variable; temporal and spatial clustering studies by Doherr et al.[18] revealed an incubation period of 7 to 28 days. Bacteria are phagocytosed after entry into the host but continue to replicate. Intracellular survival of *C. pseudotuberculosis* has a key role in the formation of abscesses and is possibly mediated by two virulence factors: bacterial cell wall lipids and phospholipase D (PLD) protein exotoxin. The bacterial cell wall lipids may facilitate survival in macrophages, whereas the PLD exotoxin has profound effects on survival and multiplication within the host. The PLD toxin may directly affect phagocytic cells or inactivate complement and reduce opsonization of the bacteria. The exotoxin also increases vascular permeability, enhancing the spread of infection both locally and through the lymphatics. The subsequent vascular changes permit bacterial spread to additional locations, including regional lymph nodes. Humoral and cell-mediated immune responses ultimately develop, clearing the bacterial infection.[23]

Recovery generally is complete within 2 to 4 weeks after abscess maturation, although rarely horses develop persistent or recurrent infections lasting for more than 1 year. In one study, 91% horses had complete recovery with no recurrence of infection in subsequent years, implying a long-lasting immunity.[13] In 9% of affected horses, however, infections persisted more than 1 year or recurred as external or internal abscesses.[13] In sheep and goats, studies have shown that acquired humoral and cellular immune responses develop after infection and that macrophages acquire the ability to kill the organism.[23] Similar studies have not been performed in horses.

Corynebacterium pseudotuberculosis produces various exotoxins, which play a role in virulence; the most studied is PLD. Phospholipases are a heterogenous group of enzymes that share the ability to hydrolyze one or more ester linkages in glycerophospholipids. Although all phospholipases target phospholipids as substrates, each enzyme has the ability to cleave a specific ester bond. Thus, qualifying letters (e.g., A, B, C, D) are used to differentiate among phospholipases and to indicate the specific bond targeted in the phospholipid molecule. PLD is important in the pathogenesis of the disease by its action on cell membranes, causing hydrolysis and degradation of sphingomyelin in endothelial cells and increasing vascular permeability.[24] The bacterial PLD is similar to the PLD of the brown recluse spider, which explains the presence of pain and edema at the site of infection. Targeted mutagenesis of PLD in *C. pseudotuberculosis* reduced the ability of this bacterium to establish a primary infection or cause chronic abscess formation in regional lymph nodes. These results indicate that PLD is a virulence determinant of *C. pseudotuberculosis*, increasing the persistence and spread of the bacteria within the host.[25] The synergistic activity of *C. pseudotuberculosis* exotoxins with the exotoxins of *Rhodococcus equi* in lysing red blood cells in agar forms the basis for the synergistic hemolysis inhibition test.[26]

Clinical Findings

External Abscesses

External abscesses may occur anywhere on the body but most frequently develop in the pectoral region and along the ventral midline of the abdomen (see Fig. 45-1). This form of infection is commonly known as "pigeon fever," because of the large size of the pectoral abscesses with the appearance of a pigeon's breast, or "dryland distemper," because of its prevalence in arid geographic regions. Abscesses contain tan, odor-free, purulent exudate and are usually well encapsulated. Additional sites with a predilection for abscess formation include the prepuce, mammary gland, axilla, triceps, limbs, and head. Other less common areas are the thorax, neck, parotid gland, guttural pouches, larynx, flanks, umbilicus, tail, and rectum. Septic joints and osteomyelitis have been reported.[13] Horses may have an abscess involving a single site or involving multiple regions of the body. It is common to observe multiple subcutaneous abscesses coursing along a suspected lymphatic.

Clinical signs most frequently associated with external abscesses are edema, fever, and nonhealing wounds. Other clinical signs include lameness, ventral dermatitis, weight loss, depression, anorexia, and mammary gland or preputial swelling. Generally, horses with external abscesses do not develop signs of systemic illness, although one-quarter will develop fever.[13] If signs of systemic illness are present, further diagnostic testing to rule out internal infection is warranted. In cases of external abscessation, a large area of edema is often observed in the area of abscess formation. As the abscess matures, this area becomes hard and painful. Some abscesses become quite large, particularly in the pectoral region. Abscesses typically have a thick capsule and can cause severe lameness if located in the axillary, triceps, or inguinal region.[13] Maturation can be slow and drainage difficult to establish if the abscess lies deep to muscle.

After drainage is established, either by spontaneous rupture or lancing, most horses recover within 10 to 14 days without complications. The abscesses may contain from 5 to 400 mL of thick, tan, purulent exudate. Ultrasonography may aid in determining the best location for drainage of external abscesses (Fig. 45-4). The case fatality for horses with external abscesses is very low (0.8%).[13]

Clinical pathologic abnormalities that may be observed include anemia of chronic disease, leukocytosis with neutrophilia, hyperfibrinogenemia, and hyperproteinemia. These hematologic parameters can occur with either internal or external abscesses but are more consistently observed with internal abscesses.

Internal Infection

Approximately 8% of affected horses develop internal infection, which is associated with a case-fatality rate of 30% to 40%.[13,15] In a retrospective study, infection was localized to a specific organ(s) in 90% (27/30) of horses. Involvement of multiple internal organs was identified in 37% (10/27) of horses. The organs most often involved were liver and lungs, with kidney and spleen being affected less often. Abdominal ultrasonography was a useful diagnostic tool to identify affected abdominal organs specifically[15,21] (Figs. 45-5 to 45-9).

A diagnosis of internal infection is based on clinical signs, clinicopathologic data, serology, diagnostic imaging, and bacterial culture. The most common clinical signs are concurrent external abscesses, decreased appetite, fever, lethargy, weight loss, and signs of respiratory disease or abdominal pain. Other signs observed in horses with internal abscesses include ventral edema, ventral dermatitis, ataxia, hematuria (caused by renal abscesses), and infrequently, abortion. The median age in two studies was 7 and 8 years, with a range of 1 to 23 years.[13,15]

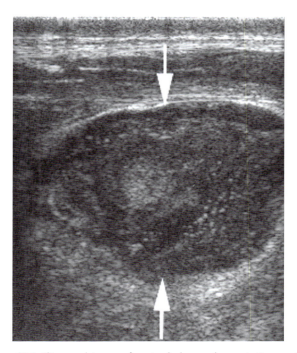

Figure 45-4 Ultrasound image of pectoral abscess demonstrating exudate with mixed echogenicity surrounded by thin hyperechoic capsule (*arrows*). The absecess is approximately 3 to 4 cm in diameter.

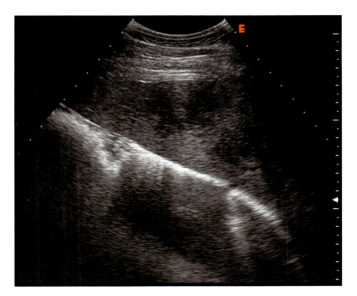

Figure 45-5 Abnormal right liver lobe showing multiple, irregularly shaped, hypoechoic areas in a horse with diffuse hepatic infection. Recheck ultrasound at 60 days showed significant improvement after antimicrobial treatment. Ultrasound image was obtained from the right 11th intercostal space with a 4.0-MHz curvilinear transducer at a scanning depth of 16 cm.

Anemia of chronic disease, leukocytosis with neutrophilia, and elevated fibrinogen are common features of infection, particularly in horses with internal abscesses[13] (Table 45-1). Leukocytosis with neutrophilia was seen in 36% and 76% of horses with external and internal abscesses, respectively. Hyperproteinemia, caused by increased serum globulin concentrations, was observed in 38% and 59% of horses with external and internal abscesses, respectively.[13]

Peritoneal fluid is frequently abnormal in horses with abdominal abscesses. However, peritoneal fluid analysis may be

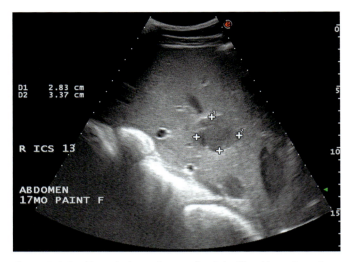

Figure 45-6 Focal hepatic abscess in a yearling Paint filly with persistent fever and poor body condition. Multiple (5-6) additional abscesses were seen throughout the right liver lobe. Ultrasound-guided aspirate from another abscess on the liver surface (not shown) yielded a positive diagnosis. Ultrasound image was obtained from the right 13th intercostal space using a 4-MHz curvilinear transducer at a scanning depth of 18 cm.

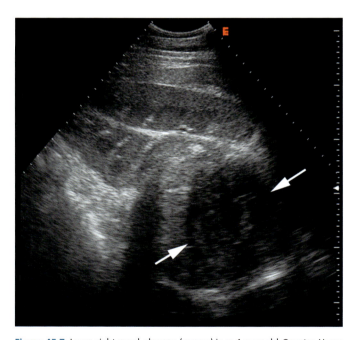

Figure 45-7 Large right renal abscess (*arrows*) in a 4-year-old Quarter Horse mare with recent onset hematuria and a previous history of external abscessation 6 months prior. Ultrasound-guided aspiration and gentle lavage yielded nearly 1 L of purulent material on 2 subsequent days. The abscess resolved after 10 weeks of antimicrobial therapy. Ultrasound image was obtained from the right 14th intercostal space using a 2.5-MHz curvilinear transducer at a scanning depth of 27 cm.

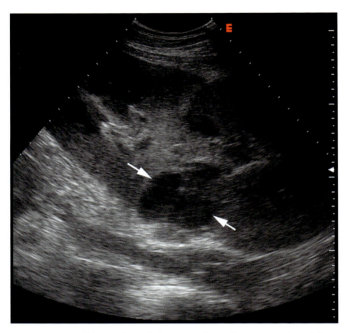

Figure 45-8 Small (2-4 cm) renal abscess involving the cortex and medulla in a 12-year-old Arabian mare with anorexia and weight loss. Extensive infection within the right liver lobe was also found. Both sites of infection responded to long-term antimicrobial therapy. Ultrasound image was obtained from the right 17th intercostal space using a 4.0-MHz curvilinear transducer at a scanning depth of 20 cm.

Table 45-1 Values of Key Clinicopathologic Data in 30 Horses with Internal *Corynebacterium pseudotuberculosis* Infection

Clinicopathologic Data	Mean ± SD	Range
Hematocrit (%)	33.9 ±7.2	23.4-50.0
Total white blood cell (WBC) count (cells/μL)	19,297 ± 9485	6400-53,420
Neutrophil count (μL)	16,080 ± 9109	2944-49,627
Platelet count (cells/μL)	228,967 ± 86,280	15,000-449,000
Fibrinogen (mg/dL)	670.0 ± 306.4	100-1600
Total protein concentration (g/dL)	8.7 ± 1.5	6.3-12.1
Globulin concentration (g/dL)	6.7 ± 1.8	3.5-10.5
Synergistic hemolysis inhibition (SHI) titer	2611	64-20,480

normal if abscesses are located retroperitoneal in the kidneys without involvement of other abdominal structures. *Corynebacterium pseudotuberculosis* was isolated from 32% of samples of peritoneal fluid from affected horses.[13] Failure to isolate the organism from peritoneal fluid does not rule out the disease. The organisms could be located retroperitoneal, sequestered within a thick capsule, or suppressed by local factors or nucleated cells.

Some horses develop C. *pseudotuberculosis* abscesses deep in musculoskeletal structures associated with the limbs and are presented for evaluation of acute or chronic lameness. Affected horses typically have an inflammatory leukogram with anemia and hyperglobulinemia. Increased synergistic hemolysis inhibition titers (SHI) are common and ultrasonography may be useful to assist with localization of lesions and to facilitate surgical drainage to alleviate lameness.[27]

Ulcerative Lymphangitis

Ulcerative lymphangitis is the least common form of C. *pseudotuberculosis* seen in horses in North America, although this form of disease has been reported worldwide. Limb swelling, cellulitis, and draining tracts following lymphatic vessels are seen. Horses often develop severe lameness, fever, lethargy, and anorexia. Aggressive medical therapy is necessary, or the disease may become chronic, resulting in limb edema, lameness, weakness, and weight loss.[1]

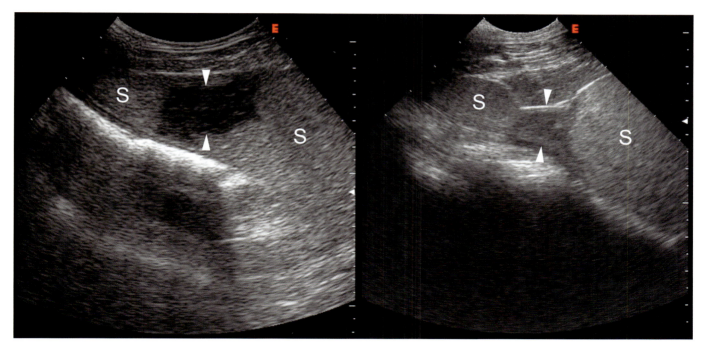

Figure 45-9 Ultrasonographic progression of a splenic abscess *(arrowheads)* in a 15-year-old Arabian gelding referred for anemia and hyperfibrinogenemia. Initial exam revealed a nearly anechoic area of splenic abscessation *(left image)*. Recheck ultrasound at 6 weeks showed improved echogenicity and reduction in size *(right image)*. Abscessation was also found within the left liver lobe which was aspirated to confirm *C. pseudotuberculosis*. The horse fully recovered after 11 weeks of antimicrobial therapy and monitoring. Both images were obtained from the left flank region at a scanning depth of 9-10 cm. *S*, Spleen.

Diagnosis

Culture

The typical clinical presentation of single or multiple, maturing pectoral abscesses, with or without ventral midline abscesses, is highly suspicious of *C. pseudotuberculosis* infection. Culture of the characteristic tan or blood-tinged, odorless exudate is diagnostic. Bacteriologic culture of aspirates or draining abscesses readily yields growth of moderate to large numbers of organisms on blood agar in 24 to 48 hours. The colonies appear small, white, and opaque. Gram stain reveals gram-positive pleomorphic rods. Equine isolates reduce nitrate (unlike most strains from small ruminants).[12] In horses with internal infection, samples obtained by ultrasound-guided aspiration from affected organs can also yield a positive culture.[15,21-23]

Serology

Without a positive bacterial culture, the practitioner must rely on hematology, clinical chemistry, and serologic testing to support a diagnosis. Hematologic changes are nonspecific and indicative of a chronic inflammatory response. Serologic testing using the synergistic hemolysis inhibition (SHI) test can be a useful aid in the diagnosis of internal abscesses if used in conjunction with other clinical and laboratory findings.[13,26,28] The SHI test measures immunoglobulin G (IgG) to the exotoxin of *C. pseudotuberculosis* and is available through the California Animal Health and Food Safety Laboratory System in Davis, CA. Serology is generally not helpful for diagnosis of external abscesses and may be negative early in the course of disease and even at the time of abscess drainage. Positive SHI titers must be interpreted carefully, after appropriate consideration of clinical signs, to distinguish active infection from exposure or convalescence. Both published and unpublished data from the University of California suggest that a reciprocal titer of 256 or greater is indicative of active infection. Horses with internal abscesses generally have SHI titers of 512 or higher,

although horses with active external infection commonly have similar titers. In one study of internal infection, SHI titers ranged from 512 to 20,480.[15] Titers of 16 or lower are considered negative, whereas titers between 16 and 128 are considered suspicious or indicative of exposure.[29] In general, the SHI test is most useful for detection of internal abscesses attributable to *C. pseudotuberculosis* infection in the absence of detectable external abscesses.[28] There is considerable overlap in values from horses with active disease, exposure, and recovery from infection. Experimental inoculation of horses with a bacterin-toxoid developed from *C. pseudotuberculosis* produced increased SHI titers equivalent to those seen with active infection; the protection offered from this bacterin has not been proved to date.

Ultrasonography

Ultrasonography is extremely useful for diagnosis of internal infections in horses, not only for identifying affected organs but also for defining the nature and extent of involvement of abdominal viscera. Abdominal ultrasound permits documentation of involvement of specific organs in the absence of clinicopathologic evidence of disease involving these organs. Abdominal ultrasound may be used for collection of transcutaneous liver and kidney biopsies and aspirates of abscesses for a definitive diagnosis. Thoracic ultrasound should be performed in affected horses to determine the severity of pulmonary disease (Fig. 45-10). Serial examinations can be used to evaluate response to treatment. Examinations should be performed using low-frequency (2.5-3.5 MHz) and medium-frequency (5 MHz) ultrasound transducers. Complete examination of the abdomen consists of both right and left paralumbar fossa regions, all intercostal spaces from the ventral lung margins to the costochondral junctions, and the ventral abdomen from the sternum to the inguinal region. Presence of peritoneal fluid and abnormalities of the liver, spleen, kidneys, stomach, duodenum, small intestine, cecum, and large colon can be observed.

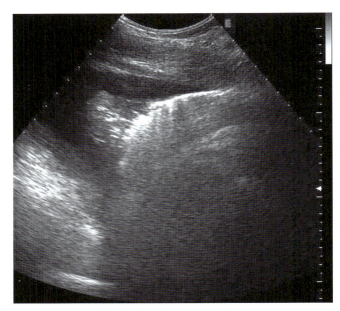

Figure 45-10 Cranioventral consolidation with moderate pleural effusion in mare with pneumonia secondary to *C. pseudotuberculosis*. The small hyperechoic areas within the consolidated lung represent air trapped within the small airways. The image was obtained from the right sixth intercostal space with a 3.5-MHz curvilinear transducer at a scanning depth of 16 cm.

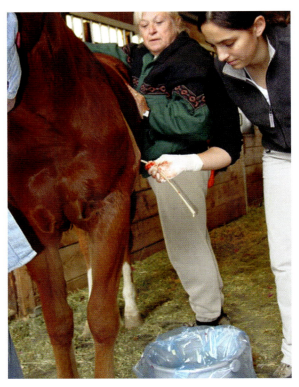

Figure 45-11 Deep abscess in left triceps muscle was causing severe lameness in this yearling gelding. The lameness was relieved after insertion of a polyvinyl chest tube to drain the abscess.

Hepatic abnormalities associated with *C. pseudotuberculosis* infection in horses include hepatomegaly, multiple small hypoechoic areas resulting in a "moth-eaten" appearance, and discrete, circular, anechoic to hypoechoic areas (see Figs. 45-5 and 45-6). Renal abscessation may appear as a single large (10-15 cm in diameter) area or multiple anechoic to hypoechoic areas involving either the cortex or the medulla[21] (see Figs. 45-7 and 45-8). Splenic abnormalities may also be observed and include small, irregularly shaped, hypoechoic areas without obvious encapsulation (see Fig. 45-9). In horses with pulmonary involvement, examination of the thorax may reveal presence of pleural defects ("comet tails"), consolidation, pleural effusion, or pericardial effusion (see Fig. 45-10).[15]

Early diagnosis of internal infection caused by *C. pseudotuberculosis* is important for a successful outcome but is often difficult because of the insidious onset and nonspecific nature of clinical signs, which may include anorexia, fever, lethargy, and weight loss. In endemic areas, horses that have had an external abscess in the previous 6 months and then develop signs of systemic illness should be suspected of having internal *C. pseudotuberculosis* infection, as should horses with compatible signs residing on a property where other horses have had external abscesses. For horses with this history, ultrasonography and serologic testing are recommended as an aid for diagnosis of internal infections.

Therapy

External Abscesses

The treatment regimen must be individualized for each horse depending on the severity of disease, including the presence of systemic illness (e.g., fever, anorexia), the extent of soft tissue inflammation, the maturity of the abscess, and the ability to establish drainage of pus. Establishing drainage is the most important treatment and ultimately leads to faster resolution and return to athletic performance. The proximity of the fibrous abscess capsule to the skin varies, often being less than 1 cm deep for ventral midline abscesses, to greater than 10 cm for

deep pectoral, axillary, triceps, or inguinal abscesses (Fig. 45-11). Aspiration and drainage of superficial abscesses are easily performed; the use of diagnostic ultrasound is helpful for localization of deeper abscesses and to judge maturity of the abscess and proximity to the skin. If the abscess is immature or cannot be safely incised, subsequent ultrasound examinations may be necessary to establish the ideal time to lance into the abscess. The abscess contents and lavage solutions (e.g., saline with or without antiseptic) should be retrieved and disposed of to prevent further contamination of the immediate environment.

Antimicrobial Therapy

Antimicrobial therapy is indicated for treatment of horses with ulcerative lymphangitis or internal abscesses. The use of antimicrobials for external abscesses is not necessary in most horses and may prolong the time to resolution.[13] Antimicrobial therapy may be justified when signs of systemic illness (e.g., fever, depression, anorexia) or extensive cellulitis are present. Horses with deep intramuscular abscesses that are lanced and draining through healthy tissue may also benefit from antimicrobial therapy.

C. pseudotuberculosis is susceptible in vitro to many antimicrobials typically used in horses, including penicillin G, macrolides, tetracyclines, cephalosporins, chloramphenicol, fluoroquinolones, and rifampin, but some isolates may be resistant to aminoglycosides.[7,30,31] Several factors should be considered when choosing an antimicrobial: the intracellular location of the organism, the presence of exudate and a thick abscess capsule, anticipated duration of therapy, cost of the drug, and convenience of administration. Despite in vitro susceptibility, the nature of the bacteria and the copious exudate render certain antimicrobials ineffective for some cases. Trimethoprim-sulfa (30 mg/kg, twice daily orally) and procaine penicillin (20,000 U/kg twice daily intramuscularly) are highly effective

Table 45-2 Antimicrobial Drugs Used to Treat 30 Horses with Internal C. *pseudotuberculosis* Infection

Antimicrobial	No. of Horses	No. Also With Rifampin
Rifampin	19	—
Trimethoprim-sulfa	11	3
Gentamicin	10	—
Ampicillin	9	4
Ceftiofur	9	7
Penicillin G	5	3
Cefazolin	2	—
Enrofloxacin	2	2
Erythromycin	2	—

for treatment of external abscesses, especially on the ventral midline. Rifampin (2.5-5 mg/kg twice daily orally) in combination with ceftiofur (2.5-5 mg/kg twice daily intravenously or intramuscularly) appears highly effective for treatment of internal abscesses. Internal abscesses have reportedly responded to procaine penicillin (dose as above), trimethoprim-sulfa (dose as above), potassium penicillin (20,000-40,000 U/kg four times daily intravenously), doxycycline (10 mg/kg twice daily orally), or enrofloxacin (7.5 mg/kg once daily orally).

Internal Infection

Antimicrobial therapy is indicated for the treatment of horses with systemic infection caused by C. *pseudotuberculosis*.[13] The median duration of antimicrobial therapy in a recent study was 36 days and ranged from 7 to 97 days. A variety of antimicrobials to which C. *pseudotuberculosis* is susceptible were used to treat these internal infections (Table 45-2). Rifampin was used in combination with another antimicrobial in the majority of horses. Rifampin alone was used for continued treatment in horses after initial treatment with a combination of rifampin and another antimicrobial.[22] Thoracic and abdominal ultrasound are useful to monitor response to therapy. Ultrasound findings, in addition to clinicopathologic data, aid in the decision-making process for continued antimicrobial therapy in these cases (see Fig. 45-10).

The overall mortality associated with internal infections is reported to be 30% to 40%,[13,15] but horses that did not receive antimicrobial therapy had a 100% fatality rate.[13] Antimicrobial therapy for treatment of internal abscesses and ulcerative lymphangitis must be continued for 1 to 6 months. Resolution of infection is determined based on clinical signs, normal clinical pathologic values, and decline in immunoglobulin concentrations. Some horses with very high SHI titers remain seropositive for up to 1 year because of the lengthy half-life of IgG (21 days) and for other reasons that are unknown. Under such situations the clinician should monitor a steady decline in serum SHI titers to C. *pseudotuberculosis*. Purpura hemorrhagica or vasculitis has been reported in horses with systemic infection requiring concurrent therapy with antimicrobials and corticosteroids.[13]

Ulcerative Lymphangitis

Horses with ulcerative lymphangitis or cellulitis should be treated early and aggressively with antimicrobials, or residual lameness or limb swelling may occur. Typically, intravenous (IV) antimicrobials (ceftiofur or penicillin G) alone or in combination with rifampin (orally) are used until lameness and swelling improves, and then therapy with oral antimicrobials, such as trimethoprim-sulfamethoxazole or rifampin, is continued to prevent relapse. The time to resolution in one study was approximately 35 days.[13] Physical therapy, including hydrotherapy, hand walking, and leg wraps, as well as administration of nonsteroidal antiinflammatory drugs (NSAIDs), are also recommended.

Prevention

Until a protective bacterin or toxoid is developed for horses, horse owners in endemic areas must rely solely on good sanitation and fly control and avoid unnecessary environmental contamination from diseased horses to prevent C. *pseudotuberculosis* infection in their horses. Presently, there is no evidence that diseased horses within a stable should be quarantined, but strict insect control should be implemented. Proper sanitation, disposal of contaminated bedding, and disinfection may reduce the incidence of new cases. Proper wound care is also important to prevent infection from a contaminated environment.

A commercial bacterin-toxoid is available for use in small ruminants (Caseous D-T, Colorado Serum Co., Denver; Glanvac 6 TM, Pfizer Animal Health, Australia).[32] The safety and effectiveness of this product has not been tested in horses. The inability experimentally to reproduce the disease as seen in horses in endemic areas and the sporadic nature of disease complicate research efforts.

Nocardiosis

Marta Gonzalez Arguedas

Nocardiosis is a localized or disseminated bacterial disease of a large variety of animals and of humans caused by *Nocardia* spp.,[33-36] which are soil saprophytes that act as opportunistic pathogens.[33,37] In humans and domestic animals, *Nocardia* causes suppurative to granulomatous tissue reactions, which are most severe in immunosuppressed individuals.[38] *Nocardia* spp. infections in horses are rare. When they do occur, they are usually associated with significant derangements in the host immune system.[38-40] The most common manifestations of disease are pulmonary and pleural disease or nodulo-ulcerative cutaneous lesions.

Etiology

Members of the *Nocardia* spp. are gram-positive, aerobic, saprophytic, nonmotile, non–spore-forming actinomycetes.[33,35,36,41,42] Nocardiae appear as long, slender, branching filaments with a tendency to fragment into rods and cocci.[42] When cultured, these organisms produce aerial filaments.[35,42] Components of the cell wall, especially mycolic acid, render *Nocardia* spp. partially acid-fast.[32,35,36,42]

Although most nocardial infections in horses are caused by *Nocardia asteroides*,[35,37,38,42] Deem and Harrington[34] reported a case of fatal pleuropneumonia in a 15-month-old Quarter Horse colt with histologic lesions characteristic of pulmonary nocardiosis in which *Nocardia brasiliensis* was isolated from the lung and bronchial lymph node.

Pathogenic nocardiae are obligate aerobes growing over a wide temperature range (10° C-50° C [50° F-122° F]).[32] *Nocardia* spp. will grow on most nonselective media used routinely for culture of bacteria, fungi, and mycobacteria.[36,41,43] However, in specimens containing mixed flora (e.g., respiratory secretions), nocardial colonies are easily obscured by those of more rapidly growing bacteria. Nocardiae normally appear within 2 to 7 days on most routine bacteriologic media.[43,44] Their relatively slow growth often results in the cultures being discarded before the nocardiae can be visualized.[35,43] The colony surface, waxy to powdery to velvety depending on the abundance of aerial growth, becomes wrinkled with age.[33,41,43,45] Although the colonies are usually white when first visible, most *Nocardia* spp. produce carotenoid-like pigments that result in colonies with various shades of yellow, orange, pink, or red.[33,35,45]

With the widespread use of molecular methods of identification, the number of recognized *Nocardia* spp. is increasing, and members of the genus *Nocardia* are becoming increasingly difficult to identify using phenotypic criteria.[46] Currently, more than 30 species are included in the genus.[33,47]

Molecular analysis demonstrates that *N. asteroides* includes several species with similar biochemistry, structure, and antimicrobial resistance: *N. asteroides, N. abscessus, N. cyriacigeorgica, N. farcinica, N. nova,* and *N. transvalensis.*[33,36,43,44,47] These species together are referred to as the *N. asteroides* complex.[33,43,44,47] It is important to note that all the literature about nocardiosis in horses was published before these species were recognized, therefore it is impossible to determine the clinical relevance of each individual species in horses. For purposes of simplicity, the discussion that follows will use the former name of *N. asteroides.*

Epidemiology

Nocardiae are present in most environments and found extensively worldwide. They are saprophytic, making up an important component of the normal soil microflora, and are often associated with water.[33,41,44] Nocardial infections may be acquired through inhalation[35,41,42,44] or by traumatic percutaneous introduction of organisms.[41,44] Dust, soil, and plant material serve as vehicles.[33,35] In humans, intestinal nocardiosis may result from ingestion of the organism[35,42]; however, this form of infection has not been reported in horses. Infection is not considered contagious.[41] Transmission between or among animals and persons has not been demonstrated to occur.[34,43,44] Nocardiosis is not considered a zoonotic disease.[41]

In the horse, pulmonary and generalized infection appears to require profound constitutional and immune disturbances and should be considered an opportunistic infection.[33,39,42] In a review of 16 horses with nocardiosis admitted to the Veterinary Teaching Hospital, University of California, Davis, over an 18-year period, almost 90% had an underlying immunosuppressive problem.[39] The two horses that survived had local infections associated with trauma. The remaining 14 cases were associated with concurrent serious systemic illnesses and compromised immune systems that would have led to the death of the horses in the absence of nocardiosis. From the same study, the prevalence of nocardiosis in equine patients from 1965 to 1983 was 16 of 180,000 (0.009%). Two entities emerged as predominant conditions linked with systemic or pulmonary nocardiosis in horses: severe combined immunodeficiency of Arabian foals and pituitary pars intermedia dysfunction.[39] It appears that the circumstances favoring nocardiosis infection in horses closely parallel those recognized in human medicine, where the majority of patients with clinically recognized *N. asteroides* infection have underlying debilitating and/or immunodepressant conditions.*

Pathogenesis

The outcome of infection with *N. asteroides* is largely determined by the ability of a given strain to resist the initial neutrophil leukocyte response and subsequent attack by activated macrophages and cell-mediated immunity.[35,43] Macrophages and neutrophils by themselves are insufficient to control infection by virulent strains of *N. asteroides.*[35] In vitro, virulent *N. asteroides* can grow within and destroy macrophages.[41] The resistance of this species to oxidative killing by neutrophils and monocytes has been attributed to nocardial catalase and superoxide dismutase.[33,35,41,43,50] In contrast, less virulent strains of *N. asteroides* are capable of surviving within macrophages in an altered cellular state called an "L-form."[35] L-forms are microbial variants that lack a structurally intact cell wall; some may revert

*References 33, 34, 39, 44, 48, 49.

to the parental form when the inducing condition is removed. L-forms of *Nocardia* spp. can be recovered from clinical material obtained from patients and may explain the occasional late relapse of nocardial infections.[35,43] The cell wall of nocardiae possesses mycolic acids that contribute to virulence by resisting killing by macrophages.[41] Several bacterial toxins, including hemolysins, have been identified in association with *N. asteroides* but are not thought to be widespread or important virulence factors.[35,43]

Nocardia spp. do not elicit an effective humoral immune response, and B lymphocytes are considered unimportant in the protective response. Protective immune responses are T-cell mediated.[35,43,50,51]

Clinical Findings

Nocardiosis can be a localized or disseminated infection.[45,48] A chronic course is usual, but in immunologically incompetent patients, disease may be acute in onset and rapid in progression.[45] Nocardiosis is infrequent in the horse; however, the following clinical forms have been recognized: pulmonary nocardiosis, disseminated nocardiosis, cutaneous and mycetomatous lesions, and rarely, abortion.[35,38,41,48]

Pulmonary Nocardiosis

Clinical signs are related to severe pulmonary infection and may include increased respiratory rate and effort, cough, and nasal discharge.[43] No specific clinical signs are diagnostic for pulmonary nocardiosis, and the clinical presentation of disease may run the full spectrum of either acute or chronic pulmonary infection. There may be pneumonia, abscess formation, or pleural involvement[35] (Fig. 45-12).

Disseminated Nocardiosis

Disseminated or systemic nocardiosis is characterized by widespread abscess formation in two or more organs of the body. After establishment of primary pulmonary nocardial infection, the organism may be disseminated hematogenously, leading to extrapulmonary disease.[35,36,43] Any anatomic location can be involved.[35] In humans, the most frequently affected sites include

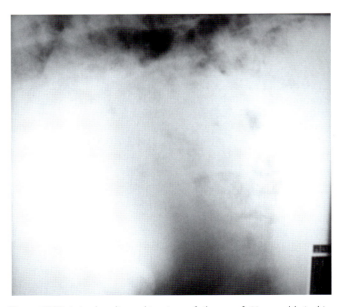

Figure 45-12 Lateral radiographic view of thorax of 21-year-old Arabian gelding with disseminated nocardiosis secondary to pars intermedia pituitary dysfunction. *(Courtesy Dr. Robert Mealey.)*

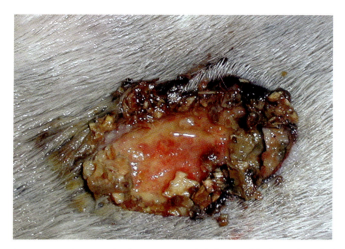

Figure 45-13 Ulcerative skin lesion on ventral abdomen of the horse described in Figure 45-12. *(Courtesy Dr. Robert Mealey.)*

the central nervous system and eyes (especially the retina), skin and subcutaneous tissues (Fig. 45-13), kidneys, joints, bone, and heart.[36,43]

Localized Cutaneous and Subcutaneous Nocardiosis

Rarely, *N. asteroides* has been reported to cause dermatitis without systemic lesions in horses.[52] This form of disease usually occurs after traumatic introduction of *Nocardia* spp. into the skin. After the organism breaches the integrity of the skin, localized bacterial growth may progress sufficiently to induce an inflammatory response with accumulation of polymorphonuclear leukocytes (PMNs), leading to cellulitis or pyoderma. Often, the infection becomes circumscribed to form an abscess.[35] Skin lesions appear as firm, painless, slow-growing subcutaneous nodules, which can occur anywhere on the body. The lesions may ulcerate and discharge a thick, odorless, grayish white or yellowish material.[52] Because the initial response to *Nocardia* is pyogenic, self-limited cutaneous lesions have the same appearance as diseases caused by other pyogenic bacteria, such as *Staphylococcus* and *Streptococcus* spp.,[35] and they may be disregarded or treated as staphylococcal in origin.[35,43]

Nocardia-Induced Mycetomas

Mycetomas are chronically progressive, destructive subcutaneous infections. Mycetomas caused by fungi are called *eumycetomas,* whereas those caused by the actinomycetes are called *actinomycetomas.* The most common bacteria isolated from equine actinomycetomas are *Actinobacillus* spp., *Nocardia* spp., and *Actinomyces* spp. Regardless of causative agent, the organism usually gains entrance to the body through traumatic inoculation. The mycetoma most often starts as a painless nodule developing at the site of the injury, days to months after the injury. This nodule increases in size and may eventually become purulent and necrotic. Pus may discharge through sinus tracts. Chronic granulomatous inflammation with concomitant swelling and enlargement of the surrounding areas occurs, with the formation of multiple secondary nodules and draining sinus tracts. The exudate from these nocardial mycetomas may contain "grains" (sandlike particles) similar to those seen in actinomycosis. The granules represent small colonies of the infecting agent surrounded by masses of inflammatory cells.[35,43,52-55]

Abortion

Nocardia spp. have been recorded among the genital flora of clinically healthy mares.[56] *Nocardia* spp. have been associated with sporadic abortions in cattle and swine but rarely are associated with abortion in horses.[38] Bolon et al[37] reported two cases of abortion in an Arabian and a Thoroughbred mare during the sixth gestational month. Both mares had a history of repeated failure to carry foals to term and were apparently healthy. Fetal necropsies revealed lesions in lung, liver, and placenta. The chorion was mottled, white and red, opaque, and in the Arabian fetus, avillar. Filamentous bacilli within the lungs of both fetuses, the liver of the Arabian, and the chorion of the Thoroughbred were gram positive, silver positive, and acid-fast positive. *N. asteroides* was cultured from the uterus of the Arabian mare.[38]

Nocardioform placentitis is the term used to describe a distinct type of placentitis of horses that was first diagnosed in 1986 at the University of Kentucky, Livestock Disease Diagnostic Center[55] (see Chapter 8). Although similar to members of the genus *Nocardia* in morphology, the cause of this condition is one of several genera of gram-positive, branching, filamentous actinomycetes. The most common isolates in clinical cases of abortion are *Crossiella equi,* a microorganism unrelated to *Nocardia,*[33,57] and *Amycolatopsis* spp.[58,59] Recently, another filamentous actinomycete, *Cellulosimicrobium (Cellumonas) cellulans* (formerly *Oerskovia xanthineolytica*), has also been associated with nocardioform placentitis.[60]

Pathologic Findings

Nocardiosis is a predominantly suppurative process, but granulomatous or mixed responses may occur. Tissue destruction with the formation of abscesses is characteristic of all clinical forms of nocardial disease.[35,43-45] Exudates are sanguinopurulent and sometimes may contain small (<1 mm in diameter), soft granules consisting of bacteria, neutrophils, and debris.[33] *Nocardia asteroides* is isolated most often from the lungs (Fig. 45-14). Other tissues from which *N. asteroides* has been isolated or identified are tracheal fluid, cornea, skin lesions, brain, spleen, peritoneal fluid, pleural fluid, lymph nodes, pericardial abscess, uterus, incision from repaired rectal tear, liver, and kidney.[38,39,61] Pulmonary lesions grossly resemble those described for nocardial infections in humans and other primates.[61] There may be necrotizing abscesses that are not encapsulated or sharply circumscribed, solitary masses, reticulonodular infiltrates, large irregular nodules (frequently with cavitation), interstitial infiltrate, and pleural effusion.[35] The most frequently observed change is fibrinohemorrhagic pleuritis.[61] Other gross and histopathologic findings may include necrosuppurative lymphadenitis, necrosuppurative nephritis, and ulcerative suppurative dermatitis.[41]

Diagnosis

Confirmation of a diagnosis of nocardiosis depends on the cytologic and bacteriologic evaluation of appropriate specimens[44] (Fig. 45-15). Clinical laboratory findings are not specific and may include evidence of an inflammatory or infectious process, as well as evidence of immunosuppression. Thus lymphopenia, left shift, toxic neutrophils, neutrophilia, hyperfibrinogenemia, and hyperglobulinemia or hypoglobulinemia are possible.[34,61]

Direct Examination

Gram-stained smears of *Nocardia*-infected samples reveal rod-shaped to coccoid forms and gram-positive branching filaments. Most strains are partially acid-fast.[33,41,50] Gram staining is the most sensitive method by which to visualize and recognize nocardiae in clinical specimens.[44] Modified acid-fast staining is not reliable (may vary with the strain and culture media used) and should be used only to confirm the acid fastness of organisms detected by Gram staining.[43,44]

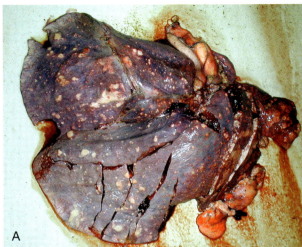

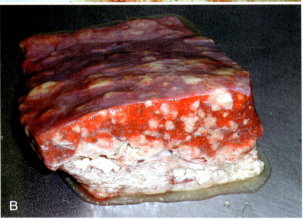

Figure 45-14 **A,** Gross appearance of lungs of the horse desribed in Figure 45-12. Note the abscessation. **B,** Cut section through an affected area of lung. *(Courtesy Dr. Robert Mealey.)*

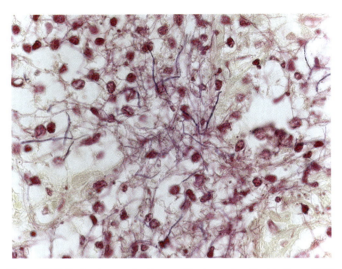

Figure 45-15 Photomicrograph of lungs of the horse described in Figure 45-12. Note the numerous long, red-shaped to filamentous bacteria typical of *Nocardia*. *(Courtesy Dr. Robert Mealey.)*

Isolation and Identification

Standard collection and transport procedures suitable for bacterial and fungal cultures are adequate for isolation of *Nocardia* (see Chapters 27 and 46), but refrigeration of specimens should be avoided because some *Nocardia* strains lose viability at low temperatures.[33,43]

Serologic Testing

Major problems arise with developing serodiagnostic methods because the host infected with nocardiae usually develops a minimal, nonspecific antibody response.[35] Serologic tests (immunodiffusion, complement fixation, enzyme-linked immunosorbent assays) and cutaneous hypersensitivity tests using extracellular antigen to detect nocardial infection in cattle and dogs are of uncertain sensitivity and are not generally available.[33,44] Currently, no serodiagnostic test is routinely used to confirm nocardial infection in human patients.[35,43]

Molecular Identification

Conventional methods for identification of *Nocardia* spp. (growth characteristics, colony and microscopic morphology, biochemical and antimicrobial susceptibility testing) are insufficient to distinguish among some members of the *N. asteroides* complex.* At present, molecular methods used to identify the nocardiae to the species level include restriction endonucle-

---

*References 33, 35, 41, 43, 44, 47.

ase analysis of an amplified portion of the 16S ribosomal ribonucleic acid (rRNA) gene, polymerase chain reaction (PCR)–restriction endonuclease analysis of the amplified 65 hsp gene, and sequencing methodologies (e.g., of 16S rRNA or DNA).[33,44,62] An experimental study demonstrated that the diagnosis of nocardiosis by seminested PCR in mice is a rapid and more sensitive test than culture for detection of *Nocardia* in blood and different visceral organs. This method has the additional advantage over culture techniques of being able to detect L-forms of *Nocardia* in clinical specimens, which otherwise fail to grow on routine isolation medium.[63]

Therapy

Clinical experience has shown that successful therapy of nocardiosis requires the use of antimicrobial drug(s) in combination with appropriate surgical drainage.[43,48] When possible, abscesses, empyemas, and serosal effusions are treated by surgical debridement, drainage, and lavage. Granulomatous proliferations require excision.[33,34,41,43] Initial selection of a therapeutic regimen should take into account the site and severity of infection, host immune status, potential drug interactions or toxicity, and the species of *Nocardia*. Antimicrobial susceptibility testing is recommended as a guide to therapy, but such testing may be misleading, and discrepancies between in vitro data and clinical outcome are well documented.[41,43,44]

In horses the selection of antibiotic and duration of therapy are based on human medicine. In human patients, sulfa-containing antimicrobials are the treatment of choice for nocardiosis caused by *N. brasiliensis* and *N. asteroides* complex and have resulted in substantial improvement in outcome.[36,41,43,44,48] In human patients with primary cutaneous infection, trimethoprim-sulfa is sufficient in combination with appropriate surgical debridement. In severely ill or immunosuppressed patients, two or more drugs, which usually include a sulfa-containing agent, are frequently prescribed despite a lack of clinical data supporting the efficacy of combination therapy.[43,44] Amikacin has been used successfully, usually in combination with other agents, including sulfonamides, in patients with nocardiosis involving several different body sites and in immunocompromised patients. Synergy between trimethoprim-sulfa and amikacin has been demonstrated in vitro.[43] Other potentially efficacious choices include amoxicillin-clavulanate, third-generation cephalosporins, newer macrolides, imipenem, and other aminoglycosides.[43,44,48]

Clinical improvement is generally evident within 5 to 10 days after initiation of therapy.[43] In human medicine, recommendations on the duration of therapy are empiric and based on reports of relapse after sulfonamide therapy of different duration. Long-term antimicrobial treatment (6-12 months) may be necessary to avoid relapses.[34,41,43-45] The clinical outcome depends on the site and extent of disease and underlying host factors.[36] For horses with pulmonary and disseminated nocardiosis, the prognosis is poor because most of these patients are severely immunocompromised or debilitated. Prognosis is usually good in patients with only skin involvement.[39]

Public Health Considerations

As noted earlier, intestinal nocardiosis in humans may result from ingestion of the organism.[35,42] Transmission between or among animals and humans has not been demonstrated.[34,43,44] Nocardiosis is not considered a zoonotic disease.[41]

Anthrax

Maureen T. Long

Bacillus anthracis has a special place in world history and microbiology because anthrax was the first disease for which a causal relationship to a bacterium was demonstrated.[57,64,65] In 1877, Robert Koch injected a pure culture of sporulated organisms into animals and caused lethal anthrax. In 1881, Pasteur successfully demonstrated the ability of attenuated organisms to protect sheep from clinical anthrax. Before the widespread availability of a vaccine in the 1930s, anthrax was one of the most important causes of mortality in herbivores worldwide.

Etiology

Bacillus anthracis is a large, gram-positive rod (3-5 μm long) that forms spores and is cultivated both aerobically and anaerobically. This organism is often confused with *Bacillus cereus* and must be differentiated by morphologic and biochemical characteristics.[57] Specifically, *B. anthracis* is nonhemolytic, has a capsule, and is nonmotile.[57,66] Gamma phage will lyse the organism, and *B. anthracis* is positive on a "string of pearls" test.[57,67]

Epidemiology

Bacillus anthracis has a vegetative and a spore state.[57,68] Classic theory maintains that sporulation provides a state of low nutrient requirement for the organism, allowing maintenance in the environment, usually soil, for decades.[68-70] In general, spores can survive temperature extremes and favor alkaline conditions. They also survive tanning and processing of hides.[68]

The most common route of natural infection for animals is thought to be ingestion, but inhalation and skin penetration may also occur.[70] There may be concomitant damage to mucous membranes. Mechanical infection by biting flies has been demonstrated experimentally; this transmission likely occurs seasonally in areas with high incidence and has been particularly associated with outbreaks of anthrax in wildlife in Russia and Australia.[68,71-74] Climatic stressors allow reliable prediction of anthrax outbreaks.[68,71,73,75-77]

With climatic change, outbreaks of anthrax occur in infection cycles. A harbinger of infection occurs with the sudden death of one or two animals that have been recently introduced into an area.[57,70] These infected carcasses contaminate the soil with *B. anthracis*.[69,71,74,76-81] The next or secondary infection cycle involves multiple animals who develop anthrax after exposure to contaminated soil (or carcasses).

Anthrax is a reportable disease in the United States; suspected or confirmed cases must be reported to the state veterinarian. In addition, *B. anthracis* is listed as a Category A bioterrorism agent. Although the fall of 2001 focused attention on human anthrax and this organism as a terror threat, animal anthrax has always been present in the United States.[68,76,77,82] The Ames strain isolated from this human outbreak originates from a trail that crosses West Texas to Mexico in which the soil is heavily laden with *B. anthracis*. In fact, 2000 and 2001 were banner years for anthrax in animals (www.aphis.usda.gov). In 2000 the North Dakota Red River Valley (80 horses and cows), South Dakota (9), Nevada (32 cows), and Minnesota (10 cows) had animal losses to anthrax. In Nebraska, several cattle deaths were suspected to result from anthrax. In June through October 2001 and 2002, deaths were reported in cattle, deer, bison, water buffalo, and elk in Texas, South Dakota, Minnesota, North Dakota, and California. Texas reported 1638 animal cases of anthrax in 2001. In 2005, 109 cases of animal anthrax cases were confirmed in 16 North Dakota counties.* In 2006, a large outbreak of anthrax in Saskatchewan, Canada affected more than 800 animals including 6 horses.[83]

Animal and human anthrax has a worldwide occurrence, and only notable recent reports are reviewed here. A large seasonal outbreak occurred in western Alberta, Canada, in 1999.[71,75] The outbreak was widespread, affecting seven cattle farms. One horse also died due to anthrax. This outbreak resulted in movement restrictions and vaccination of 650 livestock on the identified farms and 25,000 animals in the surrounding vicinity. More than 1585 bison carcasses were disposed of during 11 outbreaks that occurred in Alberta and adjacent territories.[71]

Since 1950 the U.S. Centers for Disease Control and Prevention (CDC) has been involved in the investigation of numerous anthrax outbreaks involving animals in Texas, North Dakota, Iowa, Pennsylvania, Louisiana, Wyoming, California, Connecticut, North Dakota, Missouri, New Jersey, Oklahoma, and Ohio.[68] Infection has likely occurred in many other states with animal infection only reported locally.

Risk factors associated with recent outbreaks have been identified.† In the Alberta outbreak, old anthrax graves and weather patterns were highly associated with occurrence. There was a long, dry spring followed by heavy rainfall. In this and other studies, farms with poor drainage and soil with a high degree of organic content were involved, rather than arid soil with minimal vegetative support.[76,77,86,87] During an outbreak, *B. anthracis* is found throughout the epizootic environment. Besides soil, positive samples have included hay, biting flies, and feed (from contaminated bone meal). *B. anthracis* may undergo rounds of germination and sporulation depending on soil conditions. An outbreak of anthrax in the Yamal peninsula identified blood-sucking insects and organic substances in the soil as risk factors for recurring outbreaks. Only vaccination in this region actually breaks the cycle of high numbers of wild ungulates and livestock developing disease.

Pathogenesis

The mammalian incubation period is 1 to 7 days for respiratory and gastrointestinal (GI) anthrax.[57,70,88,89] Susceptibility to disease is greatest for cattle, followed by sheep, then horses and goats.[70] These differences in susceptibility may result from differences in oral and GI physiology and frequency of transmission. Pigs frequently develop clinical anthrax after exposure to *B. anthracis* but are the only species that may spontaneously recover (many still die).[85,90]

---

*www.agdepartment.com/Progarms/lavistock/BOAH/2005 Anthrax.pdf.
†References 65, 68, 71, 73-78, 80, 81, 84, 85.

Ingestion is likely the primary route of inoculation for most animals; a break in the mucous membranes is considered important for development of disease.[65,91] There is an initial round of primary replication in the regional lymph nodes.[70] The organism enters the bloodstream through lymphatic drainage, with resultant bacteremia, septicemia, toxemia, and dissemination to all major organs. Proliferation of lethal toxin is considered the primary cause of death.

Classically, three clinical forms of anthrax are described in animals and humans. Cutaneous disease is most often observed in humans working with animal hides and hair contaminated with *B. anthracis* spores.[68,91,92] This form results in gelatinous edema, which leads to a "malignant pustule." After a necrotic ulcer forms, the organism can disseminate to give rise to classic septicemia, which is usually fatal. Pulmonary anthracic disease is common in humans or animals that inhale spores.[88,89,93-95] An acute hemorrhagic mediastinitis occurs that is rapidly fatal. Cattle and other animals may inhale spores in dusty environments, leading to a vegetative state and localized pulmonary infection that eventually disseminates. GI disease occurs from oral ingestion. In humans, confinement of infection to the GI tract is rare.[70] A process similar to cutaneous infection occurs, except that the mucosa is the site for invasion, pustule formation, and ulceration. This infection has an extremely high mortality rate.

The ability of *B. anthracis* to evade the immune system, undergo rapid vegetative proliferation, and elaborate toxin are critical steps in the pathogenesis of anthrax.[96,97] The bacterium has a poly-D-glutamyl capsule that protects against complement and phagocytosis.[66,98] Anthrax toxin has three components: protective antigen (PA), lethal factor (LF), and edema factor (EF).[96,97,99] The toxin uses the PA molecule to bind to the cell surface; because PA is important in binding, antibodies that recognize this protein usually neutralize the activity of toxins.[90,99,100] LF is required to mediate the fatal effect of *B. anthracis*. EF is required for extravasation of intercellular fluids into subcutaneous and peritoneal compartments and interstitial spaces on infection with *B. anthracis*. This toxin is an adenylate cyclase protein. Different combinations of these toxins lead to specific manifestations of pathology.[96,97] The combination of PA and LF must be present for lethality. If EF and PA are complexed, these proteins produce edema. When all three toxin components are present, the organism causes necrosis of cells with edema and is lethal.

Clinical Findings

Most of the clinical signs of anthrax, other than sudden death, have been described in cattle, the species in which anthrax is most frequently reported.* Most natural cases of anthrax in horses are associated with disease in cattle. Across all species, the predominant sign observed in outbreaks of anthrax is sudden death, bleeding from orifices, and failure of blood to clot.[83,102]

A peracute form of anthrax is most often observed early in an outbreak. Cattle are either found dead or with premonitory signs of fever (lasting 1-2 hours), muscle tremors, dyspnea, and congestion of the mucous membranes, followed by collapse and death with discharge of bloody fluid from nostrils, mouth, anus, and vulva. Animals with acute disease have a high fever lasting approximately 48 hours, increased heart rate, anorexia, and ruminal stasis. Animals are severely depressed with congested mucous membranes. Abortions can occur, or if lactating, blood-stained milk may be observed. In cattle, bloody diarrhea is common. Edema of the head, limbs, and perineum occurs. Terminally, affected animals collapse and die.

Although not as frequently diagnosed with *B. anthracis* infection as cattle, horses do develop disease and die from anthrax.* After an incubation period of about 3 to 7 days (can be as short as 1 day or as long as 7 days), horses usually develop the acute form of anthrax, although sudden death may occur. Initial clinical signs frequently include colic, with presenting signs that may resemble those of acute enteritis. These horses progress to high fever with dyspnea. Subcutaneous edema of the ventral neck, thorax, and abdomen may be seen, especially with mediastinal involvement. Ventral edema involving the prepuce and mammary gland is postulated to be secondary to local transmission from insects. Most affected horses die within 2 to 4 days of onset of clinical signs. Subcutaneous edema, especially of the inguinal, preputial, and ventral thoracic and abdominal areas, was the most common clinical sign observed in affected horses in one recent outbreak.[83] Failure of blood to clot was considered the most sensitive carcass characteristic of anthrax across all species.[83]

Pigs frequently acquire infection as a result of being fed infected carcasses.[57,85,103] Although they can demonstrate the same clinical signs as cattle with anthrax, pigs usually have a characteristic edema of the throat and head, often severe enough to obstruct the airway and throat. A blood-stained, frothy discharge occurs from the nose or mouth. There are petechial hemorrhages of the skin.

Diagnosis
Clinical Pathology

Because sudden death or a short course of fatal disease is the hallmark of anthrax, blood testing from affected horses or any other livestock species is extremely uncommon.[57,103,104] Should one have the unfortunate experience of examining a blood smear, an extremely high level of bacteremia is the most notable observation. Aspirated edema fluid also contains organisms. A new methylene blue stain performed on blood or edema fluid demonstrates chains of vegetative cells that are large, square, gram-positive rods. The nonstaining internal spores are centrally located with an ellipsoid shape.

Diagnostic Testing

If a sample for culture is obtained, initial identification of *B. anthracis* is through the basic microbiologic features discussed earlier. Inoculation of guinea pigs for lethality or fluorescent antibody testing of smears of froth, blood, or splenic aspirate is much safer for laboratory personnel.[105] Serologic and molecular-based techniques are important for identification of the specific strain of *B. anthracis*.[103,105-107] Strain typing to determine the origin of exposure in humans is a priority when bioterrorism is suspected. Molecular-based techniques have been developed for environmental monitoring and likely pose an alternative to inadvertent culture of body fluids.

Treatment

Usually, anthrax is rapidly fatal in horses, and it is unlikely that there would be an opportunity for therapy of an animal showing clinical signs at diagnosis. Careful examination of other exposed animals for disease should be performed. Close monitoring of any exposed horses may result in timely administration of antimicrobial agents. Antimicrobials recommended for prevention and treatment of anthrax include penicillin, tetracyclines, and fluoroquinolones.[57,68,108,109] Recent outbreaks in humans support the use of fluoroquinolones as a first-line antimicrobial in suspected *B. anthracis* infection.[109,110] IV administration is highly recommended. Single or short-duration administration

---

*References 69, 70, 73, 76, 77, 80, 82, 101.

*References 69, 70, 76, 77, 80, 82, 101.

of prophylactic antibiotics is recommended for exposed humans and is an option for horses.[110] Supportive care is essential and consists of cardiovascular support in the form of fluid and oncotic therapy. Intranasal oxygen may alleviate signs of dyspnea.

Pathologic Findings

If an animal dies of disease consistent with anthrax in an endemic area, it is best not to open the carcass.[68,72-74,76-79,82,111] Not only is this important for human safety, but it is also exceptionally important for long-term control by minimizing environmental contamination. Collection of blood in a closed system or a splenic aspirate obtained percutaneously is recommended to facilitate confirmation of the diagnosis. Blood clots poorly in affected animals, thus a sample may be obtained for an extended time after death.

The pathologic hallmark of anthrax is the absence of rigor mortis, with passage of blood from body orifices. Blood from these sites and blood drawn at the time of death fails to clot. Petechiae and ecchymoses are widespread, with large quantities of blood-stained serous fluid within body cavities. Severe mediastinal edema, enteritis, and splenomegaly are common. In particular, the spleen has a "blackberry jam" appearance.

Prevention

Although not routinely available in the United States, vaccines are available for prevention of anthrax in cattle in other countries.[101,110,113-116] Use of cattle vaccines in horses is controversial and is not recommended in the guidelines of the American Association of Equine Practitioners. Injection site reactions and severe edema after vaccination have been described. However, immunoprophylaxis has been demonstrated as useful in cattle and experimental models of disease.* If disease and subsequent exposure to B. anthracis are identified or suspected in horses, methods should be implemented to prevent additional disease in horses and to minimize risk of human disease. Animals should have all external debris removed by thorough bathing with soap and water. If there is gross contamination of an animal, a 0.5% hypochlorite solution can be used. The efficacy of a chlorhexidine scrub for decontamination of animal hair is unknown. Animals should be moved immediately away from sites that have been exposed to anthrax-laden carcasses.

Maintenance of the vegetative state is essential for carcass disposal.[71,79,111,119] In its vegetative form, B. anthracis is quite labile[57]; the putrefactive process actually destroys most bacteria within the carcass. Site contamination comes from body fluids that, on exposure to air, allow sporulation of bacteria in these samples.

Some controversy surrounds the optimal methods of disposal of anthrax-suspect carcasses. The World Health Organization (WHO) recommends incineration of closed carcasses as the best method. The alternative to this is heat treatment or rendering of closed carcasses. Burial is considered the final choice in disposition and should occur quickly with minimal damage to the carcass. Veterinarians and public health professionals are key personnel in determining whether a specific method is appropriate in a given situation.

Several factors should be considered if carcasses are to be incinerated. The most important aspect is ensuring complete incineration, including the ventral parts of the carcass.[79] The soil from the site can be burned separately from the carcass or actually torched. Controversy exists as to whether there are bacteria

*References 90, 101, 110, 113, 114, 116-118.

in the "updrafts" of the burned carcasses; however, most microbiologists and public health agencies discount this as a true risk for human disease or bacterial dissemination. B. anthracis has been isolated from the ashes of incinerators, but bacterial counts are very low and associated with poor incinerator hygiene.

Rendering, done properly, is analogous to autoclaving. In the nonsporulated state, this organism is susceptible. However, the processing step could result in exposure of the carcass to air. The carcass must be "broken" down in a closed system for best practices. All wastewater must be autoclaved.

Burial must be deep so that scavengers do not disturb the bodies before putrefaction has occurred. If spores are buried, climatic, geologic, animal, and human upheavals can result in exposure years later if a burial site is disturbed.

Public Health Considerations

The zoonotic risk of B. anthracis cannot be minimized, and the occupational risk of exposure in veterinarians is very high compared with the risk of intentional human-to-human transmission.[65,68,78,91] Personal protection when handling anthrax-suspect animals should be complete, including gloves, boots, protective suits, and respiratory and eye protection. This protection must be maintained throughout all environmental and equipment decontamination processes. Complete bathing is recommended after handling any tissues or animals. In some situations, prophylactic antibiotic therapy is recommended if exposure is thought to be high or inadvertent through improper attention to personal protection. Animal hide, hair, and wool can contain spores, and humans at occupational risk should seek immediate medical attention if skin or respiratory signs occur. Considerations of B. anthracis as a bioterrorist agent are discussed elsewhere.[103,106,114]

Enterococcal Infections

Debra C. Sellon and J. Lindsay Oaks

Enterococci are gram-positive bacteria that occur singly, in clusters, or in chains. In 1984, the new genus Enterococcus was proposed to include the genera Streptococcus faecalis and S. faecium.[120] There are now at least 23 species classified in the genus Enterococcus. Enterococci are more hardy and environmentally resistant than the streptococci, growing at temperatures ranging from 10°C to 45°C (50°F-113°F) and surviving for as long as 30 minutes at 60°C (140°F). They can grow in solutions up to 6.5% NaCl and at a pH of 9.6.[121]

Enterococci are normal commensal flora of the GI tract of humans and many animal species. Although present at comparatively low numbers (<1% of total adult human intestinal microflora), they are important medically because of their growing significance as nosocomial pathogens.[122-124] They are the third most common isolate from human blood infections,[125] the most frequent isolate from surgical site infections in intensive care units,[126] and the second most common nosocomial pathogen in the United States.[127] Enterococci are commonly isolated from chronic wounds of horses and appear to have a high potential for biofilm production in the wound environment.[128,129]

Enterococci have been identified as the cause of numerous types of opportunistic infections in horses and other domestic animals. However, at least at this time, equine enterococcal infections are typically sporadic. Most enterococcal strains encountered in veterinary medicine are not especially virulent, are associated with low morbidity and mortality, do not exhibit high-level resistance to antimicrobials, and are not related to outbreaks of nosocomial strains. Often, their isolation from culture of clinical samples is clinically irrelevant because the organism is merely present as an environmental contaminant rather than as a causal pathogen for infection.

At least five factors might contribute to the establishment of *Enterococcus* as a nosocomial pathogen in a patient: (1) the ability to acquire or develop resistance to many common antimicrobial drugs; (2) the ability to transfer this resistance to other, more pathogenic organisms; (3) the presence of a variety of virulence factors; (4) access to an extraintestinal site; and (5) the transmission of enterococci by the hands of health care workers or through other fomites. Growing evidence indicates that a subset of enterococcal strains may be particularly virulent and have the propensity to cause outbreaks of nosocomial disease within health care facilities. Surface virulence factors, such as aggregation substance, Ace (adhesin of collagen of *E. faecalis*), *E. faecalis* adhesion molecule, and enterococcal surface protein, may facilitate the binding of enterococci to epithelial surfaces, and the formation of vegetative lesions and may contribute to pathogenicity.[122,124] Putative secreted virulence factors include cytolysin/hemolysin and gelatinase.[124] At this time the significance of these virulence factors in vivo is uncertain because their presence does not seem to correlate with isolates from patients who have died because of enterococcal infections.[123,130,131] Antimicrobial resistance and the ability to survive in a variety of environments make enterococcal organisms particularly suited to establishment of nosocomial infections.[122]

As a group, the enterococci are intrinsically resistant to many antimicrobial agents typically used in veterinary medicine, including penicillins, cephalosporins, and low concentrations of aminoglycosides. The low level of intrinsic resistance to aminoglycosides is the result of an inability of the drug to cross the enterococcal cell membrane.[122] As a result, combination therapy with a β-lactam and an aminoglycoside is synergistic and frequently efficacious clinically. Currently, in routine antimicrobial susceptibility testing, most equine isolates are susceptible to ampicillin and resistant to aminoglycosides (because of low-level intrinsic resistance). Based on the recommendations for treatment of enterococcal infections in humans,[132] for ampicillin-susceptible enterococcal isolates, monotherapy with ampicillin is likely to be effective for superficial infections (e.g., urinary tract, soft tissue) in immunocompetent patients. However, for more serious infections (e.g., endocarditis, osteomyelitis) improved clinical responses are seen when the cell wall–active agents are combined with aminoglycosides. The β-lactam drug damages the bacterial cell membrane, facilitating uptake and microbicidal activity of the aminoglycoside.

In addition to their intrinsic antimicrobial resistance, enterococci are able to acquire genetic elements that confer high-level resistance to β-lactams, aminoglycosides, and glycopeptides (e.g., vancomycin). Vancomycin resistance was first reported in 1986 and has spread rapidly since that time.[133] In strains that exhibit high-level resistance to aminoglycosides, combination therapy with a β-lactam will not result in synergy, and there is no benefit from addition of aminoglycosides. Although no consensus exists on the optimal therapy of these resistant strains, high doses and continuous infusions of ampicillin or vancomycin are usually recommended. Therapy with cephalosporins and trimethoprim-sulfa combinations is generally ineffective against enterococci regardless of their in vitro susceptibility profiles. Acquired resistance to chloramphenicol, fluoroquinolones, rifampin, and tetracyclines is common, and these drugs appear to be only bacteriostatic and result in poor clinical responses when used to treat serious enterococcal infections.[132] Antimicrobial resistant enterococci are frequently present in the gastrointestinal tract of healthy horses[134,135] and there has been at least one report of multidrug resistant strains of *Enterococcus* causing synovial infection secondary to trauma in horses.[136]

Listeriosis

Melissa T. Hines

Listeria monocytogenes is a bacterial pathogen of worldwide distribution that causes disease in humans and a variety of animal species. In veterinary species, listeriosis is of most importance in ruminants. Clinical disease is uncommon in horses, but sporadic cases of septicemia, encephalitis, abortion, and ocular disease have been reported. Because of the small number of equine cases, specific information on equine listeriosis is limited.

Listeria bacteria are gram-positive rods that are facultative anaerobes.[137] There are several species within the genus, and although *Listeria ivanovii* has occasionally been associated with abortion in ruminants, *L. monocytogenes* is considered the only species of major clinical significance. Based on somatic and flagellar antigens, 16 serotypes of *L. monocytogenes* have been identified, with almost all cases of animal and human infection being caused by serotypes 1/2a, 1/2b, 4a, and 4b.[137,138]

L. monocytogenes is ubiquitous in the environment and has been found in a variety of samples, such as soil, water, vegetation, and silage.[121,138] The organism is frequently shed in the feces of carrier animals, and although information in horses is limited, in one study in Germany, approximately 5% of horses shed *L. monocytogenes*.[139] Fecal contamination is generally thought to be the most common source of the organism, but *L. monocytogenes* can also be found in urine, uterine discharge, aborted fetal tissues, and milk. In the environment the organism can survive for long periods, multiplying in a wide range of environmental conditions, including temperatures of 4°C to 45°C (39°F-113°F).[137,138] The organism can grow over a pH range of 5 to 9, often reaching high numbers in poorly preserved silage or decaying vegetation when the pH rises above 5.4. The association between clinical listeriosis and silage in ruminants has resulted in the disease sometimes being referred to as "silage disease." Similarly, in Iceland, an association is believed to exist between listeriosis in horses and feeding silage.[140] In three foals with listeriosis, however, none of the foals or their dams had been fed silage, and the source of infection was undetermined.[141]

The most common route of infection in listeriosis is ingestion, although infection may also occur through the nasal mucosa, conjunctiva, or wound contamination.[137,138] Some proposed routes of infection in neonatal foals include ingestion from the environment or infected mare's milk, inhalation, through the umbilical remnant, and transplacental infection.[141-144] *L. monocytogenes* is an opportunistic pathogen, and clinical disease is thought to occur when the host's resistance is decreased as a result of stress factors such as concurrent disease, climate, pregnancy, a large infective dose, or immunodeficiency. Although no specific risk factors have been identified in most equine cases, meningoencephalitis and septicemia caused by *L. monocytogenes* were reported in an Arabian foal with combined immunodeficiency, and *Listeria* keratitis was reported in a horse previously treated with topical corticosteroids.[145,146]

L. monocytogenes is a facultative intracellular organism that invades both phagocytic and nonphagocytic cells. The organism can be found in multiple tissues but has a predilection for the intestinal tract wall, reproductive tissues, and medulla oblongata. A number of virulence factors are involved in the pathogenesis of listerial infection, including listeriolysin O, a hemolysin that allows the internalized listeriae to escape from the phagosome. Once within the cytoplasm, the listeriae proliferate and induce polymerization of host cell actin, which ultimately serves to move the bacilli toward the cell's periphery, where projections of the infected cell's cytoplasmic membrane invaginate into adjacent cells, allowing the listeriae to enter that cell directly. As with many intracellular organisms, immunity to

L. monocytogenes is thought to be primarily mediated by cellular responses.[137,138]

L. monocytogenes has been reported as an uncommon cause of septicemia and systemic disease in foals from birth to 5 months of age and in adult horses.[140-145,147-149] Clinical signs include depression, anorexia, fever, diarrhea, and abdominal pain. Weakness, seizures, ataxia, jaundice, and respiratory distress have been reported as well. Abortion resulting from *L. monocytogenes* has also been reported in mares.[150,151] Bacterial ulcerative keratitis has been described in two equine cases[146,152]; these horses showed no evidence of concurrent systemic listerial infection. In most other species, ocular listerial infection is usually associated with other forms of infection, such as meningoencephalitis, but primary corneal infection has been reported.[152-154]

Diagnosis of listeriosis is generally established by microbiologic culture.[137] Polymerase chain reaction has also been described.[155,156] This technique has been used to confirm diagnosis in one case of encephalitis in an adult miniature horse at the University of Florida (Clare Ryan, personal communication). Cytologic examination of a direct smear from infected tissue, such as corneal scrapings or aborted tissue, may reveal grampositive rods consistent with *Listeria*.[137,146] At necropsy, histopathology, culture, and immunohistochemistry can be helpful in establishing a diagnosis.[137,142] It may be difficult to culture organisms from the brain in neural listeriosis, presumably because the organisms are intracellular and present in low numbers. In general, serology had not been useful in the diagnosis of listeriosis because of both the prevalence of positive titers in healthy animals and the cross-reactions with other organisms.[137,157,158]

L. monocytogenes is typically susceptible to many antibiotics. However, isolates from a corneal scraping and from blood cultures from three foals were all resistant to ceftiofur.[141,146] The isolates from the foals were susceptible to several antibiotics, including amikacin, gentamicin, ampicillin, penicillin, cephalothin, chloramphenicol, amoxicillin with clavulanate, doxycycline, erythromycin, rifampin, and trimethoprimsulfamethoxazole.[141] Because of the limited number of cases, it is difficult to give an accurate prognosis, but some foals and adults with clinical listeriosis have responded to systemic antibiotic therapy.[140-145,147,148] Listerial keratitis has resolved after topical antibiotic therapy.[146,152]

L. monocytogenes is considered a zoonotic agent.[137,138] Clinical listeriosis in humans occurs most often in pregnant women and immunocompromised patients. Possible sources for human infections include exposure to contaminated soil and food or to human and animal carriers. Most human epidemics have been traced to food sources of animal origin. In a study in Brazil, 9 of 121 samples (7.4%) of horsemeat for human consumption were positive for *L. monocytogenes*.[159] Direct transmission from animals to humans is uncommon.

Anaerobic Infections

J. Lindsay Oaks* and Debra C. Sellon

Obligately anaerobic bacteria, referred to here as "anaerobes," are common opportunistic pathogens. Veterinary clinicians and microbiologists have historically been aware that these organisms can cause significant pathology, often requiring specific antimicrobial therapy. Traditionally, little effort has been devoted to specific detection or identification of these bacteria. Anaerobes usually require specialized equipment to culture and have been inherently difficult to identify accurately once isolated. Historically, identification of an anaerobe did not alter therapy because anaerobes were, and in most cases remain,

*The authors acknowledge and appreciate the original contributions of these authors, whose work has been incorporated into this chapter.

predictably susceptible to many of the antibiotics already being used to treat concomitant infection with facultatively anaerobic or aerobic bacteria. (The facultative anaerobe group, which includes most of the common veterinary bacterial pathogens, and the obligately aerobic bacteria are typically referred to as "aerobes," and this colloquial nomenclature is used in this chapter.)

More recently, innate or acquired antimicrobial resistance in anaerobes has been observed in human isolates, providing more incentive to detect and identify these pathogens. Studies in human hospitals investigating the value of anaerobic microbiology show both medical and financial benefits.[160] Although such economic analyses are not available for equine medicine, the specific detection and treatment of anaerobic bacterial infections improve clinical outcome in equine cases. To realize these benefits, it is incumbent on veterinary diagnostic laboratories to provide accurate and clinically timely results of anaerobic testing. This chapter addresses nonenteric infections caused by obligately anaerobic bacteria. Enteric and systemic/myonecrotic diseases caused by *Clostridium* spp., are discussed in Chapters 41 and 42, respectively.

Etiology

The anaerobic bacteria are a large and taxonomically diverse group of bacteria that are unable to survive in the presence of free oxygen concentrations greater than about 5 µM.[161] Sensitivity to molecular oxygen results from their inability to detoxify reactive oxygen molecules formed as a byproduct of either respiratory metabolism or exposure to ambient levels of atmospheric oxygen. Bacteria that are tolerant of oxygen or that utilize oxygen metabolically (obligate aerobes and facultative anaerobes) typically possess enzymes such as catalase, superoxide dismutase, and peroxidases to detoxify reactive oxygen molecules.[162] These enzymes are generally absent in anaerobes because the detoxification reactions of catalase and dismutase result in formation of more molecular oxygen. To avoid the production of oxygen, the predominant metabolic pathways for obligately anaerobic bacteria are fermentative, and they utilize organic molecules as electron acceptors in energy production. The metabolic end products of carbohydrate and amino acid fermentation include volatile fatty acids, alcohols, indole, and sulfur compounds that are foul smelling, one of the hallmark clinical signs of anaerobic infections.[163]

Anaerobes have limited protection from exposure to oxygen by alternate detoxification pathways such as superoxide reductase. This enzyme produces hydrogen peroxide, which is detoxified into water by reductase and rubrerythrin pathways.[162,164] Aerotolerance is also quite variable among what are classified as obligate anaerobes, and growth of some obligate anaerobes such as *Bacteroides* may even be enhanced by low levels of oxygen (about 300 nM). Some obligate anaerobes may metabolically utilize, and detoxify, oxygen with cytochrome oxidase systems and oxygen-dependent respiratory chains.[161,162] These features may allow *Bacteroides*, as well as other obligate anaerobes with similar systems, to colonize mucous membranes or establish infections without prior colonization of and reduction of oxygen by facultatively anaerobic bacteria such as *Escherichia coli*.[161]

The taxonomy of anaerobic bacteria is complex and currently undergoing major revisions; this trend is likely to continue for the foreseeable future.[165-168] Although these taxonomic revisions are primarily of academic interest, they do reflect the difficulty in obtaining accurate identification of anaerobic isolates and may complicate the optimal selection of appropriate antimicrobial therapy. This also makes it difficult to compare the results of older studies to newer studies. The primary basis for this ongoing taxonomic reorganization is

Table 45-3 Clinically Significant Obligately Anaerobic Bacteria of Humans, Horses, and Other Mammals

Organism Group	Genera
Gram-negative rods	Bacteroides
	Campylobacter
	Capnocytophaga
	Fusobacterium
	Porphyromonas
	Prevotella
	Selenomonas
	Wolinella
Gram-negative cocci	Veillonella
Gram-positive rods	Actinomyces
	Bifidobacterium
	Clostridium
	Eubacterium
	Lactobacillus
	Mobiluncus
	Propionibacterium
Gram-positive cocci	Gemella
	Peptostreptococcus

the use of nucleotide sequence-based phylogenetic analyses, particularly of the 16s rDNA gene, in place of the previously used, less reliable analyses based on phenotypic and biochemical characteristics.[166,168]

For the aerobic and facultatively anaerobic bacteria, taxonomy based on phenotypic and biochemical characteristics correlate relatively well with genetic analyses. However, for anaerobes, schemes based on phenotypic and biochemical characteristics result in much greater discrepancies, including misclassification of organisms with regard to highly fundamental traits such as Gram-staining properties, morphology, aerotolerance, and spore formation.[165,166,168] Despite the dramatic changes in the classification of anaerobes and the great diversity of this group of bacteria, most of the clinically significant anaerobic pathogens of humans and other mammals, including horses, belong to a limited number of genera[166-175] (Table 45-3).

Epidemiology

Anaerobic bacteria are ubiquitous members of the normal flora of the skin and mucous membranes of all mammals,[166,171,176] and the major genera found as normal flora of horses appear to be similar to the clinically significant and normal flora anaerobes of humans and other mammals. It may seem somewhat counterintuitive that obligately anaerobic bacteria are found in high numbers at sites that are exposed to ambient air, such as the skin or oral cavity. However, in addition to the inherent aerotolerance that some obligate anaerobes possess, anaerobic microenvironments are created in these areas by the presence of facultatively anaerobic bacterial flora (including many of the other bacteria familiar to clinicians, such as staphylococci, streptococci, pasteurellas, actinobacilli, and members of the Enterobacteriaceae) that consume free oxygen.[177] Anaerobes are also frequent opportunistic pathogens that cause infections when these bacteria gain access to anaerobic conditions in tissue, usually resulting from the presence of necrotic tissue and co-infection with facultatively anaerobic bacteria. Although anaerobes may cause infections by themselves, in most cases anaerobic infections are polymicrobic, with multiple obligately anaerobic bacteria as well as facultatively anaerobic bacteria.

Although most of the clinically significant anaerobes can be found on most sites of the body, certain genera are more common in certain sites. In humans the genera that predominantly colonize a given site are also those most likely to be found in infections associated with those anatomic areas, and

detection of certain genera in the blood can predict the part of the body where the infection originates. Although this association has not been well demonstrated for horses, this most likely reflects the lack of information about normal equine anaerobic flora and routine anaerobic blood culturing rather than lack of such a correlation.

The most clinically important equine infections caused by obligately anaerobic bacteria are pneumonia and pleuropneumonia (see Chapter 1). Anaerobes that are reported from the equine oral and respiratory tracts include *Bacteroides, Clostridium, Eubacterium, Fusobacterium, Peptostreptococcus,* and *Veillonella,* as well a number of other, unidentified anaerobic gram-positive rods and cocci.[169,178,179] In one series of studies, 37% to 68% of lower respiratory tract infections had involvement of anaerobes, usually *Bacteroides;* 68% to 81% were mixed with facultative anaerobes such as streptococci, pasteurellas, actinobacilli, and Enterobacteriaceae; and 85% had multiple anaerobes.[173,174,180,181] The most frequently reported anaerobes from cases of equine respiratory disease include *Bacteroides, Clostridium, Eubacterium, Fusobacterium, Peptostreptococcus,* and *Veillonella.*[169,173,174,179-186] The clinical significance of the anaerobic component of these infections is suggested by studies that found the presence of anaerobes was associated with decreased survival,[173,174,181,185] and horses treated with metronidazole showed improved clinical responses and survival rates.[174,183] The anaerobic bacteria involved in equine respiratory infections most likely arise from aspiration of normal oral flora, because most of the respiratory anaerobic pathogens are also found on the pharyngeal tonsillar surfaces.[169] Anaerobes are also often associated with a variety of paraoral infections, including submandibular abscesses, mandibular osteomyelitis, sinus infection, and dental abscesses. The predominant anaerobes involved in these infections are very similar to those found in respiratory infections and as normal flora of pharyngeal tonsillar surfaces,[169] and they presumably arise by extension from normal flora opportunistic infections.

Anaerobes are also common flora of the equine reproductive tract (see Chapter 8). In normal stallions, 96% of samples collected from the urethra, urethral fossa, smegma, and preejaculatory fluid contained *Bacteroides, Clostridium, Fusobacterium, Peptococcus,* and *Peptostreptococcus.* In normal mares, 100% of clitoral swabs, 24% of endometrial swabs, and 40% of endometrial washes contained *Bacteroides, Clostridium, Fusobacterium, Peptococcus,* and *Peptostreptococcus* spp.[187] Anaerobes, including *Bacteroides, Clostridium, Fusobacterium,* and *Peptostreptococcus* spp., can also be isolated from uterine samples from mares with cytologic evidence of acute endometritis. Presumably, anaerobes may contribute to uterine pathology during active infection, but the ability to culture anaerobes from clinically normal mares illustrates the difficulty in interpreting the significance of anaerobic bacteria identified in mucosal samples.

Anaerobic bacteria are also frequently associated with intraabdominal infections, such as abscesses and cholangiohepatitis.[188-190] The genera of anaerobic bacteria associated with these infections are similar to those found as normal flora in the equine colon and include *Bacteroides, Bifidobacterium, Clostridium, Eubacterium, Lactobacillus,* and *Peptostreptococcus.*[191-194] A variety of other opportunistic infections, including orthopedic,[177] mammary, cutaneous, and muscular infections,[195] may involve anaerobes. As a general rule, any wound or sterile site, especially when infection is caused by contamination with bacteria from the skin or mucous membranes, may potentially involve anaerobic bacteria.

Pathogenesis and Clinical Signs

Although it is uncommon for anaerobic bacteria to be the primary or sole pathogen in an infection, when this is the case, they contribute significantly to the pathology and clinical signs. Any infection in which the source of bacteria is skin or mucosal flora may be complicated by anaerobic involvement under appropriate conditions. The presence of necrotic tissue and co-infection with facultatively anaerobic bacteria are the two main predisposing factors.[177,196] Necrotic tissue will have a compromised blood supply and thus decreased levels of oxygen. Facultatively anaerobic bacteria will reduce the oxygen tension sufficiently through aerobic metabolism to allow anaerobes to proliferate. Concomitant infection with the obligately anaerobic bacteria benefits survival of facultative anaerobes by providing nutritional or growth factors, suppression of antibacterial responses such as leukocidins, suppression of neutrophil chemotaxis, suppression of phagocytosis, and impairment of opsonization.[177,197] This mutually beneficial relationship likely explains the high frequency of co-infection with both obligate and facultatively anaerobic bacteria.

Anaerobic infection, once established, results in extensive tissue necrosis and pus formation. Although a very diverse group, many of the pathogenic anaerobes have similar types of virulence factors. Many anaerobes produce a number of potent exotoxins, including collagenases, proteases, DNases, heparinases, and leukocidins, that result in necrosis of tissue and localization of leukocytes.[177,198] Other important virulence factors are structural molecules, including the presence of a polysaccharide capsule, pili, and endotoxin. Capsule formation is classically associated with *Bacteroides fragilis* but may also be found with other anaerobic bacteria.[197,198] Capsules on bacteria may increase tissue adherence and may be chemotactic for neutrophils, which favors abscess formation, and capsular material from *B. fragilis* has been shown to be able to induce abscess formation in the absence of any viable organism.[177,197-199] The increased recruitment of neutrophils does not necessarily result in clearance of the bacteria because these encapsulated bacteria are also more resistant to killing by neutrophils.[177,197] In addition, the gram-negative anaerobes also produce endotoxin.[198]

No clinical signs or lesions definitively differentiate infections with anaerobic bacteria from infections with, or infections that include, facultative bacteria. Moreover, because most anaerobic infections are co-infected with facultative bacteria, most anaerobic infections will have the typical suppurative and inflammatory lesions that are associated with bacterial infections in general. However, two products of the fermentative metabolism utilized by most anaerobic bacteria, foul-smelling compounds and gas, produce clinical signs that, when present, are highly suggestive of anaerobic involvement. As previously mentioned, many of the metabolic end products of carbohydrate and amino acid fermentation are foul smelling,[163] and clinical samples from anaerobic infections will have a foul odor. In one study of equine pleuropneumonia, 62% of horses with anaerobic involvement had putrid breath or pleural samples.[181] Putrid-smelling breath and clinical samples are also frequently noted in other reports of equine anaerobic respiratory infections.[173,183,185] Free-gas echoes detected by ultrasound within pleural or abscess fluids have also been shown to be a sensitive and specific indicator of anaerobic infections.[185]

Diagnosis

The diagnosis of anaerobic infections is made primarily by culture and identification. Gram-stained cytology slides may assist in making a presumptive diagnosis of anaerobic involvement, although the morphology of anaerobes is not generally unique enough to be able to differentiate them definitively from other types of bacteria. However, the visualization of multiple types of bacteria in a suppurative lesion, with isolation of fewer types of bacteria on aerobic culture, may suggest the presence of anaerobes. Gram-negative rods with tapered ends may suggest *Fusobacterium* spp.

The primary requirement for the isolation of anaerobic bacteria is the ability to create an oxygen-free environment. This is usually accomplished with either anaerobic chambers for large caseloads or benchtop jars or bags for smaller-scale use. Initial isolation is made on a variety of nonselective and selective agar-based media formulations. Subsequent identification is usually based on phenotypic and biochemical characteristics. However, accurate identification to the species level is often difficult. Fortunately, for clinical purposes, identification to the genus level is generally sufficient to document anaerobic involvement or to make decisions regarding antimicrobial therapy or the need for antimicrobial susceptibility testing. If further identification is required, this may be done by analysis of short-chain fatty acid profiles, using liquid chromatography or capillary electrophoresis, or by molecular methods, such as 16s rDNA sequencing.[166,200] Because many anaerobes are fastidious and relatively slow growing, identification even to the genus level generally takes 4 to 7 days, and clinicians should be aware that anaerobic culture results will take longer than those for most facultative or aerobic bacteria.

One of the greatest challenges for the clinician in the diagnosis of anaerobic infections is to maintain the viability of these bacteria in clinical samples between collection and receipt by the laboratory. Anaerobic bacteria in general are fragile and highly susceptible to inactivation by adverse environmental conditions; thus proper sample collection, storage, and transportation are essential to obtain good results from the laboratory. The first priority is to prevent exposure of the bacteria in the sample to oxygen. During collection, the length of time that the sample is exposed to ambient air should be minimized. As a general rule, tissue samples with a volume of 1 cm^3 or greater or fluid samples with a volume of 1 mL or greater submitted in a sterile, airtight container will effectively maintain an anaerobic environment and anaerobe viability for several hours.[201] However, volumes greater than 2 cm^3 or 2 mL are optimal. Smaller samples should be collected into anaerobic transport systems that are designed to maintain a low oxygen tension and prevent desiccation. Although there are anaerobic transport systems designed for use with swabs, another important general rule to observe whenever possible is that samples of tissue or fluid are preferable to swabs because of the larger volume of material available for culture, as well as the improved ability to prevent exposure to ambient air. Samples for anaerobic culture should be submitted to the laboratory as quickly as possible; even with properly collected samples in anaerobic transport systems, the recovery rates begin to drop after 24 hours.[202] The optimal temperature at which to hold and transport samples is room temperature.[201] Samples should not be frozen or refrigerated (4° C) because this will decrease recovery rates.[203]

Proper sample selection and collection is also very important for interpretation of laboratory results. Samples for anaerobic culture should be collected from normally sterile sites. Because of their ubiquitous presence and very high numbers (up to 10^9-10^{12} bacteria per gram), it is generally inappropriate to request anaerobic cultures from sites that have normal anaerobic flora, such as the skin, oral cavity, nasopharyngeal cavity, genital mucous membranes, feces, or intestinal lumen.[201] When sample collection requires bypassing areas with normal flora, such as with bronchoalveolar lavage, great care should be taken to avoid contaminating the sample with normal flora. Because most anaerobic infections are acquired from normal flora, any degree of contamination will potentially result in misleading results.[169,181] A number of anaerobic pathogens, including *Bacteroides*, *Clostridium*, *Fusobacterium*, and *Peptostreptococcus*, are present in the lungs of dead horses without respiratory disease.[179]

This indicates that, as with interpretation of other types of microbiology findings, anaerobic bacteriology results must be interpreted with regard to other clinical and laboratory evidence that supports a diagnosis of infection.

Therapy

Treatment of anaerobic infections is similar to that of other bacterial infections, with debridement and antimicrobial drugs being the most important components of therapy.[180,204,205] Removing necrotic debris by either surgical debridement or drainage of pus is crucial for increasing blood supply and oxygen tension, improving host antibacterial immune responses, and improving the access and function of antimicrobials at the site of infection.[204]

A number of antibiotics have good activity against obligate anaerobes, including penicillins, cephalosporins, carbapenems, chloramphenicol, lincosamides, metronidazole, macrolides, glycopeptides, tetracyclines, and the newer quinolones (which does not include the earlier quinolones labeled for veterinary use, such as enrofloxacin).[204,206,207] Many of these antimicrobials are not used routinely in horses for reasons of safety (lincosamides) and expense (carbapenems, macrolides, glycopeptides, quinolones). Consequently, the drugs most often used in the treatment of anaerobic infections in horses are penicillins, cephalosporins, chloramphenicol, metronidazole, and tetracyclines. In human medicine the resistance of a number of anaerobes, including *Bacteroides*, *Fusobacterium*, *Prevotella*, and *Porphyromonas*, to penicillins, cephalosporins, and tetracyclines is reported to be increasing.[176,206,208] Accurate or recent comparative data on the prevalence of antimicrobial resistance in veterinary medicine in general, and equine medicine in particular, are lacking.[209] However, even older equine literature reports significant rates of resistance of *Bacteroides* spp. to penicillins (18%-68% of isolates), cephalosporins (17%-62% of isolates), and tetracyclines (2%-36% of isolates), indicating that these drugs should not be regarded as predictably effective against anaerobic infections.[173,207,209,210] Lower rates of resistance to penicillins and tetracyclines are also reported for *Fusobacterium*, *Prevotella*, and *Porphyromonas*.[173,210] More recent literature examining human isolates of these organisms indicates that their rate of resistance to tetracyclines is much higher (33%-50%).[176] The variable susceptibility of multiple anaerobic bacteria to these antimicrobials indicates that their use should always be based on susceptibility testing.

At present, the drug that remains a good empiric choice for treatment of anaerobic infections is metronidazole. Metronidazole is able to reach plasma levels above the 90% minimal inhibitory concentration for anaerobes when given intravenously, orally, or rectally. It also appears to be safe and improves survival in equine patients with pleuropneumonia.[181,183,186,211] Resistance to metronidazole remains rare in human medicine[176,206,208,212] and equine medicine but has been reported for up to 10% of *Prevotella* spp. and 17% of *B. tectum* isolates.[173] Metronidazole resistance is also reported in an approximately 10% to 15% of *Sutterella* spp.,[176] organisms that have not been reported from horses.

Although there are safety concerns for humans who handle chloramphenicol, this antibiotic also remains a good empiric choice that is predictably effective against most of the common anaerobic pathogens, including *Bacteroides* spp.[209,210] Trimethoprim-sulfamethoxazole is reported to have good in vitro activity against anaerobes; however, its activity in vivo may be limited by the presence of purulent material, and clinically it does not appear to be highly effective in the treatment of lower respiratory tract infections.[174,182,213] Because most anaerobic infections are polymicrobic, antimicrobials directed against facultative bacteria are also usually required, especially when using metronidazole, which does not have activity against aerobic or facultatively anaerobic bacteria.

Public Health Considerations

There are no public health concerns with the anaerobic bacteria because none of these bacteria are regarded as zoonotic pathogens.

Mycobacterial Infections

J. Lindsay Oaks* and Debra C. Sellon

The mycobacteria comprise the only genus in the family Mycobacteriaceae and are a large group of aerobic, non–spore-forming bacterial rods. Bacteria in this group retain arylmethane dyes such as fuschin when mixed with phenol to allow uptake of the dye (e.g., carbolfuschin), then resist decolorization with acid alcohols or inorganic acids. This is the basis for their designation as "acid-fast." The ability to stain acid-fast results from the high cell wall content of hydrophobic mycolic acids and other complex lipids and waxes. In general, mycobacteria have long generation times and thus are slow growing compared with other bacterial pathogens. Although growth rates vary widely, most of the significant human and veterinary mycobacterial pathogens take 14 to 60 days of culture to detect visible growth.[214,215]

Mycobacterial infections generally result in either multifocal pulmonary or disseminated granulomatous disease ("tubercles") or localized subcutaneous infections. Pulmonary or disseminated tuberculous disease is typically caused by the obligate pathogens *Mycobacterium tuberculosis* and *Mycobacterium bovis*, the classic agents of human and bovine tuberculosis, respectively.[214,216] Multifocal to infiltrative disease in ruminants is caused by another obligately pathogenic organism, *Mycobacterium avium* subsp. *paratuberculosis*, the causative agent of Johne's disease.[217] These particular mycobacteria are relatively unusual in that they are primary pathogens in mammalian hosts, and host immunodeficiency is not a prerequisite for disease.[214,216-218] Other mycobacteria are environmental organisms, ubiquitous in soil and water, that cause sporadic and opportunistic infections that present as either disseminated disease in immunocompromised hosts or localized infections in immunocompetent hosts. The only environmental mycobacterium frequently associated with disseminated granulomatous disease in veterinary medicine is *Mycobacterium avium* subsp. *avium* (MAA), sometimes referred to as "atypical tuberculosis" or "avian tuberculosis." Many mycobacteria are entirely saprophytic and nonpathogenic. These become an issue when encountered in diagnostic samples, and caution needs to be used in ascribing significance to them.[219]

Although disease caused by *M. bovis* and to a lesser extent *M. tuberculosis* has been reported in horses, equine tuberculosis is uncommon even in areas where the disease is prevalent in humans and other animals.[220-222] Infection with *M. avium* subspp. *paratuberculosis* (Johne's disease) can be induced experimentally in horses.[223] The recent literature also describes a single case in a Sicilian ass from North America, although the diagnosis was not confirmed by culture.[224] Consequently, naturally occurring equine Johne's disease, if it truly occurs at all, appears to be exceedingly rare.

The most common mycobacterial disease observed in horses is disseminated disease caused by MAA, which has been reported sporadically from North America and Europe.[220,225-232]

*The authors acknowledge and appreciate the original contributions of these authors, whose work has been incorporated into this chapter.

Other than a single case in which MAA was associated with septic arthritis,[233] all MAA infections described in horses have been disseminated disease. Although little is known about the source of equine MAA infections, the cases are very sporadic, and there is no evidence that these infections are contagious among horses. In other species, including humans, the source of infection is environmental.[216,234-237] Granulomatous disease in horses has also been described in association with other *M. avium* subspecies.[238-240]

Localized infections with other species of mycobacteria have also been described in horses but are surprisingly rare. These include a single case of abortion caused by *Mycobacterium terrae*,[241] a recent case of fetal disseminated granulomatous disease and abortion from which a pure culture of *Mycobacterium holsaticum* was obtained from fetal tissues (Slavic D, Shapiro J, Animal Health Laboratory, University of Guelph, unpublished data), and a single case of subcutaneous infection caused by *Mycobacterium smegmatis*.[242]

The predominant lesions in horses are respiratory and enteric, suggesting that the entry of MAA is by aerosol or ingestion of environmental organisms, respectively. Once in the intestine, MAA initially infects enterocytes, and to a lesser extent M cells, overlying intestinal lymphoid tissue. After extrusion from the intestinal epithelium into the submucosa, MAA is scavenged by local macrophages where it replicates as a facultative intracellular organism. The host immune response to infected macrophages results in granuloma formation by activation and recruitment of macrophages into the affected area.[243]

Clinical disease resulting from MAA is the result of organ dysfunction from infiltration and destruction of tissue by granulomatous inflammation. Weight loss is frequently observed in MAA-infected horses and is attributed to intestinal malabsorption and disruption of hormonal regulators of metabolism.[244] MAA exposure is most likely ubiquitous and probably occurs in all horses, suggesting that most MAA infections are subclinical and easily eradicated by host immune responses. Equine MAA infections are not associated with overt congenital or acquired immunodeficiency syndromes. However, more subtle defects that predispose horses to MAA infections may go unrecognized.

MAA infections in horses are typically diagnosed only after disease is highly advanced, and such infections have been uniformly fatal.[220,225-232] The clinical presentation varies depending on the organ system(s) affected. Cases of MAA are most common in horses between 1 and 6 years of age.[220,225-232] There does not appear to be a gender or breed predisposition.

MAA is a chronic disease, with most affected horses having clinical disease histories of 2 to 12 months. Presenting complaints typically include depression, intermittent fever, and weight loss. Many, but not all, infected horses have mild neutrophilia. In some cases, anemia is present. One of the most consistent clinical presentations of equine MAA infections is chronic diarrhea caused by involvement of the small intestine, cecum, or colon.* Many of these horses also have hypoalbuminemia from malabsorption and protein-losing enteropathy, which may result in ascites, pleural effusion, and edema. Although pulmonary involvement is common, overt respiratory signs such as dyspnea and coughing are uncommon. Similarly, although the liver is usually affected, and increased liver enzyme activities may be seen on clinical chemistries, overt liver disease is uncommon.[220,225-232] Thoracic and mesenteric lymphadenopathy is usually present. Involvement of the axial skeleton, particularly the cervical vertebrae, is frequently described and results in lameness, neck or back pain or stiffness, and occasionally spinal cord signs.[220,229] Other clinical lesions reported in conjunction with disseminated MAA infection

include abortion,[228] oral ulcers,[228] ocular infection,[231] guttural pouch masses and ulcers,[227] dermatitis,[225,232] abscessation, and mastitis.[220]

Localized infections with other mycobacteria are generally the result of traumatic injuries that inoculate environmental mycobacteria into lesions. These infections are rare but should be suspected with nonhealing granulomatous or pyogranulomatous wound infections that do not respond to conventional drainage and antimicrobial therapy. In other animals and humans, cutaneous mycobacterial infections typically present as nodular, ulcerated, fistulous draining tracts.[245]

The antemortem diagnosis of MAA may be challenging because of nonspecific clinical signs. Examination of biopsy specimens should reveal the characteristic granulomatous lesions and presence of acid-fast organisms. The absence of visible acid-fast organisms does not rule out mycobacterial infection, however, since smears or sections from culture-positive samples may be negative.[220,225,230,233] Because of their hydrophobicity, mycobacteria generally will not stain with Gram stain or Romanowsky-type stains (e.g., Diff-Quik).[214,245] Intradermal tuberculin testing with *M. bovis* or MAA antigens appears to lack specificity, with up to 70% of apparently uninfected horses giving positive reactions.[221,246] However, a negative test may suggest that a horse is not infected. Gross necropsy findings are often highly suggestive, and histopathology is generally suggestive or diagnostic of a mycobacterial infection.

Culture of tissue or fluid samples remains the "gold standard" for detection of mycobacterial pathogens. Mycobacteria are environmentally hardy, and thus they can be shipped to the laboratory with only minimal precautions to prevent desiccation of the sample.[214] Samples for culture should be stored and shipped at 4° C (39° F). It is essential to inform the laboratory that mycobacteria are suspected because they require specialized media and prolonged incubation for successful isolation.[247] Mycobacteria generally are slow growing, but quite variable. *M. bovis* or *M. tuberculosis* require 6 to 8 weeks to detect visible growth, whereas *Mycobacterium fortuitum* or *M. smegmatis* may be visible after only 2 to 3 days.[214,245,247]

Polymerase chain reaction (PCR) assay techniques to amplify species-specific target DNA sequences or to amplify genes for sequencing and genetic analysis may be used to confirm mycobacterial infections in clinical samples. Analysis of the 16S rRNA gene has become the gold standard for bacterial phylogenetics, and analysis of this region has proved to be very useful for definitive identification of mycobacterial isolates.[248,249] This approach has also been used successfully for identification of veterinary mycobacterial pathogens,[250-252] including MAA in a horse.[233] PCR methods, including sequencing, have the advantage of rapid results (2-3 days). PCR methods can be performed directly on clinical samples, eliminating the need for culture and greatly reducing the time required for a diagnosis.[250-253] In cases where fresh tissue samples are not available, PCR methods can also be used on formalin-fixed, paraffin-embedded samples.[252] The primary disadvantage of direct detection of mycobacteria in clinical samples is that it precludes evaluation of biologic properties, such as antimicrobial resistance. However, susceptibility testing and other phenotypic information often are not essential for the diagnosis or treatment of mycobacterial infections.

Horses with disseminated MAA are typically thin to emaciated. Gross necropsy findings typically include multifocal to miliary nodules, ranging in size from microscopic up to about 4 cm in diameter in affected organs.[220,225-232] Any portion of the gastrointestinal tract may be affected, but the cecum and colon appear to be most frequently involved.* In severe cases the large numbers of coalescing nodules may give the appearance of an

---

*References 220, 225, 226, 228, 230, 232.

*References 220, 225, 226, 228, 230, 232.

infiltrative disease similar to bovine Johne's disease.[225,229] Another prominent feature of intestinal infection is the presence of ulceration or crateriform lesions in the mucosa.[226,228,230] Ulceration may also be seen when lesions are present on the skin[225,232] or other mucosal surfaces, such as the guttural pouch[227] or oral mucosa.[228]

Microscopically, the nodules are granulomatous inflammation, with the primary inflammatory cells consisting of macrophages, epithelioid macrophages, and multinucleated giant cells (Langhans' cells).[220,225-232,243] Variable numbers of lymphocytes, neutrophils, plasma cells, and fibrosis may also be present. Caseous or liquefactive necrosis may be observed in some nodules. With ulcerative lesions, suppurative inflammation may be seen at the ulcerated surface,[227] most likely from secondary infections by other bacteria. Acid-fast bacilli can generally be demonstrated in the cytoplasm of macrophages within lesions.[225,226,229,231,232] However, in a significant proportion of culture-confirmed cases described in the literature, acid-fast organisms were not detectable.[220,230]

In the previously reported cases, MAA-infected horses were presented with either very advanced or terminal disease, and treatment was not attempted.[220,225-232] Based on the experience with treatment of MAA-infected humans, therapy with drug combinations that are highly effective for treating *M. tuberculosis* (ethambutol, isoniazid, rifampin, streptomycin) are ineffective for treating MAA. Recent incorporation of the newer macrolides azithromycin and clarithromycin into MAA treatment regimens has vastly improved the success rates.[247,254] These macrolides are more effective against MAA because of their low minimum inhibitory concentrations (MICs) and ability to achieve high concentrations in macrophages and tissues. Monotherapy with macrolides is not recommended, and azithromycin or clarithromycin should be combined with other drugs, such as ethambutol or rifampin, for additive or synergistic efficacy and to prevent development of resistance.[247,254] Human patients are treated for up to 1 year after conversion to culture-negative status for MAA pulmonary disease and lifelong for disseminated MAA disease.[247]

Combinations of azithromycin (10 mg/kg every 24 hours [q24h]) or clarithromycin (7.5 mg/kg q12h) with rifampin (5-10 mg/kg q12-24h) have been used safely and successfully to treat *Rhodococcus equi* pulmonary infections in foals.[255] Toxicity was limited to mild and self-limiting diarrhea in 5% to 28% of these foals. Therefore, it may be theoretically possible to treat selected MAA-infected horses with some expectation of success. However, the long-term treatment of an adult horse with these drugs may be prohibitively expensive, and no data are available on toxicity with prolonged therapy or the actual clinical efficacy of these drugs for equine MAA infections.

Treatment of cutaneous or other localized infections caused by other environmental mycobacteria is much more likely to be successful. In the single described case in which treatment of a subcutaneous *M. smegmatis* abscess was attempted, the infection was successfully resolved with surgical debridement and 18 days of trimethoprim-sulfonamide (30 mg/kg q12h), followed by 28 days of oral enrofloxacin (5 mg/kg q12h).[242] In treatment of these types of mycobacterial infections in dogs, cats, and humans, the role of surgical debridement of deep-seated infections and removal of any associated foreign bodies is strongly emphasized for success.[235,245,247]

In general, the environmental mycobacteria most often associated with localized infections in other animals and humans—*Mycobacterium abscessus, M. chelonae, M. fortuitum, M. marinum, and M. smegmatis*—are predictably susceptible, as well as predictably resistant, to certain antibiotics, including amikacin, cefoxitin, clarithromycin, doxycycline, enrofloxacin, and sulfonamides.[235,247,256] Because patterns of susceptibility are characteristic for different mycobacterial species, accurate identification of isolates is necessary for selecting appropriate antimicrobials. Based on published susceptibility data for a given mycobacterium, it is usually possible to select an appropriate drug regimen empirically.[235,245,247,256] For equine cases, cost and route of administration will also likely be factors in selecting a feasible course of therapy. Acquired resistance may also occur, particularly to fluoroquinolones, and it is generally recommended that all clinically significant isolates of environmental mycobacteria be susceptibility tested.[235,245,247]

Control strategies in the form of disinfection, quarantine, or vaccination are neither required nor likely to be helpful because MAA and other environmental mycobacteria are ubiquitous in the environment, and disease in horses is not defined by exposure.[216] The exceptions would be infections with *M. bovis* or *M. tuberculosis*. Although treatment of these infections is theoretically possible and has been accomplished successfully in other veterinary species, the public health implications and poor prognosis are likely to make attempted therapy prohibitive or impractical.[218]

Mycobacterium bovis is a well-documented zoonotic disease that may be acquired by drinking contaminated milk or through inhalation of, or wound contamination with, infected tissues.[218] Although there appear to be no documented human cases of *M. bovis* acquired from infected horses, no theoretic reason exists why this cannot occur, and appropriate safety precautions should be observed if working with an infected horse. Human cases of *M. tuberculosis* acquired from domestic animals have not been documented, and indeed most infections in animals appear to be acquired from humans.[218,257] Nevertheless, if an infected horse is encountered, due caution would be prudent, and any humans who may have been the source of infection should be referred to their physician for tuberculosis screening. As eradicated or regulated diseases, detection of either *M. bovis* or *M. tuberculosis* has significant public health and agricultural implications, and these are reportable diseases in most developed countries.

MAA and other environmental mycobacteria are not regarded as zoonotic organisms. Susceptibility to disease is not defined by exposure, which for most humans and animals is continuous. Although both humans and animals develop MAA disease, molecular epidemiologic analysis of the isolates from human and animal MAA cases indicates that human cases are not acquired from animals.[216,219,234,235,247]

The complete reference list is available online at www.expertconsult.com.

CHAPTER

46 Laboratory Diagnosis of Fungal Diseases

Barbara A. Byrne

Introduction to Fungi

Fungi are eukaryotic organisms, unlike prokaryotic bacteria. Fungi are characterized by cellular organelles, such as a nucleus; however, they have several important differences from mammalian eukaryotic cells. Fungi have a cell wall that contains the sterol ergosterol and many carbohydrates such as glucan and galactomannan. The metabolic pathways for synthesis of these unique structures are the primary targets of antifungal therapy.

Fungi have a variety of morphologic structures and forms in vivo and in vitro. The terminology describing fungal morphology and taxonomy can be complex. Additionally, fungal names and structures will vary depending on whether asexual or sexual reproduction is being observed; the asexual forms most often are clinically relevant. Box 46-1 provides a primer for fungal terminology.

Whether opportunistic or primarily pathogenic, fungi occur as yeasts (e.g., *Candida* spp.) or molds (e.g., *Aspergillus* spp.). Yeasts generally exist as single-celled organisms that multiply through budding. Molds, or filamentous fungi, form hyphae or elongated structures that may or may not be septate. Reproduction of filamentous fungi can occur through several mechanisms. Dermatophyte hyphae within the host may fragment to become arthroconidia, which are easily spread to other animals and the environment. Hyphomycetes, such as *Aspergillus* spp., can form complex asexual reproductive forms often called fruiting structures. Zygomycete asexual reproduction occurs

---

Box 46-1 Definitions of Common Terms Used in Mycology

Arthrospore Asexual condidium formed by fragmentation of the hyphae usually found in vivo; often seen indermatophytosis; arthrocondia are a type of conidium.

Chromoblastomycosis Fungal infection of the skin and subcutaneous tissue characterized by brown sclerotic bodies; also caused by dematiaceous fungi such as *Fonsecaea*.

Conidium Asexual reproductive cell formed from hyphae or phialides by budding or division; an infectious unit; plural *conidia*.

Dematiaceous Descriptive term for fungi with melanin pigment that gives hyphae a brown or black color.

Dermatophytosis Infection of the hair and superficial skin by fungi of the genera *Microsporum* and *Trichophyton* in animals.

Dimorphic Structural term for fungi that can convert between two different morphologies (e.g., yeasts and molds); temperature is one factor that triggers the conversion; examples include *Coccidioides immitis* and *Blastomyces capsulatum*.

Ectothrix Arthroconidia that are outside the hair shaft in dermatophytosis.

Endothrix Arthroconidia that are inside the hair shaft in dermatophytosis.

Fungus Eukaryotic cell (or groups of cells) with cell walls that are nonmotile and do not photosynthesize.

Hyalohyphomycosis Fungal infection caused by any mold that forms colorless, septate hyphae (e.g., seen with *Aspergillus*).

Hyphae Elongated filaments seen in molds; can be septate or nonseptate; singular *hypha*.

Hyphomycete Filamentous fungus with uncolored hyphae; asexual reproduction occurs through formation of conidiophores, phialides, and conidia; hyphae are frequently septate; examples include *Aspergillus* and *Acremonium*.

Macroconidia Large, multinuclear conidia that form from hyphae; seen only in culture, not in animal; basis for identification of many fungi, particularly dermatophytes.

Microconidia Small, single-celled conidia that form directly off hyphae.

Molds Multicellular fungi that can form mycelium; they are a subset of fungus.

Mycelium Grossly visible mat or accumulation of hyphae; plural *mycelia*.

Mycetoma General term for a tumor-like lesion that has granule-containing pus; granules of a *eumycotic* mycetoma contain fungi; an *actinomycotic* mycetoma is caused by bacteria such as *Actinomyces* and *Nocardia*.

Phaeohyphomycosis Fungal infection caused by dematiaceous fungi (e.g., *Phaeoacremonium parasiticum, Alternaria*); usually found in the skin or subcutaneous tissues, but infection can also be internal or disseminated.

Phialide Cell that produces and pushes out conidia.

Pseudohyphae Filamentous elongation of budding cells (e.g., *Candida*) that do not separate to form chains; generally the pseudohyphae narrow at the point of attachment.

Septae Divisions between hyphae or cross-walls of hyphae.

Spherule Sac-like structure that contains many endospores; characteristic of *Coccidioides immitis* in vivo.

Spore Infectious unit that results from sexual reproduction in fungi; often used improperly when referring to conidia.

Vesicle Oval structure bearing phialides and conidia (e.g., seen in *Aspergillus*).

Yeasts Unicellular fungi that do not produce mycelia and reproduce by budding.

Zygomycete Filamentous fungus that has asexual reproduction through sporangia and sporangiospores; generally considered a lower form of fungi; hyphae are frequently nonseptate; examples include *Rhizopus* and *Mucor*.

Zygomycosis Fungal infection caused by a zygomycete (e.g., *Rhizopus, Mucor*).

through a sporangium that contains sporangiospores. Fruiting structures and sporangiospores are rarely found within tissues unless exposed to air such as in the sinus or guttural pouch. These reproductive structures can occasionally be observed histologically and are essential to fungal identification in culture. Other fungi, such as *Coccidioides immitis*, are dimorphic, having different structures in vivo (e.g., spherules) and in vitro (hyphae).

This chapter provides the clinician with the necessary information regarding basic sample collection, culture techniques, morphology, identification, and antifungal susceptibility testing to ensure optimal sampling for fungal culture and accurate interpretation of results.

Host Susceptibility

Fungal infections, with the exception of dermatophytosis, are generally rare in equine species, but they still represent important pathogenic processes. Disease caused by fungal infection depends on many factors, primarily host susceptibility, pathogenicity of the fungal species, and dose of fungal organisms. Fungal infections, such as candidiasis, can be observed in neonatal foals that are often immunocompromised through failure of passive transfer, have increased susceptibility because of alterations in normal flora from antibiotic use that decreases colonization resistance, and may have poor physical defenses resulting from indwelling medical devices and wounds or abrasions. These foals illustrate the major host factors contributing to fungal infection.

Sources of Fungal Pathogens

Most fungal infections are opportunistic and originate from the environment, transient contamination of the host, or normal flora. Fungi that survive and reproduce in the environment are termed *saprophytes;* they can be opportunistic pathogens. Some fungi utilize host substances without causing harm; these are commensal fungi. Many saprophytic fungi can be found on body surfaces without causing damage or utilizing host substances; these are termed *transients.* Some fungi require an animal host for survival, cause host damage, and are considered obligate pathogens; for example, the zoophilic dermatophytes require an animal host but are transmissible from animal to animal and to humans.

Knowledge of the source of agents can be important for interpretation of fungal culture results. Because most fungal infections arise from the environment, they can be a frequent contaminant in samples collected for fungal culture. Samples, such as skin, can have a large number of transient fungal species that can be detected in the laboratory. Transient fungal organisms are also common in the upper respiratory tract, where conidia are filtered from inspired air by nasal turbinates and mucus. Feeds, such as hay and alfalfa, will often have high numbers of molds, which can easily contaminate the nasal passages and upper trachea. Many saprophytes will grow on conventional agar used to isolate and identify fungi, leading to false-positive results on fungal culture.

Laboratory Safety

Although safety is an important concern when working with any infectious agent, fungal pathogens require special consideration, especially in the laboratory. Filamentous fungi cultured in the laboratory produce millions of conidia that are easily aerosolized when a culture plate is opened. This leads to widespread contamination of the laboratory that can be introduced into other cultures and expose laboratory personnel to large numbers of infectious fungi. Even saprophytic fungi can cause

disease in healthy adults if sufficient numbers of conidia are present. The systemic dimorphic fungi, such as *Coccidioides immitis*, are generally not infectious from the patient but are highly infectious when they are in mold form in the laboratory (see Chapter 47). *Coccidioides immitis* is one of the most common and dangerous of laboratory-acquired infections. Consequently, manipulation of all fungal cultures should be carried out in a biosafety hood, and plates should be sealed to prevent aerosolization of hyphae and conidia. The clinician should always inform the laboratory when a fungal infection is suspected, especially the dimorphic fungi as some may grow on conventional bacterial agars.

Specimen Collection and Transport

Aspirates, tissues, and hair or scales can be appropriate for fungal culture. Fungal organisms do not withstand extreme heat or cold and should be protected appropriately during storage and transport to the laboratory. Almost all samples can be collected as they would for bacterial culture (see Chapter 27). Because some pathogenic fungi may be present in small numbers within a tissue, a swab does not provide an adequate sample size for optimal detection of fungi; a biopsy sample or fluid aspirate is preferred. In general, samples do not require refrigeration if they are to be placed on culture media within a few hours. If transportation to the laboratory for primary cultures will take longer, they should be stored and shipped at 4°C (39°F) to prevent overgrowth by bacteria and contaminating fungi.[1]

Skin

The skin has many fungi on its surface, and cleaning with 70% ethanol before sample collection can help remove these superficial contaminants (see Chapters 7 and 50). Hair and scales from a suspected ringworm lesion should be collected using forceps or by skin scraping. The leading edge of the lesion is best for culture because it will contain the most fungal elements. Collected specimens should be placed in a dry container for transport to the laboratory. It is not necessary to store skin scrapings and hair at cool temperatures as long as the sample can be inoculated on fungal culture media within 72 hours. If a deeper infection is considered likely, a punch biopsy is a preferred sample.

Eye

Fungal infections of corneal tissue are common, particularly in neonatal foals or as a complication of corneal ulceration (see Chapter 10). As for bacterial culture, the cornea should be scraped gently. Scrapings should be placed in a sterile container and can be left on the instrument used for scraping. Alternatively, the scrapings can be placed directly on an agar suitable for fungal growth provided the agar is immediately transported to the laboratory where the sample can be streaked for isolation and incubated. A sample should be placed immediately on a slide for cytologic examination.

Blood

The lysis-centrifugation method or broth medium for blood culture can be used for fungal culture (see Chapter 27). The pellet resulting from centrifugation or media from the blood culture broth should be inoculated to the appropriate fungal culture medium.

Fluids

Fluids collected by aspiration are appropriate for fungal isolation and identification. The volume collected should be enough to represent the lesion present and should allow for inoculation of multiple media and for cytologic examination. If the sample also contains bacteria, such as a transtracheal aspirate, it should be kept cold (4° C [39° F]) and shipped on wet ice or gel packs to minimize overgrowth of the bacteria.

Tissue

Ideally, a biopsy of affected tissue should be collected for fungal culture and cytologic examination. Swabs may be used for diagnosis of oral lesions of suspected candidiasis (see Chapter 49).

Direct Examination

Cytology and histopathology are essential components for diagnosis of fungal disease. Fungal elements can be rare and localized within a lesion, so samples submitted for culture may not contain fungal organisms. Thus cytologic and histopathologic examination may increase sensitivity of testing for fungal organisms. It will also allow detection of unculturable agents or those that are very difficult to isolate. Unfortunately, a specific etiologic diagnosis usually cannot be made from filamentous fungal elements observed histologically, although a presumptive identification of many yeasts is possible (see section on Gram Stain). Culture of the organism or use of molecular techniques will be necessary for definitive identification of the causative agent observed microscopically.

Fungal infection is almost always accompanied by inflammatory cells. In most tissues, granulomatous inflammation along with some suppuration is typically seen. One exception is infection caused by *Cryptococcus* spp. Often, minimal to no inflammation is present, most likely because of the antiinflammatory effect of the fungal capsule.

Potassium Hydroxide Treatment

Potassium hydroxide (KOH) can be used on clinical specimens to clear cellular material and better visualize fungal elements. This method is used most often when examining skin scrapings or flakes and hair for the presence of hyphae and arthroconidia in suspected dermatophyte infections, but KOH can be used on many sample types (see Chapter 50). The specimen is placed in a few drops of 10% to 20% KOH and incubated for 5 to 10 minutes; gentle heating can clear samples more quickly. A coverslip is placed over the KOH-digested sample, and the slide is examined microscopically without staining. Alternatively, a variety of stains can be used after KOH treatment. In dermatophytosis, arthrospores develop and form as hyphae break apart and appear as a linear chain of small, round to rectangular, highly refractile structures. Ectothrix, when arthrospores are present on the outside of the hair shaft, is consistent with most animal dermatophyte infections. When arthrospores are found within hairs, it is termed endothrix.

India Ink

India ink is most useful for identification of *Cryptococcus neoformans* or *C. gattii* in fluids or tissues (see Chapter 53). A drop of India ink is placed on a slide with a drop of water and then the fluid or tissue is added. The ink will stain the background dark, leaving the abundant capsular material unstained (Fig. 46-1). The "soap bubble" appearance is pathognomonic for *Cryptococcus*.

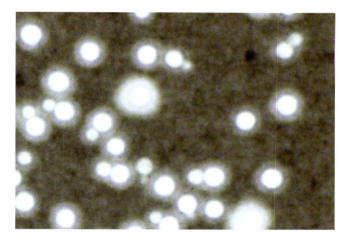

Figure 46-1 India ink stain of *Cryptococcus neoformans*. The unstained halo around the yeast is capsular material consistent with this yeast. Budding organisms are present (600×).

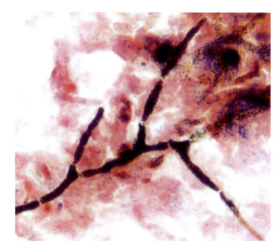

Figure 46-2 Gram stain of fungal hyphae in clinical specimen, *Aspergillus* spp. (1000×).

Gram Stain

The Gram stain is very good for demonstrating the presence of yeasts. The yeast organisms will stain dark blue/purple, and budding will be easy to detect. Other fungal structures, such as hyphae, may stain variably or even poorly with Gram stain.

Some of the structures seen during a direct microscopic examination include hyphae when a filamentous fungus is present, yeasts, and spherules in the case of coccidioidomycosis. Occasionally, when a filamentous fungus is present in a body space where there is free air or oxygen, a conidial head may form with phialides and conidia. Otherwise, this structure is usually only observed when the fungus is cultured in vitro.

The fungal features present can help narrow the list of possible fungal species present. Colorless septate hyphae branching at 45-degree angles with parallel walls and septae are suggestive of *Aspergillus* (Fig. 46-2). Broad (5-20 μm) hyphae with few to no septae and walls that are not parallel are most consistent with zygomycosis. Septate hyphae that are black or brown color are most likely a dematiaceous fungal species that contains melanin as a component of the fungal cell wall. This condition is called phaeohyphomycosis. The presence of sclerotic bodies

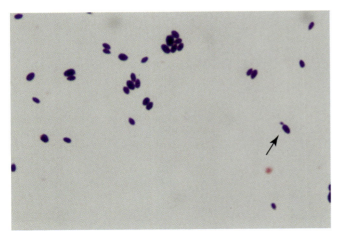

Figure 46-3 Gram stain of *Candida* spp. The arrow points to a budding yeast (1000×).

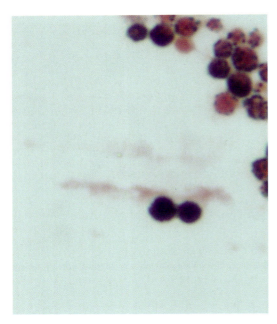

Figure 46-4 Gram stain of *Cryptococcus neoformans*. The yeast can have stippled staining. Note very narrow ("wasp-waist") budding (1000×).

that appear brown with both horizontal and vertical septations is most similar to chromoblastomycosis.

Yeasts can be partially differentiated on the basis of size, shape, and budding characteristics. *Candida* are round to oval (Fig. 46-3); they can form pseudohyphae in tissues. Pseudohyphae are an elongated outgrowth from the yeast cell and tend to narrow at the cellular divisions. *Cryptococcus*, in addition to its abundant capsule, exhibits narrow-based budding; *Cryptococcus neoformans* and *C. gattii* can stain somewhat poorly and can have a stippled appearance (Fig. 46-4). *Coccidioides immitis* forms spherules within the host tissue. These are large, 10 to 100 μm in diameter, containing multiple round endospores. *Sporothrix schenckii* organisms are oval yeasts that have elongated or cigar-shaped budding.

Artifacts can occur with the Gram stain. Linear strands of fibrin or degenerate cells will stain pink and can appear similar to fungal hyphae.

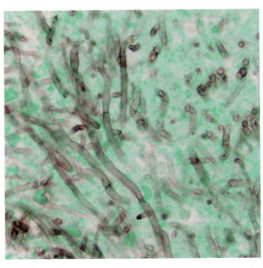

Figure 46-5 Gomori's methenamine silver stain of biopsy from ethmoid turbinate of horse. The hyphae stain gray-black. *Aspergillus* was isolated from the sample (1000×).

Other Stains

Two common stains used to identify fungi in clinical specimens are Gomori's methenamine silver (GMS) and periodic acid–Schiff (PAS). The GMS stain is very useful for detection of both yeasts and filamentous fungi, but it is generally reserved for histology laboratories and fixed-tissue sections because the staining procedure is specialized. GMS stains fungi gray or black (Fig. 46-5). Periodic acid–Schiff stains the fungal cell wall, and fungi appear pink. The PAS stain is very useful for detection of yeasts and hyphae.

Many other staining techniques are available, including methylene blue, Giemsa, and calcofluor white stains. Methylene blue can be useful to identify the intracellular yeast *Histoplasma capsulatum*. Calcofluor white staining is rapid but requires a fluorescent microscope for viewing, and artifacts can make interpretation difficult.

Culture and Identification

Specialized media are required for fungal isolation and identification; consequently, fungal culture should be specifically requested when samples are submitted to the microbiology laboratory. Some fungi may grow on conventional blood agar used in bacteriology; this method is not reliable for identification, however, and fungal growth should be subcultured to appropriate fungal culture medium. All cultures should be incubated at 30° C (86° F); if no suitable equipment is available, samples should be cultured at room temperature (about 25° C [77° F]). Culture plates should be sealed to minimize evaporation but allow air exchange. Agar plates should be examined every few days for 4 weeks before considering them as negative for fungal growth. Growth of yeasts usually occurs within a few days to 1 week. Growth of molds can take days to weeks.

Dermatophyte Culture

Collection of hair or scales from suspected dermatophytosis lesions and culture probably represent the most common and easiest fungal detection method used by equine practitioners (see Chapter 50). Hair and scales should be placed on suitable media, such as dermatophyte test medium (DTM) or dermatophyte identification media, and incubated in the dark at room temperature or 30°C (86°F). Dermatophyte test medium contains chloramphenicol, gentamicin, and cycloheximide to inhibit bacteria and some saprophytic fungal growth. Dermatophytes will turn the media alkaline, resulting in a color change to red. Some type of medium that encourages sporulation (e.g., rapid sporulation medium) should be inoculated at the same time because dermatophytes grown on DTM may not have adequate conidial production for identification. DTM cultures should be examined daily for fungal growth and color change; the red color should appear before or when fungal growth is evident to be consistent with a dermatophyte (Fig. 46-6). Some saprophytic fungi will grow on DTM and may cause a red color. Regardless of the color change, the mold should be examined for macroconidia and microconidia to confirm the isolate as a dermatophyte rather than a saprophytic contaminant (Fig. 46-7).

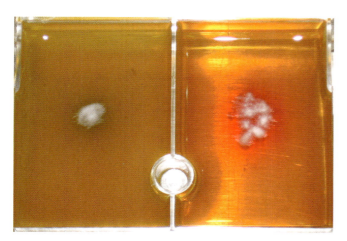

Figure 46-6 Inoculated rapid sporulation media *(left)* and dermatophyte test media (DTM; *right*) on split plate. The DTM medium has turned red, with growth of *Microsporum gypseum.*

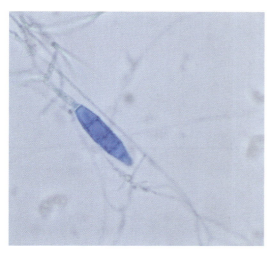

Figure 46-7 Tape preparation of fungal growth of *Microsporum gypseum* stained with lactophenol aniline blue. The large structures are macroconidia. The rough outer wall of the macroconidia and few (or no) microconidia are consistent with the genus *Microsporum* (600×).

Culture of Fluid or Tissue

Any fluid samples, such as urine, bronchoalveolar lavage (BAL), or transtracheal aspirate (TTA), should be centrifuged and the resulting pellet used to inoculate media. Tissue samples should be macerated by chopping with a scalpel blade or stomacher to release fungal elements. Generally, samples will be plated initially on some type of fungal agar. If the sample is likely to have bacteria, it will be cultivated on a medium containing antibiotics, such as inhibitory mold agar (IMA), which contains chloramphenicol. If no contaminants are expected, the sample can be inoculated onto a noninhibitory medium such as Sabouraud dextrose agar or potato dextrose agar. Although the IMA will inhibit growth of contaminating bacteria, many molds will not have their characteristic gross and microscopic morphology, necessitating subculture to a noninhibitory medium and delaying definitive identification. Some fungi will grow on blood agar used for bacterial isolation and identification but will also need subculture to a noninhibitory fungal agar for identification.

Identification of Fungal Species

Identification of the fungal species causing an infection is both art and science. Much of identification is based on fungal morphology in vitro but also can rely on biochemical testing. The first step in identification depends on the morphologic differentiation between yeast and mold; often this can be done based on the initial direct examination of the submitted sample.

Yeasts will appear as regular colonies on inoculated plates and as single-celled organisms with budding on Gram stain. Their shape and budding characteristics can be used for preliminary identification of the genus. Definitive identification will depend on additional biochemical testing. Kits are available for identification of many pathogenic yeasts, including the API Microbial Identification Strips 20C AUX, Yeast (bioMérieux Vitex, Hazelwood, MO) and RapID yeast plus panel (Remel Labs, Lenexa, KS). Additionally, selective agar that produces a characteristic color change (CHROMagar Candida) can be used for both genus and species identification of *Candida*. Although identification to the genus level is often sufficient for treatment, many yeasts, particularly certain species of *Candida* (e.g., *C. glabrata*), have shown resistance to common antifungal agents. Thus speciation can aid selection of the appropriate drug for treatment.[2]

Molds are identified based on macroscopic appearance, such as color, rapidity of growth, and diffusible pigment in the agar, and microscopic features, such as hyphal morphology, with or without septae and asexual reproductive structures. Algorithms are available for fungal identification.[3] When microscopic morphology does not allow definitive identification, molecular techniques can be used for species identification. As for yeasts, definitive identification of molds to the species level can be helpful for choosing the most appropriate treatment, particularly with *Aspergillus* spp. (Fig. 46-8), because some species have known resistance to certain antifungal drugs.[2,4]

Pneumocystis carinii (P. jirovecii)

Pneumocystis carinii is an organism with uncertain taxonomic position; it has frequently been categorized as either a fungus or a protozoan (see Chapter 53). Ribosomal ribonucleic acid (rRNA) sequencing suggests that *P. carinii* is most closely related to fungi, particularly *Saccharomyces cerevisiae.*[5] This agent does not grow in routine bacterial or fungal cultures. Consequently, it is detected using a variety of stains. A Giemsa or Papanicolaou stain demonstrates abundant foamy material in BAL or alveolar spaces. *Pneumocystis carinii* is better visualized with a GMS stain or immunohistochemical staining to detect *Pneumocystis* antigen. Alternatively, molecular methods can be used to detect *Pneumocystis* deoxyribonucleic acid (DNA).[6]

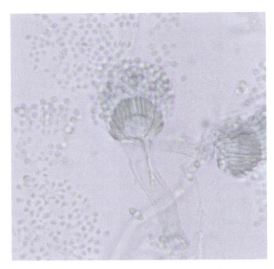

Figure 46-8 Tape preparation of fungal growth of *Aspergillus* spp. stained with lactophenol aniline blue demonstrating characteristic fruiting structures (600×).

Interpretation of Culture Results

Interpretation of a positive fungal culture from a site that is often contaminated with saprophytic fungi can be difficult. Therefore it is important to include a cytologic or histologic examination of the tissue to document the presence of fungi, such as yeasts or hyphae, in the tissue. Isolation of common saprophytic fungi that are often not pathogenic, such as *Mucor* or *Rhizopus*, is more consistent with contamination. Furthermore, inflammation almost always accompanies fungal infection and would help support the interpretation.

Probably the most common samples from which fungi are isolated are TTAs and skin scrapings or biopsies. Isolation of an opportunistic fungus must always be interpreted cautiously because these sites frequently have transient fungi that can contaminate the sample. The patient should have other clinical, cytologic, or histologic evidence that a fungus is present before interpreting the isolate as a true infecting agent.

Finally, because fungi can be found in small numbers within lesions, samples submitted to the laboratory may not contain fungal elements that are sufficiently viable for isolation. Consequently, a negative fungal culture does not rule out the presence of a fungal infection.

Molecular Diagnosis of Fungal Infections

General molecular methods used to identify pathogenic organisms are described in Chapter 27. This section identifies specific fungal organisms for which molecular methods could be used for diagnosis and addresses issues that apply directly to fungal pathogens.

The polymerase chain reaction (PCR) is the most common method used to detect fungal DNA in samples. Primers can be designed to recognize fungi at many levels of identification. For example, universal primers detect virtually all species of fungi; genus-specific primers identify fungi belonging to a single genus as in detection of all *Aspergillus* spp., and species-specific primers may be used for detection of a single species. Most PCR tests used for fungal detection are directed toward rRNA genes or the spacer regions between the genes. The polymerase chain reaction using universal fungal primers can be helpful when the histologic examination suggests a fungal infection, including hyphae, but isolation was not successful. However, this test should be used only on samples that do not have any chance of saprophytic contamination, or a false-positive result will be obtained. If a sample is positive, further testing (e.g., sequencing of PCR product, DNA probe) can be used to identify the genus and species present.

The polymerase chain reaction can also be used to identify a fungus after growth is observed in the laboratory. Because morphologic identification can take days to weeks, PCR amplification can provide a rapid result and lead to more rapid, definitive treatment.

Molecular methods for detection exist for many fungi.[7] Most frequently these techniques are used to detect *Aspergillus* spp., *Cryptococcus* spp., and *Candida* spp.[8-11] Polymerase chain reaction methodology is also available for diagnosis of *Pythium insidiosum*[12] (see Chapter 51).

One disadvantage of using molecular methods for diagnostic testing is that fungal cells can be scarce in infected tissues, making detection difficult. Molecular methods should not replace primary culture, isolation, and identification, but rather supplement these standard diagnostic techniques to provide the quickest and most accurate diagnosis.

Fungal Antigen Detection

Testing for fungal antigen is available to aid diagnosis of fungal infections in humans and animals. The most frequently used methods are latex agglutination and enzyme immunoassay (EIA) for detection of *Cryptococcus* spp. capsule. Large amounts of capsule are released into the systemic circulation; this allows detection of fungal antigen in serum or exudate from the site of suspected infection. The result is reported as a "titer" but is a measure of antigen not antibody. Because this test is quantitative, it can be used during treatment to evaluate response. A declining antigen titer indicates a positive response to treatment.

Several antigen-based tests exist to detect invasive *Aspergillus* spp. infection in humans.[7] These methods most often use EIA to measure galactomannan, a component of the *Aspergillus* fungal cell wall, in body fluids or serum.[13] These tests have not been validated in horses to diagnose aspergillosis, and even in human patients, they are controversial because cutoff values are not universally agreed on.[7] Another but less specific cell-wall component measured to detect fungal infection is (1→3)-β-D-glucan.[14] This substance is present in the most pathogenic fungi, including *Aspergillus* and *Candida*. Thus the β-D-glucan assay has the potential to detect a number of invasive fungal infectious agents. However, like the galactomannan assay, it has not been validated for use in horses.

Antifungal Susceptibility Testing

Testing of fungal isolates for susceptibility to antifungal drugs is becoming more widely available, and many human and veterinary laboratories will perform testing on yeasts. Determination of a minimum inhibitory concentration (MIC) for filamentous fungi is more difficult to perform and standardize; consequently, this testing is limited to a few laboratories. Traditionally, few equine isolates are tested for antifungal drug susceptibility because many antifungal drugs are prohibitively expensive for use in large species. However, as more drugs become available in the less expensive generic formulations, use of these drugs to treat horses will become more widespread. An understanding of the advantages and limitations of antifungal sensitivity testing is important for the equine clinician to ensure optimal use of antifungal drugs.

The Clinical and Laboratory Standards Institute (CLSI) has standardized testing of antifungal drugs against yeasts since 1997 and molds since 2002.[15,16] Standardization of methodologies is necessary for reproducibility and comparison of results within and between laboratories and assessment of the clinical utility of this testing. Establishment of an MIC or zone of inhibition of growth to indicate that an organism is susceptible or resistant to a particular drug is in its infancy and is only available for some yeast and a few species of filamentous fungi.

The usefulness of antifungal drug susceptibility testing is the ability to use the result to predict clinical outcome. In general, the clinician should remember that (1) in vitro measurement of susceptibility does not guarantee clinical success, (2) finding an organism to be resistant in vitro should predict therapeutic failure, and (3) host factors can be the most important component for a positive clinical outcome.[17] Interpretation of an MIC as susceptible or resistant depends on two criteria: (1) whether the MIC measured in vitro meets or exceeds the drug concentrations found within the animal and (2) reliable clinical data that demonstrate successful treatment of the respective fungal infection at or below the MIC.[17] Interpretive criteria are best established for yeasts, particularly *Candida* spp., with the antifungal drugs amphotericin B and the azole class. Unfortunately, few data exist in the human literature for mold susceptibility interpretations, and few to no studies have been performed in common veterinary species such as the horse. Thus the use and interpretation of MIC values for fungi are controversial.[18]

However, a number of yeast and mold isolates have demonstrated both in vivo and in vitro resistance to common antifungal drugs. Some of these species, such as *Aspergillus terreus*, *Aspergillus fumigatus*, *Paecilomyces lilacinus*, *Candida* spp., and *Cryptococcus neoformans*, do cause infections in veterinary species.[2,4,19] Consequently, more laboratories are using fungal susceptibility testing.

The two major methods for antifungal susceptibility testing are agar diffusion using either discs or ETest (an antifungal impregnated strip that allows determination of fungal MIC on agar media) and broth dilution. Most testing evaluates the ability of the drug to inhibit fungal growth (80% reduction), rather than determining fungicidal activity.[20]

Although all laboratories do not currently offer antifungal susceptibility testing, several commercial broth-based systems are available for yeast MIC determinations. The Sensititre Yeast One Colorimetric Antifungal Panel (Trek Diagnostic Systems, Thermo Fisher Scientific, Westlake, OH) has a fairly wide range of drug concentrations and has at least 85% agreement with reference methods.[21]

Serology

Serologic testing can be used to confirm fungal infection in horses, although its use has been limited. Serology for *Aspergillus* infection has been performed for horses using agar gel immunodiffusion, immunoblot, or enzyme-linked immunosorbent assay (ELISA).[22,23] This testing has been helpful in diagnosing systemic aspergillosis but has had variable results in detecting *A. fumigatus* infection of the guttural pouch. The ELISA test does not seem to differentiate normal from diseased horses, but detection of antibody directed toward two *Aspergillus* proteins of 22 and 26 kDa did identify diseased horses in immunoblot tests.[23]

Serology has helped identify horses with coccidioidomycosis (see Chapter 47). Only 4% of normal horses have a positive titer, and this titer remains stable or decreases with time.[24] Thus a positive test result should be highly suggestive of infection and can be used prognostically.[25]

The complete reference list is available online at www.expertconsult.com.

CHAPTER

47 Coccidioidomycosis

Maureen T. Long, Demosthenes Pappagianis,* and Jill Higgins*

Coccidioidomycosis is an infectious disease caused by primarily two species of *Coccidioides, C. immitis* and *C. posadasii*.[1-3] In the literature, the former species is often designated the Californian and the latter the non-Californian *Coccidioides*. *Coccidioides* spp. reside in the soil and cause disease in mammalian hosts after being inhaled primarily through contaminated dust or very rarely through skin puncture.[3]

Coccidioides fungi are part of the large order of mostly saprophytes, the *Onygenales*. However, this particular genus tends to associate with pathogenic infections in animals, including equids (Box 47-1). The first reported case of coccidioidomycosis was described in a human in Argentina by Posadas in 1892.[4] In 1894, Rixford[5] reported a human case in California, which was the forerunner of thousands of additional cases occurring in the southwestern United States. Both Posadas and Rixford carried out experiments involving injection of *C. immitis* into experimental animals, although this did not include equids.

Naturally occurring coccidioidomycosis in nonhuman mammals was reported in cattle by Giltner[6] in 1918. The disease was not reported in equids until the 1940s, according to Maddy.[7] Wilding et al[8] alluded to the disease in burros. In the earliest report, 13 of 22 horses raised near Phoenix and a

*The authors acknowledge and appreciate the original contributions of these authors, whose work has been incorporated into this chapter.

burro near Mesa, Arizona were reactive to intracutaneously injected coccidioidin, indicating prior infection with *C. immitis*.[8]

Deliberate infection of horses by intravenous injection of live *C. immitis* was carried out by Smith et al[9] to induce antibodies that could serve as standardized serologic controls (particularly for the diagnosis of coccidioidomycosis in humans). Neither the size of the inoculum nor the clinical outcome was described, although serum from these horses was satisfactory as an antibody-positive serologic control. The earliest cases of equine

---

Box 47-1 Equids with Naturally Acquired Coccidioidomycosis

Burro (Equus asinus)
Horse, domestic (Equus caballus)
Horse, Przewalski's (Equus przewalski)
Kiang (Equus hemionus kiang)
Onager (Equus hemionus onager)
Zebra, Grévy's (Equus grevyi)
Somali wild ass (Equus africanus somaliensis)

---

coccidioidomycosis were reported by Zontine,[10] Rehkemper,[11] and Crane.[12]

Etiology

Coccidioides immitis is a diphasic and pleomorphic mold/fungus with a (saprobic) growth phase in nature or in usual laboratory culture that differs morphologically from the (parasitic) growth phase usually seen in the tissues of an infected host (Fig. 47-1). The saprobic form consists of filaments (hyphae) 2 to 3 μm in diameter, some of which can differentiate into a chain of thick-walled arthroconidia ("spores"). These conidia can be barrel shaped or cylindrical, 2 × 5 μm in size, and often alternate with empty, degenerate "disjunctor" cells that readily fracture, permitting airborne dispersion of the arthroconidia, which are highly infectious. Clinicians who suspect the presence of *C. immitis* in material submitted to the laboratory must inform laboratory personnel of the potential hazard of handling such samples.

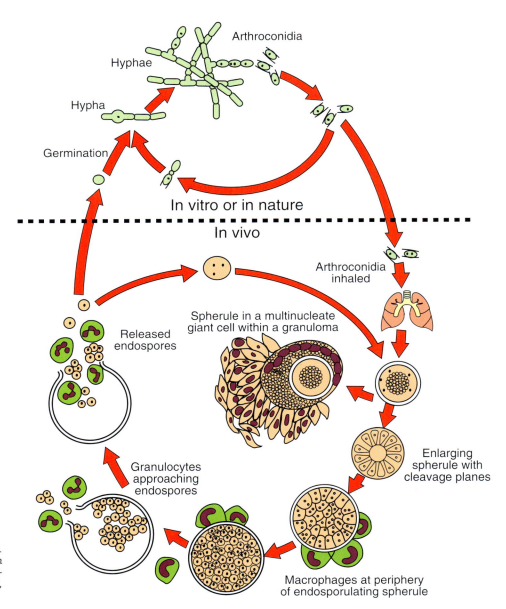

Figure 47-1 Life cycle of *Coccidioides immitis*. (Modified from Collier L, Balows A, Sussman M, et al, editors: Topley & Wilson's microbiology and microbial infections, ed 9, London, 1998, Hodder Arnold.)

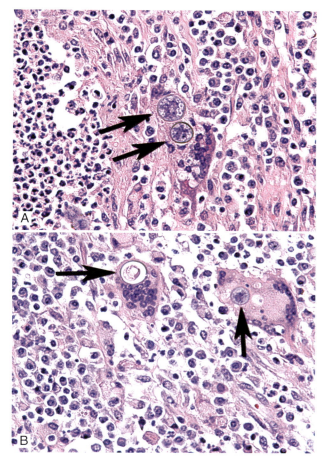

Figure 47-2 Histopathologic appearance of *Coccidioides immitis* in an equine spleen. **A,** Two endosporulating spherules *(arrows)* in area containing plasma cells, lymphocytes, and portion of multinucleated giant cell near abscess containing abundant neutrophil granulocytes. **B,** Two nonendosporulating spherules *(arrows)* in multinucleated giant cells. *(Courtesy Suzanne Johnson, PhD.)*

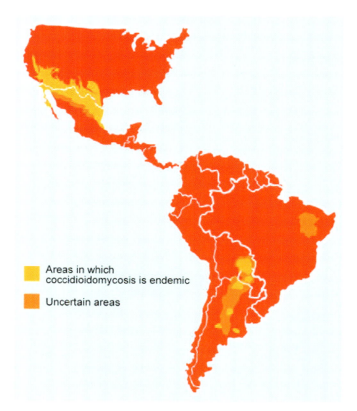

Figure 47-3 Geographic distribution of *Coccidioides immitis* sites where coccidioidomycosis is usually acquired. *(Illustration courtesy of Margaret Shear. In Hector RF, Laniado-Laborin R: Coccidioidomycosis—A fungal disease of the Americas. PloS Med 2:e2, 2005.)*

When inhaled or otherwise introduced into the tissue of a mammalian host, the arthroconidia become rounded and enlarge to become spherules (20-100 μm in diameter), which undergo internal division of cytoplasm and nucleus. This results in the production from a single cell (arthroconidium) of hundreds of endospores in one generation. Each released endospore can then enlarge to become a spherule, which releases more endospores. The conversion from arthroconidia to spherules is influenced by elevated (body) temperature, increased carbon dioxide (CO_2), and perhaps surface-active agents; the in vivo process appears to be influenced by presence of inflammatory leukocytes (Fig. 47-2). The released endospores evoke a polymorphonuclear leukocyte (PMN) response, whereas the spherules evoke a macrophage response. Thus mixed suppurative-granulomatous inflammation is characteristic of coccidioidal lesions. In chronic lesions, caseation and hyalinization (fibrosis and collagen deposition) are seen.[13]

The wall of C. *immitis* contains the polysaccharides chitin, glucan, and mannosyl (proteins)[14]; these impart toughness to the exterior. During the growth of the spherule-endospore phase, enzymes, such as chitinase, glucanase, and proteases, likely participate in changing the cellular structure during the morphologic changes. With the maturation of the spherule and its release of endospores, chitinase is released.[15] This enzyme is the antigen to which the infected host responds by production of complement-fixing immunoglobulin G (IgG).[16]

Epidemiology and Epizootiology

C. *immitis* resides in soils of the Western Hemisphere and is present in North, Central, and South America (Fig. 47-3). The fungus is indigenous to California, Arizona, Utah, Nevada, New Mexico, Texas, and adjacent areas of Mexico.[1]

Persistence of this fungus in the soil and arrival of previously uninfected individuals (human and nonhuman) ensure continued occurrence of coccidioidomycosis. Many, but not all, of the areas to which the organism is endemic correspond to the Lower Sonoran Life Zone, characterized by hot, dry summers; relatively mild winters; and moderate rainfall. The number of cases of coccidioidomycosis is influenced by rainfall in at least two ways: (1) rainfall wetting the soil can reduce dust and airborne arthroconidia, suppressing the number of infections; or (2) rainfall, by moistening the soil, can lead to growth of the hyphal/arthroconidial form, increasing the subsequent risk of exposure to infectious arthroconidia and therefore more cases. In the late summer and in the fall, there is usually a progressive increase in the number of cases until the rainy season begins. In Arizona, a dry period is followed by summer "monsoon" rains, then followed by another dry season, resulting in essentially two annual seasons of coccidioidomycosis.

C. *immitis* does not appear uniformly distributed throughout endemic areas; rather, it exists in scattered pockets of soil. The characteristics of the soils have not provided a specific, clear reason for the restricted distribution and persistence of the organism. The soil often is alkaline, may contain ash from the ancient campsites of Native American Indians, and often contains concentrations of certain salts, such as calcium, sulfate, and sodium chloride, which can inhibit microorganisms that can compete with (or inhibit) *Coccidioides*. These competing organisms probably decrease as the soil water evaporates, increasing the concentrations of salt but still permitting survival of *Coccidioides*.

Recent genetic analyses that compared the two *Coccidioides* spp. to nonpathogenic and pathogenic relatives of the *Onygenales* found that *Coccidioides* diverged to acquire genes that indicate nutritional reliance on animal based (keratin-rich) protiens.[17] This finding may also explain the nonuniform geographic distribution since it was hypothesized that this divergence, from pure soil and plant-based saprophytic fungi that of acquire characteristics of true pathogens using animals and their carcasses, allowed a unique environmental niche for survival. Thus the indigenous sites where *Coccidioides* occurs may reflect the presence of degenerating mammalian carcasses that have provided a nutrient rich environment in addition to the physical soil conditions.

Annual human infection is not insubstantial due to *Coccidioides* spp., with approximately 15,000 cases now occurring in the United States annually.[18] Northern Mexico is reported to have the highest number of human cases; the overall prevalence of infection based on skin reactivity testing is between 10% and 40%.[18]

Equine cases of coccidioidomycosis have been reported mainly in the southwestern United States, although in some cases, equid acquisition of C. *immitis* may have occurred at a location remote from the home area. Indeed, horses not residing in coccidioidal areas may be exposed to products (e.g., alfalfa, grass hay) exported from endemic areas. For example, a man who resided in London was exposed when unpacking pottery from Arizona through finely shredded packing material,[19] and a man in North Carolina was exposed to C. *immitis*–contaminated cotton from California. Cases of coccidioidomycosis in horses are usually sporadic. However, a cluster of cases occurred at the same site in a compound holding several Przewalski's horses.[20] It was proposed that this herd of young males, intimidated by more dominant adult males, may have been stressed, increasing their susceptibility to develop clinically apparent coccidioidomycosis.

Transmission from one host to another does not ordinarily occur, except rarely from a mother to a fetus[21,22] or from an infected organ donor to organ recipient (see sections on Prevention and Public Health Considerations).

Pathogenesis

Inhaled arthroconidia can be deposited in large or small airways. The arthroconidia shed an outer wall layer that is antiphagocytic and, under the influence of leukocytes, increased CO_2, elevated (body) temperature, and surface-active agents, become rounded and enlarge to produce the spherule. Enzymes, such as serine and aspartyl proteases, urease, alkaline phosphatase, and chitinase, are released during the morphologic evolution of *Coccidioides*. At least some of these enzymes may contribute to the pathogenesis. Urease is reported to alkalinize the phagosome of leukocytes, thereby impairing phagocytic destruction of the fungus.[23] Proteinases may exert damaging effects on the host tissue components or leukocytes. Chitinase, a potent antigen,[15] may contribute to pathogenesis through formation of antigen-antibody complexes.[16]

The usual respiratory route of infection can lead to asymptomatic, subclinical infection (60% of infected people). The symptomatic infection (40% of infected people) can be variable. Most infected individuals recover after weeks to months. Complete recovery leads to immunity against a second "primary" (pulmonary) infection. From 5% to 10% of symptomatic human

patients will have a residual pulmonary lesion (e.g., cavity, solitary nodule). Approximately 5% to 7% of symptomatic patients have dissemination outside of the thorax; this is influenced by innate factors, including racial derivation, presence of certain human leukocyte antigen (HLA) tissue markers, and blood group B. Dissemination also is increased by certain acquired states: immunosuppression by human immunodeficiency virus (HIV) or medication for organ transplantation and by pregnancy.

Early infection is endobronchial or pneumonic, often accompanied by hilar lymphadenopathy. Extrathoracic dissemination can involve virtually any tissue or organ, an exception being the rare involvement of the mucosal surface of the alimentary tract or of the endocardium.

A broad range of animals (over 64 different species) have been infected with *Coccidioides*. The spectrum of the disease varies among and within species. Dogs appear to fit a clinical range similar to that of humans. Cattle and sheep, on the other hand, are resistant, rarely exhibiting illness despite coccidioidal lesions in the thoracic lymph nodes. The equids that have been infected included domestic and wild species (see Box 47-1).

Clinical Findings

In humans, most disease is subclinical with spontaneous recovery resulting in life-long immunity.[18] Multiple manifestations of coccidioidomycosis have been reported in horses, with a wide range of severity and effect on survival. Various anatomic sites are affected (Fig. 47-4). Once thought to be a universally devastating disease, some forms of coccidioidomycosis may now be amenable to successful treatment or even spontaneous recovery. As in other species, equine exposure usually occurs

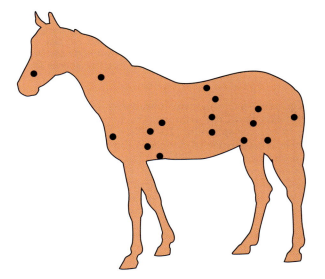

Cervical vertebrae	Pleura (effusion)
Nasal tissue	Tracheobronchial lymph nodes
Skin over xiphoid	Patella
Pectoral abscesses	Liver
Lung	Peritoneum (effusion)
Lumbar vertebrae	Mammary gland
Pelvis	Pericardium (effusion)
Hind limb muscle	Spleen
Placenta/uterus	Kidney
Fetus	Abdominal lymph nodes

Figure 47-4 Anatomic locations of coccidioidomycosis reported in the horse.

through inhalation of airborne arthroconidia. Because of this common exposure route, the disease often affects the respiratory tract; however, lymphohematogenous dissemination can occur, leading to foci of infection in various organs such as bone, skin, and abdominal viscera.[24,25] Rarely, inoculation occurs percutaneously, leading to localized subcutaneous infections.[26] The multiple clinical syndromes have been described as miliary or interstitial pneumonia[27-29] (Fig. 47-5), pneumonia with pleural effusion[24] (Fig. 47-6), osteomyelitis,[30,31] mastitis,[32] abortion,[21,22]

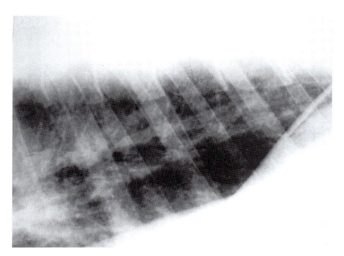

Figure 47-5 Radiograph showing multiple small nodular lesions in lung of horse with coccidioidomycosis.

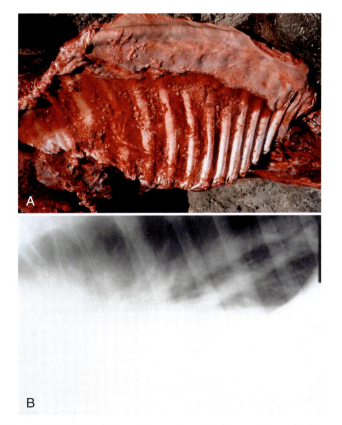

Figure 47-6 **A,** Parietal pleura with granulomata in horse with coccidioidomycosis. **B,** Radiograph indicating pleural effusion in horse with coccidioidomycosis. *(Courtesy Richard Mansmann, VMD, PhD.)*

and various sites of superficial or internal abscessation.[25] An obstructive nasal coccidioidal granuloma in an Arabian gelding was excised[33] and recurred 5 years later.[34]

Clinical signs vary with the form of disease; however, common signs include fever, significant weight loss, and current or historical respiratory signs (adventitial lung sounds, increased respiratory rate, coughing, evidence of pleural fluid). Other signs may reflect the specific organ system involved, including musculoskeletal pain with osteomyelitis, abortion with placental infection, colic and peritoneal effusion with abdominal involvement, or chronic draining tracts with peripheral lesions.

In horses with pulmonary coccidioidomycosis, thoracic ultrasound may identify "comet tail" artifacts consistent with pleural roughening, areas of pulmonary consolidation, and accumulations of pleural fluid. Common thoracic radiographic abnormalities include diffuse interstitial/miliary pattern (see Figs. 47-5 and 47-6) consistent with a granulomatous pneumonia, pleural fluid lines, dorsal displacement of large airways by hilar lymphadenopathy, and large mass lesions in the mediastinum or small focal abscesses throughout the lung field.[25,29]

Hematologic abnormalities in horses with coccidioidomycosis include an inflammatory leukogram with hyperfibrinogenemia, leukocytosis with mature neutrophilia and hyperglobulinemia, as well as mild anemia.[25]

A recent retrospective study showed different survival trends for different clinical syndromes.[29] For example, all six mares that aborted an infected fetus had a low serum coccidioidal IgG titer by quantitative immunodiffusion (≤ 8) and showed no signs of systemic infection. All survived, and one mare reportedly had several healthy foals subsequent to the abortion. Conversely, the disease in horses with massive dissemination or pneumonia with thoracic effusion (mean serum titer of 176 and 332, respectively) was overwhelmingly fatal (19/21) despite treatment in some cases. Serologic data have recently confirmed that subclinical infection with natural resolution occurs in horses living in endemic areas (previously associated also with positive skin tests[7]), further supporting the wide spectrum of infection and disease exhibited in horses.[35] Prognosis should be assessed individually for each horse on the basis of chronicity of infection, severity of clinical signs, organ systems involved, dynamics of titer over time, initial response to treatment, and immune status of patient.[29]

Some trends have been identified regarding the signalment of affected horses. They tend to be young to middle aged when presented, 6.3 years in one retrospective study[25] and 8.1 years in another.[29] Serologic data suggest that horses in endemic areas are exposed to the pathogen at a young age.[35] Older horses likely were previously exposed to the fungal pathogen and have overcome the infection. Those that develop clinically apparent disease will likely do so at the initial exposure. Coccidioidomycosis does not appear to be a disease of older or debilitated horses; this is similar to trends reported in dogs[36] and people[37] (mean age of 5 and 40.3 years, respectively). Females have been overrepresented (66%[29] and 76%[25]) among affected horses in both equine retrospective studies. Pregnancy has been postulated to have an effect on severity of clinical signs in mares, as it does in humans.[38] However, no conclusion has been made as to whether this contributes to the overrepresentation of clinical female equine patients. Arabians were significantly overrepresented as clinical patients in one retrospective study[25] and made up a high proportion of healthy horses carrying a positive titer.[35] However, numbers are still too small to ascribe a greater susceptibility to this breed. A seasonal trend has been identified, with 72% of clinical cases presenting from late fall into winter (October through March), possibly following exposure during the dry, dusty months of late summer and early fall.[29] Heightened awareness is appropriate for diagnosticians during this time of year.

Nondomestic horses display a range of clinical presentations. Although disseminated coccidioidomycosis was reported to have a high incidence in Przewalski's horses,[20] seropositive, apparently healthy Przewalski's horses have also been detected. A Grévy's zebra in southern California had disseminated coccidioidomycosis affecting the cervical vertebrae and internal organs.

Diagnosis and Pathologic Findings

Confirmation of coccidioidomycosis requires laboratory support. However, diagnosis depends on suspicion and awareness of the provenance (residence and travel) history of the horse, appreciation of the varied clinical patterns of disease, estimation of the time of onset of illness, and the usefulness of laboratory tests.

Direct demonstration of *Coccidioides* in tracheobronchial washings, exudates, or tissues, as stained by hematoxylin and eosin (H&E) and periodic acid–Schiff (PAS), Papanicolaou, or calcofluor white for detection of chitin in the fungal wall, can secure the diagnosis promptly (see Chapter 46). Potassium hydroxide digestion of host cell tissue components is withstood by the *C. immitis* cell. Detection of an unequivocal endosporulating spherule establishes the diagnosis. Usually the coccidioidal cells are visible in H&E-stained tissue (see Fig. 47-2), but cells can be sparse and are more readily visualized with PAS or methenamine silver stains that can detect the polysaccharides of fungal cell walls. Occasionally, clinicians may not observe the pathognomonic endosporulating spherules (20-100 μm in diameter) but will see immature spherules with rather thick, double-contour walls (15-50 μm) that can be confused with other fungi (e.g., *Blastomyces dermatitidis*).

Attempts to recover the fungus by culture should be made for confirmation of the diagnosis and should it become necessary during treatment, for the assay of the susceptibility to antifungal agents. Culture of infected tissues or exudates on conventional culture media (blood agar, Sabouraud glucose agar) or media containing cycloheximide (to inhibit nonpathogenic fungi) and chloramphenicol or other antibacterial antibiotics can enhance recovery of *Coccidioides*. Mycelial growth can become visible in 2 to 3 days and can yield a sufficient amount of the organism to permit application nucleic acid testing via either the Hybridization Protection Assay (Gen-Probe) for specific identification of ribonucleic acid (RNA) of a suspected *C. immitis* isolate or polymerase chain reaction (PCR) within hours. Inoculation of mice with the unknown culture usually requires growth of the organism for approximately 1 week to yield sufficient cells of the organism to replicate in the animal and to produce the characteristic endosporulating spherules.

Even while attempting to recover and identify the infecting organism, serum samples should be tested for antibody.[16] In general, a consistent, sequential serologic response occurs after infection with *Coccidioides*: early, there is an IgM response, and later, an IgG antibody response (IgA can also be detected, but its usefulness has not been clearly established). The IgM is produced in response to polysaccharide/peptide antigen, and the IgG is induced by chitinase (Fig. 47-7).

Various tests can be used to detect IgM, IgG, or both. Screening for antibody can be carried out by immunodiffusion (ID), enzyme immunoassay (EIA), or antigen-coated latex particle agglutination (LPA). The role of EIA or LPA in equine serology is unknown. Because of false-positive reactions for IgM by EIA or LPA, reactive sera should be tested for confirmation by ID (Table 47-1). Careful observation reveals that in ID, some equine sera produce a confusing line of reaction with human serum. Once a qualitative test is positive for coccidioidal

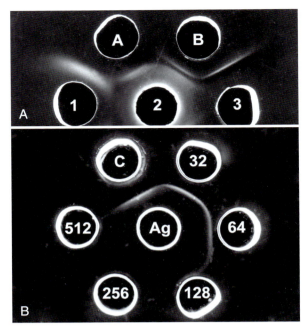

Figure 47-7 Immunodiffusion serologic test for coccidioidomycosis. **A,** Qualitative test with serum from horse with coccidioidomycosis in central well. Left well contains control human serum positive for immunoglobulin M (IgM). Right well contains control human serum positive for IgG. Left upper well contains coccidioidal antigen (heated) reactive with IgM. Right upper well contains coccidioidal antigen (unheated) reactive with both IgM and IgG. The equine serum was positive for both IgM and IgG. **B,** Quantitative test in which center well contains coccidioidal antigen. Left upper well contains control (human) serum positive for IgG. Right upper, right middle, right lower, and left lower wells contain equine pleural fluid diluted 1:32, 1:64, 1:128, and 1:256, respectively. The line of antigen-antibody precipitation indicates that the titer is 1:128.

Table 47-1 Current Application of Serologic Tests in Coccidioidomycosis

Test	Detection of IgM	Detection of IgG
Immunodiffusion (ID)	Yes	Yes
Enzyme immunoassay (EIA)	Yes*	Yes†
Complement fixation (CF)	No (rare‡)	Yes
Latex (antigen-coated) agglutination	Yes*	No

IgM, Immunoglobulin M; IgG, immunoglobulin G.

*These tests, intended for detection of IgM, have a substantial proportion of false-positive reactions.

†Occasionally, EIA positive for IgG has only IgM demonstrable by ID.

‡Rarely, serum positive by CF contains only IgM detectable by ID.

antibody, usually little is gained by repetition of the qualitative tests. However, because a recognized correlation exists between the titer (concentration) of IgG and the severity and extent of coccidioidal disease, quantitative serologic tests (complement fixation or quantitative ID) should be performed to obtain a titer of antibody.[29] By experience, titers greater than 1:16 have been associated with pulmonary and/or thoracic coccidioidomycosis.[29] Horses with localized involvement such as the mammary gland or with extrapulmonary lesions, such as kidney, bone, or other soft tissue such as skin, have demonstrated lower titers.[29] Testing sequential sera, initially at 1-month intervals (later at longer-spaced periods), permits comparison of titers. A rising or very high titer is usually indicative of worsening disease and poor prognosis, whereas a falling titer indicates improvement.[29] All serologic results must be interpreted with all clinical findings, including a pyogranulomatous process.

Presence of antibody in the serum of horses usually indicates past or current coccidioidomycosis.[16] In a recent study, in which healthy horses residing in a residential area and with no known history of disease were tested by serology, only 4% were positive.[35] However, the authors have recently detected coccidioidal antibody in the serum of a 2-day-old foal that did not have coccidioidomycosis, but the dam was known to be seropositive. Apparently, the antibody in the foal was derived from colostrum. In humans, transplacentally transferred antibody can be detected in newborn infants without coccidioidomycosis, but whose mothers had coccidioidomycosis.

Detection of coccidioidal antigen[39] or deoxyribonucleic acid (DNA)[40] may allow infection to be detected earlier than antibody, but these tests have not yet achieved full clinical utility. Direct amplification of *Coccidioides* spp. antemortem from clinical specimens has had mixed success. Both conventional and real-time PCR protocols have been described for diagnosis. In addition, protocols have been developed that differentiate *C. immitis* from *C. posadasii*.[40-42] These techniques have epidemiologic value, especially for determining the geographic range of these organisms because of their utility for testing soil.[43] In humans, PCR diagnostic techniques for pulmonary *Coccidioides* infection are reported to have a sensitivity of 75% and specificity of 99% with 60% and 90% positive and negative predictive values, respectively, compared to culture of specimens.[44,45] In one case report, PCR was successful in detecting the agent in 2/2 human cerebral spinal fluid (CSF) samples.[46] Little is published regarding the antemortem utility of PCR testing in horses, however, real-time PCR is available commercially for animals and can differentiate between *C. immitis* and *C. posadasii* (Pusterla N, personal communication). Testing thus far has successfully detected *Coccidioides* spp. infections in tissues, including lung, spleen, and placenta, and in clinical fluids consisting of pericardial effusion and CSF (Pusterla N, personal communication).

Therapy

Therapy of coccidioidomycosis can be conservative (supportive), surgical, medical, or a combination of medical/surgical modalities, depending on the extent of the disease and the intent of the owners. Coccidioidomycosis can be chronic, necessitating treatment lasting for months or years. Systemic antifungal therapy in horses is expanding as newer and generic agents have become available and financially feasible for many horse owners. Therapy that was considered cost prohibitive because of the price of drugs and duration of treatment is now considered a reasonable option.

The conservative approach may be attempted for mild forms of the disease (e.g., placentitis, abortion) or other forms that are accompanied by a low titer (<8) and mild clinical signs. A small proportion (4.1%) of healthy horses in endemic areas may carry a titer of up to 8 at a given time.[35] These horses are subclinically infected and may not require treatment. Because of the possibly devastating nature of disease; however, all cases should be monitored closely (clinically, serologically, and hematologically) to allow for early detection of disease progression and to institute antifungal therapy before disease has become too severe. In horses with a low titer, a decision for antifungal medical intervention should be based on hematologic evidence of inflammation, weight loss, clinical signs of active infection (e.g., fever), and a rising IgG titer over time.[35]

Surgical therapy can be applied to various tissues. If the disease is limited to peripheral and cutaneous tissues, excision could be curative. Limited osseous disease can be approached surgically, but this is appropriately carried out with accompanying systemic antifungal medication.

Medical therapy can include parenteral or oral medications. Currently, two main classes of antifungal medications are used to treat coccidioidomycosis: polyenes and azoles.

Amphotericin B (AMB) and its lipid formulations are administered parenterally, particularly by intravenous (IV) or intrathecal route. The polyenes interact adversely with ergosterol in the fungal cell membrane. The increased availability of azole antifungal agents has resulted in a decrease in the use of AMB both because of ease of administration and because of the nephrotoxic, hematopoietic toxic, and vasculopathic effects of AMB. In some cases, however, such as rapidly progressing coccidioidomycosis, AMB may remain the first-choice antifungal.

Ketoconazole and the triazoles itraconazole, fluconazole, and voriconazole are currently available to treat fungal infections. These drugs are usually administered orally, although some IV preparations are available. The azoles inhibit the synthesis of ergosterol, leading to faulty sterol in the fungal cell membrane. Toxicity of the azoles is relatively greater for fungal cells than for the mammalian cells. Oral ketoconazole is poorly absorbed in the horse[47] and usually requires co-administration of an acidifying agent to enhance alimentary absorption. Fluconazole and itraconazole are practical for long-term oral administration but with a possible side effect of dose-dependent hepatotoxicity. There is a report of successful treatment of coccidioidal osteomyelitis in a horse with oral itraconazole[31] and a recent report of two horses with pulmonary coccidioidomycosis treated successfully with fluconazole.[27] Fluconazole possesses a superb pharmacokinetic profile in horses, with a high oral bioavailability, a high volume of distribution, and a long elimination half-life.[48] Thus fluconazole should be considered as a favorable agent to treat equine coccidioidomycosis. Because of its long half-life, fluconazole may show a cumulative effect, and therefore therapeutic drug monitoring throughout the course of treatment is warranted to facilitate adjustment of the dose if necessary.[27] Periodic blood tests to monitor hepatic parameters is also recommended.

Previously reported dosing regimens for mycotic infections in the horse include fluconazole at a loading dose of 14 mg/kg orally (PO), followed by 5 mg/kg PO once daily[27,48]; itraconazole at 2.6 mg/kg PO twice daily[31]; and AMB intravenously daily or every other day to a cumulative dose of 12 mg/kg over 1 month[49] or a cumulative dose of 6.75 mg/kg over 5 weeks.[50]

Sufficient duration of treatment is often a dilemma when treating any horse with coccidioidomycosis. In the recent cases of pneumonia, discontinuation of treatment at 5 to 6 months was based on complete resolution of signs and hematologic abnormalities, as well as a decreasing IgG titer.[27] In both of these horses, clinical signs resolved within 2 weeks of initiation of treatment; however, chronic inflammation evidenced by leukocytosis and hyperfibrinogenemia persisted for 2 to 4 months after resolution of signs. Serial titers should be used to follow response during the course of treatment and for early detection of relapse in the posttreatment period.[16] Long-term, intermittent serologic testing of recovered horses may be indicated until their titers have become low, 1:2 to 1:4, but clinical assessment should be foremost.

Prevention and Public Health Considerations

Minimizing exposure to soil dust containing *C. immitis* in endemic areas may reduce the risk of infection. Efficacious experimental vaccines (thus far effective in mice and monkeys, but not in humans) may be forthcoming.[51,52]

Horses and other species acquire coccidioidal infections by inhalation of arthroconidia (rarely through the skin). Horse-to-horse and horse-to-human (or human-to-human) transmission, in general, does not occur. However, following a report of ultimately fatal coccidioidomycosis in a veterinarian who was present during a necropsy of a horse with disseminated coccidioidomycosis,[53] some owners and veterinary personnel became concerned that the disease might be acquired by proximity to an infected horse. (The veterinarian may have been exposed not only during the necropsy but also through contaminated artifacts, including the mane and tail of the index infected horse.) Natural transmission of the spherule/endospore phase (which would be the usual morphologic form expressed in the infected host) from host to host has not been demonstrated, except from infected organ donors to organ recipients.[54,55]

An interesting interhuman transmission of C. immitis (other than maternal to fetus) has been reported.[56] A patient with coccidioidal osteomyelitis of the right knee and left ankle underwent curettage and irrigation of the wounds. Plaster casts were applied to immobilize the limbs. Windows cut in the plaster casts permitted placement of dressings in the wound sites. Subsequently, several medical personnel, who were near or involved in removing dressings, developed coccidioidomycosis. The exudates from the infected limbs contaminated the plaster casts on which C. immitis grew in the hyphal/arthroconidial form and became aerosolized when the dressings were changed.

In the laboratory, infectious arthroconidia are produced in about 5 days. Therefore Coccidioides-containing body fluids,

exudates, or dressings used to cover lesions should be changed in less than 48 hours. Moistening dressings before removing them will help to minimize the risk of formation and aerosolization of the infectious arthroconidia. Contaminated dressings and body fluids should be treated with bleach disinfectant (0.5% sodium hypochlorite) for at least 30 minutes before discarding. The arthroconidia are also readily killed by heating at 60°C (140°F) for 30 minutes.

There is a theoretic risk that exudates (or an infected placenta) deposited in the soil of a corral or paddock could contaminate the soil with C. immitis. In an endemic area, however, infectivity of the environment already exists for the human owners and horses. If a horse has acquired the infection while in an endemic area but is then transported to a nonendemic area, it is unlikely that conditions would be suitable for the propagation of C. immitis in the soil in the new location.

In the performance of a necropsy on a horse with putative or proven coccidioidomycosis, it would be prudent to wear a gown, gloves, and a mask and to decontaminate the postmortem site with 0.5% sodium hypochlorite.

Acknowledgments

Spencer Jang, University of California, Davis, provided the discussion on histology.

The complete reference list is available online at www.expertconsult.com.

Sporotrichosis

48

Robert J. MacKay

Sporotrichosis is a chronic, progressive, lymphocutaneous infection of horses and other animals caused by members of the *Sporothrix schenckii* complex. The disease in horses and mules was first reported in 1909[1] and in donkeys in 1941.[2]

Significant genetic variability has been shown in S. schenckii by molecular analysis, suggesting that this fungus is not a single species but rather a group of cryptic species known collectively as the S. schenckii complex.[6]

Etiology

Sporothrix schenckii is a geophilic, dimorphic fungus, growing in a yeast form in tissue and in culture at 37°C (98.6°F) but as a filamentous fungus at 30°C (86°F).[3,4] The mycelial form has fine, septate, branching hyphae that carry perpendicular ovoid roseate conidia. The organism converts to the yeast form at 37°C when grown on rich media such as blood agar in 10% carbon dioxide. Yeast colonies are cream colored, moist, and smooth, whereas mycelial colonies are initially small, glabrous, and white-gray, then after 7 days are wrinkled and leathery with gray-to-black surface coloration.[5] *Sporothrix schenckii* is a common saprophyte of decaying plant material and hay but also can live on (but not parasitize) sphagnum moss and other living plants.

Epidemiology and Pathogenesis

Sporotrichosis is an uncommon disease of the horse, humans, and other animals.[7] The organism and disease occur worldwide but are more common in tropical, subtropical, and temperate climates than they are in cold climates.[3] Sporotrichosis in working horses in the United States during the early twentieth century occurred most commonly on newly deforested land in the catchment areas of rivers, with cases occurring progressively less frequently toward the river mouths.[8] Although 24, 11, and 36 cases were seen annually in northwest Pennsylvania in 1910, 1911, and 1912, respectively, there was never more than a single case on a property.[8] A rare departure from the typical sporadic nature of sporotrichosis is a large and continuing outbreak that began in Rio de Janeiro in 1998 and by 2004 had affected 1503 cats, 64 dogs, and 759 humans.[6] Cats with sporotrichosis have unusually large amounts of fungus in tissue exudates and are thought to have transmitted the infection to humans and dogs in the Rio outbreak via bite and scratch wounds.

Disease occurs when fungal mycelium is traumatically inoculated into the dermis and converts to the yeast morphotype.[6] Although infection can be passed between animals, Meyer[9] identified only two instances of likely horse-to-human transfer out of hundreds of cases examined. After 3 to 5 weeks,[3] the infection establishes in the skin and subcutis and can spread in lymphatics, expanding the infection to other parts of the skin, with resultant lymphangitis. Proximal lymph nodes may become involved in this manner, and rarely, the infection can be disseminated to other organs. Virulence factors are not well understood but reflect genetic variability among strains of *S. schenkii*.[9] Suspected virulence factors include thermotolerance in culture, capacity for melanin synthesis, potential for adhesion to tissue macromolecules, ergosterol peroxide production, and expression of virulence proteins.[9,10] Agglutinins to the yeast form are produced during infection and are detected in various diagnostic tests.[11]

Clinical Findings

Lesions most often begin on the distal limb, although the face, neck, or torso can also be the initial site of infection (Fig. 48-1).[4,5,11-14] There are single to multiple, firm, well-demarcated (0.5-5 cm in diameter), nonpruritic, nonpainful cutaneous nodules. Lesions enlarge slowly and usually ulcerate and drain a creamy red-brown to yellow purulent discharge. The infection may stay localized or spread along lymphatics (see Fig. 48-1). In cases involving the pelvic limbs, lesions typically extend from the distal limb to the region of the external inguinal lymph node.[5] The lymphatics appear corded and are interrupted by indurated nodules that ulcerate and drain. Linearly arranged lesions thus may have a "beads on a necklace" appearance. Cycles of healing and recurrence of lesions may continue for months or even years.

Diagnosis

The finding of ulcerative lymphangitis is highly suggestive of the diagnosis of sporotrichosis.[4] Other diagnostic considerations are undifferentiated bacterial lymphangitis, glanders/farcy *(Burkholderia mallei)*, epizootic lymphangitis *(Histoplasma farciminosum)*, ulcerative lymphangitis *(Corynebacterium pseudotuberculosis)*, and leishmaniasis. Strong supportive evidence for the diagnosis is the finding of characteristic budding, spheric to cigar-shaped yeast bodies in exudate, tissue fluid, or biopsies.[3,4,11] Organisms can be found either extracellularly or within neutrophils, macrophages, or multinucleate giant cells.

In horses, organisms are sparse, so diagnosis by cytology and histology may be difficult. Predigestion with diastase and staining with periodic acid–Schiff (PAS), Gomori's methenamine silver (GMS), Gridley's, or Giemsa stains or polyclonal anti-*Mycobacterium bovis* (BCG) antibody may improve sensitivity of these techniques.[5,6,9] Specific immunostaining of cytologic or histologic preparations allows differentiation of *S. schenckii* from other parasitic yeasts.[6] Definitive diagnosis is by culture of the organism on Sabouraud agar or equivalent at 30°C or room temperature.[3] Final identification of the organism requires demonstration of either mycelium-to-yeast conversion in culture or pathogenicity for mice.[15] A nested polymerase chain reaction (PCR) assay has been designed and validated for the detection of *S. schenckii* in clinical samples or cultures.[16] This assay targets the small-subunit ribosomal ribonucleic acid (RNA) gene and has a sensitivity of 40 fg of *S. schenckii* deoxyribonucleic acid (DNA).

A procedure used successfully for culture of *S. schenckii* from three horses and a donkey has recently been reported.[5] In brief, samples were inoculated onto and grown on sheep blood agar at 35°C to 37°C (95°F-98.6°F) for 1 week, inhibitory mold agar at 25°C to 30°C (77°F-86°F) for 3 weeks, and potato flake agar (PFA) at 25°C to 30°C for 1 week. Characteristic conidial morphology was identified in wet mounts of PFA colonies and dimorphism was confirmed by subculture on sheep blood agar.

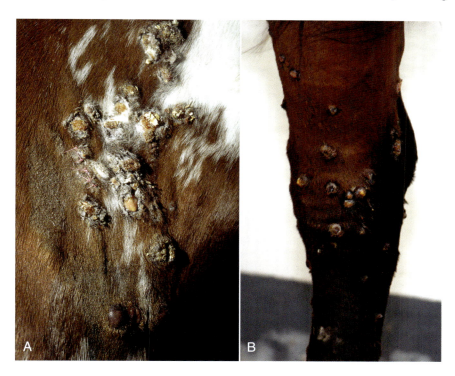

Figure 48-1 **A,** Typical subcutaneous nodules with ulceration and cording of lymphatics in shoulder of 16-year-old Paint Horse mare with sporotrichosis. **B,** Sporotrichosis on distal limb of horse. (**A,** *Courtesy Dr. Debra Sellon;* **B,** *courtesy Dr. Bonnie Rush.)*

Slide latex agglutination and tube agglutination tests for serum antibodies against *S. schenckii* are available. Titers greater than or equal to 8 are supportive of the diagnosis.

Therapy, Prognosis, and Prevention

Most cases of sporotrichosis will resolve spontaneously after very prolonged courses but may leave disfiguring scar tissue or in rare cases, disseminate to internal organs. Iodine is the traditional treatment of choice for equine sporotrichosis.[5,11-14] The mechanism of action is unknown but is presumed to involve enhancement of innate inflammatory responses. Regimens that have been used successfully in horses include sodium iodide (20-40 mg/kg intravenously [IV], daily as a 20% solution, then orally [PO] at the same dose), potassium iodide (10 mg/kg PO, once or twice daily) and ethylenediamine dihydriodide (1-2 mg/kg of the *active ingredient* given once to twice daily for the first week, then 0.5-1.0 mg/kg once daily).[4] Organic iodide is considered by some authors to be more effective than inorganic iodides. Lesions typically resolve over a period of weeks. To prevent relapses, it is recommended that treatment continue for 4 weeks beyond the resolution of clinical signs. Iodide should not be given to pregnant mares and should be discontinued in any horse with signs of iodism such as scaling and alopecia, fever, anorexia, coughing, lacrimation, nasal discharge, nervousness, or cardiovascular dysfunction.

The Clinical and Laboratory Standards Institute (CLSI) has standardized a microdilution assay for filamentous fungi to be used for determination of minimal inhibitory concentration (MIC) values for prospective antifungal agents.[17] Breakpoints proposed for *S. schenckii* on the basis of MIC results are *susceptible* (≤1 μg/mL), *intermediate* (2 μg/mL), and *resistant* (≥4 μg/mL). For at least the last decade, itraconazole has been the treatment of choice for human sporotrichosis.[6,9] A recent analysis of 16 different MIC studies confirmed the in vitro potency of this drug, with reported MICs for *S. schenckii* ranging from 0.03 to more than 16 μg/mL and geometric means from 0.4 to 4.08 μg/mL.[9] The surveyed strains of *S. schenckii* were also generally susceptible to amphotericin B and terbinafine, variably susceptible to voriconazole and micafungin, but almost uniformly resistant to fluconazole. This last result is surprising in light of the reported clinical effectiveness of fluconazole in dogs and cats with sporotrichosis.[5] Because generic itraconazole capsules are available in many parts of the world, it is now possible to treat a 500-kg horse at the recommended dose rate of 5 mg/kg orally once daily for less than $20 per day. In light of the fact that this dose rate only achieves reported mean maximal plasma concentration of 0.15 μg/mL in experimental horses,[18] it is not clear that itraconazole treatment of sporotrichosis would be more effective than traditional iodide therapy.

The prognosis for full recovery from sporotrichosis in otherwise healthy horses is good to excellent.

Because of the potential for transfer of infection to humans, gloves should be worn during handling of an infected horse.

Public Health Considerations

Sporothrix schenckii is pathogenic to humans, although horses are not considered a high-risk source of infection. Human disease is characterized by skin infections (rose handler's disease) and can rarely progress to lymphangitis or disseminated disease. This infection is especially dangerous for immunocompromised people, and laboratory infections have occurred, including infection by an equine isolate.[8,19]

The complete reference list is available online at www.expertconsult.com.

Candidiasis

Susan E. Barnett and Natalie Ann Carrillo*

49

Etiology

Members of the genus *Candida* are dimorphic fungi that belong to the family *Cryptococcaceae*; they are small (2-6 μm), thinwalled, ovoid yeasts that reproduce by asexual multilateral budding.[1,2] They are ubiquitous, are found on many plants, and are considered part of the normal flora of the alimentary tract, upper respiratory tract, and genital mucosa of mammals. *Candida* spp. are opportunistic pathogens, and *Candida albicans* is the most common species isolated from healthy and diseased people and animals (Fig. 49-1). Other common *Candida* spp. include *C. glabrata*, *C. parapsilosis*, *C. tropicalis*, and *C. krusei*.

*The authors acknowledge and appreciate the original contributions of these authors, whose work has been incorporated into this chapter.

Epidemiology

Candida is first acquired by neonates during passage through the birth canal, subsequently colonizing the mucosal and mucocutaneous surfaces of the gastrointestinal (GI), respiratory, and genitourinary tracts.[1] Opportunistic infections and life-threatening pathology can occur in neonatal and adult patients whose immune defenses have been altered by disease or various interventional strategies.[2]

Risk factors for candidiasis include prolonged broad-spectrum antibiotic therapy;[1,3-5] disruption of cutaneous or mucosal barriers by burns, surgery, cytotoxic agents, or trauma[1]; prolonged immunosuppression by disease states such as sepsis[5]; and administration of drugs such as glucocorticoids.[1,2,4] Other risk factors identified are low birth weight[5] (e.g., in premature foals), long-term placement of indwelling intravenous (IV) and urinary catheters,[1,3,5] long-term endotracheal tubes,[1,5] prolonged parenteral nutrition,[1,3,5] persistent neutropenia,[1,2] and severe primary immunodeficiency (e.g., agammaglobulinemia, selective immunoglobulin M [IgM] deficiency), and acquired immunodeficiency (e.g., failure of passive transfer).[6]

Pathogenesis

Under most circumstances, overgrowth of *Candida* spp. is inhibited by the normal microflora of the GI and respiratory tracts, genitalia, and skin. When the mammalian host is compromised by any of the previously mentioned risk factors, *Candida* can readily become pathogenic. Local proliferation in wounds or mucosal surfaces is often the first step in spread of infection.[1] The organism often invades through breaks in the skin or mucosa; electron microscopic studies have implicated mechanical and enzymatic factors in the invasion of the oral epithelium.[4]

Once in the body, circulating neutrophils appear to be an important determinant of further spread of candidal infec-

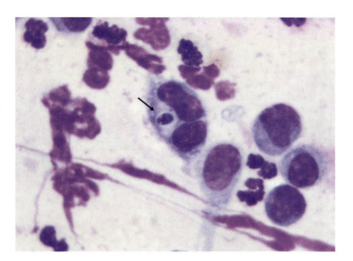

Figure 49-1 Binucleated, macrophage-engulfing yeast *(arrow)*, later identified as *Candida albicans*. Sample was taken from the left tibiotarsal joint of a neonatal foal. *(Courtesy Heather L. Wamsley, Department of Clinical Pathology, University of Florida, College of Veterinary Medicine.)*

tion.[1,2,4] Immunosuppressed patients and those with persistent neutropenia are at greater risk for developing candidiasis.

The microcirculation of tissues (e.g., lung, kidneys, joints, eyes, liver, brain, myocardium) acts to filter and clear the blood of pathogens. When systemic candidiasis is present, this activity results in embolic colonization and microabscess formation at these sites,[1] leading to the different presentations of candidal disease.

Candida albicans appears to have a number of virulence factors that promote successful parasitism such as rapid germination on seeding of tissue from the bloodstream, protease production to help invade tissues, surface integrin-like molecules for adhesion to extracellular matrix proteins, phenotypic switching and surface variation to avoid clearance by the immune system, and hydrophobicity.[2] *Candida* also has several mechanisms by which it can develop resistance to several antifungals, thereby increasing its pathogenicity.

Clinical Findings

Thrush

Thrush is a local overgrowth of *Candida* spp. in the oral mucosa and tongue that manifests as white plaques on these areas (Fig. 49-2). Oral colonization with infection is the most common presentation in immunosuppressed human patients, especially those with human immunodeficiency virus (HIV) infection.[7] This is likely the most common presentation in horses as well, although epidemiologic studies are lacking. Mucocutaneous forms of candidiasis such as thrush are often related to defects in cell-mediated immunity, whereas systemic spread is generally associated with neutropenia.[2] Oral candidiasis is a clear indication for initiation of antifungal therapy and pursuit of further diagnostic testing to determine systemic involvement.

Systemic Candidiasis

Clinical manifestations of systemic candidiasis are often nonspecific, with unresolved fever the only clinical sign in many cases.[8] Hematogenous candidiasis can occur after colonization of the oral mucosa or GI tract or can be acquired through the introduction of venous (and urinary) catheters. Administration of total parenteral nutrition is a risk factor for human patients, and this association appears likely in the foal.[1,3,5,7]

The hematogenous spread of *Candida* can lead to meningitis, omphalophlebitis,[5] pneumonia,[5,6] and arthritis.[3,5,6,9] Fungal

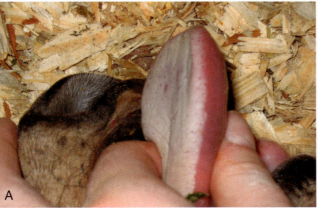
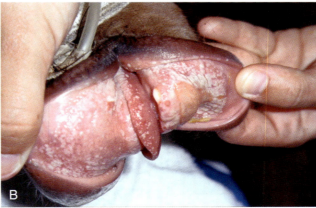

Figure 49-2 Foal with thrush. Note the white plaques on the tongue **(A)** and mucous membranes **(B)**. *(Courtesy Dr. Clare Ryan and Dr. Steeve Giguére, Department of Large Animal Clinical Sciences, University of Florida, College of Veterinary Medicine.)*

keratitis and panophthalmitis have been reported in a foal with systemic candidiasis.[5] In human patients, endophthalmitis is considered pathognomonic for systemic candidiasis.[10]

Septic arthritis caused by *Candida* spp. can present as two clinical syndromes: (1) an isolated monoarthritis caused by direct intraarticular inoculation of commensal fungi, by means of an injection, laceration, or during surgery[11] or (2) a monoarthritis or polyarthritis from hematogenously disseminated candidiasis.[9] In either case, treatment is difficult, and prognosis is guarded. Clinical signs of septic arthritis caused by *Candida* spp. are clinically indistinguishable from those of infectious arthritis caused by other, more common bacterial pathogens.[9,12] Affected animals present with synovial effusion with or without lameness and fever (Fig. 49-3). Nucleated cell counts in synovial fluid of human patients with *Candida* arthritis more often resemble noninfectious inflammatory arthritis than acute bacterial arthritis, and routine culture does not readily detect these organisms.[12]

The role of *Candida* spp. in the pathogenesis of gastric ulcers remains to be determined. In one study, however, *Candida* spp. colonized the keratinized layers of gastric mucosa surrounding ulcers in foals that died or were euthanized because of gastric rupture. This finding suggests that this pathogen plays a predisposing role in the pathogenesis of gastric ulcers in some foals.[4]

Fungal endometritis is present in 1% to 5% of mares diagnosed with endometritis.[13] Repeated iatrogenic invasion of the reproductive tract, decreased ability to clear fluid and organisms, pneumovagina, poor conformation, and administration of progesterone may be involved in the pathogenesis. Because yeasts are considered commensal organisms of the urogenital tract, the presence of *Candida* is insufficient to support a diagnosis of fungal endometritis. Concurrent evidence of an inflammatory response must be obtained on cytology or biopsy.[13] *Candida albicans* vulvovaginitis has also been reported following progestogen treatment in mares.[14]

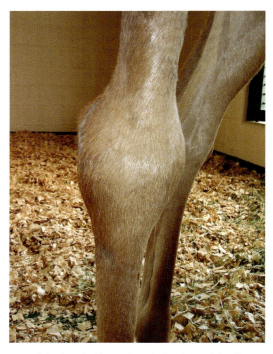

Figure 49-3 Left hock with effusion from foal with *Candida albicans* arthritis. *(Courtesy Dr. Steeve Giguére, Department of Large Animal Clinical Sciences, University of Florida, College of Veterinary Medicine.)*

Diagnosis

A diagnosis of candidiasis is supported by isolation of the organism from appropriate clinical samples such as blood cultures, synovial fluid, surgically resected umbilical structures, and cerebrospinal fluid (CSF). Caution must be exercised when *Candida* spp. are isolated from transtracheal washes and uterine biopsies because of the commensal nature of these organisms in the more external portions of the respiratory and urogenital tracts, respectively.

Therapy

Antifungal Therapy

Polyenes

Amphotericin B is an antifungal agent produced by *Streptomyces nodosus*. This drug targets the membrane of the fungal cell by binding to ergosterol (principal sterol in cell membrane), increasing membrane permeability, allowing leakage of intracellular contents, and causing cell death. The in vitro spectrum of activity includes *C. albicans*, *Mucor* spp., and *Aspergillus fumigatus*. Other *Candida* spp., *Fusarium*, and other *Aspergillus* spp. are resistant to amphotericin B.[8] Amphotericin B deoxycholate has been available for more than 40 years, but its clinical usefulness is limited by nephrotoxicity and infusion-related toxic effects. The agent binds to sterols on the cholesterol-rich lysosomal membranes of the distal renal tubular cells, with resultant increased cell permeability and cell death. Infusion-related toxic signs in horses include anorexia, dysrhythmias, anemia, fever, hypersensitivity reactions,[15] and thrombophlebitis.[11] Dose reduction to ameliorate adverse effects can lead to treatment failure.[8] The dose recommended for treatment of adult horses and foals is 0.1 to 0.6 mg/kg administered in a 5% dextrose solution IV over 30 minutes, 1 to 3 times per week.[15] One report described daily administration of 0.1 mg/kg for 30 days to an adult horse without serious side effects.[16]

Amphotericin B is also available in several lipid-based formulations, including amphotericin B lipid complex (ABLC), amphotericin B colloidal dispersion (ABCD), and liposomal amphotericin B (L-AB). These formulations are less nephrotoxic and are associated with fewer infusion-related toxic events.[8] No information is currently available regarding their use in horses.

Azoles

Azole antifungal agents target the membrane of the fungal cell by inhibiting cytochrome P-450 enzymes necessary for the biosynthesis of ergosterol, a main component of the fungal cell membrane structure.[8] Ketoconazole was the first available azole antifungal agent. Oral bioavailability in the horse is poor but can be increased to approximately 23% when the drug is acidified with hydrochloride (HCl).[17]

Fluconazole is active against *Candida* spp. and *Cryptococcus*, but molds such as *Aspergillus* and dimorphic fungi, such as *Histoplasma* and *Blastomyces*, are usually resistant. The pharmacokinetics for fluconazole outlined in the horse demonstrate that it is well absorbed after oral administration and distributes well into CSF, synovial fluid, aqueous humor, and urine, obtaining concentrations similar to those found in serum.[18] A loading dose of 14 mg/kg orally (PO) is recommended, followed by 5 mg/kg every 24 hours (q24h).[19] Fluconazole is considered the drug of choice for treatment of equine candidiasis, but some strains of *C. albicans* and many other *Candida* spp. may be resistant to fluconazole in human patients.[7,8,19]

Itraconazole has been reported as successful for treatment of several horses at a dose of 3 mg/kg for mycotic rhinitis caused by *Aspergillus* spp. and *Conidiobolus.*[20] The suspension appears to be better absorbed than the capsule form of itraconazole, and a dose of 5 mg/kg PO q24h has been suggested.[21] Itraconazole has been successfully used in combination with dimethylsulfoxide (DMSO) to treat fungal keratitis, but even in this combination does not reach measureable concentrations in the aqueous humor.[21,22] Local treatment of keratitis with chelating agents enhances in vitro sensitivity of itraconazole against *C. albicans.*[23]

The triazole antifungal agent voriconazole is effective against both yeasts and molds[8] in human patients, and in horses, voriconazole demonstrates excellent oral bioavailability and safety. Although fungicidal against many organisms, it is fungistatic against *C. albicans.* Cerebrospinal fluid concentrations are reportedly approximately 30% to 50% of plasma concentrations.[24] A suggested dose in adult horses is 3 mg/kg PO q12h,[24] although a dose of 10 mg/kg PO q24h has been reported and used in a foal with apparent safety.[25,26]

Other antifungal agents, such as posaconazole and micafugin, have been studied in humans and mice and as yet have not been investigated in horses.[27,28]

Topical Therapy

In the treatment of oral candidiasis, which occurs commonly in human denture-wearers and immunocompromised individuals, oral rinses are frequently employed. Chlorhexidine rinses (0.12-0.2% chlorhexidine gluconate, 30-60 second rinse twice daily) appear to be effective in reducing *Candida* colonization of the oral cavity and may be considered as adjunctive treatment for cases of thrush.[29]

Supportive Therapy

In addition to targeted antifungal therapy, affected foals and adult horses should receive appropriate supportive therapy. Treatment of septic arthritis caused by *Candida* spp. must be aggressive and should include successive joint lavages with at least one arthroscopic flush to facilitate physical removal of accumulated fibrin. This fibrin will hide and harbor the organism and potentially perpetuate the infection.

The complete reference list is available online at www.expertconsult.com.

50 Dermatophytosis

Rosanna Marsella

Dermatophytosis (ringworm) is a superficial cutaneous fungal infection caused by keratinophilic fungi that are able to invade the stratum corneum of the skin, the hairs, and other keratinized structures. Several dermatophytes are reported to induce cutaneous disease in horses. Clinically, dermatophytosis induces folliculitis and presents as a crusting and scaling disease, similar to bacterial folliculitis.

Etiology

Trichophyton equinum is the most common causative agent of dermatophytosis of horses.[1,2] Two varieties of *T. equinum* have been reported, *T. equinum* var. *equinum* and *T. equinum* var. *autotrophicum.* Other, less common agents are *Trichophyton verrucosum, T. mentagrophytes, Microsporum equinum, M. canis, M. gypseum,* and *T. bullosum.*[3-5] In one study, *T. equinum* var. *autotrophicum, M. canis,* and *M. equinum* were reported to be restricted to racing horses only, whereas *M. gypseum* occurred in racing, riding, and breeding horses.[6]

Epidemiology

Dermatophytes are highly contagious. Transmission occurs by either direct contact between horses or through contact with contaminated equipment. Infection can be readily transmitted, particularly by infected saddle-girths, on which the fungus can survive for 12 months.[7] Insects are also reported to play a role in the transmission of disease.[8,9] The source of infection varies, depending on the dermatophyte. Some dermatophytes are zoophilic, and the source of infection may be another infected animal such as a horse (e.g., *T. equinum*), a cat (e.g., *M. canis*), cattle (e.g., *T. verrucosum*), or a rodent (e.g., *T. mentagrophytes*). Other dermatophytes are geophilic (e.g., *M. gypseum*), and the source of infection is infected soil. Exposure to dermatophytes does not always lead to the establishment of the infection. Some individuals appear to be more predisposed than others, possibly related to the type of immune response mounted by the individual (see section on Pathogenesis).

The prevalence of ringworm varies greatly, depending on geographic location and husbandry conditions. In one epidemiologic study conducted in Egypt, 42% of horses with skin disease were positive for dermatophytes.[10] Horses less than 2 years old were more susceptible to infection. Fourteen species belonging to nine genera of keratinophilic and cycloheximide-resistant fungi were recovered from collected specimens. Trichophyton was the dominant genus, and *T. equinum* was the most frequently identified dermatophyte.

In a study of 200 horses in Italy, only 9% of horses were positive for *T. equinum.*[11] Although the clinical diagnosis of ringworm is quite common, many cases that clinically resemble ringworm may be bacterial folliculitis. At the University of Florida, only 5% of all the horses with skin disease that have cultures for dermatophytes are confirmed to have ringworm. The majority of horses that clinically appear to have ringworm are instead diagnosed with bacterial infections, either *Staphylococcus* or *Dermatophilus* spp.

Pathogenesis

Exposure to dermatophytes does not always result in clinical disease in horses. The outcome after exposure depends on the virulence of the dermatophyte, the conditions of the skin, environmental conditions, and the immune status of the host.

Virulence Factors

Dermatophytes produce enzymes such as keratinases that enable invasion of the hair and the stratum corneum and facilitate establishment of infection.[12,13] *Trichophyton equinum* produces urease, gelatinase, protease, hemolysins, and keratinase.[14] Some differences in enzyme production have been found between *T. equinum* and *T. mentagrophytes*. *Trichophyton mentagrophytes* may have stronger enzymatic properties, which clinically lead to more inflammatory reactions. Hemolytic activity and the ability to induce hypersensitivity reactions are also important virulence factors, especially for *Trichophyton* spp.[15,16]

Host Factors and Immune Response

The conditions of the skin and immune system of the host play a crucial role in determining whether infection is established and how readily it is eliminated. Any impairment of the barrier function of the skin may foster establishment of infection. In particular, abrasions can facilitate the development of lesions and prolong the recovery period; abrasions are an important risk factor for infections in the girth area.[6,7] Allergic individuals appear to be at increased risk, possibly a result of the self-trauma caused by the underlying allergy, as well as other immunologic factors such as their propensity to build a humoral response rather than a more protective cell-mediated response.

Young horses (<3 years of age) are at increased risk for developing dermatophytosis.[6,7] Stress, such as training, also predisposes to the development of ringworm. In one study, 32% of horses in training were clinically affected, whereas only 1.1% of breeding horses were affected with pathogenic dermatophytes.[6] Concurrent diseases that may compromise the immune response can predispose to the development of dermatophytosis.[17]

Immunity is acquired by active infection. Both nonspecific and specific immune responses are important for clearing dermatophyte infections. Serum inhibitory factors deprive dermatophytes of iron, which is an essential nutrient. Both humoral and cell-mediated immune responses are elicited, but cell-mediated immunity appears to be most important for resolution of infection.[18,19] The development of cell-mediated immunity correlates with the development of an inflammatory response and is associated with clinical cure, whereas the lack of or a defective cell-mediated immunity predisposes the host to chronic or recurrent dermatophyte infection.[20] The inflammatory reaction also promotes keratinocyte proliferation, which facilitates the elimination of the fungus from the skin surface.

Horses that self-clear dermatophyte infections develop immunity and rarely experience recurrence of infection. Some horses because of either a defective immune response or a concurrent illness fail to develop long-term immunity and are prone to recurrent infection, unless the dermatophyte is completely eliminated from their environment.

Environmental Factors

Environmental conditions, such as high temperature, humidity, and insect exposure, also play a role in pathogenesis of dermatophytosis.[15,21] Interestingly, bedding and hygiene do not correlate with dermatophytic infections of the hooves.[22]

Clinical Findings

Primary lesions of dermatophytosis consist of follicular papules and pustules. Individual lesions may present as spreading circular patches of alopecia (Figs. 50-1 and 50-2), surrounded by erythema and scaling (epidermal collarettes). Urticaria-like lesions can be observed in early stages of the disease. As the infection progresses, crusting and scaling (seborrhea) develop. Pruritus is usually absent but may be present in some cases. Hair is epilated easily in affected areas. In some horses, nodular lesions can develop as the result of ruptured follicles (furunculosis), which elicits a strong inflammatory response, intense erythema, and suppurative exudate.

The most frequently affected sites are the girth and the shoulder area, usually from use of contaminated equipment. A

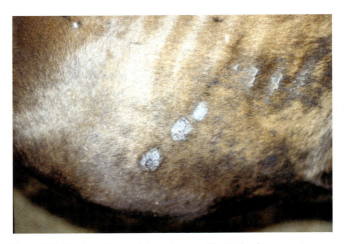

Figure 50-1 Circular patches of alopecia caused by Trichophyton equinum on shoulder of horse. In this case, pruritus was present and lesions were excoriated.

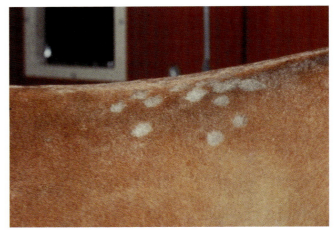

Figure 50-2 Circular patches of alopecia on back of horse, most likely caused by contaminated saddle pad. Lesions showed minimal inflammation. No pruritus was present.

survey of 568 horses in training and 2535 horses on breeding farms showed that the majority of lesions on racing horses were located on the girth areas.[6] Other frequently affected areas are the muzzle and the pastern region.

Dermatophytosis is overdiagnosed when only clinical signs are used to make the diagnosis.

Diagnosis

Diagnosis of dermatophytes should be based on positive culture followed by identification of the dermatophytes.

Wood's Lamp

Examination with a Wood's lamp is commonly used but not recommended as a diagnostic tool for equine dermatophytosis because only a few strains of dermatophytes show positive fluorescence. Positive fluorescence is indicated by apple green color on the hairs themselves. This finding is not very common. To complicate the assessment, topical therapy may cause false-positive reactions. Since most cases have been treated topically, false results are frequently seen (e.g., blue fluorescence on scales).

Direct Examination of Hair

Arthrospores can be detected by direct examination of hair. This test requires experience and is time-consuming. Positive results have been reported in approximately half of affected horses; therefore direct examination is not considered a sensitive diagnostic test.[25]

Culture

Fungal culture is the most reliable diagnostic test for dermatophytosis and should be used in cases in which bacterial folliculitis has been ruled out. The area should be gently swabbed with alcohol to decrease contamination by saprophytic fungi. After the alcohol has evaporated, hairs should be plucked, ensuring that the roots are included. Dermatophyte test medium (DTM)

is often used, although demonstrated to be inferior to Sabouraud dextrose agar.[26] It is important to note that *T. verrucosum* may not grow on DTM, requiring Sabouraud dextrose agar for a positive diagnosis.[27] At the optimum incubation temperature of 27° C (80.6° F), a color change to red can be observed in DTM only a few days after inoculation with infected hairs (Fig. 50-3). This color change requires approximately 3 days with *M. canis*–infected hairs, 4 days with *T. equinum*, and 5 days with *T. mentagrophytes*.[28] It is important that the growth of the colony and the change of the color of the media occur at the same time to be a positive culture. Other fungi can induce a color change, but it typically takes a longer time than the time required by a dermatophyte. Once the colony growth is observed, identification should be done to confirm the diagnosis and identify the source of infection.

Dermatophytes are positively identified by morphologic and biochemical characteristics.[29,30] *Trichophyton equinum* is identified by its morphology, dependency on nicotinic acid, hair perforation, and enzyme production. The type of culture medium influences growth and appearance of the *T. equinum* colonies. On solid Sabouraud agar, two types of colonies may be observed. Colonies with characteristic radial folds and grooves in the paracentral zone and umbilical elevation in the center are the most common. Typical features of *T. equinum* include dark-red pigmentation of the reverse side of the colony in the culture on solid Sabouraud medium with glucose and yellow-orange pigmentation on the same medium with no glucose.[31] Importantly, *T. equinum* strains cannot grow in the absence of vitamins, whereas they reveal rapid growth when nicotinic acid is added.[32] Most of the organic nitrogen sources are stimulatory for spore germination, which occurs within 24 hours.[33] Isolates of *M. equinum* produce typical macroconidia, are negative in the hair perforation test in vitro, and are urease positive.[34]

It is important to note that false-positive results with DTM can also occur. In specimens obtained from horses, a high contamination rate (36%), mostly from molds, was found with a cycloheximide-supplemented medium, making the examination of these cultures for the growth of dermatophytes impossible.[35] For this reason, it is important to use alcohol before plucking hairs to submit for culture. Also, it is important to realize that some animals may be carriers of dermatophyte organisms without associated clinical signs. Culture results

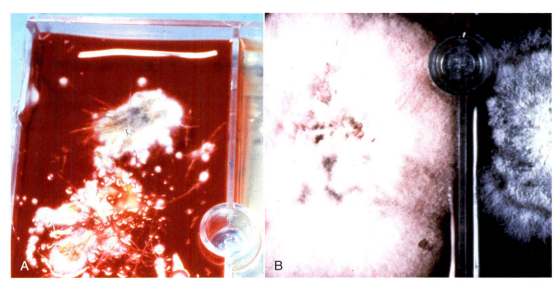

Figure 50-3 A, Dermatophyte test medium (DTM) plate demonstrating red color change in conjunction with growth of Trichophyton. **B,** Nondermatophyte fungal growth on DTM agar.

should always be interpreted in conjunction with history and clinical signs.

Differential diagnoses should include other, more common causes of folliculitis such as bacterial infections (e.g., staphylococcal pyoderma, dermatophilosis). Therefore cytology should be done in all suspected cases. Cytology allows assessment for the presence of bacteria and yeast and diagnosis of secondary bacterial infections. Although not as common, parasitic diseases should also be considered. Skin scraping should be performed in all cases. Although a negative scraping does not always rule out the possibility of parasitic infections, it may provide information regarding the presence of *Demodex* and other mites.

Other diseases that may present with crusting and scaling include contact allergy, sarcoids, and autoimmune diseases such as pemphigus foliaceus or systemic lupus erythematosus.[23] Importantly, acantholytic cells can be found on cytology in horses with dermatophytosis.[24] This is caused by the severe inflammatory response triggered by dermatophytes and the release of enzymes that may break desmosomal attachments between keratinocytes. Therefore the identification of acantholytic cells on cytology should not be considered pathognomonic for pemphigus foliaceus, and a definitive diagnosis should be made only after histopathologic evaluation. This is particularly important because the therapy for pemphigus foliaceus (e.g., glucocorticoids) would be highly contraindicated in horses with dermatophytosis. In older horses, neoplastic diseases, such as mycosis fungoides, should also be considered as differential diagnoses for patches of alopecia and scaling. In these cases as well, biopsies are necessary for a definitive diagnosis.

Pathology

Biopsy findings consistent with a diagnosis of dermatophytosis include luminal folliculitis and pyogranulomatous furunculosis. Biopsy can be helpful in cases when the culture results are equivocal. The presence of follicular arthrospores in conjunction with an inflammatory reaction is proof of clinically relevant infection. Superficial perivascular dermatitis with neutrophilic exocytosis and pustule formation is also often present. Palisading crusts are similar to those observed with dermatophilosis. As previously mentioned, acantholysis can be observed in some cases.

Therapy

Because most horses spontaneously resolve dermatophyte infections, many treatments have been advertised as a "cure" for dermatophytosis. Very few controlled studies have been performed to assess scientifically the efficacy of these therapies. As a general rule, therapy is aimed at reducing contagion to the environment and facilitating the resolution of lesions, usually with topical therapy.

Topical Therapy

Topical therapy should be considered for all horses with dermatophytosis.[36,37] A variety of such treatments have been recommended. Currently, one of the most frequently used treatments in clinical practice is 2% lime sulfur (LymDyp, Teva Animal Health, Saint Joseph, MO).[38,39] Disadvantages of this treatment include the smell and the temporary yellow discoloration of white areas. Lime sulfur can also permanently damage jewelry and clothes. Rinses of 0.2% enilconazole,

although not approved for use in horses, are reported to be effective for treatment of equine dermatophytosis when used once or twice weekly.[40] Shampoos are less desirable than rinses because of the lack of residual activity. Commonly used ingredients for "antifungal" shampoos include miconazole, ketoconazole, and chlorhexidine (e.g., Nizoral, [McNeil Consumer Healthcare, Fort Washington, PA] KetoChlor, Virbac, Fort Worth, TX). No controlled studies have evaluated the efficacy of these products in equine dermatophytosis.

All animals in contact with horses with dermatophytosis should receive topical therapy because they may be carriers without any evidence of cutaneous lesions. Treatment of large numbers of horses should be primarily aimed at reducing the spread of infection. In clinically affected horses, hair regrowth should not be used as an indication of cure because regrowth can occur while animals remain infected. It is therefore important to reculture the animal and demonstrate a lack of dermatophyte growth. Horses with low numbers of arthrospores on their coat may fluctuate between positive and negative cultures, so three consecutive negative cultures at 2-week intervals are recommended for confirmation.

Systemic Therapy

Although various dosages of griseofulvin have been recommended for the treatment of equine dermatophytosis, no published studies support this drug's efficacy and appropriate dose. Similarly, there are no studies on the pharmacokinetics and efficacy of other systemic antifungal treatments (e.g., ketoconazole, itraconazole, fluconazole, terbinafine). The lack of information together with the cost of treatment prevents the recommendation of these therapies.

Environmental Control

Environmental control relies mostly on the use of diluted bleach (1:40) and elimination of infected tack. An enilconazole-based product (Clinafarm EC) available for use in poultry hatchery facilities may be considered for use in highly contaminated barns, although it is not specifically approved for this use. All animals must be evacuated during treatment.

Prevention

Vaccine

Vaccines have been used in the past in small and large animals to manage endemic dermatophytosis.[41-43] Immunity obtained after vaccination appears to be cross-reactive.[44] Currently, however, there are no commercially available vaccines for prevention of equine dermatophytosis in the United States.

Public Health Considerations

Equine dermatophytosis can be contagious to humans, as documented by several case reports.[45-47] Infection is caused by direct contact with affected horses, including bareback riding.[48] Infections in humans are either self-limiting or responsive to antifungal treatment.[49]

The complete reference list is available online at www.expertconsult.com.

51 Pythiosis and Zygomycosis

Amy M. Grooters

Although the oomycete *Pythium insidiosum* and the zygomycetes *Conidiobolus* spp. and *Basidiobolus ranarum* fall into two taxonomically distant groups of organisms, they are typically grouped together by equine clinicians and pathologists because they share similar clinical and histologic characteristics. Both cause cutaneous lesions characterized by pyogranulomatous and eosinophilic inflammation associated with broad, sparsely septate hyphae. Because of these similarities, pythiosis and zygomycosis have been referred to collectively as "phycomycosis." Despite remaining a convenient label for cases without a definitive, culture-based diagnosis, "phycomycosis" is no longer an appropriate taxonomic designation and should be replaced in current literature with the more specific terms *pythiosis* and *zygomycosis*. Clinically, differentiating between these infections is important because of differences in epidemiology, choice of therapy, and prognosis.

Pythiosis

Pythiosis, a pseudofungal infection caused by the oomycotic pathogen *Pythium insidiosum*, is best known as a cause of cutaneous and subcutaneous disease in horses[1] and of gastrointestinal (GI) or cutaneous disease in dogs.[2] It has also been described as an uncommon cause of cutaneous and subcutaneous lesions in cats and calves[3,4] and of arteritis, keratitis, or periorbital cellulitis in humans.[5,6] In older literature, *P. insidiosum* has been referred to using the now-outdated synonyms *Hyphomyces destruens*,[7] *Pythium destruens*,[8] *Pythium* spp.,[9] and *Pythium gracile*.[10]

Clinical manifestations of pythiosis have been recognized in horses for more than a century and variably referred to as "kunkers," "Florida horse leeches," "bursatti," and "swamp cancer," as well as "phycomycosis." The disease was first noted in the mid-nineteenth century when British veterinarians working with horses in India observed a chronic granulomatous cutaneous disease that they termed *bursautee*. A fungal etiology for this disease was suspected on the basis of histologic findings in the late nineteenth century,[11] and the pathogen was isolated as early as 1901 by Dutch investigators working with horses in Indonesia.[12] However, it could not be induced to sporulate using standard fungal media and was thus assumed to be a sterile zygomycete or "phycomycete" fungus based on the morphologic characteristics of its vegetative hyphae. It was not until 1974 that Austwick and Copland[13] were able to produce biflagellate zoospores from isolates obtained from horses in New Guinea, identifying the pathogen as an oomycete that was likely a member of the genus *Pythium*. The species name *Pythium insidiosum* was introduced in 1987 by De Cock,[14] who was able to produce sexual reproductive structures from pathogenic isolates and who found the morphologic characteristics of several isolates from horses and dogs to be identical.

Etiology and Epidemiology

The causative agent of pythiosis is the aquatic oomycete *P. insidiosum*, a member of the kingdom Stramenopila that is more closely related to algae than to true fungi.[15] The taxonomic differences between oomycetes and fungi are reflected on the cellular level by differences in cell membrane and cell wall composition. Ergosterol, an essential component of the fungal cell membrane and a common target of antifungal drugs, is not a principal sterol in the oomycete cell membrane.[16] In addition, oomycetes generally lack chitin, which is an important structural component of the fungal cell well.

The infective stage of *P. insidiosum* is thought to be the biflagellate zoospore, which is released into warm-water environments and swims in a helical pattern as part of a complex homing sequence that allows it to locate, move toward, and encyst on specific host tissues.[17] *Pythium insidiosum* zoospores are attracted to animal hair, as well as to cut edges of skin, and likely cause infection by encysting in damaged skin or GI mucosa.[18] Although many infected horses have a history of recurrent exposure to standing fresh water,[19,20] other risk factors for the development of pythiosis have not been identified. Affected animals are immunocompetent and otherwise healthy. Given the affinity of *P. insidiosum* zoospores for damaged skin, it seems likely that animals with cutaneous wounds or parasite-induced injury to GI mucosa would be more likely to become infected. However, documented epidemiologic evidence to support this assumption is lacking. The presence of a traumatic wound before the development of cutaneous pythiosis has been reported in a small number of canine and equine cases. Because traumatic incidents are rarely observed by the owner, however, it is often difficult to determine whether lesions noted early in the course of disease resulted from trauma or from early infection.

In the United States, pythiosis is encountered most often in the Gulf Coast states but has been recognized in animals living as far north as New Jersey, Virginia, North Carolina, southern Illinois, southern Indiana, and Kentucky and as far west as Oklahoma, Missouri, and Kansas. Although GI pythiosis has recently been documented in dogs living in Arizona and northern California, no reports of equine pythiosis have been made from these regions to date. Globally, pythiosis is most often encountered in Southeast Asia (especially Thailand and Indonesia), eastern coastal Australia, New Zealand, and South America (especially Brazil and Costa Rica), but it has also been recognized in Korea, Japan, and the Caribbean (Haiti).

Clinical Findings

Pythium insidiosum infection in horses most often causes large, ulcerative, proliferative granulomatous lesions involving cutaneous or subcutaneous tissues of the distal limbs (generally below the knee and hock), ventral abdomen (Fig. 51-1), ventral thorax,

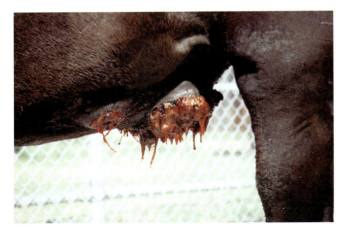

Figure 51-1 Large, ulcerative, draining granulomatous lesion caused by *Pythium insidiosum* infection on ventrum of mare. Note the presence of a stringy, viscous fluid hanging in strands from the surface of the lesion.

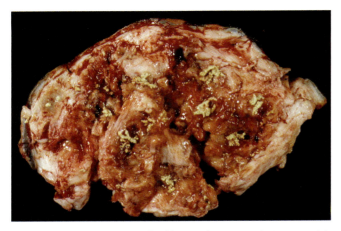

Figure 51-2 Necropsy photograph of large subcutaneous lesion caused by *Pythium insidiosum* infection in horse. Note the presence of multiple, tan to yellow, branching, coral-like masses, commonly referred to as "kunkers." *(Courtesy Dr. Corrie Brown, University of Georgia.)*

or face.[1,7,21,22] Less frequently affected areas include the dorsum and external genitalia.[20] Solitary lesions are most common,[21] but multiple lesions have been reported.[7,20,21,23] Intense pruritus is typically associated with cutaneous pythiosis and often results in self-mutilation of the affected tissues. Lesions typically appear as circular masses that are rapidly expanding, ulcerative, and necrotic and that contain multiple fistulous tracts that drain a serosanguineous, hemorrhagic, or mucopurulent fluid.[1] In addition, a characteristically stringy, viscous fluid may be observed hanging in strands from ventral abdominal lesions (see Fig. 51-1) or matting the hair around extremity lesions.

Sinus tracts in *P. insidiosum* lesions contain multiple, 1-mm to 10-mm, tan to yellow, branching, coral-like firm masses or coagula that are commonly referred to as "kunkers" or "leeches" (Fig. 51-2). Histologically, these kunkers are composed of hyphae, inflammatory cells (especially eosinophils), collagen, and necrotic debris, and they are especially prevalent deep to the junction of the ulcerated portion of the lesion and the intact epidermis.[24] Kunkers are often extruded from draining tracts and may be found in bandage material. Other diseases that can cause similar cutaneous lesions in horses include cutaneous habronemiasis; excessive granulation tissue; bacterial

granulomas; sarcoid, squamous cell carcinoma; and zygomycosis. Both habronemiasis and zygomycosis can produce tissue grains, but in habronemiasis, they are usually smaller and lack the typical coral-like shape of kunkers associated with pythiosis.[24,25]

Although most *P. insidiosum* lesions are confined to cutaneous and subcutaneous tissues, long-standing infections may sometimes invade deeper tissues. Extension of pythiosis through fascial planes resulting in infection or inflammation of an underlying tendon sheath, joint, or bone has been described in horses with extremity lesions present for longer than 2 months.[23,26,27] Horses with bone involvement are often presented with lameness (which may be non–weight-bearing) and edema of the affected limb. Radiographic findings are characterized by extensive, disorganized bony proliferation with variable osteolysis and cortical erosion.[26-28] Bones in which infection has been observed include the phalanges, the third metacarpal and metatarsal bones, and the proximal sesamoid bones. Periostitis resulting from adjacent soft tissue infection may cause significant periosteal proliferation without actual invasion of the periosteum; therefore, in cases with radiographic changes that are limited to proliferative changes of the periosteum, differentiation between periostitis and osteomyelitis cannot be made without a biopsy.[28]

In addition to local invasion of deeper tissues, dissemination of chronic cutaneous *P. insidiosum* infection to regional lymph nodes and lung has been reported in a small number of horses. Infection of an inguinal lymph node has previously been described in four horses with cutaneous hindlimb lesions.[24,29] Likewise, pulmonary lesions have been described in three horses with preexisting cutaneous lesions.[1,30,31] In one of these cases, however, the organism was not isolated, and the gross and microscopic characteristics of the lesions were not described.[31]

Intestinal granulomas similar to the enteric lesions found in dogs with GI pythiosis have been described in four horses.[32-35] Clinical signs in these horses included colic, and in each case a jejunal mass was detected during abdominal exploratory (three horses) or necropsy (one foal). Two of these horses had no recurrence of pythiosis after resection of the jejunal lesion; a third horse was euthanized at surgery because of extensive jejunal infarction thought to have resulted from prolonged intestinal distention.[35]

Diagnosis

The clinical manifestations of equine pythiosis were recognized for more than a century before the pathogen itself was conclusively identified; the definitive diagnosis of pythiosis has historically been challenging because of difficulties associated with isolation and morphologic identification of the pathogen. As a result, a presumptive diagnosis is often made on the basis of typical clinical and histologic findings. However, a number of recently developed serologic, immunohistochemical, and molecular-based tools are likely to make the definitive diagnosis of pythiosis possible in a greater number of affected animals, even when culture is unsuccessful.

Although cytologic and histologic findings may be supportive of a diagnosis of pythiosis, they do not allow differentiation of pythiosis from infections caused by the zygomycetes *Conidiobolus* and *Basidiobolus*, which have similar histologic and cytologic characteristics.

Cytology

Cytologic examination of exudate from draining tracts often reveals pyogranulomatous, eosinophilic, and suppurative inflammation. Hyphal structures are not usually visualized in exudate. However, macerated tissue fixed in 10% potassium hydroxide (KOH) for 30 minutes may be examined microscopically for the presence of typical, wide, sparsely septate, branching hyphal elements.

Culture

Isolation of *P. insidiosum* from infected tissues is not difficult when appropriate sample-handling and culture techniques are employed. However, because these techniques are fairly specific, it is important to use a laboratory with expertise in the isolation of pathogenic oomycetes. Kunkers are more likely than tissues to provide a positive culture and are the preferred source of inoculum.[36] For best results, unrefrigerated kunkers should be wrapped in a sterile, saline-moistened gauze sponge and shipped at ambient temperature to arrive at the laboratory within 24 hours of collection. However, when samples cannot be processed for more than 2 days after collection, they should be shipped with ice packs, stored in the refrigerator, or stored at ambient temperature in an antibiotic solution to decrease proliferation of bacterial contaminants.[36]

The use of selective media significantly increases the likelihood of isolating pathogenic oomycetes, especially from lesions with secondary bacterial infection. The author routinely uses vegetable extract agar[37] amended with streptomycin (200 µg/mL) and ampicillin (100 µg/mL) for the isolation of *P. insidiosum*. As a commercially available alternative, Campy blood agar (Remel, Lenexa, KS), which contains trimethoprim, vancomycin, polymyxin B, cephalothin, and amphotericin B, is also effective. Small pieces of fresh kunkers should be placed directly on the surface of the agar and incubated at 37° C (98.6° F); growth is typically observed within 24 hours.

Although the identification of oomycetes is generally based on morphologic features of sexual reproductive structures, such as oogonia and antheridia, isolates of *P. insidiosum* rarely produce these structures in vitro. Therefore identification of *P. insidiosum* should be based on colonial and hyphal characteristics; growth at 37° C; production of motile, reniform, biflagellate zoospores; and, if possible, specific polymerase chain reaction (PCR) amplification or ribosomal ribonucleic acid (rRNA) gene sequencing. Colonies on vegetable extract or Sabouraud dextrose agar are typically submerged and white to colorless and have an irregular radiate pattern.[14,38] Microscopically, hyphae are broad (4-10 µm in diameter), hyaline, and sparsely septate and tend to branch at right angles. Zoospores can be readily produced by placing boiled grass blades on the surface of a 1- to 2-day-old colony growing on 2% water agar, incubating at 37° C for 18 to 24 hours, and then placing the infected grass blades in a dilute salt solution.[39-41] After 2 to 4 hours of incubation at 37° C, terminal vesicles from which zoospores are released can be visualized extending from the cut edges of the infected grass blades. Although the production of zoospores is an important supporting feature for the identification of pathogenic oomycetes, it is not specific for *P. insidiosum*. It does, however, rule out zygomycosis.

Serology

Both immunoblot[42] and enzyme-linked immunosorbent assay (ELISA)[43,44] have been used successfully to demonstrate the ability of sera from *Pythium*-infected horses to recognize soluble mycelial antigens of *P. insidiosum*. Unfortunately, the only assay currently available to practicing veterinarians has not been tested for specificity using serum from horses with basidiobolomycosis or sporotrichosis or from healthy horses that are regularly exposed to nonpathogenic oomycetes in pasture environments; therefore its rate of false-positive results is unknown. In the author's experience, the specificity of immunoblot serology for the diagnosis of pythiosis in horses is not as high as in dogs and cats; occasional false-positive results are observed in horses with other types of fungal, as well as nonfungal, inflammatory diseases.

Molecular Assays

To circumvent the difficulties associated with obtaining a culture-based diagnosis of pythiosis, a *P. insidiosum*–specific PCR assay was developed.[45] This assay can be applied to deoxyribonucleic acid (DNA) extracted from either cultured isolates or appropriately preserved, infected tissue samples.[46] In addition, the author has successfully applied this technique to DNA extracted from paraffin-embedded tissue sections.[47] The major advantage of this assay is its high specificity.

Immunohistochemistry

Immunohistochemical (IHC) techniques using polyclonal antibodies, developed first by Brown et al[48] and later by Patton et al,[49] have previously been used as confirmatory tests for pythiosis. These techniques have the advantage of being applicable to paraffin-embedded tissues. However, at least one of these antibodies has demonstrated cross-reactive staining of *Conidiobolus* and *Lagenidium* hyphae in canine tissue.[50,51] Therefore the specificity of this antibody for the IHC diagnosis of pythiosis is questionable. A newer polyclonal anti–*P. insidiosum* antibody raised in chickens and adsorbed with sonicated *Lagenidium* and *Conidiobolus* hyphae appeared to be highly specific for the IHC detection of *P. insidiosum* hyphae in both equine tissues (Fig. 51-3) and canine tissues,[52] but it is not currently available.

Pathologic Findings

Histologic findings associated with pythiosis are characterized by eosinophilic granulomatous to pyogranulomatous inflammation with necrosis and fibrosis. Infected tissues typically contain multiple foci of necrosis or coagula that contain amorphous eosinophilic material, hyphae, collagen, and degenerate eosinophils and are surrounded and infiltrated by neutrophils, eosinophils, and macrophages.[24] Some of these coagula are organized and large enough to be grossly visible as kunkers. Discrete eosinophilic granulomas may also be observed. The area between the necrotic foci or discrete granulomas is characterized by granulomatous and granulocytic inflammation and often

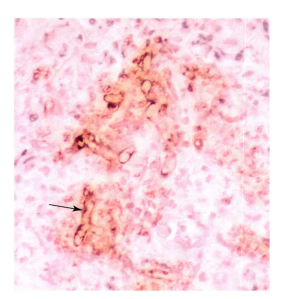

Figure 51-3 Photomicrograph showing immunohistochemical stain of tissue excised from cutaneous lesion in horse with pythiosis. Note the presence of multiple, broad *Pythium insidiosum* hyphae *(arrow)* with nonparallel walls and rare septation. (Avidin-biotin-peroxidase method with polyclonal anti–*P. insidiosum* antibody; Mayer's hematoxylin counterstain; 40×.)

contains epithelioid macrophages, lymphocytes, plasma cells, and mast cells. Vascular changes, including vessel wall invasion, vasculitis, thrombosis, and intimal changes, are variably present. In chronic lesions, fibrosis becomes more predominant, and the number of inflammatory cells is reduced.

Hyphal structures are usually found within areas of necrosis or at the center of discrete granulomas. Although *P. insidiosum* hyphae are difficult to visualize on hematoxylin and eosin (H&E)–stained sections, they may be identified as clear spaces ("hyphal ghosts") surrounded by a band or sleeve of eosinophilic material. Hyphae are easily visualized in sections stained with Gomori's methenamine silver (GMS) but not with periodic acid–Schiff (PAS). They are broad (mean, 4 µm; range, 2-7 µm), rarely septate, and occasionally branching.[24]

Therapy

Current recommendations for the treatment of equine pythiosis include surgical removal of as much infected tissue as possible, combined with immunotherapeutic injection of *P. insidiosum* antigens. In horses with nonresectable lesions, immunotherapy alone may be curative or may cause the lesion to regress to a size that is amenable to resection. Because the success of either surgery or immunotherapy depends on initiating therapy early in the course of disease, biopsy should be performed without delay in horses that develop lesions suggestive of pythiosis. Unfortunately, lesions caused by pythiosis (especially those that have been present for several months before diagnosis) may not resolve despite aggressive surgical and immune therapy.

Surgery

Complete surgical resection of infected tissues provides the best opportunity for cure of equine pythiosis. Whenever feasible, surgical excision of *P. insidiosum* lesions should be performed with 2- to 3-cm margins.[1] Unfortunately, the location (e.g., distal limb), size, and invasiveness of lesions often make complete removal of infected tissue difficult and necessitate leaving the incision open to heal by second intention.

Laser photoablation has recently been recommended as an adjunctive tool for reducing the risk of postsurgical recurrence in horses with cutaneous or subcutaneous pythiosis.[53,54] By inducing collateral thermal necrosis, photoablation acts to kill hyphal organisms that may have infiltrated surgical tissue margins. Photoablation with carbon dioxide (CO_2) or neodymium:yttrium-aluminium-garnet (Nd:YAG) lasers has previously been used in human patients for adjunctive therapy after partial resection of bacterial and neoplastic lesions.[55-57] Sedrish et al[54] described the use of Nd:YAG laser to photoablate the tissue bed after mass removal in two horses with cutaneous pythiosis. A defocused beam of 80 W, continuous power, and a noncontact fiber was used in a cross-hatch pattern, resulting in an energy density of 300 to 500 J/cm². Because Nd:YAG lasers create greater thermal damage, they may be more effective than diode or CO_2 lasers for postoperative photoablation treatment of *P. insidiosum* infection. Surgeons using laser photoablation for the treatment of cutaneous pythiosis should keep in mind that the laser plume is a potential vector for transmitting infectious materials[58] and should strictly adhere to laser safety protocols.

Immunotherapy

Immunotherapy, in the form of parenteral administration of water-soluble antigens extracted from an isolate of *P. insidiosum*, has been used successfully for more than 20 years for the treatment of equine pythiosis. The effectiveness of this form of treatment is likely related to stimulation of changes in the cell-mediated immune response to infection. Because immunotherapy with *P. insidiosum* antigens is not effective in horses with

zygomycosis or other cutaneous diseases, a definitive diagnosis based on culture or molecular identification of the pathogen, in addition to histopathology, is needed before initiating treatment.

A therapeutic *P. insidiosum* vaccine consisting of killed, sonicated mycelium was first developed by Miller[59] in the early 1980s and was found to be effective in resolving pythiosis in approximately 50% of equine patients. Cure rates were even higher when vaccination was used in conjunction with surgical debridement. In animals that responded favorably to the vaccine, signs of improvement (decreased exudate, resolution of pruritus, stabilization of lesion size) were first noted 5 to 10 days after the first of three or more weekly injections. Epithelialization, closure of draining tracts, and reduction in inflammation and lesion size were observed 14 to 28 days after initiation of immunotherapy. Adverse effects associated with immunotherapy using this vaccine preparation included development of a severe, local tissue reaction, with pain, edema, and sterile abscesses at the injection site. Two patients with extremity lesions developed osteitis and septic arthritis despite apparent resolution of the *P. insidiosum* infection.[59,60]

A second type of *P. insidiosum* vaccine, developed by Mendoza, consisted of secreted antigens of *P. insidiosum* precipitated from broth culture medium.[61] When evaluated in 41 *P. insidiosum*–infected horses from Costa Rica, Mendoza's vaccine was found to have efficacy similar to that achieved with Miller's vaccine but with less severe tissue reactions at the injection site. Mendoza also found that lesion duration was an important factor in predicting response to immunotherapy, with cure rates of 100% in horses with lesions that had been present for 15 days or less but no cures in horses with lesions present for more than 2 months. In addition, the stability of the exoantigen vaccine preparation was reported to be superior to Miller's sonicated mycelial preparation, allowing Mendoza's vaccine to be stored at 4°C (39°F) for up to 18 months without loss of efficacy. Further work with both types of vaccines by Newton and Rosa[62] in the early 1990s supported Miller and Mendoza's findings.

More recently, another therapeutic vaccine that contains both secreted antigens and soluble mycelial antigens was described by Thitithanyanont et al,[63] who used it successfully to treat *P. insidiosum* infection causing arteritis in a young boy in Thailand. Subsequently, Mendoza[64] evaluated the efficacy of this vaccine for the treatment of equine pythiosis and found that it effectively resolved *P. insidiosum*–induced lesions in 13 of 18 horses that had failed to respond to surgical and medical therapy. The protocol for immunotherapy using this vaccine consists of an initial intradermal administration of 0.1 mL of a 2-µg/mL antigen preparation, followed by subcutaneous administration of a second dose 15 days later. If a poor clinical response is observed, the vaccine is readministered on a weekly basis for up to 2 months. The local inflammatory response of the patient to the initial injection appears to be an important prognostic factor; animals that produce a large (>30 mm) wheal with erythema and edema are more likely to be cured eventually than those that have a minimal local response. This vaccine product is available through Pan American Veterinary Laboratories (www.pavlab.com, 800-856-9655).

Medical Therapy

The administration of traditional antifungal drugs, such as amphotericin B, ketoconazole, and iodides, is typically ineffective for the treatment of pythiosis. For amphotericin B and the azoles, this is likely because ergosterol is not an important component of the oomycete cell membrane. However, there are sporadic reports in the equine veterinary literature of response of *P. insidiosum* lesions to systemic treatment with amphotericin B, sodium iodide, or potassium iodide.[1,31] In addition, topical therapy with either amphotericin B or a combination of keto-conazole and dimethylsulfoxide (DMSO) has been recommended for adjunctive therapy, although information regarding efficacy is largely anecdotal.[1] In general, medical therapy is not recommended for the treatment of pythiosis in horses except as an adjunct to surgical resection and immunotherapy.

Zygomycosis

The term *zygomycosis* refers to infections caused by fungi in the class Zygomycetes, including the genera *Basidiobolus* and *Conidiobolus* in the order Entomophthorales, and the genera *Rhizopus, Absidia, Mucor, Saksenaea,* and others in the order Mucorales. In human and veterinary patients, the Mucorales fungi tend to cause acute, rapidly progressive disease in debilitated or immunocompromised individuals, whereas the Entomophthorales fungi typically cause chronic localized infections in subcutaneous tissue or nasal submucosa of immunocompetent patients.[65,66] Culture-confirmed infections caused by pathogens in the order Mucorales have not been well documented in equine patients, with only three case descriptions in the literature to date. However, *Basidiobolus ranarum* and *Conidiobolus* spp. have been well documented in horses as causes of cutaneous and nasopharyngeal lesions, respectively.

Etiology and Epidemiology

Basidiobolus ranarum (previously *B. haptosporus*), *Conidiobolus coronatus, C. incongruus,* and *C. lamprauges* are saprophytes that are widely distributed in nature. Both *Conidiobolus* and *Basidiobolus* spp. are found in soil and decaying plant matter, and *Basidiobolus* spp. are also frequently isolated from insects and from the feces of amphibians and reptiles.[65] Cutaneous infection with *Basidiobolus* or *Conidiobolus* spp. likely occurs by percutaneous or submucosal inoculation of soil-borne spores through minor trauma or insect bites. Infection may also result from inhalation or ingestion of spores. Affected animals are typically immunocompetent. Zygomycosis caused by the Entomophthorales occurs most often in tropical and subtropical regions of the world, with most human cases reported from Africa and Asia.[65] In veterinary patients, basidiobolomycosis and conidiobolomycosis have been encountered throughout the southeastern United States, as well as eastern and northern coastal Australia.

Clinical Findings

Basidiobolomycosis

Basidiobolus ranarum infection in horses causes cutaneous and subcutaneous lesions that are grossly similar to those caused by pythiosis but are most often found on the lateral aspects of the head, neck, chest, or trunk[21] (Fig. 51-4). This distribution may reflect a higher likelihood for these areas to come into contact with spore-containing soil or organic material when the animal lies on the ground.[67] Lesions are single, roughly circular, ulcerative, granulomatous masses with an edematous and hemorrhagic surface[68,69] (Fig. 51-5). As with pythiosis, these lesions are pruritic and often associated with self-trauma. Kunkers are often present but are smaller than those associated with pythiosis (usually <2 mm)[67] and lack the discrete, coral-like shape of *P. insidiosum* kunkers.[24]

Conidiobolomycosis

In horses, sheep, dogs, humans, and other mammalian species, conidiobolomycosis occurs most often as a nasopharyngeal infection with or without local dissemination into tissues of

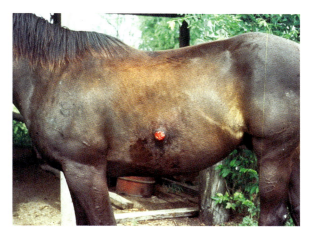

Figure 51-4 Ulcerative cutaneous lesion on trunk of horse caused by *Basidiobolus ranarum* infection. *(Courtesy Dr. Carol Foil, Louisiana State University.)*

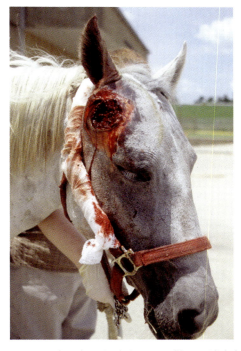

Figure 51-5 Large, circular, ulcerative lesion caused by *Basidiobolus ranarum* infection on head of 19-year-old mare.

the face, retropharyngeal region, retrobulbar space, or cerebrum.[2,65,70-72] Infected equine patients typically exhibit multiple ulcerative granulomas or lobulated to pedunculated nodules involving the external nares, nasal cavity, or nasopharynx[21] (Fig. 51-6). Lesions may be either unilateral or bilateral and may extend into maxillary sinuses. Thickening of the nasal septum and narrowing of the nasal passages often lead to dyspnea and noisy respiration, and blood-tinged mucopurulent nasal discharge is a common historical finding. Exudate-containing kunkers may accumulate in the guttural pouches.[73] As with basidiobolomycosis, the kunkers associated with conidiobolomycosis are typically smaller than those associated with pythiosis and are of no particular shape. In an unusual presentation, a mare with harsh respiratory sounds and bilateral nasal discharge was found to have multiple tracheal granulomas caused by *C. coronatus* infection but no lesions in the nasal passages.[74]

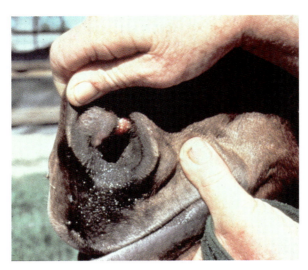

Figure 51-6 Nasal polyp caused by conidiobolomycosis in a horse. *(Courtesy Dr. Carol Foil, Louisiana State University.)*

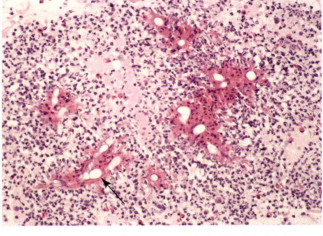

Figure 51-7 Photomicrograph of tissue excised from basidiobolomycosis lesion shown in Figure 51-5. Note the presence of large, sometimes bulbous hyphae *(arrow)* surrounded by a thick eosinophilic sleeve. (Hematoxylin and eosin [H&E] stain; 20×.)

Mucormycosis

Absidia corymbifera has been described as a cause of mucormycosis in three horses. One of these horses presented with an extensive left forelimb lesion consisting of an ulcerative, granulomatous mass that contained draining tracts.[75] Culture of distilled water flushed through the draining tracts yielded *A. corymbifera*. Treatment with amphotericin B administered parenterally, as well as topically, was unsuccessful. In two other horses kept in the same paddock, *A. corymbifera* was diagnosed on the basis of IHC staining of tissues with a monoclonal antibody.[76] One of these horses had disseminated disease, with lesions in the stomach, intestine, lungs, and brain. In the second horse, only skin lesions were noted, characterized as large ulcers that initially developed as erythematous indurated areas, with subsequent central necrosis. Lesions were located on the muzzle, nostrils, lips, knees, and hocks.

Pathologic Findings

The histologic features of zygomycosis are similar to those associated with pythiosis.[24] Distinct eosinophilic and necrotic foci centered on hyphal structures and surrounded by pyogranulomatous and eosinophilic inflammation are typically observed (Fig. 51-7). Large, well-organized coagula of eosinophils and hyphae can be seen grossly as kunkers. Multinucleated giant cells, plasma cells, lymphocytes, and mast cells are common in the granulomatous tissue surrounding the eosinophilic foci. Lesions associated with mucormycosis are more likely to demonstrate vascular changes (e.g., thrombosis, vascular invasion by hyphae, infarction) than those associated with entomophthoromycosis.

On GMS-stained sections, hyphae appear broad, thin walled, and occasionally septate. The histologic hallmark of zygomycosis is the presence of a wide (2.5-25 μm) eosinophilic sleeve surrounding the hyphae and making them easily located on H&E–stained sections (see Fig. 51-7). This finding helps to differentiate zygomycosis from pythiosis, in which eosinophilic sleeves tend to be thin or absent. In addition, the hyphal diameter tends to be significantly larger for *Basidiobolus* spp. (mean, 9 μm; range, 5-20 μm) and *Conidiobolus* spp. (mean, 8 μm; range, 5-13 μm) than for *P. insidiosum* (mean, 4 μm; range, 2-7 μm).[24]

Diagnosis

Because serologic and IHC techniques are not currently available for the diagnosis of zygomycosis in veterinary patients, a definitive diagnosis must be based on isolation and identification of the pathogen. The Entomophthorales fungi typically grow well on media routinely used for the isolation of pathogenic fungi such as Sabouraud dextrose agar, potato flakes agar,[77] potato dextrose agar, and cornmeal agar. The author routinely uses potato flakes agar amended with ampicillin (100 μg/mL) and streptomycin (200 μg/mL) for initial isolation of *Conidiobolus* and *Basidiobolus* spp.

Identification of zygomycetes in the laboratory is generally based on morphologic characteristics of asexual reproductive structures (conidia) and sexual reproductive structures (zygospores).[78] *Conidiobolus* isolates on potato flakes agar or half-strength cornmeal agar readily produce primary conidia that are forcibly discharged and can be visualized on the underside of the Petri dish lid. Primary conidia of *C. coronatus* are spherical and 40 μm in diameter and have a prominent basal papilla. Because *C. coronatus* is a heterothallic species, zygospores are not observed in clinical isolates. *Conidiobolus incongruus,* however, is a homothallic species that produces large (15-25 μm), round, smooth, thick-walled zygospores without beaks. Reproductive structures of *B. ranarum* are readily produced after 3 to 5 days of incubation on half-strength cornmeal agar. Zygospores are easily identified as large (20-50 μm), thick-walled, round intercalary structures with beaklike protuberances that represent the remains of copulatory tubes. Primary conidia (often with a hyphal tag still attached), secondary conidia (morphologically similar to primary conidia but often smaller), and capilliconidia (oval to elongate spores with a terminal adhesive knob that develops at the end of a thin supporting hypha) may all be visualized on the inside of the Petri dish lid.

Therapy

Because it causes locally invasive lesions that rarely disseminate, the treatment of choice for cutaneous and subcutaneous zygomycosis is complete surgical resection of infected tissues. However, because lesion location and extent often preclude complete surgical excision, medical therapy with potassium iodide is often used either alone or in conjunction with surgical debulking of the lesion. Although the mechanism for the antifungal activity of iodides is unknown, they have been used with variable success for the treatment of both basidiobolomycosis[69] and conidiobolomycosis[70,74] in horses and have the advantage of relatively low expense. Iodides are typically administered orally as potassium iodide (10-40 mg/kg orally [PO] every 24 hours [q24h]) or organic iodide (1-2 mg/kg PO q24h). Parenteral sodium iodide (20% solution at 20-40 mg/kg intravenously q24h for 7-14 days) may be used in combination with oral iodide therapy for the first 1 to 2 weeks of treatment. Patients should be monitored for signs of iodide toxicity, which include excessive lacrimation, nonpruritic generalized alopecia with scaling, anorexia, depression, serous nasal discharge, cough, salivation, and nervousness.[79] If signs of iodism occur, medication should be stopped until signs resolve, then restarted at a lower dose. Administration of iodides to pregnant mares is not recommended.

Theoretically, as true fungi, zygomycetes should be more likely than *P. insidiosum* to respond to antifungal medications that target ergosterol such as amphotericin B, itraconazole, ketoconazole, and fluconazole. Amphotericin B has been administered with variable response as an intralesional injection with DMSO or as part of a topically applied solution that also contains DMSO and ketoconazole.[1,80] McMullan et al[31] reported resolution of suspected nonresectable nasal conidiobolomycosis after intralesional injection of amphotericin B (50 mg in 10 mL 5% dextrose administered 4 times at 5-day intervals) combined with topical application of amphotericin B in DMSO.

The use of oral ketoconazole to treat zygomycosis in horses has not been reported. However, because ketoconazole has poor absorption from the GI tract and may need to be administered by nasogastric tube,[81] its usefulness is limited. Itraconazole was used unsuccessfully at a dose of 3 mg/kg PO q12h to treat one horse with nonresectable nasal conidiobolomycosis.[82] Although the lesion showed a 50% reduction in size after 12 weeks of therapy, it relapsed 2 weeks after medication was discontinued, and the horse was euthanized. However, because serum levels of itraconazole were undetectable in this horse, treatment failure may have been partly caused by inadequate dosage.

Fluconazole is one of the few antifungal drugs for which detailed pharmacokinetic data are available for horses. Its bioavailability after oral dosing is high, and a long-term oral treatment protocol consisting of a loading dose of 14 mg/kg followed by 5 mg/kg q12h maintains plasma and body fluid concentrations greater than 8 μg/mL.[83] Fluconazole has been used successfully to treat nasal conidiobolomycosis in two mares in which pregnancy precluded the use of iodide therapy.[84] One mare received 2 mg/kg PO q12h for 8 weeks, and the other received a loading dose of 14 mg/kg PO followed by 5 mg/kg q12h for 6 weeks. Nasopharyngeal signs improved within 2 weeks of initiating treatment in both mares, and lesions were not detectable by endoscopic examination in either mare when treatment was discontinued. Unfortunately, long-term follow-up for potential recurrence of lesions after discontinuation of therapy was not reported.

Regardless of the choice of therapy, owners of horses with zygomycosis should be warned that the prognosis for response to therapy is guarded, and recurrence of lesions is common. Animals treated early in the course of disease are more likely to have a successful outcome. Therefore pursuing appropriate diagnostic testing soon after lesions are detected is imperative.

The complete reference list is available online at www.expertconsult.com.

CHAPTER

52 Aspergillosis

Debra C. Sellon and Catherine Kohn*

Aspergillus species are among the most common fungal organisms. These saprophytes are widely distributed in the environment in soil, decaying vegetation, and organic debris. The members of this genus are opportunistic invaders of animal tissues, and healthy animals are resistant to infection unless exposed to a massive number of conidia or mycelia. Risk of disease caused by *Aspergillus* spp. is thought to be increased in immunodeficient horses and in horses with concurrent, severe enterocolitis or hematopoietic neoplasia. Transmission is usually by aerosol; guttural pouch mycosis and pulmonary disease are recognized manifestations of *Aspergillus* infection in horses. Pulmonary lesions are characteristically granulomatous. Keratomycosis caused by *Aspergillus* spp. is also common in horses.

Etiology

The classification and identification of *Aspergillus* species are based primarily on morphologic characteristics of the organism in culture. The genus *Aspergillus* is in the family Trichocomaceae of the order Eurotiales in the class Plectinomycetes of the phylum Ascomycota.[1] Fungi of the phylum Ascomycota are characterized by telomorphic (sexual) reproduction. Some textbooks[2] classify *Aspergillus* in the phylum Deuteromycota (fungi imperfecta), probably because this phylum contains anamorphic organisms, for which sexual reproduction has not been identified. The sexual state is found in very few species of *Aspergillus*, and the anamorphic (asexual) state is usually encountered in cultures from clinical patients.

Morphologic characteristics of *Aspergillus* spp. vary in culture. In general, *Aspergillus* spp. spread rapidly over the medium, forming a mycelium of flat to aerially branching and interlacing hyphae and conidiophores. The mycelium may be powdery white, greenish yellow, brown, or black.[1] The hyphae are nonpigmented and septate. Conidiophores (stalks) are characterized by a vesicle at the tip. The vesicle bears papillae (phialides) that give rise to unicellular conidia (cells produced by asexual reproduction) that are arranged in chains (Fig. 52-1). The characteristic shape of the conidiophore and spore heads is responsible for the name *Aspergillus*, which was conferred on the organism by an eighteenth-century priest who noted

---

*The authors acknowledge and appreciate the original contributions of these authors, whose work has been incorporated into this chapter.

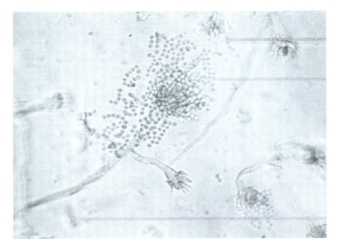

Figure 52-1 Photomicrograph of *Aspergillus* conidiospores. *(Courtesy Dr. Joseph Kowalski, The Ohio State University College of Veterinary Medicine.)*

the resemblance of this pattern to that of a holy water sprinkler ("Aspergillum").[1] Conidia may be colorless or darkly pigmented.

Approximately 180 species of *Aspergillus* are currently recognized, of which about 40 species have been identified in opportunistic infections of humans. Clinical studies of aspergillosis in horses usually report the presence of *Aspergillus* spp., and many do not identify the particular species involved. *Aspergillus fumigatus* is the most common species identified. *Aspergillus niger*[3,4] and *Aspergillus versicolor*[5] have also been reported to cause disease in horses. One case of keratomycosis caused by *Aspergillus oryzae* has been reported.[6] Mycotoxins produced by *Aspergillus flavus* cause equine aflatoxicosis.[7]

Virulence Factors

Because of their small size (2-3 μm in diameter), conidia of *Aspergillus* spp. remain in suspension in air for a long time, and these respirable particles can efficiently penetrate to the alveoli.[8] *Aspergillus* spp. are ubiquitous. The environment of the horse and particularly the "breathing zone" are almost continually rich in hyphae and conidia of *Aspergillus*, and people and horses constantly inhale fungal elements. In healthy horses and persons, fungi are cleared from the respiratory tract by pulmonary defense mechanisms (mucociliary clearance, phagocytosis by pulmonary macrophages). *Aspergillus* spp. are thermotolerant. The organisms thrive at 37° C (98.6° F), are able to grow at 55° C (131° F), and are reported to survive at temperatures up to 75° C (167° F).[9] These fungi are thus able to grow rapidly in body tissues of immunoincompetent hosts.

Aspergillus spp. survive in the bloodstream and tissues by being able to find and assimilate essential growth nutrients in these alien environments. The ability of these organisms to sense nitrogen sources in the environment and to regulate nitrogen utilization is essential to their survival.[10] Other fungal attributes that support the acquisition of essential nutrients include siderophores, phosphatases, and phospholipases. Fungal organisms require iron for growth, and blood is "fungistatic" because most iron is bound to transferrin.[9] *A. fumigatus* produces at least six siderophores that are able to remove iron from transferrin in vitro.[8,9] *A. fumigatus* has a high phosphate requirement. Phospholipases and phosphatases allow the organism to recover phosphate from environments that are not phosphate rich, such as blood, and to utilize inorganic phosphates.

Aspergillus spp. may act as allergens. Allergic bronchopulmonary aspergillosis, allergic rhinosinusitis, asthma, and aspergilloma have been reported in immunocompetent human patients.[8] Inhalation challenge with extracts of *A. fumigatus* in horses with recurrent airway obstruction can induce signs of this disease.[11]

Gliotoxin and other toxins are putative virulence factors produced by *A. fumigatus*.[12] These factors may have direct toxic effects on tissues, and many are immunosuppressive.

A number of fungal characteristics assist *Aspergillus* spp. in evading host immune responses. Melanin pigment on the surface of conidia can neutralize reactive oxygen species and protect the organisms against attack by macrophages and neutrophils.[9] *Aspergillus* spp. have extensive antioxidant capabilities and many efflux pumps to facilitate export of toxins. Hydrophobins form part of the external layer of the cell wall of the conidia and may protect them from destruction by alveolar macrophages.[9] In vitro, conidia and hyphae may be phagocytosed by endothelial cells and tracheal or alveolar epithelial cells.[8] In theory, fungi sequestered in these cells could evade immune surveillance. Some investigators speculate that *Aspergillus* organisms may be able to "direct" their phagocytosis by these "nonprofessional" phagocytic cells during times of environmental stress.[8] This ability to invade endothelial and epithelial cells may be a mechanism that facilitates angioinvasion and thrombosis by *Aspergillus* spp. in vivo.[8]

Epidemiology

Aspergillus spp. are ubiquitous in the environment of horses, as previously discussed. In one study, 67.8% of the fungi recovered from air and surface samples taken in three stables in the winter were *Aspergillus* spp.[13] Fungal contamination can be reduced by management changes; more environmental fungi were recovered from stables with wooden stalls, dirt floors, and straw bedding than from hospital stalls with masonry walls, synthetic flooring, and bedding composed of wood shavings.[14] Not surprisingly, *Aspergillus* spp. may be encountered in the conjunctiva[15-20] (50% of 43 horses sampled in one study[20,21]) and in airway fluid samples obtained by transtracheal aspiration of healthy horses.[22] Conidia may be found free in the transtracheal wash fluid or within large mononuclear cells. *Aspergillus* can also be routinely cultured from the ingesta,[23] the skin, and the caudal reproductive tract, including the external genitalia.[24]

Universal exposure of horses to *Aspergillus* and other fungi confounds attempts to document that these agents are the cause of disease. It is important to demonstrate the presence of conidia or hyphae in diseased tissues to substantiate the diagnosis. Body fluid samples and culture plates may be easily contaminated with aspergilli or other fungi.

Mycotic Keratitis (Keratomycosis)

Aspergillus spp. are the most common cause of keratomycosis in horses. Case review studies have shown that this organism can be isolated from 33% to 77% of horses with keratomycosis[25-31] and 2% to 22% of eyes from horses with external eye disease.[17] *Fusarium* spp. are also encountered frequently (10 of 39 horses [26%] with keratomycosis in one study[32]), whereas *Alternaria*, *Cladosporium*, *Pseudallescheria*, *Geotrichum*, *Scedosporium* spp., *Stemphylium* spp., *Penicillium*, *Cylindrocarpon*, *Scytalidium*, and *Torulopsis* are infrequently reported.[26,32] Nonseptate filamentous fungi, such as *Mucor*, and yeasts, such as *Candida*, may also be associated with mycotic keratitis. The mycology of keratomycosis may vary with the geographic region. Mycotic keratitis is thought to be rare in the United Kingdom, although a recent report documented six cases (1998-2002).[33]

Although mycotic keratosis may occur more frequently during the summer and fall in some regions, cases are seen year-round in Florida, where the majority of cases are reported to occur October through January.[32] No apparent age, breed, or gender predisposition exists for mycotic keratitis.

Endometritis and Placentitis

The most common causes of mycotic endometritis are *Aspergillus* spp. and *Candida* spp.[24,34] Mycotic infections account for 1% to 5% of cases of endometritis in mares.

Aflatoxicosis

A. flavus and *A. parasiticus* produce toxic metabolites known as aflatoxins. Corn, peanuts, peanut meal, and cottonseed meal are the most frequently contaminated sources of aflatoxins. The toxins are also found in other nuts (pecans, walnuts, almonds, hazelnuts).[7] Ambient temperatures between 78°F and 90°F (25.5°C-32°C), drought stress, and high relative humidity or grain moisture favor production of aflatoxins.[35] Factors that reduce protection of the seed or damage the seed coat, such as shortened husks or insect damage, also enhance the risk of aflatoxin production.

Pathogenesis

The virulence of *Aspergillus* organisms is usually a function of the immune incompetence of the host, rather than the presence of specific virulence factors intrinsic to the fungus.[9] Because this fungus is ubiquitous, it is frequently inhaled, ingested, or contacted directly (e.g., corneal surface) by potential hosts. Those hosts with weakened innate or acquired immune responses are at risk for colonization by this opportunistic organism. Invasive aspergillosis has become an important disease in patients with acquired immunodeficiency syndrome (AIDS) and in other human patients who are severely granulocytopenic because of their disease or from immunosuppressive treatment with anticancer drugs or corticosteroids. Invasive aspergillosis has been reported to occur in 70% of patients who remain granulocytopenic for 34 or more days.[36] A CD4 lymphocyte count less than 50 cells/mm^3 is a risk factor for invasive aspergillosis in AIDS patients.[36] Leukopenia and neutropenia are often associated with enterocolitis and typhlitis in horses.

In horses, immune incompetence is assumed to be an important risk factor for invasive aspergillosis, an otherwise uncommon disease. Pulmonary aspergillosis has been reported in a horse treated for ill thrift and intestinal malabsorption with corticosteroids[23] and in another with dysfunction of the pars intermedia of the pituitary.[37] Hyperadrenocorticism in horses with hyperplasia of the pars intermedia may be immune suppressive.[38] Invasive aspergillosis has been reported in four horses with hemolymphatic neoplasia (three with myelomonocytic leukemia and one with disseminated hemangiosarcoma).[23,39,40] Several investigators have noted an association between invasive aspergillosis and antecedent enterocolitis.[4,23,38,41-43] In one study, pulmonary aspergillosis developed in a mean of 11 days after enterocolitis in 16 horses (14 with salmonellosis).[23] In another study, 25 of 29 horses with pulmonary aspergillosis had evidence of primary or secondary disease that caused loss of the integrity of the bowel wall; 12 of these horses were leukopenic.[38] Loss of integrity of the bowel mucosa likely provided a portal for absorption of fungi from the bowel lumen, allowing embolic spread of the organisms to other organs, particularly the lungs, but also kidney and brain.[4,44] Broad-spectrum antibiotic therapy may contribute to the problem by destroying symbiotic bacteria that balance the gastrointestinal flora, preventing growth of potential pathogens.

Aspergillosis is occasionally reported in immunocompetent horses.[3,45,46] Fatal pneumonia caused by *A. niger* and *Rhizopus stolonifer* was diagnosed in two young horses recently moved to an unused, unclean stable.[3] The organisms were recovered from the lungs of affected horses and from the stable bedding. A third case of fatal invasive pulmonary aspergillosis was reported in an immunocompetent horse housed in a bank barn.[45] These authors hypothesize that affected horses were exposed to overwhelmingly large aerosol doses of fungi. *Aspergillus* spp. were isolated from a large, well-encapsulated mediastinal mass at the base of the heart in an otherwise healthy horse.[46,47]

Antigens of *A. fumigatus* have been implicated in the pathogenesis of recurrent airway obstruction (RAO) in horses. Inhalation challenge with an extract of *A. fumigatus* induced increased pulmonary resistance in horses with RAO[48] and caused signs of airway obstruction in RAO-affected horses in remission, but not in healthy control horses.[11] Serum allergen-specific immunoglobulin E (IgE) concentrations suggest that horses with RAO are more often sensitized to some allergens associated with *A. fumigatus* than are healthy control horses.[49,50] In addition, bronchoalveolar lavage fluid concentrations of IgE and IgG directed against antigens of *A. fumigatus* were greater in RAO-affected horses than in control horses,[51] and extracts or whole preparations of *A. fumigatus* induced greater in vitro histamine release from degranulating mast cells of RAO-affected horses than from healthy horses.[52] RAO has been extensively reviewed elsewhere.[53,54]

Keratomycosis

Aspergillus spp. are destructive pathogens in the eye. The propensity for horses to develop mycotic keratitis may be related to the fact that *Aspergillus* spp. and other fungi are usually among the commensal conjunctival flora, and horses are constantly exposed to fungi in fodder, bedding, and stable dust. A warm, humid environment (e.g., heated barn, ambient conditions) may predispose horses to fungal keratitis. Frequent treatment of bacterial keratitis with topical antibiotics may reduce the numbers of nonpathogenic bacteria while favoring multiplication of pathogenic bacteria and fungi.[15,55] The use of ophthalmic antibiotics is associated with a shift in the population of ocular flora from predominantly gram positive to gram negative.[56] Commensal flora of healthy eyes may produce antimicrobial substances that limit the population of pathogenic organisms.[14,15,55] For example, *Streptomyces natalensis*, a conjunctival commensal organism in healthy horses, produces the antifungal natamycin.[14,57] In one study, affected eyes of 32 of 39 horses with fungal keratitis (82%) were treated intensively with topical ophthalmic antibiotics before entry into the study, suggesting that this treatment may have been a risk factor for developing keratomycosis.[27]

Topical corticosteroids may enhance fungal replication and reduce corneal tissue resistance to fungal invasion, resulting in enhanced penetration of the cornea.[26,58] However, Andrew et al[27] documented prior treatment with topical corticosteroids in only 6 of 39 horses with keratomycosis, whereas 5 of 23 affected horses had prior treatment with topical corticosteroids in another study.[59] These findings collectively suggest that, although treatment with corticosteroids increases the risk of keratomycosis, other factors are likely important in the pathogenesis.

The equine eye is prominent, and the cornea has a large surface area, putting this structure at risk for trauma. Any epithelial defect can provide entry for fungi into the deeper layers of the cornea, or penetrating trauma may seed deeper layers of the cornea with fungi. Fungal replication and dead fungal hyphae induce a severe polymorphonuclear neutrophil (PMN, leukocyte) inflammatory reaction. Local release of proteases from fungi, leukocytes, and keratocytes destroys stroma.[27,57,60] Once established in the corneal stroma, fungi tend to burrow toward Descemet's membrane, where they are poorly responsive to medical treatment.[57] Corneal avascularity and the absence of corneal lymphatics may slow the response to deep infection. Healing depends on neovascularization arising from the limbus. Stromal abscesses may result from penetrating corneal wounds that seed the deeper corneal tissues, although other factors may be important, particularly where clusters of cases are identified.[57] A breach in Descemet's membrane by a penetrating wound or fungal-induced inflammation may allow *Aspergillus* organisms access to the anterior chamber, resulting in endophthalmitis.

Deficiencies in the immunoprotective qualities of tear film and the cornea in some horses may predispose them to keratomycosis.[32] Gliotoxin and other putative fungal virulence factors may inhibit corneal vascularization, reduce PMN cell infiltration, suppress cell-mediated phagocytosis, reduce cytolytic T-cell proliferation and activation, and decrease leukocytic antifungal proteinase activity.[57] *Aspergillus* and *Fusarium* isolates from equine patients with keratomycosis inhibited angiogenesis in an in vitro model in which fungi inhibited differentiation of capillary-like tubules from human umbilical vein endothelial cells.[61] Corneal healing in horses depends on neovascularization by endothelial budding and subsequent corneal invasion of limbal vessels. Inhibition of this process could impair corneal healing.

Endometritis and Placentitis

Common factors that increase uterine exposure to the ubiquitous aspergilli include frequent uterine lavage (which may introduce fungal organisms), poor vaginal conformation, pneumovagina, cervical adhesions, and urine pooling (see Chapter 8). Increased exposure to *Aspergillus* organisms increases the risk of infection.

Aflatoxicosis

Of the four types of aflatoxins, B_1 is the most abundant.[35] Aflatoxins are metabolized in the liver by mixed-function oxidases. One of the metabolites is a highly reactive oxide that binds with deoxyribonucleic acid (DNA), messenger ribonucleic acid (mRNA), and proteins, impairing protein synthesis and inducing cancer in some species.[35] Impaired protein synthesis results in necrosis, particularly in the liver, and improper antibody formation. Acute intoxication with large doses of aflatoxin leads to liver damage and death. Chronic exposure to sublethal doses may be asymptomatic in horses or may induce immune suppression and ill thrift with poor feed conversion.[62] Cumulative exposure increases the risk of liver and lung cancer in humans.[62] Dietary deficiencies in protein, selenium, and vitamin E increase susceptibility to aflatoxicosis.[35]

Clinical Findings

Despite *Aspergillus* spp. being opportunistic organisms, they have been reported to cause a diverse array of clinical disease in horses, including keratomycosis, nasal plaques, guttural pouch mycosis, RAO, pneumonia, pulmonary or mediastinal masses, placentitis, endometritis, endocarditis, vasculitis and cerebral infarction, and aflatoxicosis.

Mycotic Keratitis

Aspergillus spp. may colonize corneal erosions, producing lesions ranging from superficial abrasions with associated pain, miosis, blepharospasm, epiphora, and photophobia[60,63,64] to severe interstitial keratitis of varying depths.[63] These lesions usually develop rapidly, although indolent infections may occur.[65] Focal or diffuse corneal opacity and edema may be present (Fig. 52-2). Ulcers may appear raised and are often characterized by roughened borders, with surrounding radiating lines of leukocyte infiltration.[65] As fungi proliferate, dry, white to grayish, fluffy lesions may be observed, and the corneal surface may appear slightly green.[65] As the fungi invade the corneal stroma, neovascularization, microabscesses, and stromal malacia may be observed. Secondary anterior uveitis with aqueous flare will ensue, and corneal rupture and endophthalmitis may be sequelae.[65] Reliable signs that indicate healing of mycotic keratitis include clearing of the corneal edema, progressing from the periphery toward the lesion, in association with abundant, deep stromal vascularization that extends to the margin of the opacified stroma.[25] As the stromal opacification decreases in size, it may become more dense because of fibrosis.

Corneal stromal abscesses are characterized by a yellow-white opacity deep to intact (non–fluorescein-staining) corneal epithelium or a relatively small corneal defect[57,64] (Fig. 52-3).

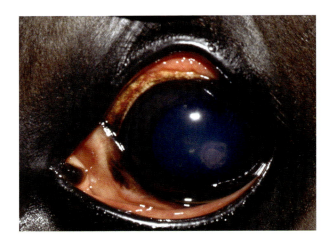

Figure 52-2 Keratomycosis in a horse. *(Courtesy Dr. Anne Metzler, The Ohio State University College of Veterinary Medicine.)*

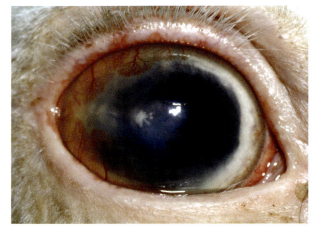

Figure 52-3 Mycotic stromal abscess in a horse. *(Courtesy Dr. Anne Metzler, The Ohio State University College of Veterinary Medicine.)*

Satellite lesions are often observed, and associated corneal edema may be prominent.

Mycotic keratitis should be suspected in corneal lesions that respond poorly or worsen during antibiotic therapy and in those that show improvement followed by deterioration when treated with topical corticosteroids.[66] Differential diagnoses include bacterial keratitis (especially caused by *Pseudomonas* spp. and β-hemolytic streptococci), equine recurrent uveitis, bacterial stromal abscesses, viral keratitis, corneal dystrophies or degeneration, and indolent ulcers.[65]

Pulmonary Aspergillosis

In the early stages of infection, clinical signs of respiratory disease may be absent or mild.[40] Advanced or extensive pulmonary disease may be associated with nasal discharge, nasal plaques, abnormal breath sounds (crackles, wheezes, pleural friction rubs), tachypnea, dyspnea, and pleural hemorrhage.[38,44] A history of vague respiratory signs that respond poorly to antibiotic therapy should suggest the possibility of fungal infection. In one retrospective study, 4 of 29 horses with pulmonary aspergillosis had a history of intermittent treatment with moderate doses of corticosteroids, and 23 of 29 (79%) had been previously treated with antibiotics.[38]

Nasal or Sinus Aspergillosis

Mycotic plaques caused by *Aspergillus* spp. may occasionally occur on the mucosa of the nasal passages in the absence of *Aspergillus* infection elsewhere, or these plaques may be present in horses with concurrent pulmonary aspergillosis. Three horses with unilateral aspergillosis of the middle meatus had unilateral, foul-smelling nasal discharge and intermittent epistaxis, and two of three had submandibular lymphadenopathy.[67] Affected horses may have multiple mycotic plaques, and nasal discharge may be continuous or intermittent. In a retrospective and prospective study of 277 cases of sinonasal disease, 13 horses had intranasal mycotic lesions, mycotic sinusitis, or mycotic lesions at the sinonasal ostium.[68] Most of these lesions were caused by *A. fumigatus*. Lesions of the nostrils were often ulcerative granulomas.[69] An ulcerated mycetoma at the commissure of the upper lip of one horse was caused by infection with *A. versicolor* that extended through to the buccal mucosa.[5]

Central Nervous System Aspergillosis

A. niger caused necrotizing vasculitis with cerebral infarction in an 18-year-old Morgan mare with a 10-day history of diarrhea.[4] The mare was depressed, incoordinated, and dysphagic and died after 4 days of treatment with fluids and trimethoprim-sulfamethoxazole and pyrimethamine.

Endometritis and Placentitis

Mares with fungal endometritis typically have a white to gray vaginal discharge. The uterus contains variable amounts of fluid that may induce distention and flaccidity.[24,70] *Aspergillus* has also been reported to cause severe focal placentitis, resulting in abortion.[71]

Aflatoxicosis

Ingestion of aflatoxin (500-1000 parts per billion [ppb]) by mature horses decreased feed intake, with resultant weight loss and induced liver damage.[7] In other horses, ingestion of feed containing 900 ppb or more than 6500 ppb of aflatoxin caused death, with brain, liver, kidney, and heart damage in affected horses.[7] Aflatoxins, fed at doses greater than 2 mg/kg, were uniformly fatal in weanling ponies.[72] Aflatoxin B_1 was found at a concentration of 114 μg/kg in corn fed to horses that died (three) or became ill.[73] Chronically affected horses show a spectrum of clinical signs, including weight loss, behavioral changes (somnolence, yawning, aggression, head pressing, circling, blindness) associated with liver impairment, or death.[7,74]

There are a few reports of naturally occurring aflatoxicosis in horses.[74-78] Clinical signs included soft feces, anorexia, icterus, and rapid weight loss. Necropsy findings in affected horses included centrilobular hepatic necrosis, bile duct hyperplasia, fatty liver, and hemorrhagic enteritis.

Diagnosis

The diagnosis of aspergillosis must be based on identification of the organism in tissue such as the cornea. The organism grows well on most commercially available fungal culture media.[2] Isolation of fungi from the conjunctiva, proximal airway, or other tissues that could collect environmental contaminants is not sufficient to establish a definitive diagnosis. Culture and cytologic evaluation of infected tissue or exudates should be attempted. Specimens should be obtained from several areas of the lesion, including deeper tissues, to maximize the possibility of finding fungal organisms if they are present.

Serology

Attempts to diagnose invasive aspergillosis based on serology have been unrewarding. Anti-*Aspergillus* antibodies can be detected in healthy, as well as diseased, horses, likely because of constant environmental exposure to these fungi.[38,42] Counter immunoelectrophoresis and enzyme-linked immunosorbent assay (ELISA) using complex antigenic mixtures did not discriminate between healthy and diseased horses.[79] However, immunoblotting analysis based on reactivity to low-molecular-mass antigens was positive in diseased horses but not in healthy horses of the same study. This assay is not commercially available.

Real-Time Quantitative Polymerase Chain Reaction

A real-time (RT) quantitative polymerase chain reaction (PCR) test evaluates the number of copies of DNA from fungi in corneal tissues of horses with mycotic keratitis.[80] Horses with confirmed fungal disease had a significantly greater number of copies of fungal DNA than horses with healthy eyes. Four of five horses with fungal keratitis had more than 1000 copies/25 ng of DNA, whereas healthy horses had 5 to 321 copies/25 ng of DNA in their corneal tissue.[80] This assay is commercially available at the author's institution. This approach to diagnosis holds promise for quantifying fungal load and may prove useful to monitor response to therapy.

Culture

Confirmation of identification of the genus and species of the fungus requires culture of tissue or fluid samples. *Aspergillus* spp. will grow readily on most fungal media.[2] Although cultures may be positive in as little as 3 days, an average of 25 days was required to identify the isolates in one study.[81] It is not practical to wait for culture results before beginning treatment.

Susceptibility Testing

Antifungal susceptibility testing (measuring the inhibitory activity of the tested antimicrobial agent) and correlations between in vitro susceptibility and clinical outcome of invasive fungal diseases in human patients have been the subject of intensive research.[81] Many factors other than susceptibility of the etiologic agent to the chosen drug affect clinical outcome, including host immune status, location of the infection, duration of the infection, drug pharmacokinetics, and patient compliance.[82] Standardized methods of assessment of in vitro susceptibility of yeasts and filamentous fungi to some common antifungal drugs have been developed.[83] Tentative "breakpoints" for fluconazole, itraconazole, and 5-fluorocytosine against *Candida* spp. have been established, and breakpoint values for fluconazole and flucytosine are useful in predicting clinical outcome.[72] Meaningful correlations between in vitro susceptibility test results and clinical outcome for most filamentous fungi and yeasts have not been established.[82-85]

Current recommendations to physicians managing patients with fungal diseases are to (1) identify a fungal isolate at the genus and species level if possible; (2) perform in vitro susceptibility testing (using approved methods) only for fluconazole and flucytosine susceptibility of *Candida* isolates from sterile sites; (3) attempt susceptibility testing for *Candida* spp. and amphotericin B; *Cryptococcus neoformans* and fluconazole, flucytosine, or amphotericin B; and *Histoplasma capsulatum* and fluconazole for patients in whom initial antifungal therapy has failed; and (4) select therapy for all other fungal isolates based on guidelines or survey data.[83,86]

Antifungal sensitivity testing is difficult to obtain in the veterinary clinical setting,[20] and results of in vitro susceptibility testing often do not correlate well with clinical response to treatment.[32] In particular, fluconazole may demonstrate low activity with in vitro test systems but high activity in vivo, possibly due in part to the drug's excellent tissue solubility.[87] Troke et al[88] demonstrated that fluconazole was fifteenfold more potent than ketoconazole in a model of vaginal candidiasis in mice, despite being eightyfold less active in vitro. The value of in vitro antifungal susceptibility testing in veterinary medicine is unproved.

Currently, determination of fungicidal activities of antimicrobial agents against yeasts and molds holds promise for the development of clinically relevant correlates of in vitro susceptibility. In vitro studies employing minimum fungicidal concentration (best assessed in animal models) or "time-kill" methods (ability of antimicrobial agent to kill fungal isolate over time) have predicted in vivo response.[89] To date, these methods have not yet been standardized, and their use in the veterinary setting has not been explored.

Biopsy

Aspergillus organism are readily identifiable in infected tissues. Typical hyphae in tissue are 2 to 5 μm in diameter and branch dichotomously at 45-degree angles (Fig. 52-4). Hematoxylin and eosin (H&E) stain will identify the hyphae, although periodic acid–Schiff (PAS) and silver stains, such as Gomori's methenamine silver (GMS), are reported to be particularly useful in demonstrating the organisms.[24,44]

Immunohistochemical Techniques

Immunofluorescent techniques using genus-specific conjugates have been described to identify *Aspergillus* spp. in tissues.[44] These techniques do not allow speciation. A three-layer indirect enzyme immunohistochemical technique uses polyclonal rabbit antibodies raised against somatic antigens of *A. fumigatus*, *A. flavus*, and *A. niger* in a peroxidase-antiperoxidase system.[4] This latter technique distinguished *A. niger* in brain tissue of an affected horse.

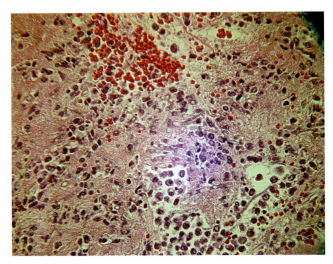

Figure 52-4 Photomicrograph of branching hyphae of *Aspergillus* in kidney of horse with disseminated aspergillosis and hemolytic anemia.

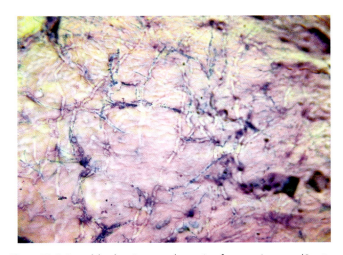

Figure 52-5 Fungal hyphae in corneal scraping from equine eye. *(Courtesy Dr. Anne Metzler, The Ohio State University College of Veterinary Medicine.)*

Mycotic Keratitis

Cytologic Examination

Identification of fungal hyphae in corneal scrapings is considered diagnostic (Fig. 52-5). In one study, 86% of 36 corneal scrapings from horses with keratomycosis were positive for fungal hyphae.[81] If the cornea has reepithelialized, deeper scrapings must be carefully obtained because fungi tend to invade deeply, and examination of scrapings of superficial layers of the cornea may yield false-negative results. Histology of corneal tissue obtained by keratectomy may be helpful in establishing a diagnosis.

Culture

Brooks et al[32] found that 84.6% of 39 horses with keratomycosis had positive cultures. From 30% to 50% of horses with keratomycosis are reported to have concurrent bacterial keratitis. In healthy equine eyes, gram-positive cocci and rods predominate on the conjunctiva, although gram-negative organisms may be present.[64] In one study, 90% of bacterial isolates from horses with keratomycosis were gram-positive organisms,[81] whereas a second study showed gram-positive organisms in 5% to 45% of isolates and gram-negative organisms in 2% to 45% of isolates from affected eyes.[64] Topical antibiotic treatment induces a shift from a predominance of gram-positive to an increasing proportion of gram-negative organisms.[28] Antimicrobial sensitivity patterns of bacterial agents may change during treatment, and secondary cultures may be necessary to guide adjustment of therapy.[28]

Corneal Biopsy and Staining

Examination of corneal biopsies was diagnostic in all six horses with keratomycosis in one study.[32] Histopathologic examination revealed edema, loss of epithelialization, necrosis of the corneal collagen, interstitial keratitis, and fungal organisms that tended to penetrate toward Descemet's membrane.[81]

Multifocal punctate corneal erosions may be caused by *Aspergillus* spp. but may be mistaken for viral lesions. Fungal microerosions may not take up fluorescein stain but will be visible with rose bengal staining.[90]

Pulmonary Aspergillosis

Antemortem diagnosis of pulmonary aspergillosis may be difficult. In one study of 29 horses subsequently shown to have pulmonary aspergillosis at necropsy, only 1 horse was diagnosed antemortem.[38] Pulmonary ultrasonography and radiography may be useful. Radiographs may demonstrate a diffuse interstitial and peribronchiolar pattern,[43] and ultrasonography may reveal a pleural effusion. The presence of many characteristic fungal hyphae in fluids obtained by transtracheal aspiration, bronchoalveolar lavage, or thoracocentesis supports the diagnosis of pulmonary aspergillosis. Positive cultures of these fluids also support the diagnosis, particularly when positive results are obtained on several occasions or when growth is rapid and exuberant and the predominant or only organism present is *Aspergillus*. Nevertheless, because healthy horses may harbor *Aspergillus* organisms in the airways, results of cytologic examination and culture of airway fluids should be corroborated by positive cultures of affected tissues. Lung biopsy may provide tissue for culture.

At necropsy, pulmonary pathology is characterized by fibrinonecrotic, hemorrhagic pneumonia with congestion or edema. Lesions are often found around large blood vessels. In more chronic cases a miliary distribution of nodules (granulomas) and fibrosis may be identified.[38,43,44] Histologically, multiple, septate, branching hyphae are found in pulmonary lesions (Fig. 52-6). *Aspergillus* organisms are angioinvasive, with hyphae possibly found radiating from the center of blood vessels,[38] and are associated with extensive vasculitis and thrombosis.[3,4]

Nasal and Sinus Aspergillosis

Endoscopy usually provides the diagnosis, although in some horses, endoscopy with the patient under anesthesia may be required to see the lesion. Radiographs of the skull and surgical exploration of the affected sinus are useful in defining the extent of nasal or sinus aspergillosis. Disease caused by plaques of *Aspergillus* spp. in the guttural pouch is described in Chapter 1.

Central Nervous System Aspergillosis

The diagnosis of central nervous system (CNS) aspergillosis is often made at necropsy. In one case report the horse's right cerebral cortex had a malacic focus 2.5 cm in diameter, with extensive hemorrhage predominantly involving gray matter.[4] Histologically, the lesion was characterized by fibrinoid necrotizing vasculitis and thrombosis with many fungal hyphae. The cecum and large colon showed large foci of severe necrosis and

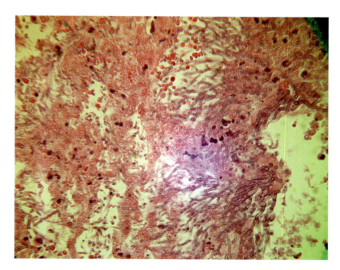

Figure 52-6 Photomicrograph of branching *Aspergillus* hyphae in a radiating pattern typical of invasive aspergillosis in lung of horse with large-colon volvulus, diarrhea, and *Aspergillus* pneumonia.

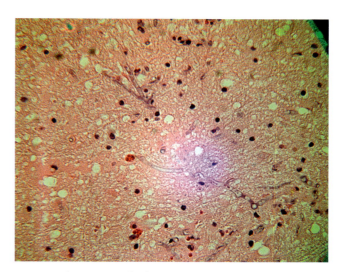

Figure 52-7 Photomicrograph of *Aspergillus* hyphae in brain of 4-month-old Morgan colt with ileus, hypoproteinemia, hemolytic anemia, and focal necrosis of cortical white matter.

hemorrhage. No fungal hyphae were found in the bowel tissues; however, systemic infection likely resulted from translocation of fungi from the bowel lumen. Acute focal coagulation necrosis of the cortical white matter with hemorrhage and intralesional *Aspergillus* hyphae were observed in a 4-month-old Morgan colt with a 1-week history of hypoproteinemia and hemolytic anemia (Fig. 52-7).

Endometritis and Placentitis

Aspergillus organisms can be identified by cytologic evaluation of uterine fluid obtained with guarded culture swab, in cultures of uterine fluid, and in appropriately stained biopsy tissue from the uterus or placenta. An accompanying inflammatory response should also be identified.

Aflatoxicosis

Clinical signs and associated serum chemistry abnormalities consistent with liver disease (increased hepatic enzyme activities and concentrations of bile acids and ammonia) suggest the possibility of aflatoxicosis. Feed should be tested to confirm the presence of aflatoxins. Aflatoxins exhibit bright–greenish yellow fluorescence, best observed in damaged grain under ultraviolet light. Thin-layer chromatography and ELISA, among other techniques, can be used to identify the aflatoxin.[35,74]

At necropsy, acute aflatoxicosis is characterized by centrilobular hepatic necrosis and hemorrhage with ascites. In subacute cases, hepatic lipidosis may be present. Histologic abnormalities of the liver include hepatocyte degeneration and necrosis, lipidosis, bile duct proliferation, and fibrosis.[35,74]

Therapy

Except for dermatomycosis and mycotic keratitis, fungal diseases in horses are relatively uncommon. Chemical, biochemical, and pharmacologic aspects, as well as practical uses of antifungal agents for treating animals, have been recently reviewed.[91-93] Studies of the pharmacokinetics of antifungal agents in horses are limited, and meaningful studies of treatment and outcome are lacking. The choice of a drug for treating fungal diseases in horses is largely guided by personal opinion informed by anecdotal accounts reported in the literature regarding treatment of a small number of equine patients and inferred from the literature concerning fungal diseases of humans. Fungal diseases have become increasingly common in human patients with cancer or AIDS, and the literature pertaining to treating mycoses in human patients is vast.

The systemic antifungal drugs most often used in horses include the polyene agent amphotericin B and the azole agents: the imidazole derivatives miconazole, enilconazole, and ketoconazole and the triazole agents itraconazole, fluconazole, and voriconazole. Dosage recommendations for systemic therapy in horses vary (Table 52-1), based on empiric experience, limited pharmacokinetic data, or extrapolation from recommendations for treating humans. Recommendations for ophthalmic therapy are discussed separately (Table 52-2).

Polyene Antifungal Drugs

Amphotericin B (AMB) is a product of the soil actinomycete *Streptomyces nodosus*. The drug is insoluble in water, is poorly absorbed after oral administration, and is administered intravenously (IV) or topically. AMB exerts its antifungal effect by binding to ergosterol in the fungal cell wall. Ergosterol is not a component of mammalian cells. Binding results in increased porosity of the fungal cell membrane, resulting in loss of essential intracellular substances and eventually cell death.[94] Reactive forms of oxygen also play a part in the lethal or cellulitic action of AMB.[91] One mechanism proposed is the autooxidation of AMB, resulting in the formation of free radicals.[95,96] The spectrum of action of AMB is reported to include *H. capsulatum*, *Blastomyces dermatitidis*, *C. neoformans*, *Candida* spp., *A. fumigatus*, and *A. flavus*.[97] Fungicidal or fungistatic activity depends on the concentration of the drug at the site of infection.[91] There are reports of successful use of AMB to treat systemic candidiasis in foals,[98] candidal arthritis,[99] fungal pneumonia,[100] phycomycosis,[101-103] pulmonary cryptococcosis,[104] and pulmonary histoplasmosis.[105] Long-term treatment with AMB failed to cure one horse with cryptococcal meningitis.[106]

Resistance to AMB among fungal isolates from animals and humans is relatively rare.[107] Some intrinsic resistance is observed among *Pseudallescheria boydii* and many *Aspergillus* spp.[91] The nephrotoxicity of this drug has limited its systemic use in horses. Adverse reactions reported in horses treated with AMB include depression, fever, lethargy, restlessness, tachycardia,

tachypnea, polyuria, anorexia, collapse, phlebitis, weight loss, anemia, and uremia.[108]

Lipid-encapsulated formulations of AMB have been developed to reduce the drug's toxicity in human patients. In the clinical setting, these formulations are at least as effective as the deoxycholate conjugate of AMB.[109] Lipid-encapsulated AMB has not been evaluated in horses, and the expense will likely preclude its use, except possibly in foals. Of more practical interest are recent studies demonstrating that mild heating of AMB (70° C [158° F] for 20 minutes) reduces the toxicity of the drug to human and pig cells in vitro and to mice in vivo.[110-112] Reduced toxicity resulted in a larger therapeutic index for AMB, allowing administration of a higher dose of the drug to experimental mice with cryptococcal or candidal infections. Reduced toxicity was not associated with a reduced effectiveness of heat-treated AMB in prolonging survival of mice with experimental cryptococcosis or candidiasis.[111]

Azole Antifungal Drugs

The azole antifungal drugs act by reducing ergosterol biosynthesis. Drugs of this class variably inhibit mammalian oxidative drug-metabolizing enzymes, and therefore the metabolism of concurrently administered drugs may be affected.[113] The imidazoles have a higher affinity for mammalian cytochrome P-450 enzymes than the triazoles.[113] Drug interactions with H_2 blockers, proton pump inhibitors, phenytoin, rifampin,[114] and sulfamethoxazole[91] have been described in humans. The azoles also variably reduce gonadal and adrenal steroidogenesis.[108] This effect is most prominent for the imidazole derivatives miconazole, enilconazole, and ketoconazole, particularly miconazole, and is negligible for the triazole fluconazole. All the azole drugs except fluconazole are immunosuppressive in people, especially with respect to lymphocyte function.[115] This attribute may reduce the host inflammatory response to fungi but may also limit the efficacy of these antifungal drugs. Antifungal drugs should be used only when evidence of fungal infection is strong.[57] This issue has not been studied in horses.

In general, the azoles are active against *Candida albicans*, *C. neoformans*, *B. dermatitidis*, *H. capsulatum*, *Coccidioides immitis*, and dermatophytes.[108] *Aspergillus* spp. are often less susceptible to ketoconazole.[108]

Miconazole (MICON) is poorly soluble in water. Oral MICON has poor bioavailability, and the topical form does not penetrate tissues well.[91] Poor bioavailability and an anecdotal report of anaphylactic reactions after systemic administration[57] limit MICON to topical use in horses. MICON is reported to be fungistatic for *Aspergillus* and the mycelial phase of *H. capsulatum*.[91] One horse with nasal plaques caused by *Pseudallescheria boydii* was successfully treated with MICON.[116]

Topical enilconazole (ENIL) was used successfully to treat a case of guttural pouch mycosis caused by *Aspergillus* spp. When nebulized, ENIL, in combination with oral ketoconazole, was successful in the treatment of a horse with *Scopulariopsis* pneumonia.[117]

Ketoconazole (KETO) is a lipophilic imidazole derivative. Systemic absorption is reported to be poor in horses after oral administration of 30 mg/kg every 24 hours (q24h); serum concentrations of the drug were undetectable.[118] Oral absorption of KETO depends on gastric acidity, and concurrent administration of 0.2-N hydrochloride (HCl) (q12h) resulted in detectable levels of the drug in serum in the same study. The bioavailability of KETO was 23% in one horse. Successful treatment of one horse with oral KETO (in combination with nebulized ENIL) for *Scopulariopsis* pneumonia has been reported.[117] Oral KETO therapy failed to cure three horses with coccidioidomycosis in one study.[119] KETO should not be administered to pregnant mares.[108]

Table 52-1 Systemic Antifungal Therapy in Horses

Drug	Dose	Route	Duration	Indication	Outcome*	Reference
Amphotericin B (AMB) deoxycholate	Day 1: 0.1-0.3 mg/kg, then ↑0.1-0.5 mg/kg daily or EOD	IV or IA in 5% dextrose over 1-4 hours	Variable; several weeks	Systemic candidiasis in foals	S	97
				Fungal pneumonia	S	100
				Candida arthritis	S	103
AMB	100 mg, then ↑50 mg/day, up to 200-250 mg/450 kg	IV (?) Intrathecal		Cryptococcal meningitis	F	106
AMB	0.1-1.5 mg/kg EOD			Phycomycosis	S	101
				Phycomycosis	S	102
				Candida arthritis	S	99
AMB		Topical, intralesional		Phycomycosis		101
AMB		Intralesional		Conidiobolomycosis		152
AMB (mg/kg)	Day 1: 0.3 Day 2: 0.45 Day 3: 0.6 Days 4-7: none Days 8-30: 0.6 EOD	IV, diluted		Pulmonary histoplasmosis	S	105
AMB (mg/kg)	Days 1-3: 0.35 Days 4-5: 0.4 Days 6-31: 0.6 3 g total dose	IV diluted Pretreat with flunixin meglumine	31 days	Pulmonary cryptococcosis	S: 1 case	104
Miconazole	5 g q12h, 2% solution	Topical	4 weeks	Nasal *Pseudallescheria boydii*	S: 1 case + Na iodide IV + K iodide PO	116
Enilconazole (ENIL)	33.3 mg/mL 60 mL	Topical	2 weeks	Guttural pouch aspergillosis	S: + ITRA PO	122
ENIL	0.9% or 1.7% solution q24h	Topical	9-13 days	Atypical guttural pouch mixed mycosis, including *Aspergillus*	S: 3 cases + debride	153
ENIL		Nebulized		*Scopulariopsis* pneumonia	S: + KETO	117
Ketoconazole (KETO)	3.6 mg/kg q24h	PO		Coccidioidomycosis	F	119
KETO	30 mg/kg q24h	PO		Pharmacokinetics: undetectable in blood and tissues		118
KETO	30 mg/kg + 0.2-N HCl q12h	PO	5 doses	Pharmacokinetics: 23% bioavailability		118
Itraconazole (ITRA)	3 mg/kg q12h	PO	3-4.5 months	Nasal aspergillosis	S: 2/2 cases + surgery for 1 case	120
ITRA	q12h	Topical	14 days	Nasal aspergillosis	S	121
ITRA	5 mg/kg q24h	PO	3 weeks	Guttural pouch aspergillosis	S: 1 case + topical ENIL	122
ITRA	2.6 mg/kg q12h	PO		Osteomyelitis, coccidioidomycosis	S: 1 case	123
Fluconazole (FLUC)	9-11 mg/kg loading dose 4-55 mg/kg q24h	PO		Systemic candidiasis (foals)	S	97
				Disseminated candidiasis	S	125
FLUC	14 mg/kg loading dose 5 mg/kg q24h	PO		Pharmacokinetics		141
Voriconazole	4 mg/kg q24h	PO		Pharmacokinetics		131
Voriconazole	10 mg/kg q24h	PO	24 days	Pulmonary aspergillosis (neonatal foal)	S	47

EOD, Every other day; *IV*, intravenous; *IA*, intraarterial; *PO*, oral; *q12h*, every 12 hours; *Na*, sodium; *K*, potassium; *HCl*, hydrochloride.

*S, Successful treatment; F, failure of treatment.

Itraconazole (ITRA) is a lipophilic triazole that is well absorbed and provides high tissue concentrations in human patients after oral administration. The pharmacokinetics of ITRA have not been established for horses. ITRA has a wider spectrum of activity than KETO and is effective against *C. albicans*, *Aspergillus*, *B. dermatitidis*, *C. immitis*, *C. neoformans*, and *H. capsulatum*.[108] Oral and topical ITRA has been used successfully to treat two horses with nasal aspergillosis,[120,121] one horse with guttural pouch aspergillosis (concurrently treated with topical ENIL),[121] and one horse with osteomyelitis caused by coccidioidomycosis.[122] One horse with guttural pouch aspergillosis was treated successfully with ENIL, using an indwelling catheter.[123]

Fluconazole (FLUC) is a triazole that is water soluble. In horses, FLUC is rapidly and well absorbed after oral administration (systemic availability of 101 ± 28%).[87] The harmonic mean elimination half-life was 37.8 hours after oral administration. Using the recommended dosing regimen (see Table 52-1), plasma FLUC concentrations are maintained at greater than 8.0 μg/mL, and FLUC is detectable in cerebrospinal fluid (CSF), synovial fluid, aqueous humor, urine,[87] vitreous, choroids, retina, iris, conjunctiva, cornea, and lung tissues[124] of healthy horses.[87] FLUC is excreted primarily in the urine, and the dose should be adjusted in horses with renal compromise. In vivo responses of fungal pathogens to FLUC may be good despite a poor response in vitro.[88,91] *Aspergillus* spp. and other molds are reported to have some intrinsic resistance to FLUC.[91] Foals with systemic candidiasis have been treated successfully with oral FLUC.[97,125] Few adverse effects of FLUC treatment are reported in humans.[91] Use of FLUC in the management of fungal diseases of horses is likely increasing, although reports evaluating clinical efficacy are lacking.

Table 52-2 Common Topical Antifungals Used to Treat Keratomycosis in Horses

Antifungal Drug	Topical Formulation and Frequency
Natamycin	5% every 6 hours
Miconazole	1% every 6 hours
Itraconazole	1% with 30% dimethyl sulfoxide (DMSO) every 6 hours
Fluconazole	0.2% every 6 hours
Ketoconazole	Not available
Amphotericin B	0.15% every 6 hours
Povidone-iodine	2% solution every 12 hours
	0.1% solution every 2-4 hours*
	7% solution to cauterize after corneal scraping*
Silver sulfadiazine[†]	Dermatologic cream 1% every 12 hours*

Data from Brooks DE: Inflammatory stromal keratopathies: medical management of stromal keratomalacia, stromal abscesses, eosinophilic keratitis, and band keratopathy in the horse. Vet Clin North Am Equine Pract 20:345, 2004.

*Data from Barton MH: Equine Keratomycosis. Compend Equine Pract 14(7):936, 1992.

[†]Efficacy against *Candida* spp. but not recommended for use in horses.

Voriconazole is a second-generation azole antifungal drug that is effective against *Aspergillus* spp. isolated from people and in the treatment of some patients with invasive aspergillosis.[114,126] Voriconazole can be given IV or orally in human patients, for whom the oral bioavailability is excellent. A single oral dose of 4 mg/kg resulted in a mean concentration of 0.86 ± 0.22 µg/mL in the aqueous humor of four healthy horse eyes.[127,128] No adverse effects were noted. Systemic absorption and distribution of voriconazole is good in horses after either intravenous or repeated oral dosing.[129-131]

Chitin Synthesis Inhibitors

These newer antifungal drugs inhibit the synthesis of chitin, an important component of the cell wall of many fungi but not of mammals. Chitin synthase inhibitors have a narrow spectrum of antifungal action.[132]

Lufenuron, a nonspecific chitin synthase inhibitor, was administered by the intrauterine route at a dose of 540 mg in 60 mL of sterile water in four mares with mycotic endometritis.[70] Based on empiric observations, the authors concluded that lufenuron contributed to the recovery of these mares. In contrast, lufenuron had no effect on the in vitro growth of *Aspergillus* and *Fusarium* spp. isolated from the corneas of horses with keratomycosis.[133] In the same study, 21 healthy adult horses were given lufenuron orally at dosages of 5 mg/kg q24h for 3 days, 20 mg/kg q24h for 3 days, or 60 mg/kg q24h for 1 day. Blood concentrations of lufenuron were lower than the ineffective concentrations achieved in vitro. Lufenuron was detected in blood samples from 20 of 21 horses. Currently, minimal data support the efficacy of lufenuron in the treatment of fungal diseases in horses.

Nikkomycin Z is a competitive inhibitor of chitin synthase. In experimental models of fungal infection, this drug has poor antifungal activity against many opportunistic fungi, including *A. fumigatus*.[126] In vitro, nikkomycin Z is synergistic with ITRA against *A. flavus* and *A. fumigatus*.[95,134] This drug has not been evaluated for use in horses.

Mycotic Keratitis

The goals of therapy are to sterilize the cornea, control secondary anterior uveitis, maximize retention of vision, speed corneal healing, and control ocular pain. Initial choice of an antifungal agent is largely based on clinical signs, results of cytologic evaluation of corneal scrapings, and knowledge of the epidemiology of fungal keratitis in the locale where the affected horse is living.

Because most reported cases of fungal keratitis in horses are caused by *Aspergillus* spp., initial treatment for this organism is recommended. Delaying therapy until culture results are reported is not in the patient's best interests because of the long time frame required to obtain results. Treatment should be suitably modified when culture results are available. Antifungal sensitivity testing may be useful in horses that respond poorly to initial antifungal therapy (see previous discussion).

A limited number of antifungal drugs are available for ocular use. These include the polyene antifungal drugs natamycin and AMB; the azoles MICON, ITRA, and FLUC; the antibiotic heavy metal combination drug silver sulfadiazine (as a 1% cream); 2% povidone-iodine solutions; and an ophthalmic ointment containing 1% ITRA and 30% dimethyl sulfoxide (DMSO).[135]

Corneal penetration of the antifungal drug is a key factor in the success of treatment. The concentration of drug in the cornea depends on the molecular mass of the drug, route of administration, ability of the drug to penetrate the corneal tissues, and duration of contact with the cornea.[115] Larger compounds, such as AMB and natamycin, barely penetrate the intact corneal epithelium after topical administration. ITRA is lipophilic and readily penetrates cell membranes. Contact time with the cornea can be increased by frequent application of drugs (hourly or q2h), by constant infusion via a subpalpebral lavage system, or by superficial keratectomy. Application of occlusive ointments also increases contact time. When the corneal epithelium is no longer intact, these factors may be less influential in the success or failure of topical treatment.[115] Long-term treatment is usually necessary to resolve the fungal infection and the attendant inflammatory reaction. Appropriate systemic antifungal therapy in conjunction with topical antifungal treatment may be beneficial in many cases.

Polyene Antifungal Drugs

Natamycin is fungicidal and available in an ophthalmic preparation for topical use. It is the least irritating of the polyene antibiotics. Natamycin has poor solubility and is administered to human and equine patients as a 5% suspension that adheres well to ulcerated corneal tissues.[65,115] Recent studies have shown that the drug penetrates the cornea well after topical application.[115] It is a broad-spectrum antifungal with favorable activity against *Fusarium* and *Aspergillus*, but it is expensive. A formulation for systemic use is not available.

AMB, also fungicidal, can be used topically in the eye as a 0.15% solution (prepared with sterile water and refrigerated in a dark bottle). AMB generally has poor corneal penetration after topical or systemic administration and is irritating. AMB has been demonstrated experimentally to impair reepithelialization of defects in rabbit corneas when applied topically as a 1% solution,[136] and it may be toxic to corneal tissue,[115] although 0.15% solutions are well tolerated by human and equine patients. AMB is reported to be irritating if used at concentrations above 0.3%,[64,137] and subconjunctival administration of more than 125 to 300 mg may induce tissue necrosis and ulceration.[64] An ophthalmic preparation of AMB is not available commercially.

Nephrotoxicity of AMB has limited its systemic use in horses. This drug can be used when other antifungal agents have failed or are suspected to be ineffective. AMB is antagonistic to MICON, and the two drugs should not be used concurrently.[56] Recently developed lipid formulations of AMB have greatly reduced toxicity in humans; however, these have not yet been studied in horses and at present are prohibitively expensive. Heat-treated AMB is less toxic than other formulations and may be useful in horses, although it has yet to be studied in this species. AMB is light sensitive and requires refrigeration for storage.[64]

Azole Antifungal Drugs

Clotrimazole is one of the first imidazole derivatives developed for topical, broad-spectrum antifungal therapy. In vitro, clotrimazole is active against dermatophytes, *Candida* spp., *Aspergillus* spp., *C. immitis*, and *C. neoformans*.[91] Three of six horses with keratomycosis were successfully treated with topical clotrimazole in the United Kingdom.[33] The use of clotrimazole to treat keratomycosis in horses is seldom reported, however, and the efficacy of the drug in the clinical setting is unknown.

Miconazole has a broad spectrum of antifungal activity that includes *Aspergillus*. In a rabbit model, topical MICON was reported to produce corneal concentrations of 10 µg/g in undebrided corneas and 93 µg/g in debrided corneas, suggesting that topical use could be effective in the treatment of keratomycosis.[115,138]

KETO is reported to induce high corneal concentrations after experimental topical administration. Although corneal toxicity is not associated with topical use, a topical formulation of this drug is not available.[115]

After oral administration in people, ITRA produces lower corneal concentrations than those induced by oral FLUC or KETO.[115] Some success in treatment of keratomycosis in horses with oral ITRA in conjunction with topical natamycin has been anecdotally reported, although approximately 50% of these equine patients required surgical treatment of their ocular fungal diseases.[139] Topical use of ITRA may also be associated with poor corneal penetration. Recently, an ointment containing 1% ultramicronized ITRA and 30% DMSO has been shown to induce equine corneal ITRA concentrations of 7.9 ± 0.33 µg/g, a value that is approximately seven times greater than that achieved by topical administration of ITRA alone.[139,140] Brooks et al[32] showed that 64% of all fungal isolates and all nine *Aspergillus* isolates in one study were susceptible to ITRA.

FLUC is minimally protein bound and highly water soluble, and it distributes well in body tissues and fluids. FLUC readily penetrates all ocular tissues and fluids in rabbits after oral administration[115] and reaches concentrations of 11.39 ± 2.83 µg/mL in the aqueous humor of healthy horses after oral administration.[87] Corneal concentrations are reported to be highly correlated with serum concentrations.[115] FLUC also achieves relatively high corneal concentrations after topical administration in rabbits,[115] but it is undetectable in equine corneas after 10 days of oral treatment (14 mg/kg loading dose, then 5 mg/kg q24h).[141] FLUC has a wide therapeutic margin of safety, and this broad-spectrum antifungal agent is fungicidal for *Aspergillus* spp.[28] In one study, however, all nine *Aspergillus* isolates were resistant to FLUC, and 21 of 22 total fungal isolates were resistant to the drug.[32] The authors recommended against the use of FLUC for mycotic keratitis in horses based on its demonstrably poor in vitro activity against equine ocular pathogens. Despite these findings, there are numerous anecdotal reports of good response of horses with keratomycosis to treatment with FLUC.[64]

Topical voriconazole, administered as 0.5% and 1% solutions to four healthy equine eyes, penetrated the corneas and induced mean aqueous humor concentrations of 1.43 ± 0.37 µg/mL and 2.35 ± 0.78 µg/mL, respectively.[127,128] Topical 3.0% solutions caused blepharospasm, epiphora, and chemosis. In vitro studies suggest that *Aspergillus* and *Fusarium* spp. isolated from horses in the United States with ulcerative keratomycosis are likely to be highly susceptible to voriconazole.[142] Topical voriconazole has been described for treatment of horses with keratomycosis.[29] Voriconazole solution (1%) was successful in treatment of two horses with corneal stromal abscessation when administered by intracorneal and subconjunctival injection.[143]

Silver Sulfadiazine

Available as a cream, silver sulfadiazine is a combination sulfonamide and heavy metal that functions as a heavy metal donor.[141] Liberated silver binds to microbial DNA and prevents replication but does not interfere with epithelial cell regeneration.[115] The drug is effective against *Aspergillus*, *Fusarium*, and yeasts.[65] An isolated report suggested that silver sulfadiazine has broad antifungal activity and is useful for the treatment of human keratomycosis.[144,145] An in vitro study showed that silver sulfadiazine was fungistatic and fungicidal for six *Aspergillus* spp. and 11 other fungal isolates from diseased eyes of horses.[144] The drug is inexpensive and has been used for the treatment of equine keratomycosis, although it is not labeled for ophthalmic use.[28] Topical application four to six times daily may be useful as initial therapy for a penetrating corneal injury with suspected plant contamination, when fiscal issues limit therapeutic options, and for follow-up treatment after intensive therapy has been completed.[64] The efficacy of silver sulfadiazine for the treatment of equine keratomycosis has been questioned.[57]

Povidone-Iodine Solution

Dilute (0.1%[65] or 2%[57]) povidone-iodine solutions may be used topically for treatment of equine keratomycosis. The efficacy of these solutions is not documented. More concentrated solutions or Lugol's iodine solution (2%-7%) should be reserved for cauterizing the cornea after corneal scraping.[65]

Thiabendazole

Thiabendazole, a thiazolyl benzimidazole anthelmintic, is reported to have fungistatic and fungicidal properties and has broad-spectrum in vitro activity against many pathogenic fungi.[145,146] Some studies showed no correlation between in vitro activity and clinical outcome.[91] Washing skin lesions caused by *Trichophyton equinum* with a thiabendazole suspension did not prevent subsequent isolation of fungi from the lesions.[92,147] This compound has been available as a 14.29% paste for deworming pigs. Joyce[146] reported treatment with thiabendazole paste of 11 horses with nonulcerative keratitis of presumed mycotic origin. Five horses treated twice daily for 30 days recovered and had no recurrence of disease for 12 months. Thiabendazole caused no ocular irritation in any of the 11 treated horses. This modality of therapy is inexpensive but of unproven efficacy.

Choice of Antifungal Medication

Aggressive treatment of equine keratomycosis should begin immediately (before culture results are available).[66] In vitro susceptibility testing suggests that voriconazole and miconazole are likely to be the most effective antifungal agents in treating ulcerative keratomycosis in horses.[142] Topical administration of voriconazole, MICON, FLUC, or ITRA is reported to be successful in treating mycotic keratitis in horses.[29,57] Topical ITRA and 30% DMSO resolved keratomycosis in 8 of 10 equine eyes (4 were positive for *Aspergillus* spp.), with a mean duration of treatment of 34.6 days (range, 16-53 days).[135] The addition of systemic antifungal therapy may be beneficial.

Brooks et al[32] reported susceptibility patterns based on minimum inhibitory concentration (MIC) and 50% inhibitory concentration (IC$_{50}$) for *Aspergillus* spp. isolated from equine cases of keratomycosis. Breakpoints for determining susceptibilities were provided. In this study, all nine *Aspergillus* isolates were resistant to FLUC and seven of nine were resistant to KETO. All nine isolates were susceptible to ITRA, MICON, and natamycin, and the authors recommend the use of MICON or natamycin, but recommended against the use of FLUC, for horses with *Aspergillus* keratitis.

Unfortunately, in vitro susceptibility information may correlate poorly with the clinical response of patients to treatment, and these relationships require further study.[17,88,115] Standard methods for susceptibility testing of filamentous fungi have been developed recently but are not universally employed or accepted.[83] In addition, criteria for determining susceptibility are often not reported. Choice of antifungal therapy for keratomycosis in horses is often based on personal preference of the attending clinician and expense of the available drugs (see Tables 52-1 and 52-2).

Duration of Therapy

Medical treatment must provide a long duration of exposure of the cornea to antifungal drugs to promote resolution of fungal infection.[57] The mean duration of successful treatment in two studies was 27 (range, 12-82) days and 48 (range, 31-192) days.[27,65] When clinical signs have improved, the frequency of treatment may be decreased. Signs of improvement include healing of the corneal epithelium (no fluorescein uptake) and diminished signs of uveitis (absence of aqueous flare, reduced ocular pain resulting in absence of blepharospasm and photophobia). Deep stromal neovascularization changes in color from deep red to pale pink or white,[57] and the corneal scar becomes more dense from fibrosis as the lesion contracts during healing. Antifungal therapies may be fungistatic rather than fungicidal, and intact fungi may remain indolent in corneal tissue. Evidence of worsening of clinical signs should prompt return to aggressive, frequent medical treatment.

Surgical Treatment

Deep or rapidly progressing corneal infections, especially those characterized by keratomalacia or that respond poorly to medical treatment, and stromal abscesses that do not respond to medical treatment in 48 to 72 hours usually require surgical intervention.[27,57,148] Necrotic corneal tissue and associated fungal organisms are debrided. Cytologic examination and culture of material obtained by surgical debridement may provide a definitive diagnosis. Debridement and keratectomy increase drug penetration into infected corneal tissue and reduce collagenolysis.[59] Subsequent application of a flap or graft improves corneal integrity and supplies vascular access to fungal ulcers or stromal abscesses. The use of conjunctival pedicle grafts, bridge grafts, hood grafts, island grafts, and full-thickness penetrating keratoplasty has been reported.[17,27,57] Postsurgical corneal scarring may be extensive; however, early surgical intervention may speed recovery and improve the prognosis for saving the globe and for sight.[27,57]

Medical therapy should continue for several weeks after surgery, depending on clinical signs.[17] Six to 8 weeks after placement of a conjunctival flap, the limbal attachment may be severed.

Other Treatments

Atropine sulfate and flunixin meglumine for control of uveitis and ocular pain, topical antiproteinase therapy, and prevention of collagenolysis have been recently reviewed.[57] Flunixin meglumine may reduce the rate of corneal vascularization and therefore impair healing.[57,149] Nonsteroidal antiinflammatory drugs (NSAIDs) that reduce iridocyclitis and anterior uveitis, which are potentially blinding complications, must be employed in the context of careful assessment of the rate of corneal vascularization. Phenylbutazone may have a less negative effect on corneal vascularization than flunixin meglumine and may be a good choice when corneal vascularization is proceeding slowly.[57,149] Bacterial keratitis may complicate keratomycosis, and concurrent topical antibiotic therapy is recommended.[20,27,59,60,65]

Fibrosis and scar formation after successful treatment of mycotic keratitis may reduce vision and can be aesthetically unappealing. Cyclosporin A, an agent that inhibits proliferation of fibroblasts and increases fibroblast apoptosis, may be useful to reduce corneal scarring, although this treatment modality has not been studied in horses.[57] Topical antibiotic-steroid therapy at this time may help to reduce vascularization and corneal scarring,[17] although treatment with corticosteroids is risky if viable fungi remain in the cornea.[57]

Corticosteroid Treatment Contraindicated

Corticosteroid drugs should never be employed by any route in the treatment of equine keratomycosis.

Prognosis

Potential complications of keratomycosis include corneal scarring and pigmentation, iris prolapse, uveitis, synechia, cataract formation, rupture of the eye, endophthalmitis, phthisis bulbi, and blindness.[65] After medical treatment, 43% to 56% of horses have some vision, approximately 10% have a nonvisual eye, and 25% to 48% require enucleation.[64] The prognosis can be substantially improved by a combination of intensive medical treatment and timely surgical intervention. In one study, 63% of horses treated with combined medical and surgical therapy were "visual"[59]; in a second study, 92% of treated horses retained sight.[27]

Pulmonary Aspergillosis

There is only one report of successful treatment of pulmonary aspergillosis in a horse.[47] Invasive pulmonary aspergillosis represents a serious therapeutic challenge in human patients as well.[150] *Aspergillus* spp. are often sensitive to ITRA and are variably sensitive to AMB and FLUC.[97] Voriconazole is likely to be effective,[47,114] but to date, clinical experience with this second-generation azole in horses is limited, and its expense may preclude its use except in neonatal foals.[47]

The prognosis for horses with pulmonary aspergillosis is extremely poor. The disease was fatal for all 29 affected horses in a retrospective study,[38] as well as for all affected horses in other reports.[3,41-43] The single report of a surviving horse was a neonatal foal treated with oral voriconazole.[47] The poor prognosis may reflect the difficulty in making an early diagnosis of pulmonary aspergillosis and the severity of other concurrent disease. The ability to diagnose this disease reliably in its early stages may improve success in treatment. Real-time PCR may permit earlier diagnosis; however, the methodology has not yet been validated in this clinical setting.

Nasal and Sinus Aspergillosis

When the lesions of nasal aspergillosis represent focal disease, the prognosis for recovery is good with aggressive therapy, usually a combination of surgical debulking and topical antifungal drugs. Horses with nasal and pulmonary aspergillosis have a poor prognosis because of the devastating nature of the pulmonary disease.

Three horses with nasal aspergillosis responded to topical treatment with natamycin (25 mg/100 mL sterile water) followed by insufflation of natamycin powder, although the condition did recur in one horse.[67] Lavage with 1% natamycin solution after transendoscopic removal of large mycotic plaques was successful in treating 10 of 11 horses with mycotic sinonasal disease.[68] Debulking facilitates medical management. Of eight horses with nasal rhinitis associated with *Aspergilllus* spp. and treated with topical enilconazole, seven horses recovered and no adverse effects were noted.[151] Horses were treated topically via a catheter placed through the nasal meatus or through the lateral nasal wall for a mean of 3.8 weeks with each treatment consisting of 25 to 100 mL of a 0.2% to 2% solution of enilconazole.

Endometritis and Placentitis

Treatment of endometritis caused by *Aspergillus* spp. has included copious lavage of the uterus followed by instillation of AMB (in sterile water or saline), clotrimazole, nystatin, or FLUC; lavage with dilute iodine solutions; and intrauterine plasma.[24,34] Results of treatment are often suboptimal. Iodine solutions may cause irritation and fibrosis. Systemic treatment with FLUC has also been suggested for mares that do not respond to repeated uterine lavage and topical antifungal therapy.[24] In one study, intrauterine lufenuron showed promise for the treatment of fungal endometritis,[70] although the efficacy of lufenuron in this clinical setting has not been critically evaluated.

The prognosis for recovery from fungal endometritis is poor. Fungal endometritis and frequent lavage, particularly with iodine solutions, may result in adhesions of the uterus, vagina, or cervix.[34] Fertility may be reduced.

Aflatoxicosis

No specific antidote exists for acute aflatoxicosis, and supportive therapy (fluids, analgesics, sedatives as needed) should be instituted. In subacute intoxication, gastrointestinal absorption of aflatoxins can be reduced by oral administration of sodium calcium aluminosilicate, an agent that adsorbs aflatoxins.[35] Supplementary vitamin E and selenium may be beneficial. Prevention of ingestion of contaminated grains is imperative.

The complete reference list is available online at www.expertconsult.com.

---

53 Miscellaneous Fungal Diseases

Debra C. Sellon, Maureen T. Long, and Catherine Kohn*

Blastomycosis

Blastomycosis is an extremely rare disease in horses. Fatal disseminated infection has been reported in two horses and a miniature horse, and fatal subcutaneous infection was reported in a third horse. *Blastomyces dermatitidis* is not contagious or zoonotic. Clusters of cases occur in persons and dogs as a result of exposure to a common environmental source of the fungi. The ecology of this fungus is still incompletely understood.

Etiology

The thermally dimorphic ascomycete *B. dermatitidis* is the cause of all manifestations of blastomycosis. Conidia, measuring 2 to 10 μm in diameter, are the infectious agents. The yeast form is thick walled and usually 8 to 15 μm in diameter, although yeasts as large as 30 μm have been reported.[1] In tissues, yeast cells display characteristic broad-based buds.

Virulence Factors

Several factors contribute to the virulence of *B. dermatitidis*.[2] In tissues the organism converts to a yeast form that is more resistant to phagocytosis and killing than are conidia. The yeast cell wall may have antiphagocytic properties, and cell wall phospholipids may contribute to virulence.[3] The BAD1 antigen (formerly called *WI-1*), a cell wall surface antigen, is an important factor for the adherence of yeasts to macrophages and to lung tissue. Loss of the antigen results in impaired binding and entry into macrophages and in diminished capacity of the yeast to adhere to the lung. A strain of *B. dermatitidis* experimentally deprived of this antigen by gene deletion was avirulent in mice.[4] BAD1 has other antiinflammatory effects that include influencing the profile of proinflammatory cytokines, such as suppressing tumor necrosis factor alpha (TNF-α) release by host macrophages.[5]

Epidemiology

The ecology of the filamentous form of *B. dermatitidis* in nature has proved challenging to define, and the organism is difficult to isolate from environmental sources. Based on environmental isolates in two outbreaks of human and canine disease, the mycelial form of *B. dermatitidis* is thought to be a saprophyte found in moist soil of acid pH and high organic content, usually in wooded areas near water.[1,2] Optimal conditions for growth of the mycelia in its natural microenvironment may be short lived, and the organism may be present in large numbers only transiently. *B. dermatitidis* is endemic in the Mississippi, Missouri, and Ohio River watersheds; the Great Lakes regions of the United States and Canada; and the St. Lawrence River Valley[1,2] (Fig. 53-1). The disease is also found in Africa but is seldom reported from other parts of the world.

Blastomycosis has been reported in many species, most often in dogs and humans,[6] but rarely in horses. Dogs are considered sentinel animals for human infections. Blastomycosis is not contagious or zoonotic among infected persons or animals. The disease occurs sporadically, although clusters of cases have been described and are likely associated with an increase in infective conidia in an environment that is transiently optimal for mycelia growth. *B. dermatitidis* was isolated from soil on the banks of a beaver pond near a camp in Wisconsin; 48 people who visited the camp developed blastomycosis.[7] Most infections occur during the cooler and wetter months of the year. Agricultural workers, hunters, campers, and their canine companions are particularly at risk for infection.[1]

The prevalence of asymptomatic pulmonary infections is unknown. Spontaneous recovery from an identified blastomycosis infection in humans is uncommon, and mortality rates in

*The authors acknowledge and appreciate the original contributions of these authors, whose work has been incorporated into this chapter.

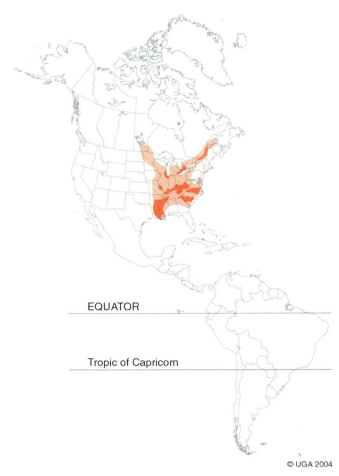

EQUATOR

Tropic of Capricorn

© UGA 2004

Figure 53-1 Shading indicates area of endemic blastomycosis. Darker shading indicates areas of higher incidence. *(From Greene C: Infectious diseases of the dog and cat, ed 3, Philadelphia, 2006, Saunders.)*

untreated persons with chronic blastomycosis may be as high as 60%.[2] *B. dermatitidis* organisms are not among the flora of healthy persons. These findings suggest that the incidence of asymptomatic infection may be low.

Pathogenesis

Blastomycosis is a disease of immunocompetent persons and is relatively infrequently reported as an opportunistic infection in immunocompromised patients.[2] In patients with acquired immunodeficiency syndrome (AIDS), the neurologic form of blastomycosis is more common, and the disease is more severe and more often fatal than in immunocompetent patients.[8] Infection most often occurs by inhalation of aerosolized conidia. In the lungs the conidia are phagocytized by neutrophils, monocytes, and alveolar macrophages. Macrophages may inhibit the conversion of conidia to yeasts, but conidia that remain viable in tissues rapidly transform into the more resistant yeast. A robust cellular immune response is crucial in the host's defense against the organism. *B. dermatitidis* has a predilection for bone and skin and may reach these organs by dissemination from the lungs. Infection may also occur by direct inoculation through the skin.

Intravenous inoculation of one horse with *B. dermatitidis* caused chronic inflammatory foci in the lungs.[9] Subcutaneous

inoculation did not produce disease. No further details of these studies are available.

Clinical Findings

Clinical signs in human patients with blastomycosis are variable and often nonspecific; weight loss, fever, malaise, and fatigue are common to many diseases. The onset is usually insidious, and the clinical course is often chronic. Pulmonary, cutaneous, osseous, genitourinary, and central nervous system (CNS) abnormalities, as well as sporadic disease of almost any organ, have been reported in humans.[2] Forty percent of dogs with blastomycosis have ocular lesions.[6] Misdiagnosis is common in human patients, possibly because the index of suspicion for this disease is low, but also because blastomycosis can mimic many other diseases. For example, pulmonary manifestations of blastomycosis can be easily confused with bacterial pneumonia, tuberculosis, or neoplasia.[2]

Several equine cases have been reported in the literature,[10-14] and the author has seen one additional case.[15] One horse had cutaneous blastomycosis,[10] one had cutaneous disease with concurrent osteomyelitis,[13] three had cutaneous and disseminated disease involving lung and multiple other body sites,[12,14] and two horses had fatal disseminated blastomycosis without cutaneous disease.[11,15] Cutaneous disease was the primary presenting complaint when present, and cytologic evaluation of exudate typically revealed yeast-like organisms identified as *Blastomyces*. In horses without cutaneous disease the primary complaint was lethargy, weight loss, and cough and *B. dermatitidis* yeast forms were seen in peritoneal and pleural fluid. The identity of the observed yeast was confirmed by culture or molecular techniques.

In this small case series, blastomycosis in horses tended to be a disseminated or locally aggressive and fatal disease. Two of the affected horses resided in the Ohio River Valley, one horse was from eastern Pennsylvania, and two were from Minnesota. Although rare, blastomycosis should be considered a differential diagnosis for horses with pneumonia, pleuritis, peritonitis, or skin disease that is poorly responsive to antibiotic therapy, particularly if the affected horse resides in a region where blastomycosis is endemic.

Diagnosis

Radiography and ultrasonography may be helpful in determining the location and extent of abscesses caused by *B. dermatitidis*. Evaluation of the hemogram, serum chemistry profile, and serum fibrinogen aid in evaluating the systemic effects of infection.

Cytology

Cytologic examination of body fluids (transtracheal aspirate, bronchoalveolar lavage, pleural, peritoneal, cutaneous exudate) often allows identification of typical, thick-walled yeasts that are 8 to 15 μm in diameter with broad-based budding.[1] The sensitivity of cytologic examination for diagnosis of blastomycosis in human patients was 93% in one study.[16]

Ancillary Diagnostic Testing

In biopsies of tissues from affected humans, epithelioid granulomata, pyogranulomatous inflammation, necrosis, and fibrosis may be seen.[1] Yeasts are usually plentiful in infected tissues (Figs. 53-2 and 53-3). The thick-walled yeast cells are generally of uniform size (8-15 μm in diameter), although large cells (20-30 μm) have been described. Broad-based budding is the identifying feature and must be seen to have strong evidence of the presence of *B. dermatitidis*. The yeast wall may not stain with hematoxylin and eosin (H&E), and the cytoplasm may

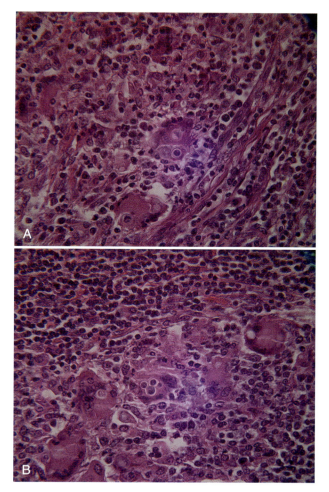

Figure 53-2 Photomicrographs of *Blastomyces dermatitidis* in lymph node of the horse described by Toribio et al.[11] **A,** Note broad-based bud. **B,** Note multiple giant cells.

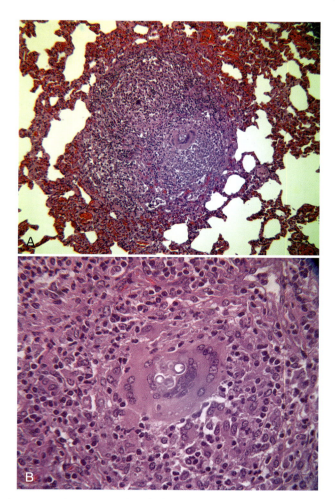

Figure 53-3 Photomicrographs of *Blastomyces dermatitidis* in the lung of 3-year-old Rocky Mountain mare with disseminated blastomycosis. **A,** 30×. **B,** 40×.

shrink away from the wall, leaving a space.[1] The sensitivity of histopathologic testing for the diagnosis of blastomycosis in persons in one study was 81.5%.[16]

Culture

Samples of infected body fluids or tissues usually produce characteristic yeasts within 2 to 4 weeks in cultures incubated at 37° C (98.6° F).[2] Culture is still considered the "gold standard" for the diagnosis of blastomycosis in human patients, although the sensitivity of this test in one study was 66.4%.[16]

On Sabouraud dextrose agar incubated at 25° C (77° F), the growth rate of the filamentous fungi is variable and slow, and cultures should be held for 2 months or more.[1] Colonies may be flat and glabrous (described as "skinlike") or may be fluffy white to brownish tan, sometimes with concentric rings. The appearance of the conidia is not distinctive, and identification of *B. dermatitidis* depends on observing the characteristic yeasts that appear within days to weeks when subcultures are incubated at 37° C.[1]

Molecular Identification of Yeasts

Molecular techniques for identification of the yeast form of *B. dermatitidis* in culture and fixed tissues are commercially available.[17] The application of deoxyribonucleic acid (DNA) amplification techniques to samples of body fluids or fresh tissues from clinical patients requires further study.

Serology

Antibody Detection

Serology has not proved to be a sensitive or specific method of diagnosing blastomycosis in humans. Immunocompromised persons may produce low concentrations of antibodies. A comparison of results from enzyme-linked immunosorbent assay (ELISA), complement fixation (CF), and immunodiffusion (ID) tests for antibody to *B. dermatitidis* in persons with documented blastomycosis showed that the assays had diagnostic sensitivity of 80%, 40%, and 65%, respectively.[18] Cross-reactions with other fungi (particularly *Histoplasma capsulatum*) are common.[2] An agar-gel immunodiffusion (AGID) test currently used in the diagnosis of canine blastomycosis has a sensitivity and specificity of greater than 90%. However, positive serologic testing alone is not considered sufficient to establish the diagnosis.[6]

When purified WI-1 (BAD1) antigen was used in a radioimmunoassay (RIA) to detect serum antibodies to *B. dermatitidis*, 85% of 68 persons known to have the disease were identified.[19] The RIA also detected 3% of patients with histoplasmosis, coccidioidomycosis, sporotrichosis, or candidiasis. All healthy persons had negative tests. In another study, anti–WI-1 serologic testing identified 75% of 32 human patients with blastomycosis.[20] Testing by RIA detected anti–WI-1 antibodies in 92% of infected dogs,[21] and RIA titers declined during treatment, suggesting that the RIA might be useful in monitoring the progress of therapy in affected dogs. AGID detected antibodies against the A antigen of *B. dermatitidis* in 41% of dogs with blastomycosis.[21]

Antigen Detection

Detection of *B. dermatitidis* antigen in the urine of persons and dogs with blastomycosis has been reported. Durkin et al[16] used antibodies to mold antigens in an immunoassay and showed that the sensitivity of the test in patients with blastomycosis was 92.9% and the specificity 79.3%. Cross-reactions occurred in 96% of patients with histoplasmosis, 100% of those with paracoccidioidomycosis, 2.9% of those with cryptococcosis, and 1.1% of patients with aspergillosis. Shurley et al[22] used a competitive-binding inhibition ELISA test with antibodies raised against yeast-phase lysates and detected antigen in the urine of 100% of 36 dogs with blastomycosis. Unfortunately, cross-reactivity with *H. capsulatum* and elements in urine from healthy dogs were observed in this study. The sensitivity and specificity of tests for antigen determination should be optimized before these assays can be used reliably in the clinical setting. These tests may be useful in combination with results of physical examination, cytology, and culture in patients with suspected blastomycosis.

Therapy

Antifungal treatment of horses with blastomycosis has not been attempted. Recommendations for treatment of humans with blastomycosis are based on limited data.[2] Amphotericin B (AMB) (0.5-0.6 mg/kg/day until the disease is controlled) is the treatment of choice in patients with life-threatening disease. After the disease has been controlled, an oral azole drug can be substituted for AMB. Itraconazole is the drug of choice for patients who have non–life-threatening disease that does not involve the central nervous system (CNS). Recent reviews suggest that voriconazole may also be an effective treatment alone or in combination with AMB, especially in patients with CNS blastomycosis.[23-25] Ketoconazole can be used for pulmonary infections that are not life threatening, although there are reports of CNS blastomycosis in patients who were successfully treated with ketoconazole for chest disease.[2] Ketoconazole distributes poorly to the CNS. Fluconazole is reported to have efficacy comparable to ketoconazole, is less toxic, and achieves good concentrations in the CNS. Fluconazole is an alternative in patients who cannot tolerate itraconazole.

Prevention

Recent studies have demonstrated that mice can be protected from an intrapulmonary challenge of *B. dermatitidis* by subcutaneous injection of a mutant strain of the fungus.[5] The mutant strain lacks the BAD1 gene and therefore the BAD1 cell surface antigen, previously shown to be a virulence factor. Mouse protection was characterized by the induction of a strong cell-mediated immune response. Because blastomycosis occurs rarely in the horse, it is unlikely that development of an effective vaccine would be warranted for this species. However, for persons or horses in endemic regions, vaccination might be a consideration in the future.

Cryptococcosis

Cryptococcosis is an uncommon disease in horses, although the incidence of asymptomatic infection is unknown. Among approximately 40 horses reported to have cryptococcal infection, respiratory and CNS diseases were the most common clinical manifestations. Cryptococcus is not contagious, and cases occur sporadically. Clustering of cases in Australia may be related to the fact that ubiquitous eucalyptus trees are known to harbor cryptococci. Few horses with cryptococcosis have been treated, and there is little information in the literature to guide judgments on prognosis (usually considered to be poor) and therapy.

Etiology

Cryptococcus neoformans and *Cryptococcus gattii*, formerly known as *C. neoformans* var. *gattii*,[26] are the cause of virtually all cryptococcal disease in mammals.[27] Because of the recent change in classification of *C. gattii*, most of the literature refers to this organism as a variant of *C. neoformans*. Consequently, in this chapter, unless otherwise stated, comments regarding *C. neoformans* can be taken to refer also to *C. gattii*. *C. neoformans*, classified in the phylum Basidiomycotina, is a spherical to ovoid, budding yeast 3 to 25 μm in diameter[28] that possesses a capsule 1 to 30 μm in thickness composed of at least three heteroglycans.[29] The heteroglycan composition of the capsule is the basis for distinguishing the many species of *C. neoformans*, of which two (in addition to *C. gattii*) are the cause of most diseases: *C. neoformans* var. *grubii* and *C. neoformans* var. *neoformans*. In animal tissues and fluids the yeast reproduces by typically narrow-based budding.[29]

Virulence Factors

C. neoformans has three genetically controlled characteristics largely responsible for its virulence: the ability to produce a capsule, melanin formation, and the ability to grow at 37° C.[30]

Capsule

The distinctive polysaccharide capsule of the yeast affords several modes of protection from the host's immune response. The capsule blocks phagocytosis, masks ligands on the fungal cell surface to which antibodies might bind, reduces the respiratory burst of phagocytes, downregulates production of protective cytokines (T helper cell type 1 [Th1] response), and upregulates production of Th2 cytokines.[27,30] Mutant cryptococcal organisms that have deficient capsules are less virulent than their parent strains, and increases in virulence have been associated with structural changes or increased thickness of the capsule.[30,31] The capsules of the yeast may enlarge during infection.[30,32] Circulating solubilized capsular polysaccharide antigens in human patients with disseminated cryptococcosis may inhibit leukocyte migration to the site of cryptococcal infection.[33]

Melanin

Cryptococcus organisms are efficient producers of melanin through the enzyme phenol oxidase.[31] Melanin scavenges oxygen free radicals derived from leukocytes, and this antioxidant effect contributes to virulence.[30,33] Melanin also impairs antibody formation, depresses lymphoproliferation, and downregulates TNF-α production.[27] Because it contributes to the negative charge of *C. neoformans*, melanin may also impair phagocytosis of the organism.[33]

Thermotolerance

The ability to live and replicate at mammalian body temperature (37° C) is a characteristic of invasive fungal pathogens in general. Temperature-sensitive mutant strains of *C. neoformans* are avirulent in mammalian models of cryptococcal disease. The ability to grow at high temperature is under the control of multiple genes in *C. neoformans*.[30]

Epidemiology

C. neoformans is an opportunistic, saprophytic yeast that is ubiquitous worldwide. Bird manure, particularly pigeon droppings, and bat guano harbor *C. neoformans* var. *grubii* and *C. neoformans* var. *neoformans*, which can remain viable for up to 2 years in fecal material.[1] Purines, urea, and creatinine are present in high concentrations in bird excreta and readily used by the yeast as substrates for metabolism.[34,35] The pigeon may be the most important vector for dispersing *C. neoformans* and maintaining it in the environment.[1] *C. neoformans* is also found in rotting wood, and *C. gattii* has been associated with flowering red and river gum trees (species of Eucalyptus trees) in Australia, Columbia, India, and southern California.[29] The prevalence of eucalyptus trees in the environment may explain the relatively frequent occurrence of cryptococcosis in horses and other species in western Australia.[36,37] *C. gattii* is endemic in Australia.[26] Admixture of soil with contaminated feces or rotting material from trees results in a reduction in numbers of organisms, possibly because of ingestion by soil amebae.[1] The yeast can also be isolated from ripe fruits, rotting vegetables, and dairy products.[1] High humidity fosters growth of *C. neoformans*, whereas exposure to direct sunlight can kill the yeast.[1]

Disease caused by *C. neoformans* usually occurs sporadically. Outbreaks comprising multiple cases of affected persons or animals, presumably exposed to the same source of the organism, are infrequently reported, and transmission of disease among affected animals or humans has not been described.[31] A large outbreak of *C. gattii* in humans, dogs, cats, ferrets, llamas, and porpoises was reported in British Columbia.[38] Vancouver Island was found to be heavily colonized with *C. gattii*, an organism formerly thought to be restricted to warm and tropical climates. The worldwide distribution of this pathogen may be changing.[26] Although *C. neoformans*, and particularly *C. gattii*, cause disease in immunocompetent people, these yeasts are primarily opportunistic pathogens, and most affected humans and animals are immunocompromised, such as from human immunodeficiency virus (HIV) infection, corticosteroid treatment, chronic leukemia, lymphoma, sarcoidosis, and Cushing's disease.[1,30,31] Men are more frequently infected than women, and most cases occur in postpubertal persons.[31] *C. neoformans* infection has also been associated with pregnancy in women.[1]

Although *C. neoformans* is an opportunistic pathogen, it can be recovered from healthy persons on the skin or in sputum, where it may be an incidental or transient colonizer.[1] Most adults possess antibodies to this organism,[30] and the incidence of asymptomatic infection is unknown. In a preliminary study, 3% of 61 healthy horses in New South Wales had serum antibodies to *C. neoformans*, suggesting previous exposure to or latent infection with cryptococci.[37,39] In southwestern British Columbia, Canada, an area where *C. gattii* is emerging as an important human and animal pathogen, 4 of 260 horses tested had nasal colonization with *C. gattii* but none had a serum cryptococcal antigen titer.[40]

Pathogenesis

The pathogenesis of cryptococcal infections in human patients has been reviewed,[27,30,31,33] but very little is known about the pathogenesis of infection in horses. Cryptococcal disease in healthy people or animals may result from exposure to a large dose of the yeast or to a particularly virulent strain.[31] Initial exposure to the organism occurs by ingestion, contact through abraded skin or mucous membranes, or most often, inhalation of either desiccated yeast cells or (more likely) basidiospores. Basidiospores are produced in the environment by the sexual form of the *C. neoformans*, *Filobasidiella neoformans*, or from monokaryotic hyphae that develop under appropriate conditions, in the absence of mating.[33] Desiccated, poorly encapsulated yeast cells usually have a diameter greater than 2 µm (too large to be easily aerosolized and readily respirable) and reduced viability, whereas basidiospores, with a diameter of 2 µm, are small enough to reach the distal airways when inspired[33] and are resistant to desiccation. Mucociliary responses clear healthy airways of most inhaled infectious fungal propagules, and those that reach the alveoli are controlled by local host inflammatory responses, resulting in elimination of the fungi by alveolar macrophages, lymphocytes, neutrophils, and activated T cells. A robust cell-mediated immune response is essential to successful host defense against cryptococci, and Th1 immune responses are important for protective immunity.[30]

Antibodies to *C. neoformans* may be detected in human patients with early or focal infections.[8] During active disseminated infection, antibodies are usually not detectable, perhaps as a result of forming complexes with circulating capsular cryptococcal antigens or inhibition of antibody synthesis by these antigens.[8,31] In some human studies, antibody titers increase as capsular antigen titers decrease, and the patient improves clinically.[39] The presence of antibody in the serum of infected persons may be an indication for an improved prognosis.[8,39]

Yeasts that are not destroyed by the immune inflammatory response are segregated by a chronic inflammatory process that produces granulomas. The presence of a large granuloma reflects a robust cell-mediated immune response to cryptococcal organisms.[37,41] In one study, three of seven horses with *C. neoformans* infection had large granulomas in the dorsocaudal lung.[36] The same three horses had evidence of exercise-induced pulmonary hemorrhage (EIPH), and the investigators suggested that EIPH may predispose affected lung to colonization by inhaled cryptococci.[36] The dorsocaudal region of the lung receives air through the terminal ramifications of the principal bronchus and is a likely site for deposition of inhaled particles.[36,42] In addition, this is a common site in which to find evidence of EIPH.

In immunocompetent persons, *C. neoformans* may persist indefinitely in a latent state within a granuloma.[30] In theory, subsequent reactivation of latent infection may be associated with immune suppression or concurrent disease and may result in a disseminated cryptococcal infection, without evidence of recent infection.

In immunocompromised hosts, particularly those with CD4+ T-cell deficiency, cryptococcal infection disseminates within the lung and is translocated across the gastrointestinal (GI) wall after ingestion of infectious propagules or swallowing of infected nasal or pulmonary secretions and then disseminates hematogenously to other tissues, with a predilection for the leptomeninges and CNS. Dissemination from the lung may take weeks or months in human patients.[8] The reason this organism favors the CNS has not been documented. Infection of the nasal cavity and the maxillary and frontal sinuses in the horse could result in meningitis and CNS invasion by direct extension through the cribriform plate.[36,38] Hematogenous dispersion to the CNS has also been suggested.

Cryptococcal endometritis may be associated with chronic yeast colonization of the clitoral sinus.[44]

Clinical Findings

A review of 44 cases of cryptococcosis in horses reported since 1902 showed that 16 horses had pneumonia or pleuritis,[34,36,37,45,46] 12 had upper respiratory tract infections (nasal plaques, sinus infections),[34,47-49] 11 had CNS disease,[34,43,50-53] three had abdominal disease,[34,36,54] two had endometritis,[44,45] one had a locally aggressive subcutaneous mass,[55] and one had disseminated disease with osteomyelitis.[56] One horse had both pneumonia and CNS disease,[52] and another had a nasal granuloma and jejunal lesion.[54] McGill et al reported an additional 20 horses with cryptococcosis in Western Australia with affected horses tending to have lower respiratory tract involvement.[57]

Onset of disease is often insidious, with a slow progression characterized by vague signs. Purulent nasal discharge often creamy white in color, cough, and weight loss were common signs in horses with respiratory disease. Two foals aborted by mares with cryptococcal placentitis or endometritis had cryptococcal pneumonia.[58] Violent dementia, head tilt, ipsilateral weakness, unilateral blindness, ataxia, and weight loss were clinical signs of the neurologic form of cryptococcal disease. A pregnant mare with a large, abdominal cryptococcal granuloma had weight loss and poor fetal growth.[36] Another horse had colic resulting from an intraluminal jejunal cryptococcal granuloma within an intussusception.[34] A jejunal lesion was an incidental finding in a horse with a cryptococcal nasal granuloma.[54] One horse had a large, nonhealing skin lesion that extended into the subcutaneous tissues, invading through several intercostal spaces to the pleura.[55]

Diagnosis

Clinical Diagnostic Testing

Endoscopic examination of the nasal passages permits close evaluation of cryptococcal lesions in the upper airways.[48,49] The nasomaxillary ostia and the ethmoturbinate regions should be carefully examined. Tissue for cytology, culture, and histopathology can often be obtained endoscopically. Tracheoscopy may be useful to observe exudates, and bronchoscopy may help to localize the lesions and to obtain samples through bronchoalveolar lavage (BAL).

Radiography and Computed Tomography

The extent of cryptococcal infection in the nasal passages, the maxillary and frontal sinuses, and the ethmoid region should be evaluated radiographically.[48,49] Computed tomography (CT) may be useful to define these lesions further, although it remains to be determined if CT will provide more information than radiography, which has the advantage of ready availability in the standing horse.

Ancillary Diagnostic Testing

Cryptococci can be seen in clinical specimens (cerebrospinal fluid [CSF], abdominal or pleural fluid, transtracheal aspirates, BAL fluid, aspirates from infected lesions) when stained with new methylene blue, Gram stain, or Romanovsky-type stains[29,36,53,56] (Fig. 53-4). Wright's stain is frequently used but may distort the capsule and shrink the organism.[59] India ink preparations demonstrate the capsule and may be especially useful for samples of CSF. A drop of the specimen is deposited on a drop of India ink on a slide and then covered with a coverslip.[60] The yeast (unstained) is silhouetted against a black background, and the capsule appears as a large, transparent halo[59] (Fig. 53-5). In wet preparations the cell wall is refractory, and the capsule varies in thickness from a few micrometers to a diameter greater than that of the yeast cell.[31] Yeast cells are spherical and may appear with a single bud, attached by a thin connection. Care should be taken in examining India ink preparations. When budding is not seen, lymphocytes, fat droplets, and aggregated droplets of India ink may be mistaken for yeasts.[8,59,61] Inability to visualize yeasts in cytologic preparations does not rule out infection. Yeast cells with small capsules or present in small numbers are easily overlooked.[59]

Biopsy

Impression smears from biopsy specimens can be rapidly evaluated by cytology. In tissues the yeast capsule does not stain well

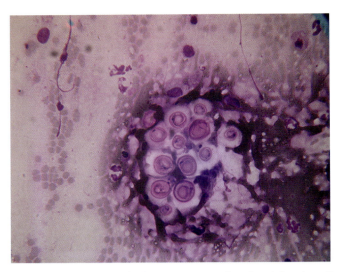

Figure 53-4 Photomicrograph of cryptococci in exudates from infected maxillary sinus in horse.

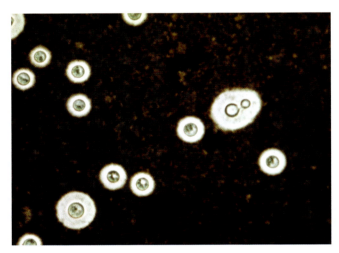

Figure 53-5 Cryptococci in India ink preparation. The infected material was obtained from a cat. *(Courtesy Dr. Joe Kowalski, The Ohio State University College of Veterinary Medicine.)*

with periodic acid–Schiff (PAS), Gomori's methenamine silver (GMS), or Masson-Fontana stains that show encapsulated yeast cells (often distorted or collapsed) with a thin cell wall, surrounded by apparently empty space[31,59] (Fig. 53-6). Mayer's mucicarmine, which stains the capsule rose-red and the cell pink, is the best choice and does not stain other fungal organisms that might be confused with cryptococci such as *Blastomyces* or *Coccidioides*.[59] The associated inflammatory response may be minimal or granulomatous.[31]

Culture

C. neoformans is easily cultured on standard fungal media that do not contain cycloheximide. Large, cream to yellow-colored colonies appear in 3 to 5 days when the yeast is cultured on Sabouraud dextrose agar.[29] Encapsulated colonies are mucoid.[59] Mycelia are rarely observed in culture. Colonies produce urease, assimilate D-proline, and grow readily at 37° C.[29] A generous inoculum may increase the likelihood of a positive culture. Sedimentation of 15 to 20 mL of CSF is reported to facilitate culturing cryptococci in other species,[59] and collecting such a large sample from an adult horse would be feasible.

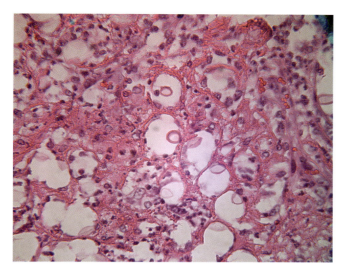

Figure 53-6 Photomicrograph of cryptococci in meninges of horse. Note the clear halo of the unstained capsule surrounding the yeast cell (40×).

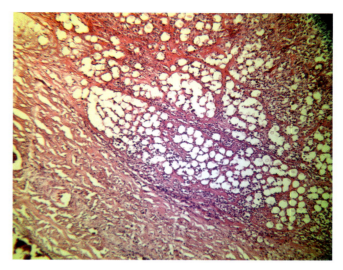

Figure 53-7 At higher magnification, *Cryptococcus neoformans* are characterized by a "soap bubble" appearance.

C. neoformans can be distinguished from most other species of *Cryptococcus* by its ability to produce melanin through phenol oxidase. When cultured on Staib's birdseed agar, colonies acquire brown to black pigment.[31] Several commercial methods are available to identify the species of the isolate. For epidemiologic studies, individual strains of *C. neoformans* can be biotyped or fingerprinted.[31]

Cultures may require several weeks for a positive result and thus are not helpful in the immediate management of clinical patients. A rapid urease test is used for expedient identification of *C. neoformans* in human patients.[31]

Serology

Assays for Cryptococcal Antigens

In persons and cats with cryptococcosis, the capsular polysaccharide antigen glucuronoxylomannan is not rapidly cleared from circulation and may be identified by a latex agglutination assay that utilizes specific rabbit hyperimmune immunoglobulin coating the latex particles.[8] Five immunodiagnostic kits for identification of cryptococcal antigen are commercially available in the United States.[31,59] Depending on the particular kit, these tests can detect as little as 10 ng of capsular polysaccharide.[31] Elimination of most interfering substances can be accomplished by digesting the test serum or CSF with pronase.[31,62] In humans a positive agglutination at a dilution of 1:4 is strongly suggestive of cryptococcal infection, whereas a titer of 1:8 is usually an indication of active infection.[31] Infected cats may display very high dilution titers (1:10,000), and a titer greater than 1 is considered positive.[47] Antigen detection is more sensitive (about 95%) than culture (about 75%) or India ink preparation in people[31] and is reported to have a sensitivity of 95% and a specificity of 100% in the cat.[63] False-positive tests may result from rare cross-reactions with antigens from other microorganisms (e.g., *Trichosporon asahii*, formerly *T. beigleii*) or contamination with agar or agarose.[8,31] False-negative tests may arise as a result of low levels of antigen, interfering immune complexes, a prozone effect (high titers of antigen), or infection with a strain that is poorly encapsulated or unencapsulated.[31] Pretreatment of the sample with pronase eliminates the immune complexes, and the effect of antigen excess is ameliorated by dilution.[8]

Changes in capsular antigen titer have proved useful in monitoring response to treatment in cats and humans.[31,59] Successful treatment is associated with a reduction in antigen titer, although decreases in antigen titer may lag behind clinical response.[59] Because results from test kits may vary, it is important to use the same methodology for successive tests.

In the few reports of measurement of serum cryptococcal antigen titers in horses, this test appears to be useful in the diagnosis and management of cryptococcal disease in this species. Serial evaluation of serum cryptococcal antigen concentrations using latex agglutination titer methodology[39] (Wampole Crypto LA, Wampole Laboratories, Cranbury, NJ) during successful treatment of a pony for cryptococcal pneumonia showed that the initial titer was 1:4096. When recovered, the pony's titer was 1:256.[37] The pericardial fluid cryptococcal antigen titer was 1:1024 in a foal with cryptococcal pneumonia.[44]

Enzyme immunoassays (EIAs), employing monoclonal antibodies for recognition of serotypes, have been developed to detect cryptococcal capsular polysaccharide antigen and anticryptococcal antibodies. EIAs have several advantages over latex agglutination tests; EIAs are less subjective, are unaffected by prozone reactions, are more sensitive, may detect antigen earlier, and may have fewer false-positive results.[31] EIAs should not be used for urine.[8] To date, use of EIA has not been reported in the diagnosis of cryptococcosis in horses.

Molecular typing and immunocytochemistry were used to identify one isolate from a horse as *C. gattii*.[37]

Antibody Detection

In other species, anticryptococcal antibodies are not usually detected during active infection, and assessment of serum antibody concentrations is not useful for diagnosis. Serial assessments of serum antibody concentrations may be useful in monitoring therapy because the appearance of serum anticryptococcal antibodies may be a good prognostic sign. Antibody has been detected in healthy horses that were previously infected or were sequestering a latent infection.

Pathologic Findings

C. neoformans causes both focal and disseminated disease in horses. Although clinical signs referable to one organ system may be prominent, widespread pathologic lesions may be discovered at necropsy. Histologically, typical lesions are characterized by a "soap bubble" appearance resulting from aggregation of many cryptococcal organisms with unstained capsules[64] (Fig. 53-7). Cellular reaction is usually minimal and characterized by relatively small numbers of variably degenerated macrophages, neutrophils, and lymphocytes. Other, likely more chronic lesions may be granulomatous, with multinucleate giant cells and epithelioid cells, and fibrous tissue surrounding the yeast cells.

Upper Respiratory Tract

Gross lesions may vary from nodular and granulomatous to gelatinous. Endoscopically, the lesions appear as fleshy, firm, yellowish, discrete or lobulated masses of irregular contour, sometimes associated with yellow mucinous exudate.[48,49] The lesions may invade adjacent bone.

Lower Respiratory Tract

Gross lesions vary from discrete nodules to large, caseous masses that may replace a major portion of the lung. Few or many nodules may be present and widely disseminated in the lung. Calcium deposition may be evident in some nodules, and hemosiderin deposition may be obvious. In more severely affected horses the lung may be swollen or diffusely consolidated with many viscous, mucopurulent abscesses. The caseous material may be yellow and gelatinous.[65] When the cryptococcal capsules are large, the lesions may have a grossly mucinous texture.[64] Variously extensive fibrosis may be present in other areas of the lungs. Hilar lymph nodes may be enlarged and reactive or caseous. Pleuritis and pleural effusion may be present.

Central Nervous System

Cryptococcus has a predilection for the meninges in horses, although lesions in the brain and spinal cord have also been observed.[43,50,53,66] Gross lesions may appear as discrete gelatinous foci with thickening of the meninges or as cystlike cavitations in brain tissue. Histologic examination of the tissues is often required to identify lesions because they may not otherwise be apparent.[64]

Gastrointestinal Tract

GI localization of cryptococcal organisms is rarely reported in horses. One of the three horses reported to have abdominal manifestations of cryptococcal infection had large cryptococcal abscesses of mesenteric lymph nodes that were adherent to adjacent segments of large colon, duodenum, ileum, and uterus.[36] Another horse had a polypoid cryptococcal granuloma attached by a narrow stalk to the mucosal wall of the jejunum at the site of an intussusception.[34] The third horse had a small, intramural cryptococcal granuloma in the jejunum that was an incidental finding at necropsy.[36]

Reproductive Tract

Two mares were reported to have cryptococcal placentitis and endometritis. Placentitis was characterized by diffusely distended stroma of the allantochorion, with associated yeasts and mild infiltration of neutrophils on the chorionic surface.[44,58] Two mares that aborted foals with cryptococcosis had endometrial biopsies characterized by clusters of giant cells within the stratum spongiosum and individual multinucleate giant cells within the stratum compactum. Giant cells contained cryptococci.[58]

Subcutaneous Tissue

An extensive ulcerating cryptococcal mass involving the skin and subcutaneous tissues was found at necropsy adherent to the parietal pleura and adjacent lung.[55]

Therapy

Treatment of horses with cryptococcal disease has been infrequently attempted and has been unsuccessful with the exception of five cases described above.[34,37,48,49,53] The survivors included one pony treated successfully with AMB for a large pulmonary cryptococcal granuloma[37]; a horse with surgical resection of a jejunal intussusception involving an intraluminal cryptococcal granuloma[34]; two horses with sinonasal cryptococcal granuloma treated with multimodal therapy consisting of surgery, intravenous AMB, oral fluconazole, or topical enilconazole[48,49]; and a horse with cryptococcal meningitis and optic neuritis treated with oral fluconazole.[53] The decision not to treat affected horses is often made because of the expense of therapy, the invasive and frequently extensive nature of cryptococcal lesions, and the poor prognosis.

Histoplasmosis

Histoplasmosis is an uncommon disease of horses, although serologic studies suggest that in endemic areas, many horses have been exposed to the pathogen *Histoplasma capsulatum*. The fungus can cause disease in immunocompetent animals and humans, particularly after exposure to a large, usually inhaled, amount of fungus. In immunocompromised humans a life-threatening, disseminated manifestation of infection is common. Reports of histoplasmosis in horses are too limited to warrant drawing conclusions about epidemiology, treatment, or prognosis in this species, except with respect to *Histoplasma farciminosum*.

Etiology

Three varieties of the dimorphic ascomycete *H. capsulatum* are identified: (1) *H. capsulatum* var. *capsulatum*, the cause of histoplasmosis in animals and humans; (2) *H. capsulatum* var. *duboisii*, the cause of a distinct variant form of disease in humans, African histoplasmosis; and (3) *H. capsulatum* var. *farciminosum* (HCF), the agent causing enzootic lymphangitis in horses in Africa, the Middle East, and parts of Asia. Only *H. capsulatum* var. *capsulatum* is found in North America. *H. capsulatum* var. *farciminosum* is discussed in a separate section following this discussion of *H. capsulatum*. In nature, *H. capsulatum* var. *capsulatum* (hereafter referred to as *H. capsulatum*) is a filamentous fungus. It colonizes moist soil with high nitrogen content and is found in bat and bird guano, particularly the excreta of chickens and starlings.

In culture on Sabouraud dextrose agar the fungus grows in 2 to 3 weeks as white or brown colonies.[8] The mycelia produce macroconidia (8-16 µm in diameter) and microconidia (2-5 µm in diameter). Because of their small size, microconidia are readily aerosolized and respirable and are the primary etiologic agents of disease. At 37°C, microconidia germinate and form mycelia that are transformed into small (2-5 µm in diameter), budding, oval yeasts. Budding occurs at the narrow end of the yeast cell, forming a narrow, often long and threadlike, distinctive neck.[1] Three to 6 weeks is required for the process of conversion to the mycelia and then to the yeast form of the organism in culture.[8]

Virulence

A variety of factors contribute to the virulence of *H. capsulatum*. The conidia of the filamentous fungus are infectious, but conversion to the yeast form is a requirement for virulence in the host. *H. capsulatum* is not an obligate intracellular parasite, but it lives within cells of the reticular endothelial system and is disseminated by them within the host.[67] The yeast is phagocytized by macrophages after opsonization with antibody or complement. The yeast binds to integrins on the surface of mononuclear cells through a recently discovered ligand (HSP60) on the yeast cell surface. *H. capsulatum* also binds to a specific receptor on the surface of dendritic cells. Dendritic cells have substantially greater anti–*H. capsulatum* activity than macrophages. The nature of these yeast/host phagocytic cell interactions, the subject of ongoing research, may influence the ability of the yeast to remain viable once engulfed by the phagocytic cell. Viable intracellular yeasts inhabit phagolysosomes with a higher pH than those containing dead *H. capsulatum* organisms. The yeast may be able to alter the intracellular environment to permit survival and growth. Production of calcium-binding protein by yeast cells is controlled by expression of the CBP1 gene. Expression of this gene during host cell infection is another requirement for virulence.[68]

Limiting availability of free iron is one mammalian host defense against invasion by bacterial and fungal pathogens, including *H. capsulatum*. The yeast has three mechanisms for acquiring iron that is essential for pathogenicity: (1) secretion of low-molecular-weight iron-chelating siderophores that scavenge ferric iron; (2) the ability to reduce ferric to ferrous iron and thereby utilize iron from ferric salts; and (3) acidification of transferrin-containing microenvironments in the host cell, releasing bound iron.[68]

Epidemiology

Histoplasmosis is the most common endemic mycosis of humans.[8] *Histoplasma* spp. are distributed worldwide. The fungus thrives in microclimates where the ambient temperature varies from 22°C to 29°C (80°F-90°F), the annual precipitation is 35 to 50 inches per year, and the relative humidity is 67% to 87%.[1] *H. capsulatum* is endemic in the Mississippi, Missouri, and Ohio River valleys; southwestern and eastern Ontario to Montreal, Ottawa, and the St. Lawrence River Valley; some regions of South America; and focal regions around the world where the climate is optimum for growth (Fig. 53-8). Within a favorable climatic zone, the fungi may be focally concentrated in locales where wild or domestic birds congregate. Infection in humans is associated with disturbance of soil that contains the fungus. Infection is not transmissible from host to host, but epidemics may occur after exposure to a common source (e.g., bird roosts, old houses or barns, contaminated soil disturbed during excavation or farming).[66] The organisms may be disseminated by prevailing winds and by migratory birds, particularly the starling.

Clinical disease is relatively uncommon in immunocompetent humans and very uncommon in horses; however, exposure to infectious propagules and asymptomatic infection are common. From 50% to 80% of healthy persons in endemic areas are reported to have positive delayed hypersensitivity reactions to intradermal histoplasmin, a filtrate of broth containing the fungal mycelia.[8,67,70] Of 467 healthy horses in central Kentucky, 50% reacted positively to histoplasmin in one survey,[71] whereas 8.7% of 51 horses in Uruguay were positive,[72] 7.9% of 2221 horses in Mexico were positive,[73] and 73% of 44 horses were positive in Missouri.[71,74]

Pathogenesis

Inhaled microconidia reach the small airways, where the spores germinate into the yeast form of the organism. Phagocytic cells of the reticuloendothelial system, particularly pulmonary macrophages and dendritic cells, engulf the yeast. Parasitized phagocytes efficiently disseminate the yeast to tissues rich in reticuloendothelial cells such as lymph nodes, spleen, liver, and bone marrow. Occasionally, the yeast may localize in the CNS. Reticuloendothelial cells throughout the body ingest and sequester the yeasts.[69] In immunocompetent hosts, a robust cell-mediated immune response occurs in 10 to 14 days. Antigen-specific T-lymphocyte–mediated immunity develops,

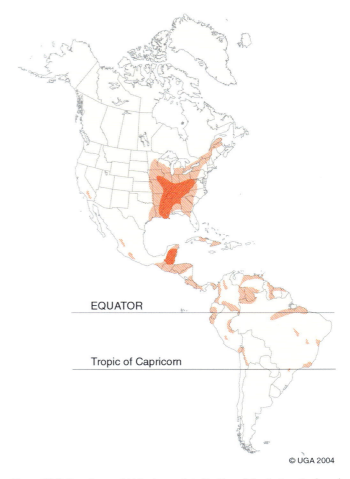

© UGA 2004

Figure 53-8 Prevalence of histoplasmosis in North and South America based on seropositivity in people. Shading indicates areas of endemic histoplasmosis. Darker shading indicates areas of higher incidence. *(From Greene C: Infectious diseases of the dog and cat, ed 3, Philadelphia, 2006, Saunders.)*

and macrophages become fungicidal and kill the intracellular organisms.[67] Necrotic foci may develop at the site of infection. These foci become abscesses that are soon encased in a fibrous capsule. Calcification may occur over the ensuing several years.[69] Clinical signs of disease are often not observed when the fungal load is light and the invading yeasts are well controlled by the host's immune system. Viable yeast cells may be sequestered within granulomata and may subsequently be reactivated by the onset of another debilitating disease or by immunosuppression.

Exposure to a large inoculum may induce disease in immunocompetent hosts. Clinical signs in persons usually develop approximately 3 weeks after inhalation of the microconidia.[8] Recovery from natural infection confers some immunity. Persons may become hypersensitive to the yeast and may experience a severe or even fatal anaphylactic reaction on reexposure.[1] A poor cell-mediated immune response allows progressive dissemination of the yeast that may result in fatal disease.[69] Disseminated histoplasmosis usually occurs in persons with T-cell deficiencies.

Lymphatic tissue in the GI tract may be a destination of disseminated yeasts. Additionally, the host may cough up and swallow infectious material from the lung. Resultant ulcerative enterocolitis and typhlitis in horses may be associated with protein-losing enteropathy, panhypoproteinemia, edema, diarrhea, or intestinal perforation.

Clinical Signs

Clinical manifestations of *H. capsulatum* infection in humans depend on inoculum size and the immune competence of the affected person. Immunocompetent patients may have asymptomatic infections or mild, flulike disease. In the latter case, thoracic radiographs may show a focal or miliary distribution of small, calcified nodules. Recovery may take weeks to months. Healthy or immunocompromised persons may develop chronic lung disease characterized by transient signs of pneumonia. This is followed by chronic indolent lung disease in immunocompetent persons or signs of progressive fibrosis, cavitation, necrosis, and death in patients who are or become immunocompromised.[8]

Surveys of the response to intradermal histoplasmin suggest that many horses residing in endemic areas have been exposed to the fungus, but disease is reported infrequently, suggesting that horses are relatively resistant to histoplasmosis. Among 23 cases of equine histoplasmosis reported in literature, 14 horses had pulmonary disease, 9 had abdominal or GI disease, and 1 foal had CNS disease. Five mares aborted as a result of *Histoplasma*-induced placentitis or histoplasmosis in the foal.[75-88] Some horses had more than one affected organ system, and one adult horse had disseminated histoplasmosis.[67] Clinical signs among infected horses include chronic weight loss, depression, fever, dyspnea, anorexia, edema, diarrhea, colic, abortion, and neonatal death. *H. capsulatum* was isolated in cultures of the spleen from a clinically normal mare and from the fetal membranes of her foal.[83,89]

Gastrointestinal histoplasmosis is uncommon in humans and usually occurs in persons with mediastinal histoplasmosis or progressive disseminated disease.[90] Intestinal histoplasmosis has been described in two horses[78,83] and was found at necropsy in an additional five horses.[82] Both of the reported horses had a history of chronic weight loss and progressive anorexia. Diarrhea, edema, and in one horse progressive toxemia resulted in the demise of these two horses.

Mycotic Keratitis

Keratitis caused by *Histoplasma* spp. was reported in a horse from Germany.[91] The horse displayed blepharospasm and endophthalmitis. A white opacity located ventrally and centrally in the cornea contained several subepithelial bullae and diffusely stained with fluorescein. The rest of the eye was not affected.

Diagnosis

Clinical Diagnostic Testing

Pulmonary disease is common in horses with histoplasmosis, and thoracic radiographs may demonstrate isolated, sometimes calcific nodules; multiple miliary nodules; diffuse interstitial densities; or focal cavitating lesions.

Cytology

Yeast cells may be identifiable in smears from transtracheal wash, BAL, peritoneal fluid, or blood specimens and in impression smears of tissues. Cytologic examination of bone marrow aspirates may also be helpful. The material should be fixed on a slide with methyl alcohol and stained with Wright's or Giemsa stain. The ovoid cells, 2 to 4 μm in diameter with a bud at the narrow end, are seen within macrophages or free in fluid or tissue. The yeast cell wall appears as an unstained halo around the cell.[1] Small, atypical *Blastomyces* or acapsular *C. neoformans* (among other agents or artifacts) may be mistaken for *H. capsulatum*.[8] Cytology is an insensitive method of detecting *Histoplasma*, and confirmatory tests are required to establish the diagnosis.

Ancillary Diagnostic Testing

Assessment of a serum chemistry profile may be helpful, particularly in horses with GI histoplasmosis that are likely to have panhypoproteinemia associated with protein-losing enteropathy. Leukopenia and neutropenia may be evident if bowel wall integrity is lost. Other agents that could induce inflammatory bowel disease or diarrhea should be sought. One horse was reported to have concurrent salmonellosis with histoplasmosis.[83]

Culture

Culture of the organism remains the gold standard for diagnosis of histoplasmosis. The fungus will grow on Sabouraud dextrose agar or blood agar without antibiotics at 25°C under moist conditions to prevent the plates from drying out. Colonies that appear on blood agar are initially glabrous, pink to reddish brown, and develop into mycelia that are white to brownish. These colonies are very similar to those of *B. dermatitidis* and other fungi. Incubation at 37°C and demonstration of the characteristic yeast cell are required for identification of *H. capsulatum*. Cultures should be kept for 6 to 12 weeks.[1]

Limitations to the use of a positive culture as the basis for diagnosis and management of affected persons include (1) human patients with mild forms of histoplasmosis usually have negative cultures, (2) about 20% of patients with disseminated and 50% of those with chronic pulmonary histoplasmosis have false-negative cultures, (3) the slow growth of cultures precludes using culture results as a basis for therapy, (4) antibody production may be poor in immunocompromised hosts, and (5) invasive procedures may be required to obtain samples for culture.[70] An exoantigen test or molecular characterization may also be used for identification.

Histopathology

Tissue samples should be stained with GMS or PAS stains (Fig. 53-9). Experience is required to identify the yeast cells reliably in tissues and to distinguish them from other organisms. The sensitivity of histopathology for the diagnosis of human histoplasmosis is low (<50%).[70]

Serology

ID and CF tests are standard for diagnosis of histoplasmosis in humans.[70] The ID test, which recognizes the H and M antigens of *H. capsulatum*, is less sensitive than CF. Host CF response is greater to the mycelial than to the yeast antigen. Positive CF titers are found in about 95% of persons with histoplasmosis, although only weakly positive titers (1:8 or 1:16) may be found in 25% to 33% of patients. Cross-reactions can occur in patients with blastomycosis, aspergillosis, coccidioidomycosis, or candidiasis. Chronic histoplasmosis is associated with persistent antibodies, and prolonged exposure or latent infection may result in detection of antibodies for several years. Results of serologic testing do not provide a definitive diagnosis and should not be used as a basis for determining appropriate treatment. Antibodies to *H. capsulatum* were identified by AGID in one horse with pulmonary histoplasmosis.[81]

Antigen Detection

Antigens are released from yeast cells during active infection and may be detected in blood, urine, and other body fluids, particularly in human patients with disseminated or acute pulmonary histoplasmosis after inhalation of a large number of microconidia. For patients with acute pulmonary disease, BAL fluid antigen titers may be higher than serum or urine titers. In general, antigen detection is more sensitive in urine than in serum. False-negative tests may occur, probably because of low fungal burden. Serial determination of antigenemia or

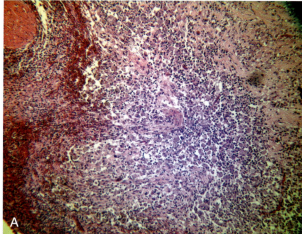

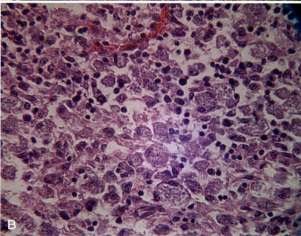

Figure 53-9 A, Photomicrograph of *Histoplasma* yeast cells in spleen of weanling Standardbred filly with disseminated histoplasmosis. **B,** Photomicrograph of *Histoplasma* yeast cells in giant cells in spleen of weanling Standardbred filly with disseminated histoplasmosis.

Table 53-1 Sensitivity (% Positive) of Laboratory Tests for Diagnosis of Pulmonary Histoplasmosis in Humans

Test	Acute or Subacute Pulmonary,* Pericarditis, Rheumatologic	Chronic Pulmonary	Mediastinal
Antigen	25-75	15	0
Fungal stain	10	40	<25
Culture	15	50-85	<25
Serology	95	100	67

From Wheat LJ: Trends Microbiol 11(10):488, 2003.

*In acute pulmonary, the sensitivity of antigen detection ranges from about 25% in patients with local manifestations to greater than 75% in those who present within the first month of exposure.

Table 53-2 Sensitivity (% Positive) of Laboratory Tests for Diagnosis of Disseminated Histoplasmosis in Humans

Test	Not Immune Suppressed	Immune Suppressed
Histology	40-61	57-64
Serology	85-100	82
Immunodiffusion*	71-100	57-77
Complement fixation†	85-97	60-79
Culture	86-90	82-89
Antigen Detection		
Urine	80	82
Serum	67	60
Either	82	82

*For H and M bands.

†With yeast and mycelial antigens.

increases serum antibody concentrations, further confounding the diagnosis.[70]

Pathology

Gross necropsy findings in affected horses include enlarged, firm lungs; swollen, mottled, yellow-tan liver; dilated, thickened, ulcerated, or hemorrhagic intestine; enlarged tracheobronchial lymph nodes; and focal placental necrosis.[82] One horse with GI histoplasmosis had widespread, deeply ulcerated lesions in the cecum and colon.[83]

Histopathology of tissues from affected horses showed focal or coalescing pyogranulomatous inflammation with many macrophages and giant cells. In tissues from aborted fetuses and neonatal foals, focal infiltration with multinucleate giant cells containing yeast cells was seen in lung, liver, lymph nodes, and intestines.[82] In placental lesions the subchorionic stroma adjacent to blood vessels, the surface of the allantois, and chorionic villi were most prominently affected and were sites where organisms could be detected.[82] The submucosa of the cecum and colon was diffusely infiltrated with lymphocytes and macrophages laden with yeast cells (pyogranulomatous inflammation) in one horse with intestinal histoplasmosis.[83]

Tables 53-1 and 53-2 summarize the sensitivity of selected diagnostic tests for pulmonary and disseminated histoplasmosis, respectively, in human patients.

Mycotic Keratitis

In one horse with keratitis, a smear of a specimen obtained by corneal brushing and stained with Wright's stain showed intracellular and extracellular, spherical, globular structures up to 4 µm in size that were surrounded by an unstained halo. A

antigenuria is useful in monitoring response to therapy and in detecting relapse in human patients because reductions in antigenemia/antigenuria are associated with successful treatment, whereas increasing values suggest recrudescence of disease. False-positive tests are rare in people, but cross-reactions may occur in patients with blastomycosis and other fungal diseases.[70]

Antigen detection would likely be useful in confirming a diagnosis of histoplasmosis in horses. To date, there are no reports of attempts at antigen detection in horses with histoplasmosis.[70]

Molecular Identification

Polymerase chain reaction (PCR) and DNA probe methods for detecting *H. capsulatum* in tissues have shown some promise and are currently under development. DNA probes are commercially available for identification of culture isolates.[70]

Intradermal Testing

Intradermal testing with histoplasmin is of no use diagnostically because of the large number of persons and horses in endemic areas with positive reactions to histoplasmin from exposure to *H. capsulatum*. False-positive results are observed in human patients with other fungal diseases. Exposure to histoplasmin presumptive diagnosis of histoplasmosis was made based on cytology. Fungal cultures were negative.[91]

Therapy

Histoplasmosis is a rare disease in horses, and data are insufficient to draw conclusions about equine treatment. Treatment of affected horses has been infrequently attempted because of the severity of clinical signs, failure to make the diagnosis, expense of treatment, and concerns of a poor prognosis for recovery from fungal disease.

One 2-year-old filly was successfully treated for *Histoplasma* pneumonia.[81] The horse was treated with AMB (Fungizone) using an escalating dosage regimen.[92] The horse made a full recovery to athletic use.

AMB followed by itraconazole is the recommended therapeutic regimen for acute or chronic pulmonary or disseminated histoplasmosis in humans. Prolonged treatment is required. Recommendations include 6 to 12 weeks of treatment with itraconazole for immunocompetent persons with acute pulmonary histoplasmosis and 12 to 24 months of itraconazole (up to lifelong therapy) for immunocompromised patients with disseminated histoplasmosis.[69]

Mycotic Keratitis

One horse with an ulcer putatively caused by *Histoplasma* spp. was treated with topical fluconazole and 1% atropine for about 5 weeks.[91] To reduce the potential for developing iridocyclitis caused by rapid death of fungi in the stroma, treatments with fluconazole were introduced gradually and increased from twice daily to 4 times daily over a 4-day period. The cornea over the bullae was scarified to improve penetration of fluconazole. The horse recovered completely except for a faint corneal scar.

Histoplasma capsulatum var. farciminosum

HCF is the cause of epizootic lymphangitis of horses in the Middle East, Asia, and Africa. Infection results in ill thrift and decreased ability to work and is a source of major economic loss in countries where the horse is relied on for transport. HCF is not found in North America.

Etiology

As with *H. capsulatum* var. *capsulatum*, HCF is a thermally dimorphic organism. The saprophytic mycelia and the yeasts found in tissues can be cultivated on Sabouraud dextrose agar enriched with 2.5% glycerol, but PPLO dextrose glycerol agar may be the most useful medium.[93] At 25° C, mycelial colonies appear after 4 to 8 weeks of incubation. The mycelial colonies are yellow to light or deep brown, convoluted, waxy, and cauliflower-like.[93,94] Mycelia produce several types of conidia. Incubation of the mycelial colonies at 35° C to 37° C on brain-heart infusion (BHI) agar with 5% blood results in transformation to the yeast form. In one study, transformation required four or five serial transfers to fresh media, performed at intervals of 8 days.[93] Transformation of the mycelial to the yeast phase was achieved within 3 to 4 weeks in another study.[95] The yeast cell closely resembles that of *H. capsulatum* var. *capsulatum*.

Epidemiology

Epizootic lymphangitis occurs in horses, mules, and donkeys, particularly in Egypt and India and in North Africa, the Middle East, southern Asia, southern Europe, and parts of Russia. It is endemic in countries that border the Mediterranean.[94] Of 2907 Ethiopian cart horses, 26% were infected with HCF based on clinical examination and culture.[96] In contrast, 83 (2.8%) of 3000 horses at a large racing facility in Iraq had enzootic lymphangitis during a 6-month period of observation.[95] Cases were more common in fall and early winter in Iran[85] and in January in Egypt.[1]

The disease is both contagious from equid to equid and zoonotic. Although the route of infection has not been definitively established, direct inoculation of infective propagules through abraded skin or mucous membranes is suspected to be common. Fomites, including harness, mangers, water buckets, and wound dressings, and flies also transmit the organism. Stallions may transmit HCF to mares during breeding. The less common respiratory manifestation of the disease may result from inhalation of HCF when dust is heavily contaminated.

Pathogenesis

After invading the skin, HCF disseminates through the lymphatics to regional lymph nodes or, in severe cases, to other organs.[94] Clinical signs are observed several weeks to 6 months after infection. Nodular lesions develop in the skin along the lymphatics and in the lymph nodes. These lesions eventually ulcerate and drain a thick, mucopurulent material containing yeast cells. Nodules occur wherever there is skin trauma (particularly under the harness and on the extremities). Horses that have a heavy systemic burden of fungi may succumb to pneumonia or failure of other affected organs. Some horses are asymptomatic carriers of HCF, based on the presence of calcified skin lesions, serologic evidence of antibodies, and positive reactions to intradermal tests. These methods do not distinguish exposure from chronic infection.

Clinical Signs

Affected horses display clinical signs referable to cutaneous (most common), ocular, or respiratory disease. In cutaneous disease, granulomatous, often ulcerated masses are seen in chains following lymphatic vessels[94] (Figs. 53-10 and 53-11). Draining ulcerated nodules eventually heal and scar, as others form. The forelimbs, neck, and head are common sites. After about 6 months, few new lesions develop. Mortality is not high

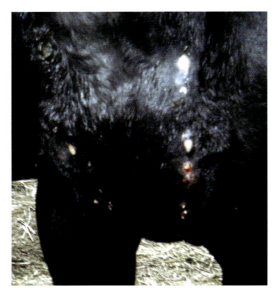

Figure 53-10 *Histoplasma capsulatum* var. *farciminosum* in pectoral lymphatics of horse. (*Courtesy Dr. John Barnes, North Carolina State University.*)

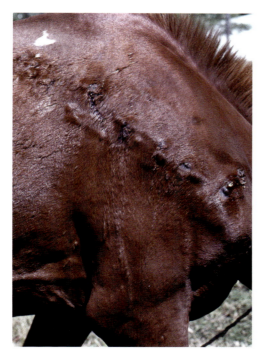

Figure 53-11 *Histoplasma capsulatum* var. *farciminosum* in lymphatics of shoulder and neck of horse. *(Courtesy Dr. John Barnes, North Carolina State University.)*

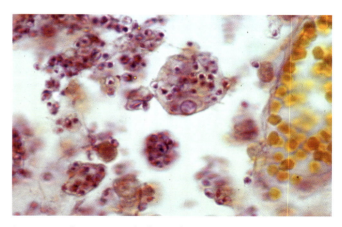

Figure 53-12 Photomicrograph of *Histoplasma capsulatum* var. *farciminosum* in an infected nodule. (Periodic acid–Schiff stain; 400×.) *(Courtesy Dr. John Barnes, North Carolina State University.)*

Pathology and Histology

Typical lesions are pyogranulomatous nodules that may be seen in lymphatic vessels, pleura, spleen, liver, bone marrow, and lung. Interstitial pneumonia may also be recognized. Lymphatic vessels may be thickened or fibrotic in chronic or locally resolved infections. Histologically, granulomas are characterized by the presence of many large macrophages, often containing yeast cells that are seen after staining with PAS or GMS stain.[94]

Serologic Tests

Tube agglutination and passive hemagglutination tests have been reported to identify increased titers in horses with epizootic lymphangitis,[99] and this assay can be used as a practical screening test. A serum agglutination titer of 1:80 or higher is reported to be positive.[94] Fluorescent antibody,[100] AGID, and ELISA[99] tests have also been described. ID and CF tests were positive in 26.5% of 200 horses from a farm where epizootic lymphangitis had previously been diagnosed, whereas 3% of horses on the farm were showing clinical signs of the disease when the blood samples were taken.[101] These findings suggest that serologic testing may not have a high degree of specificity for active disease, but it may reflect past exposure or asymptomatic infection.

Animal Inoculation

Immunosuppressed mice are susceptible to HCF and are suitable for diagnostic testing.[94]

Intradermal Testing

Intradermal histofarcin (a soluble antigen) induced a local reaction in all serologically positive horses in one study.[101] Intradermal testing may have low specificity for active disease.

Therapy

In many places, horses with epizootic lymphangitis must be reported to regulatory agencies, and a policy of slaughter and eradication is in effect. In endemic areas where treatment is allowed, oral and IV iodide[102,103] or AMB have been administered. A combination of topical application of an extract of crude dried ground berries of *Phytolacca dodecandra* with intramuscular administration of penicillin/dihydrostreptomycin was reported to be as effective as intravenous/oral administration of sodium iodide with intramuscular penicillin/dihydrostreptomycin for treatment of cart horses in Ethiopia.[103]

(10%-15%), but inability to work because of these painful nodules results in significant economic hardship in countries where the horse is an important beast of burden. In the ocular manifestation of this disease, conjunctivitis, nodular enlargements over facial lymphatics, and nasolacrimal lesions are noted.[97] Serous ocular discharge and swelling of the eyelids are associated with the development of nodules on the conjunctiva or nictitans. Lacrimal and conjunctival lesions are reported to be the only clinical abnormalities noted in some horses in Egypt.[95,97] In the upper respiratory tract, usually near the external nares, HCF forms yellowish papules or nodules that ulcerate and bleed. Pulmonary granulomata may eventually cause fatal disease.[1,98] Disseminated disease has been infrequently reported.[1]

Diagnosis

Pattern recognition of clinical signs in horses in endemic regions is often the basis of diagnosis. Several confirmatory tests have been described. Culture of HCF from body fluids or tissues is the "gold standard" for confirming the diagnosis but may be impractical.

Cytology

Cytologic examination of material aspirated from a nodule that has not yet drained usually shows typical yeasts (Fig. 53-12). Giemsa or Gram staining demonstrates round cells 1 to 5 μm in diameter, usually within macrophages. In one study, direct microscopy yielded positive results in 79% of cases.[95]

Culture

The organism may be difficult and time-consuming to grow from body fluids and tissues, and false-negative results are likely. Samples can be cultured at 26°C to induce growth of the mycelial phase of the organism. Subsequent transformation to the yeast form is required to substantiate the diagnosis. In one study, HCF was isolated from 58% of infected horses.[95]

In conjunction with removal of crusts and exudates from cutaneous lesions, AMB treatment is reported to be successful.[94] In vitro tests have shown that nystatin is more effective than AMB and 5-fluorouracil in inhibiting growth of HCF,[104] and the author suggests using parenteral AMB and concurrent topical nystatin. In another in vitro study, clotrimazole was more effective than AMB at inhibiting the growth of four HCF isolates from sick horses. The minimum inhibitory concentration (MIC) of clotrimazole for the mycelial and yeast forms of HCF was 1.25 µg/mL, whereas the MIC for AMB was 100 µg/mL.[105] There are no reports of clinical trials using either of these two therapeutic regimens.

Large lesions can be surgically debrided and packed with iodine.

Prevention

A killed vaccine prepared from the yeast and given subcutaneously to horses has been reported to provide protection. A modified live vaccine is reported to be in use for horses in China. Little information is in the accessible literature concerning these vaccines.

Pneumocystis Infections

Maureen T. Long

Etiology

Pneumocystis organisms are a group of pathogenic fungi, some of which are host adapted.[105,106,107] Structurally, this is a thin-walled, "trophozoite-like" form with a single nucleus, as well as a typical thick walled, cyst-like organism with multiple (usually eight) inner bodies. The procyst is considered either a product or a subtype of the trophozoite stage. Pneumocystis is evolutionarily placed between the sister groups of fungi, Ascomycota and Basidiomycota.[108] The Ascomycota are the very large group of fungi that vary from the sexual *Saccharomyces* to the asexual *Aspergillus* and *Candida*. The Basidiomycota include the edible and inedible mushrooms, rusts, and pathogens such as *Cryptococcus neoformans*. In the absence of the ability to culture Pneumocystis in vitro and confirm species by cross-mating of isolates, a trinomial nomenclature evolved in which forma specialis (f. sp.) is used to designate each type or variety until formally designated which has since evolved separate species names.[108-112] *Pneumocystis carinii* f. sp. hominis is now *Pneumocystis jirovecii* and is thus far the only Pneumocystis species that has been found in humans.[113] *Pneumocystis carinii* f. sp. *carinii*, or *P. carinii* and *P. wakefield* are the host-adapted species for the rat with *P. murina* named for the mouse species and *P. oryctolagi* named for the rabbit. A specific subtype associated with equine infection was identified by sequencing of the mitochondrial ribosomal ribonucleic acid (rRNA) gene.[114] Samples from four foals were sequenced and demonstrated 85%, 84%, and 78% agreement with human and ferret, SCID-mouse, and rat sequences, respectively.[115] As of this publishing, the equine, dog, pig and ferret sequences have not been named.

Epidemiology

Historically *Pneumocystis* spp. infection and disease have been considered a problem primarily in immunocompromised hosts. Recent evidence supports the hypothesis that this organism is either a component of normal respiratory flora or a primary upper respiratory component of immunocompetent animals.[105,116,117] Exposure and infection with Pneumocystis occurs during childhood, often during the neonatal period.[117-122] The syndromes associated with Pneumocystis infection in immunocompetent children include asymptomatic infection, mild upper respiratory infection, and bronchiolitis. Several studies suggest an association between this organism and sudden infant death syndrome yet a causal relationship between *Pneumocystis* spp. infection and primary disease in the immunocompetent host is questionable.[123-126] Pneumocystis is common in samples from the upper respiratory tract or by bronchoalveolar lavage (BAL) in asymptomatic animals and people with no identifiable immunologic risk.[120,127-129] Some of these carriers may have chronic lung disease. Pregnancy, concomitant medications (not classified as immunosuppressive agents), or undiagnosed immune compromise may have affected the frequency of detection of Pneumocystis DNA in these studies. Asymptomatic Pneumocystis colonization has also been demonstrated in mice, rats, and ferrets.[127,130-133] Recent epidemiological investigations in the United Kingdom demonstrate a yearly increase of 7% per year from 2000-2010 and this was primarily associated with non-HIV persons suffering with chronic lung disease.[134] Evidence from environmental, animal, and human molecular epidemiologic studies suggests that the fulminant syndrome, *Pneumocystis carinii* pneumonia (PcP), is not be the result of reactivation of a latent infection that was acquired earlier in life.[133] Initial infections likely originate from direct transmission of the organism from an immunocompetent carrier to an immunocompromised individual.[111,122,130,131,133-138]

Pneumocystis infections have been detected in many other animals. Immunodeficient dogs die from overwhelming *Pneumocystis* infections, and the organism has been detected sporadically in dogs with interstitial pneumonia.[117,115,139-150] Young swine develop a fatal interstitial pneumonia and can be concomitantly infected with Pneumocystis.[151-153] Cattle, goats, and sheep have reportedly been infected with Pneumocystis and infected goats and sheep are likely to have a pneumonitis type of disease.[108,147]

Pathogenesis

Pneumocystis infection is associated with two disease conditions in horses: acute, fulminant PcP and secondary infections with pulmonary fibrosis (pneumocystosis).[154-160] When an overwhelming alveolar infection occurs in the immunocompromised horse, the ensuing PcP is life–threatening, and the organism is readily found in the alveoli of the lung.[161-162] It resides extracellularly in alveolar spaces, adhering to alveolar type I cells, and causes a severe exudative disease process. The tissue reaction is moderate and characterized by lymphocyte and plasma cell localization within the alveoli and mild thickening of the interstitium surrounding the alveoli. Foals with severe combined immunodeficiency (SCID) develop classical PcP in which alveoli are packed with *P. carinii* (Fig. 50-13).[161] The alveolar spaces become moderately thickened with inflammatory cells. Severe accumulations of proteinaceous debris create dyspnea and hypoxia.

Pneumocystis infections in immunocompetent humans and horses with normal numbers of CD4+ T cells have been described. However, the requirement of CD4+ T cells for protection against disease has been demonstrated in murine models and in human patients with acquired immunodeficiency syndrome (AIDS).[111,117,162-164] Loss of CD4+ cells and susceptibility to disease can be reversed by interferon-gamma (IFN-γ).[165] Nonspecific CD8+ effector cells actually increase lung injury.[166,167] Macrophages are considered important in the killing of *Pneumocystis* organisms; however, these cells must be augmented by T cells, IFN-γ, and granulocyte colony-stimulating factor (G-CSF).[167] Other effector molecules are likely also important and have yet to be identified.

Localization of Pneumocystis to the alveoli results in accumulation of a proteinaceous fluid, causing severely impaired

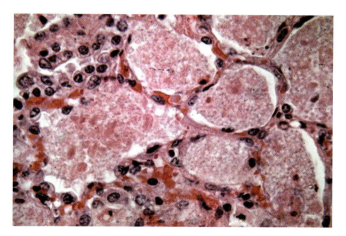

Figure 53-13 Photomicrograph of section of lung, stained with hematoxylin and eosin, from foal with severe combined immuno–deficiency (SCID). The alveoli are moderately thickened and contain small numbers of mononuclear inflammatory cells with occasional neutrophils. The alveoli are lined with epithelium that is cuboidal, consistent with pneumocyte type I hyperplasia. The alveoli are filled with pink-staining, granular fluid (highly proteinaceous). Distinct areas along the alveoli do not pick up stain. *(Courtesy Lance Perryman, Colorado State University.)*

oxygenation.[168,169] This condition has been compared to a disease called alveolar proteinosis. Pulmonary alveolar proteinosis is characterized by insidious onset of exercise intolerance and dyspnea. The proteinaceous material is thought to be alveolar secretions consistent with surfactants. In idiopathic disease, lack of clearance rather than overproduction of proteinaceous fluid is considered the pathogenesis. Granulocyte-macrophage colony-stimulating factor (GM-CSF) is necessary for activation of pulmonary macrophages and removal of the pulmonary surfactant. The exact pathogenesis of proteinaceous accumulations in PcP is not known.

In many animals and humans with signs or symptoms of pulmonary disease, *Pneumocystis* organisms have been detected with BAL. Many of these reports describe the presence of chronic fibrosing lung pathology.[169] In these equine cases, Pneumocystis may not be the inciting cause of pulmonary disease but may have colonized the compromised lung secondary to another disease process.[158-160] This condition is referred to as pneumocystosis to differentiate it from acute, overwhelming PcP as previously described. Pneumocystosis in immunocompetent humans and rabbits has been associated with severe malnutrition.[111,170]

Clinical Findings

The primary immunodeficiency of horses associated with PcP is the SCID syndrome in which Arabian foals are born without functional B cells and T cells.[161] Onset of PcP is insidious, with foals presenting in moderate to poor body condition with other systemic signs such as anorexia and depression. These foals usually have intermittent fever and nasal discharge that may initially respond to antibiotic therapy. Foals become increasingly dyspneic, with persistent fever, tachycardia, and tachypnea. Upon auscultation, foals have bilateral crackles and moist rales in the trachea. Eventually an abdominal breathing pattern ensues, and foals exhibit signs of respiratory compromise and hypoxemia. These foals frequently develop infections of other body systems (e.g., joint ill, diarrhea), which may also ultimately result in their demise.

Pneumocystis has been isolated from presumably immunocompetent foals (4 months to 1 year of age) and adult horses

with severe, atypical interstitial pneumonia.* Affected animals present in acute respiratory distress with exceptional abdominal effort. Usually these animals are persistently febrile. Lymphadenopathy may be present. A dry, harsh cough is common, and wheezes and crackles are audible over both thoracic cavities. Therapy is unrewarding, and horses often die within 1 week. Sudden collapse and death have also been described. Whether or not there is an underlying acquired or other immunodeficiency in affected equids is unknown; however, when investigated, most of these horses have either normal lymphocyte or CD4+ T cells. Evidence of other immune compromise has been demonstrated in several case reports in cases where severe immune deficiency is not apparent. These include splenic and lymphoid hypocellularity (Paso Fino foal),[174] decreased immunoglobulins (Warmblood foal),[171,174,] and the use of corticosteroids.[175] Recently, an adult Paso Fino mare was reported to have a syndrome consistent with common variable immunodeficiency consisting of decreased IgM and IgA with decreased expression of major histocompatibility complex (MHC) class II antigens.[173,176] This horse also had proliferative pneumonia attributable to *Pneumocystis* infection and had marked liver changes consistent with pyrrolizidine alkaloid toxicity.

Diagnosis

Clinical testing for Pneumocystis infection is similar to that described for other types of respiratory infection, including complete blood count, serum biochemistry, transtracheal wash (TTW), and BAL. Abnormalities of leukocyte counts are not consistent unless animals have the SCID defect, in which case a total lymphocyte count of less than 1000 cells/mL is present. Immunocompetent animals may have decreased, normal, or increased white blood cell counts, characterized predominantly by changes in neutrophil numbers. Serum biochemical analysis may be normal or may demonstrate hypergammaglobulinemia unless there is a concomitant gastrointestinal disorder allowing loss of protein or horses are SCID and have minimal gammaglobulin production. Hyperfibrinogenemia is also common. Affected foals may be severely hypoxemic and hypercapneic. In equine infections with Pneumocystis, BAL is essential for detection of fungal elements. Cellular analysis of the BAL is more consistently mononuclear than observed with TTW samples, consisting of macrophages and giant cells. Areas of negative staining are frequently observed within the foamy eosinophilic background. Staining of these specimens with Gomori's methenamine silver (GMS) demonstrate the oval to crescent-shaped organisms in the areas that were originally negatively stained (Fig. 50-14). Transtracheal washes usually reveal the presence of increased mucin and neutrophils. Fungal elements may or may not be observed; usually the *Pneumocystis* organism is not detected in these samples. Bacteria are frequently observed and isolated by culture.

Foals with Pneumocystis infection have a mixed alveolar and interstitial pattern on thoracic radiography. The interstitial pattern in these foals has been described as a reticulonodular pattern.[156] Air bronchograms indicate the presence of an alveolar pattern. The presence of abscessation is highly associated with concomitant *R. equi* infection. Ultrasound evaluation reveals consolidation characterized by a "comet tail" appearance of the parietal pleura throughout all lung fields. Abscesses identified concomitantly with this modality also indicate *R. equi* infection.

Molecular diagnostic techniques performed on respiratory secretions are considered confirmatory for a diagnosis of *Pneumocystis* infection in an animal with compatible respiratory signs and appropriate cellular responses. These molecular

---

*References 155, 156, 157, 159-160, 171, 172, 173.

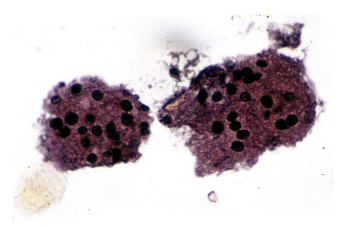

Figure 53-14 BAL fluid obtained from horse in respiratory distress. BAL was centrifuged, and cells stained with GMS demonstrate many organisms approximately 6 mm in diameter, consistent with the fungus Pneumocystis.

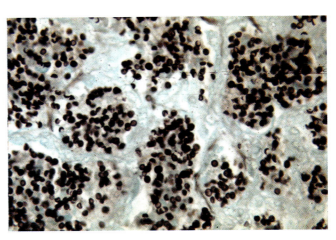

Figure 53-15 Photomicrograph of section of lung, stained with Gomori's methenamine silver (GMS), from foal with SCID. The alveoli are filled with approximately 6-mm organism that pick up GMS stain (black refractile bodies), consistent with Pneumocystis. *(Courtesy Lance Perryman, Colorado State University.)*

techniques primarily consist of polymerase chain reaction (PCR) performed on either BAL samples, fresh lung tissue, or fixed lung tissue.[139] PCR performed on nasal swabs is of value for epidemiologic purposes; positive results obtained from the secretions of the lower respiratory tract indicate pulmonary colonization with Pneumocystis.

Infections with Pneumocystis or other opportunistic pathogens should prompt investigation of the immune status of the affected horse. This should include quantification of Ig classes, immunophenotyping of circulating lymphocytes, and in situ evaluation of cell phenotypes in lymphoid organs. Immune function tests, such as lymphocyte blastogenesis testing, may be considered.

Pathologic Findings

Grossly, the lungs of affected horses are firm and dark red (hepatized).[155,156,159,172,175] Fluid may run from cut surfaces. Histopathology associated with alveolar infection of immunocompromised horses is similar to that of other species. Alveolar changes consist of proliferation of the alveolar epithelia resulting from type II pneumocyte hyperplasia (see Fig. 50-13). Within the alveoli, there is accumulation of pink or acidophilic cellular fluid. This edema fluid frequently fills the alveolar space and has a "honeycomb" appearance with accumulations of karyorrhectic nuclei, neutrophils, and giant cells. Neutrophils may be increased in the bronchi and bronchioles. Where the alveoli are not completely occluded, the "trophozoite-like," thin-walled form resides. The walls of the alveoli are only moderately thickened and contain infiltrates of plasma cells and lymphocytes. GMS staining demonstrates the organism within tissue sections (Fig. 50-15). "Cysts with parenthesis-like bodies" are considered diagnostic for Pneumocystis infection.

When associated with atypical interstitial pneumonia, the primary lesion is a severe histiocytic, proliferative interstitial pneumonia.[158]

Therapy

Limited reports of successful treatment of Pneumocystis infection in horses are available.[161] One horse with a transient CD[4+] and CD[8+] lymphopenia responded to traditional therapy with potentiated sulfonamides (trimethoprim-sulfamethoxazole,

30 mg/kg every 12 hours for 30 days). This foal was also treated with interferon-alpha (100 units) orally every 24 hours for 5 days. Dapsone (3 mg/kg orally every 24 hours), a sulfone antimicrobial that inhibits folic acid, has been used as a follow-up treatment in a foal with acute *Pneumocystis* infection.[178] A short course of corticosteroid therapy may be considered for affected horses. There is evidence of increased survival with the use of corticosteroids in children and AIDs patients with PcP.[179] This course of corticosteroid therapy is used in children irrespective of immune status.

Prevention

Because of the sporadic nature of PcP and pneumocystosis, preventive strategies are not available. The cause of underlying pulmonary fibrosis is not known, although viral infection has been suggested as a cause thus immunoprophylaxis against respiratory pathogens should be performed. Second, control of dust and ammonia within the environment will contribute to overall respiratory health. Third, exposure to plants containing pyrrolizidine alkaloids should be minimized. Exposure to plant or environmental toxins has been proposed as a cause for underlying interstitial pneumonia in horses (see Chapter 1). The stall of any immunocompromised horse should be disinfected, and environmental decontamination with sodium hypochlorite is advised.

Public Health Considerations

Because of the recent identification of a host-adapted species of Pneumocystis, previous designation of these infections as "zoonotic" has been removed.[110,113] However, because the organism may be capable of infecting humans, especially immunocompromised humans, personal protection consisting of gloves, boots, gown, and possibly mask is recommended when performing necropsies, handling respiratory secretions, or performing invasive pulmonary techniques.

The complete reference list is available online at www.expertconsult.com.

CHAPTER

54 Laboratory Diagnosis of Parasitic Diseases

Ellis C. Greiner

Some helminth and protozoan parasites are easily diagnosed because the diagnostic stages passed in the feces are readily detected and identified. Other parasites require more effort to identify because the eggs are not distinguishable; larval fecal cultures are needed to determine the species or groups of nematodes present, and some require special procedures to enhance diagnosis. This chapter assists the equine clinician in sample selection and interpretation of results to facilitate rapid and accurate diagnosis of helminth and protozoan parasitic diseases of horses.

Helminth Diagnosis

Some helminth parasites of horses have complex life cycles, and immature stages may go on circuitous journeys through viscera before arriving at the site where the adult worms will develop and produce offspring. Sometimes, these worms do not follow the correct route and migrate to the central nervous system (CNS), where they may cause severe damage. These conditions are usually confirmed at necropsy, when the parasites may be recovered and identified.

When larval stages of parasites migrate through tissues, normal parasite diagnosis by fecal examination is not possible because the mature adults have not developed and have not begun to produce and release the eggs or larvae. This interval is referred to as the prepatent period.

Diagnosis of helminth infection based on observation of eggs or larvae is facilitated by examination of fresh fecal samples. Some parasites are common in horses at any age, whereas others are restricted to the foals because the adult horses mount a sufficient immune response to prevent the adult worms from developing.

A large variety of nematode parasites infect horses. Most reside in the gastrointestinal (GI) tract and are detected by fecal examination; examples include the strongyles (Fig. 54-1), ascarids (Fig. 54-2), threadworms (Fig. 54-3), pinworms (Fig. 54-4), lungworms (Fig.54-5), and stomach worms. Some nematodes reside in solid tissues and do not pass any stages in the feces; these include the filarial worms, *Onchocerca cervicalis*, *O. reticulata*, and *Parafilaria multipapillosa*, which are detected by discovery of microfilariae, which are motile embryos (Fig. 54-6). Some worms cause severe problems but do not produce any stages that leave the host, such as *Halicephalobus deletrix*, which is usually diagnosed by histopathology at necropsy. Summer sores are caused by larval stomach worms which produce no eggs or larvae and are species of *Draschia* and *Habronema*.

The diversity of flatworms is rather depauperate compared with the nematodes. Three species of tapeworms develop as adults in the intestines (*Anoplocephala perfoliata* [Fig. 54-7], *A. magna* and *Paranoplocephala mamillana*), and the larval cyst of one tapeworm (hydatid cyst of *Echinococcus*) rarely develops in the liver. Two flukes, *Fasciola hepatica* in the liver (Fig. 54-8) and *Heterobilharzia americana* in mesenteric veins (Fig. 54-9), rarely infect horses because the horse is not the normal host for either. These flukes develop to adults that shed eggs in the feces, which could be detected by fecal sedimentation.

Protozoan Diagnosis

Very few protozoal organisms infect the GI tract of horses, and some are believed to be beneficial as the ciliate fauna of the large bowel. Others are pathogenic or potentially pathogenic, including flagellates, such as *Giardia* (Fig. 54-10) and possibly *Leishmania* (Fig. 54-11), and coccidians, such as one species of *Eimeria* (Fig. 54-12) and *Cryptosporidium* (Fig. 54-13).

Laboratory Procedures

Procedures that are used to diagnose parasitic infections in horses include gross fecal examination, fecal flotation, fecal culture, fecal sedimentation, direct smear, Baermann procedure, cellophane (Scotch) tape test, McMaster's counts, stained fecal smears, impression smears, skin biopsy examination, and blood smears. It is highly desirable to have a compound microscope calibrated with an ocular micrometer to facilitate precise measurement of ova or other parasite structures.

Gross Fecal Examination

Before altering the feces for diagnostic purposes, examination without magnification for consistency, evidence of blood, and the macroscopic presence of worms should be performed. If the horse is impacted or there is delayed movement of ingesta, parasite ova may be more developed than normal. Conversely, if there is diarrhea, ova may not be as developed as expected. Blood might indicate high numbers of strongyles migrating within the intestinal mucosa, with resultant petechial hemorrhages and frank hemorrhage.

Fecal Flotation

Fecal flotation techniques use a variety of solutions, including sodium nitrate, zinc sulfate, sucrose, and sodium chloride, to identify parasite ova or larvae. The author prefers sodium nitrate as a fecal flotation solution because it will concentrate most nematode eggs and larvae, tapeworm eggs, flagellate cysts, and coccidian oocysts, as well as parasitic mites consumed when the host is trying to alleviate mite-associated pruritus. The goal is

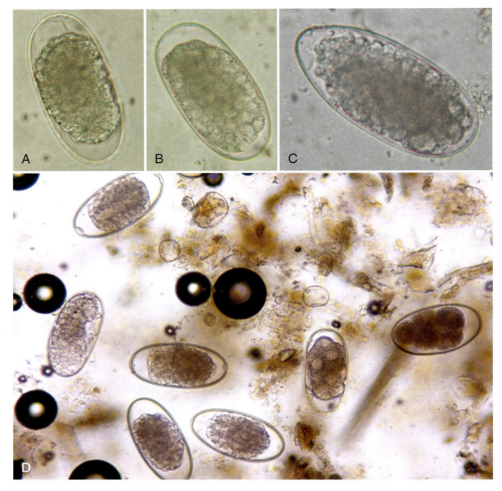

Figure 54-1 **A,** Strongyle egg (112 × 54 μm). **B,** Strongyle egg (104 × 51 μm). **C,** Strongyle egg (90 × 69 μm). **D,** Strongyle eggs.

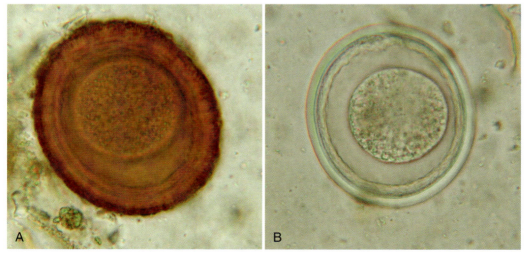

Figure 54-2 **A,** *Parascaris equorum* egg (88 × 77 μm). **B,** *P. equorum* infertile and atypical egg (80 × 66 μm).

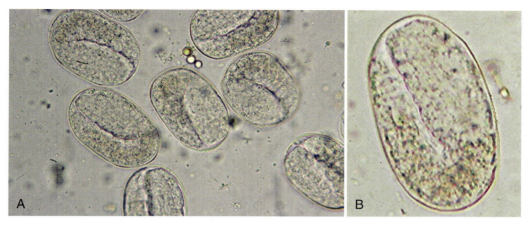

Figure 54-3 **A,** *Strongyloides westeri* eggs. **B,** *S. westeri* egg (58 × 33 μm).

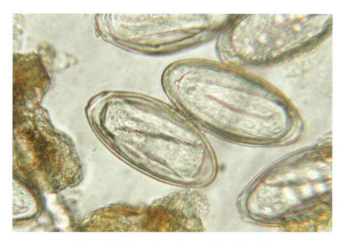

Figure 54-4 *Oxyuris equi* eggs (88 × 42 μm).

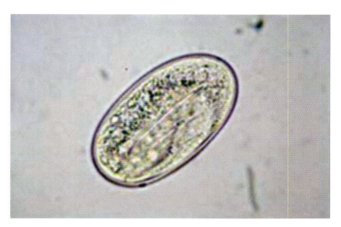

Figure 54-5 *Dictyocaulus arnfieldi* egg (92 × 58 μm).

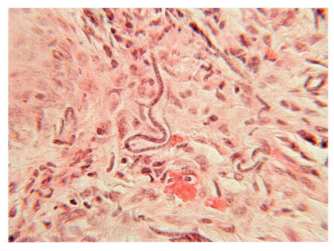

Figure 54-6 *Onchocerca cervicalis* microfilariae in skin section (width, 3.5 μm).

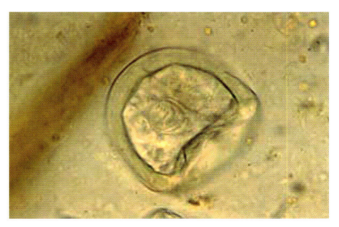

Figure 54-7 *Anoplocephala perfoliata* (72 μm).

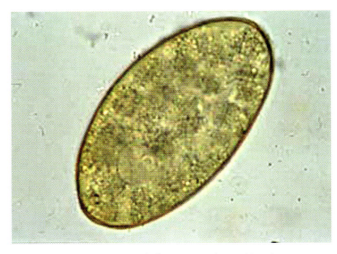

Figure 54-8 *Fasciola hepatica* egg (134 × 66 μm).

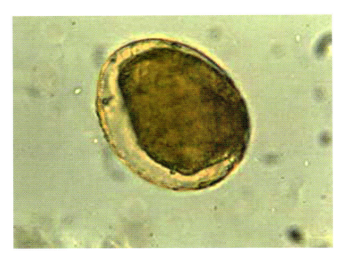

Figure 54-9 *Heterobilharzia americana* (94 × 76 μm).

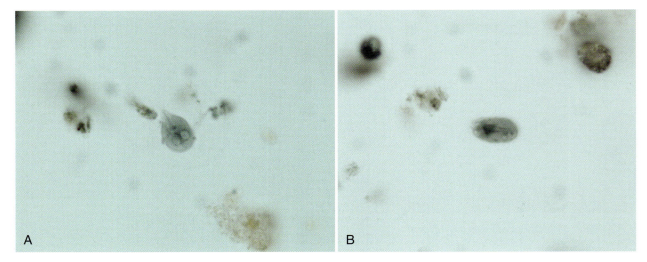

Figure 54-10 **A,** *Giardia intestinalis* trophozoite (iron hematoxylin stain; 11 × 7 μm). **B,** *G. intestinalis* cyst (iron hematoxylin stain; 8 × 6 μm).

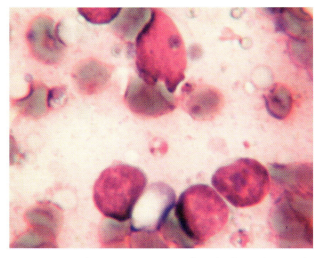

Figure 54-11 *Leishmania* sp. amastigotes from skin lesion (3 × 3 μm).

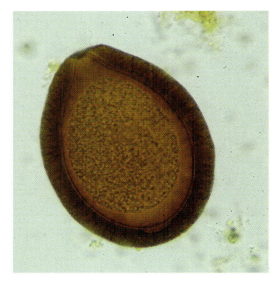

Figure 54-12 *Eimeria leuckarti* unsporulated oocyst (88 × 69 μm).

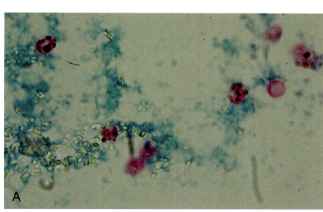
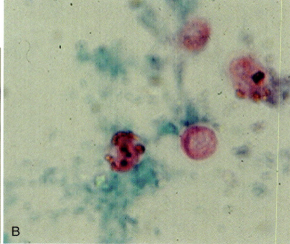

Figure 54-13 A, *Cryptosporidium parvum* oocysts (Kinyoun acid-fast stain; 4.5 μm). **B,** *C. parvum* oocysts (Kinyoun acid-fast stain).

to establish a solution with a specific gravity that will allow the eggs to float to the top of a liquid column, effectively concentrating and cleansing them in the process. The feces (preferably at least 2-4 g) should be homogenized thoroughly in the medium of choice in less volume than will fill the tube in which the flotation will be done. The fecal solution is then poured into the tube through a layer or two of gauze to eliminate large pieces of debris. The tube is topped off with more flotation medium until there is a slight positive meniscus in the tube opening. A 22 × 22 mm coverslip is placed on top of the tube, which is allowed to stand for at least 10 minutes. Alternatively, the tube may be centrifuged with the coverslip in place for 10 minutes. Most of the diagnostic stages will adhere to the surface film on the underside of the coverslip.

The coverslip is carefully removed and gently placed on a labeled microscope slide. The slide is first scanned systematically using the 10× objective using a good quality microscope. High magnification may be used to clarify the identity of detected eggs. It is important to optimize light transmission through the slide by appropriately adjusting the substage iris diaphragm of the microscope.

Fecal Cultures

The largest and most diverse group of parasites in horses is the strongylate nematodes, referred to as "small" strongyles (cyathostomes) and "large" strongyles. Because more than 40 species of strongyles are found in horses and their ova have a similar microscopic appearance, specific species of strongyle ova cannot be identified by microscopy with any reliability. Fecal culture by an experienced parasitologist can facilitate species diagnosis if this level of identification is considered necessary.

The feces are cultured for 10 to 12 days to obtain the infective third-stage (L_3) larvae to allow differentiation of some of the strongyle species present. A sample of 5 to 10 g of fresh feces is mixed with an equal quantity of vermiculite and formed into a ball in two layers of gauze. The top of the ball is tied closed with a piece of string, and the ball is moistened and placed into a jar with a lid that contains water about 5 to 10 mm deep. The string is held so the fecal ball is just above the surface of the water while the lid is screwed down to hold the string in place and secure the ball. The jar is labeled and placed into a dark chamber for 10 to 12 days at room temperature. When opened, the water at the bottom may be placed into a Petri dish and examined with a stereoscope to detect and

Box 54-1 Key to Identification of Nematode Larvae from Equine Feces		
1.	Esophagus with obvious midlevel constriction (rhabditiform).	Free-living trematodes
	Esophagus without such a constriction.	2
2.	Body not enclosed in sheath; tip of tail has V notch.	*Strongyloides westeri*
	Body not enclosed in sheath.	3
3.	Containing fewer than 16 distinct gut cells.	Cyathostomes
	Body with more than 16 gut cells.	4
4.	Body with 16 gut cells.	5
	Body with more than 16 gut cells.	7
5.	Sheath tail is short and rounded.	*Trichostrongylus axei*
	Sheath is long and whiplike.	6
6.	Very large larvae with well-defined triangular cells.	*Oesophagostomum* spp.
	Medium-sized larvae with rectangular gut cells.	*Posteriostomum* spp.
	Long, thin, larvae; poorly defined gut cells; small trilobed process on posterior end.	*Strongylus equinus*
7.	Larvae with 28 to 32 well-defined gut cells.	*Strongylus vulgaris*
	Larvae with 18 to 20 gut cells.	8
8.	Broad larvae, medium length, with well-defined gut cells.	*Triodontophorus* spp.
	Small, slender larvae with blunt tail and poorly defined gut cells.	*Strongylus edentatus*

recover larvae. Alternatively, if few larvae are present, a Baermann procedure may be used to concentrate the larvae from the fecal ball. The motile larvae may be inactivated and stained slightly to better visualize the morphology with the addition of a drop of Lugol's iodine to the edge of the coverslip of the wet mount containing living larvae. Box 54-1 provides a key to the infective L_3 larvae.

Fecal Sedimentation

Fluke eggs do not rise in normal flotation media, thus the sedimentation procedure may be used to cleanse and concentrate such eggs. A simple procedure with soapy water (1 mL of inexpensive dish detergent in 500 mL of water loaded into a squeeze bottle) may be used. Two to 4 g of feces is placed into a sample cup and mixed thoroughly with approximately 40 mL of sedimentation solution. The solution is poured through a double layer of gauze into a vertical 50-mL centrifuge tube. After standing for 5 minutes, the solution is decanted or aspirated. The process is repeated with soapy water. The third resuspension uses fresh water. After the eggs have been cleaned and concentrated by these sedimentation steps (water remains clear), the sample of the sediment is placed on a glass slide and examined microscopically.

Direct Fecal Smear

A small amount of feces is placed on an applicator stick and mixed thoroughly in normal saline on a microscope slide. A coverslip is placed and the preparation examined using a compound microscope to identify flagellated and ciliated protozoa. This procedure is not as sensitive as fecal flotation or sedimentation because there is no cleansing or concentration of potential diagnostic stages present in the sample.

Baermann Procedure

The Baermann procedure is used to search for motile nematode larvae or tiny adult nematodes. It uses a simple device consisting of a funnel mounted vertically, a rubber tube that fits on the stem of the funnel, and a clamp to close off the tubing. The funnel is filled with warm water, and the clamp is shut to hold the water within the funnel. It is helpful to squeeze the tubing to express air trapped inside the tube or funnel stem. The feces or larval culture material is placed in a few layers of gauze, and the gauze is wrapped around the sample to make a ball. A hardware cloth support should be cut to fit in the funnel reservoir to act as a support for the ball of feces. The feces are added to the reservoir and allowed to stand from 2 hours to overnight. The fluid is then drawn into a small Petri dish, and the contents are examined under a stereomicroscope. If nematode larvae or tiny adults (e.g., *Probstmayria*) are seen thrashing back and forth, some of these are placed onto a microscope slide with a drop of Lugol's iodine solution and a coverslip added. Nematodes lack circular muscles and thus cannot change the length of the body. They can only flex one way and then the other in a characteristic manner. The larvae may be examined and compared to standard larval diagrams to facilitate taxonomic identification (Fig. 54-14).

Cellophane (Scotch) Tape Test

The cellophane (Scotch) tape test is the preferred test for detection of pinworm *(Oxyuris equi)* ova (see Fig. 54-4). These ova adhere to the perineum and are rarely observed in routine fecal flotation or sedimentation samples. A length of clear cellophane tape is wrapped around three or four fingers with the sticky side out, and the tape is pressed against the perineum, then placed onto a glass slide. Saline or water may be placed over the tape and a long coverslip added to facilitate visualization of the ova (Fig. 54-15).

McMaster's Procedure

The McMaster's procedure is used to estimate the level of fecal contamination with parasite ova. Because it is a dilution technique, it may produce a false-negative result if low numbers of ova are present in a sample. Therefore it is best used in combination with an initial standard flotation. The McMaster's technique is often used to determine whether an anthelmintic treatment was effective. Pretreatment results are compared to results from samples collected 10 to 14 days after therapy.

A 4-g sample of fresh feces is added to a 120-mL screw-cap sample cup with sufficient sodium nitrate solution (fecal flotation medium) to bring the total volume to 30 mL and is mixed thoroughly. The solution is poured through one layer of gauze into another cup. After thorough mixing, the solution is used to fill the McMaster chamber. After standing for 10 minutes, the slide is placed on a compound microscope with the 10× objective in place. The width of each of the six lanes of the McMaster chamber is equal to the diameter of the field of view. The slide is systematically scanned to count the total number of each type of egg present on both sides of the chamber. If the counts between sides vary more than 20%, it is considered evidence of insufficient mixing of the sample, and the procedure should be repeated. The total count by parasite type present is multiplied by 25 to determine the eggs per gram (EPG) of feces. (NOTE: The volume of fluid and the weight of feces used can vary and are based on the following: the volume under each grid is 0.15 mL, thus the volume under both grids is 0.3 mL. This is $\frac{1}{100}$ the volume used [30 mL], thus the number of eggs would be multiplied by 100; if 4 g of feces were

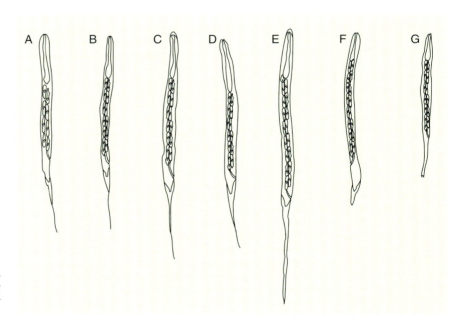

Figure 54-14 Infective larvae of strongyles. **A,** Cyathostome; **B,** *Posteriostomum*; **C,** *Strongylus equinus*; **D,** *Strongylus edentatus*; **E,** *Strongylus vulgaris*; **F,** *Trichostrongylus axei*; **G,** *Strongyloides westeri*.

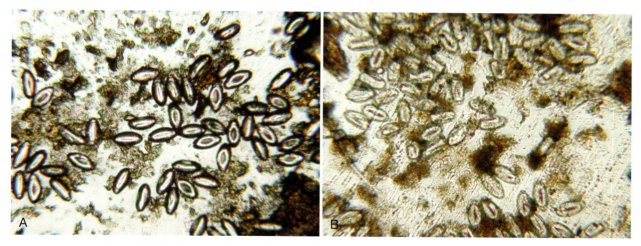

Figure 54-15 **A,** *Oxyuris equi* eggs under tape without saline. **B,** *O. equi* eggs under tape with saline.

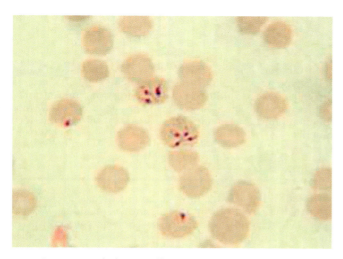

Figure 54-16 *Theileria equi* (formerly *Babesia equi*) piroplasms.

Box 54-2 Modified Key to Microfilariae of Horses

1. Microfilariae encased in membranous   *Setaria equina*
   sheath; found in blood.
   Microfilariae not enclosed in sheath.   2
2. Microfilariae with round posterior ends,   *Parafilaria*
   200 μm long and present in hemorrhagic   *multipapillosa*
   nodules in dermis.
   Microfilariae with pointed posterior ends,   3
   greater than 200 μm.
3. Tail is short.   *Onchocerca cervicalis*
   Tail is long and whiplike.   *Onchocerca reticulata*

Modified from Soulsby EJ: Textbook of veterinary clinical parasitology, Philadelphia, 1965, FA Davis.

---

used, this would be divided by 4 to obtain EPG. This is the same as multiplying by 25.)

Impression Smears

When horses are suspected of having cutaneous lesions attributable to *Leishmania*, a deep scraping that draws blood from the lesion is made. Smears of the exudate are stained with Wright's or Giemsa to reveal the presence of amastigotes. Impression smears of biopsies from spleen, liver, or bone marrow would reveal visceral amastigotes about 2 μm in length with recognizable nucleus and kinetoplast (Fig. 54-16).

Skin Biopsy Examination

For diagnosis of microfilariae of *Onchocerca* spp., dermal biopsies are obtained from the unpigmented area of the ventral abdomen. These may be either fixed for histologic examination or teased apart in saline. If the latter approach is used, begin with warm saline and allow the teased preparation to stand for approximately 15 minutes before examining for motile microfilariae that have emerged from the tissue. Histologic sections will reveal the microfilariae in the superficial dermis (see Fig. 54-6). Box 54-2 provides a key to the microfilariae of the filarial nematodes of horses.

Blood Smears

Blood smears may be used to facilitate diagnosis of equine piroplasmosis and rarely microfilariae of *Setaria*. The microfilariae will be free in the blood, but the piroplasms of *Theileria equi* (see Fig. 54-16) and *Babesia caballi* will be in erythrocytes (see Chapter 56).

Isolated Worms Recovered from Necropsy or Passed in Feces

Proper fixation of parasites will make identification easier for the parasitologist examining the specimens. Although most veterinary practices have formalin for fixing tissue, this is not the ideal solution to fix nematode, cestode, or trematode parasites. Nematodes should be fixed in stock glacial acetic acid if they are medium to small in size, then transferred and stored in 70% ethanol with glycerin (90 parts 70% ethanol, 10 parts glycerin). Flatworms should be relaxed about an hour in water, then fixed as flat as possible in AFA (85 parts 85% ethanol, 10 parts stock formalin, 5 parts glacial acetic acid). Some trematodes may need to be placed between two microscope slides and slight pressure applied, allowing AFA to diffuse around the specimens. Maintain pressure for a few minutes, then place the specimens into a vial with AFA. Maggots should be dropped into boiling water for a minute and then placed in 70% ethanol. Lice, ticks, and mites may be placed directly into 70% ethanol.

When shipping parasites to an identification service, provide appropriate contact information, including your e-mail or contact address, the host species, the location from which the specimens originated (organ), and any other pertinent clinical information.

The adult helminths passed in the feces and large enough to see with the naked eye include *Anoplocephala magna* (see Fig. 58-1, *B*), *Anoplocephala perfoliata* (see Fig. 58-1, *A*), *Parascaris* (see Fig. 57-6), *Oxyuris equi* (see Fig. 57-10), and nematodes observed on the sleeves of gloves used in rectal palpations include species of *Strongylus* (see Fig. 57-4) and cyathostomes (see Fig. 57-3).

Suggested Readings

Bowman DD: Georgi's parasitology for veterinarians, Philadelphia, 2009, Saunders.

Jacobs DE: A color atlas of equine parasites, Philadelphia, 1986, Lea & Febiger.

Lichtenfels JR: Helminths of domestic equids, Proc Helm Soc Wash 42, Special Issue 92, 1975.

Manual of veterinary parasitological laboratory techniques, Technical Bulletin 18, London, 1979, Ministry of Agriculture, Fisheries and Food.

Soulsby EJ: Textbook of veterinary clinical parasitology, vol 1, Helminths, Philadelphia, 1965, FA Davis.

CHAPTER

Equine Protozoal Myeloencephalitis

55

Sharon Witonsky, Debra C. Sellon,* and J.P. Dubey*

In 1970, Rooney et al[1] reported 52 cases of focal myelitis-encephalitis in horses from Kentucky and Pennsylvania, with the highest incidence in young Standardbreds. Horses were presented for evaluation of progressive spinal ataxia of one or more limbs. At necropsy, focal lesions of vascular damage, hemorrhage, mononuclear cuffing, gliosis, and neuronal and axonal degeneration were observed in one or more segments of the spinal cord. This report is now thought to be the first published description of equine protozoal myeloencephalitis (EPM).

In 1974, separate reports by Beech and Dodd,[2,3] Dubey et al,[4] and Cusick et al[5] described 14 horses in the United States with focal malacia and hemorrhage in the white and gray matter of the brain and spinal cord. Protozoal organisms observed in the central nervous system (CNS) tissues of each horse resembled *Toxoplasma gondii* but differed in several respects, including an absence of *T. gondii* antibody responses in affected horses. A subsequent serosurvey of horses revealed that 20% of 1294 serum samples tested by microtitration and indirect hemagglutinin test were positive for antibodies to *T. gondii*.[6] Attempts to induce disease in healthy ponies by oral administration of infective *T. gondii* oocysts with concomitant corticosteroid injections were unsuccessful,[7,8] and the etiologic agent of EPM remained a mystery for almost 20 years.

In 1991, a protozoan apicomplexan parasite was successfully cultured from the spinal cord of a horse with EPM,[9] and Dubey et al[10] proposed the name *Sarcocystis neurona* for the parasite associated with encephalomyelitis in horses in North America. Subsequently, other investigators were able to isolate *S. neurona* from affected horses,[11] and the phylogenetic relationship of the organism to members of the family *Sarcocystidae* was confirmed based on small, ribosomal ribonucleic acid (rRNA) gene sequence.[12] Because of greater than 99.5% homology within a 742–base pair (bp) segment of the 18S rRNA gene, investigators mistakenly suggested that *S. neurona* was synonymous with *Sarcocystis falcatula*.[13] The opossum is the definitive host for *S. falcatula*, and birds are intermediate hosts. However, *S. neurona* is distinguishable from *S. falcatula* on the basis of its genetic composition, structure, biology, and ability to infect horses, and the two parasites are now recognized as separate species.[14-19]

In the past 15 years, numerous studies have advanced our understanding of the life cycle and epidemiology of *S. neurona* and enhanced our abilities to diagnose, treat, and prevent EPM. Despite these advances, however, EPM remains one of the most common infectious neurologic diseases of horses in North America.

Etiology

Sarcocystis neurona is the most common etiologic agent identified as a cause of EPM, but similar parasites, including *Neospora hughesi*, have been incriminated as etiologic agents in a few horses.[20-25] In this chapter, EPM refers to disease caused by infection of the equine CNS with *S. neurona* unless specified otherwise.

Sarcocystis neurona has a complex life cycle involving both sexual and asexual stages (Fig. 55-1). The definitive hosts for *S. neurona*, the opossums (*Didelphis virginiana* and *D. albiventris*),[26] become infected through ingestion of mature sarcocysts containing bradyzoites in tissues of intermediate hosts such as the skunk,[27] raccoon,[28] nine-banded armadillo,[29,30] domestic cat,[31] and sea otter.[32] Bradyzoites are released from the sarcocysts in the gut lumen of opossums and transform directly in the small intestine into male and female gamonts without any replication.[33,34] The male gamonts divide into several gametes. An oocyst is produced after the fertilization of the female gamont by the male gamete; the entire process can be completed in the small intestine of the opossum within 24 hours of ingestion of sarcocysts. Oocysts sporulate in the lamina propria, producing two sporocysts, each containing four sporozoites. Fully sporulated oocysts or sporocysts are excreted in the feces of the opossum. *Sarcocystis neurona* sporocysts from opossum feces are approximately 10 × 8 μm in size.[35]

After ingestion of sporocysts by an intermediate host, sporozoites are released, invade the intestinal epithelium, and undergo asexual multiplication in many tissues. The number of asexual generations (schizogony) has not been determined. Studies in interferon-gamma (IFN-γ) knockout mice suggest that *S. neurona* multiplies in visceral tissues, lungs, and heart before invading the CNS. *Sarcocystis neurona* multiplies in the CNS and visceral tissues by a specialized form of schizogony, called *endopolygeny* (Fig. 55-2). In endopolygeny the nucleus

*The authors acknowledge and appreciate the original contributions of these authors, whose work has been incorporated into this chapter.

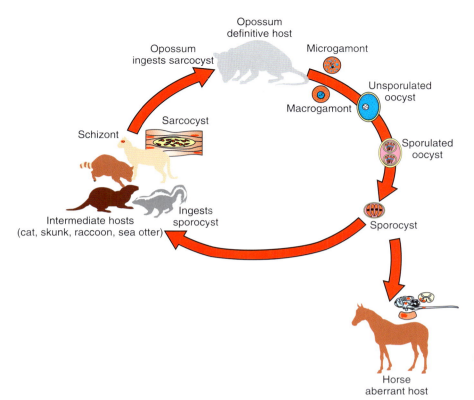

Opossum
definitive host

Opossum
ingests sarcocyst

Microgamont

Macrogamont

Unsporulated
oocyst

Sarcocyst

Sporulated
oocyst

Schizont

Sporocyst

Intermediate hosts
(cat, skunk, raccoon, sea otter)

Ingests
sporocyst

Horse
aberrant host

Figure 55-1 Proposed life cycle of *S. neurona*. *(From Dubey JP, Lindsay DS, Saville WJ, et al: A review of Sarcocystis neurona and equine protozoal myeloencephalitis (EPM). Vet Parasitol 95:89–131, 2001.)*

becomes lobulated.[34] The lobes are connected by chromatin strands and may be arranged in groups. In early stages the uninucleate schizont sometimes resembles a macrophage or a degenerated host cell (Fig. 55-2, C). Finding multiple nucleoli in a nucleus helps to distinguish *S. neurona* from degenerating host cells. Several merozoites may develop within the same host cell[10,34] to become mature schizonts and produce merozoites without leaving the host cell; thus the developmental cycle may be asynchronous. Merozoites are formed centrally or peripherally in the schizont, often around a residual body (Fig. 55-3). Schizonts and merozoites are periodic acid–Schiff (PAS) reaction negative. Mature schizonts in the CNS are up to 30 μm long and may be oval, round, elongated, or irregular in shape.[34] The mechanism by which *S. neurona* is transported is unknown, but it has been proposed that it may reach the CNS protected in mononuclear cells (Fig. 55-4).[36]

Both neural and inflammatory cells in the CNS may be parasitized. Several hundred merozoites may be present in a single neuron.[4] In histologic sections of CNS, individual merozoites are about 3 to 5 μm long and contain a single, centrally located, vesicular nucleus.[34]

Ultrastructurally, schizonts and merozoites are located in the host cell cytoplasm without a parasitophorous vacuole at any stage of development (see Figs. 55-2 and 55-3). Fully formed merozoites have the same organelles as found in most coccidians (except that rhoptries are absent in *Sarcocystis* merozoites).[37] Merozoites released from schizonts eventually give rise to encysted stages (sarcocysts).[31] The earliest sarcocysts consist of a tissue cyst wall enclosing a few round forms, called *metrocytes*. Metrocytes divide into two organisms that eventually become bradyzoites. Unlike schizonts, sarcocysts are located in a parasitophorous vacuole inside host cytoplasm. It takes approximately 2 months or more for sarcocysts to mature in the intermediate hosts.[34] Sarcocysts observed in experimentally infected cats and raccoons were approximately 700 μm in length with a cyst wall 1 to 3 μm thick.[31,34,38] Bradyzoites are

slender and approximately 5 μm in length. Intermediate hosts do not usually exhibit recognizable clinical signs as a result of *S. neurona* infection, but encephalomyelitis has been documented in the cat, raccoon, mink, skunk, sea otter, Pacific harbor seal, Canadian lynx, fisher, and dog.[39] Horses are considered aberrant intermediate hosts for *S. neurona* in which only schizonts have been identified with certainty. Raccoons, armadillos, sea otters, skunks, cats, and possibly other mammals are intermediate hosts of *S. neurona*.[27-31,39-41] In the intermediate hosts, sarcocysts are microscopic; bradyzoites are slender and tiny. The villar protrusions on the sarcocyst walls are up to 2.5 μm long and have microtubules that extend into the ground substance.[34]

There have been numerous reports of myeloencephalitis in horses associated with *Neospora* spp. infection.[20-23,25,42] A new species, *Neospora hughesi*, was isolated from infected horses and is considered distinct from *Neospora caninum* based mainly on genomic analysis of the first internal transcribed spacer (ITS-1) region of the rRNA gene[23] and amino acid differences in two immunodominant surface antigens.[24]

Epidemiology

In North America, the opossum *(Didelphis virginiana)* is the only known definitive host for *S. neurona*.[26] Opossums in North America may be simultaneously infected with several *Sarcocystis* spp., including *S. neurona*, *S. falcatula*, *S. speeri*, and others.[34,43,44] Risk factors associated with the presence of *S. neurona* sporocysts in opossums include season and higher body condition score.[45] Approximately twice as many opossums trapped in spring were positive for sporocysts as opossums trapped in fall or winter. These investigators found no association between sporocyst presence in trapped opossums and age, gender, or the presence of young in the pouch of females.[45]

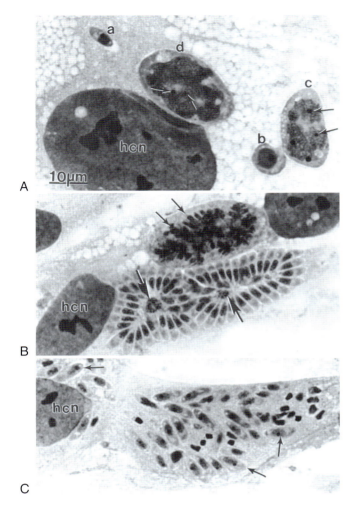

A

B

C

Figure 55-2 Schizogonic stages of S. neurona in bovine turbinate cells (Giemsa stain; hcn, host cell nucleus; bar applies to all figures). **A,** Differentiation of merozoite nucleus into schizont nucleus. Note a merozoite with enlarged nucleus (a), globular schizont with nucleus containing one nucleolus (b), lobulated nucleus (c) with five nucleoli (arrows), and a schizont with large nucleus with two nucleoli (arrows) (d). **B,** Three schizonts. Note merozoites budding at the surface (small arrows) and residual bodies (large arrows) in two mature schizonts. **C,** Development of second generation of schizonts without merozoites of the first generation leaving the host cell. Arrows indicate merozoites transforming to schizonts. (From Dubey JP: J Vet Parasitol 15:91–102, 2001.)

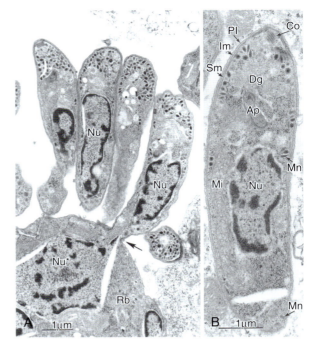

A 1µm   **B** 1µm

Figure 55-3 Transmission electron micrographs of S. neurona in brain of horse; S. neurona (isolate SN7) was obtained from this horse.[31] **A,** Portion of schizont showing several budding merozoites, one of which still attached (arrow) to the residual body (Rb). Nu, Nucleus of merozoite; Nu*, nucleus of schizont still in residual body. **B,** Merozoite. Ap, Putative apicoplast (Golgi adjunct); Co, conoid; Dg, dense granule; Im, inner membrane complex; Mi, mitochondrion; Mn, microneme; Pl, plasmalemma; Sm, subpellicular microtubule. (From Dubey JP, Lindsay DS, Saville WJ, et al: A review of Sarcocystis neurona and equine protozoal myeloencephalitis (EPM). Vet Parasitol 95:89–131, 2001.)

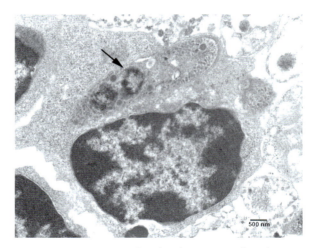

Figure 55-4 Equine monocyte infected 24 hours previously with merozoites of SN-37R isolate of S. neurona. Arrow indicates a single merozoite that is free in the cytoplasm of the monocyte.

A similar study of opossums in southern Michigan revealed that 31 of 206 opossums examined (15%) were infected with S. neurona.[46] This study confirmed that summer season was a risk factor for infection, but body condition score was not a factor. A higher frequency of S. neurona infection was observed in adult animals (12.6%) and females (9.2%) than in juveniles (2.4%) and males (5.8%). Multivariate analysis suggested that concomitant infection with other Sarcocystis spp. and presence of young in the pouch of females were risk factors for S. neurona infection in opossums.[46]

Armadillos,[29,30] raccoons,[28] skunks,[27] sea otters,[43] cats,[31,47] and possibly horses[48] have been identified as natural intermediate hosts for S. neurona. Dubey et al[28] demonstrated the presence of S. neurona sarcocysts in muscle of naturally infected raccoons. When these muscles were fed to opossums, S. neurona sporocysts were shed in the feces. Feeding sporocysts to IFN-γ knockout mice resulted in classic protozoal myeloencephalitis. After experimental infection by feeding of S. neurona sporocysts,

raccoons developed schizonts and merozoites in many tissues, including the brain, and sarcocysts in skeletal muscle, especially the tongue.[38]

The raccoon is probably the most important intermediate host for S. neurona in the United States because it is found throughout the country and is often infected with S. neurona. The role of the domestic cat and other intermediate hosts in the natural epidemiology of EPM is controversial, but most researchers consider it unlikely that the cat plays a major role.[49]

Fourteen of 35 cats (40%) from horse farms in southwestern Ohio with prior *S. neurona* infections in horses on the premises were seropositive for *S. neurona*. Horses from the same premises had a 93% seropositive rate. In contrast, the seroprevalence rate among general cat populations in the Eastern United States is estimated to be between 5% and 10%.[50-52]

The geographic range of clinical EPM in horses is defined by the range of the opossum, the definitive host of *S. neurona*. In areas where the opossum is common, approximately 50% of horses are seropositive, indicating exposure to *S. neurona*.[53-59] In central Wyoming and Montana, outside the natural range of opossums, only 6.5% and 0%, respectively, of wild horses are seropositive.[60,61] The South American opossum, *Didelphis albiventris*, is also a definitive host for *S. neurona*. Approximately 65% of horses in Brazil are estimated to be seropositive to *S. neurona* and 2.5% are estimated to be seropositive to *N. hughesi*.[62-64] *Sarcocystis neurona* isolates from North America are genetically similar, regardless of the host, but differ from South American isolates.[65]

The horse is the most common species in which myeloencephalitis caused by *S. neurona* infection is identified. In 1998, the U.S. Department of Agriculture (USDA) estimated the incidence of EPM to range from 0.06% in the southern states to 0.43% in the central United States, with a national average of 0.014%.[66] Clinical cases of EPM have been diagnosed in native horses of Panama[67] and Brazil,[68] but the incidence of EPM in seropositive horses in those countries is unknown. Horses in Europe, South Africa, and Asia diagnosed with EPM have invariably been imported from the Western Hemisphere.[69-73] Although serologic evidence indicates exposure of other equid species to *S. neurona*, with a recent study demonstrating 3% to 4% seroprevalence in horses from Spain,[74] the only reports of clinical disease in these species are in a single pony and a Grant's zebra.[75-77]

Most clinicians consider clinical EPM as a sporadic disease.[78] However, prior diagnosis on a premises is a risk factor for diagnosis of future cases of EPM,[79] and clusters of disease over a short period have been reported on single farms.[67,80] In 1990, Fayer et al[81] reported on 364 histologically confirmed cases of EPM from many areas of the United States. Thoroughbreds, Standardbreds, and Quarter Horses were the breeds most often affected. There were no obvious patterns of infection based on geographic location, gender, or season. Also in 1990, Boy et al[82] reported that the risk for EPM among 82 horses in Pennsylvania was higher in male and Standardbred horses. Neither study had control populations to confirm the significance of the demographic observations.

In 2000, Saville et al[79] reported the results of a case control study of 251 horses diagnosed with EPM at Ohio State University on the basis of positive immunoblot or polymerase chain reaction (PCR) of cerebrospinal fluid (CSF). These horses were compared to a control group of 225 horses with neurologic diseases other than EPM and a control group of 251 horses admitted to the hospital for evaluation of nonneurologic disorders. In the final multivariable logistic regression analysis of EPM horses versus neurologic control horses, factors associated with increased risk of EPM included admission in the fall season, hay storage not secure from wildlife, wooded terrain around the premises, previous diagnosis of EPM on the premises, and a recent (< 90 days) adverse health event for the horse.[79] Adverse health events included lameness, parturition, accident or injury, management changes, lacerations, surgical procedures, colic, and other medical problems. In the final multivariable logistic regression analysis of EPM horses versus nonneurologic control horses, factors associated with increased risk of EPM included admission to the hospital during the spring/summer/fall season, hay storage not secure from wildlife, use of the horse for racing or showing, age 1 to 5 years, previous

diagnosis of EPM on the premises, and a recent adverse health event for the horse. Protective risk factors included age less than 1 year, use for breeding, and observation of birds, but not opossums, on the premises.[79]

In 2003, Rossano et al[83] reported on a study of EPM in 1121 equids in 98 horse herds in Michigan. Serum samples were tested by immunoblot for presence of antibodies to *S. neurona*. Samples were stratified based on relative opossum abundance and herd size. Management factors such as age, fly control, wildlife control, and type of feed containment were examined. No single management factor was associated with herd seroprevalence. The authors speculate that it is difficult to restrict exposure of horses to *S. neurona* on farms located in areas with an abundance of opossums.[83]

Sarcocystis neurona has been associated with CNS infection and disease in many nonequid mammalian species, including southern sea otters,[84-86] Pacific harbor seals,[87,88] skunks,[75,89] mink,[75,90] raccoons,[91-93] dogs,[39,41] and cats.[75,94,95] An unconfirmed *S. neurona*–like infection has also been reported in a rhesus monkey[96] and Canadian lynx.[97] The presence of antibodies to *S. neurona* is a risk factor for myocarditis in southern sea otters.[98] Strains of *S. neurona* isolated from opossums and sea otters are morphologically and molecularly indistinguishable from equine isolates.* Rejmanek et al[101] further defined the association between *S. neurona* in opossums and sea otters and horses when they determined that, in a small group (10 opossums, 6 horses, 1 cat, 23 sea otters, 1 porpoise) of naturally infected animals in California, using 15 genetic markers, the *S. neurona* strains were identical. These data suggest that *S. neurona* from opossums was the cause of disease in both encephalitis and EPM in sea otters and horses, respectively. Additional studies in sea otters[102,103] demonstrated that both *S. neurona* and *T. gondii* are capable of undergoing self-mating as a mechanism of persistence and possibly virulence because outbreaks of disease were identified with single clones of *T. gondii* and *S. neurona*. The implications for self-mating and disease, as well as the role of *S. neurona* infection in these species and its impact on the natural history of EPM in horses, are still being defined.

Pathogenesis

The only known method of transmission of *S. neurona* to horses is through ingestion of sporocysts in opossum feces. Merozoites and schizonts may be observed in a variety of cell types in the CNS of horses with EPM, including neurons, mononuclear cells, and glial cells.[4] Only asexual stages of the parasite have been isolated from horses and, in the absence of evidence that sarcocysts form in the muscle of horses, equids are considered aberrant or "dead-end" hosts.

Several investigators have reported clinical signs of disease in one or more horses after experimental infection with *S. neurona* sporocysts or merozoites.[104-108] To date, however, none has successfully fulfilled Koch's postulates by isolating the organism from the experimentally infected horse and subsequently reproducing disease in another horse with that isolate.

It has been difficult to consistently reproduce neurologic disease with demonstrable histopathologic lesions in experimentally infected horses by feeding or oral administration of *S. neurona* sporocysts even when horses are immune suppressed with dexamethasone.[104,107-109] In 2001, Saville et al[107] used a model of transport stress immediately before inoculation with *S. neurona* sporocysts. All infected horses developed clinical signs of disease as early as 9 days after infection, with the most

---

*References 14, 32, 65, 86, 88, 99, 100.

severe signs in horses infected immediately after transport, but the histologic lesions observed in infected horses were minimal. All tissue sections from infected horses were negative for *S. neurona* by immunohistochemistry (IHC), tissue culture, and bioassay in IFN-γ knockout (GKO) mice.[107]

After oral infection with sporocysts, microscopic lesions consistent with *S. neurona* can be identified in experimentally infected horses as early as 7 days after infection, suggesting that *S. neurona* can migrate to other organs and to the CNS more quickly than initially predicted.[110]

Ellison et al[111] has also developed an experimental model of infection in which horses are injected with autologous lymphocytes infected with *S. neurona* merozoites. Using *S. neurona* merozoites isolated from a naturally occurring EPM horse, all three infected horses developed clinical signs consistent with EPM, developed antibodies in the serum and CSF against *S. neurona*, and *S. neurona* was isolated from postmortem tissue in all three infected horses. No histopathologic changes were provided in the report.

Because of the difficulties in developing a consistent and reproducible experimental model, as well as to understand the etiology and immune response to infection, investigators have employed both immunodeficient and immunocompetent horse and mouse models. *Sarcocystis neurona* has been isolated from the blood and tissues of immunodeficient and immunocompetent horses after experimental infection.[105,112,113] The parasite was isolated from the blood of an Arabian foal with severe combined immunodeficiency (SCID) at 21 days after oral infection with *S. neurona* sporocysts.[113] Parasitemia after infection was confirmed in a larger study in which six immunocompetent foals and three SCID Arabian foals were infected either orally with *S. neurona* sporocysts or intravenously (IV) with *S. neurona* merozoites.[105] Foals were stressed by weaning immediately before infection. Despite prolonged parasitemia and persistent infection of visceral tissues (skeletal muscle, cardiac muscle, lung, liver, and spleen), as demonstrated by PCR and culture, SCID horses did not develop neurologic signs after oral or IV infection.[105] In contrast, although parasitemia was undetectable, four of six orally infected immunocompetent foals developed neurologic signs consisting of ataxia and proprioceptive deficits. Parasites were detectable by PCR or culture in the CNS tissues of immunocompetent foals with neurologic signs. These studies demonstrate that specific immune responses (B and T cell mediated) are required to control parasitemia and infection of visceral tissues of horses. However, these responses are often unable to control neuroinvasion and prevent development of clinical signs.[105] In 2005, Rossano et al[112] confirmed the presence of parasitemia in immunocompetent horses after oral infection with *S. neurona* sporocysts by culturing the organism from blood of experimentally infected weaning horses.

Murine models of *S. neurona* infection provide additional clues to the pathogenesis and immune control of *S. neurona* in mammalian hosts. Infection of immunocompetent mice is not associated with disease; however, infection of GKO mice, incapable of producing IFN-γ, with either sporocysts or merozoites, consistently results in fulminant neurologic disease and death, regardless of the genetic background of the mice.[18,114-116] Examination of the CNS of infected GKO mice that die after *S. neurona* infection reveals inflammatory infiltrates consisting mostly of neutrophils and macrophages, fewer eosinophils, rare multinucleated giant cells, scattered subacute perivascular cuffing, and intralesional protozoa.[117] Lesions and organisms are most common in the caudal brain, especially the cerebellum, and equally distributed in white and gray matter of the brain and spinal cord.[117]

In 2001, Dubey[118] described the pathogenesis of *S. neurona* infection in GKO mice fed sporocysts. Parasitemia was demonstrable by bioassay at 1 to 8 days after infection. Sporozoites were observed in histologic sections of all regions of the small intestine and in cells in Peyer's patches of a mouse killed 6 hours after ingesting sporocysts. At 1 day after infection, organisms were present in all regions of the small intestine and in mesenteric lymph nodes. Parasites were visible in extraintestinal tissues by 3 days after infection and in the brain within 2 weeks after infection.[118,119] Parasites could be found in the brain, liver, lung, heart, and eyes of mice examined at 20 to 62 days after infection.[119] Witonsky et al[120] described splenomegaly, lymphadenopathy, mixed inflammatory infiltrate in the liver, perivascular infiltrate in the liver and lung, and interstitial pneumonia in GKO mice at 14 days after infection.

Although there is a paucity of specific information regarding the pathogenesis of *S. neurona* infection in horses, the information gleaned from pathologic and epidemiologic reports of natural infection, results of experimental equine infections, and extrapolation from murine models of disease suggest a likely theory for the pathogenesis of EPM.

After ingestion of sporocysts from opossum feces, *S. neurona* replicates to a limited extent in equine gastrointestinal epithelial cells.[121] Cell-associated parasitemia provides the parasites with access to visceral and CNS tissues where subsequent rounds of asexual reproduction occur. After hematogenous spread to the CNS, *S. neurona* may localize in any area, from cerebrum to spinal cord, but is not found in peripheral nerves. Specific immune responses limit parasitemia and visceral organ infection but do not always prevent CNS invasion and disease. The exact location of parasite replication in the CNS of an infected horse determines the type and severity of clinical signs that are observed. Some types of immune suppression and stress may increase the likelihood of neurologic disease after infection with *S. neurona*.

Most information regarding host immune response to *S. neurona* infection has been gained from murine models of infection. The consistent induction of disease in GKO mice clearly demonstrates the importance of IFN-γ in disease control.[18,114-116] Interferon-gamma is released in the mammalian brain in response to a variety of infectious agents and is considered an essential component of host immune response to CNS infection.[122] In C57Bl/6 mice, protection from neurologic disease is mediated by CD8 T lymphocytes.[120,123,124] Mice lacking these cells develop clinical signs of meningoencephalomyelitis with typical histopathologic lesions.[115] The relevance of this observation to equine disease is uncertain because of reports that SCID foals (lacking B and T cells) do not develop neurologic disease after infection with *S. neurona* sporocysts or merozoites, despite persistent parasitemia and widespread replication of parasites in visceral tissues.[105]

Genetic background also influences development of clinical disease in mice.[114,125] Marsh et al[125] reported that C57Bl/6 nude mice (lacking T cells) developed neurologic disease after experimental infection with *S. neurona*, but ICR SCID mice (lacking B and T cells) did not. This apparently contradictory observation remained unexplained until Ahlgrim et al[114] demonstrated that nude and SCID mice with a C57Bl/6 genetic background develop severe neurologic disease and die after experimental infection with *S. neurona*, whereas nude and SCID mice on a BALB/c background consistently survive infection without clinical signs. Resistance to clinical disease in BALB/c mice appears to be related to a component of innate immunity other than natural killer (NK) cell function.[114,126] When BALB/c SCID mice were infected with *S. neurona* they failed to develop neurologic disease even when NK cells were depleted. However, these mice did develop fulminant neurologic disease when IFN-γ function was blocked.[126] These data suggest that BALB/c mice may have a cell type, other than B cells, T cells, or NK cells, that secretes more IFN-γ than secreted by similar cells in C57Bl/6 mice. The relevance of this observation to equine disease is uncertain, but it may indicate genetic differences in susceptibility to CNS infection and disease in horses.

Relatively little is known about immune responses to *S. neurona* infection in horses. Two surface proteins of *S. neurona*, Sn14 and Sn16, are expressed in vivo in the horse and are strong immunogens.[127] However, many horses readily develop clinical disease despite the presence of specific antibodies, suggesting that humoral responses are not protective. Specific B-cell and T-cell responses limit and control parasitemia and replication of parasites in visceral tissues of horses, but, in this model, these responses cannot prevent neuroinvasion and neurovirulence.[105] By contrast, Ellison and Witonsky[128] demonstrated that antibodies to surface antigen 1 (SAG1) did significantly enhance protection against *S. neurona* SAG1 challenge based on daily and cumulative clinical signs. Vaccinated horses had significantly increased SAG1 antibody titers versus controls. With this model, there are likely multiple mechanisms of protection, but there was an association between significantly higher serum antibody titer in the vaccinated groups with significantly decreased clinical signs.[128] Parasites may be able to induce an immunosuppression toward parasite-derived antigens, including suppression of IFN-γ production, facilitating parasite survival in the horse.[129] Yang et al[130] and Witonsky et al[131] did demonstrate that both naturally and experimentally *S. neurona* infected horses had decreased proliferation responses to nonspecific mitogen phorbol myristate acetate and ionomycin. Although the exact mechanism is not known, it does suggest that *S. neurona* may be capable of limiting the immune response. The limited available data suggest that both innate and adaptive immune responses are important for control of infection of *S. neurona* in horses. Additional information is needed to determine better the nature of protective immune responses and guide production of better vaccines for prevention of disease.

Clinical Findings

Clinical signs of EPM vary greatly because of the diffuse or multifocal localization of parasites and inflammatory lesions in gray or white matter of the brain, brainstem, or spinal cord.[78,132-134] Onset of disease may be acute or insidious, and signs may progress rapidly or remain stable for long periods. Most affected horses are bright and alert with normal vital signs, but focal asymmetric muscle atrophy may be obvious on initial examination (Fig. 55-5). Muscle atrophy is most common in the gluteal or quadriceps muscles but may also mimic sweeny, radial nerve paralysis, or polyneuritis equi.[134] Occasionally, affected horses exhibit more generalized, mild muscle atrophy. Complete blood count (CBC) and serum biochemical profile are usually unremarkable.

Initial reports of EPM described horses with progressive neurologic disease that might include ataxia and conscious proprioceptive deficits of one or more limbs, cranial nerve deficits, or cerebral signs.[1-5,135] In 1978, Mayhew et al[136] reported that 8 of 32 horses (25%) with EPM had signs of brain disease. MacKay[137] reported in 1997 that a survey of 158 cases of EPM from Ohio State University revealed that 126 (80%) had spinal cord signs alone, 10 (6%) had only brain signs, and 22 (14%) had both brain and spinal cord signs. In 2000, Saville et al[138] reported the frequency of specific clinical signs in 251 horses diagnosed with EPM. Spinal ataxia was observed in 88.8% of 251 horses with EPM, weakness in 80.5%, spasticity in 56.2%, muscle atrophy in 14.3%, cranial nerve dysfunction in 11.6%, and seizures in 6%. More than 74% of affected horses had clinical signs involving both front and rear limbs, 0.4% involved front limbs only, and 19.9% had signs only in the rear limbs. Severity of gait deficits ranged from mild (grade 1-2, 19.9%) to

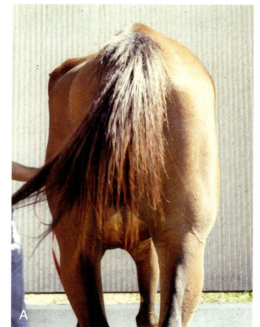

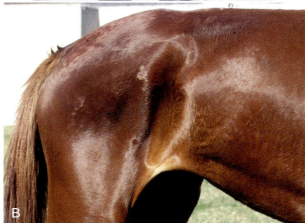

Figure 55-5 Asymmetric muscle atrophy resulting from *S. neurona* infection. **A,** Atrophy of left gluteal muscles. **B,** Atrophy of right quadriceps, tensor fascia lata, and biceps femoris. *(Courtesy Dr. Robert MacKay.)*

severe (grade 4-5, 22.2%). Clinical signs were asymmetric in 68.9% of horses.[138]

Gait abnormalities are the most common presenting complaint for horses with EPM. Ataxia, spasticity, weakness, and conscious proprioceptive deficits of one or more limbs indicate spinal cord involvement. Mild conscious proprioceptive deficits and weakness resulting in an asymmetric gait are easily confused with lameness, occasionally resulting in misdiagnosis or delay in treatment. Some neurologic lesions may manifest as behavioral or training problems or injuries resulting from the abnormal gait. Examples of performance problems that have been attributed indirectly to EPM include frequent bucking, head tossing, excessively high head carriage, difficulty maintaining a specific lead, back pain, upward fixation of the patella, and difficulty negotiating turns.[132,137,139] Areas of hyporeflexia, hypalgesia, hyperhidrosis, or complete sensory loss may be identified.[133] Most horses with EPM exhibit gradual progression of the severity and range of clinical signs, but some horses may experience a sudden exacerbation in severity.[133] Occasionally, horses exhibit

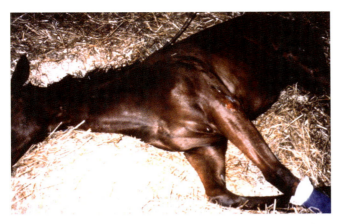

Figure 55-6 Horse presenting with acute onset of recumbency and inability to rise caused by equine protozoal myeloencephalitis (EPM). Note the decubital ulcers after just 48 to 72 hours of recumbency.

acute recumbency and inability to rise as the initial clinical sign recognized by owners (Fig. 55-6).

The most common signs of brain or brainstem involvement in horses with EPM are depression, head tilt, facial paralysis, and difficulty swallowing[133] (Fig. 55-7). Affected horses may also exhibit seizure activity, dementia, head shaking, amaurosis (central blindness), or narcolepsy-like activity.[78,132,134,140] Some horses with EPM have abnormalities of the upper airway, including laryngeal hemiplegia or dorsal displacement of the soft palate as a result of involvement of the nuclei of the vagus, glossopharyngeal, accessory, or hypoglossal nerve.[132] Difficulties with prehension, mastication, or deglutition of food may result from involvement of the nuclei of the facial, trigeminal, glossopharyngeal, hypoglossal, or vagus nerve. Head shaking, responsive to antiprotozoal therapy, has been reported in horses with EPM.[139] Urinary incontinence reported in horses with EPM presumably results from damage to sacral spinal cord segments.[141] Affected horses had normal anal reflexes and normal anus and tail tone.

In a longitudinal retrospective study of 251 horses with EPM, Saville et al[138] reported a 55.4% survival rate. Approximately 90% of horses in the study were treated for EPM, and 65% of treated horses showed some improvement in clinical signs. Of horses that improved after treatment, horses with mild neurologic deficits had a 92.3% survival rate, horses with moderate neurologic deficits had a 72.2% survival rate, and horses with severe neurologic deficits had a survival rate of 55.6%. The likelihood of improvement in clinical signs after diagnosis of EPM was lower in breeding and pleasure horses than in racing and show horses, possibly as a result of age or exercise factors.

Diagnosis

The considerable variability in presenting complaints and progression of neurologic disease in horses with EPM and the high prevalence of antibody to *S. neurona* in horses in North America make this disorder inherently difficult to diagnose definitively. A number of antemortem diagnostic tests for EPM, most of them based on detection of antibody to *S. neurona* in the serum and/or CSF, have been described. None of these tests is currently considered definitive when used alone, and the "gold standard" for diagnosis remains postmortem identification of characteristic lesions and parasites within the CNS.

In 2002 a consensus panel of experts was convened by the American College of Veterinary Internal Medicine to review

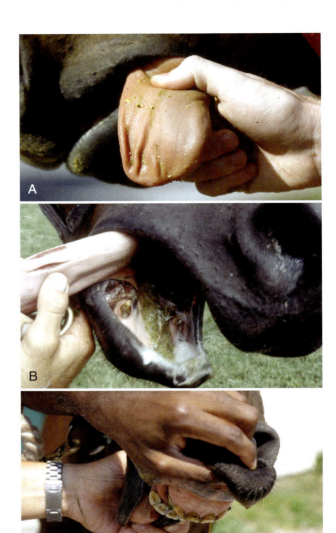

Figure 55-7 Cranial nerve abnormalities in horses with EPM. **A,** Unilateral atrophy of tongue caused by impaired hypoglossal nerve (cranial nerve XII). **B,** Self-mutilation of tongue secondary to loss of trigeminal nerve (cranial nerve V) sensory function. **C,** Deviation of mandible to the right secondary to a loss of trigeminal nerve motor.

available information related to diagnosis of EPM. The final published statement from this consensus panel recommends a systematic approach to diagnostic testing, beginning with a thorough physical and neurologic examination.[142] This examination should affirm the presence of neurologic abnormalities, and the absence of musculoskeletal disease, as the primary cause of the presenting complaint. The neurologic examination should localize probable neurologic lesion(s) and facilitate construction of an accurate list of differential diagnoses. The next step in the diagnostic process is to perform appropriate laboratory or other diagnostic tests to rule out as many differential diagnoses as possible, given limitations appropriate to the individual client and patient. In many cases the necessary diagnostic testing will require access to facilities, equipment, and laboratories capable of supplying specialty services. After exclusion of reasonable differential diagnoses, specific diagnostic tests for EPM may be considered. In some cases, response to antiprotozoal therapy is considered the diagnostic test of choice after excluding appropriate differential diagnoses.[142]

Routine laboratory testing, including CBC and serum biochemical profile, is within normal limits in most horses with EPM. CSF analysis may be helpful in ruling out other differential diagnoses. Horses with EPM do not consistently have changes in CSF color, clarity, cell counts, protein concentration or cytology, although some horses do have mildly increased mononuclear cells and protein. Iatrogenic contamination of CSF with even small quantities of peripheral blood can confound interpretation of immunoblot tests described below.[143]

The introduction of the Western immunoblot by Granstrom et al[144] in 1993 offered a dramatic advance in antemortem diagnosis of EPM. Before that time, diagnosis was based solely on the presence of neurologic disease and exclusion of other differential diagnoses. In recent years, investigators have described modifications to the original procedure,[145] as well as other serologic tests for immunoglobulin G (IgG) antibodies to S. neurona, including direct agglutination test,[146] indirect fluorescent antibody test (IFAT),[147] and enzyme-linked immunosorbent assay (ELISA).[148-150]

The standard Western immunoblot test (IBT) detects the presence of S. neurona–specific antibodies in the serum or CSF of horses.[144] Proteins from cultured S. neurona merozoites are separated by polyacrylamide gel electrophoresis. Antibody responses to three proteins (14.5, 13, and approximately 7 kDa) are specifically assessed in interpretation of IBTs (Fig. 55-8). A modification of IBT that eliminates cross-reactivity with S. cruzi, a parasite of cattle, and assesses reactivity to 30-kDa and 16-kDa bands as the criteria for a positive test is reported to have enhanced sensitivity and specificity.[145] However, since horses are not infected with S. cruzi, this modification seems irrelevant.[34]

Approximately 50% of clinically normal horses in many parts of the United States are seropositive for S. neurona, indicating exposure to the parasite. As a result, IBT of serum samples lacks specificity for diagnosis of clinical EPM. Granstrom[151] compared results of CSF IBTs from 254 horses with neurologic disease. A postmortem diagnosis of EPM was made in 124 horses. Sensitivity and specificity of immunoblot analysis of CSF samples were each reported to be approximately 89%. Positive and negative predictive values in this population were 85% and 92%, respectively. These results prompted the recommendation of IBT of CSF samples as a standard for antemortem diagnosis.[137]

Subsequent studies assessing the accuracy of IBT of CSF for diagnosis of EPM using postmortem evaluation as a "gold standard" concluded that IBT had a relatively low specificity with numerous false-positive results.[152-154] Daft et al[154] compared CSF Western blot results to histopathologic evaluation of CNS tissues and reported that the IBT had a sensitivity of 87% and a specificity of 44% for diagnosis of EPM in 65 horses with neurologic disease. In horses without neurologic disease, sensitivity was 88% and specificity 60%. The high sensitivity in both groups of horses suggests that IBT of CSF is useful for ruling out EPM in horses when the prevalence of infection is low or moderate. However, IBT should not be used as the sole diagnostic criterion for confirmation of EPM and is inappropriate as a screening test for EPM in neurologically normal horses.[155]

False-positive immunoblot results may occur because of laboratory error, iatrogenic blood contamination of the CSF at sampling, alterations in the permeability of the blood-brain barrier, normal presence of low levels of specific antibody in the CSF, or after passive transfer of colostral antibody to neonatal foals. Miller et al[143] demonstrated in 1999 that false-positive immunoblot results may occur after introduction of microscopic quantities of seropositive blood into the sample.[143] Cytologic evaluation of CSF obtained for IBT analysis may aid in interpreting results by enabling the clinician to assess the degree of iatrogenic blood contamination at the time the sample was obtained. A total red blood cell count in the CSF of less than 50 cells/μL, if the serum is at least moderately positive, is recommended for accurate interpretation of immunoblot results.[143]

For several years the calculation of albumin quotient and IgG index was recommended to assist with interpretation of IBT for EPM.[156,157] However, the immunoblot can be falsely positive because of blood contamination despite a normal albumin quotient, and these indices are no longer widely used.[143]

Presence of S. neurona–specific antibody in the CSF of foals after ingestion of colostrum from seropositive mares suggest that antibody can cross the intact equine blood-brain barrier in sufficient quantities to result in a positive IBT.[158] This conclusion is supported by the observation that antigen-specific antibodies are detectable in the CSF of adult horses after vaccination with ovalbumin.[159] Most foals ingesting colostrum containing S. neurona–specific antibodies are seronegative by 9 months of age.[158]

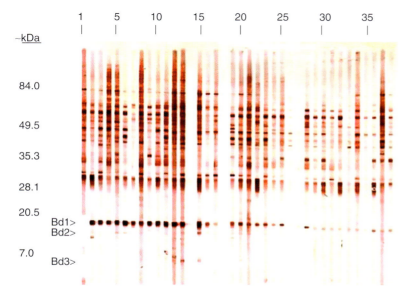

Figure 55-8 Immunoblot of equine serum samples. The *Sarcocystis neurona*–specific bands are designated by the numbered arrows to the left of the first lane, and their approximate molecular weights are based on the migration of standards of known molecular weight *(far left)*. Band 1 = 14.5 kDa; band 2 = 12 kDa; and band 3 <7 kDa. Lanes 15, 16, and 17 contain positive, diluted positive (for assessing lower detection limit), and negative sera, respectively. Lanes 14 and 18 are blank. Lanes 1 through 13 contain sera that tested positive by immunoblot test (IBT). Lanes 19 through 23 contain sera with equivocal IBT reactivity. Lanes 24 through 38 contain sera that tested negative by IBT. *(From Dubey JP, Mitchell SM, Morrow JK, et al: Prevalence of antibodies to Neospora caninum, Sarcocystis neurona, and Topxoplasma gondii in wild horses from central Wyoming. J Parasitol 89:716–720, 2003.)*

False-negative serum or CSF immunoblot reactions are uncommon but may occur, especially if a horse is recently exposed to *S. neurona*. In a study by Rossano et al,[160] horses with a negative serum immunoblot result were highly likely to have a negative CSF immunoblot test as well. Approximately one-third of seropositive horses in that study had negative CSF immunoblot results. The high negative predictive value of the IBT using either serum or CSF samples makes it a valuable tool for eliminating EPM as a differential diagnosis for horses with neurologic disease.

Other available diagnostic tests, which have been described for diagnosis of EPM in experimentally and naturally infected animals, include a direct agglutination test,[135] an IFAT,[147,161] and SAG-based ELISAs.[148,149,162,163] The direct agglutination test has been used primarily for detection of *S. neurona* antibodies in the serum of experimentally infected mice, with a reported sensitivity of 100% and specificity of 90%.[146] The accuracy of the IFAT using serum and CSF of horses naturally and experimentally infected with *S. neurona* was assessed by comparison to histopathologic diagnosis. Sensitivity and specificity of the IFAT using serum were 83.3% and 96.9%, respectively. Using CSF, the sensitivity and specificity were reported to be 100% and 99%, respectively.[147] A comparison of IFAT results with results from two types of immunoblot showed that the IFAT was more accurate for serologic diagnosis of EPM.[161]

Because diagnosing EPM cases is challenging with these tests, newer assays that assess antibody specific responses to specific proteins have been developed. They include SAG1, SAG2, SAG4/3 fusion protein, and SAG6.[148,149,162,163] Howe demonstrated that strains either express SAG1 or SAG5.[164] Horses, while not developing clinical disease, can produce antibodies following exposure to *S. fayeri*, which can cross-react with SAG2, if the serum dilution is <1:250.[150] Thus the IFAT has demonstrated cross-reactivity in *S. fayeri* infected horses.[147] SAG6 is predominantly expressed in sea otters, and it has an unknown role in EPM horses.[181,192] A SAG4 and SAG3/SAG4 fusion protein demonstrated the best correlation with IBT.[149] Because individual horses express varied responses to SAG2, 4/3, all three antigens are used in the commercial assays.[165] Results of the SAG2, 4/3 ELISAs are reported as titers or serum: CSF titer ratios when both sample types are tested.[165] Serum antibodies diffuse across the blood brain barrier at a normal rate.[159] When intrathecal antibody production occurs, the ratio of serum:CSF antibodies becomes proportionately smaller. For the commercially available assays, the basis for the SAG2, 4/3 serum:CSF titer ratios are that ratios that are less than 100 are predictive of an EPM diagnosis. These guidelines are based on an unpublished data set of 129 necropsy cases with paired serum and CSF samples (Morrow, personal communication; Reed, Howe, Morrow, et al, manuscript under review). With the development of these assays, there is less reliance on the IgG index, a calculated measure of intrathecal antibody production, based on total IgG and the albumin quotient (AQ). It is now possible to calculate antigen specific antibody indexes or a C-value, which are likely more accurate in determining intrathecal antibody production.[159]

Few published studies are available that compare SAG-based diagnostic tests. Surface antigen 1 was compared with the IFAT using a small number of horses, some of which were confirmed positive, confirmed negative, suspect positive, and suspect negative.[166] Johnson et al found that using a cutoff of 1:32 on serum, the SAG1 sensitivity was 12.5% and specificity was 97.1%.[166] For the IFAT, with the cutoff being 1:80 on serum and 1:5 on CSF, the sensitivity and specificity on serum was 94.4 and 85.2% and on CSF the sensitivity and specificity were 92.3 and 89.7%, respectively.

Polymerase chain reaction testing of CSF to detect the presence of *S. neurona* deoxyribonucleic acid (DNA) has a high specificity for EPM, but sensitivity is quite poor.[12,167] Merozoites rarely enter the CSF, and free parasite DNA is destroyed by enzymatic action, resulting in a very large number of false-negative results. Diagnosis of EPM in horses that have died may be facilitated by immunohistochemical studies to detect antigens in CNS tissue.[168,169]

Pathologic Findings

At necropsy, gross lesions of the CNS may or may not be visible. The brainstem and spinal cord are more often affected than the cerebrum. When present, lesions usually consist of multifocal hemorrhagic foci varying from clearly demarcated areas of discoloration to larger lesions affecting the brain or multiple segments of the spinal cord[2,4,5,136,170] (Fig. 55-9). Microscopically, hemorrhage, nonsuppurative inflammation, and small areas of necrosis may be seen (Figs. 55-10 through 55-13).[34,133] Perivascular cuffing with mononuclear cells is common. Giant cells, gitter cells, and eosinophils are frequently observed in inflammatory foci and in the meninges overlying the lesion.[133]

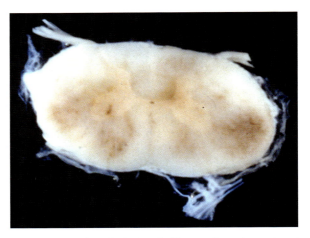

Figure 55-9 Cross-section of spinal cord of horse with equine protozoal myeloencephalitis (EPM). Focal areas of discoloration indicative of necrosis. (Unstained.) *(From Dubey JP, Lindsay DS, Saville WJ, et al: A review of Sarcocystis neurona and equine protozoal myeloencephalitis (EPM). Vet Parasitol 95:89–131, 2001.)*

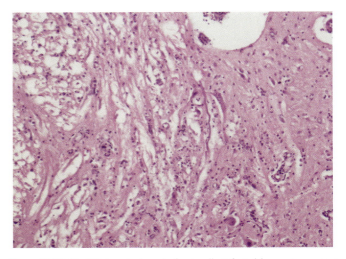

Figure 55-10 Myelitis in spinal cord of naturally infected horse; *S. neurona* was named based on the organism in this horse.[10] Focal necrosis with numerous basophilic merozoites scattered throughout the neural parenchyma.

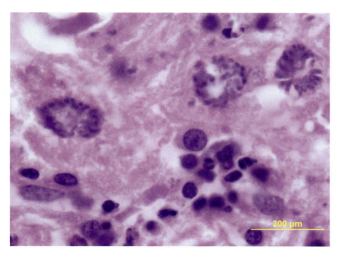

Figure 55-11 Hematoxylin and eosin (H&E)–stained section of neural tissue from the same horse as described in Figure 55-6. Higher-power magnification shows developing stages of the parasite.

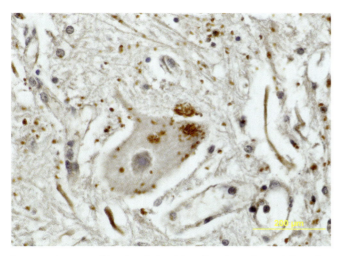

Figure 55-12 Immunohistochemical staining of sections of neural tissue from the same horse as described in Figure 55-9. Numerous *S. neurona* organisms inside and outside neurons.

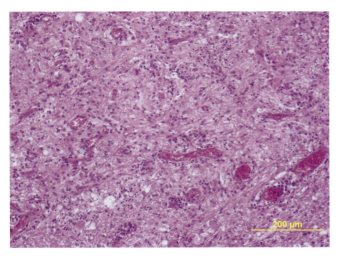

Figure 55-13 Focus of mononuclear cell infiltration in spinal cord of another naturally infected horse.

Organisms are seen in association with lesions in fewer than half of cases. Organisms are infrequently found in sections stained with hematoxylin and eosin. Prior administration of corticosteroids did not influence the likelihood of observing parasites in association with CNS lesions in a study by Boy et al,[82] but prior treatment with trimethoprim-sulfonamide alone or with pyrimethamine significantly decreased the likelihood of observing parasites. Merozoites may be observed singly or in groups (schizonts) up to 20 µm in diameter. Parasites may be observed either free in tissues or within neurons, macrophages, glia, eosinophils, or vascular endothelium.[134] When observed, they are strongly basophilic, PAS negative, and agyrophobic.[133] Visualization of organisms may be improved with immunohistochemical staining using an *S. neurona*–specific antiserum (Fig. 55-12) that does not cross-react with closely related species.[168,169]

In most naturally infected horses, macroscopic or microscopic lesions caused by *S. neurona* are not observed in any tissues other than the CNS. However, Mullaney et al[48] identified mature sarcocysts in the tongue and skeletal muscle of a 4-month-old Shire filly with neurologic disease consistent with EPM. This horse also had schizonts in the brain and spinal cord.

Therapy

Antiprotozoal Drugs

Four antiprotozoal drugs or drug combinations are approved by the U.S. Food and Drug Administration (FDA) for use in the treatment of EPM in horses: ponazuril, nitazoxanide, diclazuril, and a combination of pyrimethamine and sulfadiazine.

Ponazuril

Ponazuril (Marquis, Bayer Corporation, Kansas City, MO) is a primary metabolite of toltrazuril, a member of the triazine family of chemotherapeutic agents. Ponazuril has anticoccidial activity against a variety of parasites, including *S. neurona*, and was the first approved medication for treatment of EPM.[171] Toltrazuril, the parent drug, has activity on the mitochondria and respiratory chain of some avian coccidian parasites. Ponazuril may also have activity against the plastid body, an organelle of apicomplexan parasites that functions in amino acid synthesis, electron transport, and energy metabolism.[171] A chlorophyll complex of coccidian organisms, not found in mammals, appears to serve as the receptor for this drug.[172] Because ponazuril is a weak acid with high lipid solubility, it is able to cross the intact blood-brain barrier and enter the CSF, most likely by passive diffusion.

Ponazuril is absorbed well in horses after oral administration at 5 mg/kg body weight in a 15% paste formulation.[173] Concentrations of drug in the serum and CSF during a 28-day course of daily treatment were 4.33 ± 1.10 mg/L and 0.162 ± 0.05 mg/L, respectively. The terminal elimination half-life of ponazuril in serum was 4.3 ± 0.6 days.[173] At 1 µg/mL, ponazuril inhibits growth of *S. neurona* in vitro by 98.6%; at 0.1 µg/mL, growth is inhibited by 94.4%.[174]

Kennedy et al[175] reported that administration of ponazuril 15% oral paste to 24 horses at 0, 10, or 30 mg/kg for either 28 or 56 days resulted in minimal changes in serum biochemical profiles, coagulation profiles, or hematology parameters. Uterine edema was observed at necropsy of three of four mares treated with ponazuril at 30 mg/kg. At 10 times the label dose (50 mg/kg) for 10 days, adverse effects included intermittent anorexia, weight loss, and mild colic.

In a field trial of ponazuril 15% oral paste, 101 horses with EPM were randomly allocated to treatment at either 5 or 10 mg/kg for 28 consecutive days.[176] Diagnosis of EPM was made based on a neurologic gait abnormality of grade 2 or greater, normal cervical radiographs, and the presence of *S. neurona*–specific antibodies in the CSF by immunoblot analysis. Treatment success was defined as conversion to a negative CSF immunoblot or demonstrated improvement of at least one neurologic grade on day 118 compared with findings on day 0. The outcome was considered successful for 63 horses (62%) and unsuccessful for 38 horses (38%). The majority of treatment successes (76%) demonstrated improvement by the end of the 28-day treatment period. Some horses (15 of 63) did not show improvement until after conclusion of therapy on day 28. Of the 38 horses with unsuccessful outcomes, 8 showed noticeable improvement during the treatment period and then regressed during the 90-day follow-up period, suggesting that a longer period of treatment may have been needed. Possible adverse effects observed in a low number of horses during the field trial included blisters on the nose and mouth, skin rash or hives, loose feces, and mild colic. One horse, with a prior history of seizures, experienced a seizure while being treated. In experimentally infected horses, prophylaxis at 5 mg/kg starting 7 days before and continuing 28 days after inoculation with *S. neurona* sporocysts reduced clinical EPM in horses but did not eliminate infection.[177]

Furr et al[178] assessed the ability of daily feeding of ponazuril to horses to prevent or limit clinical signs of EPM after experimental infection. A transport stress model of infection was used. All untreated horses developed signs of neurologic disease consistent with EPM; only 71% and 40% of horses in the 2.5 and 5.0 mg/kg ponazuril groups, respectively, developed neurologic abnormalities. In a separate study, Dirikolu et al demonstrated that DMSO increased the oral bioavailability of toltrazuril sulfone (ponazuril).[179]

Diclazuril

Diclazuril (Protazil, 1.56% diclazuril, Merck Animal Health, Summit, NJ) is available as a top-dress feed, to be administered at 1 mg/kg for 28 days.[180] In vitro studies determined that 1 ng/mL inhibited *S. neurona* merozoite proliferation by greater than 95%. Two safety studies were performed, one of which assessed mean steady-state plasma concentrations between 2000 to 2500 ng/mL, and one which determined a linear relationship between plasma and CSF concentrations of diclazuril. Predicted CSF concentrations were 20 to 70 ng/mL, exceeding the minimum 1 ng/mL in vitro IC95, when fed 1 mg/kg diclazuril daily for 28 days. A multicenter clinical field study was performed using 214 horses. The effect of treatment using 1 mg/kg, 5 mg/kg, or 10 mg/kg for 28 days on horses diagnosed with EPM based on grade 2 or greater ataxia in at least 1 limb and antibodies present in the CSF for *S. neurona*. Horses were examined, and Western immunoblot was performed on serum and CSF at days 0, 27, and 48. Clinical success, based on investigator detected improvement of at least 1 grade in ataxia score, was 67% (28/42 horses) in horses given 1 mg/kg.

Folate Inhibitors

Folate inhibitors, the first drugs described for treatment of EPM in horses, are still widely used. The combination of sulfadiazine and pyrimethamine blocks successive steps in protozoal folate synthesis. The recommended dosage is 20 mg/kg of sulfadiazine and 1 mg/kg of pyrimethamine once daily at least 1 hour before feeding with hay or grain for at least 3 to 9 months.[133,137] This drug combination is now approved by the FDA for treatment of horses with EPM.

In vitro studies demonstrate that pyrimethamine is coccidiocidal for *S. neurona* at 1.0 μg/mL and trimethoprim is coccidiocidal at 5.0 μg/mL.[181] None of the sulfonamides has activity against *S. neurona* in cell culture on its own at 50 or 100 μg/mL. However, combinations of sulfonamides (4 or 10 μg/mL)

with 0.1 μg/mL of pyrimethamine had improved coccidiocidal activity.[181] Pharmacokinetic studies of pyrimethamine showed that repeated dosing at 1 mg/kg body weight is unlikely to produce sustained CSF drug levels greater than 0.1 μg/mL. Failures observed with sulfonamide/pyrimethamine treatment may be related to a failure to obtain sustained coccidiocidal concentrations of drugs in the equine CNS.[181,182] However, because pyrimethamine concentrates in the CNS tissue rather than plasma, the concentration at the desired site of action may be more than 0.1 μg/mL.[133,183]

The peer-reviewed veterinary literature contains very little information regarding the efficacy of folate inhibitors for treatment of EPM in field cases. A multicenter trial of 105 horses treated for 90 to 210 days reported that 66% of horses responded favorably to treatment. Treatment response was defined as improvement of two grades or more in evaluation of gait or reversion to negative immunoblot status.[133] Recommendations for duration of therapy are varied, and minimal data support them. Horses with a negative immunoblot when folate inhibitor therapy is discontinued are reportedly unlikely to relapse. Unfortunately, most horses do not obtain CSF immunoblot-negative status with treatment.[133]

Folate synthesis inhibitors are generally considered to be safe therapeutic options when administered for short periods. However, prolonged therapy, as is frequently needed for treatment of horses with EPM, has been associated with a variety of adverse effects in a few horses, including fever, depression, anemia, leukopenia, neutropenia, sexual dysfunction in stallions, abortion, and teratogenesis.[133,184-188]

In a report by Fenger[188] in 1998, 15.4% of 13 horses treated with standard doses and 50% of 12 horses treated with double doses of sulfadiazine/pyrimethamine developed anemia.[188] Neutropenia was reported in 7.7% of horses receiving standard-dose therapy and 50% of horses receiving double-dose therapy. An increase in mean corpuscular volume (MCV) of red blood cells was reported in 25% of standard-dose horses and 66.7% of double-dose horses. Hematologic abnormalities associated with prolonged sulfadiazine/pyrimethamine therapy in horses have been attributed to folate deficiency, and folic acid supplementation has been recommended.[132] However, subsequent reports suggest that folate supplementation paradoxically exacerbates folate deficiency in treated horses, and its use cannot be justified.[184,186]

Caution should be exercised in the treatment of pregnant mares with EPM because of the risk of teratogenic effects associated with folate synthesis inhibitor therapy. Foals born to mares treated with sulfonamides, trimethoprim, pyrimethamine, folic acid, and vitamin E orally during pregnancy have exhibited a fatal syndrome of myeloid, erythroid, and lymphoid aplasia and hypoplasia with epithelial dysplasia and renal nephrosis or hypoplasia.[133,186] Serum folate concentrations in affected mares and their foals were lower than those reported for normal broodmares.

Supportive Therapy

A variety of ancillary and supportive therapies may be indicated for the treatment of some horses with EPM. Short-term antiinflammatory therapy may be beneficial for treatment of moderate to severely affected horses during the first few days of antiprotozoal therapy or when the onset of signs is acute and rapidly progressive.[132,133] Nonsteroidal antiinflammatory drugs (NSAIDs), such as flunixin meglumine at 1.1 mg/kg IV twice daily or phenylbutazone at 2.2 to 4.4 mg/kg IV or orally twice daily, are frequently used. For horses with moderate to severe clinical signs, dimethylsulfoxide (DMSO) at 0.5 to 1 g/kg as a 10% solution IV or by nasogastric tube once or twice daily may be beneficial. Use of corticosteroids, such as dexamethasone, in horses with EPM is controversial because of the potential of these drugs to suppress immune responses to the parasite. However, judicious short-term use in horses with severe clinical signs may be beneficial in reducing CNS inflammation and associated clinical signs while waiting for antiprotozoal drugs to begin working.[133]

Many clinicians recommend supplementation of vitamin E 6000 to 10,000 IU orally daily for antioxidant effects throughout the course of therapy and rehabilitation.[133] Biologic-response modifiers have been recommended for treatment of horses with EPM because of the possibility that affected horses may be immunocompromised. Drugs that have been used include levamisole (1 mg/kg orally twice daily for 2 weeks), killed Propionibacterium acnes (Eqstim, Neogen, Lansing, MI), and mycobacterial cell wall extract (Equimune IV, Vetrepharm, London, Ontario, Canada).[133] No experimental or field trial data exist to support the efficacy of these drugs in the treatment of EPM.

General supportive care is indicated for horses with neurologic dysfunction that significantly impairs ability to stand and move, eat, drink, or perform other vital functions. This may include provision of appropriate fluid and nutritional support, deep bedding, sling support, and protective headgear.

Prevention

The only known route of transmission of S. neurona to horses is through ingestion of sporocysts shed in the feces of opossums. Therefore, prevention strategies are aimed at minimizing opossum access to horse feeds and pastures. Whenever possible, feed should be protected from wildlife access through use of enclosed facilities and containers with tight-fitting lids.[132,133] After feeding, scattered grain should be swept from aisleways and other areas near horses. Cat, dog, and bird food should not be left out overnight in barns or near pastures. Insects, birds, and rodents may mechanically transfer sporocysts in barn areas, and control of these species may help reduce the incidence of EPM on a farm.[133] Risk factors associated with EPM include recent adverse health events.[79] Prompt treatment of illness and injury, close monitoring of pregnant mares, and minimizing stress associated with these events may be beneficial. Proximity of a creek or river to the premises where the horse resides is associated with a reduced risk of EPM. This may provide a preferred habitat for opossums, decreasing their presence near barns and equine feed supplies.[79]

The most effective means to kill S. neurona sporocysts in feed or in the environment is heat treatment. Heating to 55°C (131°F) for 15 minutes or 60°C (140°F) for 1 minute or more renders sporocysts noninfective to GKO mice.[189] Treatment with bleach (10%, 20%, and 100%), 2% chlorhexidine, 1% povidone-iodine, 5% o-benzyl-p-chlorophenol, 12.56% phenol, 6% benzyl ammonium chloride, or 10% formalin was not effective in killing sporocysts.[189]

Pyrantel tartrate kills merozoite and sporozoite stages of S. neurona in vitro.[190] However, the drug was ineffective in preventing infection in GKO mice.[191] In 2005, Rossano et al[192] reported that daily feeding of pyrantel tartrate failed to prevent seroconversion associated with daily low-dose oral administration of S. neurona sporozoites to horses. Feeding diclazuril at 50 ppm was able to prevent infection in GKO mice fed sporocysts of S. neurona.[193] Similar studies have not been performed in horses.

A killed whole-parasite vaccine prepared from S. neurona merozoites was marketed in the United States under a conditional license for the prevention of EPM in horses (EPM Vaccine, Fort Dodge Animal Health, Fort Dodge, KS) but is no longer available. Administration of this vaccine results in an antibody response that is purported to inhibit parasite replication in vitro. The antibody response induced by vaccination is indistinguishable by IBT of serum or CSF from the response to natural infection.[194] Intradermal skin testing of vaccinated horses suggests that some degree of cell-mediated immunity is also induced by vaccination.[195] Data demonstrating in vivo efficacy of the vaccine for prevention of EPM in horses was not demonstrated, and the vaccine was removed from the market.

Public Health Considerations

To the authors' knowledge, there are no reports of human disease caused by infection with *Sarcocystis neurona*.

The complete reference list is available online at www.expertconsult.com.

CHAPTER

56 Piroplasmosis

L. Nicki Wise, Donald P. Knowles, and Chantal M. Rothschild*

Equine piroplasmosis (EP) is an infectious, noncontagious, tick-borne disease caused by the hemoprotozoan parasites, *Theileria equi* (previously *Babesia equi*) and *Babesia caballi*.[1-3] This disease, which is historically described in the literature as equine malaria, equine biliary fever, and horse tick fever, affects all equid species, including horses, donkeys, mules, and zebras.[3,4] Infection with either or both of these obligate, intraerythrocytic organisms causes varying degrees of hemolytic anemia and associated systemic illness. Without treatment, horses infected with *T. equi* maintain lifelong persistent infection; horses infected with *B. caballi* harbor the infection for extended periods and can with unknown efficiency eliminate the infection without chemotherapeutic intervention.[2,5,6] Horses chronically infected

*The authors acknowledge and appreciate the original contributions of these authors, whose work has been incorporated into this chapter.

with either parasite rarely exhibit clinical signs of disease yet can transmit disease to other horses. Equine piroplasmosis is found globally where tick vectors are present and is endemic in tropical, subtropical, and some temperate regions.[6-8] Several countries, including the United States, Canada, England, and Australia, are officially considered EP free, which presents ongoing economic and regulatory challenges regarding international horse transport.[9] Economic losses in endemic countries associated with EP are significant and include the cost of treatment, abortions, death, and restrictions on international exportation and participation in international equestrian events.[10] The goals of control and disease eradication vary tremendously between endemic and nonendemic nations.

Etiology

The genera *Babesia* and *Theileria* belong to the family *Piroplasmidae* within the phylum Apicomplexa. *Babesia caballi* is regarded as a true Babesia because it exclusively replicates within erythrocytes in the vertebrate host (Fig. 56-1).[11-13] Currently, there is uncertainty as to the appropriate taxonomic classification for *T. equi*. Although long considered a "small *Babesia*," *T. equi* has several characteristics that distinguish it from other species within the genus, including initial development in peripheral blood mononuclear cells before erythrocyte invasion (as occurs with *Theileria* spp.), division into four merozoites within the erythrocytes (forming the "Maltese cross," Fig. 56-2), and resistance to some babesicidal drugs.[11,12,14] Molecular phylogenetic investigations indicate that this organism possesses characteristics of both *Babesia* and *Theileria* lineages, placing it between the two.[15,16] Recently completed genomic sequencing data indicate that *T. equi* may represent a new genus altogether.[17] Additional research is needed to determine the impact of such a taxonomic reclassification, but for the remainder of this chapter, the organism will be referred to as *Theileria equi*. Because both *Babesia* and *Theileria* are piroplasms, the disease termed *equine piroplasmosis* conforms to either classification.

Piroplasmosis occurs in most countries, and with over 850 tick species worldwide, the potential for transmission is high.[18,19] However, the presence of a competent tick-vector and infected horses within the same area does not always lead to further infection or disease. Many factors must be considered, including season, climate, host-specificity, and the particulars of a competent tick's life cycle.[19,20] For *T. equi*, the reservoir of infection is the persistently infected equid; however, for *B. caballi*, both the infected horse and the primary tick vector, *Dermacentor nitens*, serve as reservoirs for transmission. Tick transmission can occur via three forms: intrastadial, transtadial, or transovarial. Intrastadial transmission occurs when acquisition and transmission of the parasite occurs within one life stage (no stage transition before transmission). Transtadial describes acquisition of infection in one stage and the ability for the same tick to transmit the infection during subsequent life stages. The parasite is maintained within the tick as it develops. Transovarial transmission occurs when the female acquires parasites that enter the ovaries and are transmitted to offspring, allowing maintenance of the parasites across tick generations.[19]

Multiple ixodid tick species have been identified as either natural or experimental vectors of EP. *Babesia caballi* is transmitted by 15 separate species (seven *Dermacentor [Anocentor]* spp., six *Hyalomma* spp., and two *Rhipicephalus* spp.) and *T. equi* by 14 species (four *Dermacentor* spp., four *Hyalomma* spp., five *Rhipicephalus [Boophilus]* spp., and *Amblyomma cajennense*).[10,21-23] *Babesia caballi* is transmitted transtadially and transovarially by its vectors, thus allowing the infected horse and the tick to serve as a source of infection.[23] Conversely, the infected horse is the only reservoir of *T. equi* infection because it is transmitted through transstadial methods. Recently, intrastadial transmission of *T. equi* has been demonstrated experimentally and was a likely mode of transmission during the recent reemergence of *T. equi* in Texas.[22] Transovarial transmission of *T. equi* has also been reported, although the importance of these occurrences in natural transmission has not been detailed.[21,24] Because of their longevity and mobility, male ticks can transmit *T. equi* to multiple horses.[2] In 2009, an outbreak of *T. equi* was identified on a large ranch in Southern Texas involving over 400 horses.[22,61] An investigation of this property allowed the identification of two previously unrecognized competent vectors of *T. equi* within the United States, *Amblyomma cajennense* and *Dermacentor variabilis*. It was demonstrated that the ticks collected from the infected horses on the premises were capable of transmitting disease to naïve horses.[22]

Parasitemia typically does not exceed 1% in *B. caballi* infections and may be as low as 0.1%, even in clinical cases.[3] Reported parasitemia in natural infection with *T. equi* usually ranges from 1% to 7%.[2] Infection with *B. caballi* has been said to be self-limiting, lasting up to 4 years after infection, although this is not always the case.[3,8] Asymptomatic carrier horses represent a reservoir for maintenance and dissemination of parasites to

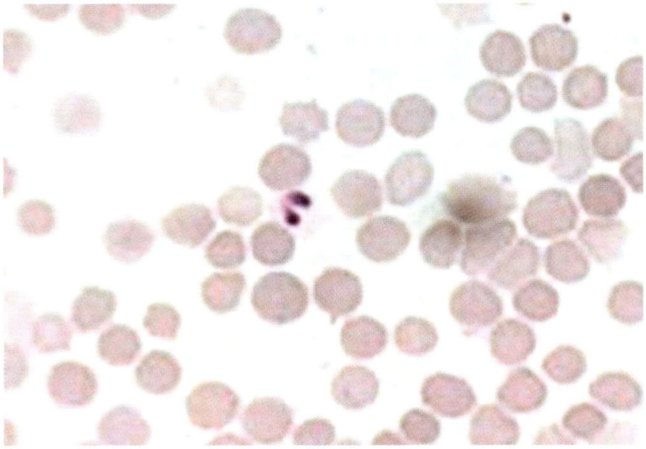

Figure 56-1 Equine erythrocyte containing *Babesia caballi* merozoites. Diff-Quik, 100× oil magnification. *(Image courtesy Peter Awinda.)*

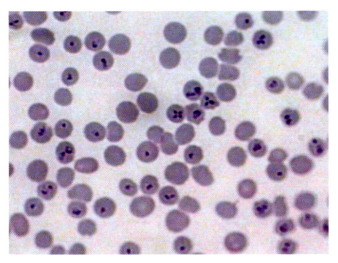

Figure 56-2 Equine erythrocyte containing *Theileria equi* merozoites in characteristic Maltese cross formation. Diff-Quik, 100× oil magnification.

ticks and horses.[20,25] Because new tick species capable of transmitting equine piroplasms are being recognized and reliable control methods do not currently exist, it is important to prevent the introduction of both infected horses and ticks into EP-free areas.

Transmission can also occur iatrogenically through inappropriate use of equipment contaminated with blood. This occurs most frequently during the practice of needle sharing between positive and naïve horses, but any contaminated equipment, such as dental tools, nasogastric tubes, and tattooing tools, may result in transmission.[26,27] Infection can also be caused when chronically infected horses serve as blood donors to naïve horses. The illegal practice of "blood doping" (prerace blood transfusions) was implicated in the 2008 Florida outbreak.[27]

Life Cycles

The life cycles of both *B. caballi* and *T. equi* involve distinct stages that occur in both the host and the tick. Both parasites progress through three life stages, the sporozoite (asexual transmission stage), the merozoite (asexual blood stage), and the gametocyte (sexual blood stage).[11,13] The development of these parasites within the tick varies, depending on species of tick involved. Regardless of species variation, for both *B. caballi* and *T. equi*, infectious sporozoites are transmitted through the tick saliva to the equid host. The precise incubation periods are not defined for *B. caballi* or *T. equi*.

Babesia caballi

The life cycle of *B. caballi* is typical of most *Babesia* spp. in that only erythrocytes are targeted in the mammalian host (Fig. 56-3). Natural infection is initiated by feeding of infected ticks on a naïve equine host. Sporozoites enter the host and directly invade erythrocytes. Within the erythrocyte, the parasite develops from a small trophozoite into larger pyriform merozoites measuring approximately 2 to 5 μm long and 1.3 to 3 μm in diameter.[5] When an uninfected tick feeds on the infected horse

and ingests parasitized erythrocytes, merozoites survive and penetrate the epithelial cells of the tick midgut where multiple fissions occur. This is followed by infection of a variety of the tick's tissues, including (depending on the specific tick species) the ovaries of the female, leading to transovarial transmission. Small pyriform bodies produced in the salivary glands of the larvae, nymphs, and adults of the next tick generation are infective to the naïve horse.[26,28] The large, paired merozoites joined at the posterior ends in the equine erythrocytes as visualized on a blood smear are a diagnostic feature of *B. caballi* infection (see Fig. 56-1).[2]

Theileria equi

The details of the life cycle of *T. equi* have not been fully elucidated and may vary, depending on the tick species involved (Fig. 56-4).[24,29-31] Infected ticks feed on horses and inject *T. equi* sporozoites into the new mammalian host with their saliva. As with other theilerial species, it is speculated that these sporozoites first invade peripheral blood mononuclear cells (PBMCs), which can be detected in these cells 2 to 3 days after transmission. Asexual reproduction gives rise to approximately 200 merozoites per cell, each measuring approximately 2 μm in length, which rupture out the PBMC and enter the circulation to invade erythrocytes.[11,12] Inside the erythrocyte, they again reproduce asexually, forming additional larger merozoites, which can appear in the distinct "Maltese cross" formation (see Fig. 56-2). After rupture of infected erythrocytes, merozoites enter the circulation again and invade new erythrocytes where replication continues. Some merozoites become spheric in shape, forming ring forms within the erythrocyte, termed *gamonts*. Ticks can ingest gamonts, where they grow in the tick's midgut and fuse, forming zygotes (sexual replication). Inside the zygote a kinete is formed, which will later penetrate into salivary gland cells of the tick. In these cells, sporonts, sporoblasts, and then sporozoites are formed (sporogony). Sporozoite development is typically complete between day 6 and 24 after completion of tick feeding.[12]

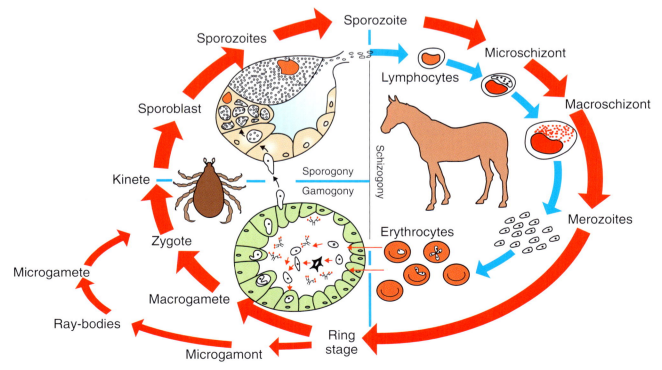

Figure 56-3 Life cycle of *Babesia caballi*. (*Illustration by Massaro Ueti.*)

Theileria equi

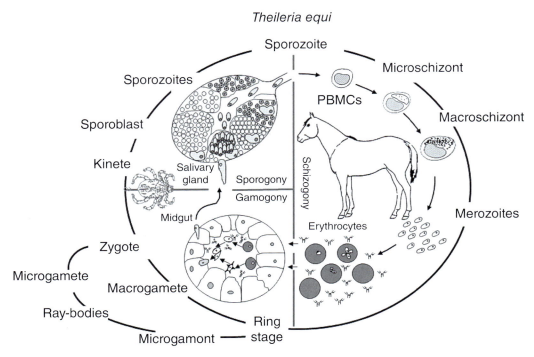

Figure 56-4 Life cycle of *Theileria equi*. (Illustration by Massaro Ueti.)

Epidemiology

Numerous studies have been published regarding the local epidemiology and distribution of EP within specific countries and regions.[32-54] These publications should be interpreted and compared with caution given the profound variation in experimental design, sample population, and diagnostic methods. Few countries in the world are free from EP. Epidemiologic data is not available for all nations, but the countries currently recognized as nonendemic by the Office International des Epizooties (OIE) include Australia, Canada, United States, England, Iceland, Ireland, and Japan. The OIE Web site, www.oie.int/wahis/public.php, is consistently updated to provide the most up-to-date international information. Most of the areas currently deemed free of EP are climatically suitable for appropriate tick vectors or already possess competent tick vectors, thus there is the continual possibility of introducing *T. equi* and *B. caballi* into free areas either by infected horses or infected ticks.

Babesia caballi and *T. equi* are usually present in the same geographic regions (tropical and subtropical climates), can share vectors, and frequently co-infect horses.[5] In most regions, however, infections with *T. equi* are more common than infections with *B. caballi*.[2,3,14] Most horses in these endemic areas are infected within the first year of life, but outbreaks of overt clinical disease are uncommon in these areas.[5] Acute clinical disease is most often observed when naïve horses are moved into endemic areas, yet in some regions, such as South Africa, horses commonly present to veterinarians for emergency treatment related to infection.[41,42]

Theileria equi and *B. caballi* are endemic in almost all of Latin America, with the exception of the southern parts of Chile and Argentina. Almost all horses in Brazil, Colombia, Puerto Rico, and Mexico are seropositive for *T. equi* and *B. caballi*.[2,6,32-35,43] Despite the widespread distribution of infection and the intense tick infestation of the horse population in many parts of Latin

America, data are limited regarding which ticks are responsible for transmission of EP in these countries. The most common species of ticks found on horses in Brazil are *D. (Anocentor) nitens* and *A. cajennense*.[35,44,45] Intense infestation by these ticks is observed in horses at a young age in many regions of the country. In 1995, Barbosa et al found that 100% of foals in southeastern Brazil seroconvert to *T. equi* by 127 days of age and to *B. caballi* by 150 days.[35]

These parasites are also widely present in Portugal, Spain, France, Switzerland, Greece, and Italy.[46-50] Piroplasmosis is also endemic in the Balkan Peninsula, Hungary, Romania, and the states of the Caucasus region.[51,52] Both parasites are widespread in the horse populations of Mongolia, China, and many parts of Southeast Asia and Asia.[37-39,53] Historically considered free of infection, sporadic reports of both *T. equi* and *B. caballi* seropositive horses have been documented in Japan.[36] High infection rates have also been reported in the Middle East, including Kuwait, Oman, and India, where *T. equi* is reported more commonly.

Morocco, Republic of South Africa, Madagascar, and nearly all other parts of the African continent are also considered endemic for *T. equi* and *B. caballi*.[5,6,34,54-56] Two tick species, *R. evertsi evertsi* and *H. truncatum*, are considered the primary vectors within this region.[5] In South Africa, almost all clinical cases of EP are due to *T. equi*, and although the exact economic impact of this disease on South Africa is unknown, one survey found that infection with *T. equi* was the most commonly treated infectious disease of horses in that country.[5]

Although *T. equi* was introduced into Australia in the 1950s and 1960s by contaminated needles and instruments, the organism did not become established.[3,6,14,57,58] *Boophilus microplus* is present in parts of Australia, so the potential for disease introduction and transmission exists.

Recent outbreaks within the United States have placed the EP-free status of this country under scrutiny.[18,27] The first case of *B. caballi* was identified in a horse in 1961 in southern Florida; the source of infection was never definitively determined, although it was speculated that it was caused by importation of horses from Cuba.[8,10,60] During the following decade in extensive surveillance programs, several hundred total cases of both *B. caballi* and *T. equi* were diagnosed in seven states. *Dermacentor nitens* was identified in large numbers in the affected Florida counties, yet this vector's role in disease transmission was never determined. All infected horses were deported, quarantined, or treated until negative on serology. Intense surveillance of horses and ticks continued in Florida until 1988 when the United States was deemed free of disease.[10] To maintain this status, the USDA APHIS improved restrictions on importation of horses from endemic areas. It was later determined that the serologic tests previously used for diagnosis of infection were not sensitive enough, which may have contributed to the influx of positive horses into the country. Prior to availability of more sensitive diagnostic tests, most cases of piroplasmosis in the United States were sporadic and linked to illegal importation of horses and often the inappropriate use of blood-contaminated equipment between horses.[18]

In 2008, twenty *T. equi* infected horses were identified on seven separate premises in Florida.[27] All affected horses were associated with horses that had been imported from Mexico, and all were engaged in illegal horse racing. Given the history and distribution of infected horses, inappropriate management practices were assumed to be the mode of transmission. No natural vectors were identified despite aggressive surveillance. In 2009, an outbreak of *T. equi* involving more than 400 horses was identified on a large ranch in Southern Texas.[22,61] All infected horses resided on the premises or had been associated at some time with the ranch. The outbreak was immediately addressed by the OIE and APHIS, and all horses were quarantined, euthanized, or entered into a USDA-Washington State University led research program.

Pathogenesis and Immunity

Although some details of pathogenesis remain unclear, infection with either parasite causes erythrocyte lysis, resulting in variable degrees of hemolytic anemia. Hemolysis results from the physical rupture of erythrocytes during release of merozoites (intravascular), as well as from removal of infected erythrocytes from the circulation by the spleen (extravascular).[26] Nonparasitized erythrocytes are also removed from circulation, but the reason for this phenomenon is unknown. Data from experimentally infected splenectomized donkeys indicate that the biochemical structure of erythrocyte membranes changes significantly during infection with *T. equi*.[62] It was suggested that this conformational change could lead to decreased deformability of red cells, which may cause reduced blood flow in the microvasculature. Both parasites also cause thrombocytopenia and alter coagulation in infected horses through unknown mechanisms.[63,64] Hypotheses regarding the pathogenesis of this phenomenon include immune-mediated destruction, splenic sequestration, and/or excess consumption as is observed in disseminated intravascular coagulation. *Babesia caballi*–infected erythrocytes can cause the formation of microthrombi within small vessels, leading to venous stasis and vasculitis.[65,66] Rarely, severe EP can result in hypercoagulability, systemic inflammatory response syndrome, and subsequent multiorgan system dysfunction.[26]

Placental transmission from infected mares to their fetuses also occurs.[67-71] Infection of a fetus can result in abortion (late gestation most common), stillbirth, or birth of an infected foal (neonatal piroplasmosis). This transmission has been documented to occur across placentas that are histologically normal. Not all foals from infected mares are affected, thus the mechanism and prevalence of this type of transmission is unclear.

Investigation of the natural outbreak in Texas identified infection in a number of pregnant mares yet no abortions or related complications were observed. Conversely, *T. equi* has been reported to be responsible for 11% of all abortions in South Africa.[72] Based on the variation of reported occurrence, it is likely that individual horse variation or geographic strain differences could influence the prevalence. Exposure to semen from an infected stallion is not considered to be a means of transmission, although blood exposure during breeding practices technically could pose a risk of transmission.[73]

Immune responses to infection remain poorly defined. It is widely accepted in endemic areas that protective immunity is present after an initial infection with the parasite, yet no studies directly addressing this phenomenon have been performed. The resistance to clinical disease acquired by previously infected horses could be a result of continued stimulation of the immune system by the persisting parasite, continuous reexposure to the parasite (in endemic areas), or persistence of protective antibodies. It has been reported that horses infected with *B. caballi* can clear the infection over a period of years if reexposure does not occur. It is not understood how and why this clearance can occur, and it is also unknown if these horses can be reinfected once "cleared." There is no evidence for cross-immunity between *T. equi* and *B. caballi*.[12,26] A horse can simultaneously be infected with both parasites.[26,37]

Innate immunity plays a central role in control of some *Babesia* and *Theileria* parasites, although its importance in EP is unclear.[74-76] The spleen is important in eliminating most hemoprotozoan parasites, and equids with intact spleens are typically able to control *T. equi* and *B. caballi* infections and survive. However, splenectomized horses infected with *T. equi* develop high levels of parasitemia and invariably succumb to the infection.[77-79] Inapparent carriers of *T. equi* will also develop fatal disease on surgical removal of the spleen.[80] Depending on the infectious dose and other factors, splenectomized horses experimentally infected with *B. caballi* can survive, but fatalities have also been reported.[54] Despite its important role, the spleen and innate immune system are insufficient for protection against *T. equi* in the absence of adaptive immunity. Knowles et al demonstrated that foals with severe combined immune deficiency (SCID) infected with *T. equi* are unable to control parasite replication and become severely anemic.[79] SCID foals lack mature T and B lymphocytes and are incapable of antigen-specific immune responses but have intact spleens and a competent innate immune system.[81-85] This demonstrates that the spleen is unable to control *T. equi* infection in the absence of parasite-specific immune responses and that erythrolysis caused by *T. equi* does not require a specific immune response. Considering the importance of cell-mediated immune responses to other parasites, such as *T. parva* and *B. bovis*, it is possible that cell-mediated immunity plays a key role in immunity against *T. equi* and *B. caballi*.[79,86] Only limited information is available demonstrating the contribution of cellular immunity to control of EP.[87,88]

The correlates of the adaptive immune responses to either parasite are unclear. Horses infected with *T. equi* produce antibodies against merozoite surface proteins, termed *equi merozoite antigens* (EMAs).[89,90] High antibody titers to these proteins have been correlated with parasite control.[91,92] The nomenclature of equine immunoglobulin G (IgG) has recently been adjusted to accommodate the seven unique IgG heavy chain genes identified in the equine genome.[93] During acute stages of infection with *T. equi*, high levels of IgGa (now IgG1) and IgGb (IgG4 and 7) correlate with control, and IgG(T) (IgG3 and 5) levels increase during chronic infection.[92] Specific antibodies to EMA proteins are first detected 7 to 11 days after experimental infection in ponies and reach a peak 30 to 45 days after infection.[94] Passively transferred colostral antibodies to *T. equi* and

B. caballi may persist in the foal for 4 to 5 months.[95] Foals from endemic areas are particularly resistant to clinical disease, yet it is unclear if this is due to the presence of low level parasite presence or protective antibodies from the dam.[5,32] Donkeys vaccinated with *T. equi* immunogen were able to mount a protective response characterized by high antimerozoite antibody titers and merozoite-specific lymphocyte proliferation.[91] Recently, it was documented that foals with SCID received repeated infusions of *T. equi* hyperimmune plasma prior to inoculation with the parasite were able to delay the time to peak parasitemia.[96]

Even less is known about protective immune responses against *B. caballi* infection. Infected horses produce antibodies to rhoptry associated protein 1 (RAP 1), which is utilized on serologic detection of infection.[97] This conserved apical merozoite protein remains partially uncharacterized in *B. caballi*, but in *B. bovis* plays a pivotal role in induction of humoral immunity.[98] Overall, additional research is needed to define the protective roles of antibody and cellular adaptive immune responses against these parasites.

Clinical Findings

Variation in severity of clinical disease depends on the region, strain of the parasite, and overall health of the horse. Details of strain variation are lacking, yet on comparison of disease severity across the globe, significant differences exist. For example, in South Africa, acute infection often requires emergency therapy, and one report indicated that EP was the most commonly encountered infectious equine disease in South Africa.[5,42] Conversely, the outbreak in Texas in 2009 that identified infection in over 400 horses resulted in virtually no clinical signs of disease.[22,61] Horses infected with either parasite can present with similar clinical signs, but uniformly, infection with *T. equi* typically results in more severe clinical disease than *B. caballi*.[1] After transmission, depending on factors including dose and immunity, clinical signs develop within 10 to 30 days for *B. caballi* and 12 to 19 days for *T. equi*.[3] Clinical infections may be acute, chronic, or most commonly, inapparent.

Acute Equine Piroplasmosis

Acute infection is often initially characterized by nonspecific signs of infection, including pyrexia (often exceeding 40°C [104°F]), lethargy, decreased appetite, and peripheral edema. Petechiations due to profound thrombocytopenia may be observed on mucous membranes including the third eyelid. Signs of hemolytic anemia follow with pale or icteric mucous membranes, tachycardia, tachypnea, weakness, and pigmenturia (hemoglobinuria and/or bilirubinuria).[1,3,99,100] More severe signs are rare with *B. caballi* infection. Petechiations may be observed on mucous membranes, including the third eyelid. Less common complications include pneumonia, pulmonary edema, central nervous disease symptoms, colic, impactions, diarrhea, and catarrhal enteritis.[5] In severe cases, systemic involvement results in disseminated intravascular coagulopathy, renal failure, liver disease, and multiple organ dysfunction. With appropriate treatment and a competent immune system, most horses survive acute infection.

Fulminant, often fatal infection, termed *peracute*, has also been described. Horses may be found dead with no premonitory signs or progress quickly to signs of multiple organ dysfunction and are unlikely to respond to therapy. Foals infected in utero (neonatal piroplasmosis) may initially exhibit nonspecific signs of disease, including weakness and decreased suckling, but signs often progress to resemble those of an acutely infected adult.[3,70,72,101] Some foals are apparently normal at birth but develop clinical signs of EP 2 or 3 days later. Affected foals have a poor prognosis without therapy, and the infection can be fatal. Neonatal piroplasmosis may appear similar to equine neonatal isoerythrolysis, but differentiation is important so that adequate therapy can be implemented.[71,101] Adult horses suddenly introduced into areas with large numbers of infected ticks can present with this form of the disease as well.[41]

Chronic Equine Piroplasmosis

Chronically infected horses generally exhibit signs of nonspecific chronic inflammatory conditions, including weight loss, poor body condition, partial anorexia, malaise, and decreased performance.[26] General physical examination is unlikely to aid in diagnosis, but rectal examination may reveal splenomegaly.[2,3,65] Horses may also be mildly anemic.

Inapparent Carrier

Importantly, the vast majority of *B. caballi* and *T. equi* seropositive horses are inapparent carriers. These horses have low levels of parasitemia and no obvious clinical signs. Carriers are reservoirs for the parasites and have the potential to disseminate infection with iatrogenic blood transfers or where appropriate vectors are present.[25] These carriers represent the largest risk for introduction of disease into nonendemic nations and regulatory testing to enter nonendemic areas is enforced in an attempt to prevent such occurrences. These horses are also at risk of developing a relapse in clinical illness if immunocompromised, stressed, splenectomized, or on steroid administration.[80,96,102-104] A report from Jordan documented five presumed inapparent carriers participating in strenuous exercise that immediately after completion of the exercise, developed profound weakness, with two dying suddenly.[104] Recrudescence of marked *T. equi* parasitemia was assumed. Experimental therapy with beclomethasone before and after inoculation with *T. equi* resulted in a 50% increase in parasitemia as compared to controls.[102] These relapses have not been reported for *B. caballi*.

Pathology

Results of clinical pathologic laboratory analyses may aid in diagnosis. Most horses, regardless of clinical syndrome, exhibit some degree of anemia characterized by decreased packed cell volume (PCV), hemoglobin, and erythrocyte count.[62,65,66,105] Red blood cell indices, mean corpuscular volume (MCV), mean corpuscular hemoglobin (MCH), and MHC concentration (MCHC) are variable.[62] Thrombocytopenia is commonly reported, and one report noted a decrease in platelet count in 39% of *T. equi* infections, 80% of *B. caballi* infections, and 100% of dual infections.[3,63-66] Clotting times may be prolonged or normal. Acute infections can be characterized by lymphopenia and neutropenia with occasional left shift, but the leukogram often varies, depending on infection stage and severity.[64,106] Fibrinogen may be elevated or decreased, and albumin level can vary, depending on hydration status, chronicity of disease, and any associated conditions that result in protein loss.[63,100] Hyperbilirubinemia is often observed and the liver enzymes, alkaline phosphatase (ALP), sorbitol dehydrogenase (SDH), aspartate aminotransferase (AST), and gamma-glutamyl transpeptidase (GGT), may be elevated.[64] These elevations are attributed to reduced blood flow to the liver, which can result in centrilobular necrosis in severe cases. Concurrent with ongoing hemolytic events, pigmenturia caused by either hemoglobinuria or bilirubinuria occurs.

With severe systemic involvement, renal insufficiency can lead to azotemia and abnormalities in urinalysis consistent with alterations in kidney function. Infected erythrocytes can be identified in sternal bone marrow aspirates of asymptomatic horses, but the utility of this test as a diagnostic tool is limited.[107]

Gross and histopathologic findings depend on the clinical presentation, severity of disease, and associated complications. Gross examination may indicate evidence of anemia, as well as variable degrees of icterus, edema, and splenomegaly. Other findings may include pulmonary edema and congestion, cardiac hemorrhages, hydropericardium, hydrothorax, hepatomegaly, ascites, enlarged discolored kidneys, and lymphadenopathy. Histopathologic findings may include centrilobular necrosis of the liver, renal tubular necrosis with hemoglobin casts, and microthrombi within the liver and lungs.[5] Pulmonary tissue examination can demonstrate congestion, edema, and hemosiderin-laden macrophages within the pulmonary alveolar walls.[3,100,108,109] Parasitized erythrocytes can also be observed within vessels and macrophages, and hemosiderosis in the liver and spleen can be observed secondary to erythrolysis.[5,108,109]

Diagnosis

An appropriate list of differential diagnoses should be developed based on whether the horse resides in or has visited an endemic region. In general, acute onset of the aforementioned clinical signs could also be caused by equine infectious anemia virus, equine viral arteritis virus, equine ehrlichiosis, purpura hemorrhagica, African horse sickness, leptospirosis, immune-mediated hemolytic anemia (possibly the result of severe infection [i.e., clostridial myonecrosis]), and red maple leaf toxicity.

Various diagnostic modalities can be used alone or in combination to diagnose infection, but the most appropriate test varies, depending on phase of infection, access to diagnostic laboratories, and whether the horse resides in an endemic or nonendemic region. Diagnosis of acute EP can be made on the basis of clinical signs and the careful examination of blood smears.[1,3] Serologic testing is necessary to diagnose chronically infected horses and for regulatory purposes. The rules and regulations in place vary for each country, and it is important to review these guidelines prior to collecting or submitting any samples from suspect animals. Careful and secure handling of samples is necessary, and samples should only be submitted to an authorized laboratory. In the United States, the Federal authorities (Area Veterinarians-in-Charge) can be found at http://www.aphis.usda.gov/animal_health/area_offices/ and the State veterinarians can be found at http://www.usaha.org/Portals/6/StateAnimalHealthOfficials.pdf. Information for all countries can be found on the World Organization for Animal Health (OIE) Web site (http://www.oie.int).

Microscopy

Diagnosis by microscopic examination of blood smears is possible only in the acute phases of EP. If present in high enough numbers in the circulation, parasitized erythrocytes can be observed in blood smears. In inapparent carrier and chronically infected horses, the low number of parasites in circulation decreases the sensitivity of this technique. The piroplasms of T. equi and B. caballi can be easily distinguished from one another. Within the erythrocyte, B. caballi typically appears as two large pyriform (pear-shaped) merozoites that measure approximately 2 to 5 μm in length.[26] During clinical infection with B. caballi, the percentage of erythrocytes parasitized is

typically less than 1% and may be less than 0.1%. *Theileria equi* merozoites occur within erythrocytes as polymorphic, small piroplasms, occasionally arranged in a distinct Maltese cross formation. The *T. equi* merozoites are smaller and typically measure 2 to 3 μm in length.[11,12] The percentage of infected erythrocytes during clinical disease as the result of *T. equi* is usually between 1% to 5% but in severe cases can exceed 20%.[26]

Serology

Several serologic tests were developed to increase diagnostic sensitivity especially in those horses exhibiting no clinical signs. These tests include the complement fixation test (CFT), indirect fluorescence antibody test (IFAT), competitive enzyme-linked immunosorbent assay (cELISA), and western immunoblot.

The CFT was historically the accepted regulatory method for control of movement of horses between nonendemic and endemic nations. The underlying principle of the CFT is the fixation of complement during the reaction between specific parasite antigen and antibody from infected horse sera.[2,14] Horse serum samples that react at a dilution of 1:5 are considered positive. Antibodies against the parasites can be detected on CFT approximately 8 to 11 days after infection, with titers beginning to decline at 2 to 3 months.[14] The CFTs for *B. caballi* and *T. equi* are very specific tests yet lack sensitivity, especially in the chronic stage of infection or after treatment.[90] It is reported that horses may transiently go negative 3 to 15 months after treatment for *B. caballi* and 24 months for *T. equi*.[105,110] The subisotype IgG(T), now classified as IgG5 and to a lesser extent IgG3, remains elevated in chronic *T. equi* infections.[92] Recently, it was demonstrated that although IgG3 fixes complement, IgG5 does not, supporting the historical finding that IgG(T) was incapable of complement fixation.[93,111] Therefore it is not unexpected that the CFT lacks sensitivity for diagnosis of chronic or inapparent *T. equi* infection. Cross-reactivity between antibodies against *T. equi* and *B. caballi* when using the CFT has been reported.[14,95] Regardless of the fact that the CFT was previously the official regulatory test for establishing piroplasmosis status prior to travel to a nonendemic country, the CFT is not considered the diagnostic test of choice for chronic infection.

The IFAT is also a very specific test that lacks sensitivity. It is, however, considered more sensitive than the CFT and is used when CFT results are inconclusive.[2,14] In this assay, parasite antigens are bound to glass slides and allowed to react with sample horse sera. These reactive antibodies are fluorescently labeled, and serum is considered positive if this specific reaction is noted under ultraviolet (UV) light at a dilution of 1:80 and higher. The earliest antibody responses in horses experimentally infected with *B. caballi* and *T. equi* are noted at 3 to 20 days after infection, with positive titers still detectable in the chronic phase of infection. Titers were more consistently detected and remained elevated longer with the IFAT versus the CFT.[94] IFAT is typically reserved for confirmation of CFT results and use in laboratory settings not as a regulatory test, given the inherent subjective nature of result interpretation.

Since 2004, the cELISA has been the regulatory test required by the OIE for international horse transport.[9,10] The *T. equi* cELISA is currently considered to be the most sensitive means of detection of chronic or inapparent infection.[90] This test utilizes recombinant EMA-1 and specific monoclonal antibodies; EMA-1 is an immunodominant antigen unique to *T. equi*.[89,90,112] Horses infected with *T. equi* generate a positive result on the cELISA as early as 21 days after experimental infection and approximately 5 weeks after tick transmission. The EMA-1 cELISA is validated for use against multiple different strains of *T. equi* found around the world.[90]

The *B. caballi* cELISA utilizes a recombinant form of the RAP1 protein, and this test, when compared with CFT using 300 equine serum samples from around the world, was able to diagnose infection in 25% more cases than with the CFT.[97] However, the currently available RAP-1 cELISA relies on the recognition of epitopes that are not present in all *B. caballi* strains. Because of subtle genetic differences between the recombinant RAP-1 used in the cELISA and South African isolates of *B. caballi*, the test is unable to detect all infected horses in South Africa.[113] Although similar differences exist between the recombinant EMA-1 used in the *T. equi* cELISA and South African *T. equi* isolates, the cELISA continues to detect infected horses in South Africa.[114]

In general, the cELISA has improved performance compared with CFT and IFAT.[10,94] The use of recombinant proteins and monoclonal antibodies allowed for standardization of these tests and markedly increased sensitivity as compared to the other serologic tests.[90,97,115] Both cELISA tests are marketed by VMRD (Pullman, WA) and are currently not available to general practitioners. Kumar and others also reported field validation of an ELISA using whole *T. equi* merozoite antigen in India, and the results indicated this test to be an easy, economical, and reliable means of *T. equi* diagnosis.[116]

Recently, with increasing use of PCR in laboratory settings (see later), the validity of a positive cELISA result has come into question. Despite treatment and apparent clearance of *T. equi*, as demonstrated by negative PCR and transmission studies, cELISA results remain positive, sometimes for up to 24 months after clearance.[61] The reason for this persistence of antibodies is unclear, but the transmission risk that these PCR-negative, seropositive horses pose must be determined.

Western blot (or immunoblot) has been previously utilized only in a research setting for diagnosis of *T. equi* and *B. caballi*. The National Veterinary Services Laboratory in Ames, Iowa, is now offering an immunoblot as an adjunct diagnostic tool for detection of *B. caballi* infection.[117] Research is underway to validate these tests for use in *T. equi* diagnosis.

Other Diagnostic Methods

Polymerase chain reaction (PCR), which detects the presence of parasite deoxyribonucleic acid (DNA), is a technique currently used only in research settings. The PCR for *T. equi* is an incredibly sensitive method utilized to clarify confounding test results and for confirmation of clearance success.[61] Evidence exists that *T. equi* strains from around the world are not 100% genetically identical, making standardization of this test difficult.[114,118] Polymerase chain reaction for *B. caballi* has thus far proved to be inconsistent. As it is currently performed, it is unlikely that PCR will be standardized and commercially marketed for detection of *T. equi* or *B. caballi* infection.

Therapy

Strategies for therapeutic intervention should be based on whether the horse resides in an endemic or nonendemic area. Horses in endemic regions should only be treated in an attempt to alleviate clinical signs and decrease recovery time. Aside from permanent movement of an infected horse, clearance of these organisms serves little purpose in these areas because lifelong immunity is assumed to be conferred with chronic infection. In nonendemic regions, attempting to remain EP free, treatment of infected horses with the intent of clearance (chemosterilization) is desired. Numerous drugs have been tested both in cell culture and *in vivo*, but variable methods and confounding findings make interpretation of results difficult. It is widely assumed that *T. equi* infections are more difficult to eliminate than

B. caballi. It has been reported that horses with *B. caballi* infection may self-clear the infection over a period of years, but this does not always occur.[3,6] Until recently, it was widely accepted that chemosterilization of a *T. equi* infected horse was unachievable. Clearance of *T. equi* was previously reported, yet the research was conducted prior to the development tests with increased sensitivity for parasite persistence.[119,120] Data collected during the natural outbreak in Texas indicate that *T. equi* can be eliminated from an infected horse with appropriate dosing of imidocarb dipropionate (ID).[61]

For alleviation of clinical signs related to either parasite, ID is considered the drug of choice. This drug, marketed as Imizol (Merck Animal Health, United States) is only safe when administered intramuscularly (IM), yet local injection site reactions do occur. Reported dosages for alleviation of clinical signs vary; most sources indicate that 2.2 to 4.4 mg/kg of body weight given IM once or twice is effective.[61,119,121-123] If necessary, lower dosages can be repeated at 24 to 72 hour intervals for two to three treatments. In nonendemic nations where chemotherapeutic clearance of the organism is desired, animals infected with *B. caballi* can be cleared with a dosage of 4.4 mg/kg IM every 72 hours for four treatments.[123] For clearance of *T. equi*, preliminary indicate that the same dosage is effective.[61,123a] Currently, in the United States, if a horse tests positive for *T. equi*, the owner can enroll the horse in the APHIS-controlled ID treatment program.[18] Equine practitioners are advised not to treat any infected horse without clearance from appropriate state and federal authorities.

Imidocarb dipropionate acts as an anticholinesterase, thus adverse reactions to the drug often present as sweating, agitation, colic, and diarrhea.[124,125] Typically, these signs are transient and rarely life threatening. Adverse effects can potentially be prevented with an intravenous (IV) dose of glycopyrrolate at 0.005 mg/kg once or reversed with a single IV dose of atropine at 0.1 mg/kg. Both of these anticholinergic drugs can also cause serious adverse effects. Administration of the anticholinergic *N*-butylscopolamine (Buscopan, Boehringer Ingelheim, Germany) at 0.3 mg/kg IV immediately prior to imidocarb administration treatment can also lessen clinical signs without addition of adverse side effects.[61]

Because ID undergoes hepatic and renal clearance, necrosis in both of these organs has been documented to occur with intoxication.[124,125] Horses undergoing ID therapy should be carefully monitored for development of complications. Transient azotemia and/or elevations in urinary GGT/creatinine ratios and transient elevations in liver enzymes may be observed during the course of treatment but usually resolve with discontinuation of the drug. Donkeys and mules are incredibly sensitive to ID, therefore its use in these species is not recommended.[119] Information regarding treatment of *T. equi*–infected neonatal foals with ID is limited with only one case report.[126] Imidocarb is detectable in the milk 2 hours after administration to a lactating mare as a single dosage of 2.4 mg/kg IM.[127] Although not reported, it is unclear if levels in the milk could potentially cause toxicity in the suckling foal. On administration of ID to pregnant mares followed by induced abortion, circulating levels of ID comparable to the dam's serum concentrations were detected in each fetus.[72]

Diminazene aceturate and diminazene diaceturate have been used with success for alleviation of clinical signs due to *T. equi* and *B. caballi* at a dosage of 3.5 mg/kg IM every 48 hours for two treatments.[128] Efficacy of both drugs increases with the second dose, yet no successful chemosterilization attempts have been reported. Other drugs are reported to have efficacy in treatment of EP, but these drugs are no longer commonly utilized in equine practice.[26,122,129] Oxytetracycline, when administered IV at 5 to 6 mg/kg once daily for 7 days, is effective against *T. equi* but not *B. caballi*.[64]

Prevention

Prevention of disease in endemic areas is virtually impossible, especially since some regions report close to 100% infection of all horses. For these populations, it is essential for foals and young horses to be infected early in life. It is assumed that the immunity conferred with initial infection acts to protect the horse from recurrent disease on subsequent exposures. For nonendemic nations, the foundation of protection is regulation of horse movement to and from endemic nations. Depending on the nonendemic country, horses must test negative for *T. equi* and *B. caballi* on the designated serologic test.[9] Positive horses are generally denied entrance unless for tightly regulated events, and these horses undergo strict quarantine measures and are examined thoroughly for ticks prior to shipment.[10] Careful acaricide application is generally mandated immediately prior to travel to ensure ticks are not introduced with the horses. The regulatory system put in place by the OIE and nonendemic nations has been successful, although isolated cases continue to occur in these areas. These isolated cases are rarely caused by tick transmission and are most often linked to the use of blood-contaminated equipment and practices involving needle sharing or blood transfusions from untested donors.[58,59] In the United States, a horse that is identified as positive on cELISA must be immediately quarantined and the state and federal authorities must be notified. The most appropriate action is determined by the state and federal regulatory officials on a case by case basis.

Nonendemic areas that border endemic areas cannot prevent introduction of ticks so diligent actions must be taken to reduce horses' contact with ticks. These measures include routine application of acaricides, surveillance for the presence of ticks, and reduction in vegetation.[18] A variety of chemicals and are available to reduce tick exposure, including carbamates, natural and synthetic pyrethrins. Being aware of the habitat and the seasonality of ticks in the area of interest is important.

No vaccine is currently available for prevention of infection or disease from *T. equi* or *B. caballi*. Immunization studies have utilized several approaches but since the correlates of protective immunity in horses are unknown developing an effective vaccine will be difficult. Immunization with whole merozoites induced protection in four donkeys.[91] Vaccines directed against tick antigen are available for cattle but not for horses.[130]

Public Health Considerations

Although a strain of *T. equi* has been implicated in rare human cases, there have been no confirmed reports of human infection with either *B. caballi* or *T. equi*.[131] A few *Babesia* species can be transmitted to humans including the bovine pathogens *B. bovis* and *B. divergens*, the canine pathogen *B. canis*, and the white-footed mouse and white-tailed deer pathogen *B. microti*. Reportedly transmission can occur through infected ticks or as a result of contaminated blood transfusions.[132]

The complete reference list is available online at www.expertconsult.com.

57 Nematodes

Martin K. Nielsen, Craig R. Reinemeyer, and Debra C. Sellon*

Numerous nematode parasites infect horses. The first section of this chapter describes the important nematodes of the gastrointestinal tract of horses. Nematode infections with clinical manifestations affecting the skin (onchocerciasis, habronemiasis) and the respiratory tract (lungworm infection) are discussed later in this chapter. Chapter 4 discusses nematode infection of neural and somatic tissues (*Halicephalobus* spp.); Chapter 10 discusses infection of ocular tissues (*Thelazia* spp.).

Gastrointestinal Nematodes

Martin K. Nielsen and Craig R. Reinemeyer

Strongylosis

The term *strongylosis* refers to infection with any of dozens of species of similar nematodes that reside as adults within the large intestine of equids. These parasites are classified in the family Strongylidae and are commonly known as "strongylid nematodes" or "strongyles." Differences in morphology, biology, pathogenicity, anthelmintic susceptibility, and management strategies support the practicality of discussing the strongyles as two major groups: the subfamily *Strongylinae* ("large strongyles," strongylins) and the subfamily *Cyathostominae* ("small strongyles," cyathostomins, cyathostomes).[1]

Strongylinae (Large Strongyles, Strongylins)

Etiology

The *Strongylinae* have become quite rare in managed horse populations but can still be encountered. The overwhelming majority of strongyle species infecting the horse belong to the cyathostominae covered later in this chapter. The large strongyles occurring in North America belong to four genera: *Strongylus*, *Triodontophorus*, *Craterostomum*, and *Oesophagodontus*. Compared with small strongyles, the large strongyles possess substantial, globular, buccal capsules (oral cavities) by which they can attach firmly to the mucosa of the cecum or colon.

*The authors acknowledge and appreciate the original contributions of these authors, whose work has been incorporated into this chapter.

Specimens of the genus *Strongylus* are large, stout nematodes (~1.5-4.5 cm × 2 mm), whereas *Triodontophorus*, *Oesophagodontus*, and *Craterostomum* are smaller and resemble the cyathostomins in size.

All strongyles invade gut tissues after initial infection, but only larval stages of the genus *Strongylus* migrate to organs beyond the alimentary tract. Larvae of *Strongylus vulgaris* wander within the vascular system; those of *Strongylus edentatus* invade the liver and retroperitoneum; and *Strongylus equinus* larvae migrate within the liver and pancreas[2] (see section on Pathogenesis). Because of their protracted migration, members of the genus *Strongylus* have long prepatent periods ranging from 5.5 to 12 months, depending on the species.

Epidemiology

The role of the environment in the transmission of strongylosis is virtually identical for large and small strongyles. The cycle of transmission begins when strongylid eggs are passed in the feces of an infected host. Strongylid eggs are homogenous, and large strongyle eggs cannot be differentiated from those of cyathostomins. Equine feces usually contain adequate levels of moisture (>24%)[3] and oxygen to support hatching and development of larval stages, and eggs are able to hatch when environmental temperatures exceed 8°C (46°F).[4,5] The first larval stage (L$_1$) hatches from an egg, feeds on organic material in the manure, molts to the second larval stage (L$_2$), and eventually develops into an infective, third-stage larva (L$_3$). Rates of egg hatching and larval development increase in direct proportion to environmental temperatures. Under field conditions, the minimum interval between egg passage and development to the infective stage is approximately 1 week. Rates of development from eggs to L$_3$ are very low if not completely impaired during winters in colder climates, so parasite transmission generally does not occur at a significant level except during the typical grazing season.

After larvae reach the infective, third stage, prolonged survival is fostered by a different set of environmental conditions, and larvae persist better at low temperatures. Third-stage strongylid larvae are surrounded by a durable sheath that protects them from desiccation but does not allow them to feed. Accordingly, infective larvae survive by metabolizing energy reserves that are stored within intestinal epithelial cells. These limited energy stores are depleted more rapidly at higher temperatures, so infective larvae can survive only briefly in hot weather. Because larvae persist well in cold conditions, the concept of a "killing frost" does not exist. Horses can acquire strongyle infections while grazing pastures during winter and through the subsequent spring.

Environmental conditions during spring and autumn are ideal for strongyle transmission in all regions. However, geoclimatic variations result in seasonal differences in strongyle transmission patterns during winter and summer. In northern temperate climates (above ~40 degrees north latitude), summer is a favorable season for hatching of strongyle eggs and development into infective larvae.[6] Northern winters are too cold for eggs to hatch, but larval survival is excellent. In contrast, southern temperate summers are too hot and dry for sustained larval persistence, but winter conditions are mild enough to allow some egg hatching, as well as excellent survival of existing larvae.[3,7] In terms of transmission potential, horses in southern temperate regions experience substantial risk during autumn through spring, whereas transmission in pastured, northern horses is virtually perennial.

In northern temperate climates, migrating *Strongylus* larvae return to the gut and begin egg production during spring.[8] Third-stage larvae develop during spring and summer, and ingestion by grazing horses completes transmission. Adult large strongyles survive in the host through summer and autumn,

become senescent during winter, and are replaced in the following spring by a new population.[8] The annual epidemiology of *Strongylus* infection has not been studied in southern temperate regions.

Pathogenesis

Large strongyles damage the host as both larval and adult stages. Within days of infection, L$_3$ *S. vulgaris* larvae invade the submucosa of the small intestine and molt to the L$_4$ stage.[9] These larvae enter local arterioles, burrow beneath the intima, and migrate proximally to the root of the anterior mesenteric artery (AMA).[10] A proportion of *S. vulgaris* larvae continue to wander past this site, and migratory lesions have been observed in the root of the aorta and in other arterial branches.[11] Larvae within the intima of the proximal AMA cause severe local arteritis, accompanied by focal enlargement, thrombi within the vessel lumen, and hypertrophy of the medial layer (Fig. 57-1). This lesion is classically described as a "verminous aneurysm," although the arterial walls are neither thin nor dilated. Verminous arteritis is associated with an increased incidence of colic, although the pathophysiologic mechanisms are unknown. The simplest hypothesis is that emboli from the thrombus are carried distally and occlude the arterial supply of the gut. This so-called thromboembolism will then result in ischemic segments of the intestine, which may cause very painful colic manifestations in the horse. However, a necropsy survey of ischemic bowel lesions of horses failed to demonstrate emboli in the majority of cases.[12] Other hypotheses for inducing colic include primary changes in gut motility[13] and interference with local neurologic control.[14]

Migrating larvae of *S. edentatus* and *S. equinus* have been associated with hemorrhagic and inflammatory lesions in the liver, pancreas, and retroperitoneal tissues. These lesions do not cause distinct clinical signs but may contribute to the general inflammatory component of strongylosis. In the final stage of migration, all *Strongylus* larvae return to the large intestine and form nodules within the gut wall.[15] Adult large strongyles emerge from these nodules to take up residence within the gut. The parasitic nodules can be greater than 1 cm in diameter and often are filled with purulent material whether occupied or vacant.

Adult large strongyles can use their buccal capsules to attach firmly to the mucosa of the cecum or ventral colon. These worms are said to "plug feed," drawing small amounts of gut mucosa into the oral cavity and presumably ingesting tissue

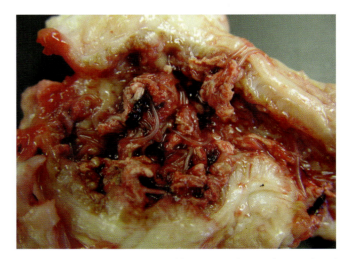

Figure 57-1 Verminous arteritis caused by migrating larvae of *Strongylus vulgaris*. (*Courtesy Dr. Charles Faulkner, Department of Comparative Medicine, University of Tennessee College of Veterinary Medicine, Knoxville.*)

proteins. Rupture of local vessels may cause focal hemorrhage, but the consequences of adult feeding activities are only a minor component of strongylosis. One noteworthy species of large strongyle, *Triodontophorus tenuicollis*, feeds in colonies of 20 or more adults and causes large (1-3 cm), deep ulcers in the dorsal colon.[2]

Clinical Findings

Strongylosis is characterized by nonspecific signs of weight loss and poor growth, rough hair coat, and compromised performance.[16] Experimental infections caused pyrexia, tachycardia, anorexia, diarrhea, and listlessness.[17] Larval *S. vulgaris* infections do not cause distinct clinical signs but are associated with an increased incidence of colic. When infarction of the large intestine occurs, these cases invariably have a fatal outcome.

Diagnosis

Infection with adult strongyles is easily demonstrated by using a variety of concentration techniques to detect strongylid eggs in the feces (see Chapter 54). Concentration techniques include simple fecal flotation using saturated salt or sugar solutions, as well as quantitative procedures such as the McMaster's, modified Wisconsin, or modified Stoll technique.[18] Regardless of methodology, the presence of strongyle eggs in the feces of grazing horses is ubiquitous, so the diagnostic value of fecal examination is not robust. Even quantitative techniques that calculate the numbers of eggs per gram of feces have limited interpretive value because strongylid egg counts are not correlated to the numbers of parasites that produced them, and they are not predictive of the severity of clinical parasitism.[19-21]

Strongylid eggs are homogenous, and those of cyathostomins cannot be differentiated from large strongyle eggs (Fig. 57-2). In mixed infections, more than 95% of strongyle eggs passed in the feces are produced by cyathostomins. Proportional contributions of various strongylid genera or subfamilies to the total egg count can be determined by fecal culture, which requires that feces containing strongyle eggs be kept moist, aerated, and incubated at room temperature for 10 to 14 days. The L3 larvae that develop in these conditions are collected and examined, and the proportional contributions by cyathostomins (Fig. 57-3) and the various genera of large strongyles (Fig. 57-4) can be calculated.[18]

A polymerase chain reaction-enzyme-linked immunosorbent assay (PCR-ELISA) for identifying six species of cyathostomins has proved reliable and applicable for detecting the presence of these species in fecal samples.[22] Similarly, a reverse line blot assay capable of detecting 21 species of cyathostomins and all three species of *Strongylus* has been developed and validated.[23,24] Recently, a real-time PCR assay has been developed for the detection and semiquantification of *S. vulgaris* DNA in fecal samples.[25] Such assays are currently available for research purposes only, but it is possible that molecular tests will be made available for routine usage in the future. Hematology and serum chemistry of horses with strongylosis often indicate mild anemia, leukocytosis with eosinophilia, hypoalbuminemia, beta-globulinemia, and elevations of IgG(T) antibodies.[15,26] Essentially all abnormalities are consequences of inflammation and protein-losing enteropathy.

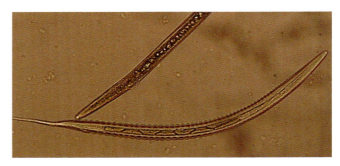

Figure 57-3 Third-stage larva (L3) of cyathostomin nematodes. *(Courtesy Dr. Martin K. Nielsen, M.H. Gluck Equine Research Center, Department of Veterinary Science, University of Kentucky, Lexington.)*

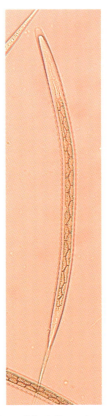

Figure 57-4 Third-stage larva (L3) of *Strongylus vulgaris*, a large strongyle. *(Courtesy Dr. Martin K. Nielsen, M.H. Gluck Equine Research Center, Department of Veterinary Science, University of Kentucky, Lexington.)*

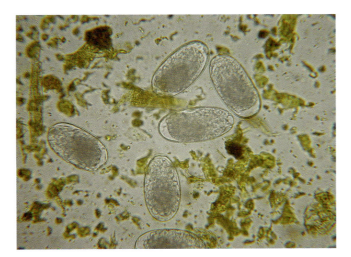

Figure 57-2 Photomicrograph of typical strongylid eggs passed by large strongyles and cyathostomins. *(Courtesy Dr. Charles Faulkner, Department of Comparative Medicine, University of Tennessee College of Veterinary Medicine, Knoxville.)*

Pathologic Findings

Discrete hemorrhages, approximately 1 cm in diameter and occurring beneath the serosa of the ileum, have been termed *hemomelasma ilei* and are considered indicative of recent *S. vulgaris* infection.[11] The pathologic lesions caused by fourth-stage and fifth-stage *S. vulgaris* larvae within blood vessels have been characterized by scanning electron microscopy.[27] Typical lesions consist of large thrombi surrounding larvae located within vessels with dilated lumens and thickened walls. Active coagulation is evident on the surfaces of larvae, thrombi, and vascular endothelium, where aggregations of red blood cells, platelets, and fibrin can be observed. The concurrent existence of a mature thrombus with additional, active thrombi indicates cumulative formation over time. The arterial walls become thickened by fibrosis and occasionally by dystrophic calcification.[15] After thrombotic lesions are fully developed, the artery may never return to normal.[28]

On rare occasions, migrating *Strongylus* larvae have been associated with cerebrospinal disorders.[15] More common are eosinophilic lesions in the pancreas[29] or eosinophilic granulomas in the liver and epicardium.[30]

Therapy

Several anthelmintics belonging to three chemical families are effective for treatment of adult large strongyles, but migrating larvae are susceptible to only three anthelmintic regimens (Table 57-1). Because of the inflammatory nature of lesions associated with migrating larvae, specific chemotherapy cannot be expected to result in immediate alleviation of clinical signs of strongylosis. Anthelmintic resistance has not yet been convincingly documented for any of the large strongyle genera.

If large strongyles are suspected of causing clinical disease, it is recommended to treat with one of the larvicidal formulations. However, in case of *S. vulgaris*, the damage in the AMA will already have occurred, and it is not certain if removing the parasites will resolve the condition. Nevertheless, it has been shown that the endarteritic lesions are capable of healing considerably upon anthelmintic treatment.[31]

Prevention

General approaches to strongyle control are discussed in greater detail in the next section on *Cyathostominae*. Chemotherapeutic approaches to control large strongyles include daily administration of pyrantel tartrate (2.64 mg/kg), which kills ingested strongylid larvae before they can invade gut tissues and establish infection.[32] Unlike some populations of cyathostomins, resistance to pyrantel tartrate has not been demonstrated in large strongyles to date.

Elimination of large strongyles from a herd is not only feasible, it has been accomplished at a majority of well-managed horse farms in North America.[33] However, recent studies illustrate that *S. vulgaris* can reemerge, whenever anthelmintic treatment intensities are reduced to a level below two dewormings per horse per year.[34] Because larvicidal anthelmintics (see Table 57-1) can kill all stages of *Strongylus* larvae within the host, at least 6 months would be required after treatment before another adult population could develop and begin to contaminate pasture with eggs. By repeating larvicidal treatments at intervals of no greater than 6 months, new infections could not arise on a farm where all animals had been maintained on this program. Also, because the maximum duration of survival of free-living stages in the environment is approximately 1 year, no infective large-strongyle larvae could remain on pastures where this program had been maintained for 18 months or longer.[35]

Public Health Considerations

The large strongyles have no zoonotic potential and cannot infect any domestic animals other than equids.

Cyathostominae (Cyathostomes, Cyathostomins, Small Strongyles, Trichonemes)

Etiology

The *Cyathostominae* found in North America belong to eight genera: *Cyathostomum, Cylicocyclus, Cylicodontophorus, Cylicostephanus, Coronocyclus, Parapoteriostomum, Poteriostomum,* and *Petrovinema*.[36] Another genus, *Gyalocephalus*, has been assigned to a different taxonomic group, but it behaves biologically as a cyathostomin. In contrast to large strongyles, cyathostomins have shallow or cylindrical buccal capsules with which they attach weakly to the mucosa of the large intestine. Most small strongyle species are moderately sized nematodes, less than 1.5 cm in length by about 1 mm in diameter.

After ingestion by a grazing horse, L_3 cyathostomins invade the mucosa of the cecum, ventral colon, or to a minor extent, the dorsal colon.[37] Within 1 to 2 weeks after infection, a fibrous capsule develops around the larva,[38] which is now said to be "encysted." Small-strongyle larvae develop through multiple, sequential stages. The invading stage (early third-stage larva, or EL_3) grows into a late third-stage larva (LL_3), then molts into an early fourth-stage larva (EL_4) and ultimately a late fourth-stage larva (LL_4). All larval growth and maturation occur within the confines of a mucosal or submucosal cyst. The LL_4 stage emerges from the cyst into the lumen of the large intestine and develops into a reproductive, adult nematode. Larval

Table 57-1 Spectra of Various Anthelmintics Labeled for Efficacy against Strongylid Nematode Parasites of Horses

Chemical Class	Compound	Dosage	Large Strongyles		Cyathostomins	
			Adults	**Migrating Larvae**	**Adults and Luminal Larvae**	**Encysted Larvae**
Benzimidazoles	Fenbendazole	5 mg/kg	Yes	Yes*	Yes	Yes*[†]
	Oxfendazole	10 mg/kg	Yes	No	Yes	No
	Oxibendazole	10 mg/kg	Yes	No	Yes	No
Heterocyclic compounds	Piperazine	88 mg/kg	No	No	Yes	No
Macrocyclic lactones	Ivermectin	0.2 mg/kg	Yes	Yes	Yes	No
	Moxidectin	0.4 mg/kg	Yes	Yes	Yes	Yes[‡]
Tetrahydro-pyrimidines	Pyrantel pamaote	6.6 mg/kg	Yes[§]	No	Yes	No
	Pyrantel tartrate[¶]	2.64 mg/kg/day	Yes	No	Yes	No

*Requires a regimen of 10 mg/kg daily for 5 consecutive days.

[†]Label claims for efficacy against early third-stage (EL_3), late third-stage (LL_3), and fourth-stage (L_4) cyathostomin larvae.

[‡]Label claims for efficacy against late third-stage (LL_3) and fourth-stage (L_4) cyathostomin larvae.

[§]Efficacy against *Strongylus edentatus* is less than 90%.

[¶]When fed daily, aids in the control of certain nematode parasites.

development may be progressive, producing an adult worm in as quickly as 5 to 6 weeks, or larvae may arrest development in the EL_3 stage,[39] and not undergo further maturation for up to 2.5 years.[40]

Epidemiology

The bionomics of cyathostomin development and persistence in the environment are virtually identical to those of large strongyles, discussed previously. An annual cycle has been hypothesized for cyathostomin populations within the host.[26] A large proportion of encysted larvae emerge from gut tissues during late winter or early spring and mature into adult cyathostomins. The reproductive activity of this new population is manifested by the spring increase in fecal egg counts.[41] This population continues to reproduce through the summer months, when conditions are favorable for egg hatching and larval development. In northern climates, a second generation of adult cyathostomins may arise in late summer as a direct product of infection earlier in the grazing season. The majority of larvae ingested during autumn are destined to undergo arrested development within the host. This population overwinters within host tissues and emerges in the following spring to initiate another annual cycle.

Arrested development is a strategy employed by many nematode species to avoid unfavorable environmental conditions. Cyathostomin larvae specifically interrupt their development at the EL_3 stage and can remain encysted in tissues for 2 years or longer.[39,40] Small strongyle populations in northern climates undergo arrested development during winter, presumably to avoid environmental conditions that are unfavorable for egg hatching. Similarly, cyathostomin populations in the south would arrest during summer to evade hot, dry weather, which favors neither larval development nor persistence.

Pathogenesis

Cyathostomin third-stage larvae cause mucosal inflammation of the cecum and ventral colon when they first invade the gut after ingestion.[42] Within a few weeks, these larvae become surrounded by a fibrous capsule within the mucosa or submucosa of the host organ.[38] The capsule protects the horse from the parasitic products inside the cyst, but it also shields the nematode from inflammatory and immune responses of the host. Minimal inflammation is observed around encysted larvae as long as the cysts remain intact (Fig. 57-5). Rupture of the cysts during larval emergence releases excretory and secretory products that have accumulated over time. Larval excystment results

in lesions of focal edema, congestion, and hemorrhage, with accompanying leakage of tissue fluids into the bowel lumen. The cumulative severity of the lesions and their effect on the host are correlated to the numbers of larvae emerging. Adult small strongyles are ineffective plug feeders and cause minimal damage as mature parasites.[43]

Clinical Findings

Strongylosis is characterized by weight loss and poor growth, rough hair coat, and compromised performance.[16] Cyathostomins can cause these general clinical signs in the absence of a large-strongyle component. One specific syndrome, larval cyathostominosis, is a seasonal condition caused by synchronous emergence of large numbers of encysted cyathostomins.[26] This syndrome is characterized by severe diarrhea, rapid weight loss, marked hypoproteinemia, and passage of numerous larval cyathostomins in the feces. In the acute phase, this condition has been associated with a case-fatality rate of around 50%.[44] However, cases of larval cyathostominosis are rare, given the ubiquity of these parasites. In northern climates, larval cyathostominosis occurs most frequently in late winter, when encysted larvae are expected to emerge from arrested development. In southern regions, larval cyathostominosis is most common in late summer and autumn for the same reasons.[45]

Diagnosis

Diagnosis of the nonspecific aspects of strongylosis is discussed in the section on *Strongylinae*. Strongylid eggs are homogenous, and those of cyathostomins cannot be differentiated from large-strongyle eggs. In mixed infections, more than 95% of strongyle eggs passed in the feces would be produced by cyathostomins, and this proportion can be confirmed by coproculture, as discussed previously.

Recent attempts to develop serologic assays to detect infection with encysted larval cyathostomins have shown great promise.[46,47] Such assays would be of great value in equine practice because these stages cannot be detected by fecal examination, yet clearly are the most pathogenic. In addition, a molecular assay has been validated for identifying 21 different species of cyathostomins by fecal analysis.[24] This technology allows parasitologists to study the relative impact of individual species in natural infections, as well as to identify species with higher levels of anthelmintic resistance.

Pathologic Findings

Soon after larval ingestion, L_3 cyathostomins penetrate the basement membrane of the epithelial cells of the tubular glands in the large intestine, where they provoke a fibroblastic reaction. This increases as the larvae grow, eventually leading to goblet cell hyperplasia and hypertrophy and distortion of the glands. Modest infiltration with lymphocytes and (in some cases) eosinophils occurs below and around the encysted larvae.[42]

The major lesions of cyathostomin infection occur during larval emergence and include typhlitis and colitis, which contribute to protein-losing enteropathy.[48] Intense, focal eosinophilia may develop when the cyst wall is breached by an emerging larva.[42]

Therapy

Anthelmintic resistance is widely documented in cyathostomin parasites, and all equine establishments should be expected to have at least some level of resistance to one or more drug classes. In the absence of resistance, adult cyathostomins were susceptible to several anthelmintics belonging to four chemical families, and two anthelmintic regimens demonstrate activity against encysted larvae (see Table 57-1). The efficacy of a dewormer against adult cyathostomins can be evaluated simply with a fecal egg count reduction (FECR) test (Box 57-1).

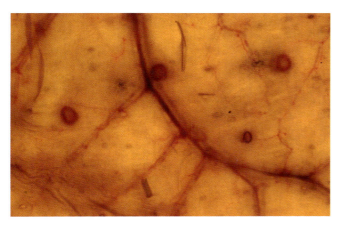

Figure 57-5 Cyathostomin larvae encysted in mucosa of cecum. *(Courtesy Dr. Andrew Peregrine, Department of Pathobiology, Ontario Veterinary College, University of Guelph, Ontario, Canada.)*

Box 57-1 Fecal Egg Count Reduction (FECR) Test

Fecal samples are collected from individual horses before treatment and examined by a quantitative egg-counting technique. The results are reported as strongyle eggs per gram (EPG). An accurate dose of the product to be tested is administered, based on a current body weight and consistent with label recommendations. Ten to 14 days after treatment, another fecal sample is examined from the same animal, and the percentage reduction of egg counts is calculated, using the following formula:

$$\frac{\text{EPG (pretreatment)} - \text{(posttreatment)}}{\text{EPG (pretreatment)}} \times 100 = \text{FECR}$$

It is recommended to use an egg counting technique with a detection limit of 25 eggs per gram (EPG) or less. Always use the same technique consistently. Include horses with the highest possible pre-treatment egg counts, and never use horses with counts below 200 EPG.

The FECR test should be established on the farm level by calculating the FECR for a number of individual horses and then subsequently calculating the average FECR for the treated group. It is recommended to include at least 5 to 10 horses on each farm if possible.

Suggested cut-off values for resistance depend on the drug tested and the number of horses investigated, but for the range of 5 to 10 horses, the following cut-off values are recommended as general guidelines for strongyle nematodes:

- Benzimidazoles: 95%
- Pyrantel: 90%
- Ivermectin: 95%
- Moxidectin: 95%

If the farm average FECR falls below these values, anthelmintic resistance should be suspected. However, it is important to rule out other causes of decreased efficacy such as misdosing, inadequate storage, etc. One must also consider how many horses were tested and how high the starting FEC were. Due to inherent variability in the measurement of FEC when performing FECR test, interpretation of the data can sometimes be difficult when results fall into the borderline zones. In such cases, it is recommended to repeat the FECR test.

Most equine anthelmintics are labeled only for removal of adult and larval cyathostomins from the lumen of the gut; larvae encysted in the gut wall may not be affected. When mature worms are killed by deworming, larval stages emerge from tissues at varying intervals thereafter, apparently to reestablish reproducing populations. Anthelmintic treatment purportedly can even induce parasitic disease by promoting the synchronous emergence of arrested cyathostomin larvae from tissue cysts.[49] In addition to the endogenous supplementation of adult populations, horses grazing on infective pastures rapidly acquire a new generation of larvae to maintain the cycle.

Previously, recommended treatment regimens for larval cyathostominosis consisted of 70 days of alternation between ivermectin, fenbendazole, and corticosteroids.[50] However, with the introduction of moxidectin, treatment of this syndrome became much simpler; a single administration of this drug (400 μg/kg) should be regarded as the drug of choice for this condition and can be combined with oral administration of corticosteroids. In addition, acute cases of larval cyathostominosis require intensive fluid therapy and shock management, and patients must therefore be hospitalized.

Prevention

Strongyle infection is ubiquitous in grazing venues, so the major objective of control is to limit pasture contamination with feces containing strongylid eggs. This can be accomplished by targeting the general fecal component. In fact, the use of commercial vacuum units to remove manure from pastures at biweekly intervals was very effective for controlling the transmission of strongyles in the United Kingdom.[51] However, pasture hygiene is labor intensive and requires expensive machinery and relatively flat paddocks for effective implementation. For grazing horses, pasture rotation has not been a successful control strategy because it is extremely complicated and requires extensive monitoring beyond the capacity of laypersons.

Rather than limiting fecal contamination, most strongyle control programs attempt to reduce the numbers of parasite eggs contained in the feces. This requires chemical intervention, so anthelmintics are the keystone of almost all strongyle control programs for horses. Administering pyrantel tartrate (2.64 mg/kg) daily in the feed is a preventive, chemical approach because it kills ingested strongylid larvae before they can invade gut tissues and establish infection. One concern about this program is that perennial use could interfere with the development of acquired immunity, especially by younger horses. In addition, populations of cyathostomins can develop resistance to pyrantel tartrate, rendering its daily use ineffective.[52]

A common strategy is to administer anthelmintics at a frequency that removes reproducing adults but also limits cumulative egg production by the herd over the course of a grazing season. Egg counts should decrease by more than 90% after the successful removal of a small-strongyle population. Ultimately, however, adult populations are replaced, reproduction resumes, and egg counts return to previous levels. The interval between effective treatment and resumption of significant egg production is known as the egg reappearance period (ERP).[52] Formerly, ERPs were quite predictable for various classes of equine anthelmintics, but this appears to be changing due to emergence of drug resistant populations. Originally, benzimidazole or pyrantel pamoate treatments typically provided an ERP of 4 weeks, ivermectin prevented contamination for 6 to 8 weeks after treatment, and the ERP of moxidectin was approximately 12 weeks. The ERPs were initially used to define the intervals between anthelmintic treatments, but this is now considered an unsustainable approach for parasite control. Instead the ERPs can be used to measure emerging levels of anthelmintic resistance. Suppressive treatment tends to select for anthelmintic resistance, or at least for populations that reproduce faster and have shorter ERPs. Cyathostomin populations that are resistant to benzimidazole anthelmintics were first identified in the 1960s and are now widespread in most countries. Resistance to pyrantel salts is found both in Europe and North America, where it was documented on approximately 40% of horse farms in one survey.[52] Levels of pyrantel resistance appear to be higher in the United States than elsewhere in the world, but it remains unknown whether this is due to usage of pyrantel tartrate or other factors.

Until recently, the macrocyclic lactones ivermectin and moxidectin remained the only anthelmintics that were fully effective against equine strongyles. But recent findings clearly illustrate that ERPs for both drugs have been dramatically reduced to about 4 to 5 weeks.[53,54] These findings are ascribed to survival of premature stages of cyathostomins in the large intestinal lumen and have been interpreted as resistance by this particular stage.[53,54] Because no new classes of equine anthelmintics are anticipated in the near future, current control strategies must be revised to preserve the efficacy of available drugs for as long as possible.

Biologic control with nematode-trapping fungi has potential as a nonchemical approach to equine parasite control.[55] These fungi are natural predators of nematodes and kill free-living larvae by trapping them in a network of hyphae. Fungal spores can be fed to animals so that they pass though the alimentary tract and inoculate the feces. Fungi trap nematode larvae as they develop in the feces and significantly reduce the numbers of larvae on pasture. At present, fungal products are not commercially available.

Modern approaches to cyathostomin control emphasize the use of effective drugs, high levels of parasite surveillance, and decreased intensity of treatment within the herd. These approaches can maintain health, limit pasture contamination, and decrease selection pressures for anthelmintic resistance. One such approach, termed *selective treatment*, is based on characterizing the contaminative potential of each horse in a herd, then designing control programs based on individual characteristics.[56-59] The magnitude of strongylid egg counts of horses after a long sojourn from deworming can be used to classify individual animals as low, moderate, or high contaminators. Horses that are "low contaminators" apparently control parasitism on their own and do not contribute significantly to overall contamination of the premises. Such animals do not need to be dewormed at all if only cyathostomins are present on the premises. If large strongyles are a potential threat, low contaminators only need to be dewormed twice annually with a larvicide, at the beginning and end of a grazing season, to prevent reestablishment of large strongyles. Horses that are "high contaminators" should be the major focus of control and probably need repeated anthelmintic treatment throughout the grazing season. Finally, those horses that are "moderate contaminators" can be dewormed on a schedule that is intermediate between the two extremes. Eradication of cyathostomins is not a realistic goal for any control program.

Public Health Considerations

The cyathostomin nematodes that infect horses have no zoonotic potential and cannot infect any domestic animals other than equids.

Parascarosis

Etiology and Epidemiology

Parascaris equorum (ascarids, roundworms), as with other members of the superfamily *Ascaridoidea*, resides as an adult in the small intestine of its host. *P. equorum* is the largest nematode that infects horses, growing to approximately the size of a pencil when mature (Fig. 57-6). Thick-walled eggs are passed in the feces 10 to 15 weeks after infection[60-62] (Fig. 57-7). Development of eggs to the infective stage in the environment requires about 10 days at optimal temperatures (25°-35° C [77°-95° F])[63] and probably several weeks in cool conditions. The infective stage is an egg containing a second-stage larva (L_2).[2] Larvated eggs are ingested from the environment, hatch in the small intestine, and the liberated L_2 ascarids enter the portal circulation and are carried to the liver. Larvae are migrating through the liver within 24 hours of infection.[61] After approximately 1 week, larvae are carried to the lungs, where they break out of the vasculature and enter alveoli. These larvae migrate up the airways or are coughed up into the pharynx, where they are swallowed and return to the small intestine to complete maturation.

The major features of the epidemiology of parascarosis are the extreme persistence of the infective stage in the environment and the predominance of infection in juvenile horses. Larvated *Parascaris* eggs remain viable for 10 years or more, so one patent infection on a premise can affect several future generations of foals. Susceptible animals acquire infection by ingesting larvated eggs from the environment. Unlike strongylids, ascarid infections can be transmitted in confinement venues as well as on pasture. *Parascaris* eggs possess a sticky, protein coating[64] that allows them to adhere to a variety of surfaces, including vertical walls and the hair coat or udder of a mare. *Parascaris* infection is found almost exclusively in juvenile horses less than 18 months of age.[65] Horses develop extremely effective acquired immunity against *Parascaris*, and it is unusual to see patent infections in mature horses. Infections in juvenile horses often involve hundreds of worms, comprising a liter or more of parasites. Weanlings and yearlings ultimately lose their ascarid infections, probably through a combination of acquired immunity and senescence of the adult worm population. *Parascaris* is transmitted solely by equids; no alternate definitive hosts exist.

Pathogenesis

The pathogenesis of adult ascarid infections is poorly understood, but parasitized foals exhibit reduced weight gain and inferior body composition, with elevated total body water and decreased total body solids. The simplest explanation for their impact is that the large mass of worms in the small intestine competes with the host for digested nutrients, especially amino acids. This hypothesis was supported by an experiment showing that ascarids absorbed radiolabeled methionine after oral administration to foals.[66] In addition to competition for amino acids, reduced dietary intake by infected foals can result in hypoproteinemia.

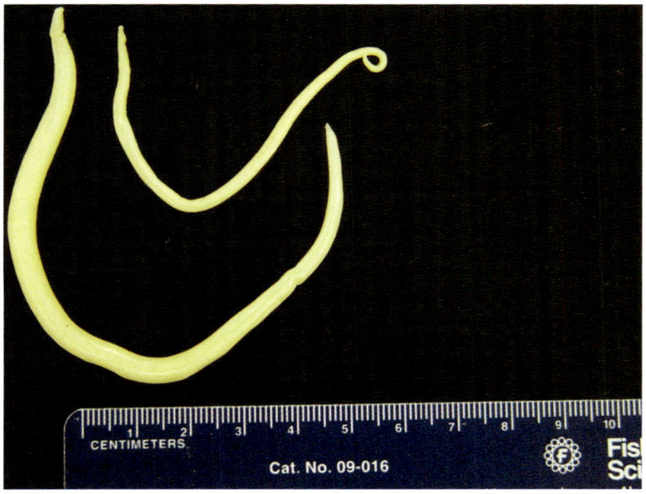

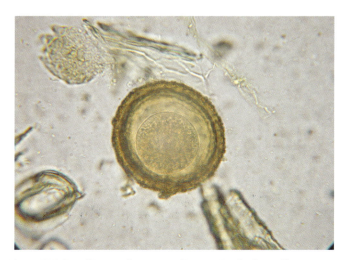

Figure 57-6 Parascaris equorum adults; male *(top)* and female *(bottom)*. *(Courtesy Dr. Charles Faulkner, Department of Comparative Medicine, University of Tennessee College of Veterinary Medicine, Knoxville.)*

Figure 57-7 Egg of *Parascaris equorum*. *(Courtesy Dr. Charles Faulkner, Department of Comparative Medicine, University of Tennessee College of Veterinary Medicine, Knoxville.)*

Clinical Findings

Hepatic migration (1 week after infection) is not accompanied by apparent clinical signs. Invasion of the lungs (2-4 weeks after infection), however, can cause frequent coughing and a grayish white, purulent nasal discharge.[65,67] This exudate may also be visualized within the trachea by endoscopic examination. Affected foals often experience secondary bacterial infection, especially with *Streptococcus equi* subsp. *zooepidemicus*. Weanlings or yearlings infected with adult ascarids may exhibit poor growth, ill thrift, rough hair coats, and a pot-bellied appearance, but juveniles with modest worm burdens often appear normal. A large mass of ascarids can cause impaction of the small intestine, with accompanying colic and eventual intestinal rupture if not relieved. The likelihood of intestinal rupture is not directly correlated to worm numbers. In addition to signs of abdominal pain, foals with ascarid impaction may have gastric reflux (containing intact worms) and shock secondary to possible toxic or hypersensitivity reactions to parasite antigens.

In a retrospective study of foals with ascarid impaction that were treated surgically, the median age at presentation was 5 months (range, 4-24 months).[68] Males were affected more often than females (67% and 33%, respectively). Approximately 75% of cases occurred during the fall season (late August to early November). At presentation, foals tended to be tachycardic and febrile, with injected and toxic mucous membranes and a prolonged capillary refill time. Gastrointestinal tract sounds were often reduced or absent.

Diagnosis

Patent ascarid infections are easily detected by fecal examination using one of the qualitative or quantitative concentration techniques discussed previously. Egg counts were recently found to have a high diagnostic specificity and a moderate sensitivity, but no correlation was found between egg counts and the number of worms in the small intestine.[21] Infections involving immature (i.e., nonreproducing) worms in the intestine, lungs, or liver, however, cannot be detected by this method. Infected horses often pass intact ascarids in the feces, especially within 1 to 2 days after anthelmintic treatment. Endoscopic and radiographic findings for the pulmonary stage of infection have been described.[67,69]

Foals with ascarid impactions often have abnormal abdominal fluid ranging from serosanguineous to purulent in nature.[68] Definitive diagnosis before surgery or necropsy may be difficult. However, presence of intact parasites in feces or gastric reflux of a foal or horse 4 to 24 months of age with acute colic suggests the diagnosis. A history of recent anthelmintic treatment also supports a diagnosis of ascarid impaction in foals. In a retrospective study of 11 foals treated surgically for ascarid impaction, three were dewormed less than 24 hours before the onset of colic signs and three were dewormed 2 to 5 days before the onset of signs (54% dewormed <6 days before onset of colic). Of those cases, in which the type of anthelmintic was identified, almost all foals had been treated with ivermectin or pyrantel pamoate prior to onset of disease.[68,70] Ultrasound examination of the abdomen may facilitate presurgical or antemortem diagnosis by visualization of worms within dilated segments of the small intestine (Fig. 57-8).

Pathologic Findings

Hepatic migration during the first week after infection is accompanied by focal hemorrhage beneath the hepatic capsule and eosinophilic tracts within the parenchyma.[71] The hemorrhages heal by fibrosis, leaving depressed, white areas under the hepatic capsule. Pulmonary migration initially causes petechial hemorrhages and inflammatory changes. Four to six weeks after infection, lymphocytic nodules develop beneath the pleura.[72] These gray-green nodules may contain remnants of dead larvae

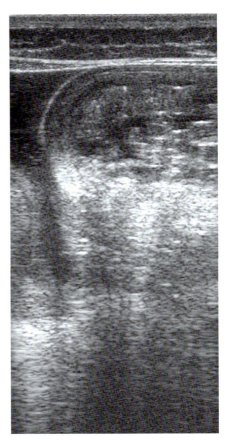

Figure 57-8 Ultrasound image of ascarids within lumen of small intestine of foal with signs of colic. *(Courtesy Dr. Maureen T. Long.)*

and are more numerous after reinfection than after primary exposure.

Therapy

Parascaris is the dose-determining parasite for some equine dewormers, especially the benzimidazoles. This means that a higher dosage of a given anthelmintic is required to kill ascarids than other internal parasites, and this parameter often determines the approved label dosage of an equine parasiticide. Adult and juvenile ascarids in the lumen of the small intestine are susceptible to numerous anthelmintic products (Table 57-2). The ascaricidal efficacy of an anthelmintic can be evaluated by FECR testing (see Box 57-1) based on pretreatment and posttreatment counts of *Parascaris* eggs. Interpretation of FECR for ascarids, however, has not been characterized as well as for strongyles. In recent years, ascarid populations at some breeding farms in several different countries have developed apparent resistance to the macrocyclic lactone anthelmintics moxidectin and ivermectin, as indicated by poor FECR.[73-75] In 2005, Kaplan et al reported that ivermectin failed to reduce egg counts or worm counts in foals that had been inoculated with a purportedly resistant strain of *Parascaris* from Canada.[76] Anecdotal reports of ivermectin resistance in *P. equorum* are countless in Europe and North America, and resistance should generally be expected till proved otherwise.

Foals that are suspected to have heavy ascarid burden should not be treated immediately with highly efficacious antihelminthics. Initial administration of a drug with lesser efficacy, specifically fenbendazole (5 mg/kg), may lessen the risk of posttreatment ascarid impaction. If ascarid impaction is suspected,

Table 57-2 Spectra of Various Anthelmintics Labeled for Efficacy against Nonstrongylid Nematode Parasites of Horses

Chemical Class	Compound	Dosage	Parascaris equorum	Strongyloides westeri	Oxyuris equi
Benzimidazoles	Fenbendazole	5 mg/kg	Yes*	No	Yes
	Oxfendazole	10 mg/kg	Yes	No	Yes
	Oxibendazole	10 mg/kg	Yes	Yes[†]	Yes
Heterocyclic compounds	Piperazine	88 mg/kg	Yes	No	Yes
Macrocyclic lactones	Ivermectin	0.2 mg/kg	Yes	Yes	Yes
	Moxidectin	0.4 mg/kg	Yes	NA[‡]	Yes
Tetrahydro-pyrimidines	Pyrantel pamaote	6.6 mg/kg	Yes	No	Yes
	Pyrantel tartrate[§]	2.64 mg/kg/day	Yes	No	Yes

NA, Not applicable.

*Requires a dosage of 10 mg/kg.

[†]Requires a dosage of 15 mg/kg.

[‡]Moxidectin may not be used in foals less than 6 months of age.

[§]Aids in the control of certain nematode parasites when added to the feed daily.

treatment should include administration of mineral oil by nasogastric tube, appropriate supportive care to maintain hydration and treat shock, and analgesic therapy.

If medical therapy fails to relieve the impaction, surgical exploration with small intestinal enterotomy to remove worms may be attempted. In a retrospective study of 11 horses presented for surgical treatment of ascarid impaction, only 1 horse survived.[68] Another retrospective study reported the long term survival rate to be 27%.[70] Impactions in these horses were usually at multiple sites, and postoperative complications leading to death included colic, endotoxemia, fever, adhesions, severe peritonitis, focal necrotizing enteritis, intestinal perforation, and abdominal incision infections.[68]

Prevention

The objective of an ascarid control program is to limit environmental contamination with reproductive products (i.e., passage of eggs in feces). Contamination can have far-reaching effects because of the extreme persistence of the infective stage in the environment. In contrast to strongylids, ascarid control efforts must be applied to the entire farm premises, not only pasture venues.

If administered daily in the feed, pyrantel tartrate (2.64 mg/ kg) kills ingested ascarid larvae after they hatch from the egg but before they can invade the tissues of the small intestine. This approach can be very effective in horses that reliably ingest the pelleted product. Ascarid resistance to pyrantel pamaote has been reported in one study.[77]

Control recommendations for breeding farms are based on a prepatent period of approximately 70 days or longer. It is recommended that treatments for ascarid infection begin when foals are about 60 to 90 days old and that benzimidazole type drugs should be preferred over other drug classes. Acquired immunity usually develops well before a horse's second birthday, and ascarid control efforts are not required for mature equids.

Because resistance to at least one drug class (macrocyclic lactones) has been reported, it is an excellent recommendation to monitor fecal samples of foals for ascarid eggs during the intervals between regularly scheduled treatments. The presence of large numbers of eggs 2 to 4 weeks after treatment suggests that the previous deworming was ineffective, and anthelmintic resistance could be confirmed with a standard FECR test.

Because ivermectin has some activity against larval ascarids migrating in the liver or lungs,[78] many breeding operations use it at monthly intervals in foals. This frequency is excessive, and most premises with documented *Parascaris* resistance to macrocyclic lactone anthelmintics had a history of using ivermectin or moxidectin at frequent intervals.

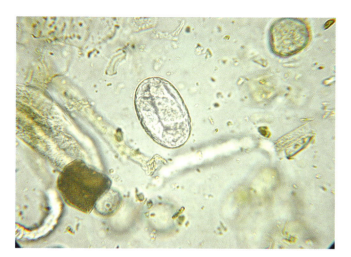

Figure 57-9 Egg of *Strongyloides westeri*. (Courtesy Dr. Charles Faulkner, Department of Comparative Medicine, University of Tennessee College of Veterinary Medicine, Knoxville.)

Ancillary ascarid control efforts are directed at reducing exposure to infective stages from the environment. These measures include rigorous hygiene of foaling stalls or other housing areas to be occupied by suckling foals. Numerous disinfectants, including Lysol, phenol, chlorine bleach, and even live steam, have been evaluated in the field.[63] None has been entirely successful in eliminating infective eggs. Because ascarid eggs can adhere to the hair coat of a horse, a standard practice at many breeding farms is to bathe mares thoroughly before introducing them to foaling stalls, with particular efforts to clean the udder.

Public Health Considerations

Parascaris equorum has no zoonotic potential and does not infect other domestic animals.

Strongyloidosis

Etiology and Epidemiology

Strongyloides westeri is a small, thin nematode (<1 cm × 1 mm) that resides in the proximal small intestine of foals. Only females are parasitic, and they reproduce by parthenogenesis. Thin-walled, oval eggs containing a coiled larva (Fig. 57-9) are passed in the feces. In the environment, *Strongyloides* undergoes a complex life cycle with alternating free-living and parasitic generations.[2] Eggs hatch and larvae develop to become either free-living males and females or infective third-stage larvae.

Sexual reproduction by free-living stages produces only larvae that are destined for a parasitic existence. Environmental development requires moist conditions and warm temperatures. Horses are infected when third-stage larvae penetrate the skin or mucous membranes. In immune adult horses the infective larvae migrate to somatic tissues and suspend further development. In mares the hormones of pregnancy and lactation apparently stimulate the arrested larvae to mobilize and migrate to the mammary gland. Third-stage larvae are passed in the milk of mares within a few days after foaling, and foals ingest infective larvae while they suckle.[79] Within the foal, larvae undergo pulmonary migration and return to the small intestine. Egg production by adult females usually begins in foals at 10 to 14 days of age,[2] but patent infections have been observed in foals as young as 5 days.[80]

Most foals develop permanent immunity against reinfection with *Strongyloides* by 5 or 6 months of age. However, foals with no prior exposure to *Strongyloides* may be susceptible to primary challenge.[81] A recent, coprologic survey of foals from central Kentucky revealed a prevalence of *Strongyloides* infection (1.5%) that was much lower than historical observations in a similar population.[82]

Pathogenesis

Strongyloides westeri occasionally causes diarrhea in infected foals,[81] but mechanisms other than simple enteritis have not been described. Although *S. westeri* patency and foal heat diarrhea both occur contemporaneously during the second week of life, no causal relationship has been established. Foal heat diarrhea continues to be common despite the declining prevalence of *Strongyloides* infections.

Clinical Findings

The most common clinical sign of strongyloidosis is diarrhea during the first month or two of life. Heavily infected foals may become emaciated, listless, and dehydrated from enteritis. This clinical syndrome must be differentiated from other causes of diarrhea in foals.

A syndrome of "frenzy" (hyperactivity and extreme discomfort) has been reported in foals that were confined on moist soil, sand, or sawdust with an acid pH.[80,83] Affected animals exhibited swelling of the lower legs within 2 days of an attack, and some developed skin lesions. This clinical manifestation was attributed to percutaneous invasion by third-stage *S. westeri* larvae. Exposed foals developed patent infections within 1 week after a frenzied episode, and *Rhodococcus equi* was recovered from regional lymph nodes.[80]

Diagnosis

Infection is confirmed by demonstrating small, thin-shelled, oval eggs containing a coiled larva in the feces of foals from 1 week to about 5 months of age (see Fig. 57-9). The observation of *Strongyloides* eggs in the feces of a diarrheic foal, however, does not necessarily implicate the nematode as the cause of the diarrhea. In a case-control study of foal diarrhea in the United Kingdom, the presence of *Strongyloides* eggs was significantly correlated to clinical diarrhea only when egg counts were very high (>2000 EPG), suggesting the presence of large numbers of adult parasites.[84]

Pathologic Findings

Little is known about the pathologic lesions associated with *Strongyloides* infection in foals. Enteritis in the proximal small intestine is the most common lesion, but edema of the entire alimentary tract was described in one severe case.[81] Systemic migration during the prepatent period may be accompanied by petechial hemorrhages and inflammatory foci in pulmonary tissues.

Therapy

Only two currently marketed equine anthelmintics have label claims for efficacy against *S. westeri*. Oxibendazole (15 mg/kg) and ivermectin (0.2 mg/kg) are both effective after oral administration (see Table 57-2). Another macrocyclic lactone, moxidectin, is also effective, but this compound is not labeled in the United States for use in foals less than 5 months of age. There are no reports of anthelmintic resistance in *S. westeri*.

Prevention

Attempts to minimize lactogenic transmission by deworming the mare with ivermectin during the last weeks of gestation have not been completely effective.[85] Environmental hygiene to remove foal feces and application of basic chemicals to adjust the pH of moist confinement areas may reduce percutaneous transmission. Many breeding farms routinely deworm foals at about 2 weeks of age with one of the products listed previously to reduce transmission and obviate clinical disease. However, the incidence of *S. westeri* infection has declined so dramatically in recent years that many breeding operations would be justified in deleting specific *Strongyloides* control measures from the facility herd health program.

Public Health Considerations

Although human lesions of cutaneous larva migrans resulted from an accidental laboratory exposure to infective larvae of *S. westeri*,[86] this parasite is generally considered to have little zoonotic potential. Humans and all domestic mammals serve as definitive hosts of various *Strongyloides* spp. other than *S. westeri*.

Oxyurosis

Etiology and Epidemiology

Oxyuris equi is a fairly large nematode (~1-6 cm in length) that resides as an adult in the small colon and dorsal colon of equids.[2] *Oxyuris* is known as a pinworm because the tail end of the female is sharply pointed. Pinworm eggs are rarely passed in feces because gravid females protrude from the anus and deposit eggs in a sticky film directly onto the anus and perianal tissues. Development is facilitated by proximity to a warm host, and eggs become infective in about 5 days. The masses of infective eggs flake off into the environment, and transmission to other horses is accomplished by ingestion. As with ascarids, pinworms can be transmitted in confinement venues, as well as on pastures. When an infective egg is ingested, a third-stage larva hatches out and invades the mucosa of the large intestine. These molt to fourth-stage larvae, which are small, wedge-shaped worms that attach to the mucosa of the proximal large intestine. Larvae ultimately molt into adults, which live in the distal colon to reduce the commuting distance for nocturnal oviposition by females. The prepatent period of *O. equi* is approximately 5 months. Equine pinworms apparently invoke acquired immunity because the prevalence of patent infections is much lower in mature horses. Adult horses can develop oxyurosis, however, if never previously infected. Recent observations suggest that the parasite is changing its pattern by more readily infecting mature horses.[87]

Pathogenesis

Larval pinworms attach to the mucosa of the cecum and ventral colon, where their plug-feeding activities may cause superficial typhlitis or colitis. Adult pinworms apparently do not have any primary pathologic impact.

Clinical Findings

As a consequence of anal pruritus associated with the egg-laying activity of female worms, affected horses rub their rumps against stall fixtures, trees, and fence posts, causing hair loss of

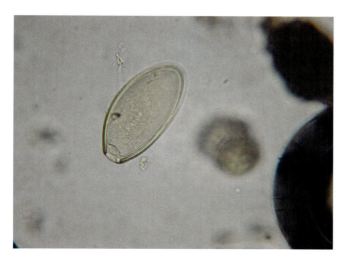

Figure 57-10 Egg of *Oxyuris equi*.

the tail and abrasions to the perianal region.[2] Adult pinworms occasionally are observed in freshly passed feces or adhering to a rectal palpation sleeve, and adult females may be observed protruding from the anus. Fresh or dried egg masses can be observed on the anus. The fresh material is greenish yellow and pasty, and the dried masses are gray, yellow, or green.

Diagnosis

Diagnosis is confirmed by recovery of *Oxyuris* eggs in samples collected from around the anus of a suspected host. Typical *Oxyuris* eggs are oval, flattened on one side, have a single operculum, and contain a coiled larva (Fig. 57-10). Various techniques can be used to collect perianal samples. In the cellophane (Scotch) tape technique, the sticky side of a small piece of adhesive tape is applied to the perianal area and then attached directly to a glass slide for microscopic examination. Diagnostic material can also be collected by scraping the perianal region with a tongue depressor dipped in mineral oil or lubricant and transferring the scrapings to a microscope slide for examination.

Pathologic Findings

Mild, superficial colitis has been attributed to attachment of fourth-stage larvae on the mucosa of the proximal large intestine. In one case, lesions of *hemomelasma ilei* on the serosa of the ileum were found to contain eggs of *O. equi*.[88]

Therapy

Virtually all broad-spectrum equine anthelmintics have efficacy against adult and larval *O. equi*. These include drugs of the benzimidazole, tetrahydropyrimidine, and macrocyclic lactone classes. Any of these products could be used as a specific therapy when the objective is to alleviate clinical signs caused by adult pinworm infection.

Prevention

Environmental hygiene would be beneficial for pinworm control but would not be expected to eliminate infective stages completely. The routine use of anthelmintics in horses less than 2 years of age should provide adequate control of pinworm infections. Because of the long prepatent period of *Oxyuris*, routine strategies for strongylid control are sufficient against pinworms as well. Since 2004, numerous reports have circulated of adult horses with pinworm infections that were refractory to treatment with macrocyclic lactone anthelmintics, even with frequent treatments and increased dosages. Macrocyclic lactones are not 100% effective against adult *Oxyuris*,[89,90] so

these observations should not be construed as unequivocal evidence of resistance, but it cannot be ruled out that it may be developing.

Public Health Considerations

O. equi has no zoonotic potential and does not infect other domestic animals. Humans serve as definitive hosts of *Enterobius vermicularis*, a pinworm that is unique to primates.

Nonenteric Nematodes

Debra C. Sellon

The adult stages of most nematode parasites that affect horses reside within the gastrointestinal tract. However, a few parasites cause significant disease within other body systems, including the skin (*Onchocerca, Habronema/Draschia*), respiratory tract (*Dictyocaulus*), eye (*Thelazia;* discussed in Chapter 10), and central nervous system (*Halicephalobus;* discussed in Chapter 4).

Onchocerciasis

Etiology and Epidemiology

At least three species of nematode parasites from the genus *Onchocerca* are associated with cutaneous and ocular lesions in horses. *Onchocerca gutturosa* affects cattle and horses in North America, Africa, Australia, and Europe.[91] Adult worms are up to 60 cm in length and live in connective tissue of the ligamentum nuchae of horses. Adult parasites produce microfilariae (200-230 μm in length) that are most numerous in the dermis of the face, neck, back, and ventral midline.[92] A number of *Simulium* spp. and *Culicoides* spp. may serve as intermediate hosts.[93-95]

Onchocerca reticulata infects horses in Europe and Asia. Adult worms may be up to 50 cm in length and live in the connective tissue of the flexor tendons and the suspensory ligament of the fetlock, especially in the front legs. Microfilariae are 310 to 395 μm in length and are most numerous in the dermis of the legs and ventral midline. *Culicoides* spp. act as intermediate hosts.[91]

Onchocerca cervicalis causes a nonseasonal dermatitis in horses worldwide.[91,96-98] Clinical disease occurs year-round but may be worse in the spring and summer. The small, threadlike adult nematode is approximately 30 cm in length and resides in the ligamentum nuchae. Microfilariae migrate to the dermis of the ventral midline, pectoral area, withers, inguinal region, and eyelids,[99] with highest numbers in the spring, when *Culicoides* spp., the predominant intermediate host, are most active.[100] Mosquitoes may also serve as vectors in some geographic areas. Microfilariae undergo development to infective larval stages over a 25-day period within the *Culicoides* vector. The estimated prevalence of *O. cervicalis* infestation in clinically normal horse populations in the United States varies from 25% to 100%.[91,101] There are no apparent breed or gender predilections for onchocerciasis, but affected horses are usually older than 4 years.[91] Because *O. cervicalis* is the most common member of the *Onchocerca* genus to affect horses, the remainder of this discussion focuses on this parasite unless otherwise indicated.

Pathogenesis

Cutaneous lesions related to *O. cervicalis* are thought to result from type I and type III hypersensitivity reactions to microfilariae.[91,96,98,102] The severity of the reaction varies between horses, and many horses have dermal microfilariae without any evidence of reaction. Ocular lesions are the result of

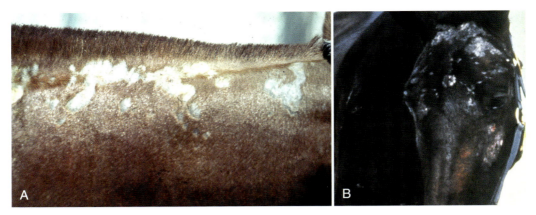

Figure 57-11 Thinning of hair and hair loss caused by *Onchocerca cervicalis* microfilariae in neck **(A)** and head **(B)** of horse. Note the inflammation and ulceration secondary to pruritus. *(Courtesy Dr. Melissa T. Hines.)*

microfilariae in the eyelids, conjunctiva, cornea, anterior chamber, uvea, and fundus. Concurrent uveitis, presumably an immune-mediated event, may be observed. In either cutaneous or ocular lesions, sudden death of parasites with chemotherapy may produce a severe exacerbation of disease, presumably as a reaction to antigens released by dead and dying microfilariae.

Clinical Findings

Lesions of cutaneous onchocerciasis secondary to *O. cervicalis* microfilariae begin as areas of thinning hair, with or without mild scaling or crusting. These areas are observed most often on the face, neck, chest, withers, and ventral midline and usually are accompanied by mild to moderate pruritus[91,96,98,102] (Fig. 57-11). Over time, lesions progress to areas of alopecia with scaling, crusting, and plaques. Chronic lesions become ulcerated and excoriated with crusts and lichenification. Depigmentation eventually occurs and is irreversible.[91,97,98] Affected horses may exhibit extreme pruritus and attempt to rub lesions on the face and ventral abdomen. However, tail rubbing is seldom seen with onchocerciasis, helping to differentiate this disorder from *Culicoides* hypersensitivity reactions.[98]

The most common clinical abnormality associated with ocular onchocerciasis is depigmentation (vitiligo) of the bulbar conjunctiva at the temporal limbus.[98] Sclerosing keratitis originating at the temporal limbus and extending toward the center of the eye may be observed.[91] Other clinical signs and lesions may include conjunctivitis, chemosis, blepharospasm, lacrimation, corneal edema, and faint multifocal corneal deposits. Signs of concurrent uveitis may be observed in some horses. Chronic infection may result in formation of nodules 0.5 to 1 mm in diameter in the pigmented conjunctiva of the temporal limbus. Peripapillary choroidal sclerosis (round or crescent-shaped area of depigmentation bordering the optic disc) has been described in some affected horses.[91,98]

Clinical signs of *O. reticulata* infestation of horses include subcutaneous nodules overlying or within the flexor tendons and suspensory ligaments around the fetlock, especially in the front legs. Severely affected horses may have associated swelling and lameness.[91]

Diagnosis and Pathologic Findings

Differential diagnoses for cutaneous onchocerciasis include summer eczema (*Culicoides* hypersensitivity), dermatophytosis, fly-bite dermatoses, mite infestations, and food hypersensitivity. Skin scrapings and direct smears of blood or cutaneous lesions are unreliable for diagnosis. Diagnosis is most easily confirmed by identification of microfilariae in minced skin biopsy preparations from horses with compatible history and clinical signs (Fig.

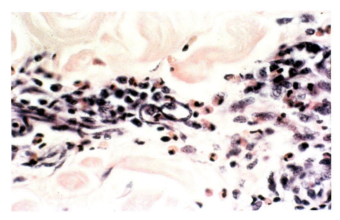

Figure 57-12 Photomicrograph of skin biopsy specimen from horse with *Onchocerca cervicalis*. Note the numerous eosinophils and presence of microfilariae. *(Courtesy Dr. Melissa T. Hines.)*

57-12). A standard 4- or 6-mm skin punch biopsy specimen is minced with a sharp blade and mixed with physiologic saline in a Petri dish. After incubation at room temperature for 30 minutes, the specimen is examined under a microscope for identification of rapidly moving microfilariae.[91,98] Routine skin biopsies reveal superficial perivascular eosinophilic dermatitis, often with visible microfilariae in the superficial dermis surrounded by degranulating eosinophils.[91,103] Chronic lesions may have evidence of fibrosis. Occasionally, necrosis of hair follicle epithelium, focal areas of collagenolysis in the superficial dermis, or lymphoid nodules in the deep dermis or subcutis may be observed.[91] Because microfilariae may be observed in the skin of normal horses, diagnosis cannot be made solely on the basis of observation of these parasites in a biopsy specimen. The final diagnosis can only be made after consideration of biopsy results, history, and clinical signs and observation of a positive response to appropriate therapy.

Therapy

Ivermectin at a dose of 200 µg/kg orally is the treatment of choice for elimination of microfilariae in the skin or ocular tissues.[104,105] A single dose may result in improvement in clinical signs within 2 to 3 weeks, with complete resolution in 2 months.[104] One study suggested that some horses may remain free of cutaneous microfilariae for 4 to 5 months or longer after treatment with injectable ivermectin. Some horses may require two or three monthly treatments before clinical signs resolve.

Approximately 10% to 25% of horses with onchocerciasis have an adverse reaction (e.g., ventral midline edema or pruritus) to ivermectin treatment within 7 to 10 days. In rare cases, severe ventral midline or eyelid edema and fever may develop. Anecdotal reports suggest that treatment may precipitate uveitis in horses with ocular microfilariae.[97] These horses should be treated with corticosteroids before or during ivermectin therapy to decrease the likelihood or severity of adverse reactions. There is no known therapy to eliminate adult *O. cervicalis* from the ligamentum nuchae of horses. Therefore affected horses will need periodic re-treatment with ivermectin to prevent or control recurrence of clinical signs.[97-99]

Alternative drugs that have been recommended for treatment of equine onchocerciasis include diethylcarbamazine at 5 mg/kg orally (PO) for a minimum of 5 consecutive days or levamisole at 10 mg/kg PO daily for 7 to 10 days. With the widespread availability of ivermectin, however, these drugs are now rarely used.

Habronemiasis

Etiology and Epidemiology

Habronemiasis, also known as "summer sores," bursatti, "swamp cancer," and granular dermatitis, is caused by a reaction to larvae of the equine stomach worms *Habronema muscae, Habronema majus (Habronema microstoma)*, and *Draschia megastoma*.[106] Adult *H. muscae* and *H. majus* are 1 to 2.5 cm in length and can be found free in the mucus covering the glandular area of the stomach.[106] They are rarely pathogenic, although large numbers may cause nonspecific gastritis or ulceration of the gastric mucosa.[107] In contrast, adult *D. megastoma* worms are 0.5 to 1.25 cm in length, invade the gastric mucosa, and cause granulomatous masses up to 10 cm in diameter. Large *D. megastoma* granulomas within the stomach contain colonies of adult parasites and have a central opening through which larvae pass into the lumen of the stomach (Fig. 57-13). Occasionally, these lesions may be large enough to obstruct the flow of ingesta or may perforate the stomach wall, resulting in diffuse or localized peritonitis, occasionally fatal.[106]

Regardless of species, adult worms produce first-stage larvae (L_1) that are passed in feces. The L_1 stages are ingested by fly maggots. The housefly *(Musca domestica)* is an intermediate host for *H. muscae* and *D. megastoma*; the stable fly *(Stomoxys calcitrans)* is the intermediate host for *H. majus*.[91] After maturation, infective third-stage larvae (L_3) on the mouthparts of adult flies are deposited around a horse's mouth or in horse feed; the larvae are ingested; and the life cycle is complete. Cutaneous habronemiasis occurs when infective L_3 parasites are deposited on wounds or other moist areas of the body such as the penis, prepuce, or periocular tissues. Occasionally, the parasite may penetrate unbroken skin to cause lesions.

Cutaneous habronemiasis has been reported in horses from most parts of the world as a seasonal, sporadic, recurrent disease.[106-120] Lesions are most frequently observed in the spring and summer and may regress in the winter. Larvae do not appear to overwinter in the skin.[91] No breed, gender, or age predilection exists. Some horses appear to have particular susceptibility to disease and have recurrent lesions each year, whereas other horses on the same premises never exhibit lesions.

Pathogenesis

The characteristic ulcerative granulomatous lesions of cutaneous habronemiasis are probably the result of a hypersensitivity reaction to parasite larvae. Evidence for the role of hypersensitivity reactions in the pathogenesis include the seasonal recurrent nature of lesions, predilection of some horses for lesions, and response to systemic glucocorticoids as a sole treatment.[91,106] The reaction of specific immunoglobulin E (IgE) with larvae is speculated to result in mobilization of eosinophils; peripheral eosinophilia may reach 15% to 20%.[106]

Clinical Findings

Cutaneous habronemiasis is characterized by large, granulomatous, ulcerative lesions most often observed in areas of wounds or on moist areas of the body such as the penis, prepuce, periocular tissues, or distal limbs (Figs. 57-14 and 57-15). Early lesions often appear as slow-healing wounds that gradually enlarge and develop the typical appearance of exuberant granulation tissue.[121] They may be solitary or multiple and can affect more than one part of the body in a single horse. The ulcerated granulomatous tissue frequently exudes a serosanguineous exudate. Pruritus varies from mild to severe. Small (1-mm) yellow granules consisting of caseation, calcification, fibrosis, and necrosis surrounding dead larvae may be observed. As lesions enlarge, they frequently take on a circular shape. These granules must be differentiated from the "leeches" observed in lesions of phycomycosis and zygomycosis (see Chapter 51). Lesions of the urethral process may obstruct urine flow, with resultant dysuria and pollakiuria.[122]

Ocular lesions are most frequently observed as yellowish, gritty plaques in the conjunctiva of the medial canthus. Lesions may also involve the conjunctival sac, the lacrimal duct, or the third eyelid (see Fig. 57-15). Lesions of the nictitans may be more proliferative. Lacrimal duct lesions typically result in a circular lesion from a few millimeters up to 2 cm in diameter, approximately 2 to 3 cm below the medial canthus.[91,106,121,123]

Pulmonary habronemiasis is uncommon and rarely associated with clinical respiratory disease. Nodular granulomas with central necrosis are present in the interstitial and peribronchial areas of the lung.[91,124-126] One foal had a *Rhodococcus equi* pulmonary abscess from which *D. megastoma* larvae were recovered.[127] Another report described small, white, necrotic foci containing *D. megastoma* in the liver of a horse.[120] It has been proposed that these types of lesions represent aberrant dissemination of larvae through the blood or lymphatic circulation; the horses in these reports did not have concurrent cutaneous lesions.[106]

Diagnosis and Pathologic Findings

A presumptive diagnosis of habronemiasis can often be made on the gross appearance of the lesions. Differential diagnoses should include bacterial granulomas, phycomycosis, zygomycosis, other fungal granulomas, exuberant granulation tissue, squamous cell carcinoma, sarcoid, and other neoplastic lesions. Definitive diagnosis is confirmed by direct smears or biopsy.

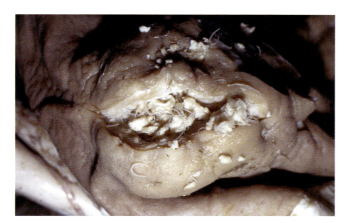

Figure 57-13 Large granuloma containing *Draschia megastoma* parasites in stomach of horse. *(Courtesy Dr. John Barnes.)*

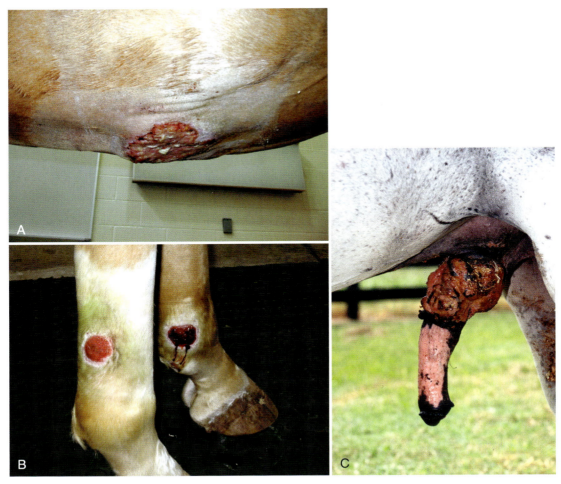

Figure 57-14 Equine habronemiasis of **A,** ventral abdomen; **B,** distal limbs; and **C,** penis. (**A,** Courtesy Dr. Steeve Giguere; **B,** courtesy Dr. Robert MacKay; **C,** courtesy Dr. Margo Macpherson.)

Deep scrapings or smears of lesions, especially from lesion granules, may reveal nematode larvae.[91] These larvae are typically large (2-3 mm wide and 60 mm long) with a large, spiny process on their tails.[121] Caution should be exercised in interpreting these types of smears because they may be negative despite the presence of the parasite, and larvae may be present in other ulcerative lesions of equine skin, including those differential diagnoses previously listed. Biopsy usually reveals varying degrees of nodular to diffuse dermatitis, numerous eosinophils and mast cells, areas of coagulative necrosis that may contain nematode larvae, and palisading granuloma formation around necrotic foci.[91]

Therapy

A wide variety of therapeutic strategies have been described for treatment of habronemiasis in horses. An individual therapeutic plan should be developed for each horse, taking into consideration the site of the lesion, size of the lesion, number of lesions, financial concerns, and practical considerations. Medical therapy alone may be efficacious for many horses; however, horses with large or refractory lesions may benefit from surgery to debulk the lesion before initiating medical therapy. Cryosurgery may also be performed with a double freeze-thaw cycle.[128]

A variety of topical preparations for treatment of habronemiasis have been described. Most of these contain some combination of organophosphates plus corticosteroids and/or dimethylsulfoxide (DMSO). Also, antimicrobial drugs are often included. These preparations were usually applied daily and covered with a bandage. Injectable or oral ivermectin therapy is also indicated for its larvacidal effects. Organophosphates have been used orally or intravenously (IV) for treatment of equine habronemiasis. Historically, trichlorfon was the most commonly used agent and was administered IV at 25 mg/kg in 1 L of 5% dextrose or physiologic saline.[129] The solution was autoclaved before use and repeated at 1- to 2-week intervals if necessary.[121] Adverse effects could occur, including restlessness, pawing, and colic. Organophosphates are no longer available for treatment of horses, and macrocyclic lactones are now recommended as the drug of choice.

Systemic corticosteroids are indicated for primary treatment of many horses with habronemiasis and to minimize hypersensitivity reactions to dead or dying parasites. These drugs have been used successfully as sole therapy for some horses with habronemiasis, supporting the theory that lesions are the result of a hypersensitivity reaction.[121] Prednisolone at 1 mg/kg PO once daily for 7 to 14 days is reported to be effective for treatment of many horses.[91,121]

Conjunctival habronemiasis may be treated topically with 0.03% echothiophate drops twice daily in combination with an antimicrobial/dexamethasone ophthalmic ointment.[91] Occasionally, conjunctival granulomas require excision or curettage.[121]

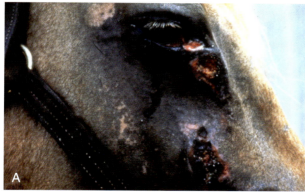

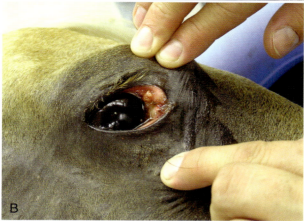

Figure 57-15 A, Typical lesions of ocular habronemiasis involving lacrimal gland at medial canthus of eye. **B,** Ocular habronemiasis involving nictitans. (**A,** *Courtesy Dr. Melissa T. Hines; **B,** courtesy Dr. Alison Morton.*)

Prevention

Regular deworming of horses with ivermectin will kill adult stomach worms and minimize larval contamination of manure. Regular removal of manure, prompt treatment of wounds, and appropriate use of insecticides will also aid in the control and prevention of cutaneous habronemiasis in susceptible horses.[121]

Lungworm Infection

Etiology, Epidemiology, and Pathogenesis

Donkeys and mules are the reservoir hosts for *Dictyocaulus arnfieldi*, the equine lungworm.[130] Infestations in the reservoir hosts do not cause clinical signs even when large worm burdens are present.[131] Prevalence of lungworm infection is estimated to be approximately 68% to 80% in donkeys, 29% in mules, and 2% to 11% in horses.[132,133]

Infection is initiated by ingestion of second-stage larvae (L_2), which migrate through the gut wall and are carried to the lungs through the lymphatics. After 13 weeks of maturation in the peripheral bronchioles, parasites begin to shed ova that are transported by mucociliary clearance to the pharynx, swallowed, and passed out in feces to become infective within 4 days. First-stage larvae (L_1) can survive up to 7 weeks in warm soil but do not tolerate cold weather well.[134] In most horses and ponies, infection is arrested at the L_5 stage and is usually nonpatent, although ova may be passed in the feces of some horses.[131] Because lungworms have been identified in horses with no known contact with donkeys or mules, it is assumed that direct horse-to-horse spread is possible.[132,135]

Experimental studies suggest that *Pilobolus* fungi may facilitate the spread of lungworm infection in a manner similar to that which occurs in cattle lungworm infections.[136] Infective larvae invade the sporangia of the fungi as they grow on manure and are dispersed in the environment when sporangia rupture.[135]

Clinical Findings

Horses with lungworm infections frequently present with signs of coughing and increased expiratory effort that may mimic the signs of reactive airway obstruction (chronic obstructive pulmonary disease [COPD]).[134,137] Auscultation frequently reveals crackles and wheezes, most often over the dorsocaudal lung fields.[137] Infected donkeys rarely show clinical signs of respiratory disease.

Diagnosis and Pathologic Findings

Diagnosis should be suspected in horses with typical clinical signs and history of exposure to donkeys or mules. Endoscopic examination usually reveals large quantities of exudate in the large airways,[135] with a preponderance of eosinophils. Diagnosis can be confirmed by visualization of the parasite, identification of ova on fecal examination with the Baermann technique, or response to appropriate therapy. It should be noted that *D. arnfieldi* rarely reaches sexual maturity in the horse, thus fecal examination is often useless. The Baermann procedure is therefore recommended for the donkeys and mules only. Occasionally, larval stages of the parasite may be observed in tracheal wash or bronchoalveolar lavage samples or in centrifuged mucus.[134,138] Iodine may be useful to stain larvae and facilitate their visualization. On rare occasions, adult lungworms may be visualized endoscopically in the bronchi. These parasites may be up to 16 cm in length.[135] At necropsy, adult lungworms are most often found in the peripheral bronchi. Circumscribed, pale, overinflated areas may be observed in lung parenchyma, especially in caudal lung regions.[131]

Therapy and Prevention

Ivermectin at 200 μg/kg PO is effective for treatment of *D. arnfieldi* and is not associated with significant adverse effects.[139,140] Moxidectin was 99.9% effective for treatment of lungworm infections in donkeys.[141] Benzimidazoles may also be effective for treatment of lungworms. In donkeys, however, fenbendazole only transiently suppressed fecal larval counts.[142]

Lungworm infections may be prevented by housing horses in areas where no donkeys or mules are present. It is advisable to avoid areas where donkeys and mules have previously been housed, unless a freeze has occurred since last habitation.

The complete reference list is available online at www.expertconsult.com.

Cestodes

Heather Stockdale Walden, Merijo Eileen Jordan,* and Joseph A. DiPietro*

58

Etiology

Three species within the family *Anoplocephalidae* (Kholod-kovskii, 1902) infect the gastrointestinal (GI) tract of horses and donkeys: *Anoplocephala perfoliata* (Goeze, 1782; Blanchard, 1848), *Anoplocephala magna* (Abildgaard, 1789; Sprengel, 1905), and *Anoplocephaloides mamillana* (Mehlis, 1831; Rausch, 1976; Schmidt, 1986). All members of the family *Anoploce-phalidae* are similar in that the scolex is unarmed and devoid of rostellum, hooks, or hooklets during all stages of development.[1,2] Within this family, four subfamilies have been described based on type of uterine development.[2] All members of the subfamily *Anoplocephalinae* (Blanchard, 1891), including the three equine tapeworm species, can be defined by the following characteristics: morphologically, the uterus persists in gravid proglottids, and biologically, members have a cysticercoid larval stage that occurs within the hemocele of oribatid mites.[2,3]

Of the three tapeworm species infecting horses, *A. perfoliata* is the most prevalent and the most frequently associated with clinical disease and is the primary focus of this chapter.

Morphology

Distinguishing characteristics of adult *Anoplocephala perfoliata* (Fig. 58-1, *A*) include the following: (1) the length of gravid adult specimens is usually 25 to 40 mm but may reach 80 mm; (2) the width of the body is generally between 8 and 14 mm; and (3) the scolex or holdfast organ is distinct and much smaller than the body, measuring only 2 to 3 mm.[1]

The scolex of *A. perfoliata* has four ear-shaped lappets measuring 0.5 to 1.0 mm that are situated posterior to the four apical muscular suckers (Fig. 58-2).[4] In contrast, *A. magna* is generally larger, measuring up to 80 cm in length and 2.5 cm in width, with a scolex 4 to 6 mm wide (Fig. 58-1, *B*), and *Anoplocephaloides mamillana* is smaller, measuring 6 to 50 mm in length and 4 to 6 mm in width.[3] The scolices of the latter two species do not have lappets as does *A. perfoliata*.

The morphology of proglottids of *A. perfoliata* has been described extensively.[1] Individual proglottids are always much wider than long. Each proglottid is hermaphroditic, containing a single set of both male and female reproductive organs. Each proglottid also contains a muscular system, a tegument, and an excretory system.

The morphology of mature eggs of *A. perfoliata* is unique (see Fig. 54-7). The eggs are 65 to 80 μm in diameter, whereas eggs of *A. magna* measure 50 to 60 μm in diameter and *Anoplocephaloides mamillana* measure about 51 by 37 μm.[3] *Anoplocephala perfoliata* eggs are round to D shaped, with an outer vitelline membrane and a thick (8-10 μm), dark, albuminous middle shell. The innermost membrane is flame or pear shaped and consists of a chitinous pyriform apparatus. The length of

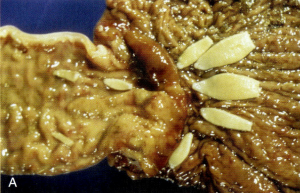
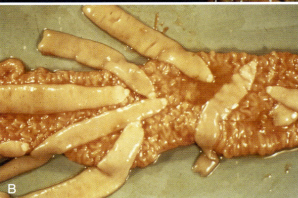

Figure 58-1 A, Mature *Anoplocephala perfoliata* attached to gastrointestinal mucosa of horse at level of ileocecal valve. **B,** Mature *Anoplocephala magna*. *(Courtesy Dr. William Foreyt.)*

the pyriform apparatus is approximately equal to the radius of the egg, measuring about 48 μm. This pyriform apparatus in turn contains the hexacanth embryo characteristic of cyclophyl-lidean cestode eggs.[1,5] The diameter of the embryo measures approximately 16 μm. Eggs seen on fecal flotation often have an amber cast resulting from contact with excreta; however, eggs dissected from gravid proglottids of the adult tapeworm are colorless.[1]

The morphology of anoplocephalid larval development is very similar among many species. In fact, it is impossible to determine the genus from studying the cysticercoid.[1] The morphology of the larval stages of *A. perfoliata* within the intermediate host has been described.[6] However, literature generally presents a detailed ontogenesis of the tapeworm of sheep and goats, *Moniezia expansa*, rather than this parasite[1,7] Briefly, the stages of ontogenesis of *A. perfoliata* begin after the tapeworm egg has been ingested. The oncosphere emerges and penetrates the intestinal wall of the oribatid mite. The oncosphere appears in the mite's body cavity within 48 hours and is very motile

*The authors acknowledge and appreciate the original contributions of these authors, whose work has been incorporated into this chapter.

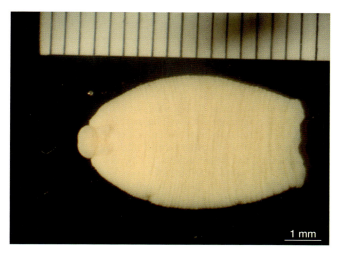

Figure 58-2 Adult *Anoplocephala perfcliata*. Note the lappets.

and active for several days to weeks. The second stage of development is the "large sphere" stage, in which the oncosphere form is lost and the larva becomes immobile. The third stage of growth within the mite's hemocoele is the "extended larva" stage, in which the body lengthens. The fourth stage is called the "segmented larva" stage. In this phase of development, the body continues to elongate but also divides into two parts that are separated by a constriction. The portion anterior to the constriction has four suckers, which are implicated in pathogenesis and which will become the scolex of the tapeworm, and the portion posterior to the constriction is a spherical capsule. Embryonic hooks are positioned caudal to the capsule and are shed. During the fifth stage of larval development, the anterior portion of the larva invaginates into the posterior capsule portion. The "cysticercoid stage" is the final stage of larval development. Morphologically, the body is spherical with a dense cuticle. Within the cuticle is the scolex, with four suckers, and the wall of the cyst is stratified. At this phase of development, the larva is infective for the final host.[8]

Life Cycle

The life cycle of the three tapeworm species that infect the GI tract of horses and donkey is indirect because these species require an intermediate, as well as a definitive, host. Stunkard[9] completed the developmental cycle of Anoplocephaline cestodes in 1937 when he discovered that certain members of one genus of oribatid mites (Acari: Oribatida), *Galumna* spp., could serve as the intermediate hosts of the sheep tapeworm, *Moniezia expansa*, a closely related cyclophyllidean that infects ruminants. A few years later, Bashkirova[6] determined the complete developmental cycle of *A. perfoliata*. With an indirect life cycle, the prevalence of cestode infection in the intermediate host is low, whereas it is high in the definitive host.[10] Intermediate host specificity is low in the various anoplocephaline cestode species, and many species of oribatid mites may become infected.[11]

Adult *A. perfoliata* parasites attach near the ileocecal valve of horses, whereas *A. magna* and *Anoplocephaloides mamillana* attach in the small intestines of the horse's digestive tract. Horses with patent infections shed tapeworm eggs in their feces. The proglottids of *A. perfoliata* are broken up by digestion during transit through the large intestines, thus only eggs are passed in the feces.[12,13] After a gravid proglottid is shed, more than 48 hours may elapse before its ova are passed in the feces.[13]

Survival time of an infective egg on pasture is important because it potentially allows for an improved chance of exposure to the intermediate host. Little is known about the longevity of *A. perfoliata* eggs in the environment, but it has been hypothesized that cestode egg survival may be shortened in tropical climates.[14] However, the infectivity of cestode eggs over time in natural conditions has not been determined. Stunkard[15] wrote that the redistribution of the anoplocephaline tapeworm eggs by rain into the upper layers of the soil would allow the eggs to remain viable for a longer period and enable the intermediate hosts in the soil to encounter the eggs and ingest them.

The life cycle continues when oribatid mites ingest viable eggs of *A. perfoliata* on the pasture. Oribatid mites are free-living mites found on herbage and in the soil of pastures. Because the cestode eggs are presumably too large to be accidentally eaten, the intermediate host may interpret them as prospective or preferred food.[16] Mackiewicz[10] hypothesized that Anoplocephaline tapeworm eggs may use chemoattraction to increase the likelihood of being eaten by the oribatid mites. This would especially hold true if the tapeworm eggs were eaten as a food item rather than as a food contaminant. On the other hand, the oribatid intermediate hosts and *A. perfoliata* eggs may be so abundant that chance encounters between the egg and mite may be the sole strategy of transmission.[10,11]

Whatever the transmission strategy, once ingested by the intermediate host, the larva or oncosphere is freed from within the tapeworm eggshell or embryophore, presumably through digestion. Activation factors that stimulate the oncosphere to tear through the intestinal wall using its hooks are unknown.[17] Once in the mite's body cavity, the development time to an infective cysticercoid within the invertebrate intermediate host is variable. Growth of the cysticercoid within the mite's hemocele depends on environmental conditions, especially temperature. The infective cysticercoid stage is formed within 8 to 20 weeks under natural conditions. Once the cysticercoid is fully developed and infective within the oribatid mite, it is ingested by a grazing horse.

The infective cysticercoid has a scolex with four fully developed suckers. It is assumed that the excysted larvae of *A. perfoliata* move along the GI tract with ingesta until reaching the ileocecal valve area, at which point the larvae attach to the GI mucosa. Behind the scolex of the larvae, germinal cells will multiply through proglottid development or asexual reproduction to produce the proglottids of the adult tapeworm.[15,18,19] The caudal end of the larvae contains the excretory pore that becomes the terminal segment of the adult tapeworm.[15] The prepatent period following ingestion of an infected oribatid mite is 6 to 16 weeks.[5,20-22]

No actual data are available on the life span of adult *A. perfoliata*, but the life span of an adult cestode may vary from a few months to several years.[18,23] A basic cestode life cycle strategy, based on repeated production of egg-laden proglottids, infers a long adult cyclophyllidean life span that often lasts for years or as long as the definitive host lives.[10,18,24] Furthermore, there is selection for repeated production of proglottids and eggs and high fecundity when the prereproductive life span is long.[18] In the case of *A. perfoliata*, this prereproductive life span may be 1 to 1½ years while the cysticercoid is in the oribatid mite.[25,26]

Epidemiology

The distribution and prevalence of *A. perfoliata* are high enough to cause concern among both horse owners and veterinarians. *Anoplocephala perfoliata* is found worldwide and is currently accepted as the most common and the most pathogenic of the equine tapeworm species.[3,22,27-31]

Box 58-1 Prevalence (%) of *Anoplocephala perfoliata* in States in the United States (U.S.) and in Other Countries*

North Carolina (U.S.)	13%
Kentucky (U.S.)	52%-54%
Louisiana (U.S.)	47%
New England (U.S.)	53%
Ohio (U.S.)	18%
Canada	14%
New Zealand	81.5%
England	31%-69%
The Netherlands	21%
Sweden	65%

*Data from references 20, 21, 27, 33-42.

The prevalence of *A. perfoliata* in North America has been reported extensively. Many epidemiologic studies report prevalence of infection at necropsy. In 1979, necropsy data collected from eight states, including Kentucky, found that 18% of foals and 26% of adult horses were infected with tapeworms.[32] The most common tapeworm identified was *A. magna*. Other studies reported prevalences of *A. perfoliata* in the United States that vary from 13% to 54% and worldwide from 14% to 81.5%[20,21,27,33-42] (Box 58-1). This geographic variation has not been explained; however, the differing rates could be caused by differences in pasture type (thus creating a better or worse environment for the intermediate hosts), pasture stocking rates, climate, or other management or environmental factors. Even with the variation in prevalence, there seems to be a trend toward higher prevalence of infection in countries with temperate climates.[13]

Many parasitologists have speculated about the factors that may have caused an increase in reports of *A. perfoliata* infection. Edwards[43] and Geering and Johnson[44] proposed that extensive use of ivermectin, which was new to the market, removed the nematode parasites with greater efficacy than drugs previously available. This selective removal of other intestinal parasites allowed tapeworms to flourish because of lack of competition, thus the increase in prevalence of *A. perfoliata* in recent decades. This hypothesis was refuted by French et al,[45] who reported that the use of ivermectin for 5 years did not promote increase of *A. perfoliata*. Others propose that antiparasitic drugs, such as pyrantel pamoate and fenbendazole, used before ivermectin was available may have had some cestocidal activity.[39,46,47] Other hypotheses include changes in climactic factors, which may in turn have a positive influence on intermediate host numbers, and changes in stocking rates and other pasture management practices.[44] However, no unequivocal data indicate that a true increase in the prevalence of *A. perfoliata* over time has occurred. Lyons et al[29] reported that the prevalence of tapeworm remained essentially unchanged in necropsies of Thoroughbred horses conducted from 1951 to 1990.

Equids of all ages can be infected with tapeworms, and unlike cattle and small ruminants, there is no acquired or age resistance.[22,29,31] Living in the lumen of the gut usually does not trigger pronounced immune responses. This allows the same host to be repeatedly infected over the course of its life.[10]

Horses of all ages, and as young as weanlings, can have patent infections with tapeworm species. The prepatent period is between 6 and 16 weeks. Adult horses as old as 40 years reportedly have been infected with *A. perfoliata*.[31] Prevalence is lower in foals younger than 1 year of age (30%-31%) than in animals that are yearlings or older (52%-60%).[31,48] No gender-related difference in the prevalence of *A. perfoliata* has been reported. In foals, prevalence was similar for colts and fillies, at 33% and 24%, respectively. In adult horses, prevalence between genders was similar, at 59% to 61% in mares, 43% to 57% in geldings, and 41% to 57% in stallions.[31,48]

Pathogenesis

Much has been published regarding the pathology associated with *A. perfoliata* infection. Although the mechanisms are not completely understood, presumably both mechanical damage and parasite antigens play a role in the process.[13] The four unarmed suckers on the scolex of *A. perfoliata* cause pathologic changes at the attachment site. The anatomy of the scolex can be directly related to the features of the lesion when viewed with a scanning electron microscope, in that pegs of mucosa are pulled up into the four suckers.[49] The distance between the tissue pegs corresponds to the distance between the suckers. Long before scanning electron microscopy was available, Skrjabin and Spasskii[1] described ulceration caused by the scolex of *A. perfoliata* embedded in the intestinal wall. These ulcers were inflamed and contaminated with food and intestinal microflora. Perforation, peritonitis, and death resulting from infection with *A. perfoliata* have been reported.[1]

Adult *A. perfoliata* cestodes inhabit the intestinal tract, attaching in clusters primarily at the ileocecal junction, in the cecum near the ileocecal junction, and less often in the terminal ileum and ventral colon[49,50] (see Fig. 58-1, *A*). This clustering of the adult tapeworms can greatly exacerbate the lesions associated with tapeworm attachment. In areas of tapeworm clustering, lesions were found to extend into the submucosa and therefore were more likely to disrupt intestinal blood supply and the nervous regulation.[50] There is no scientific explanation for the clustering of the tapeworms at or near the ileocecal junction, but it may be caused by the production of an aggregation pheromone. There has been documentation and study of an aggregation pheromone, nippolure, secreted by the female of the nematode *Nippostrongylus brasiliensis*.[51,52]

Clinical Findings

Clinical signs, such as poor body condition,[50] poor growth or chronic ill thrift, recurring diarrhea, progressive weight loss, and anemia, have been associated with infections by *A. perfoliata*.[5] These parasites do not appear to cause blood loss that would result in anemia. The anemia could be an anemia of chronic or inflammatory disease.[53]

The literature throughout the 1980s contains many clinical reports of intestinal crises in horses, such as intussusception, cecal perforation, and cecal torsion, that were circumstantially related to concurrent infection by *A. perfoliata*.[43,54,55] Barclay et al[54] associated intussusception with *A. perfoliata* in five cases admitted to the Illinois Equine Hospital, which accounted for 55% of the intussusceptions seen during a 1-year period at that clinic (Fig. 58-3). The intussusceptions all involved the ileum or the cecum (ileoileal, ileocecal, or cecocecal). The association between *A. perfoliata* and acute GI crisis was described in three reported cases of peritonitis. The peritonitis was attributed to perforation of the cecum, which in all cases was associated with infection by *A. perfoliata*.[55] Horses described in these 3 cases of peritonitis harbored high numbers of the parasite, up to 300 worms. In contrast, as few as two adult tapeworms were observed during laparotomy or necropsy of horses with intussusception.[54]

Even after an extensive review of the literature, Owen et al[56] could make no direct conclusions as to the role of tapeworms in association with equine intestinal disease. This interpretation began to change in the early 1990s when Proudman and Edwards[57] demonstrated an association between the presence of equine tapeworms and ileocecal colic. Although the association was not very strong, they found that the risk of ileocecal

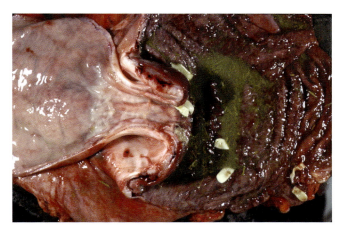

Figure 58-3 Ileocecal intussusception in horse with adult *Anoplocephala perfoliata* attached to mucosa at ileocecal junction. *(Courtesy Dr. William Foreyt.)*

colic was increased by the presence of tapeworms. More recently, *A. perfoliata* was determined to be a significant risk factor for spasmodic colic and ileal impaction, with the risk of spasmodic colic increasing with the numbers of parasites.[58] Twenty-two percent of the spasmodic colic cases and 81% of ileal impactions were tapeworm associated based on serologic and coprologic diagnoses. Their matched case-control studies suggested a dose-response link between infection intensity (as revealed by enzyme-linked immunosorbent assay [ELISA]) and risk of clinical disease.[13,58]

It is possible to relate the gross and microscopic pathology caused by *A. perfoliata* to factors predisposing horses to intussusceptions involving the ileocecal area of the GI tract, the most common site of intussusception in horses.[59] Two factors, segmental atony and hyperperistalsis, are thought to be necessary for intussusception to occur.[60] Lesions associated with tapeworm attachment may alter the pattern of intestinal motility and thus may be a potential cause of intussusception.[43] Other tapeworm-associated changes that may predispose to intussusception include local inflammatory changes at the site of parasite attachment and changes in bowel wall diameter at the ileocecal junction.[61]

Diagnosis

Diagnosis of infection by *A. perfoliata* can be made at necropsy. Location and appearance best identify adults of *A. perfoliata* (see Fig. 58-1). The tapeworms are found in clusters at or near the ileocecal junction. Finding eggs on fecal examination or using serologic antibody tests can facilitate an antemortem diagnosis of *A. perfoliata* infection. Additionally, an indirect ELISA that detects coproantigen[62] was recently evaluated by Skotarek et al.[63] Their study (n = 31) indicated a positive correlation between detectable *A. perfoliata* antigen levels and worm presence using the coproantigen ELISA, with a sensitivity of 74% and specificity of 92%. They found the use of coproantigen ELISA was more sensitive than fecal egg counts, which had a sensitivity of 54% and comparable to serologic ELISA with a sensitivity of 70% and specificity of 78%. These results suggest the use of coproantigen ELISA may offer early detection of *A. perfoliata* infection, providing information about the current status of the animal and possibly monitor response to therapy.

Coprologic examination for parasite eggs is the most common diagnostic technique to detect any GI parasite. Infection with equine cestodiasis is likely underestimated because veterinary practitioners use a standard flotation solution for microscopic fecal examination.[28] One study proposed that diagnosis has proved difficult because eggs levitate poorly with common fecal flotation solutions.[34] Another study found that 3% of horses were positive for eggs of *A. perfoliata* using flotation with sodium chloride solution (specific gravity of 1.18)[27] and 7% of horses were positive using zinc sulfate solution.[35] At necropsy, 54% of these same horses were infected with *A. perfoliata* adult worms. Another study found that the eggs, when present, appear to float with all the standard flotation solutions.[45] Although saturated sugar solution is the most sensitive of the standard flotation media,[21] this levitation medium is not typically used by veterinary practitioners. Sodium nitrate can also be used as a flotation media.[64]

Most flotation techniques are inconsistent primarily because of sporadic shedding of egg-laden proglottids.[28] When proglottids are shed, the structure (and eggs) may disintegrate before the feces pass from the horse's GI tract.[22,50] An alternative hypothesis is that tapeworm eggs are retained in the small, easily overlooked proglottids, making few eggs available in the feces for diagnosis.[5,65] Treating suspect animals with ivermectin is reported to increase the visualization of *A. perfoliata* eggs.[46] Elsener and Villeneuve[66] found a significant increase, by a factor of 2.04, in *A. perfoliata* egg detection using a modified Wisconsin sugar centrifugation technique 24 hours posttreatment of naturally infected horses.

Alternatives to simple flotation for fecal diagnosis of equine tapeworms are double-centrifugation techniques that use sedimentation followed by flotation. Although more time-consuming, these techniques improve diagnostic accuracy. Beroza et al[28] found that the use of double centrifugation first in water and then in sucrose solution improved the recovery of known numbers of formalin-fixed equine tapeworm eggs by 10 times over a technique using only gravitational flotation in sucrose solution. Centrifugal techniques improve accuracy, but as with other fecal diagnostic techniques, they often lack sensitivity because of the sporadic-shedding egg that is an inherent feature of equine tapeworms. Regardless of the fecal diagnostic method used, no correlation has been recognized between numbers of adult tapeworms and egg detection using these techniques.[43,67,68]

Serologic testing that measures serum antibodies specific for antigens of *A. perfoliata* have been developed. The first group to develop an ELISA used a scolex antigen of *A. perfoliata*.[69] This test did not show cross-reactivity to concurrent nematode infection. However, the specificity of the test is low.

Proudman and Trees[70] developed and validated an ELISA using excretory and secretory antigens of *A. perfoliata*. The diagnostic sensitivity of this test was 68% (n = 38). The specificity was 95% (n = 20) when helminth-naïve horses were used but fell to 71% with horses that were *A. perfoliata* negative at necropsy. These horses may have had prior exposure to the parasite, thus residual circulating antibodies were present. Antibody concentrations correlate with tapeworm infection intensity.[13] This immunodiagnostic test may improve the ability to diagnose and treat horses that have high numbers of *A. perfoliata*, allow monitoring of parasitemias, and may be used as a tool for epidemiologic studies.[13,69]

A polymerase chain reaction (PCR)-based assay was developed as a diagnostic tool using *A. perfoliata* deoxyribonucleic acid (DNA) extracted from feces.[71] This assay targets the internal transcribed spacer 2 (ITS-2) regions of the ribosomal DNA (rDNA) with a detection limit of 500 fg of genomic DNA. Traversa et al[72] evaluated the use of this PCR assay, compared to coprologic and serologic techniques, as a way to diagnose *A. perfoliata*. Further validation for PCR as a diagnostic tool for *A. perfoliata* is necessary, although it was found to be a species-specific way of detecting *A. perfoliata* infections in horses.

Pathologic Findings

Lesions caused by *A. perfoliata* account in part for the parasite's association with colic. Mild prolapse of the terminal ileum into the lumen of the ileocecal junction was observed in 5 of 50 horses examined at necropsy that had adult tapeworms attached to the mucosal surface of this area.[49] Extensive mucosal ulcerations near the ileocecal valve were found at necropsy in 63.1% of horses in a highly endemic area.[20]

Damage to the intestinal lining varies with the intensity of *A. perfoliata* infection.[30,49,50] The primary feature of the gross pathologic lesions found at the site of tapeworm attachment, either at the ileocecal junction or on the cecal wall, is mucosal ulceration.[49] The depth and severity of the ulceration increase as the numbers of tapeworms attached to the surrounding area increase. Pearson et al[30] associated the number of tapeworms with severity of damage. Superficial congestion with slightly raised focal ulceration is seen in horses infected with up to 20 tapeworms, whereas the mucosa is raised, thickened, and ulcerated, with nodular swellings at the area of worm attachment, in horses infected with more than 100 tapeworms. Other significant gross pathologic changes associated with attachment of *A. perfoliata* include a yellow diphtheritic membrane and gross edema of the mucosa.[20,49,50] A verrucose granulomatous lesion projecting from the mucosa of the ileocecal junction was described in 2 of 20 horses examined by Pearson et al[30] and in 7.8% of the 65 horses examined by Bain and Kelly.[20]

Histopathologic sections from the areas of tapeworm attachment reveal ulcerations of various depths from the superficial mucosa to the muscularis mucosa and submucosa.[30] In severe cases the mucosal damage may be so extensive that the glandular anatomy is distorted by fibrosis and infiltration of eosinophils into the lamina propria.[49] Inflammatory cells, eosinophils, and lymphocytes infiltrate the areas of damage, and in one case, a submucosal abscess was reported.[30] Verrucose granulomatous lesions are composed of granulation tissue, primarily lymphocytes, and associated fibrinoid necrosis, primarily neutrophils.[20]

Therapy

In the United States, paste dewormers containing ivermectin or moxidectin in combination with praziquantel are marketed for treatment of the equine tapeworm, *A. perfoliata*. In these products the cestocidal activity of praziquantel is combined with a broad-spectrum anthelmintic (e.g., ivermectin or moxidectin) effective against nematodes and *Gasterophilus* larvae. A high degree of efficacy was demonstrated for these products when administered at the label dose of ivermectin (0.2 mg/kg) and praziquantel (1 mg/kg) orally.[73] Cestode egg counts were reduced by 98%, and more than 96% of the horses positive for cestode eggs before treatment were negative on posttreatment fecal tests.

Historically, there is disagreement regarding cestocidal activity of pyrantel pamoate. Early studies indicate partial efficacy against cestodes. Slocombe[74] demonstrated that at 6.6 mg/kg, pyrantel pamoate was not very effective against *A. perfoliata*. Some eggs, worms, and segments were found in feces in the first, second, and third 24-hour periods post-treatment, however at necropsy this was determined to be only 15% of the total worm burden. This low dosage mainly demonstrated dislodgement of gravid segments, with retention of the scolex. In this same study, it was determined that at the double dose of 13.2 mg/kg, greater than 97% efficacy was achieved. A recent study examining a paste dewormer at the 13.2-mg/kg dose in five different U.S. locations demonstrated significant reductions in fecal egg counts 7 to 16 days after pyrantel pamoate treatment.[75] This study demonstrated greater than 95% efficacy overall.

Prevention

Good management will help prevent and control tapeworm infection by reducing both the numbers of eggs passed into the environment in equine feces and the exposure of horses to cysticercoid-containing mites. Reasonable stocking rates should be maintained on pastures. Overcrowding of pastures with infected animals in the cool, dry season, when oribatid mites may have peak populations, would likely produce heavy parasite burdens in the definitive host.[14] Rotation of pastures also has been recommended as a means of prevention. Although this could reduce egg numbers on the pasture, given the longevity of the adult mites on pastures (1-1½ years), transmission probably would not cease unless the horses were kept off the pasture for at least that time.[25,26]

One of the most important control methods is to isolate new animals on arrival at the farm. Because fecal testing may produce false-negative results, all new horses should be treated with an appropriate cestocidal drug before entering the grazing area.[73] If this recommendation is not followed, the potential for initiating the life cycle in a previously uninfested pasture is great. Resident horses should be routinely tested and dewormed as well.[20] Plowing and reseeding pastures have been suggested to reduce the number of oribatid mites.[5,20]

In reality, control of *A. perfoliata* infection by reduction of mite numbers is impractical for most horse owners because of the ubiquitous nature of these mites; thus the only viable alternative is prophylactic cestocidal treatment. Many parasites of livestock can be controlled by a limited number of strategically timed treatments,[76,77] but at present, not enough is known about the transmission of tapeworms to allow complete recommendations. If there were a seasonal fluctuation in mite numbers on pastures, strategically timed treatment of horses to reduce shedding of tapeworm eggs in feces just before the seasonal increase in mite populations would be advantageous.[14]

The complete reference list is available online at www. expertconsult.com.

59

Ectoparasites of Horses

Joy L. Barbet

This chapter discusses the major crawling and flying ectoparasites that affect horses and the pertinent etiologic, epidemiologic, pathogenic, clinical, treatment, and control factors for the particular arthropod. Ectoparasites affect Equidae worldwide. In addition to being annoying, many of these parasites are capable of transmitting infectious agents, inducing hypersensitivity reactions and toxic reactions, and even causing death, if exposure is overwhelming. Several ectoparasites are ubiquitous and found in most locations where horses and other livestock live; some are reportable in certain countries; and some are highly contagious, spreading easily from animal to animal. Increasing international movement of horses, as well as other livestock, makes it important for the veterinarian to be able to anticipate, recognize, and treat ectoparasitic conditions early, preventing the spread of equine and livestock diseases.

Ticks

Etiology

Horses are susceptible to infestations by many species of ticks that feed on wild or domestic ungulates in different regions. Both soft (Argasidae) and hard ticks (Ixodidae) feed on horses. *Ixodes* spp., *Dermacentor* spp., *Boophilus* spp., *Amblyomma* spp., and *Otobius megnini* (spinose ear tick) are most often identified. Exotic ticks, such as *Anocentor nitens* (tropical horse tick), if found on horses in the United States, are reportable.

Epidemiology

Life cycles among tick species may require one, two, or three hosts and a few weeks to 2 years to complete, depending on environmental conditions. Details of life cycles and hosts can be found elsewhere.[1] With multihost ticks, the larvae and nymphs usually require small vertebrate hosts, while the adults feed on larger animals. Tick infestations occur in spring or summer months (the exception being the winter tick, *Dermacentor albipictus*) or nonseasonally in the tropics. In warm climates, if rainy and dry seasons are distinct, ticks will be more active during the rainy season. Most ticks live in forests, grasslands, and scrub, infesting passing animals. Some live in the burrows or nesting areas of the host, enabling them to reach the host easily whenever conditions are favorable.

Pathogenesis

Clinical manifestations of tick infestation result from tick feeding, with local reactions consisting of papules, nodules, wheals, and sometimes pustules around the feeding site. Highly pruritic reactions with papular to urticarial lesions have been attributed to hypersensitivity to *Boophilus* spp. Other species of ticks, including *Otobius megnini* nymphs, *Anocentor nitens* (an important vector of equine prioplasmosis), and *Amblyomma maculatum*, feed in the ear canals of horses. The resulting irritation results in head shaking, ear rubbing, head tilt, or a lop-eared appearance and creates conditions conducive to the development of secondary bacterial otitis externa.

Infectious agents are readily transmitted by ticks for several reasons: (1) ticks feed multiple times throughout their life cycle; (2) many infectious agents are transmitted during tick maturation to the next stage in the life cycle; (3) ticks take relatively large blood meals, which are concentrated by secreting the host's own fluids back into the host directly or as coxal secretions; and (4) immunosuppressive substances are present in the tick saliva that reduce host defenses, allowing the microbe to become established.[1,2] Heavy tick infestations can result in poor nutritional and immunologic conditions and even anemia from blood loss. Tick paralysis results from salivary proteins found in females of some tick species, which secrete the neurotoxic proteins during feeding. Just one tick may cause partial paralysis, but a more severe or extensive paralysis may result from larger numbers of ticks feeding. Foals and ponies are more likely to be affected.[1,3]

Clinical Findings

Clinical syndromes resulting from tick infestation include (1) mild to severe papulonodular dermatitis, with or without pruritus; (2) otitis externa; (3) systemic infection with tick-borne agents such as *Babesia caballi* or *Theileria equi* (see Chapter 55), *Anaplasma phagocytophilum* (see Chapter 39), *Borrelia burgdorferi* (see Chapter 33), *Francisella tularensis*, and *Theileria annulata* (see Chapter 56); (4) anemia and poor condition; and (5) flaccid, ascending motor paralysis, particularly in foals or ponies.[1,4,5]

Diagnosis

Finding ticks on the horse is diagnostic. Identification of ticks is useful in determining which control measures will be most effective. Keys to aid identification can be found in parasitology texts and elsewhere.[6-8] When exotic ticks are suspected or tick management problems arise, consultation with governmental authorities or a parasitologist for proper identification is strongly recommended.

Pathologic Findings

Histopathologic findings for tick-induced papules and nodules range from eosinophilic and neutrophilic perivascular dermatitis with dermal edema to intraepidermal vesiculopustular dermatitis. Chronic, nodular lesions often contain large numbers of lymphohistiocytic cells forming lymphoid nodules or follicles.[9,10]

Therapy and Prevention

Control measures for tick infestations depend on the species involved. Topical or systemic acaricidal treatments are normally combined with management changes such as clearing brush, keeping pastures mowed, and avoiding tick habitats during the season of greatest tick activity. With multihost ticks, control of other tick hosts in the environment (rodents, mice, deer) may prove helpful when possible. Acaricides normally used include synthetic pyrethroids, organophosphates, and avermectins. Chlorinated hydrocarbons and formamidines (amitraz) are contraindicated because of environmental danger and toxicity to horses, respectively. Products are usually applied as sprays or dips or administered systemically. Resistance to acaricides varies regionally.

Public Health Considerations

Infestation of horses with ticks should alert their human owners that they too are at risk of tick exposure and thus potential exposure to tick-borne diseases. Humans in contact with tick-infested animals should inspect themselves for similar infestation and remove ticks as soon as possible before engorgement occurs. The longer a tick remains attached, the greater the likelihood for transmission of infectious agents to the host.

Mites

Sarcoptic Mange

Etiology

Sarcoptic mange, caused by the mite *Sarcoptes scabei* var. *equi*, is very uncommon in horses in Western Europe, North America, and Australia. It is a reportable disease in some countries, and regulatory authorities should be contacted for advice when it is strongly suspected.

Epidemiology

Sarcoptes scabei var. *equi* is a host-specific mite that completes its life cycle on members of the family *Equidae*, but it may survive long enough on humans and other species to induce an allergic dermatitis. The female mite lays eggs in epidermal burrows in the skin. They hatch and pass through larval and nymphal stages, reaching maturity in 2 to 3 weeks. Transmission is by direct contact between animals but may also occur by fomites (e.g., riders' clothing, stable blankets, harness). Mites can live off the host for only a few days, dying of desiccation, but survival could be prolonged in conditions of warmth, darkness, and humidity.

Pathogenesis and Clinical Findings

Irritant and hypersensitivity reactions to the burrowing mites and their excrement are thought to be the cause of the intense pruritus associated with sarcoptic mange. Clinical lesions consist of crusted papules, scaling, and alopecia beginning on the head, ears, and neck and progressing caudally to involve the rest of the body. Over time, excoriations, lichenification, and secondary infections result. Untreated, sarcoptic mange can lead to serious generalized debility, weight loss, and even death.

Diagnosis

Infestation is suspected in animals with a typical history and clinical signs. Diagnosis may be confirmed by microscopic examination of scale and debris obtained by deep and superficial scrapings of multiple affected areas. However, as in other species, negative scrapings do not completely rule out sarcoptic mange, and response to therapy is often used for diagnosis in highly suspicious cases.

Therapy

All infested animals and those suspected of infestation must be isolated; their blankets, harness, grooming equipment, and stables should be treated or disinfected. Handlers must change clothing and wash thoroughly before tending unaffected animals. Affected animals and in-contact animals may be treated topically using organophosphate, synthetic pyrethroid preparations, or 2% lime sulfur applied as a dip, spray, or wash at 7- to 10-day intervals for three or more treatments. These preparations may also be used when necessary for treatment of infested buildings, vehicles, and equipment after thorough cleaning. In chronic cases or when lichenification is excessive, it may be necessary to treat over a longer period. Although not licensed for this condition in horses, ivermectin, given orally at 200 µg/kg body weight every 2 weeks for three treatments, is effective in the treatment of sarcoptic mange in other species. Its use, however, does not eliminate the need for strict isolation of animals and environmental cleaning and treatment. A single dose of moxidectin gel at 0.4 mg/kg is reported to be effective when combined with environmental decontamination.[11]

Public Health Considerations

As with all sarcoptic mange mites, transient infestation of humans may occur. The mites do not reproduce on humans, but reinfestation may continue as long as contact with infested animals continues.

Psoroptic Mange

Etiology

Psoroptic mange in horses has been attributed to several species of psoroptic mites that may or may not be truly distinct species. *Psoroptes equi*, *P. ovis*, *P. natalensis*, and *P. cuniculi* have been implicated in equine infestations. Because *P. ovis* is reportable in cattle and sheep and because these mites are very similar to one another (possibly one species), appropriate authorities should be contacted for advice, especially if infested horses have had exposure to sheep or cattle or have been acquired recently.

Epidemiology

Mites are readily transmitted by direct contact or contact with fomites. Psoroptic mange mites live on the skin surface and feed by puncturing the epidermis, causing serous exudation, erythema, crusting, and pruritus. The female mite lays eggs in the surface debris. Eggs hatch within 2 to 3 days and develop to maturity within 11 to 14 days. Off-host survival of adult mites is shortest during periods of high temperature and low humidity. On average, survival on premises is 2 to 3 weeks but may be longer, depending on conditions.[12]

Pathogenesis and Clinical Findings

As with sarcoptic mange, pruritus from psoroptic mange is thought to be caused by irritant and hypersensitivity reactions to the presence and secretions of the mites. Papules, crusts, scaling, alopecia, and lichenification are the initial lesions. Lesions tend to be distributed around the outer ear, forelock, mane, tail, ear canal, and inguinal and axillary areas, with less involvement of the trunk and legs. Secondary bacterial infections may result.

Diagnosis

Diagnosis requires microscopic identification of *Psoroptes* spp. mites from multiple superficial scrapings and crusts obtained from lesions. Unlike sarcoptic mange, mites are found more readily with psoroptic mange.

Therapy

Treatment is similar to that for sarcoptic mange. Recently, a controlled study showed that a pour-on formulation of eprinomectin for cattle was efficacious in clearing affected horses of psoroptic mange. It was applied at a dose of 500 µg/kg once weekly for 4 weeks.[13] The long potential environmental survival time for psoroptic mites makes vacating premises for a minimum of 3 to 4 weeks advisable. Thorough cleaning of the premises should be carried out with complete removal of bedding and debris. Insecticidal premise treatment is recommended.

Prevention

Thorough physical examination and isolation of newly introduced horses should prevent introduction of *Psoroptes* mites into the herd. Fomites that could potentially transmit the infestation indirectly (e.g., buckets, tack, blankets, grooming equipment) should not be shared between new horses and other horses on the farm.

Chorioptic Mange

Etiology

The most frequently diagnosed mange in horses, chorioptic mange is caused by the surface-living mange mite, *Chorioptes bovis* (Fig. 59-1). As with the previously discussed mange mites, there is likely only one species of *Chorioptes* mites that infests several hosts.

Epidemiology

Transmission occurs by direct and indirect contact. The mite feeds on cutaneous scale and debris without burrowing or puncturing the epidermis. Mite eggs are laid and subsequently develop in skin debris, completing the life cycle in 2 to 3 weeks. Mites and mite eggs can survive on debris within buildings, bedding, and on grooming equipment for extended periods, depending on temperature, humidity, and conditions of hygiene. Asymptomatic carriage of mites is common in sheep and cattle and may occur in horses. Mite populations and subsequently clinical signs appear to increase in the winter and decrease in the drier summer months.

Pathogenesis and Clinical Findings

Because pruritus can range from severe to nonexistent in chorioptic mange, it is presumed that, as with other mite infestations, hypersensitivity plays a role in the pathogenesis of lesions. Chorioptic mites have a predilection to infest the skin of the legs from below the carpus and the hock. Chronic lesions may spread to the ventral thorax and abdomen and occasionally extend up to the tail base. Initial lesions include erythema, papules, and crusts arising on the lower limbs. With time these may progress to more extensive crusting, ulceration,

lichenification, and secondary infection. A difficult-to-treat, chronic, pastern dermatitis may result. Draft breeds with feathered (long-haired) fetlocks seem especially suited to maintaining infestations and horses presenting with hereditary lymphedema are frequently affected. Foot stamping, biting at the lower limbs, and rubbing of the lower limbs are symptoms usually noted by the owner.

Diagnosis

Diagnosis, by demonstrating the mite in superficial skin scrapings taken from multiple sites, can be difficult. Recommended techniques for catching these fast-moving mites include (1) using clear cellophane tape to pick up mites and crusts from the skin surface (although mites can be difficult to remove or position for identification, and parasitologists find such preparations frustrating); (2) adding insecticide to the oil used for the scrapings; and (3) vigorous brushing into a pan of soapy water. With the third technique, allow the mixture to settle out in a deep, narrow container. Decant and then centrifuge the settled material for microscopic examination of the pellet, or process the settled material as for fecal flotation.[10,14] Field collections of crusts and debris can be placed in a blood sample tube for transportation to the laboratory for examination. In warmer weather the mites may only be obtained from scrapings of the coronary band.[10]

Therapy

Chorioptic mange can be difficult to treat because of its superficial location on the skin and mites' ability to survive in the environment. Oral ivermectin is effective at reducing mite populations but will not eliminate them.[15] Effective topical treatments include a series of three whole-body baths, 5 days apart, using 1% selenium sulfide shampoo, and two treatments, 2 to 3 weeks apart, with 0.25% fipronil spray.[16,17] Fipronil spray should be applied to all affected areas, including both the forelimbs and the hindlimbs from above the carpus and stifles, respectively, distally to the hoof and in sufficient quantity to dampen the hair and wet the skin. Other topical products that should be effective include 2% lime sulfur, organophosphate products, and synthetic pyrethroids. Ideally, the legs of heavily feathered animals should be clipped (owners often resist this for cosmetic reasons) and the legs thoroughly washed and skin debris removed before each parasiticidal application. Dips or washes may need to be repeated at 5- to 7-day intervals for 3 to 4 weeks. Care should be taken to apply these products to all areas vulnerable to infestation, including rear quarters, tail base, ventral abdomen and thorax, and even the head, if the horse is biting at or rubbing infected forelimbs with its head. One author suggests a combined approach using ivermectin systemically in combination with topical treatment.[18] A single dose of moxidectin gel at 0.4 mg/kg was reported to be effective when combined with environmental decontamination.[11] A key component to treatment is isolation of infested horses and treatment of the environment and fomites. All bedding should be removed from the stables, followed by thorough cleaning and treatment of premises with insecticide. If stalls or paddocks can be vacated for 3 or more weeks, there is less likelihood mites will survive in the environment. All bedding for infested horses should be replaced with fresh product daily, if possible, or on treatment days, at a minimum. Grooming and feeding equipment should be segregated, cleaned, and treated.

Prevention

Prevention of chorioptic mite infestation includes examination of newly introduced horses for clinical lesions, followed by scrapings and cytologic preparations of any suspect lesions such as crusted papules or scaling of coronary bands. Isolation from other horses for 2 to 3 weeks to observe for suggestive clinical

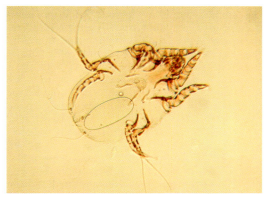

Figure 59-1 Female *Chorioptes bovis* mite. *(Courtesy Ellis Greiner.)*

signs is also helpful. Good stabling hygiene with frequent bedding changes and keeping horses in their own stalls help reduce spread. These procedures are most important in the management of breeds with heavy feathering of the lower limbs because these horses are most frequently infested.

Demodectic Mange

Etiology

Clinical demodectic mange in the horse is extremely rare. Two species, *Demodex caballi* (eyelids and muzzle) and *D. equi* (body), have been described in the horse. Disease caused by *D. caballi* has not been reported.

Epidemiology

Demodex mites are host specific and considered as normal fauna, and most animals harbor a few organisms without evidence of skin disease. They complete their life cycle within the pilosebaceous apparatus of the skin. It is thought that mites are transmitted shortly after birth by contact between the dam and foal.

Pathogenesis and Clinical Findings

Poor immune status, local changes in skin chemistry, and other unknown factors may allow mite proliferation and the development of clinical lesions. Lesions may take two forms: (1) patchy, nonpruritic alopecia and scaling of the head, neck, shoulders, and forelimbs, which may resolve spontaneously; or (2) a papulonodular form, with many mites found within follicular cysts.

Diagnosis

Microscopic examination of multiple deep skin scrapings or nodular contents should be sufficient to confirm diagnosis. Efforts should be made to detect underlying conditions that make the animal susceptible to demodectic mange. Systemic glucocorticoid treatment is the most frequently implicated cause.[10] However, endocrine diseases, other systemic diseases, nutritional factors, and immunosuppressed states should be considered.

Therapy

Some cases of demodectic mange in horses resolve spontaneously. Any underlying conditions that may weaken immune status or alter skin chemistry should be corrected if possible and this alone may result in resolution of lesions. Topical therapy to aid self-clearing includes benzoyl peroxide shampoos followed by application of 2% lime sulfur dip every 5 to 7 days and/or daily application of antibacterial ointment such as mupirocin or fusidic acid. If significant secondary bacterial dermatitis is present, a 3-week course of trimethoprim-sulfonamide or fluoroquinolone antibiotics is indicated. Most authors do not advocate attempts to treat equine demodicosis systemically. Amitraz is contraindicated in horses. Nodular lesions are refractory to treatments and may persist for years.

Trombiculid and Other Mite Infestations

Etiology

Mites inhabiting vegetation, vegetable matter, hay, straw, cereals and other stored foods, and bedding may cause dermatitis in animals contacting the infested environment or feed. These mites belong to the suborders Sarcoptiformes (Astigmata), Trombidiformes (Prostigmata), and Parasitiformes (Mesostigmata). Forage mites include mites in the genera *Acarus, Tyrophagus, , Glycyphagus, Pyemotes, Neoschoengastia, Euschoengastia, Caloglyphus, Lepidoglyphus, Cheyletus,* and *Suidasia.* Many species of larval *Trombiculidae* (harvest mites, red bugs, or chiggers) are capable of producing skin lesions and irritation in the horse. Genera represented include *Eutrombicula, Neotrombicula,* and *Leptotrombium.*

Epidemiology

Forage mites can induce dermatitis in either stabled animals or those on pasture at any time of the year, depending on their source. The source may be pasture, hay, bedding, or grain products. Trombiculid mites cause seasonal dermatitis in horses on pasture or those being housed or ridden in the natural environment. The larvae range from red to orange or yellow in color and are active in late summer and early autumn. In tropical areas, they may be present almost year-round. After feeding on lymph and disintegrated skin cells, they drop off the host and progress to free-living nymph and adult stages.

Pathogenesis and Clinical Findings

Lesions associated with these mite infestations may result from irritant, pharmacologic, or hypersensitivity reactions to the salivary secretions of the mite. Lesions caused by forage mite infestation arise in areas of primary contact: face and head for feeds and lower limbs or entire body for bedding products. Forage mite and trombiculid mite infestations contracted by horses at pasture most frequently involve the lower limbs, ventral and lateral trunk, face, and lips. Depending on the host response, a range of lesions may be observed, including a fine papulocrustous dermatitis; patches of erythema, exudation, and scaling; papular urticaria; or urticarial plaques. Pruritus may vary from absent to severe.

Diagnosis

In forage mite infestations, demonstration of the mite in the feed or the environment or from the lesions is diagnostic. One author suggests that using a flea comb is more successful than skin scrapings for finding forage mites on the skin.[10] More frequently, the mites will be found in the feed or bedding rather than on the animal. The collected material can be placed into Berlese funnels and left overnight to facilitate collection of insects and arthropods. This method was effective for retrieving *Pyemotes tritici* from hay samples in one outbreak of forage mite–induced dermatitis in horses.[19] In early cases of trombiculid infestations, it may be relatively easy to find the distinctly colored larvae attached in the center of a typical papule. Skin scrapings of lesions may dislodge enough mites for diagnosis. Later, the mites may have already detached, and the diagnosis must be based on seasonality, contact with an infested environment, and response to treatment.

Therapy

Animals infested with forage or trombiculid mites at pasture should be removed immediately from the infested environment. Although forage mites may have dropped off already, topical insecticides should be applied to kill remaining mites. Relief from pruritus may be required, using topical steroids or a brief course of short-acting systemic corticosteroids. It may require up to 8 weeks before the trombiculid mite season is finished. During this time, further contact with the infested environment should be avoided. Because infestation is likely to recur from year to year, infested pastures should be vacated at the same time in following years. Forage mite populations in the environment fluctuate significantly year to year and cannot be reliably predicted; however, it is usually safe to return animals to the same fields after 8 weeks. Forage mites are capable of massive proliferation in stored feeds and bedding when humidity and temperature are favorable. These increases in number often may be confined to one small portion of the stored product. Infested materials must be completely removed and replaced by product from a different source.

Public Health Considerations

Humans are also susceptible to forage and trombiculid mite infestations and may have lesions in areas of contact with infested vegetation or feed products at the same time animals are affected.

Pediculosis

Etiology

Horses and other *Equidae* are hosts for two species of lice: the sucking louse, *Haematopinus asini*, and the biting louse, *Bovicola (Werneckiella, Damalinia) equi* (Fig. 59-2), which is more common.

Epidemiology

Lice are host specific and survive for just a few days off the host, even under optimal conditions of high humidity and cool temperatures. The life cycle is completed on the host. Female lice produce eggs that are cemented firmly onto hair shafts. After hatching, nymphs undergo three molts, reaching maturity in 3 weeks. In temperate climates, louse activity is greatest during the autumn, winter, and early spring, coinciding with increased crowding of animals (facilitating transmission), reduced use of topical insecticides, and ideal living conditions in the horse's dense winter coat. Transmission is by direct contact with the infested animals or fomites such as brushes that contain nymphs, adults, or hair with viable louse eggs attached. Crowded, unsanitary conditions promote transmission. The sucking louse, *H. asini*, literally sucks blood from superficial vessels through a hollow tube, or stylet. Preferred feeding areas are the mane, tail, and fetlocks. Survival time off-host is shorter than that for biting lice. The biting louse, *B. equi*, feeds on superficial skin debris, hair, and secretions, using the mandibles to bite and scrape. Although preferring areas on the trunk, especially the neck, flanks, and tail base, biting lice may be found in the mane and tail as well. No known equine pathogens are transmitted by lice.

Clinical Findings

The main clinical sign of louse infestation is pruritus, manifested by biting at the flanks, kicking and stamping, restlessness and irritability, and rubbing against objects. This results in an unkempt appearance, alopecia, scaling, abrasion, and even secondary infection, if pruritus is severe. Rarely, louse infestation may be severe enough to result in poor condition or debility.

Diagnosis

Louse infestation is common in the horse and should always be a differential diagnosis for pruritus. Demonstration of fast-moving, biting lice can be difficult when numbers are low. Nits, cemented to the hair shafts, are more easily found. Under good lighting, a careful search by parting the hair coat in many places, is necessary to find adults and identify hairs bearing nits. In addition, a stiff brush may be used to collect lice by brushing hair downward, collecting hair and debris into a pan held close beneath. Lice may be observed moving among the collected debris.[14]

Therapy

Louse infestation is usually treated with applications of insecticidal shampoos, sprays, or dips applied at 10- to 14-day intervals for at least 3 to 4 weeks to eliminate newly hatching nits. Pyrethrins or synthetic pyrethroids are most often used, but organophosphate compounds and 1% selenium sulfide shampoo (left on 5-10 minutes, once lathered) are also effective.[20] Recently, imidacloprid 10% for dogs was shown to be effective for treating horses for lice. It was dosed at 1.9 mg/kg topically and repeated at 4 weeks.[21] Triflumuron, a benzoyl(phenyl)urea derivative was shown to be safe and effective in a controlled study for eliminating biting lice infestation in horses. It was applied topically on the dorsal midline at a dose of 2.5 mg/kg using a 25 mg/mL solution.[22] An observational study suggested that neem seed extract (Mite-Stop) diluted 1:20 with water and applied twice at a 7-day interval was effective in providing a clinical cure but parasitologic assessments were not performed.[23] Although not always completely effective for treating biting lice infestations, sucking lice are susceptible to oral ivermectin, 200 µg/kg, two doses administered 2 weeks apart. Tack, blankets, grooming equipment, and even the environment may harbor infective hairs. Such items should be cleaned and treated with insecticides. Particularly valuable items that may not withstand harsh treatments might be salvaged by thorough cleaning followed by placement in a sealed garbage bag and storage in a warm, preferably sunny, place for 3 to 4 weeks, allowing time for any nits present to hatch and die before the equipment is used again. All infested and in-contact horses should be treated.

Prevention

Newly acquired animals should be inspected carefully for louse infestation, treated with appropriate insecticidal products, and held in quarantine until they are ascertained to be disease free before commingling with other horses.

Biting Flies

One of the most common pests of horses and other animals, biting flies are numerous in species and found throughout the world. Lesions resulting from the bites of tabanids (*Tabanus* spp., *Haematopota* spp., and *Chrysops* spp.), stable flies (*Stomoxys calcitrans*), and black flies (*Simulium* spp.) are crusted papules that fade within a few days. Mosquito bites result in papules without crusts and also fade in a few hours to days. Hypersensitivity reactions ranging from urticaria to eosinophilic (collagenolytic) granulomas or pruritic dermatoses have been associated with the bites of these insects.[24] "Fly worry," characterized by incessant hoof stamping, tail switching, bunching, and running, can result from large numbers of biting insects. This section discusses the major types of dipterans that harass

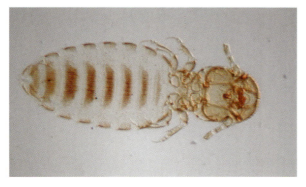

Figure 59-2 *Bovicola equi. (Courtesy Ellis C. Greiner.)*

horses, with reference to epidemiology, specific clinical syndromes, and control measures.

Tabanids

Epidemiology

Tabanid flies (*Tabanus*, *Chrysops*, and *Hybomitra* spp.), commonly known as horseflies and deerflies, serve as mechanical vectors of several livestock diseases, including *Microsporum gypseum* (see Chapter 50), equine infectious anemia (see Chapter 23), and *Trypanosoma evansi* (see Chapter 60; the causative agent of surra). These flies are mostly daytime feeders with painful bites, and they cause considerable annoyance to many species of large animals. They are not host specific, feeding on many animals and humans, although, interestingly, tabanids have been shown to preferentially feed on darker colored horses because of their attraction to the light polarizing properties of the darker coats.[25] The breeding grounds for these pests are aquatic and semiaquatic habitats, including mud and wet vegetation near bodies of water. Terrestrial species lay eggs on vegetation or in forest litter.

Therapy and Prevention

Control of tabanid flies is difficult and frequent applications of insecticides and repellents provide only short-term protection. Vegetation barriers more than 2 meters (6½ feet) in height may deter flies from entering pastures.[26] Avoiding forested pastures and daytime stabling can help reduce tabanid access to animals. Anecdotally, horse farms in Florida have relocated because of intractable tabanid activity.[14] Excessive nighttime lighting may extend tabanid feeding into the nighttime hours as well.

Stable Flies

Epidemiology

Another daytime feeder, the stable fly *(Stomoxys calcitrans)*, feeds mostly on the lower limbs, ventrum, chest, and back. A pattern of three or four bites grouped or in a chain suggests stable flies.[27] The bite is painful, and feeding is not host specific. They can cause considerable annoyance to humans. Stable flies have been implicated in the transmission of dermatophilosis (see Chapter 30) and dermatophytosis (see Chapter 50).[26] Additionally, they are a primary transmitter of the stomach worm *(Habronema microstoma)*. Stable flies breed in decaying vegetable matter, bedding, and feces, where the stomach worm larvae is ingested by the larval fly. Stomach worm larvae are deposited on the skin when the adult stable fly bites the horse. To continue the life cycle, the *Habronema* larvae must be ingested as the horse bites at the flies or at the itchy papules that result from the fly bite. These larvae also may be deposited at mucocutaneous junctions or in superficial wounds, where they migrate into the tissues, and in sensitized horses, incite the hypersensitivity reaction, resulting in proliferative lesions of cutaneous habronemiasis. Only 12 days, but usually 15 to 30 days, are required to complete maturation from egg to adult stable fly.[28] Breeding season is year-round in the tropics and the subtropics, whereas immature forms are suspected to overwinter in northern climates.

Therapy and Prevention

Control of stable flies is best accomplished by eliminating breeding grounds. Strict attention to proper removal and disposal of manure and decaying vegetation is essential. Composted manure needs to be kept hot for effective killing of eggs and larvae. Manure piles that are too large to turn regularly may be covered with weighted, black, plastic sheets to keep them hot. To prevent breeding in manure in pastures and paddocks,

breaking up and scattering of the piles should be done every 1 to 2 weeks. Topical insecticides applied to the animal are not highly effective because the stable fly spends very little time on the host, and efficacy of repellents is short lived.[28] Insecticides applied to favorite resting places of the flies (sunny walls, tree foliage), insecticide misters, and fly traps may help. Screening to exclude flies can be effective, and daytime stabling may be useful. Genes for permethrin resistance are present in stable fly populations in Florida.[29] Catnip oil and its constituent molecules are currently being studied in cattle for preventing stable fly bites and oviposition.[30]

Horn Flies

Epidemiology

Horn flies *(Haematobia irritans)* are primary pests of cattle, bison, and water buffalo but will feed on other large animals housed in proximity to these species. Infection with *Corynebacterium pseudotuberculosis*, the cause of ulcerative lymphangitis, subcutaneous abscesses, and folliculitis, is thought to be spread by biting flies, especially horn flies[28] (see Chapter 45). The eggs develop in the fresh feces of the bovine species and not in feces of other large mammals. Maturation from egg to adult may take only 9 days.[28] Adults feed on the dorsal back withers, shoulders, flank, and neck, often facing downward, or on the ventral midline of horses.

Clinical Findings

Horn flies are a common cause of ventral midline dermatitis, which often occurs in horses kept in proximity to cattle. This dermatitis is characterized by focal to multifocal areas of alopecia, crusting, depigmentation, and ulceration, usually starting at or involving the umbilical area. Because this is not considered a hypersensitivity disease, most horses on the premises will be affected. Treatment of the lesions involves cleansing and using topical antibacterial products with or without corticosteroids.

Therapy and Prevention

Control of the problem requires daily application of topical insecticides and repellents. In some areas, horn flies have developed genetic resistant to pyrethroid or organophosphate insecticides, and alternative products may be required.[31,32] For best results, appropriate horn fly control measures (sanitation, insecticide applications) applied to cattle housed in proximity to horses are recommended to reduce numbers of flies.

Black Flies

Epidemiology and Public Health Considerations

Running water is required for black fly (*Simulium* spp.) egg deposition and larval/pupal development. More than 1000 species, with differing abilities to overwinter and survive drought, are found worldwide. Equine encephalitis viruses have been found in black flies, but transmission has not yet been demonstrated. Adult flies are active in the late spring and early summer and can travel many miles from their breeding grounds. These flies inflict painful bites around the face, ears, neck, ventrum, and legs. Evidence suggests that some species of black fly are natural transmitters of vesicular stomatitis virus (see Chapter 24) and possibly other viruses.

Black flies have significant public health importance in transmitting human pathogens, causing considerable annoyance, and inducing "black fly fever," a flulike syndrome in persons with multiple bites.[33]

Clinical Findings

A crusting dermatitis on the concave surface of the ear pinnae is often attributed to bites of black flies. Also found on the concave surface of the pinna, aural plaques or aural flat warts (raised, depigmented, wartlike lesions) are likely to be caused by infection with papillomavirus, for which the black fly is the suspected vector (see Chapter 25).[34] Simulio-toxicosis is a syndrome resulting from massive attacks of black flies, which occur most often in large river basins, especially after breeding grounds are expanded by flooding.[33] Cardiotoxic or allergenic components in the saliva trigger cardiopulmonary dysfunction, possibly resulting in death of the animal. Alternatively, animals may die of blood loss from massive attacks.

Therapy and Prevention

Because black flies generally do not enter enclosed spaces, provision of shelters for animals is important. Application of permethrin insecticides to the affected horses may offer some protection. White petroleum jelly applied to the insides of horses' ears may reduce black fly feeding in that location. In some regions, environmental control of black flies has been attempted by governmental agencies.[33]

Mosquitoes

Epidemiology and Public Health Considerations

The most important species of mosquito in equine medicine are included in the genera *Culex*, *Aedes*, and *Anopheles*. Mosquitoes breed in standing water almost anywhere. Depending on the species, a film of water on leaf litter, maintained for the duration of larval and pupal periods, is sufficient.[35] They feed predominantly around dusk and dawn and continue at lower levels throughout the night. Daytime feeding may be a problem in heavily shaded, damp areas. They serve as vectors of several viruses causing equine encephalitis, including Venezuelan equine encephalitis (VEE), eastern equine encephalitis (EEE), and western equine encephalitis (WEE) (see Chapter 20), and Japanese encephalitis (JE) and West Nile virus (WNV) (see Chapter 21). Mosquitoes are unlikely to transmit equine infectious anemia virus because large amounts of blood are usually necessary for efficient transmission (see Chapter 23). In addition to their role as disease vectors, mosquitoes can cause considerable annoyance when their numbers are high, and rarely, potentially fatal anemia may result. They have been implicated in some cases of equine insect hypersensitivity.

The public health significance of mosquitoes is great because they transmit several human pathogens, including some of the same encephalitis viruses that infect horses.

Therapy and Prevention

Because the larvae develop in standing water, drainage or treatment of standing water is essential to mosquito control. If such areas cannot be eliminated, treatments to kill larvae in the water include (1) *Bacillus thuringiensis israelensis*, (2) light mineral oils, (3) organophosphate insecticides, (4) insect growth regulators such as methoprene, and (5) mosquito fish *(Gambusia)* that feed on mosquito larvae.[35,36] Environmental offices of the local government should be contacted for advice. Because of their limited duration of efficacy, repellents or insecticides should be applied to affected horses twice daily. Stabling at night in screened stalls and use of fly sheets will limit mosquito access. Propane-powered mosquito traps that produce carbon dioxide (CO_2) may be useful in limited areas of 1 acre or less.[10] Secondary attractants, such as octenol or R-octenol, are available to enhance the ability of these traps to attract no-see-ums, mosquitoes, and black flies.

Biting Midges

Epidemiology and Public Health Considerations

Species in the genera *Culicoides* and *Leptoconops* are tiny flies also known as "midges," "no-see-ums," "punkies," "sandflies" (erroneously), and other names, depending on geographic location. Despite its diminutive size, this insect inflicts a painful bite by lacerating the skin and capillaries with its mandibles. In most geographic locations, *Culicoides* spp. feed primarily at dusk and dawn, less so during the night, and sometimes during the day. However, *Leptoconops* spp., which breed in sandy or arid, alkaline soils (deserts, beaches, tidal marshes), may be active during the day as well as dusk and dawn. Most midges breed in areas of moist, muddy ground around ponds, marshes, ditches and tidal flats, standing water in tree holes, in decaying vegetation, in rotting wood, and in manure. Because they are weak fliers, windless conditions with temperatures above 10° C (50° F) are ideal for their activity, but some species tolerate cooler temperatures and winds up to 18 kph (11 mph) or higher.[37] Females of many species are able to travel an average of 2 km (1.2 miles) from their breeding grounds.[37] Midges transmit the virus causing African horse sickness (see Chapter 16), the filarial worms *Onchocerca cervicalis* and *O. reticulata* (see Chapter 57), and other important diseases in other animal species.

In addition to annoyance from being bitten, humans may develop hypersensitivity to the bites, and several human pathogens are transmitted by midges.

Clinical Findings and Diagnosis

Biting midges are the most common cause of equine insect hypersensitivity, also known as "sweet itch," "kasen," "Queensland itch," "muck itch," "dhobie itch," and "Sommerekzem." Types I and IV hypersensitivity reactions to multiple salivary antigens are implicated in the pathogenesis, and a genetic predisposition has been shown in several breeds.[38-40] It is not unusual to see the condition in related horses. Affected animals should be removed from breeding programs. In vitro immunologic studies have shown the presence of circulating immunoglobulin E (IgE) antibodies reacting to salivary antigens and that peripheral blood mononuclear cells from affected Icelandic horses have reduced T regulatory FOXP3 expression when exposed to *Culicoides* allergen as compared to cells from unaffected horses.[41,42]

Clinical signs arise between 1 and 4 years of age or 1 to 4 years after first exposure to the insects. In temperate climates, a seasonal onset is characteristic, occurring in the summer and early autumn. Horses in tropical and subtropical locations may be exposed for 9 or 10 months of the year, possibly from successive species emerging throughout the season.[43] During the first season, the condition tends to be mild, worsening each year as long as exposure to the insects continues. Pruritus is the major symptom, resulting in self-inflicted lesions. Classically, the head, ears (Fig. 59-3), mane, withers (Fig. 59-4), rump, and tail (Fig. 59-5) are affected. However, some species of *Culicoides* feed in other areas on the animal, resulting in lesions with a different distribution. A ventrally distributed form, described in the southeastern United States, involves the head and ears, the intermandibular space, chest (Fig. 59-6), upper forelegs, ventral abdomen, inguinal region, and usually the tail.[44] Rubbing and self-trauma result in alopecia, lichenification, crusting, erosions, ulcerations, and eventual wrinkling or corrugation of the skin. Secondary infections of the traumatized skin often follow.

Tentative diagnosis should be possible based on history and clinical signs. Response to appropriate insect control measures is diagnostic. Intradermal skin testing can be a useful method for confirming the clinical diagnosis. Biopsy findings of

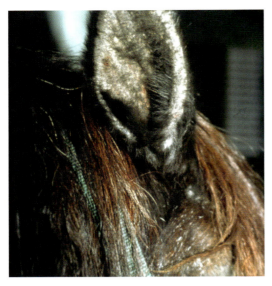

Figure 59-3 Alopecia, lichenification, and crusting of pinna typical of that seen in chronic *Culicoides* hypersensitivity. *(Courtesy Gail Kunkle.)*

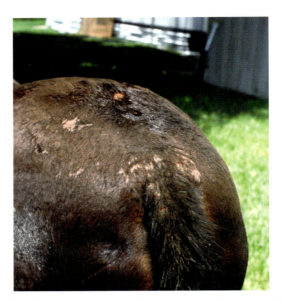

Figure 59-5 Alopecia, ulcerations, and crusts on rump with severe hair breakage and alopecia of base of tail in horse with *Culicoides* hypersensitivity.

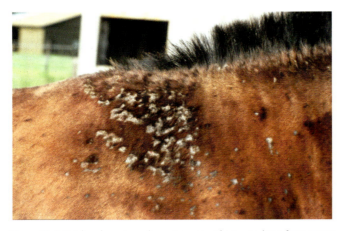

Figure 59-4 Patchy alopecia and crusting on withers, resulting from severe pruritus seen in *Culicoides* hypersensitivity.

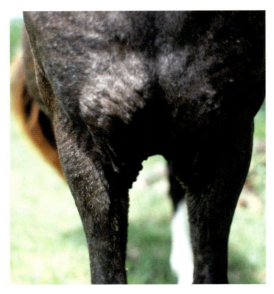

Figure 59-6 Chronic lesions of lichenification and alopecia on chest of pony with *Culicoides* hypersensitivity.

perivascular cuffs of mononuclear cells and eosinophils suggest allergic dermatitis but are not diagnostic for an etiologic agent because similar results can be seen with many ectoparasitic conditions.[24] The parasitic manges, louse infestation, other causes of allergies, and cutaneous onchocerciasis should be ruled out.

Therapy and Prevention

The only effective treatment is to prevent further exposure to the insects. Housing in insect-proof stables from late afternoon until well after dawn and daily to twice-daily application of insect repellents containing at least 2% permethrin are the minimum efforts required. Nightly stabling of affected animals should begin before the onset of the insect season and continue until the insects subside in the fall. In the author's experience, one night's exposure during the insect season can result in itching that may last as long as 2 to 4 weeks. Additionally, fine-mesh screening (32 × 32 or 2 mm × 2 mm) or netting, ceiling fans or strategically placed box fans, and automated insecticide misters may aid in situations where the stables cannot be fully

enclosed or midge populations are particularly overwhelming. Screening can be treated with insecticide to kill midges trying to pass through. Fly sheets and insect masks may be of some use if started early in the season before the horse starts to itch. After pruritus has ensued, such items will not remain on the horse for long. In selected situations where exposure is not overwhelming, CO_2 traps stationed near barn or stable areas may attract insects away from animals housed inside. One author suggests adding octenol strips to the traps to make them more attractive to midges and mosquitoes.[10] The source of these insects is usually nearby; however, because some species are able to travel more than 2 km from breeding grounds, distant sources may not be immediately obvious. Drainage of ponds, ditches, marshes, or other wet areas in the horse's immediate surroundings reduces breeding grounds, but environmental regulations may prohibit such efforts. Transfer of affected animals to higher, drier, open, and breezy pastures or to drier geographic locations often results in complete or near-complete resolution of signs.

Immediate relief from pruritus is achieved using systemic glucocorticoids. Initial doses of prednisolone required to control severe itch may be as high as 1.5 mg/kg daily, tapering to the lowest possible dose on alternating days. If insect exposure is not controlled, it is usually difficult to reduce this induction dose significantly without relapse. Should prednisolone be ineffective, oral dexamethasone, starting at 0.02 to 0.1 mg/kg every 48 hours (q48h), tapering the dose after the first week of treatment, may provide better results.[45] Additional relief of pruritus can be achieved by treating secondary bacterial infections using appropriate systemic antibiotics and weekly topical therapy with antibacterial (benzoyl peroxide or ethyl lactate) or antiseborrheic (tar and sulfur, sulfur and salicylic acid) shampoos and rinses (2% lime sulfur).

One controlled study of immunotherapy (hyposensitization) using whole-body extracts of these midges was unsuccessful.[46] In an uncontrolled study using a *Culicoides* extract with adjuvant, reduced clinical signs were reported in 9 of 10 horses.[47] Some authors report better success with immunotherapy in horses that have pollen allergies concurrent with their insect allergies, questioning the clinical relevance of positive reactions to the *Culicoides* allergen in such horses.[45,48] As possible explanations, successful immunotherapy to the relevant pollen allergens may raise the pruritic threshold in the affected horses to a level such that the insect allergy is not clinically manifested, or some positive insect allergen reactions may not be clinically relevant in some horses and may reflect insect exposure. Adjunctive treatments used by some authors include antihistamines (hydroxyzine 400 mg orally twice daily) and fatty acid supplements.[45,49,50] Results with fatty acid supplements have been inconsistent.

Nonbiting Flies

Flies in the genera *Musca* and *Hydrotaea* deposit eggs in fecal material, garbage, and decomposing organic matter. They feed on moist secretions in wounds or near mucocutaneous junctions. The housefly *(Musca domestica)*, the bush fly *(M. vetustissima)*, and the bazaar fly *(M. sorbens)* serve as developmental hosts for the horse stomach worms, *Habronema muscae* and *Draschia megastoma*, the larvae of which may induce the hypersensitivity syndrome of cutaneous habronemiasis in susceptible horses (see Chapter 57). Rarely, myiasis can result from oviposition in wounds.[51] The face fly is a developmental host for *Thelazia lacrimalis*, which is the eyeworm of horses (see Chapter 10). Similar to stable flies, removal and appropriate disposal of garbage, dung, and other decomposing organic material is essential to control fly populations. Topical insecticides and repellents reduce feeding on the animal. Good wound care and bandaging prevents secondary myiasis and cutaneous habronemiasis. Because the flies alight on sunny walls to rest, insecticidal applications to such areas are helpful. As mechanical transmitters of enteric infections in humans, these flies represent a significant public health problem.

Wound Myiasis

Etiology and Epidemiology

In obligatory myiasis, a reportable disease, the infestation of living host tissues is required for completion of the fly life cycle.[51] Species involved are the New World and the Old World screwworms of the genera *Cochliomyia* and *Chrysomyia*, respectively. Screwworm infestation of healthy tissue of wounds, fly bite lesions and dermatitis, ulcerated masses, and mucocutaneous junctions occurs in the Americas (primarily Central and South America), Africa, and Asia. The adult fly deposits eggs in the exudative lesions or moist areas. When the larvae hatch, they burrow into the healthy subcutaneous tissue, causing liquefaction and enlargement of the lesion. After 3 to 6 days, they drop out to pupate.

Myiasis caused by blowflies and fleshflies is facultative (not requiring a living host).[51] It is uncommon in horses. Genera involved are *Lucilia*, *Calliphora*, *Phormia*, *Chrysomyia*, and *Sarcophagus*. These flies lay their eggs in decomposing tissue of wounds, macerated skin lesions, and areas of fecal soiling or accumulation, as well as in carcasses of dead animals. Larvae feed on the decomposing matter and secrete enzymes that cause wound enlargement.

Accidental myiasis, a rare finding, occurs when species of the family *Muscidae* deposit eggs in decomposing tissue of wounds while feeding on exudates.[51] It is termed "accidental" because living or decaying tissues are not the normal breeding ground for these flies.

Clinical Findings

Lesions of myiasis are painful and malodorous with exudation. Exploration of the wound under sedation will reveal maggots within the necrotic tissue. Larger lesions may result in septicemia resulting from secondary bacterial infection. If untreated, screwworm myiasis almost always results in the death of the host.

Diagnosis

Diagnosis is by larval identification. If screwworm is suspected, larvae should be dropped into boiling water for 30 to 60 seconds and then preserved in 70% alcohol for official identification.[14] Appropriate authorities should be notified. In cases where tumors or granulomas are secondarily invaded, biopsy to determine the actual etiology is recommended. For best results, this should be done in an unaffected area of the mass or after the infestation and infection has been cleared.

Therapy and Prevention

Treatment includes removal of maggots, debridement and cleansing of lesions, application of topical insecticides, and administration of systemic antibiotics and other supportive therapy if septicemia is present. Avoiding surgical procedures during the fly season, prompt wound care with bandaging and application of thick topical insecticidal preparations, and keeping skin and hair free of manure deposits and soiling will prevent myiasis.

Widespread control of screwworms using sterile-male release programs and complementary insecticidal pelleted baits that attract female flies have been very successful in eliminating the problem in North America and much of Central America.[51] Similar attempts to control *L. cuprina*, an Australian blowfly, have met with some success.[51] Control of other blowflies can be aided by deep burial or cremation of carcasses and placental materials. Good sanitation practices, such as composting or spreading manure and other decaying vegetable matter and strategic use of insecticides on premises and animals, will help control flies causing accidental myiasis.

Public Health Considerations

Humans are susceptible to wound myiasis, especially those who are very young, very old, infirm, or working in or near livestock operations. Prompt and appropriate wound care and good fly control practices should minimize the risk. Blowfly maggots, particularly *P. sericata*, have been used clinically in humans to clean wounds and promote formation of granulation tissue.[51]

Hypodermiasis (Warbles)

Etiology

Warbles are caused by the larval stages of the heel flies *Hypoderma bovis* and *H. lineatum*. These are primary parasites of ruminants, and horses, a dead-end host, are only sporadically affected.

Epidemiology

Warbles flies are similar in appearance to bumblebees and fasten their eggs to hairs on the legs and ventrum. After a few days, the larvae hatch and burrow through the skin, migrating through the body via the connective tissues. *Hypoderma lineatum* migrates through the submucosa of the esophagus, and *H. bovis* migrates in the epidural fat of the spinal canal. In the spring the larvae migrate to the subcutaneous tissues of the dorsal back, where they cut an air hole and become stationary, forming a nodule. After about 2 months, they emerge through the hole and fall to the ground to pupate. The larvae fail to develop normally in the horse and are unable to complete their life cycle. Horses housed near infested cattle are at the greatest risk of developing these nodules.

Clinical Findings and Diagnosis

Although cattle can have large numbers of nodules, the horse, as an aberrant host, seldom has more than one or two nodules, usually located on the dorsal back or withers. Warbles are easily distinguished from other nodules (dermoid cysts, eosinophilic granulomas, neoplasms) by the presence of the breathing pore. Identification of the larvae removed from the cyst is confirmatory.

Therapy

The best treatment for horses is careful surgical removal of the intact larva. Care must be taken to avoid crushing the larva during surgery because leakage of its internal contents can cause an anaphylactic reaction in the host.

Prevention

Control of the warble in the primary host is important. Avermectins are effective larvicides for the control of warbles in cattle, and their use in horses for regular intestinal parasite control probably prevents many cases from developing. Before the availability of avermectins, organophosphate insecticides were used to control cattle warbles. Preventing adult flies from laying eggs on animals requires use of topical insecticides and repellents.

Miscellaneous Flies

The horse botfly (*Gasterophilus* spp.) may cause restlessness and stamping as the flies hover and lay eggs on the hair of the horse's lower limbs and head. *Dermatobia hominis*, the human botfly, may infest horses in Central and South America. The resulting nodules have breathing pores, similar to warbles.[35] Louse flies of the genus *Hippobosca* are reported in Europe, North Africa, Western Asia, and South America. Preferring perineal and inguinal regions, these flies have painful bites, causing considerable annoyance. They may be vectors of equine babesiosis, Q fever, and other rickettsial organisms.[52] In Africa, multiple species of tsetse flies *(Glossina)* bite horses, other domestic livestock, and many wild animals. They transmit nagana to livestock and horses; nagana is a chronic disease of anemia and weakness caused by protozoans in the genus *Trypanosoma*. The method of choice for control of tsetse flies is using traps baited with attractants.[53] Occasional reports of *Leishmania* in horses suggest that some species of sandflies (*Phlebotomus* and *Lutzomyia*) feed on horses, as well as humans and other animals.[54,55]

Accidental Ectoparasites

Horses can be affected by *Dermanyssus gallinae*, a mite of poultry, if housed close to poultry. Clinical signs include nocturnal pruritus, papules, erythema, and crusts on the feet and legs.[27] One author reported finding poultry lice on horses.[56] Rarely, cat fleas (*Ctenocephalides felis*) and poultry fleas or "stick-tights" *(Echidnophaga gallinacea)* have been reported on horses.[57,58] Control measures are similar to those for pets and poultry, respectively. In addition, the source of fleas, pets or poultry, should be treated.

Ants, Bees, and Spiders

In the southern United States, fire ants (*Solenopsis* spp.) are common. Horses tend to be stung by these insects on the legs, nose, or ventrum. Lesions are painful and rapidly develop a pustule, followed by crusting. Severe exposure may occur if the animal rolls on an anthill. Anaphylaxis may result, and sloughing of the epidermis may occur in the severely stung skin.[59] Bee and wasp stings result in edematous wheals or plaques at the sites of envenomation. If there has been previous sensitizing exposure, angioedema or anaphylaxis can result from stings. Spider bites, depending on the spider species involved, result in hot, painful, edematous lesions at the site of the bite, vesicular lesions, or necrotic lesions. Some spider bites progress from acute edematous lesions to necrosis and sloughing.[60] In cases of fire ant, bee, wasp, or spider envenomation, unless witnessed, it is difficult to tell after the fact which species is responsible for the lesions unless good circumstantial evidence implicates a certain species. Treatment is symptomatic and palliative.

The complete reference list is available online at www.expertconsult.com.

60 Miscellaneous Parasitic Diseases

Heather Stockdale Walden, Sally Anne L. Ness, Linda D. Mittel, Thomas J. Divers, Karl van Laaren, and Debra C. Sellon*

Trypanosomiasis

The trypanosomes are spindle-shaped protozoal parasites, most of which propel themselves with a flagellum and undulating membrane. Infection of horses with *Trypanosoma equiperdum*, *Trypanosoma evansi*, and *Trypanosoma brucei brucei* has traditionally been associated with the diseases dourine, surra, and African animal trypanosomiasis (AAT), respectively. These species make up the subgenus *Trypanozoon* (Protozoa: Sarcomastigophora: Kinetoplastida: *Trypanosomatidae*).[1] Differentiation of the parasite species in this subgenus on a morphologic, serologic, and molecular basis is unclear, and recent reports suggest that current species designations may ultimately prove to be incorrect.[1-5]

The other trypanosomes that infect horses, *T. congolense* (subgenus *Nannomonas*) and *T. vivax* (subgenus *Duttonella*), with *T. brucei brucei*, are etiologic agents of AAT. Because of the considerable confusion in nomenclature for specific trypanosomes that infect horses and the considerable overlap in clinical disease that may result from infection with these parasites, this chapter discusses the trypanosomal infections of horses as clinical syndromes (dourine, surra, and AAT) rather than individual etiologic agents.

Dourine

Etiology

Dourine is a chronic trypanosomal disease of horses that is transmitted predominantly by coitus and is characterized by genital edema, neurologic dysfunction, and death. A disease similar to dourine was described in early Arab texts[4]; the first mention of this disease in European literature was in 1796.[6] In 1894, Rouget[7] isolated *T. equiperdum* from the blood of an Algerian horse. Disease was later reproduced by subcutaneous inoculation of a horse with another isolate of the parasite, and the name *Trypanosoma equiperdum* was proposed by Doflein in 1901.[8-10]

Epidemiology and Pathogenesis

Historically, dourine has been present in Europe, North America, Asia, and Africa.[4] After World War I, the disease was eradicated from Western Europe by serologic screening, strict sanitation, and treatment of some horses with trypanosides.[4] Currently, dourine is considered a reportable disease by the World Organization for Animal Health (OIE) and is present in most of Asia, southeastern Europe, South America, and Africa. Dourine has been reported recently in Kyrgyzstan, Botswana, Lesotho, Namibia, and South Africa.[2]

Equids are considered the only natural host for *T. equiperdum*. Clinical signs are less obvious in donkeys than in horses, and these animals may be a reservoir for infection.[2] Disease is

not observed in zebras, although they may be seropositive by complement fixation test (CFT).[2] A variety of animal species, including dogs and rabbits, may show clinical signs of disease after experimental infection with *T. equiperdum*. The organism is present in the urethra of infected stallions and in vaginal discharges of infected mares. Transmission in horses primarily occurs by coitus, although mechanical transmission by arthropod vectors is also possible.[11,12] *T. equiperdum* can pass through intact mucous membranes. Transmission is considered most likely during the early stages of disease. The incubation period between exposure and initial clinical signs is highly variable; it may be as short as 1 to 2 weeks or as long as several years.[11]

Foals born to mares infected with *T. equiperdum* may be infected in utero or may become infected during parturition. Transmission to foals by ingestion of infected colostrum or milk is considered rare. Foals that ingest colostrum from infected mares will become seropositive due to passive transfer of antibodies; these foals are usually seronegative by 4 to 7 months of age.

Clinical Findings

In endemic regions, clinical signs of dourine are milder in native equids than in recently introduced breeds. The strain prevalent in southern Africa may be less virulent than the European, Asian, or North African strains, producing a very chronic, insidious disease with a long incubation period. Clinical signs may be precipitated by stress.[13] The observations of geographic differences in disease severity are supported by a recent report of genetic differences between African *T. equiperdum* isolates and isolates from China and South America.[1]

The first signs of dourine in mares are vaginal discharge, with edema of the vulva, perineum, mammary gland, and ventral abdomen. Some mares exhibit signs of vulvitis and vaginitis with polyuria or other signs of perineal discomfort. Abortion may occur if mares are infected with virulent strains. In stallions, initial clinical signs include edema of the external genitalia and perineum. Paraphimosis may occur.[13] Cutaneous plaques, when they occur, are considered pathognomonic for dourine ("silver dollar plaques"); however, these plaques do not occur with all strains of the parasite.[4] Conjunctivitis and keratitis may occur in some infected horses. Chronically infected horses develop signs of neurologic dysfunction with progressive weakness and ataxia, leading ultimately to recumbency and death. These horses usually exhibit wasting despite a good appetite and frequently have anemia. Clinical signs may wax and wane for many months or years before death, depending on the strain of infecting parasite and the host immune response.[13]

Diagnosis

In endemic regions, the diagnosis of dourine is usually made on the basis of characteristic clinical signs. Serum, whole blood in ethylenediaminetetraacetic acid (EDTA) and blood smears from affected horses may be submitted for identification of the parasite (Fig. 60-1); however, these attempts are not often

*The authors acknowledge and appreciate the original contributions of these authors, whose work has been incorporated into this chapter.

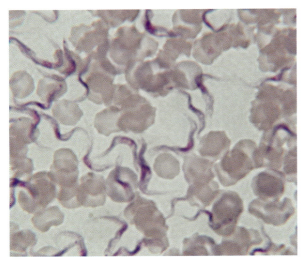

Figure 60-1 *Trypanosoma equiperdum* in blood smear from infected mouse. *(Courtesy Dr. Ellis Greiner.)*

successful. The OIE-prescribed test for diagnosis of dourine is the CFT; this test does not distinguish between infection with *T. equiperdum* and infection with the closely related *T. evansi*, *T. gambiense*, or *T. brucei*.[14,15] Despite this cross-reactivity, the CFT has been used effectively for the eradication of dourine in many countries, including Canada,[16] Ethiopia,[17] Italy,[12] Morocco,[18] South Africa,[11,19] and Russia.[20-22] An experimental chemiluminescent immunoblotting assay (cIB) was recently developed which is based on antigenic patterns recognized by immunoglobulin G (IgG) of infected horses, without cross-reacting with IgM. The cIB assay could be used as a complementary test to verify infection.[23] Alternative serologic tests include indirect fluorescent antibody (IFA), card agglutination, agar-gel immunodiffusion (AGID), arrayed immunodiffusion, and enzyme-linked immunosorbent assays (ELISA).[19,24-26]

Therapy

In most situations, treatment of horses with dourine is not recommended because it may result in an inapparent carrier state.[13] There are reports of treatment of affected horses with neoarsphenamine,[27] suramin,[28] quinapyramine dimethyl-sulfate,[29] and Bis (aminoethylthio) 4-melaminophenylarsine dihydrochloride.[30] Of these, neoarsphenamine and suramin have been used in large dourine eradication programs.[18,21,22,31] In vitro testing suggests that *T. equiperdum* is also susceptible to diminazene, melarsomine, and isometamidium.[32-34]

Prevention and Public Health Considerations

Dourine has been successfully eradicated from many parts of the world using programs based on CFT testing. The Terrestrial Code of the OIE contains recommendations for testing and quarantine of horses imported from an endemic area into a dourine-free country. Two conditions should be met before importation of semen from a stallion that resides in a country that is not considered free of dourine: (1) the stallion should be housed for 6 months before semen collection in an establishment or artificial insemination center where no case of dourine was reported during that period and (2) the stallion should be seronegative for *T. equiperdum*.

Surra

Etiology

Surra is caused by infection with the hemoparasite *Trypanosoma evansi*. The name is a Hindi word meaning "rotten."[35] Surra, the

first pathogenic trypanosome to be discovered, was originally described by Griffith Evans, a British veterinarian, who described the condition in horses and camels in India in 1880.[35] Surra is characterized by anemia, weight loss, recurrent fever, and death in a wide variety of domestic animals, including horses, cattle, buffalo, and camels, in Asia, Africa, and South America.

Epidemiology and Pathogenesis

Surra is most severe and most frequently diagnosed in horses and camels. It may also affect cattle, buffalo, llamas, dogs, cats, sheep, goats, pigs, and elephants. In some species, only occasional mild or inapparent infections are seen. The disease is seen in South America, northern Africa, the Middle East, Asia, Indonesia, and the Philippines.[36] The etiologic agent, *T. evansi*, is transmitted mechanically by hematophagous biting flies of the species *Tabanus* and *Stomoxys*. Transmission by vampire bats is also possible.[36] Mortality rate in horses can be quite high in areas where the disease has been newly introduced. Outbreaks of surra tend to occur in areas where there are large numbers of commingled horses, large numbers of appropriate vectors, and reservoir hosts. The incubation period after infection is approximately 1 to 2 weeks. There is no known age, breed, or gender predilection.

Clinical Findings

Horses with surra present with fever, progressive anemia, weight loss despite a good appetite, and neurologic abnormalities.[37] Disease is usually acute, although some horses will experience chronic manifestations. Intermittent fever correlates with intermittent episodes of parasitemia. Urticarial lesions and edematous plaques may appear on the ventral abdomen; distal limb edema and petechial hemorrhages are common. Horses with severe anemia have pale mucous membranes. Neurologic signs, when they occur, lead to progressive weakness and ataxia, most apparent in the hindlimbs.[36] Experimentally, acute infection is associated with monocytosis (up to 35%) followed by lymphocytosis.[37] In an outbreak of surra on a breeding farm in Thailand, 42% of pregnant mares aborted or gave birth to stillborn foals. On this farm, 40% (19/47) of affected horses and 10% (1/10) of affected mules died.[38]

Diagnosis

A diagnosis of surra is suspected on the basis of compatible clinical signs in a horse residing in an area endemic for this disease. In the early stages of disease, this diagnosis is confirmed by observation of typical trypanosomes in blood or tissue fluids. This approach to diagnosis is more difficult in equids with chronic disease.[39,40] Centrifugation of a blood sample and examination of the buffy coat layer may increase the sensitivity of this technique.[36] Available serologic assays include ELISA, card agglutination test, and latex agglutination test. Data on their sensitivity and specificity for the field diagnosis of equine surra are largely lacking. The mouse inoculation test[41] is considered the most accurate diagnostic test for surra but takes up to 6 weeks to complete and is therefore not practical for routine screening.[37] The mouse inoculation test and direct review of wet blood films or buffy coat preparations are accurate for diagnosis early in disease (48 and 96 hours of infection, respectively).[42,43] The reported sensitivity and specificity of other antigen detection (antigen-ELISA,[40] latex agglutination[44,45]) and antibody detection (antibody-ELISA,[40] card agglutination,[46,47] IFA[48]) methods have varied, depending on methodology and investigator.[37,42,43] Other antigen-ELISA tests developed for parasite detection in camels demonstrate high specificity and sensitivity and may be a potential future diagnostic resource for identifying infections in horses.[49] Additionally, an experimental real-time polymerase chain reaction (PCR), developed using blood from water buffaloes and horses, quantifies parasitemia of chronically infected animals with a sensitivity of 10^2 parasites/mL of blood.[50]

Therapy

Suramin is the drug that has most frequently been used for treatment of surra in horses. The recommended dose is 10 mg/kg body weight intravenously (IV), repeated 1 week later.[36] Quinapyramine sulfate at 3 mg/kg has a risk of adverse local reactions, and the dose should be divided between two or more sites.[36] Isometamidium chloride at 0.25 to 2 mg/kg intramuscularly (IM)[36] and melarsen oxide[35] have also been suggested as treatments for surra. On a breeding farm in Thailand, treatment of affected horses with diminazene aceturate at 3.5 mg/kg was initially effective in clearing *T. evansi* from the peripheral blood but was less effective with a second treatment. Approximately 50% of treated horses and mules showed moderate to severe signs of adverse reaction to the drug, including lip edema, salivation, recumbency, restlessness, and dyspnea.[38]

Prevention and Public Health Considerations

There are no vaccines for prevention of surra in horses. Prevention relies on identification and treatment of infected horses, appropriate vector control, and hygiene. Repeated treatment with antitrypanosomal medications such as suramin, quinapyramine, or isometamidium chloride has been suggested.[36]

There is a single report of human *T. evansi* infection in an Indian farmer with fluctuating parasitemia and fever who was successfully treated with suramin.[51]

African Animal Trypanosomiasis

Etiology

African animal trypanosomiasis (AAT; tsetse disease, tsetse fly disease, African animal nagana) is a disease complex caused by infection with *T. congolense*, *T. vivax*, or *T. brucei brucei*, either singly or in combination.[52-55] In East Africa, *T. congolense* is the most important cause of AAT. Cattle, sheep, goats, horses, and pigs develop significant clinical disease if infected. In West Africa, *T. vivax* is the most important cause of AAT in cattle. The polymorphic trypanosome *T. brucei brucei* causes significant disease in horses, dogs, cats, camels, and pigs.

Epidemiology and Pathogenesis

Infection of cattle, sheep, goats, pigs, horses, camels, dogs, cats, and monkeys with the etiologic agents of AAT results in disease that ranges from subclinical to mild to chronic to fatal.[52] Numerous laboratory and wild animal species may also be infected. Wild ruminants are considered reservoirs of infection.[52] In Africa, the most important biologic vectors for transmission of AAT are three species of tsetse flies: *Glossina morsitans*, *G. palpalis*, and *G. fusca*. Large hematophagous flies *(Tabanus, Haematopota, Lyperosia, Stomoxys, Chrysops)* may act as mechanical vectors in some situations.[52] The natural range of AAT infection is largely defined by the range of the principal vector, the tsetse fly, and includes the area from the southern edge of the Sahara desert to Angola, Zimbabwe, and Mozambique.[52] Only *T. vivax* occurs in the Western Hemisphere (Caribbean and South and Central America), where tabanid and hippoboscid flies probably transmit the parasite mechanically.[52]

Trypanosomes that cause AAT replicate in the skin at the site of initial inoculation, causing a sore or chancre, and then spread to draining lymph nodes and blood. Parasitemia is detectable within a few days of experimental infection. *T. congolense* localizes in endothelial cells, whereas *T. vivax* and *T. brucei brucei* localize in tissues. Antibodies to the glycoprotein coat of the parasite are produced, killing the parasite and forming immune complexes with released coat protein. Parasites are not eliminated because antigenic changes in the surface coat proteins of the trypanosome occur. The result is cycles of parasitemia, antibody production, death of parasites, immune complex formation, and glycoprotein coat antigenic changes. Many of the lesions observed in animals with AAT are probably the result of immune complex disease (e.g., anemia, glomerulonephritis).[52,56] Marked immunosuppression predisposes to secondary infections.

Clinical Findings

Clinical signs of AAT, regardless of the specific trypanosome involved, include anemia, intermittent fever, edema, and weight loss.[52,57] Abortion and infertility may be observed. Stressors, such as malnutrition or concurrent disease, increase the likelihood and severity of disease. Infection with *T. congolense* has an incubation period that varies from 4 to 24 days; it causes severe disease in horses, cattle, sheep, goats, and camels, with milder disease in pigs. In donkeys, it may cause chronic infection with longer persistence in the blood.[58] In contrast, *T. vivax* has an incubation period of 4 to 40 days and causes relatively mild disease in horses. Infection of horses with *T. brucei brucei* has a comparatively short incubation period (5-10 days) and causes severe, frequently fatal, infection of horses, camels, dogs, and cats, with mild, chronic or subclinical disease in cattle, sheep, goats, and pigs.[52] Clinical signs of trypanosomiasis may be complicated by clinical signs of secondary diseases that develop as a result of immunosuppression.

Diagnosis

A diagnosis of AAT should be suspected in horses in endemic areas with anemia and poor body condition. The diagnosis is usually confirmed by demonstration of the organism in blood or lymph node smears. Parasites, especially *T. vivax* and *T. congolense*, are readily observed in whole-blood or buffy coat smears early in infection. Stained lymph node smears are most useful for diagnosis of early infection with *T. vivax* and *T. brucei brucei* or chronic *T. congolense* infection.[52] An ELISA for detection of antigen-specific, species-specific deoxyribonucleic acid (DNA) probes for trypanosomes and PCR assays to identify specific trypanosome species have been described for diagnosis of AAT in ruminants and horses.[54,55,59-64]

Therapy

A variety of antitrypanosomal medications have been used for the treatment and prevention of AAT; however, the development of drug resistance has complicated this approach to disease control.[52,65] Quinapyramine derivatives provide effective protection against *T. brucei brucei* in horses for up to 3 months. Other drugs suggested for control of AAT include isometamidium chloride,[65,66] homidium bromide,[66] diminazene aceturate,[66] and melarsen oxide; however, potential adverse effects may limit the usefulness of some of these drugs in horses.

Prevention and Public Health Considerations

The most effective way to control AAT is to control vector populations. This may include habitat manipulation (discriminative brush clearing), sterile male eradication techniques similar to those used for eradication of screwworm in the United States, ground and aerial spraying, use of synthetic pyrethroids, and odor-baited targets impregnated with insecticides.[52]

The trypanosomes associated with AAT are considered nonpathogenic for humans.

Enteric Coccidiosis

Etiology and Epidemiology

Horses may be infected by three species of coccidia: *Eimeria leuckarti*, *E. solipedum*, and *E. uniungulsti*.[67-69] Infection with

Cryptosporidium spp., another coccidial parasite of horses, is discussed later. The most common coccidial oocyst identified in equine feces is that of *Eimeria leuckarti*. It is a rare parasite of the small intestine of horses and donkeys worldwide.[67,68,70-75] Oocysts are most frequently observed in the feces of foals and yearlings but may occasionally be detected in older horses.[68,70,72,76] Studies of oocyst shedding on Kentucky horse farms in 1986 and 2003 revealed shedding in approximately 40% of foals on more than 80% of farms.[77,78] The mean age for the first appearance of oocysts in the feces was 70 days; the age of the oldest foal shedding oocysts was 185 days. The longest oocyst shedding period was about 4 months. In a later study, the prevalence of *E. leuckarti* in foals from May to December of 2004 ranged from 0% to 54% on 6 of 7 farms surveyed in central Kentucky. Oocysts were found in fecal material through the months of May to November.[79]

Pathogenesis and Clinical Signs

The prepatent period for experimentally induced *E. leuckarti* infection in horses is approximately 35 days.[67,72] Early gametocytes of *E. leuckarti* are found in cells of the lamina propria of villi in the equine small intestine.[67] Microgametes and microgametocytes are visible by 23 days after infection; at 28 days, macrogametes have begun formation of an oocyst wall in the cytoplasm of host cells. These findings suggest that the lifespan of parasitized host cells is up to 28 days, much longer than the expected life span for normal intestinal epithelial cells (approximately 2-3 days). The host cells parasitized by *Eimeria* spp. appear to be epithelial cells that have been displaced to the lamina propria.[69] Most horses shedding oocysts of *E. leuckarti* show no clinical signs of gastrointestinal (GI) disease, and it is largely regarded as nonpathogenic in horses.[68,76,80] It has been recorded as an incidental finding in horses with diarrhea,[81,82] intestinal hemorrhage,[74] and catarrhal inflammation of the jejunum.[83] Experimental infections of ponies and foals have not been associated with any clinical signs attributable to coccidiosis.[72,84]

Diagnosis and Therapy

Oocysts can be detected in the feces of horses by standard fecal flotation with saturated sugar or sodium nitrate solution (see Fig. 54-12).[70,72,75,77,85] They are dark brown, thick walled, and ovoid and contain a prominent micropyle on the narrower end.[80] The oocysts of *E. leuckarti* are larger than those of most *Eimeria* spp. (80-90 µm × 49-69 µm).[80] Because infection with *E. leuckarti* is generally considered to be nonpathogenic, no therapeutic regimens have been reported.

Cryptosporidiosis

Etiology, Epidemiology, and Pathogenesis

Cryptosporidium spp. are apicomplexan parasites in the order *Eucoccidiorida* that infect the microvilli of intestinal epithelial cells in many domestic and wild animal species, including horses and humans. There are at least 13 species of *Cryptosporidium*, but *C. parvum* is the most widely recognized and there is new evidence of numerous genetically distinct genotypes within that species. *C. parvum* that infect calves, horses, and humans are cross-transmissible and considered a zoonotic risk. Recent reports have shown pathogenic potential of the *Cryptosporidium* horse genotype in humans,[86,87] and isolates from horses should be considered a zoonotic risk.[88-91]

Horses become infected with *Cryptosporidium* spp. by ingestion of oocysts. Oocysts are approximately 4 to 5 µm in diameter, smaller than those of most coccidia (see Fig. 54-13). Cryptosporidia develop in the apical surfaces of parasitized GI epithelial cells, beneath the limiting cell membrane, but separate from the host cell cytoplasm.[92] In contrast to most other coccidia, *Cryptosporidium* oocysts are sporulated and infectious at the time they are excreted into the feces. Some oocysts have a thick wall that enhances survival outside the host. Other oocysts have thinner walls and the potential to release sporozoites during passage through the lower gut with immediate infection of host cells and propagation of clinical disease.[80,88] Damage to intestinal microvilli results in malabsorption, maldigestion, and diarrhea.

There are relatively few studies of the prevalence of cryptosporidiosis in horses,[93-98] and the prevalence of fecal shedding of oocysts is low.[93,94,96-98] In contrast, a serosurvey of horses in England demonstrated that 91% of 22 horses were seropositive, suggesting that subclinical infection is common.[95]

A cross-sectional study of 152 horses at a large horse show, admitted to a veterinary teaching hospital, and on a breeding farm examined the prevalence and risk factors for shedding of *C. parvum* oocysts.[93] Fecal samples from only 13 horses were positive. Risk factors for fecal shedding included residence on specific breeding farms, age less than 6 months, and history of diarrhea during the preceding 30 days. Mature horses and exposure to cattle were not identified as risk factors for cryptosporidial infection of foals, suggesting that these are not important sources of infection for foals.[93]

Clinical Findings

The incubation period for *C. parvum* infection is approximately 3 to 7 days. The primary clinical sign associated with cryptosporidiosis in animals is severe, persistent diarrhea leading to dehydration, weakness, and death if untreated.[99] In immunocompetent animals, clinical signs usually last for 5 to 14 days.[80] Infection is common in foals with severe combined immunodeficiency (SCID).[100-102] *C. parvum* has also been isolated from foals that develop diarrhea while hospitalized for other problems, suggesting that the stress of hospitalization and disease may predispose to clinical cryptosporidiosis. Most reports of equine cryptosporidiosis describe the disease in foals; however, there is one report of cryptosporidial oocyst shedding in an adult Quarter Horse stallion with diarrhea.[103] The large number of seropositive horses in one serosurvey and documented shedding of oocysts in foals and horses with no clinical signs suggest that subclinical infection is common.

Diagnosis

Cryptosporidium oocysts are very small and difficult to identify by light microscopy on a routine fecal flotation. Visualization of oocysts in fecal samples can be enhanced by acid-fast or acridine orange staining. Alternatively, immunofluorescent staining or flow cytometry may be used to identify oocysts in fecal samples.[104]

Therapy

There is no known specific therapy for treatment of cryptosporidiosis. Affected animals should receive appropriate supportive care for dehydration and acid-base and electrolyte imbalances associated with severe diarrhea.

Public Health Considerations

Cryptosporidiosis is considered a zoonotic disease.[88,89,96,105-107] The strains of *C. parvum* that predominate in calves and humans are cross-transmissible,[88] and the *Cryptosporidium* horse genotype may also pose a zoonotic risk.[86,87] Because cryptosporidiosis is transmitted by a fecal-oral route, disease can be prevented by using good sanitation and hygiene practices, including appropriate handwashing. Oocysts are highly resistant to most chemical disinfectants.[108] Therefore emphasis should be placed on effective removal of all fecal material rather than use of a chemical disinfectant to kill oocysts.[88] Moist heat (pasteurization to >55°C [131°F] or live steam), freezing, or thorough drying may be the most effective means of killing oocysts.[109] Exposure to 5% ammonia solution or 10% formalin for 18 hours will also kill oocysts.[108]

Concerns have been raised regarding the potential contamination of the environment with *Cryptosporidium* oocysts shed by inapparent carrier horses. However, a study of 91 horses used for backcountry riding in California revealed that none of the horses was shedding *Cryptosporidium* oocysts.[110]

Giardiasis

Giardia duodenalis (also known as *Giardia lamblia* or *Giardia intestinalis*) is a protozoan parasite of the GI tract of many domestic and wild animals and humans. The parasite has a two-stage life cycle consisting of a trophozoite stage, which has a characteristic teardrop shape with twin nuclei and four pairs of flagella (see Fig. 54-10), and a cyst stage with four nuclei. Cysts are ingested by the host. Trophozoites excyst and reproduce by binary fission after attachment to the intestinal epithelium in the duodenum. Ultimately, trophozoites develop into inactive, environmentally resistant cysts that are excreted in feces.

There are infrequent reports of *Giardia* infection in horses; some of these reports indicate that infected horses had compatible clinical signs of diarrhea or colic.[111-118] Shedding of cysts in the feces of normal foals may be common.[119] In a survey of breeding farms in Ohio and Kentucky, shedding of *Giardia* cysts appeared to be common in apparently healthy nursing mares, the presumed source of infection for foals, leading to speculation that there may be a periparturient relaxation of immunity.[119] In one report, a 4-year-old Thoroughbred gelding with a 6-month history of intermittent diarrhea, weight loss, poor hair coat, lethargy, inappetence, and exudative dermatitis was shedding *Giardia* cysts that were detected by zinc sulfate fecal flotation.[112] Diarrhea ceased on the second day of treatment with metronidazole at 5 mg/kg three times a day for 10 days. Subsequent fecal samples obtained over a 6-week period after treatment were negative for *Giardia* cysts.

Giardia duodenalis is an important GI zoonosis. Symptoms in affected humans vary from inapparent to severe, chronic diarrhea. Symptoms begin approximately 7 days after exposure to the parasite and continue for 2 to 6 weeks or longer. Concerns have been raised regarding the potential contamination of the environment with *Giardia* cysts shed by inapparent carrier horses. However, a study of 91 horses used for back country riding in California revealed that none of the horses was shedding *Giardia* oocysts.[110]

Sarcocystosis

Sarcocystis spp. are coccidian parasites with an obligate, two-host life cycle. Intermediate hosts ingest sporulated sporocysts that are shed in the feces of definitive hosts. Mature tissue sarcocysts develop in the muscles of the intermediate host. When that host dies, ingestion of infected muscle by the definitive host completes the life cycle. The most common *Sarcocystis*

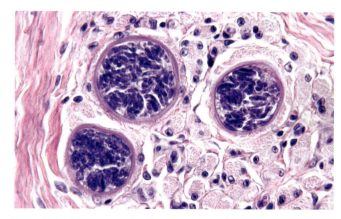

Figure 60-2 Photomicrograph of biopsy specimen from tongue of 10-year-old Thoroughbred gelding with 2-week history of extensive swelling of anterior portion of tongue. Note the large sarcocyst in the muscle and associated severe eosinophilic glossitis/myositis. *(Courtesy Dr. Kevin Snekvik.)*

infection of horses is equine protozoal myeloencephalitis (EPM) caused by *Sarcocystis neurona* (see Chapter 55).

Horses act as intermediate hosts for at least two species of *Sarcocystis: S. equicanis* and *S. fayeri*. Dogs are the definitive host for both species. Experimental infection of horses results in formation of sarcocysts in muscle, especially in the esophagus and diaphragm.[120-125] Surveys of horses at slaughter in Germany and the United States reveal that 13% to 23% of horses had sarcocysts in the muscle of the esophagus and diaphragm.[80,122,123] Fever, mild anemia, anorexia, and depression may be seen in some horses after experimental infection. In most horses, the presence of sporocysts in muscles is not accompanied by an inflammatory response. However, multifocal granulomatous myositis has been occasionally described[121,126] (Fig. 60-2). The possibility of a Sarcocystis-related toxin was suggested in one 3-year-old Quarter Horse mare with weight loss, weakness, depression, dysphagia, and large numbers of intramuscular cysts, presumed to be *S. fayeri*.[127]

A 7-year-old Quarter Horse gelding with multifocal myositis and probable *S. fayeri* cysts in the muscles was successfully treated with trimethoprim-sulfamethoxazole, pyrimethamine, and phenylbutazone. Therapeutic regimens described for treatment of EPM in horses would be reasonable for treatment of horses with myositis caused by sarcocystosis (see Chapter 55).

Aberrant Parasites

A variety of parasites that primarily infect other species have been described as causing sporadic disease in horses resulting from aberrant migration through numerous organs and tissues. This is most often described in relation to central nervous system (CNS) disease. One of the most common of these aberrant CNS parasites, Halicephalobus gingivalis, is discussed in Chapter 4.

In addition to *H. gingivalis*, several helminth and dipteran parasites have been described as etiologic agents of CNS disease in horses. These include *Strongylus vulgaris* larvae (see Chapter 57),[128-130] the filarial nematode *Setaria* spp.,[131,132] the spirurid stomach worm *Draschia megastoma* (see Chapter 57),[133] hydatid cysts of *Echinococcus* spp.,[134] and dipteran larvae belonging to the genus *Hypoderma* (see Chapter 7).[130,135-137] Clinical signs vary, depending on the affected area of the CNS and may be either acute or chronic. The diagnosis is usually made by histopathologic examination of tissues obtained at necropsy.

Adult canine heartworms, *Dirofilaria immitis*, were recovered from the heart and pulmonary vessels of one horse.[138] The ruminant liver fluke *Fasciola hepatica* has been implicated as a cause of liver disease in horses.[139-149]

Echinococcosis

Etiology and Epidemiology

Echinococcosis, or hydatid disease, is a zoonotic disease caused by infection with a metacestode of the genus *Echinococcus*. Hydatid cysts of *Echinococcus granulosus* have been reported in the liver and lungs of horses after natural or experimental infection.[150-155] The life cycle of *Echinococcus* spp. begins with passage of eggs containing a six-hooked larva (hexacanth or oncosphere) in the feces of carnivore definitive hosts. Eggs are ingested by the intermediate host. Humans may serve as accidental intermediate hosts. The larvae penetrate the intestinal mucosa and migrate via lymphatic and blood vessels to other sites, where they develop into a metacestode, forming a hydatid cyst containing numerous protoscolices. Affected tissues are ingested by a carnivore, and protoscolices develop into adult tapeworms in the carnivore's intestines to complete the life cycle.

The taxonomy of the genus *Echinococcus* is presently undergoing changes.[156-158] Currently, four species are recognized in Europe, one of which, *E. equinus*, uses equids (horses, donkeys, mules, zebras) as an intermediate host.[159] In Europe, equine echinococcosis has been described in Great Britain, Ireland, Belgium, Switzerland, Italy, and Spain.[160] The disease is also prevalent in equids in the Middle East and Africa.[161] There have been at least four reports of hydatid disease in horses in the United States.[153,155,162,163] All of the horses in these reports originated from the United Kingdom and Ireland, where hydatid disease is endemic. The prevalence of disease in horses in the United Kingdom is higher in horses used for hunting. In Ireland the prevalence in horses at slaughterhouses varies between 10% and 62%.[153,162] Disease has been correlated with the feeding of raw or improperly cooked offal from horses to dogs.[164,165]

Clinical Findings and Diagnosis

The most common site of hydatid cyst formation in horses is the liver, followed by the lung. Involvement of other organs is rare.[153] The parasite may persist for many years in some equids with no obvious clinical signs.[153,166] When clinical signs do occur, they are often related to pressure of the enlarging cyst on adjacent organs and tissues. Most cysts range in diameter from 1 to 7 cm, but they may occasionally be up to 20 cm in diameter.

There are no definitive antemortem tests for echinococcosis in equids, and the diagnosis is usually made at necropsy. However, ultrasonography of the liver of affected horses might provide evidence of cystic lesions in affected horses.

Public Health Considerations

Although humans are at risk for development of echinococcosis, the level of risk posed by equine strains of the parasite is unclear. Epidemiologic data from Europe suggest that *E. equinus* may not be infective to humans.[159] Regardless, the infective stage of *Echinococcus* is shed in the feces of the definitive host, usually a canid species, and the life cycle stages present in horses would not be directly infectious to humans.

Bots

Larvae of horse botflies are internal parasites of horses worldwide. The two species that most often infect horses are *Gasterophilus intestinalis* (horse botfly) and *Gasterophilus nasalis*. Occasional infections with *Gasterophilus haemorrhoidalis* (nose botfly) and *Gasterophilus pecorum* are reported.[167-169] Second-stage and third-stage larvae of these flies typically attach to the mucosa of the equine stomach or intestine, where they cause focal mucosal ulceration.[170]

Adult botflies are hairy and similar in size and appearance to honeybees. The common horse botfly usually lays its yellow to gray eggs on the hairs of the forelegs, mane, and flanks (Fig. 60-3). Throat botfly eggs are attached to the long hairs beneath the mandible and chin. Nose botfly eggs are deposited most often on the hairs around the muzzle of the horse. The hatching of botfly eggs is stimulated by warmth and moisture when the horse licks eggs off the hair during grooming. Larvae spend about 3 weeks migrating in the soft tissue of the oral cavity, then migrate to the stomach or small intestine, where they attach to the mucosa (Fig. 60-4). They remain in the

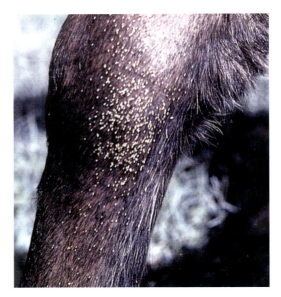

Figure 60-3 Botfly eggs on leg of horse. *(Courtesy Dr. Wendy Duckett.)*

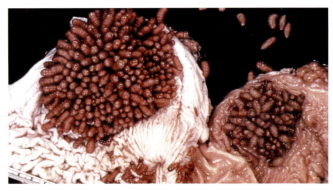

Figure 60-4 Botfly larvae attached to gastric mucosa of horse. *(Courtesy Dr. Wendy Duckett.)*

stomach until spring or early summer, when they detach, are passed in the feces, enter the soil below the manure pile, and pupate. In weeks to months, they emerge as adult flies. Non-feeding adult flies mate, and females lay their eggs during fall until the first hard frost. Adult G. pecorum bots lay eggs in batches on grass, and eggs are ingested when horses graze.

Bot larvae cause minimal pathology in most horses. The egg-laying activity of female flies can irritate horses and lead to abnormal behavior in an attempt at fly evasion. Larvae of G. nasalis burrow into the spaces around the teeth and can cause gingival irritation and necrosis. Minor irritation may be associated with attachment of larvae in the stomach or intestine. High numbers of parasites have been implicated as causes of gastric ulceration and rupture, intramural gastric suppuration, peritonitis secondary to gastroduodenal perforation, and gastro-esophageal reflux.[171-175] In a recent report, septic peritonitis in an adult mare was caused by colonic perforation associated with aberrant migration of a G. intestinalis larvae.[176] In Asia, G. pecorum has been associated with esophageal constriction and hypertrophy of the musculature of the oropharynx and esophagus with resultant dysphagia and death.[177] This species has also been associated with epidemic deaths of horses resulting from attachment of large numbers of bots to the soft palate.[167,178]

Bots can be controlled by (1) applying insecticides to prevent adult flies from laying eggs on the horse, (2) clipping hairs or removing eggs from hairs before they can be ingested by the horse, and (3) administering appropriate anthelmintic agents. Avermectin anthelmintics are highly effective for the control of bots. The most effective time to administer boticides is in the late fall after the first hard frost, when adult fly activity has ceased.

There are occasional reports of infection of humans with horse botfly larvae.[178-185] Several of these reports involved patients with known exposure to horses.[178,180,184,185] Burrowing of larvae behind the lips or inner cheek is said to elicit discomfort. Migration of first-stage larvae is associated with cutaneous and ocular myiasis in humans. The burrowing of larvae beneath the skin may produce a visible tortuous path with severe pruritus.

Besnoitiosis

SallyAnne L. Ness, Linda D. Mittel, and Thomas J. Divers

Etiology

Besnoitiosis is caused by infection with protozoan Besnoitia spp., which are cyst-forming coccidian parasites that affect multiple host species worldwide.[186] Besnoitia bennetti is the species known to infect equids and has been reported in horses and donkeys in Africa, Asia, and more recently, the United States.[187-191] Equine besnoitiosis was first reported by Bennett in 1927 in four horses from Sudan.[192,193] Currently, the only reported cases of equine besnoitiosis in North America have been in donkeys.

The Besnoitia life cycle involves both a definitive and an intermediate host. A feline definitive host has been identified for B. oryctofelisi, B. darling, and B. neotomofelis, which infect the rabbit, opossum, and southern plains woodrat, respectively.[194-196] Attempts to demonstrate the cat, or any other animal, as the definitive host in equine besnoitiosis have been unsuccessful, thus precluding researchers from elucidating the parasite's life cycle and mode of disease transmission in equine infection. In species with known life cycles, infective oocysts are ingested by the intermediate host and develop into thick-walled connective tissue cysts containing millions of bradyzoite-stage parasites.[187,194] Bovine infection with B. besnoiti produces more severe clinical disease than is observed in equine besnoitiosis, with significant morbidity and mortality reported during recent outbreaks in European cattle.[186,197,198]

Epidemiology and Pathogenesis

Much remains unknown regarding the epidemiology of equine besnoitiosis. In cattle, subclinically infected animals have been shown to act as reservoirs for infection and the introduction of an infected animal into a naïve herd is a known risk factor for development of disease within a population.[197,198] Blood-sucking arthropods (horse fly, stable fly, mosquito, and tsetse fly) have been shown experimentally to mechanically transmit B. besnoiti between cattle, but the potential for similar transmission in equids in currently unknown.[186] The potential for vertical or horizontal transmission between intermediate hosts is not known.

Clinical Findings

Clinical disease is characterized by a miliary dermatitis of pin-point parasitic cysts in the skin, mucous membranes, and conjunctiva (Fig. 60-5, A). The skin over the muzzle, nares, ears, perineum, and medial thigh appears to be preferentially affected, as does the vulvar mucosa of infected female donkeys. One of the most unique features of besnoitiosis is the development of "scleral pearls," which are cysts along the limbal margin of the sclera (Fig. 60-5, B). Cysts have also been identified in the testicles, nasopharynx, larynx, trachea, and esophagus of infected donkeys (Fig. 60-5, C), but the extensive internal involvement noted in other intermediate host species has not been documented in equids.

In a recent investigation of donkey herds in the northeastern United States, young animals (average age 2.7 years) were at increased risk for development of besnoitiosis when compared to older individuals. The most common lesions in infected donkeys were cysts in the nares (100%) and scleral pearls (83%). Only 50% of infected animals displayed nasopharyngeal/laryngeal lesions on endoscopy.[188] Some infected animals remain otherwise healthy, whereas others become cachetic and debilitated as a result of the disease. The reason for this difference in host response to infection is unknown, but similar clinical subtypes are observed with bovine besnoitiosis.

Diagnosis

The current gold standard for diagnosing besnoitiosis in donkeys is histologic identification of Besnoitia cysts within the dermis of individuals displaying clinical lesions, generally achieved via skin biopsy (Fig. 60-5, D). Studies evaluating the utility of serologic assays similar to those used to diagnose besnoitiosis in cattle are currently underway and may become available in the near future.

Therapy

There are currently no known effective treatments for equine besnoitiosis. Treatment with ponazuril for 45 days was not effective in two naturally infected donkeys.[188] Reported attempts to treat infected animals with trimethoprim-sulfamethoxazole and/or nitazoxanide have had variable success, but limited case numbers and lack of knowledge regarding clinical disease makes drawing useful conclusions from the existing literature difficult.[187,190] The potential for natural recovery from besnoitiosis and the long-term prognosis for infected animals remains to be elucidated.

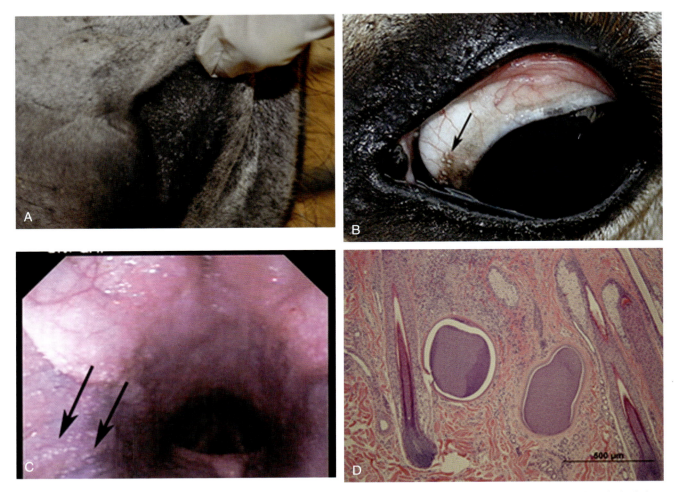

Figure 60-5 Lesions of *Besnoitia bennetti* in donkey. **A,** *Besnoitia* cysts in the nares of a donkey with besnoitiosis. **B,** Scleral pearls *(arrow)* along the limbal margin of a donkey with besnoitiosis. **C,** Endoscopic image of *Besnoitia* cysts *(arrows)* in the pharynx of a donkey with besnoitiosis. **D,** Two *Besnoitia* cysts within the dermis of a donkey with besnoitiosis. Note the surrounding granulomatous and eosinophilic inflammation. H&E 100×.

Gastrodiscus aegyptiacus

Karl van Laeren

Etiology and Life Cycle

Gastrodiscus aegyptiacus is an intestinal conical fluke of horses, zebras, pigs, and warthogs. It has been described in horses along the eastern half of Africa; however, it is likely to be present throughout Africa where wet conditions and a suitable intermediate host exist. It is particularly common in the Mashonaland area of Zimbabwe but also occurs in South Africa, Swaziland,[199] the Okavango Delta of Botswana (also recorded from Burchell's zebra in this location [KMA van Laeren, personal communication]), and Sudan.[200] Isolated cases have been recorded in Ethiopia,[201] Malawi, and Tanzania (KMA van Laeren, personal communication). However, many horse populations remain untested for its presence. It has been seen in horses in Guyana, South America, and in Cuba.[202] It is also found in India; a closely related species *Gastrodiscus secundus*, which infects equines and elephants, has also been found in India (RK Reinecke, personal communication).

Gastrodiscus spp. use snails (gastropods) as their intermediate hosts. *Bulinus tropicus* is incriminated in southern Africa,[203] whereas *Bulinus forskalii* is the prime host along the White Nile in Sudan.[200] Laboratory research has shown that *Cleopatra* spp.,

Melanoides tuberculata, Physa acuta, and *Helisoma duryi* are also susceptible. However, the latter two snails, which are exotic species to Africa (imported from North America),[204] showed high susceptibility, ranging from 96.6% to 100%.[203] This susceptibility highlights the possible spread of this parasite to other localities where potentially susceptible snails can act as new intermediate hosts. *H. duryi* has been used in some areas as a biological competitor against the snail acting as the intermediate host to bilharzia in humans.[203] Achieving infection in a host of experimental snails, however, does not necessarily imply that these snail species will play a major role in dissemination of cercaria under natural conditions. Only 12.5% of *B. forskalii* became infected under natural conditions in Sudan,[200] whereas *B. globosus* and *Biomphalaria pfeifferi* were resistant under laboratory challenge.[203]

Just as *Fasciola* spp. (liver fluke) have developed in different snail species in Europe, North America, and Australia, *Gastrodiscus* has the ability to infect and develop in a range of snails that are not the primary host. *Gastrodiscus* eggs excreted by an infected horse hatch into a miracidium. Under laboratory conditions, this takes between 12 to 14 days. The miracidium then penetrates susceptible snails, where they reproduce asexually into rediae (5 to 8 in the case of *Fasciola* but undetermined in the case of *Gastrodiscus*), daughter rediae, and finally, cercaria with an unforked tail (as for *Fasciola* and *Paramphistomes* but contrary to the forked tails of *Bilharzia cercariae*). The prepatent period is 45 days for *Melanoides tuberculata* and 53 days for *Cleopatra ferruginea;* this period for *B. tropicus* remains undetermined but is longer than 59 days.[203] Snails infected with two miricidia have been shown to produce as many as 70 cercaria per day for *M. tuberculata* and 5 cercaria per snail per day in cases in which *Cleopatra* spp. are involved. These cercaria attach to blades of grass or other plant matter just below the surface of the water, and within a few hours, they shed their tails and encyst into dark, hemispheric cysts about 0.3 mm in diameter; this is the infective stage for horses. In *Fasciola*, some cysts live on the bottom of the body of water[205] and can be consumed by drinking infected dam or stream water, but this has not been established in the case of *Gastrodiscus*. In a single case study in a donkey fed grass with encysted cercaria, the prepatent period before the eggs were passed was 115 days.

The favored habitat for these snails is dams, river banks, and seasonally flooded, poorly drained lands with a resident snail population. Horses not exposed to these habitats are not infected by this Trematode.

The ingested cyst undergoes excystation in the stomach and undergoes its entire life cycle in the cecum and large colon of its host. The adult parasite is a pink discoid structure (12 to 18 mm × 10 to 12 mm) with a conical head and rolled undersides. It can be likened to a miniature turtle-like parasite about the size of one's small fingernail.

Clinical Signs

Cow pad-like diarrhea with ill thrift is the usual presenting sign (Fig. 60-6, *A*). However, occasionally profuse colitis-like diarrhea is reported. Many horses with moderately heavy infections show weight loss without any change in the fecal appearance. Azzie[199] reported a case of per acute death after a stressful event (racing) in a heavily infected horse. Severe infections have presented with signs of colic unresponsive to medical treatment. Many of these horses with colic have turned out to have cecal-colic intussusceptions needing surgery to rectify.

Diagnosis

Occasionally, adult *Gastrodiscus* parasites can be found in the dung; however, as for most intestinal parasites, this is a rare occurrence. Laboratory diagnosis depends on a sedimentation test. Routine fecal worm egg counts (done for *Strongyles* and *Ascarids* by means of flotation principals) are inadequate to examine for *Gastrodiscus* eggs. Four grams of dung should be mixed with about 100 mL of tap water and allowed to settle. The supernatant fluid is decanted and this process is repeated four or five times. The resulting sediment is examined in a Petri dish under a dissecting microscope. The eggs are very similar to those of *Fasciola*; however, the color is the most striking feature (Table 60-1). A drop of 1% methylene blue solution (or a small drop of blue fountain pen ink) added to the sediment makes the yellowish brown color of the *Fasciola* egg become more prominent (KMA van Laeren, personal communication).

Postmortem examination of horses dying of *Gastrodiscus* show massive numbers of large conical flukes (Fig. 60-6, *B*), with a hemorrhagic edematous colitis infiltrated with lymphocytes and eosinophils. Severe anemia was noted in a horse reported by Applewhaite and Ruiz.[202]

Treatment

Even a single egg on fecal examination warrants treatment because the reproductive stage occurs in snails. The most effective treatment is with a fasciolicide drug, oxyclozanide at 8.5 mg/kg orally (PO). No side effects have been noticed with

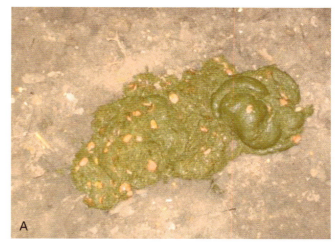

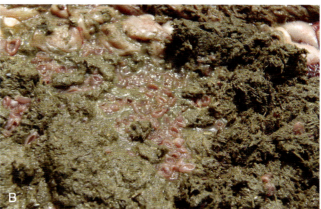

Figure 60-6 A, Gastrodiscus flukes in feces of heavily infested horse with unformed feces. **B,** Postmortem of heavily infested horses demonstrating large numbers of flukes within the colon.

Table 60-1 *Gastrodiscus* Egg Morphology Compared With *Fasciola* Egg Morphology

Gastrodiscus Eggs	*Fasciola* Eggs
Shape: oval	Shape: oval
Size: 140-170 μm × 90-100 μm	Size: 128-154 μm × 60-94 μm
Contains coarse granular material	Contains fine granular material
Color: whitish	Color: yellowish brown*
Distinct operculum	Indistinct operculum

*The color is the most striking feature. A drop of 1% methylene blue solution added to the sediment intensifies yellowish brown color of the Fasciola egg. (van Laerne personal communication).

this drug at the recommended dose rate[206] in the author's experience; however, this seems to vary between products containing oxyclozanide, with reports of anorexia after using even lower than recommended dosages. Heavily infected horses may suffer after deworming with the standard dosage with a concomitant drop in albumin levels on treatment; therefore these horses may be treated with between a third and a half of the recommended dose initially to gradually reduce the parasite burden in stages. Many of the oxyclozanide preparations available are formulated for ruminant use and are mixed with round worm remedies such as levamisole or oxfendazole. Generally speaking, the dose of levamisole that accompanies the oxyclozanide is well within safety levels for the horse, and the addition of these drugs did not pose a problem when administered to horses in the author's experience. Resorantel 65 mg/kg is also highly effective,[205] but the odd mild colic may result; the author has no personal experience with this preparation.

Other fasciolicide drugs, such as Rafoxanide (3.75 mg/kg),[205] Clorsulon, and Triclabendazole, have all been shown to be ineffective against this parasite (KMA van Laeren, personal communication).

Historically, dichlorvos (16.6 gm/500 kg) has been used[199]; however, the organophosphate family may be associated with colic or other GI side effects. Hexachlorophene has also been used in the past but with only moderate efficacy.[199] Both of these drugs have been discontinued or superseded by safer dewormers.

Usually, a single deworming annually is effective in areas like Zimbabwe where the long development period usually only produces fecal shedding many months after the rainy season has ended. In areas where horses have access to infected bodies of water, two to four dewormings per year are needed.

Prevention

As with nematode prevention practices, regular pasture cleansing appears to be more effective than any deworming programme. Infected streams, dams, and seasonally flooded areas may need to be fenced off to make them inaccessible to horses. Horses imported from known areas where the parasite is endemic should be examined by the use of a fecal sedimentation test.

The complete reference list is available online at www.expertconsult.com.

CHAPTER

61

Epidemiology of Equine Infectious Disease

Paulo C. Duarte, Ashley E. Hill, Paul S. Morley

Basics

Definition

Epidemiology is the study of the occurrence of disease in populations[1] and the application of this knowledge to control or prevent disease. The underlying tenet of epidemiology is that disease does not occur randomly in a population, which means that there are always reasons why some horses become sick and others stay healthy, even if we do not always understand those reasons. This principle has tremendous implications for veterinarians: they can identify causes and risk factors for disease and take actions to prevent or decrease the impact of a disease. In this sense, it is critical to consider more than just disease agents and hosts; it is also critical to consider the environment and management factors that impact interactions among agents and hosts. Because of this broader implication, epidemiology is also sometimes defined as "medical ecology," as will be discussed.

The mare reproductive loss syndrome (MRLS) outbreak in Kentucky in 2001 was an excellent example of epidemiology in action.[2] Even before veterinarians and producers understood the etiology of this disease, veterinarians were able to use epidemiology to identify risk factors for disease (exposure to eastern tent caterpillars[2] or pasture[3]), which allowed farm managers to implement control measures and prevent some abortions that would have otherwise occurred.

Epidemiologic Approach

A key epidemiologic approach to understanding and controlling disease involves looking for patterns of disease in the population of interest. Which horses are sick, and what do they have in common? Which horses are healthy, and what do they have in common? Which groups have been most affected? Great insight can be gained into causal mechanisms and control points that can be exploited in disease prevention efforts by (1) describing a population and identifying patterns, (2) making comparisons among different groups within a population, (3) comparing different populations, and (4) comparing the same population at different time points.

It is useful to consider the "five Ws" when trying to understand disease occurrence in a population: who, what, where, when, and why. Who is affected (and unaffected)? Include age, breed, gender, housing, water source, and vaccination status, as well as any other variables that may be relevant. What are the circumstances related to disease occurrence and has anything changed? Where are the affected and unaffected animals located? Use a map of the barn or farm with food, water, and ventilation sources marked and spatially locate the ill animals. When did each ill animal develop disease? Use this information to identify groups most affected (e.g., age groups, barns, breeds) using the tools described later in this chapter. All of this should

be interpreted with a focus on ultimately identifying "why." Why did these animals develop disease, and why were others not affected? Understanding why disease occurs allows identification of ways that disease can be prevented.

Disease Ecology

When trying to understand reasons why particular animals become diseased, it is clearly important to consider more than just an individual host and a particular agent as causes for a specific occurrence. The population to which an individual belongs must also be considered, in addition to the patterns of interactions and the environment that influences these interactions and impacts the likelihood of contagious transmission. Because of the importance of these broader considerations, epidemiology is sometimes referred to as medical ecology, or the interactions of all organisms and their environment as these pertain to health.

Mare reproductive loss syndrome, which was initially reported among broodmares in central Kentucky in 2001, is one example of disease arising from a combination of host, agent, and environmental factors. An epidemic of equine abortion, endophthalmitis, and pericarditis began in late April 2001 and lasted until June 2001[4-6]; fetal losses occurred both early and late in pregnancy[3,7] and affected more than 60% of mares on some farms.[7] Multiple bacterial species were identified[8] in tissue of aborted fetuses. The syndrome was subsequently found to be associated with ingestion of the eastern tent caterpillar,[4] and it has been proposed that bacterially contaminated barbed caterpillar hairs migrated out of the alimentary tract, spread hematogenously, and were directly responsible for the observable signs of MRLS.[9] Eastern tent caterpillars are ubiquitous in the eastern United States but were particularly abundant in Kentucky that spring because a rapid temperature increase in early spring was superimposed on an unusually dry winter and spring.[10] These climatic conditions caused an explosion of biologic activity, including growth of black cherry trees on which eastern tent caterpillar eggs are laid and larvae develop.[11] During that spring with its unusual climactic conditions, grazing on pasture[4] with black cherry trees[12] exposed horses to disease; fetuses were particularly vulnerable. The sensitivity of the fetus to disease, the environmental conditions that led to the overgrowth of caterpillars, the bacteria themselves, and the management of the broodmares all contributed to the occurrence of MRLS.

Disease Agent

Characteristics of the disease agent, including infectivity, contagiousness, pathogenicity and virulence, immunogenicity, host range, life cycle, and antimicrobial susceptibility, influence the speed and scope of disease spread. Infectiousness (infectivity) refers to the ease with which an agent infects susceptible hosts, which is sometimes quantified in relation to the amount of agent required to reliably infect an individual. Contagiousness relates to the likelihood that an agent will move between infected and susceptible hosts; it is sometimes quantified by the number of new infections that will likely result from exposure to an infected animal or as the speed with which a disease agent is transmitted through a susceptible population. Equine influenza virus and equine herpesvirus are both highly infectious, but influenza virus is more contagious. Although equine protozoal myeloencephalitis (EPM) is an infectious disease, it is not a contagious disease because the etiologic agent is not transmitted directly between horses. Pathogenicity describes the likelihood that an infected horse will develop clinical disease, and virulence describes the likelihood that disease will be severe. West Nile virus (WNV) is highly virulent in horses; more than 30% of horses with clinical disease die.[13] In contrast, EPM is not highly pathogenic; most equids exposed to the disease agent do not develop clinical disease.[14-16]

Characteristics of the disease agent that enable it to survive and spread without detection are particularly important to consider when instituting preventive or control measures. Agents that can persist in the environment, such as *Clostridium difficile*[17] or *Streptococcus equi* subsp. *equi*, require different control measures than equine influenza, which does not persist well outside the host. Some diseases spread undetected through infected horses without clinical signs of illness. Subclinically, persistently, and latently infected animals are often important reservoirs and sources of exposure for susceptible animals in a population because they go unnoticed or undiagnosed. Animals often are infected with a potentially pathogenic organism without showing clinical signs, and this can even be the predominant presentation, depending on the pathogenicity of the agent. The term *subclinical* is also used to describe animals during the induction or incubation period for infectious diseases. Animals that remain infected for extended periods are sometimes described as being "persistently infected," especially if infections continue after clinical signs of disease resolve. Persistent infection and long-term shedding of *S. equi* subsp. *equi* are common[18-20] and important to the spread of disease among populations.[20,21] In contrast, latency describes a state of dormant viral infection in which shedding stops and the virus cannot be detected until later, when the infection reactivates or recrudesces. This is a common feature among alpha herpesviruses such as equine herpesvirus (EHV) types 1 and 4.[22-29]

Host

Many host characteristics are intrinsic to the horse and relatively unchangeable such as age, gender, and breed. Other host characteristics are highly variable among individuals and can change over time, perhaps most notably, an inherent susceptibility to infectious agents or immunity. Characteristics of the host can affect both its exposure to disease and its likelihood of becoming infected if exposed. For example, geldings or spayed mares are less likely to be exposed to *Taylorella equigenitalis*, the agent that causes contagious equine metritis, and foals can be more vulnerable to disease than adults, as with *Rhodococcus equi* pneumonia.

Environment

A horse's environment includes its location, climate, and the local surroundings and interactions created by its management.[30] Characteristics of a horse's environment affect which diseases and vectors a horse is exposed to, the magnitude of that exposure, and the likelihood of developing disease if exposed. Horses that have been vaccinated with efficacious vaccines or immunized by natural exposure are more resistant to a particular disease than naïve horses. Horses that are stressed for any reason, including poor diet, concurrent disease, weaning,

transport, or mixing, are more likely to develop a disease than their unstressed counterparts. The risk of disease is not equal for similar horses when managed differently or housed in different environments.

Individual

Environmental characteristics that affect risk of disease in individual horses include climate, landscape, flora and fauna, cleanliness, air quality, housing, diet, and events that affect stress levels. Some of these factors (e.g., cleanliness, ventilation, housing, diet, stress level) are directly related to management practices and may be changeable, thus affecting risk of disease. Some management strategies (e.g., housing in open pastures, using outdoor drinking-water sources) increase potential exposure to insect vectors and also increase the risk of other diseases such as Potomac horse fever (*Neorickettsia risticii* infection) and vesicular stomatitis. On the other hand, indoor housing, especially if it is high density or poorly ventilated, can increase exposure to diseases transmitted by aerosol or oral-fecal routes, such as influenza virus and *Salmonella*. Some environments and climates support larger vector populations than others, thus increasing potential risks for diseases, such as equine infectious anemia (EIA) or the equine encephalitides, including western equine encephalitis (WEE), eastern equine encephalitis (EEE), and WNV encephalitis. Although the climate itself cannot be changed, management practices, such as using animal-safe insect repellents, treating open-water sources with larvicides, and housing horses indoors at dusk and dawn, can be used to reduce disease risk.

Population

In addition to characteristics of individuals that affect their disease risk, the aggregate characteristics of the population to which the individual belongs affects the disease risk for that individual. This aggregate of the population's susceptibility to disease is often called *herd immunity*, described as immunity of an individual that is conferred by the population to which it belongs, or the ability of a population of animals to withstand exposure without succumbing to disease because the immunity of a population is more than the sum of its parts.[31] Herd immunity is created when the likelihood is small that an infected horse shedding a disease agent will encounter a susceptible horse (Fig. 61-1). If most horses are immune or if contact among horses is heavily restricted, it is unlikely that the few susceptible horses will have contact with the infected horse sufficient to allow transmission. For example, consider a barn in

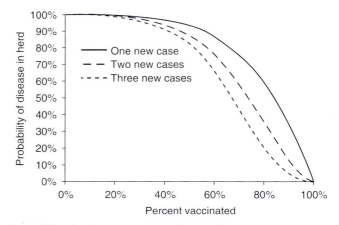

Figure 61-1 Probability of new cases of disease with 1-day infectious period as a function of percentage vaccinated in a herd of horses where each horse contacts four other horses per day.

which 90% of horses are immune to influenza virus, and each horse in the barn contacts four other horses per day. If a newly introduced horse happens to be infected with influenza virus, and conditions are adequate for transmission of virus to in-contact horses, the probability that any other horse in the barn will become infected is about 35%, and the probability that more than one horse will become infected is about 12% (Fig. 61-1). For herd immunity to be effective, the disease agent (e.g., influenza) must only reside in horses, must not have an environmental reservoir, must be transmitted directly from horse to horse, and must have a short infectious period.[32]

Disease Causation

Many veterinarians are accustomed to thinking that infectious diseases have a single cause: the disease agent. Epidemiologists think of cause in a more general sense. Any "exposure" that leads to new cases of disease can be considered a "cause" of that disease. By removing that exposure some cases of disease can be prevented. Causation has multiple levels. Again, consider MRLS. What "exposures" are associated with MRLS? The bacteria on the caterpillar hairs,[8] the caterpillars themselves,[33] exposure to cherry trees,[2] pasture grazing,[3,7] and the convergence of climatic factors resulting in caterpillar overgrowth have all been implicated in the epidemic occurrence of MRLS. Epidemiologically, all these factors are causes. Cases of disease can be reduced by removing bacteria from the caterpillars (an obviously impractical approach), minimizing exposure to caterpillars, reducing exposure to environments shared with the caterpillars (cherry trees or pasture), or returning to a more typical climate, as happened in subsequent years.

Likewise, consider encephalitis associated with WNV infection. This agent is propagated in a mosquito-bird-mosquito life cycle.[34] West Nile virus can replicate in multiple mosquito species,[35] although its primary vectors are *Culex* mosquitoes.[36] The primary hosts are birds,[37] which develop transient viremia followed by long-term (lifelong) immunity. Ticks may also play a role in maintenance of WNV.[35,38,39] New cases of equine disease can therefore be reduced by minimizing exposure to mosquitoes and ticks (e.g., controlling vector populations, using animal-safe repellents, housing horses inside at dusk and dawn) or by increasing immunity to the virus, either in birds or in horses. In birds the natural immunity that develops after initial exposure reduces the total amount of virus circulating in the mosquito population, which in turn reduces equine exposures. The increase in WNV immunity among birds is one likely reason that the number of reported equine cases of WNV-associated disease in Colorado was 378 and 426 in 2002 and 2003, respectively, and then decreased to 33 in 2004.[40]

One useful model used to understand complex causal relationships is to classify causes as component causes, necessary causes, or sufficient causes.[31] In this model, a component cause is anything that contributes to new cases of disease. Component causes can be characteristics of the host (e.g., age, vaccination status), the agent (e.g., subtype), or the environment (e.g., presence or absence of caterpillars). A sufficient cause is any set of components that, when present together, is capable of causing disease; once a sufficient cause is present or complete, disease will occur. A necessary cause is a component cause that must be present for disease to occur; without the necessary cause, disease cannot occur. For infectious diseases, exposure or infection with the infectious agent is never sufficient by itself, but it is necessary for disease to occur.

Using this model, we can see that there may be multiple sufficient causes and that disease can "flow" through any of these paths. Thus removing exposure to one component cause will only mitigate disease through the sufficient causal paths that include that particular component cause. When a particular component cause is part of a high proportion of sufficient pathways, then exposure to this particular component cause will be strongly associated with disease occurrence. The extreme of this example is when a component cause is included in all sufficient causes, in which case the component cause can also be called a "necessary cause." Necessary causes are rare among all component causes, and there are always multiple sufficient causal sets. Thus, by removing exposure to some of the component causes, we only expect to prevent some disease occurrence and not all occurrences. The objective is to maximize efficiency of disease prevention efforts by targeting component causes that are strongly associated with disease occurrence.

Identifying Causal Factors

In epidemiologic studies, a main objective is often to determine the factors (risk factors) associated with occurrence of disease so that they can be targeted in control and prevention programs. In general, we identify risk factors for a disease by comparing measures of disease frequency between different populations or groups. More specifically, this is accomplished by summarizing the occurrence of disease in the population, measuring disease frequency, and then comparing the risk of disease among horses with different exposures. By identifying differences in disease risk for groups with different exposures, we determine which exposures are associated with disease. Multiple studies are required to label exposures confidently as risk factors that are truly causal, which can then be targeted for minimizing exposure and thereby reducing the occurrence of new cases.

For example, in a study to identify the risk factors associated with EPM, horses affected with EPM and nonaffected horses were compared using a case-control study design.[41] In that study, presence of opossums on the premises, lack of feed security, and recent occurrences of major health events, among other factors, were associated with an increased likelihood of disease and thus were identified as potential risk factors for the disease.[41]

Measuring Disease

The frequency of disease occurrence is measured for different purposes, including determining and comparing the health status of populations, monitoring changes in disease occurrence over time, and establishing the risks associated with certain events in the population. For example, a practitioner might be interested in the number or proportion of diseased horses in a herd, the increase or decrease in the number of disease cases over time, or the risk of disease introduction associated with new horses introduced to the herd. Common measures of disease frequency include prevalence and incidence, as well as related measures such as attack risk, case-fatality risk, and mortality risks.

Disease can be measured in whole populations or in specific subgroups. Measuring disease in the whole population (sometimes called a "crude" measure) tells you about the overall scope of the problem. Measuring disease in subgroups (called "specific" measures) enables you to compare those groups, which is essential when attempting to identify factors affecting the occurrence of disease. For example, if you had 10 cases of neurologic disease on a farm of 100 horses, you could report that 10% of horses on the farm are affected, as a crude prevalence estimate. In contrast, you could also report that 8 of 25 (32%) horses grazing in Pasture A were affected and 2 of 75 (3%) horses in Pasture B were affected. These pasture-specific attack rates or attack risks suggest that something associated with housing in Pasture A may be the problem.

Population-at-Risk

The term *population-at-risk* refers to the group of individuals susceptible to the event of interest (e.g., infection, disease, death) at or during the time period of interest. The population-at-risk is used as the denominator in calculations of measures of disease frequency and can include the entire population or only a population subset, depending on susceptibility or specific interest in certain subgroups. For example, in describing the frequency of pneumonia caused by *Rhodococcus equi* infections, only foals would likely be included in the population-at-risk because adult horses are not considered susceptible to this disease.[42]

Types of Data

The types of data available largely determine which methods will be most appropriate for measuring disease frequency or comparing disease risk. Most data can be described as interval (measurement) or categorical data. Interval data quantify a characteristic, such as temperature, age, or weight, which can measure a large range of possible values. For example, in a group of five horses, you might take temperature measurements of 100°F, 100°F, 101°F, 101.5°F, and 102°F. Average or median values are often used to summarize interval data, and for this example, the average temperature for these five horses is 100.9°F. Interval data are often compared by subtracting one average or median from another, and differences in interval measurements among groups are often statistically tested using z-tests, t-tests, analyses of variance (ANOVA), or linear regression.

Categorical data divide groups into mutually exclusive categories (e.g., young horses versus older horses, Quarter Horses versus Thoroughbreds), and counts are used to characterize horses fitting into each category. Categorical data can be further characterized as "ordinal" if categories have an inherent order to them (e.g., young or old, light or heavy) or "nominal" if categories cannot be ranked or ordered (e.g., categories for gender or breed). Interval measurements can also be converted to ordinal measurements by dividing your range of values into categories. For example, if you wanted to describe temperature ordinally, as <101.5°F (38.6°C) versus temperature ≥101.5°F for these five horses, you would report that three horses had temperatures <101.5°F, and two had temperatures ≥101.5°F. Categories for nominal or ordinal data can be dichotomous (only two values are possible [e.g., live/dead, yes/no, sick/well]) or can have more than two possible values (e.g., breed, age group). Ordinal and nominal data are summarized using ratios, proportions, and rates. These summary measurements can then be compared using relative risks (risk ratios), odds ratios, and attributable risks. These comparisons are often tested statistically using different types of chi-square tests or logistic regression if the outcome data are dichotomous.

Generally, all characterizations of disease occurrence in populations include some type of categorical assessment of presence or absence of disease signs using a specific case definition. In summarizing these measurements, the data are standardized to account for population sizes using the number of affected animals as a numerator, and some context measurement of the "opportunity" for disease to have occurred in the population (e.g., the population at risk). The denominator that we choose greatly affects the conclusions we can draw from these measurements of disease frequency. In general, these measures of disease frequency take the form of ratios, proportions, or rates.

Using Interval Data

Interval data are usually summarized using a measure that describes central tendency (e.g., means, medians, or modes) and some measure of the variability in data such as the range of observed values, percentile rankings (e.g., values corresponding with the 25th and 75th percentiles), or the standard deviation or standard error of the mean. A simple arithmetic average summarizes the data well if the distribution of values looks like the well-recognized "normal" or "bell-shaped" curve. However, in distributions that do not have this balanced shape or in situations in which there are relatively few observations, averages can be strongly influenced by extreme values and may not represent the "center" of the data very well. In these situations, the median or mode will likely provide better measures of centrality in the data.

Using Categorical Data

Ratios, Proportions, and Rates

When using ratios, proportions, and rates to summarize disease occurrence, a count of affected animals meeting a specific case definition is used as the numerator. Do 10 affected horses represent a significant number of cases? The answer depends on the type of disease and the size of the population in which these observations were made. Are we referring to 10 sick horses in a barn of 15 horses or 10 sick horses at an entire racetrack facility with 3500 horses? The denominator provides context (e.g., is the population-at-risk 15 or 3500 horses) and improves standardization and the ability to extrapolate or make comparisons. The type of denominator we choose affects the conclusions we can draw. The ratios, proportions, and rates used as epidemiologic measures principally differ in how the denominator is calculated (e.g., which animals are included, is time considered).

Ratios

Ratios are used to express the magnitude of two events in relation to each other. Ratios vary between 0 and infinity and can also be expressed as the number of events in one group per number of events in another group. In a ratio, the numerator is not part of the denominator. For example, in a population of horses, a ratio of infectious upper respiratory tract disease (IURD) of 0.25, or 1:4, indicates that there is one diseased for every four nondiseased horses. In this case, we can also say that the odds of IURD in the population is 1:4. Ratios are also used to compare measures of disease frequency between groups.

Proportions

A proportion is a special type of ratio in which the numerator is included as part of the denominator. For disease measurement, this fraction is calculated as the number of events over the total number of possible events. A proportion varies between 0 and 1 and is usually expressed as percentage. For example, during a regular clinical examination, 10 of 100 horses examined were identified with IURD. The proportion of IURD among these 100 horses at the time of examination was 10/100, or 10%. In another situation, 100 horses were followed for 1 year. During that year, 20 new cases of IURD were identified. The proportion of new IURD cases during that 1-year period was 20/100, or 20%.

Rates

A rate is another special type of ratio. In epidemiologic terms, rate represents the average "speed" that health events will occur in a population over a specific or standardized amount of time. A rate is calculated as the number of events over the product between the total number of possible events and the time period during which each event could have occurred. A rate varies between 0 and infinity, and the units of the denominator are expressed in event-time (e.g., horse-years, horse-months). For example, 100 horses were followed for 1 year. Assume that 10 horses developed IURD in the middle of the year (0.5 year) and after this point were no longer at risk of IURD because of acquired immunity. The rate of IURD would be calculated as 10 cases/[(90 horses × 1 year) + (10 horses × 0.5 year)] and expressed as 0.11 cases per horse-year, or 11 cases per 100 horse-years. Notice that the time units of the denominator can be changed as desired, and 11 cases per 100 horse-years is the same as 11 cases per 1200 (100 × 12) horse-months, which means that you expect approximately 11 cases of IURD if you follow 100 horses for 1 year or 1200 horses for 1 month. Similarly, 33 cases of IURD would be expected to occur if 100 horses were followed for 3 years. The word "rate" is commonly used to refer to a proportion; however, rates and proportions are different quantities and are calculated differently, even though they are sometimes used as approximations of each other.

Epidemiologic Measures of Disease Frequency

Prevalence

Prevalence is the proportion of cases of disease in a population at a specific point in time[43] and is calculated as follows:

$$\text{Prevalence} = \frac{\text{Number of affected animals at a specific point in time}}{\text{Population-at-risk of being affected at that specific point in time}}$$

Prevalence is used to assess the health status of the population at a single point in time, like a snapshot. Therefore it is a static measure of disease frequency and does not allow strong inferences about previous or future occurrences of disease or how fast these occurrences accumulate over time. Prevalence measures are also used to describe the risk or probability of a condition being present in a population (Box 61-1). Note that in prevalence estimates the numerator includes all cases of disease present at the specific point in time (recent and chronic).

Cumulative Incidence

The cumulative incidence is the proportion of new cases of disease occurring in a population during a specific time period[43] and is calculated as follows:

$$\text{Cumulative incidence} = \frac{\text{Number of new cases of disease during a specific time period}}{\text{Population-at-risk of becoming a case at the beginning of that time period}}$$

Cumulative incidence is used to assess the progression of disease in the population during a specific time period and can be used to predict disease occurrence. The cumulative incidence measures the risk or probability of becoming diseased in a population during a defined time period (Box 61-2).

The cumulative incidence is an appropriate measure of disease incidence when the population is relatively "closed" (i.e., minimal movement of animals in and out of the population). When there is substantial movement of animals ("open" population), the cumulative incidence might underestimate or overestimate (bias) disease incidence,[43] and the incidence rate, also called incidence density, is a more appropriate measure of disease incidence.

Other common measures that could be described as specific types of cumulative incidence include the attack rate, mortality rate, and the case-fatality rate. The attack rate or attack risk is simply a different name attributed to the cumulative incidence in an outbreak situation and is calculated exactly as the cumulative incidence. The mortality rate or mortality risk is the proportion of all deaths ("crude" mortality rate) or deaths attributable to a specific disease ("cause-specific" mortality rate) over the total population-at-risk of death at the beginning of the time period (Box 61-3). Note that these measures are often called "rates," but in reality they are proportions because they do not include time measurements in their denominator and thus it is more precise to call them "risks."

Mortality can be calculated as a proportion, as just noted, or as an incidence using one of the methods described next. The term *mortality rate* is commonly used to describe mortality in the population, whether it is a proportion (risk) or an actual rate.

The case-fatality rate is the proportion of deaths attributable to the disease of interest during a specific period of time (Box 61-4).[43] The case-fatality rate is calculated as follows:

Box 61-2 Cumulative Incidence

A population of 100 horses was followed for 1 year to detect new cases of IURD; 20 new cases were observed during the year. The cumulative incidence of IURD in this population during that year was:

$$\text{Cumulative incidence} = \frac{20}{100} = 0.2 = 20\% \text{ in 1 year}$$

In this population, during a 1-year period, 20% of the horses developed IURD. If the conditions remain the same, we can expect 20% of the susceptible, healthy horses in that population to develop IURD in the following year. Thus the risk or probability of developing or becoming affected with IURD in that population is 20%.

Box 61-3 Mortality Rate

In a population of 100 foals followed for 1 year, 8 deaths were attributable to *Rhodococcus equi* pneumonia, one to neonatal septicemia, and one foal was euthanized because of an intestinal torsion. The crude mortality rate for this population during that year was:

$$\text{Crude mortality rate} = \frac{10}{100} = 0.1 = 10\% \text{ in 1 year}$$

The cause-specific mortality rate for deaths attributable to *R. equi* pneumonia was:

$$\text{Cause-specific mortality rate} = \frac{8}{100} = 0.08 = 8\% \text{ in 1 year}$$

In this population the risk or probability of a foal dying from any cause during that year was 10%, and the risk or probability of a foal dying from *R. equi* pneumonia was 8%.

Box 61-1 Prevalence

A population of 100 horses was examined for presence of infectious upper respiratory tract disease (IURD). At the time of examination, a total of 30 horses were diagnosed as having IURD. The prevalence of IURD in this population can be calculated as follows:

$$\text{Prevalence} = \frac{30}{100} = 0.3 = 30\%$$

In this population, at the time of examination, 30% of the horses had IURD; therefore the risk or the probability of having IURD in this population was 30%. If, for instance, someone were to buy a horse from this population without any information, the risk of buying one with IURD would be 30%.

Box 61-4   Case-Fatality Rate

A population of 100 foals was followed for 1 year. During that period, there were 20 new cases of *R. equi* pneumonia identified. Ten of the 20 affected foals died as consequence of the disease during the year. The case-fatality rate for *R. equi* pneumonia in that population of foals during that year was:

$$\text{Case-fatality rate} = \frac{10}{20} = 0.5 = 50\% \text{ in 1 year}$$

In this population, once a foal is affected by *R. equi* pneumonia, the risk or probability of dying from the disease is 50%.

$$\text{Case-fatality rate} = \frac{\begin{array}{c}\text{Number of deaths attributable to the}\\\text{disease during a specific time period}\end{array}}{\begin{array}{c}\text{Total number of cases of disease}\\\text{in that time period}\end{array}}$$

This measure of disease occurrence is often used to characterize the severity of disease and the effectiveness of treatment. Therefore the specific case-fatality rates for treated and untreated animals are often cited and compared.

Mortality rates and case-fatality rates are two of the most frequently confused epidemiologic measures, and they actually describe very different disease characteristics. Mortality rates are used to describe the risk or probability of death in a population (whether estimated by prevalence, cumulative incidence, or incidence density). This can be death attributable to all causes or death associated with a specific condition. In contrast, the case-fatality rate characterizes the likelihood of death once a condition is present. As such, the cause-specific mortality rate can be very low for a given disease, whereas the treated or untreated case-fatality rate for the same disease can be very high. For example, the mortality rate for rabies is very, very low among horses in most parts of the world. This means that very few deaths are associated with this disease in most equine populations. However, both the treated and untreated case-fatality rate is essentially 100% for rabies. This means that all horses which develop rabies can be expected to die.

Incidence Rate

The incidence rate is the number of new cases of disease per unit of animal-time. There are different ways to calculate incidence rate depending on the information available. The most accurate is as follows:

$$\text{Incidence rate} = \frac{\begin{array}{c}\text{Number of new cases of disease}\\\text{in a specific time period}\end{array}}{\begin{array}{c}\text{Sum of each individual's disease-free time}\\\text{in the population-at-risk}\\\text{in the specific time period}\end{array}}$$

The incidence rate, as the cumulative incidence, is used to assess the progression of disease in the population and can be used to predict disease occurrence. It is calculated for a specific time period, but it represents a measure of the "speed" of the disease in the population over time. In practice, incidence rate and cumulative incidence are used as approximations of each other and are given the same interpretation. The type of the population (open or closed) and the data available are what determines which is calculated. The incidence rate is not a true measure of risk but can be and is used as such (Box 61-5).

In the example in Box 61-5, we can say that, if everything remains constant, the disease is "moving" through the population at an average "speed" of 26 cases per 100 horses per year. For practical purposes, we might also say that there is a 26%

Box 61-5   Incidence Rate

A total of 100 horses were followed for 1 year. During the year, there were 20 new cases of IURD, all of which occurred in the third month of the year (0.25 year). In addition, 10 horses were sold and left the population at 6 months (0.5 year) into the year, and another 5 horses died of other causes. Among these five horses, one died at 2 months (0.2 year) into the year, two at 4 months (0.3 year), and the other two at 9 months (0.75 year) into the year. The incidence rate was:

Incidence rate

$$= \frac{20}{(65\times1)+(10\times0.5)+(1\times0.2)+(2\times0.3)+(2\times0.75)+(20\times0.25)}$$

$$= \frac{20}{77.3}$$

Incidence rate $\cong$ 0.26 cases/horse-years or 26 cases/100 horse-years
Explanation of the calculations in the denominator:
65×01 = Time-at-risk accumulated by horses that never developed IURD and were at risk for the disease for the entire 1 year (disease-free time).
10×0.5 = Time-at-risk accumulated by horses that left the population in the middle of the year and thus were at risk for IURD for 0.5 year each.
(1×0.2), (2×0.3), and (2×0.75) = Time-at-risk accumulated by horses that died of other causes and were at risk of IURD during the time they were alive: 0.2 year for one horse, 0.3 year for two horses, and 0.75 year for two horses.
20×0.25 = Time-at-risk accumulated by horses that developed IURD at 3 months into the year and were at risk for the disease for 0.25 year each.

---

risk of developing IURD in this population in 1 year, although this is a less precise interpretation.

Two other approximations can be used to estimate the denominator incidence rates when information on disease-free time for each individual horse is not available: (1) average the population-at-risk at the beginning and at the end of the time period of interest or (2) use an estimate of the total population at a certain point in time during the period of interest (usually the middle of the time period) as the average population-at-risk. In both cases, we assume that the average population represents the average number of horses at risk for a period of time equivalent to the follow-up period, and we calculate the incidence rate denominator as the product between the average population-at-risk and the follow-up period.

In these examples, we assumed that once a horse developed IURD, it also developed immunity to the disease, and thus there were no recurrences during that year. To account for recurrences, the total number of occurrences per horse would be included in the numerator, with the total disease-free time between occurrences for each horse included in the denominator.

Relationship between Prevalence and Incidence

Prevalence of disease is a function of disease incidence and duration.[43] In general, prevalence increases as the incidence and duration of disease increase, and vice versa (Box 61-6). This relationship can be used for approximation of incidence or prevalence if one measure or the other is available.

Temporal Patterns of Disease

Characterizing and understanding the occurrence of disease over time in populations are very useful and can provide great insight into the infectivity and contagiousness of disease. One standard method of graphically summarizing disease temporally is to generate an epidemic curve by plotting the number of new

Box 61-6   Prevalence and Incidence

In Box 61-2 the cumulative incidence of IURD was 20%. Assume average disease duration of 7 days (or 0.02 year). The prevalence of IURD at any given day of the year is approximately:

$$Prevalence \cong \frac{Cumulative\ incidence \times Duration}{(Cumulative\ incidence \times Duration) + 1} = \frac{0.20 \times 0.02}{(0.20 \times 0.02) + 1}$$

$$= 0.4\%$$

occurrences that develop per units of time (time is traditionally graphed on the *x* axis in whatever intervals make sense; case frequency is plotted on the *y* axis; Fig. 61-2). In general, the occurrence of disease over time can be grouped into four categories: endemic, epidemic, pandemic, and sporadic.[30]

A disease is endemic (Fig. 61-2, *A*) if it occurs at some predictable rate regardless of whether that rate is high, low, or varies during a given year or other specific time period. For example, in some regions of the United States, Potomac horse fever (PHF) is endemic because the number of new cases is relatively constant from year to year. Salmonellosis is also endemic throughout the United States, although the rates predictably increase in the summer and early fall.

A disease is epidemic (Fig. 61-2, *B*) when it occurs at a level beyond that which is typical or expected in the population.[30] For example, introduction of WNV into the United States created epidemics in horse populations throughout North America.[13,44-50] Strangles is endemic in the United States as a whole but often occurs as outbreaks or epidemics at the local level. When epidemics affect populations across multiple continents, then disease is sometimes considered pandemic (e.g., H5N1 avian influenza in 2003–2005,[51] "type 2" (H3N8) equine influenza in 1963[52-55]) (Fig. 61-2, *C*). Epidemics and pandemics occur when a highly contagious disease is introduced into a susceptible population.

A disease is considered sporadic (Fig. 61-2, *D*) if it occurs irregularly and haphazardly; sporadic disease can occur as a single case or as a cluster of cases. Vesicular stomatitis occurs sporadically in horses in the western United States.[56-58] Sporadic disease can be the result of infrequent contact between a susceptible animal and a reservoir of disease.

From a conceptual perspective, epidemics can be further separated into two general patterns: point-source and propagated (Fig. 61-3). A point-source epidemic occurs when many horses in a population are exposed at the same time to a specific disease agent. For example, a point-source epidemic might occur if a group of horses are all exposed at the same time to a toxin in the feed, such as mycotoxin-contaminated ryegrass hay.[59] An epidemic curve of a point-source outbreak (Fig. 61-3, *A*) shows a high number of initial cases, but the number of new cases often taper off quickly when the exposure to the agent is removed or disappears. Propagated epidemics occur when an infectious agent, equine influenza virus,[60] is spread from one or a few initially infected horses ("primary" cases) to other susceptible horses ("secondary" cases) that spread disease themselves (Fig. 61-3, *B*). For propagated epidemics of contagious disease, the number of new cases classically increases exponentially over days to weeks as susceptible horses become infected, then tapers off gradually as the number of susceptible horses in the population decreases and concomitantly, exposures decrease.

This conceptual model of different epidemics is very useful, but differentiating between point-source and propagated outbreaks is not always easy based on the shape of their epidemic curves. For example, a group of horses could all develop salmonellosis after consuming contaminated feed; the horses may then shed *Salmonella* in their feces, thus infecting other horses

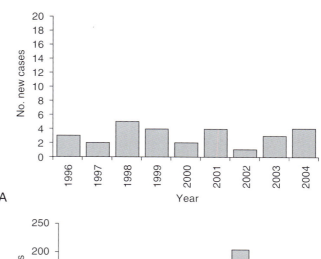

A

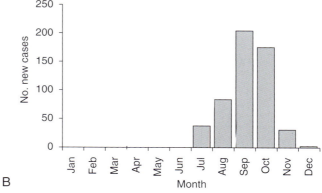

B

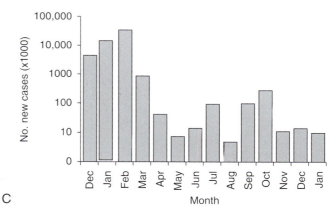

C

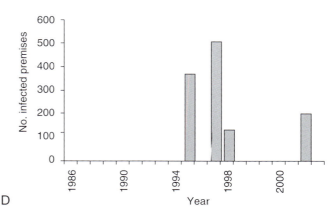

D

Figure 61-2 Epidemic curves associated with **A,** endemic disease (Potomac horse fever); **B,** epidemic disease (equine West Nile encephalitis cases in California[70]); **C,** pandemic disease (H5N1 avian influenza in Asia 2003–2005[51]); and **D,** sporadic disease (vesicular stomatitis in western United States[57,58,71-73]).

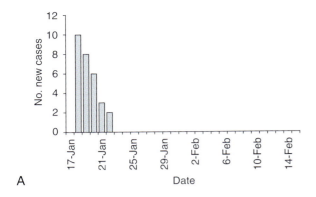

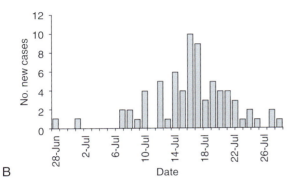

Figure 61-3 Epidemic curves from point-source outbreak of neurologic signs associated with **A,** consumption of mycotoxin-contaminated ryegrass,[59] and **B,** propagated outbreak of infectious upper respiratory disease.[60]

in their paddocks. Although the disease outbreak originated from a single source, it was then propagated through fecal-oral transmission. The shape and time scale of a propagated epidemic curve are affected by the disease incubation period, how contagious the disease is, what proportion of horses in the herd are susceptible, and how densely the horses are housed.[30]

Comparing Groups

There are two important questions to answer when comparing data from two or more groups. First, how "big" is the difference between groups? One way of evaluating how "big" is "big" is to consider whether the difference seems biologically or economically meaningful. The second question that must be considered is whether the observed difference is "real," or could it be caused more by chance variation than by a systematic difference? To quantify the size of differences between groups, typically a summary measure, such as averages or proportions, is compared or a measure of association, such as an odds ratio or relative risk, is calculated. Using this comparative information, it is necessary to evaluate whether the observed differences are meaningful or trivial. For example, in a study evaluating *Salmonella* shedding among colic patients, the association between having a fever and shedding *Salmonella* was reported[61] as an odds ratio of 9.0 with a *p* value of <0.01, indicating that horses shedding *Salmonella* were about nine times more likely to have a fever than horses not shedding *Salmonella*. This seems like a meaningful difference (i.e., nine times more likely is biologically meaningful), and the *p* value suggests that this difference is unlikely to have occurred from chance alone.

To evaluate whether there is a "real" difference versus a difference that occurred from chance variation, we typically use some type of statistical evaluation (e.g., chi-square test, z-test)

and consider the *p* value. The *p* value indicates the statistical significance of the association, or how likely we are to see results this extreme if no association existed between the factor and the disease.[62] A *p* value of <0.01 suggests that if there truly were no causal association between fever and *Salmonella* shedding, we would still see an odds ratio of 9.0 in a similar study less than 1% of the time. In other words, it is likely that the association is real, not just coincidence. The *p* value is greatly affected by the number of horses in the study (i.e., study power), the magnitude of the difference being measured (i.e., strength of association), and the degree of variation in the groups being compared (did all febrile horses and none of the afebrile horses shed *Salmonella*, or was there more variation in shedding within febrile and afebrile groups?). In general, the *p* value decreases as the number of animals being studied increases, as the magnitude of difference increases, and as the variation within each group decreases. The *p* value does not provide any information about whether the difference between groups is meaningful.

Using Measurement Data

Is the Difference Real?

If data follow a bell-shaped curve, the z-test or t-test can be used to determine how likely it is that the difference is real and not caused by chance variation. Many basic statistical packages (e.g., http://wwwn.cdc.gov/epiinfo/) will perform these simple statistical tests, or you can even use online calculators (e.g., http://www.vassarstats.net/tu.html). You can also perform this simple calculation by hand. To calculate the z-test by hand, the standard deviation (SD) of each group's data (a $5 calculator can do this for you), the number (count) of horses in each group, and the z-score values for different "confidence" levels (95% = 1.96; 90% = 1.64; 80% = 1.28) must be known. The following formula is used to calculate the limits for a confidence interval, using the 95% z-score of 1.96:

$$\text{Average1} - \text{Average2} \pm \left(\text{z-score} \times \sqrt{\frac{\text{SD1}^2}{\text{count1}} + \frac{\text{SD2}^2}{\text{count2}}} \right)$$

If the range estimated by this calculation does not include zero, there is 95% confidence that the observed difference is real and not caused by chance. If the range does include zero, the equation is recalculated using the 90% z-score of 1.64. If the new range does not include zero, there is 90% confidence that the difference is real. If the 90% range includes zero, the equation is recalculated using the 80% z-score. If the range does not include zero, there is 80% confidence that the difference is real; if the range does include zero, there is less than 80% confidence that the difference is real.

For example, if there was a concern that poor ventilation in Barn A was affecting the horses, rectal temperature data for 10 horses in Barn A and 15 horses in Barn B could be collected. If the average temperature of horses in Barn A was 102.0°F (38.8°C) with SD of 0.56, compared with 100.6°F (38.1°C) with SD of 0.71 for horses in Barn B, the limits for a 95% confidence interval for the average difference could be calculated using the following equation:

$$102.0 - 100.6 \pm \left(1.96 \times \sqrt{\frac{0.56^2}{10} + \frac{0.71^2}{15}} \right) = 1.4 \pm 0.50 = 0.9, 1.9$$

The 95% confidence interval for the difference of these average rectal temperatures is 0.9 to 1.9, which does not include zero, so there is 95% confidence that the difference is real and not caused by chance variation. Is an average body temperature difference of 1.4°F biologically meaningful? That cannot be determined by a statistical test and is better determined using clinical experience and judgment.

Using Categorical Data

In epidemiology, it is common to use the term *exposure* to refer to an individual's experience with a risk factor. In a study of EPM occurrence, lack of feed security was identified as a potential risk factor for the disease.[41] Horses "exposed" to "lack of feed security" were more likely to have EPM than horses "not exposed" to "lack of feed security" (i.e., horses that had their feed safely stored). Thus it is important to notice that "exposure" is used broadly in epidemiology and does not necessarily refer to the physical contact between the risk factor and the individual, as it might initially suggest.

Various measures of association can be used to characterize relationships between risk factors and disease. The timing of data collection relative to disease occurrence dictates to a great extent which measures of association are appropriate. If horses exposed and not exposed to a potential risk factor are followed over time to determine occurrence of disease (cohort studies), measures of incidence are obtained, and measures of association (e.g., attributable risk, attributable fraction, relative risk, odds ratio) can all be estimated. If diseased and nondiseased horses are compared in relation to their past or current exposure to a potential risk factor (case-control and cross-sectional studies), the odds ratio is the measure of association estimated.

Comparing Cumulative Incidence: Attributable Risk and Attributable Fraction

The attributable risk (AR) estimates the absolute amount of risk that is conferred or attributed to exposure in the group of individuals with the risk factor. The AR is calculated as the difference between the cumulative incidence in horses exposed and not exposed to the risk factor. Similarly, the attributable fraction (AF) is the proportion of risk attributable to exposure to the risk factor and is calculated as the AR divided by the cumulative incidence in the exposed group (Box 61-7).

In Box 61-7, 50% (10% of 20%) of the risk of IURD in horses housed in poor bedding conditions is attributable to the actual exposure to poor bedding conditions. In other words, if you could transfer all horses in poor bedding conditions to good bedding conditions, you might expect that this would prevent 50% of disease in that group. In the population there is a mixture of horses exposed and not exposed to poor bedding conditions. Therefore the reduction in disease occurrence in the population as a whole (not only in the exposed group) will depend on the proportion or prevalence of exposure in that population.

To determine the impact of control and preventive measures in the population, two other measures can be calculated: the population AR and the population AF. The population AR measures the amount of risk attributable to exposure in the population and is calculated as the product of the AR and the prevalence of exposure in the population.[43] The population AF is the proportion of risk attributable to exposure in the population and is calculated as the population AR divided by the cumulative incidence of the disease in the entire population (CI_{TP}) (Box 61-8).[43]

Comparing Cumulative Incidence: Relative Risk

The relative risk or risk ratio (RR) is the ratio between the cumulative incidence or disease risk in the exposed and nonexposed groups. It measures how large the cumulative incidence is in the exposed group compared with the nonexposed group (Box 61-9).

Comparing Prevalences: Odds Ratio

The odds ratio (OR) is the ratio between the odds of disease in the exposed group and the odds of disease in the nonexposed

---

Box 61-7 Attributable Risk

Assume that veterinarians at a racetrack believe that housing conditions contribute to the risk of IURD occurrence and that exposure to dusty environments with high levels of ammonia increase the likelihood of IURD occurrence. In other words, they believe that poor bedding (PB) conditions serve as a risk factor for IURD. A cohort study was designed to determine whether there was an association between PB conditions and occurrence of IURD. A sample of 100 horses housed in PB conditions and another sample of 100 horses housed in good bedding (GB) conditions were followed for 1 year. The cumulative incidence (CI) was calculated for both groups and compared. The data are presented below:

	Poor Bedding	Good Bedding	
IURD+	20	10	30
IURD−	80	90	170
	100	100	

$$CIPB = \frac{20}{100} = 20\% \quad CIGB = \frac{10}{100} = 10\%$$

$$\text{Attributable risk} = CIPB - CIGB = 20\% - 10\% = 10\%$$

$$\text{Attributable fraction} = \frac{CIPB - CIGB}{CIPB} = \frac{20\% - 10\%}{20\%} = 50\%$$

In this example, the attributable risk indicates that 10% of the 20% total risk of IURD in horses exposed to poor bedding conditions was actually attributable to the horses being housed in poor bedding conditions. The attributable fraction indicates that this 10% of the risk represented 50% of the total risk of IURD in the horses exposed to poor bedding conditions. Note that IURD also occurred in horses housed in good bedding conditions. Therefore, poor bedding conditions contribute to an increase in IURD but are not the only factor associated with its occurrence.

---

group. It measures how large the odds of disease are in the exposed group compared with the nonexposed group. Frequently, diseased and nondiseased horses are the groups selected in epidemiologic studies, and differences in exposure between groups are determined. In these cases, strictly speaking, the OR is the ratio between the odds of exposure in the diseased group over the odds of exposure in the nondiseased group. However, mathematically, the OR calculated as the odds of exposure in the diseased and nondiseased groups and the odds of disease in the exposed and nonexposed groups are the same (Box 61-10).

The RR and OR are also called "measures of strength of association" as they are not only indicators of whether an association exists, but also the direction and strength of the association. An RR or OR of 5 indicates a much stronger association between the risk factor and the disease than an RR or OR of 1.5. An RR or OR equal to 1 indicates no association between the risk factor and the disease. In other words, it indicates that disease is as likely to occur in the exposed as the nonexposed group. An RR or OR less than 1 indicates that the risk factor is actually protective for the disease and technically is not a risk but a protective factor. A common example is vaccination. An RR or OR of 0.5 obtained when comparing occurrence of disease in vaccinated (exposed) and nonvaccinated (nonexposed) horses indicates that disease occurrence in vaccinated horses is about half of that in nonvaccinated horses.

Outbreak Investigations: Attack Risk Table

An attack risk (attack rate) table is a quick and simple way to summarize exposures and disease occurrence and also to look for factors strongly associated with disease. It is often used to analyze data quickly during an outbreak. Consider a farm on which 10 cases of strangles are diagnosed in a population of 100

Box 61-8 Attributable Fraction

Based on the information obtained in the study described in Box 61-7, the veterinarians at the racetrack decided to implement a program to improve bedding conditions in the entire racetrack (the population). They want to know the impact such a program will have in reducing IURD in the population. According to a previous survey conducted at the racetrack, approximately 30% of the horses were housed in poor bedding conditions (exposure prevalence). Using the data from Box 61-7, the population attributable risk (PAR) and the population attributable fraction (PAF) were:

$$\text{Population attributable risk} = AR \times \text{Exposure prevalence} = 10\% \times 30\% = 3\%$$

$$\text{Population attributable fraction} = \frac{PAR}{CI_{TP}} = \frac{3\%}{13\%} = 23\%$$

Where:
CI_{TP} = Cumulative incidence of IURD in the entire population
CI_{TP} = $(CI_{PB} \times \text{exposure prevalence}) + [CI_{GB} \times (1 - \text{exposure prevalence})]$
CI_{TP} = $(20\% \times 30\%) + (10\% \times 70\%) = 13\%$
By implementing a program to improve bedding conditions at the racetrack, practitioners may expect an absolute reduction of 3% in the total IURD incidence. This reduction represents approximately 23% of the total current incidence of IURD (13%) at the racetrack. In other words, the veterinarians might expect to reduce the total incidence of IURD at the racetrack from 13% to 10%. The PAR and the PAF can also be calculated as:

$$\text{Population attributable risk} = CI_{TP} - CI_{GB}$$

$$\text{Population attributable fraction} = \frac{CI_{TP} - CI_{GB}}{CI_{TP}}$$

Where:
CI_{TP} = Cumulative incidence of IURD in the entire population
CI_{GB} = Cumulative incidence of IURD in the nonexposed (good bedding) horses

Box 61-9 Relative Risk

As in Box 61-7, a cohort study was designed to determine whether there was an association between poor bedding conditions and occurrence of IURD. A sample of 100 horses housed in poor bedding conditions and another sample of 100 housed in good bedding conditions were followed for 1 year. The cumulative incidence (CI) was calculated and compared between groups. The data are presented below:

	Poor Bedding	Good Bedding	
IURD+	20	10	30
IURD−	80	90	170
	100	100	200

$$CI_{PB} = \frac{20}{100} = 20\%$$

$$CI_{GB} = \frac{10}{100} = 10\%$$

$$RR = \frac{CI_{PB}}{CI_{GB}} = \frac{20\%}{10\%} = 2$$

A relative risk (RR) of 2 indicates that the cumulative incidence of IURD in horses exposed to poor bedding conditions is twice the cumulative incidence of IURD in horses in good bedding conditions. Horses in poor bedding conditions are twice as likely to develop IURD as horses in good bedding conditions.

Box 61-10 Odds Ratio

A study was conducted to evaluate risk factors associated with development of equine protozoal myeloencephalitis (EPM). Using a case-control study design, horses with EPM were identified for enrollment. "Security" of the hay fed to the horses from wildlife was evaluated as one of the potential risk factors.[41] Horses fed hay from "nonsecure" sources were considered "exposed," whereas horses fed hay that was protected from exposure to definitive hoses (secure hay) were considered "nonexposed."

	EPM+	EPM−	
Hay not secured	86	51	137
Secured hay	43	48	91
	129	99	228

Calculations for the odds ratio for EPM occurrence in the exposed and nonexposed groups is shown below:

$$\text{Odds ratio} = \frac{86 \times 48}{51 \times 43} \cong 2$$

An odds ratio of 2 indicates that horses exposed to nonsecure hay were approximately two times more likely to develop EPM than horses fed secure hay. Note that the interpretation of the odds ratio is similar to the interpretation of the relative risk (see Box 61-9), even though measures of disease incidence were not calculated. In epidemiologic studies the odds ratio is used as an approximation of the relative risk when the study design does not allow the calculation of measures of incidence. This approximation is more precise when the disease is rare in the population.[30]

horses. Several potential disease sources exist on the farm: a newly arrived horse, a used feed trough recently purchased from a neighbor, and participation in a recent horse show. Exposure data are collected on all horses; all horses are categorized as sick/well using a standardized case definition and as exposed or not exposed to each potential risk factor; and the attack risk table is constructed (Table 61-1).

For each potential disease source, the total number of horses exposed and unexposed should equal the number of horses on the farm. The attack risk for horses exposed to a factor is calculated by dividing the number of horses exposed and ill by the total number exposed. Likewise, the attack risk for horses not exposed to the factor is calculated by dividing the number of horses unexposed and ill by the total number unexposed. The risk ratio is calculated by dividing the attack risk for exposed horses by the attack risk for unexposed horses. The

Table 61-1 Attack Risk Table (Constructed as Described in Text)

Factor	Exposed	Ill and Exposed	Attack Risk for Exposed	Not Exposed	Ill and Unexposed	Attack Risk for Unexposed	Risk Ratio
New horse	14	3	$\frac{3}{14} = 0.21$	86	7	$\frac{7}{86} = 0.08$	$\frac{0.21}{0.08} = 2.6$
New trough	25	3	$\frac{3}{25} = 0.12$	75	7	$\frac{7}{75} = 0.09$	$\frac{0.12}{0.09} = 1.3$
Horse show	20	6	$\frac{6}{20} = 0.30$	80	4	$\frac{4}{80} = 0.05$	$\frac{0.30}{0.05} = 6.0$

Table 61-2 A 2×2 Table Constructed for Chi-Square Test (as Described in Text)

	Sick	Well	Total
Exposed	A	B	C
Unexposed	D	E	F
Total	G	H	I

Table 61-3 Example of Chi-Square Table (as Described in Text)

	Strangles	Healthy	Total
Attended horse show	6	14	20
Did not attend horse show	4	76	80
Total	10	90	100

higher the risk ratio, the stronger is the association between factor and disease. In this example, it appears the horse show was the source of the strangles outbreak. Horses that went to the show were six times more likely to have strangles than those that did not go.

Is the Difference Real?

If data can be summarized in a contingency table (e.g., a 2×2 table), a chi-square test can help determine how likely it is that an observed difference is real and not just caused by chance variation. Many basic statistical packages (e.g., http://wwwn.cdc.gov/epiinfo/) will perform this simple calculation or you can even use online calculators (e.g., http://www.vassarstats.net/odds2x2.html). You can also perform this simple calculation by hand. For hand calculation, the following chi-square values are used: 95% = 3.84; 90% = 2.70; and 80% = 1.64. Data are frequently summarized in a 2×2 table as shown in Table 61-2.

Disease categories (e.g., sick vs. well) are placed in columns and exposure status (exposed vs. unexposed) in rows. An example using data from the attack risk table on horses with and without strangles that did and did not attend a recent horse show (see Table 61-1) is shown in Table 61-3.

The chi-square value is calculated by using the following formula:

$$\frac{[(A \times E) - (B \times D)]^2 \times I}{C \times F \times G \times H}$$

$$\frac{[(6 \times 76) - (14 \times 4)]^2 \times 100}{20 \times 80 \times 10 \times 90} = \frac{[400]^2 \times 100}{1,440,000} = 11.11$$

This value can be compared to the value obtained with the 80%, 90%, and 95% chi-square values. If the chi-square value is greater than the 95% chi-square value (3.84), there is 95%

confidence that the difference is real. If the chi-square value is less than the 95% value but greater than the 90% value (2.70), there is 90% confidence that the difference is real. Similarly, if the chi-square value is less than the 90% value but greater than the 80% value (1.64), there is 80% confidence that the difference is real. In this example, the chi-square value of 11.11 is greater than the 95% value of 3.84, so there is 95% confidence that the difference in strangles occurrence between horses that did and did not attend a recent horse show is real and not caused by chance variation (i.e., $p < 0.05$).

Properties of Diagnostic Tests

In a medical context, a diagnostic test can be defined as any process or device designed to detect or quantify a sign, substance, tissue change, or body response[43] and used to gain additional information regarding the health or exposure status of an individual or population. Laboratory tests (e.g., antibody detection, cultures, polymerase chain reaction [PCR], histology) and imaging procedures (e.g., plain radiographs, ultrasonography, endoscopy, magnetic resonance imaging [MRI]) are some of the most obvious diagnostic tests used. However, a clinical examination and a questionnaire designed to obtain information about the health status of an individual can also be considered a test. This section focuses on diagnostic tests as they apply to the diagnosis of infectious disease in horses; however, the principles presented here are valid for any other type of test.

Types of Measurement

Test results can be broadly divided into qualitative and quantitative. Qualitative test results are reported in a nominal (positive or negative) or ordinal (positive, weak positive, or negative) scale and most often represent the presence or absence of antibodies or antigens in body fluids or tissues. Examples of qualitative test results in horses include the Western blot test for detection of serum antibodies against *Sarcocystis neurona*[63] and the reverse transcriptase–PCR (RT-PCR) test on nasal swabs for detection of ribonucleic acid (RNA) from equine influenza virus.[60]

Quantitative test results are reported in an interval scale (titers) or continuous scale (e.g., enzyme-linked immunosorbent assay [ELISA] optical densities, mg/dL) and usually represent direct or indirect measures of antibody, antigen, or enzyme concentrations. Examples include the indirect fluorescent antibody test (IFAT) for detection of serum antibody titers against *S. neurona*,[64] the ELISA used to detect antibody concentrations (based on optical densities) against WNV,[65] and liver function tests to detect enzyme concentrations in blood.[66] Quantitative test results are often categorized (dichotomized) into positive or negative to facilitate interpretation of test results and estimate certain test characteristics.

Test Accuracy

Test accuracy is the ability of a test to determine correctly the true status of an individual. In the context of infectious diseases of horses, test accuracy is the ability of the test to differentiate correctly between infected and noninfected horses. Test accuracy is basically determined by two characteristics: sensitivity and specificity. Test sensitivity is the proportion of infected horses correctly identified by the test as infected. Test specificity is the proportion of noninfected horses correctly identified by the test as noninfected. When sensitivity and specificity are less than 100%, their complement (1 − sensitivity and 1 − specificity) represent the proportion of false-negative and false-positive results, respectively.

Estimation of Sensitivity and Specificity

Diagnostic test sensitivity and specificity should ideally be characterized using appropriately designed, population-based studies (test validation studies).[67] There are several variations in study designs, but in general, these studies should include a representative (e.g., various ages, gender, breeds) random sample of the population of horses in which the test will ultimately be applied.[67] Typically, horses enrolled in validation studies are identified as infected or noninfected based on another diagnostic test that is considered the definitive, "gold standard" test. Traditionally, sensitivity and specificity have often been estimated by comparing test results from the test of interest (often a newly developed test) with the results from the gold standard test in the infected and noninfected groups, respectively (Box 61-11).

Estimation of sensitivity and specificity in Box 61-11 is straightforward because the test results are inherently dichotomous. In such cases the data can be simply cross-tabulated into a 2 × 2 table and the values for sensitivity and specificity calculated. However, when test results are quantitative (e.g., titers, white blood cell counts, optical densities), it is necessary to determine a cutoff value for a positive test result in order to estimate test sensitivity and specificity. The choice of a cutoff

value is somewhat arbitrary and is affected by the purpose of the testing.[68] For example, in a screening program to detect exposure to some infectious agent, the purpose is to detect all horses possibly exposed to that agent. In such cases, choosing a lower cutoff value will maximize test sensitivity and minimize the number of false-negative results. On the other hand, an equine clinician may want to determine whether a horse is infected with a certain agent, with minimal chances of misclassification. In such cases the cutoff of choice will be the one that maximizes sensitivity and specificity and minimizes the number of both false-negative and false-positive results. This cutoff value that yields the highest sensitivity and specificity is frequently the choice. To determine that cutoff value, values of sensitivity and specificity are calculated using all test results as possible cutoff values (Box 61-12).

Another option to measure accuracy of a quantitative test is the use of likelihood ratios for specific test results. Likelihood ratios measure how likely a specific test result will occur in an infected horse compared with a noninfected horse. Likelihood ratios for specific test results are calculated as the proportion of infected horses that have a certain test result over the proportion of noninfected horses that have that same test result. The

---

Box 61-11 Sensitivity and Specificity

A study was conducted to estimate the sensitivity and specificity of the Western blot test for the diagnosis of equine protozoal myeloencephalitis (EPM) caused by *Sarcocystis neurona*.[63] This study included serum samples from 63 neurologic horses necropsied at the California State Laboratory. All horses were evaluated using the "gold standard" method and classified as having or not having *S. neurona* parasites or lesions characteristic of EPM in their central nervous system. Serum samples were tested by the Western blot for detection of antibodies against *S. neurona*. The data are presented below.

		Gold Standard Test		
		Positive	Negative	
Western Blot	Positive	12	30	42
	Negative	3	18	21
		15	48	63

$$\text{Sensitivity (Se)} = \frac{12}{15} = 80\%$$

$$\text{Specificity (Sp)} = \frac{18}{48} = 38\%$$

$$\text{False-negative (1} - \text{Se)} = \frac{3}{15} = 20\%$$

$$\text{False-positive (1} - \text{Sp)} = \frac{30}{48} = 62\%$$

Box 61-12 Sensitivity and Specificity: *Indirect Fluorescent Antibody Test*

A study was designed to evaluate the indirect fluorescent antibody test (IFAT) for the diagnosis of equine protozoal myeloencephalitis (EPM) caused by *S. neurona*.[64] The study included serum samples from 109 horses necropsied at the California State Laboratory. All horses were identified as having or not having *S. neurona* parasites in their central nervous system (gold standard test). Serum samples were tested by IFAT for detection of antibody titers against *S. neurona*. The data are presented in Tables A and B below.

Table A. Frequency of IFAT Serum Titers for Horses Having or Not Having *S. neurona* Parasites in Their Central Nervous System

		Gold Standard	
		Positive	Negative
IFAT TITER	0	0	85
	10	0	6
	20	2	2
	40	0	1
	80	4	0
	160	3	2
	320	2	1
	640	1	0
	Total	12	97

Table B. Sensitivity and Specificity of IFAT Using Each Titer as a Potential Cutoff Value for a Positive Test Result

		Sensitivity	Specificity
Cutoff Value for a Positive Result	≥0	12/12 = 100%	0/97 = 0%
	≥10	12/12 = 100%	85/97 = 88%
	≥20	12/12 = 100%	91/97 = 94%
	≥40	10/12 = 83%	93/97 = 96%
	≥80	9/12 = 75%	93/97 = 96%
	≥160	6/12 = 50%	94/97 = 97%
	≥320	3/12 = 25%	96/97 = 99%
	≥640	1/12 = 8%	97/97 = 100%

In this example, an IFAT titer of 20 was the test result that yielded the lowest combined proportion of false-negative (0%) and false-positive (6%) results and is one potential choice for a cutoff value. Notice that there is a decrease in sensitivity and an increase in specificity as the cutoff value increases. The opposite occurs as the cutoff value decreases.

Box 61-13 Likelihood Ratio: *Indirect Fluorescent Antibody Test*

In the study evaluating the indirect fluorescent antibody test (IFAT) for the diagnosis of equine protozoal myeloencephalitis (EPM), titer-specific likelihood ratios were calculated.[64] Frequency of IFAT titers in *S. neurona*–infected and noninfected ("gold standard") horses and titer-specific likelihood ratios are presented below.

		Gold Standard		Likelihood
		Positive	Negative	Ratio
IFAT Titer	0	0	85	0.03
	10	0	6	0.7
	20	2	2	1.7
	40	0	1	4.4
	80	4	0	11.2
	160	3	2	28.7
	320	2	1	73.4
	640	1	0	187.8
	Total	12	97	

A likelihood ratio (LR) of 0.7 for an IFAT titer of 10 indicates that a titer 10 is 1.4 (1/0.7) times more likely in noninfected horses than in infected horses. On the other hand, an LR of 4.4 for a titer of 40 indicates that a titer 40 is 4.4 times more likely in infected horses than in noninfected horses. In this study, because of zero counts for some titers in both groups, a more sophisticated modeling technique was used to calculate the likelihood ratios and "smooth out" the data.[64] However, the basic principle of LR calculations can be illustrated using the nonzero cells as an example. For example, the LR for a titer of 20 would be calculated as the proportion of infected horses with a titer of 20 (2/12) over the proportion of noninfected horses with that same titer (2/97).

Box 61-14 Predictive Value: *Western Blot*

From Box 61-11, data on serum Western blot test results for 63 neurologic horses identified as having ("gold standard" positive) or not having ("gold standard" negative) *S. neurona* in the central nervous system are presented below.[63] Positive and negative predictive values were calculated.

		Gold Standard Test		
		Positive	Negative	
Western Blot	Positive	12	30	42
	Negative	3	18	21
		15	48	63

$$\text{Positive predictive value} = \frac{12}{42} = 29\%$$

$$\text{Negative predictive value} = \frac{18}{21} = 86\%$$

In this example, only 29% of the test-positive horses were actually infected with *S. neurona*, whereas 86% of the test-negative horses were truly noninfected.

---

advantages of likelihood ratios are that each test result has its own interpretation, and there is no need to choose a cutoff value for a positive test result. Thus there is more flexibility in test interpretation[64] (Box 61-13).

Interpretation of Test Results: Predictive Values

The ultimate question to answer after testing a horse for an infectious agent is whether or not that horse is really infected and has a particular disease. If a test could be found that was 100% sensitive and 100% specific, the answer to this question would be straightforward; a positive test result would indicate that a horse is infected, and a negative test result would indicate that a horse is not infected. Unfortunately, although some tests are more accurate than others, probably no tests truly have either 100% sensitivity or 100% specificity. In addition, regardless of how accurate a test is thought to be, the probability that tests will correctly predict disease or infection status is not the same for all populations.

Therefore we need to understand and use the predictive values to help us correctly interpret test results. Predictive values refer to the probability of being affected/infected given the test result (positive or negative). As such, the positive predictive value is the probability that a horse is infected given a positive test result. The negative predictive value is the probability that a horse is not infected given a negative test result. Predictive values are calculated as the proportion of truly infected horses among the test-positive horses (positive predictive value) and the proportion of truly noninfected horses among test-negative horses (negative predictive value) (Box 61-14).

At this point, it is important to distinguish between true prevalence (TP) and apparent prevalence (AP). True prevalence is the proportion of horses that actually have the infection or disease in the population, whereas apparent prevalence is the proportion of horses that test positive for the infection or disease.[43] True prevalence is the prevalence value used in calculating predictive values. In Box 61-14, TP was 24% (15/63), whereas AP was 67% (42/63). The TP and AP relate to each other as follows:

$$TP = \frac{AP + \text{Specificity} - 1}{\text{Sensitivity} + \text{Specificity} - 1}$$

Notice that if the sensitivity and specificity are 100%, the true prevalence and apparent prevalence are equal.

Predictive values can be directly calculated only from 2×2 tables when the study is conducted using a representative sample of the population, because in such cases the prevalence of the disease in the study group is an unbiased estimate of the prevalence of disease in the population. When this is not the case, the predictive values from 2×2 tables will be biased and should be calculated using an independent prevalence estimate by the following formulas:

$$\text{Positive predictive value} = \frac{\text{Prevalence} \times \text{Sensitivity}}{(\text{Prevalence} \times \text{Sensitivity}) + (1 - \text{Prevalence}) \times (1 - \text{Specificity})}$$

$$\text{Negative predictive value} = \frac{(1 - \text{Prevalence}) \times (\text{Specificity})}{[(1 - \text{Prevalence}) \times (\text{Specificity})] + [(\text{Prevalence}) \times (1 - \text{Sensitivity})]}$$

Predictive values are greatly affected by differences in test sensitivity, test specificity, and prevalence of disease in the population. For fixed values of sensitivity and specificity, the positive predictive value increases and the predictive value negative decreases as the prevalence increases (Fig. 61-4). This means that even when sensitivity and specificity are high, the probability of infection given a positive test result is low when the prevalence is low, and probability of infection is high when the prevalence is high. Similarly, the probability of no infection given a negative test result is high when the prevalence is low and low when prevalence is high (Box 61-15).

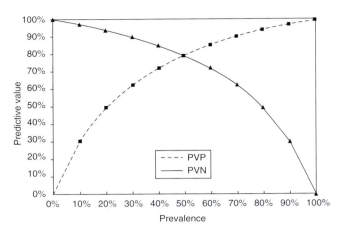

Figure 61-4 Relationship among positive predictive value *(PVP)*, negative predictive value *(PVN)*, and prevalence.

Box 61-15 Predictive Value: *Enzyme-Linked Immunosorbent Assay*

Assume a hypothetical scenario in which two populations of neurologic horses (i.e., from two veterinary hospitals in different parts of the country) were serologically tested for diagnosis of West Nile virus (WNV) infection. In Population 1, independent virus isolation studies have shown that the true prevalence of WNV is 1%, and in Population 2, the same studies have shown that WNV true prevalence is 90%. Both populations were tested with the same test, an enzyme-linked immunosorbent assay (ELISA), for detection of antibodies against WNV and determination of the infection status. Assume that the test has been shown to be 90% sensitive and 90% specific and that 1000 horses from each population were tested. The 2×2 tables below show the data for each population. The data in each cell of these 2×2 tables were distributed based on the prevalence and test characteristic information.

Population 1
Infected

		Yes	No	
ELISA	**Positive**	9	99	108
	Negative	1	891	892
		10	990	1000

$$\text{Positive predictive value} = \frac{9}{108} = 8\%$$

$$\text{Negative predictive value} = \frac{891}{892} = 99\%$$

Population 2
Infected

		Yes	No	
ELISA	**Positive**	810	10	820
	Negative	90	90	180
		900	100	1000

$$\text{Positive predictive value} = \frac{810}{820} = 99\%$$

$$\text{Negative predictive value} = \frac{90}{180} = 50\%$$

Despite the use of the same test, the probability that a test-positive horse is infected in Population 1 is only 8%, compared with the 99% in Population 2. This means that the majority (99/108) of the test-positive horses in Population 1 were actually false-positive results. Similarly, the probability that a test-negative horse is actually not infected in Population 1 is 99% versus 50% in Population 2. Therefore 50% of the test-negative horses in Population 2 were actually infected and were false-negative results.

When likelihood ratios for specific test results are used instead of sensitivity and specificity, the probability of disease for each specific test result can be calculated using the following formula:

Probability of disease given a specific test result

$$= \frac{(\text{Prevalence}/1 - P) \times \text{Likelihood ratio}}{(\text{Prevalence}/1 - \text{Prevalence} \times \text{Likelihood ratio}) + 1}$$

Using Tests in Combination

Frequently, two or more tests are used in the diagnosis of disease or infection. The tests can be used simultaneously or in sequence, and the results can be interpreted in parallel or in series. In parallel interpretation, horses testing positive in one or more tests are considered positive.[43] For example, horses might be considered infected with *Salmonella enteritidis* after testing positive in at least one of several fecal cultures performed in sequence. In series interpretation, horses are considered positive only if they test positive in all tests.[43] For example, horses tested for EPM might be considered infected only if they test positive for *S. neurona* antibodies in serum and in cerebrospinal fluid (CSF). Note that the serum and CSF tests can be run simultaneously or in sequence when a CSF test is run only in seropositive horses. When multiple tests are used, the sensitivity and specificity of the combination of tests are different than the sensitivity and specificity of each test separately. In parallel interpretation the combination of tests has higher sensitivity but lower specificity than each individual test. In series interpretation the combination of tests has lower sensitivity and higher specificity than each individual test.

Other Diagnostic Test Characteristics

Other characteristics of diagnostic tests that should be evaluated before or concomitantly with population-based accuracy studies include analytical sensitivity and specificity and reliability. Analytical sensitivity indicates the minimum detectable amount of the material (e.g., antibodies, antigens) being measured by the test. Analytical specificity indicates the potential for cross-reactivity with materials of no interest. Analytical sensitivity and specificity are assessed in laboratory conditions and affect the population estimates of sensitivity and specificity; however, they are different quantities. For example, information on the minimum amount of serum antibodies detected by an ELISA test for the diagnosis of a certain disease might be important to establish the optimum serum dilution to be used in the plaques when testing field samples. Similarly, samples from animals infected with various potential cross-reacting agents should be tested to assess occurrence of false-positive results.

Reliability is the ability of the test to produce the same results when samples are tested multiple times in the same laboratory (repeatability) or in different laboratories (reproducibility).[43] There are various measures of reliability, including the coefficient of variation and the correlation coefficient for quantitative tests and the kappa measure of agreement for qualitative tests.[43]

Overall, these measures assess how concordant test results are in multiple testing.

Strategies for Prevention of Infectious Disease

In general, prevention of infectious disease involves altering the host, agent, or environment to make it more difficult for disease to occur or spread. We usually have little control over the disease agent, so we focus on the disease host (the horse) and its environment. A herd is best able to resist infection if the horses in it are immunized, properly nourished, and minimally stressed. An environment in which new equine arrivals are quarantined, tested for disease, and immunized before mixing with the herd minimizes the likelihood of introduction of a new disease, as does an environment where contact between disease vectors (e.g., mosquitoes, ticks) and horses is minimized. Disease spread is more easily controlled in a well-ventilated environment with easily cleanable, nonporous surfaces. Standing water in which mosquitoes breed should be minimized. Water and feed troughs should be cleaned regularly; a contaminated trough can quickly amplify an outbreak of salmonellosis or strangles.

To prevent the arrival or spread of a specific infectious disease, an understanding of the disease's life cycle and risk factors is important. How do horses become infected? Through a vector, as with WNV encephalitis? By direct contact, as with equine influenza? By indirect contact, as with salmonellosis? Through aerosol spread, as with equine influenza? Minimize horses' exposure to the source of infection. How pathogenic or virulent is the disease? Does it have a lengthy incubation period, or a carrier or persistently infected state (e.g., strangles)? Identify and isolate or treat asymptomatic horses that may be sources of infection. Does the disease agent survive in the environment (e.g., *Salmonella*)? If so, institute biosecurity measures such as foot baths to minimize environmental contamination. What are known risk factors for the disease? Is it associated with pasture grazing, as with MRLS or strongyles? Change management as necessary to minimize known risk factors for the disease.

Managing an Outbreak of Infectious Disease

An outbreak investigation is a systematic approach to identifying the cause(s) and source(s) of an epidemic (see Chapter 62). The goals of an outbreak investigation are to identify the problem, identify steps that can be taken immediately to deal with the problem, and identify means by which future outbreaks can be prevented. The standard steps in an outbreak investigation are described next.

1. **Make a diagnosis.** After initial contact with the client, review relevant diagnoses before a farm visit. For each potential diagnosis, review the biology, epidemiology, diagnostic method, and treatment. At the farm, listen carefully and say nothing that might influence your client's perception of events. Take samples as needed, look for patterns that may be relevant, and define natural groups (housing, use, age, gender, or breed) that should be compared. Use clinical observations and test results to make a tentative diagnosis. If the initial diagnosis is a zoonotic or reportable disease, take appropriate action.

2. **Verify the diagnosis.** When a tentative or final diagnosis of disease has been made, ensure that it is medically sound. Use medical records, laboratory test results, and clinical examinations to confirm that the diagnosis is consistent with the information available. If the data are not consistent with the diagnosis, seek a better diagnosis.

3. **Define a "case."** To facilitate identification of cases associated with the outbreak, specify the clinical signs and test results that define a case of disease. Some illness in the population may be unrelated to the outbreak. By defining an outbreak-associated "case" of disease, unrelated illnesses may be excluded from analysis.

4. **Determine the magnitude of the problem.** Is there an epidemic? Are more horses affected by this disease than typically seen? Compute an attack risk (attack rate), as described earlier, and compare it to the normal or expected occurrence of disease, if known.

5. **Describe the outbreak temporally, spatially, and by animal characteristics.** Examine the temporal characteristics of the outbreak by creating an epidemic curve (see section on Temporal Patterns of Disease). Use the client's calendar to obtain the most accurate information on disease onset. Ask the following questions: Does it appear to be a point-source or a propagated epidemic? Does disease onset coincide with any management changes or recent additions to the farm? Describe disease spatially by making a map recording the total number of horses in each region (e.g., field, pasture, barn, farm) and the number of ill horses in each region. Be sure to record the location of feed and water sources on the map, as well as locations where horses might come in contact with wildlife or other livestock species. Record age, gender, breed, vaccination status, use, housing type, location, and feed and water sources of all animals in the population—those unaffected as well as those affected.

6. **Analyze data.** For each factor of interest (age, gender, breed, vaccination status, use, housing type, location, feed and water sources), construct an attack risk table, as described earlier. Look for differences among groups. Which factor has the strongest association?

7. **Working hypothesis.** Based on data analyses, develop hypotheses regarding the type of epidemic that is occurring (point-source versus propagated), the source of the epidemic, and possible modes of spread (e.g., direct contact, vector, fomites).

8. **Implement disease controls.** Standard disease control measures include mass treatment, quarantine, environmental hygiene, mass immunization, and applied ecology.[69] Mass treatment, such as administration of antimicrobials during a *Salmonella* outbreak, is intended to reduce transmission of disease by decreasing the amount and duration of shedding by infectious individuals and decreasing the likelihood of infection in susceptible animals. Quarantine restricts movement of horses suspected of being infectious; it is intended to reduce the likelihood that infected horses will come in contact with susceptible horses. Environmental hygiene incorporates actions that remove or prevent environmental contamination, reducing the likelihood of disease exposure for horses in that environment; use appropriate cleaning agents, and rinse thoroughly. Mass immunization (vaccination) acts to decrease the susceptibility of both the individual horse and the herd (through herd immunity). Applied ecology refers to disease control methods that target some factor other than the disease agent, such as the vector or the disease reservoir; the goal is to reduce the likelihood that horses will be exposed to disease. To apply these methods, an understanding of the disease's life cycle is important.

9. **Intensive follow-up.** Intensive follow-up includes confirmation of the diagnosis (clinical, pathologic, or microbiologic data) and confirmation of the disease source (microbiologic or toxicologic examination of feeds, fomites, or suspect carrier horses) if possible. Detailed diagrams or flowcharts of animal movements or feed preparation and distribution may be helpful in identifying points where preventive measures could be implemented.

10. **Report.** Summarize findings, and present them to the client. Colleagues and local veterinary associations may also be interested in the investigation and its results.

The complete reference list is available online at www.expertconsult.com.

Biosecurity and Control of Infectious Disease Outbreaks

62

Brandy A. Burgess and Josie L. Traub-Dargatz

Infectious diseases have spread across continents with a devastating effect on animal populations. Accordingly, the veterinarian's role in infectious disease prevention has been acknowledged for decades and is rooted in the management of rinderpest, which spread as a large epizootic in France in the mid-1700s and was the motivation for the creation of the first veterinary school, in 1762, in Lyons, France.[1] In modern times, the emergence of zoonotic diseases (e.g., Hendra virus) and multidrug resistant bacteria (e.g., methicillin-resistant *Staphylococcus aureus*) can have a significant impact on animal and public health if unmitigated.

The importance of control measures for managing infectious diseases has been acknowledged for centuries, long before the modern microbiologic era. One of the first historical figures to observe physicians transmitting pathogens to patients was Ignaz Semmelweis, a Hungarian physician (1818-1865).[2] In 1846, he deduced that medical students and physicians were transmitting pathogens to patients (puerperal fever) because of a deficiency in hygiene procedures following postmortem examinations. The problem was solved when Dr. Semmelweis instituted the use of chlorinated lime antiseptic hand washes. This was no small feat. He had surmised that puerperal fever was spread by "pathogenic" causes, before the idea of pathogens even existed. Another historical figure in infection control was Florence Nightingale (1820-1910), who observed in 1863 a very high mortality rate in London hospitals and comparatively lower mortality rates in smaller provincial hospitals.[3,4] She concluded that this difference was likely the result of patient overcrowding in London hospitals, leading to more efficient pathogen transmission. She was at the forefront of hospital surveillance for nosocomial infections.

More recently, the Study on the Efficacy of Nosocomial Infection Control (SENIC), conducted in U.S. human healthcare facilities (1970-1976), found that implementation of an infection control program reduced nosocomial infections by an estimated 32%.[5] This study specifically identified employment of trained infection control personnel, conducting surveillance activity, and having a system for reporting as important factors in the success of an infection control program. Although equivalent data for equine practices are currently not available, we can draw on the human hospital experience to improve veterinary infection control efforts.

Throughout this chapter, the term *biosecurity* is used interchangeably with *infection control* to encompass all practices intended to prevent the introduction and spread of infectious disease agents within a population, as well as the containment and subsequent disinfection to remove or inactivate infectious materials.[6] Traditionally, biosecurity focused on prevention of the introduction of an infectious agent into a population. Biocontainment, on the other hand, focused on controlling the spread of an infectious agent once it was introduced into a population. Although this distinction is reasonably straightforward, with respect to a farm or breeding facility, it is more difficult to separate biosecurity from biocontainment in the environment of an equine veterinary clinic, where disease agents are likely introduced on a daily basis, because an intended purpose of veterinary clinics is to treat sick animals. Having an infection control plan that includes screening of patients for the risk they may pose for pathogen introduction can mitigate this risk and will be a major topic discussed in this chapter.

Ethics of Infection Control

The veterinarian's oath ...

> Being admitted to the profession of veterinary medicine, I solemnly swear to use my scientific knowledge and skills for the benefit of society through the protection of animal health and welfare, the prevention and relief of animal suffering, the conservation of animal resources, the promotion of public health, and the advancement of medical knowledge. I will practice my profession conscientiously, with dignity, and in keeping with the principles of veterinary medical ethics. I accept as a lifelong obligation the continual improvement of my professional knowledge and competence.[7]

... underscores the ethical struggle of the veterinarian to protect the individual patient *(relief of animal suffering)*, protect the animal population of the present and the future *(protection of animal health and welfare)*, and protect people *(promotion of public health)*. The practice of veterinary infection control embodies many of these competing responsibilities. However, in veterinary medicine, there is very little ethical framework on which to base biosecurity decisions. A recent workshop supported by the Havemeyer Foundation brought together subject experts to address infection control concerns in equine populations.[8] Workshop participants agreed that to fulfill the ethical obligations of the profession, we must give due effort to infection control, no matter if we are practicing in a hospital or field setting or caring for an individual animal or a population of animals. Although veterinary hospital infection control is in its infancy, a survey conducted in 2004 among North American veterinary teaching hospitals found that all 30 survey respondents had some type of infection control program in their equine hospitals, as did some of the more progressive private veterinary hospitals.[3] As a profession, embracing the infection control movement allows us to meet the ethical obligations of the oath we have all taken.

Veterinarian's Role in Biosecurity

As veterinarians, we are obligated to avoid unnecessary costs and to be transparent with respect to disease risks in patients and personnel. As such, infection control is fundamental to providing excellent patient care and a safe working environment. Control of zoonotic diseases, those that can be transmitted between animals and humans, provides the opportunity for the physician and veterinarian to work together. However, opportunity does not always result in action. A study of Wisconsin physicians and veterinarians found that in general physicians are not very comfortable discussing zoonotic infections with patients; physicians felt that veterinarians should be involved in this dialogue, however, they infrequently engaged veterinarians in discussion of these diseases in their patients.[9] Research shows physicians believe it is the responsibility of public health officials or veterinarians, whereas veterinarians believe it is the responsibility of physicians or public health officials.[10] The veterinarian has a clear duty to recommend preventive measures to reduce the risk of zoonotic disease and to counsel clients to seek medical attention in the event of zoonotic disease exposure.[11]

Zoonotic diseases create the potential for liability for veterinarians when owners or personnel interact with animals in the hospital environment where the responsibility for oversight of the welfare of the people involved rests with the veterinarian. The risk of zoonotic infection is becoming greater as the percentage of the general public with compromised immune systems increases. The General Duty Clause, 5(a)(1), of the Occupational Safety and Health Act of 1970 stipulates employers be responsible for employee safety, stating an employer must "furnish to each of his employees employment and a place of employment which are free from recognized hazards that are causing or are likely to cause death or serious physical harm to his employees."[12] This includes managing the risk of exposure to zoonotic agents. In a study of veterinarians in King County, WA, 28% reported having had a zoonotic infection, yet only 31% of practices had a written infection control policy.[13] A survey of members of the American Veterinary Medical Association (AVMA) found the majority were unaware of appropriate precautions needed to reduce the risk for zoonotic disease transmission.[14] In a more recent survey of companion animal practitioners in Ontario, Canada, none of the 101 practices surveyed had a formalized infection control program and only 61% utilized control measures for infectious disease cases.[15]

Level of Biosecurity

In a recent workshop on infection control in equine populations, participants agreed that there must be a minimum standard for infection control when managing equine populations.[8] The minimum standard is unique to each facility and takes into account the level of disease risk, the risk aversion of the stakeholders, and the standards set by the rules and regulations of the state's board of veterinary medicine. It is important to recognize that disease risk, as well as risk aversion, may change through time. For example, there are periodic regional outbreaks of vesicular stomatitis (VS) in the area serviced by the Colorado State University Veterinary Teaching Hospital (CSU-VTH). During regional VS outbreaks, additional precautions are instituted with respect to history and examination of a patient prior to admission to the CSU-VTH. It is important for all veterinarians to become familiar with the rules and regulations of the state in which they practice because these in part establish a minimum standard of practice. For example, the

state of Colorado veterinary medicine rules and regulations indicate that "all veterinarians must maintain a sanitary environment in which they care for patients."[16] It further states that "if veterinarians work in clinics they do not own, they are responsible for ensuring that their work is done in a clean environment and within the standard of care." Although this seems straightforward, the standard of care relates to what a reasonable veterinary professional would do in a similar situation. The onus is on each of us to incorporate biosecurity in our practice of veterinary medicine.

Importance of Biosecurity

Infectious diseases can endanger the well-being of horses and personnel, in addition to having potentially devastating financial and emotional effects. A biosecurity or infection control program is intended to not only protect the patients and personnel but is also meant to protect the veterinary hospital or practice. A survey of infection control programs at AVMA-accredited veterinary teaching hospitals (VTHs) found that outbreaks of nosocomial infections occur frequently and identified zoonotic infections as an important occupational hazard to personnel.[17] As such, a high standard of care cannot be attained without implementing strategies to control infectious diseases (i.e., biosecurity) for the protection of the people, the patients, and the practice.

Protect Patients

There is inherent risk of nosocomial infection for any hospitalized patient. It is the veterinary hospital or practice's obligation to implement strategies to minimize that risk. It is important to recognize that all nosocomial infections are not preventable, even in facilities employing excellent infection control practices and a high level of quality care for their patients. In a survey conducted among VTHs in 1997, 67% of 18 VTHs reported outbreaks of nosocomial disease between 1985 and 1996.[6] In a more recent survey, 82% of 38 AVMA-accredited VTHs reported outbreaks of nosocomial infections in the previous 5 years.[17]

The Australian equine influenza epidemic of 2007 highlights that biosecurity is not just for protecting hospitalized patients, but it is also important for protecting animals on their home farms. During this outbreak, farms that employed some biosecurity measures, such as the use of footbaths, were less likely to experience equine influenza on their farms.[18] Ambulatory veterinarians must remain vigilant to reduce the risk of introducing an infectious pathogen onto a client's farm.

Protect Personnel

A report in 2001 indicated there are more than 1400 different infectious microorganisms known to be human pathogens, with 61% of those being zoonotic.[19] Additionally, 75% of the estimated 175 emerging infectious agents were considered to be zoonotic.[19] People working with animals, including veterinary personnel, have inherently increased risks of infection with zoonotic agents compared to the general public.[20] However, members of the general public can also be at an increased risk when attending animal exhibits.[21] Although a relatively small number of infectious diseases can be transmitted from horses to people, zoonotic infections can be devastating for those affected.[22]

Although the likelihood of acquiring a zoonotic infection from domestic animals is generally low, a number of known and emerging pathogens can affect both horses and humans. In the

United States, three agents likely to pose a threat of zoonotic infection (particularly to immune-compromised individuals) are *Salmonella enterica*, *Rhodococcus equi*, and methicillin-resistant *Staphylococcus aureus* (MRSA).[22] *Rhodococcus equi*, which is typically regarded as an equine-specific pathogen, was first reported to infect humans in 1967.[23] Since then, there have been reports of respiratory infections in humans due to *R. equi*, with the most recent being pneumonia in an immune-compromised individual.[23] It was not clear in this case if there had been any contact with horses or their environment. Methicillin-resistant *Staphylococcus aureus* infection in horses and the potential transmission between horses and people has also been described.[24,25] Several equine viruses that cause encephalitis can affect both people and horses. Horses are usually "dead-end" hosts, with the exception of Venezuelan equine encephalitis (VEE), which can be transmitted from equids to humans.[26] Although rabies occurs infrequently in horses, it should be considered a differential diagnosis in all cases of progressive neurologic disease in horses.[27,28] There have been reports of horses developing rabies while at equine events that result in exposure risk to not only the owner and the attending veterinarian but also to the public attending such events and who might have had contact with the horse while visiting the stabling area. There have been reports of zoonotic transmission from a horse of *Trichophyton equinum*,[29-31] *Microsporum equinum*,[32] and *Streptococcus equi* subsp. *zooepidemicus*,[33] further illustrating the necessity for an infection control program to include zoonotic disease agents transmitted by horses.

The emergence of Hendra virus in Australia dramatically demonstrated the importance of taking infection control precautions when working with sick horses.[34-37] One Hendra virus–associated human fatality was an individual who had assisted in the necropsy of affected horses.[38] This incident emphasizes the importance of maintaining a minimum level of infection control as standard practice because it is likely that newly emerging and reemerging infectious agents will be encountered in the future.

Protect Hospital/Practice

Numerous reports of infectious disease outbreaks among equine veterinary hospital patient populations and in equine facilities have been reported.[39-41] In a survey of infection control programs at AVMA-accredited VTHs, 58% reporting outbreaks of nosocomial infections restricted patient admissions and 32% closed part of the facility to aid in mitigation efforts.[17] One VTH, which closed because of an outbreak of *Salmonella enterica* serotype Newport, reported a financial loss of $4.12 million.[42] This estimate likely does not include indirect costs related to loss of client-provider relationships; emotional stress; lost teaching opportunities for students, interns, and residents; diminished morale of hospital staff and clinicians; and poor public relations.

Judicious Antimicrobial Use

Judicious antimicrobial use should be an adjunct to infection control measures and not relied on as a primary preventive measure. Antimicrobial resistance (AMR) is an emerging problem that affects the ability to treat individual patients and the control of disease in animal populations and has significant public health implications.[43]

Controlling the emergence of AMR involves preventing pathogenic microorganisms from acquiring resistance, as well as preventing the spread of resistant organisms.[44,45] Antimicrobial resistance arises from the interaction of bacteria and antimicrobial agents. Drug resistance can evolve through the accumulation of chromosomal mutations or resistance genes can be transferred between bacteria from different taxonomic and ecologic groups by means of mobile genetic elements such as plasmids, transposons, or bacteriophages. Theoretically, all uses of antimicrobial drugs have the potential to promote the evolution of resistance in bacterial populations. Antimicrobial drugs can provide a survival advantage for resistant bacteria, thereby propagating genetic traits conferring resistance. Genes associated with AMR to one antimicrobial can be linked to resistance genes for other antimicrobials promoting the development of multidrug resistant strains.[46] Additionally, AMR can be linked to genes conferring resistance to disinfectants.[47,48]

As noted in human hospitals,[49] many of the nosocomial pathogens associated with veterinary hospitals also are multidrug resistant.[50] This may be associated with high selection pressure applied through common use of antimicrobial drugs and disinfectants in the hospital environment.[50,51] Several actions can be taken to minimize the impact of antimicrobial use. Although antimicrobial drugs should be used when needed (e.g., to treat horses with bacterial infections), they should be used judiciously.[52,53] Inevitably, however, bacterial populations will be exposed to antimicrobial drugs and disinfectants in veterinary hospitals resulting in patient exposure to resistant microorganisms in the hospital environment. Therefore it is essential that appropriate infection control precautions be used to reduce the spread of resistance factors among microorganisms, to reduce the transmission of resistant organisms from patient to patient and between patients and personnel, and to reduce the likelihood of resistant bacteria becoming established in the hospital or farm environment.

Biosecurity Program Development

Every equine facility is unique with its own physical and operational features. As such, a specific biosecurity program needs to be tailored to each facility. Although each program will be unique with respect to its finer details, they will all be based on overarching shared infection control principles. There are general systematic approaches, such as the Hazard Analysis and Critical Control Point (HACCP) system, which can aid in program development. The application of HACCP principles to biosecurity programs in veterinary hospitals and clinics has been previously described.[6] Most of the examples in this section address veterinary clinics. However, the same general principles guiding design of a veterinary hospital infection control program can be applied to any equine facility, whether it is a boarding facility, a breeding farm, a private farm, or an equine event. Although the choice of policies governing infection control will vary between facilities, it is important that the policies are designed with all animals in mind, not only those suspected of having an infectious disease. Consideration should be given to the fact that in general the equine veterinary hospital population differs from the general equine population because hospital patients are more likely to be harboring an infectious disease and are more likely to be immune compromised. In addition, each patient is typically from a different herd, therefore, in a veterinary hospital environment, multiple herds are mixing.

Hazard Analysis/Identification

The first step in any control effort should be the identification of risks and hazards specific to the facility. Consideration should be given to pathogens that are zoonotic, foreign to the region, agents with a high nosocomial transmission risk, and those likely to have a major impact on patient management and welfare. In North America, pathogens likely to be important for equine facilities include *Salmonella enterica*, equine influenza virus, equine herpesviruses, *Streptococcus equi* subsp. *equi*, *Clostridium difficile*, rabies virus, rotavirus multidrug resistant bacteria such as MRSA, and endemic diseases considered reportable to the state or provincial animal health official such as equine infectious anemia (EIA), and those considered foreign to a region (e.g., pathogens causing equine piroplasmosis or contagious equine metritis in North America). The most important diseases will vary with the geographic location of an equine facility.

Critical Control Point Identification

The second step in designing a biosecurity program is to identify critical control points (CCP) or points at which a hazard can be prevented or minimized by applying a control measure. In an equine hospital, consider physical areas or processes in which transmission of pathogens is likely to occur and that might be preventable. Despite the existence of a large number of pathogens that pose a potential threat to the well-being of horses and personnel, there are some common features in the way these pathogens are transmitted. For example, the control of gastrointestinal and respiratory pathogens is commonly included in veterinary hospital biosecurity programs. Although there are likely multiple gastrointestinal pathogens of concern, in general, the mode of transmission is similar (i.e., fecal-oral route, contact transmission). As such, one CCP and prevention strategy may serve to mitigate the transmission risk of multiple different types of gastrointestinal pathogens. Identification of a physical area as a CCP will be facility specific. Consideration should be given to areas in which the most susceptible animals (e.g., severe disease, immune compromised, aged or young) and animals most likely to be shedding contagious pathogens (e.g., critical care or isolation units) are housed. In general, contact should be minimized between these patients and high-traffic areas such as patient receiving or examination areas. For an ambulatory practice, the CCP may be the practice vehicle and its supplies with the aim at reducing or preventing transmission of infectious agents between animals, as well as between facilities (see the section on Biosecurity in Equine Ambulatory Practice).

Critical Limits for Preventive Measures

A critical limit is a condition that must be met to prompt the preventive measure associated with a CCP. This may be as simple as requiring the isolation of a horse with diarrhea or as involved as closing a facility due to an equine herpesvirus 1 (EHV-1) outbreak. To aid in personnel compliance, consider formalizing the biosecurity program with a written document and providing training for those in the practice involved with patient care. Keep in mind that infection control procedures should be rigorous but not to the detriment of patient care and should not interfere with the ability to provide immediate medical attention to a patient.[6]

Critical Control Point Monitoring

Critical control point monitoring is essential to ensuring that a biosecurity program is effective. Monitoring can be as simple as monitoring the use of hand soap or hand sanitizer by tracking the amount of soap or sanitizer in containers provided throughout the hospital. It may entail tracking the occurrence of nosocomial infections, or it may involve active environmental surveillance. The level and type of monitoring will be specific to each facility and depend on stakeholder level of risk aversion and the available resources, both financial and personnel. It is important to note that conducting active surveillance for an organism, which survives relatively well in the environment, such as *Salmonella enterica*, not only can help identify important

pathogen reservoirs but can also indicate overall protocol compliance and effectiveness.

Corrective Action Plan

Establishing a corrective action plan in response to recognized problems is central to an effective biosecurity program, allowing for an efficient and effective response. For example, if an outbreak is recognized, the veterinary practice or hospital should have already considered the feasibility of restricting patient admission or closing the facility to aid mitigation efforts. If facility managers are unwilling to implement a corrective action then there is little purpose to having a formalized infection control program.

Evaluation of the Biosecurity Program

Determining the effectiveness of a biosecurity program will be specific to each facility. However, there are some basic principles that can be applied in all facilities. Human health care has demonstrated that conducting surveillance and providing feedback to personnel will not only enhance protocol compliance but can affect change in behavior (e.g., hand hygiene).[54] It is important for facilities to consider how important "events," such as fevers of unknown origin or catheter site infections, will be monitored to allow comparisons over time. In the age of computerized medical records, monitoring becomes much easier, especially if a facility incorporates important "events" into the record keeping system. For example, at the CSU-VTH, there is a section in the electronic medical record to note nosocomial infections, such as catheter site infections or surgical site infections, or syndromes, such as respiratory disease, diarrhea, or fever. By tracking this information and regularly summarizing and reporting it to decision makers, a hospital or practice will be able to determine the effectiveness of the program. Particularly for a hospital or practice with a large staff, instituting a program oversight group to address any issues or concerns of the facility or personnel can aid biosecurity program management. For additional information, see the section on Monitoring Biosecurity Protocol Effectiveness.

Facility managers must keep in mind that a biosecurity program is dynamic in nature. It must be pliable enough to accommodate many different situations and must evolve with the facility, its patient population, its staffing situation, and the changing risk of infectious disease. For example, VS periodically occurs in livestock in the region serviced by the CSU-VTH. As such, appropriate precautions, including education of staff new to the area, are instituted during these periodic regional VS outbreaks.

Preventive Measures

An infection control program should strive to isolate or eliminate the source of infectious agents, reduce host susceptibility, and break the cycle of microorganism transmission.[55] Unfortunately, in a veterinary hospital environment, we are generally caring for patients whose resistance to disease is compromised. As such, it becomes imperative to isolate the source of pathogenic microorganisms, thereby reducing the risk of transmission. There are several preventive measures that can be employed to this end, including rigorous hand hygiene, barrier nursing precautions, movement restriction, patient isolation, and regular environmental monitoring and sanitation, just to name a few. Standard veterinary precautionary practices have recently been published.[55] The efficacy of many of these practices in veterinary infection control have not been scientifically assessed;

nevertheless we are able to draw from knowledge gained in the field of infection control in human health care. It is important when extrapolating from human health care to keep in mind that the level of environmental contamination is typically much greater in veterinary hospitals than in human health care facilities.

Transmission Routes

In general, transmission of microorganisms can occur via contact (indirect or direct), aerosol/droplet formation, or be vector borne. Many preventive measures are intended to disrupt one or more of these transmission routes. Direct contact may involve animal to animal or animal to personnel contact. This contact can likely be prevented through the use of separation or barrier nursing precautions. Indirect contact occurs when an infectious agent is carried by personnel or an inanimate object from the infected animal to an uninfected animal or person. Prevention may include adherence to rigorous hand hygiene protocols, barrier nursing precautions, or the use of dedicated equipment for infectious disease cases. Aerosol transmission occurs with particles <5 μm in size, which can remain airborne for some time and even travel a relatively long distance.[56] Prevention of aerosol transmission can be a challenge and typically will include isolating the infected animal in its own air space. If this is unattainable, consider maintaining a significant separation between patients. Droplet transmission occurs with larger particles, which are generated during coughing and sneezing or during diagnostic procedures such as draining an abscess, wound irrigation, or performing endoscopy. Droplets generally do not remain airborne for any significant length of time and typically only travel short distances from the source. Maintaining separation between patients, using barrier nursing precautions, and performing procedures in low-traffic areas will likely be effective at preventing this type of transmission. Vector-borne transmission is associated with flies, ticks, and mosquitoes. Implementing an insect and tick control program will be important in reducing this transmission route. Patients should be examined for lice and ticks and, if found, should be treated to reduce the risk of transmission. If other health concerns preclude treatment, these patients should be segregated from the general hospital population and provided with dedicated grooming equipment.

Daily Attire

Daily attire for hospital personnel should be neat, clean, and professional. Footwear must be safe, protective, and cleanable and constructed of a nonporous material. Closed-toe footwear is strongly recommended for all hospital personnel. Standard protective outerwear (e.g., smock, coveralls) should be neat and clean, with an adequate supply on hand to allow personnel to change when outerwear becomes contaminated. Hospital attire should not be worn outside the clinic or field service environment. Personnel should be encouraged to wear hospital-dedicated clothing and footwear, especially in high-risk areas such as isolation, intensive care units, or foaling facilities. Designated surgical scrub clothes and dedicated footwear or protective shoe covers should be worn while working in surgery areas and should not be worn beyond the changing area for the surgery suite.

Hand Hygiene

Proper hand hygiene, including washing with soap and water, as well as using alcohol-based hand sanitizers, is a proven aid to preventing transmission of infectious agents and widely accepted as one of the most important infection control measures to prevent infectious disease transmission.[49,55,57,58] More detailed information on proper hand hygiene is available from the Center for Disease Control and Prevention (CDC).[59] The simple act of handwashing mechanically reduces the organic debris and transient/resident microorganisms on the skin.[55] With the addition of an antimicrobial soap, microorganisms can be killed or their growth inhibited.[55,60] Personnel in contact with horses should maintain short fingernails to minimize accumulation of contaminants underneath fingernails and to facilitate effective hand hygiene. Additionally, they should also avoid wearing elaborate jewelry on their hands for both safety and hygiene reasons. Hands should be washed before and after attending each individual animal, regardless of glove use. Gloves are an adjunct to good hand hygiene practices not an alternative to good hand hygiene practices. Common contact areas (e.g., doorknobs, drawer or cabinet handles or contents, equipment, medical records) should not be touched with contaminated hands or gloves. Although handwashing is an effective way to reduce transmission of infectious agents, doing so frequently can compromise skin integrity, increasing the risk for bacterial colonization of hands and decreasing compliance with hand hygiene protocols.[60] Consequently, it is important to provide not only soap and water but also lotions and moisturizers for application after proper handwashing to promote healthy skin.

In addition to soap and water, alcohol-based hand sanitizers can provide a practical alternative. In health care settings, the CDC recommends the use of hand sanitizers containing 60% to 95% ethyl or isopropyl alcohol.[61] Alcohol-based hand sanitizers are as effective as or more effective than handwashing at reducing bacterial contamination on hands after performing routine physical examinations on normal horses.[62] Alcohol-based hand sanitizers can also be used when soap and running water is not readily available, such as stall-side during a sporting event or during horse transit, although they are not as effective in the presence of organic debris.[55] Dispensers for hand-sanitizing solutions can be easily installed and their frequent use should be encouraged to minimize potential spread of infectious agents. Extrapolating from human health care, the costs associated with the use of alcohol-based hand sanitizers can be greater than costs associated with handwashing products, but the added benefit of enhanced compliance can be immeasurable.[63]

The bottom line is that, when hands are soiled, soap and water is recommended. In situations in which soap and water are not available or if hands are not grossly soiled, then an alcohol-based product can be used for hand hygiene. Alcohol-based products can be especially useful for frequent hand hygiene, at those times when skin is likely to become compromised as the result of frequent handwashing (i.e., chapped and cracked) or in an ambulatory practice when running water may be unavailable.

Barrier Nursing Precautions

There is evidence that barrier precautions can prevent the transmission of infectious agents[64] (Fig. 62-1). The intent is to impose a barrier between "clean" and "dirty," thereby preventing the contamination of footwear, skin, or clothing of personnel with an infectious agent found in the environment or shed by patients.[65] This may be done to minimize the spread of an infectious agent to uninfected patients/personnel or to reduce exposure of immune-compromised patients/personnel to pathogens. In most situations, barrier precautions are effective if they are implemented by informed staff and all personnel understand the rationale behind their use. In veterinary settings, barrier nursing precautions usually include the use of disposable gowns, gloves, facial protection, and implementation of footwear

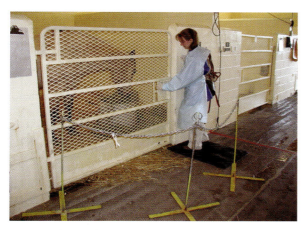

Figure 62-1 Student working with horse using barrier nursing precautions in the main hospital at the CSU-VTH. The student is wearing disposable gloves and a disposable gown. The chain barricade is placed around the stall to limit traffic, and a disinfectant foot mat is placed at the entry to the stall.

hygiene (i.e., footwear covers, rubber boots or use of footbaths or footmats).

Gowns

The use of nonsterile gowns can be an effective means to maintaining a barrier between "clean" and "dirty" or between immune-compromised patients and the rest of the hospital population. Gowns may be permeable, which are typically used for general animal care, or impermeable, which are recommended for use when splashes are expected (e.g., flushing wounds, draining abscesses, or delivering a foal). If using disposable gowns, it is not recommended to reuse them, even on the same patient. Some facilities will invest in washable fabric gowns that should be laundered before using on different patients. In general, when wearing barrier gowns, it is advisable to also wear gloves. When donning and doffing gowns, the wearer must take care to only touch the outside of the gown with gloved hands, limiting the chance for cross-contamination.

Gloves

Glove use can be an important part of creating a barrier and minimizing infectious agent transmission.[66] They are intended to be used for a single patient or patient group and should be worn when contacting feces or other bodily fluids. Gloves should be discarded and hands washed prior to accessing supply drawers, common equipment such as computers or phones, using a stethoscope, handling another patient, or touching another surface such as a doorknob. It is important to remember that gloves are not an alternative to good hand hygiene, rather they are an adjunct to hand hygiene. In human health care, it has been reported that only 22% of glove leaks were recognized by the wearer.[66] This emphasizes the need to still perform adequate handwashing after glove removal. In general, good hand hygiene will likely suffice when working with healthy horses, but gloves should be incorporated when handling a horse suspected or confirmed to have an infectious disease. Additionally, consideration should be given to double gloving when collecting samples from a patient in isolation or when glove contamination is expected. This will allow the wearer to remove the outer contaminated pair of gloves before labeling samples or removing boot covers or barrier gowns.

Facial Protection

Facial protection (i.e., face shield) is intended to prevent the exposure of mucous membranes (including eyes, nose, and mouth) to infectious materials. Consideration should be given to implementing their use anytime there may be a splash or a spray (e.g., flushing wounds, draining abscesses, performing a necropsy, or disinfecting a stall).

Footwear Hygiene

Footwear hygiene includes donning rubber overboots or disposable footwear covers and the use of disinfectant footbaths or footmats. It is imperative that footwear be clean prior to moving to a new environment, whether another area of the veterinary hospital or another equine facility when on ambulatory calls. As such, personnel should be required to wear close-toed shoes when working with animals in the practice of veterinary medicine. Footwear should also be easily cleaned, especially the soles, and there may be additional requirements for safety reasons (e.g., to wear boots that would be more protective if the person was stepped on by the patient). The policy regarding footwear type required for employment in the practice will be practice specific (see the section on Footbaths/Footmats for further information). When caring for high-risk cases, such as those in isolation, neonatal foals, or immune-compromised patients, footwear should be of a type that can be fully disinfected or dedicated to care for an individual case. Care should be taken not to contaminate one's hands or clothing when taking off protective garments. All personnel must be aware of which areas or materials are thought to have a different likelihood of contamination (i.e., the distinction between "clean" and "dirty") and make every effort to keep "clean" areas (including clothing, equipment, and supplies) free of contamination. It is equally important for all personnel to be able to recognize when contamination might have occurred so that appropriate actions can be taken to avoid transmission of the contaminants to another area (e.g., change of clothing, disinfection of contaminated supplies, and disinfection of hands).

Movement Restriction and Traffic Flow Management (Personnel, Patients, Visitors)

A very simple way to disrupt pathogen transmission is to manage traffic flow and restrict movement of both animals and humans, including personnel and visitors. In general, traffic should flow from clean areas to dirty areas and from low-pathogen risk to high-risk situations and patients. The presence of visitors in any equine facility should be assessed with regard to the risk they pose to the facility and the need for such visitation. In some areas (e.g., isolation area), it may be better to restrict visitation. In a situation in which some traffic is unavoidable, it can be minimized and more closely monitored by establishing visiting hours and requiring all visitors to check-in to the facility/hospital. Consideration should be given to implementing rules governing visitation by young children. The actions of young children can be more difficult to predict and control, and therefore they can pose more biosecurity risk, as well as be more at risk of exposure to pathogens than adult visitors. Special consideration should be given to visitors that have recently been in foreign countries (e.g., within the previous 72 hours).

Separation and Isolation

Separation and isolation are methods used to contain and disrupt the transmission of infectious agents to patients and personnel. The intent is to contain environmental contamination and reduce the likelihood of contact between patients, thereby reducing the likelihood of pathogen transmission to the general patient population. Dedicated equipment for animal management (i.e., buckets, halters), as well as for stall cleaning (i.e., pitch fork, shovel, dumpsters, or rubbish bins), is a part of maintaining separation or isolation of infectious disease cases.

Separation

Separation refers to the establishment of hospital areas with differing levels of biosecurity. This may be related to the species (e.g., horses and cattle), to the type of animal (e.g., mare or foal), to the severity of disease (e.g., colic, systemic disease, or elective surgery cases), or to the type of patient (i.e., inpatient versus outpatient). The degree of separation that can be achieved will be dictated by the physical and operational limitations of the facility. Commonly designated hospital areas include large and small animal facilities (in a mixed-animal practice), critical care units, and isolation units. Similar divisions can also be applied to home premises. For example, on a breeding farm, areas may include those that house pregnant mares, foaling mares, mares and foals, weanlings, yearlings, and horses in training or competition. Personnel and equipment movement between different hospital/farm areas should be limited or prohibited. If movement of personnel or equipment is to occur, it should be governed by clearly defined biosecurity protocols (e.g., use of protective clothing, hand hygiene, and disinfection of equipment between areas).

Isolation

Patients with suspect or confirmed infectious disease should be evaluated and managed in an area isolated or segregated from the main hospital population. In general, infectious disease cases include patients with gastrointestinal disease (e.g., colitis or enteritis), acute onset of respiratory disease (especially if febrile), abortion/fetal loss, neonatal foal death or disease, excessive salivation/oral ulceration, skin lesions with hair loss, fever with or without other clinical signs, or acute-onset neurologic disease. If it is necessary to utilize the main hospital facilities or equipment (e.g., radiology, surgery, endoscopy) for diagnostics or treatment of an infectious disease suspect, these should be done at the end of the day, thoroughly cleaning and disinfecting immediately after use. It may be helpful to establish a policy for mandatory testing of all hospitalized animals that develop specified clinical signs. A few examples include requiring *Salmonella* fecal culture of animals with fever, diarrhea, or leukopenia; rapid influenza testing of animals with fever and cough; and bacterial cultures for *S. equi* subsp. *equi* of animals with clinical signs of respiratory disease from farms with a history of strangles. It is important to gather historical information not only on the patient but also on the herd of origin. Determination of disease status will allow for more effective management of the infectious disease risk both in the hospital, as well as on the home operation.

Part of isolating an infectious disease suspect or confirmed case is to also minimize personnel traffic into isolation areas. Facilities should consider employing dedicated personnel to manage such cases. Although this is likely costly, it will greatly reduce the likelihood of contagious disease transmission caused by personnel movement. Another option is to install video surveillance systems with remote computer access. Video surveillance has the added benefit of patient monitoring without having to enter the isolation area. Reducing the number of high-risk contacts with infectious disease cases will also reduce the likelihood of pathogen transmission to personnel or patients.

Every effort should be made to minimize contact between patients with a history or clinical signs suggestive of infectious disease and the general hospital population, as well as to minimize the time spent in common areas. Acquiring a thorough history before admission can often help route a patient to the most appropriate location on arrival at the clinic. For example, the index of suspicion for infectious respiratory disease should be increased for patients with recent onset of fever, ocular or nasal discharge, or frequent coughing. This is particularly true if the animal is from a facility with a mobile equine population

such as training, breeding, or boarding facilities. It is important to identify such patients even if they are not being examined for an infectious disease problem because they may still pose a risk. For example, a foal being hospitalized for an umbilical hernia repair that has a fever, purulent nasal discharge, or enlarged submandibular lymph nodes should be handled as an infectious disease–risk patient. When referring a patient, the practitioner should inform the referral hospital of any suspected infectious diseases and clearly indicate this on patient records so appropriate precautions can be taken.

Footbaths/Footmats

Footwear hygiene is an important component of a comprehensive infection control program. Footbaths or footmats should be considered for use in traffic areas where personnel will be moving between groups of animals of different status (e.g., between colic patients and the general equine hospital population). All personnel should be instructed to use every footbath or footmat when encountered.

The use of footbaths is a common component of infection control programs in VTHs. In a survey of 31 VTHs in the United States and Canada, 97% reported using disinfectant footbaths within the facility.[67] Footbaths should be considered whenever soiling (e.g., with feces, nasal secretions, or uterine discharge) of footwear is likely and may necessitate the use of rubber boots that can readily be worn into footbaths. Footwear or rubber boots should be kept clean at all times when moving between patients. The efficacy of a footbath depends on a number of factors, including frequency of changing disinfectant, amount of organic debris on footwear, the type of disinfectant used, and compliance for use by hospital personnel. Among 30 VTHs that reported the use of disinfectant footbaths, 68% used a single type of disinfectant solution and 32% reported using more than one type of disinfectant solution (in footbaths in different locations, not mixed in the same footbath).[67] The disinfectants most often used in footbaths were quaternary ammonium compounds (42%) and phenolics (39%), followed by hypochlorite solutions (23%) and peroxygens (19%). Other disinfectants used in footbaths were povidone-iodine, chlorhexidine, and ammonia-based products (3% per each). In one study, a 1% Virkon® (Virkon-S, Antec International, a DuPont Company, Sudbury, Suffolk, United Kingdom) footbath, used under conditions typically encountered in the large animal veterinary hospital, found bacterial concentrations on contaminated rubber boots to be 67% to 78% lower than untreated boots.[67] In addition to footbaths, 26% of 31 VTHs also reported using disinfectant footmats in some locations.[67] Although more expensive than traditional footbaths, improved compliance is likely because mats can be used without the requirement for rubber boots. In a study evaluating the efficacy of a peroxygen disinfectant (Virkon S), footmats were as effective as footbaths, with mean bacterial counts 1.3 to 1.4 $\log_{10}$ lower than untreated rubber boots.[68]

Use of dedicated hospital footwear should be recommended to all those personnel with patient contact to minimize the possibility of trafficking pathogens to or from the veterinary hospital. Additionally, footwear hygiene protocol compliance may be improved because personnel may be more inclined to step onto a disinfectant mat if they are not wearing fashion or athletic footwear. Some practitioners prefer to use disposable plastic footwear covers instead of footbaths or footmats to minimize risk of spreading disease agents on footwear. Although the relative efficacy of this method has not been documented, footwear cover durability has been evaluated and was dependent on the product worn, as well as the type of surface and distance walked.[69] Most likely, any method will be effective at minimizing the movement of pathogens, provided it is properly implemented and consistently used by all personnel. Factors, such as cost-effectiveness and convenience, are likely to influence which method is preferred.

Enhancing Biosecurity Protocol Compliance

Compliance to biosecurity protocol is critical to the success of an infection control program, yet it is one of the most challenging aspects of program implementation within a veterinary practice. Providing personnel with the education and training to fully understand and practice the infection control policies is integral to program compliance. One method to encourage protocol compliance lies within the program itself. By regularly reporting results from environmental monitoring or nosocomial infection tracking, personnel will be repeatedly reminded that compliance with biosecurity protocols is critically important. Empowering personnel to become a part of program development will encourage active participation in its implementation. By creating an infection control committee, personnel will have an avenue to provide feedback, including lapses in protocol compliance, as well as recommendations for program improvement. However, there should be one individual within the practice who not only conducts a regular assessment of data but also has the ability to make decisions with respect to infection control measures in an emergency. Part of infection control program development is determining how the practice will manage protocol noncompliance: rewarding excellent compliance or penalizing poor compliance with the loss of hospital privileges, or both. Personnel should be reminded that the program has been implemented to protect people, patients, and the practice and is necessary to provide optimal patient care. A biosecurity program based on sound principles is only as good as those practicing the infection control measures agreed on by the practice decision makers.

Environmental Infection Control

Effective cleaning and disinfection are critical for breaking the transmission cycles of infectious agents. Although cleaning alone can reduce the bacterial load by 90% on a concrete surface, following up with disinfection will kill an additional 6%.[70] Cleaning and disinfection is a multistep process involving the removal of visible debris, scrubbing the area with detergent, followed by rinsing and application of an appropriate disinfectant at the correct dilution and for the recommended contact time.

Cleaning

It is imperative that all surfaces are thoroughly cleaned before any disinfectant is applied. All visible organic debris, such as feces, urine, uterine fluid, nasal exudate, and blood, should be removed prior to disinfection because their presence commonly reduces product efficacy. Many bacteria, when in the environment, are very efficient at forming biofilms (organized bacterial communities that secrete a protective extracellular matrix) that adhere to surfaces. Biofilm formation enhances bacterial survival from a variety of environmental insults, including disinfectants and other antimicrobial treatments.[71-73] Bacteria in biofilms survive well in the environment, providing a continuous source of pathogens that can cause nosocomial infections. Scrubbing surfaces with detergents will aid in removal of debris and biofilm. With this in mind, it is critical that cleanable surfaces be maintained throughout equine facilities and in particular throughout veterinary hospitals. Dirt floors or porous surfaces (e.g., untreated wood) should be avoided as these cannot be effectively disinfected.[70] If porous surfaces are present, they can be rendered less so by painting or sealing the surface.[70,74]

Disinfection

Disinfection refers to the reduction of viable microorganisms on a surface. After appropriate cleaning and rinsing, apply a disinfectant effective against the microorganism(s) of concern, ensuring that the concentration and contact time are in accordance with label directions. A number of commercial products are available for environmental disinfection. It is beyond the scope of this chapter to review all available products, but it is important for personnel responsible for choosing these products to be familiar with major classes of disinfectants, their efficacy against different pathogens, and conditions that limit their effectiveness[70] (Table 62-1). Environmental conditions, including ultraviolet (UV) light (i.e., sunlight) and temperature can greatly affect the efficacy of many products, thus consideration of these factors is important when disinfectants are applied in areas that are not climate controlled. Additionally, it is important to ensure that the products being used are registered with the U.S. Environmental Protection Agency (EPA) and that all safety precautions recommended by the manufacturer are being followed. All disinfectants should be stored in a safe place, particularly when access by children or domestic pets is possible. In addition to traditional surface disinfection, aerosol application or "directed misting" with a disinfectant can be considered for control of airborne infectious agents or difficult-to-reach areas such as ceilings or overhead areas[75,76] (Fig. 62-2). This approach is not a panacea and does not negate the importance of appropriate cleaning, but it may be a useful adjunct to cleaning and more traditional methods of disinfection. The use of aerosolized compounds should be performed with appropriate respiratory protection for personnel and compliance with all other safety recommendations.

Proper cleaning and disinfection should be employed regularly in areas used to house and manage all patients, not just areas housing patients with suspected or confirmed infectious diseases. At a minimum, all stalls should be cleaned and disinfected between patients. Routine cleaning and disinfection helps to minimize the bacterial burden in the environment and the accumulation of resistant flora that may serve as a source of antimicrobial resistance genes (see the section Antimicrobial Resistance). Special attention to cleaning and disinfection should be employed for areas known to have housed patients with suspected or confirmed infectious diseases. All areas used in the management of these patients (e.g., examination rooms, stocks, surgery suites, stalls, trailers) should be cleaned and disinfected immediately after use to minimize inadvertently tracking pathogens from contaminated to clean areas. It is critical that any equipment in contact with animals with an infectious disease be cleaned and disinfected before reuse and that these items be handled to prevent contamination of hospital surfaces. For example, a rectal thermometer used to check the temperature of a horse with salmonellosis can become contaminated, thereby contaminating the hands of personnel, as well as any surface it contacts, if not promptly cleaned and disinfected or discarded.[39]

Waste Management and Disposal

Waste management is an important part of a comprehensive infection control program. The AVMA has previously published general guidelines to aid veterinary practices in developing waste management programs.[77] However, every veterinary practice must develop a program in compliance with federal, state, and local laws and regulations.[78] The federal Medical Waste Tracking Act of 1988 (MWTA), regulated by the EPA, applies to veterinary medical waste considered to be a public health hazard. Medical and infectious waste is defined by state laws and regulations. In general, the definition will include factors such as infectivity, waste categories (e.g., sharps, tubing, fecal

Table 62-1 Common Antiseptics and Disinfectants Used in Veterinary Practice

	Activity in Organic Debris	Spectrum of Activity	Limited Activity	No Activity	Comments
Antiseptic*					
Alcohol	Rapidly inactivated	Gram-positive bacteria Gram-negative bacteria *Mycobacterium* Fungal organisms Enveloped viruses	NA	Nonenveloped viruses *Cryptosporidium* Bacterial spores (static)	Not used for environmental disinfection Minimally toxic Fast acting with no residual activity Requires water for activity (70% solution)
Biguanide (e.g., chlorhexidine)	Rapidly inactivated	Gram-positive bacteria Enveloped viruses	Gram-negative bacteria Fungal organisms	Nonenveloped viruses Cryptosporidium Bacterial spores (static) *Mycobacterium*	Not used for environmental disinfection Minimally toxic Bactericidal when used on skin Residual activity
Povidone iodine	Moderate	Gram-positive bacteria Gram-negative bacteria Fungal organisms *Mycobacterium*	Enveloped viruses	Nonenveloped viruses Bacterial spores *Cryptosporidium*	Not for environmental disinfection Useful on tissue Minimally toxic Higher concentrations have decreased activity
Disinfectant*					
Peroxygen	Very good	Gram-positive bacteria Gram-negative bacteria Fungal organisms Enveloped viruses Nonenveloped viruses Protozoa	*Cryptosporidium* Bacterial spores *Mycobacterium*	NA	Good environmental disinfectant Minimally toxic Rapid action Can be corrosive to metal/concrete
Phenol	Very good	Gram-positive bacteria Gram-negative bacteria Enveloped viruses	Fungal organisms Nonenveloped viruses *Mycobacterium*	Bacterial spores (static) *Cryptosporidium*	Environmental disinfectant Irritating to skin and mucous membranes Toxic to cats and pigs Minimal residual activity Noncorrosive
Quaternary ammonium	Moderate	Gram-positive bacteria Gram-negative bacteria Fungal organisms Enveloped viruses	Nonenveloped viruses	*Cryptosporidium* Bacterial spores (static) *Mycobacterium*	Good for environmental disinfection Minimally toxic Minimal residual activity Inactivated by anionic detergents Less effective at low temperatures and low pH Noncorrosive
Sodium hypochlorite	Rapidly inactivated	Gram-positive bacteria Gram-negative bacteria Enveloped viruses Nonenveloped viruses *Mycobacterium* Bacterial spores	NA	*Cryptosporidium*	Fair for environmental disinfection Minimal residual activity Inactivated by cationic detergents and sunlight Less effective at low temperatures and high pH Chlorine gas generated if mixed with other chemicals Corrosive to metals

Data from Block SS, editor: Disinfection, sterilization, and preservation, ed 5, Philadelphia, 2001, Lippincott, Williams & Wilkins. Linton AH, Hugo WB, Russell AD, editors: Disinfection in veterinary and farm animal practice, Oxford, 1987, Blackwell Scientific Publications. Morley PS: Vet Clin North Am Food Anim Pract 18:133, 2002; Morley PS, Weese JS: Biosecurity and infection control in large animal practice. In Smith BP, editor: Large animal internal medicine, ed 4, St. Louis, 2009, Mosby Elsevier.

NA, Nonapplicable.

*Follow label directions for appropriate dilutions and safety precautions.

waste), and which facilities are required to comply with these regulations ("the generator").[77] Veterinary hospitals should separate waste as it is generated; contain it in a manner that will protect waste handlers, the public, and patients; and label it appropriately.[77] It is important to note that according to the MWTA, waste generators are liable for medical waste from its creation to final disposal, regardless of the employ of a waste management company.

Waste from infectious patients, as well as any waste harboring an agent capable of having an adverse effect on other animals or public health, is specifically a concern for animal facilities. This can include materials such as needles, bandages, or bedding contaminated with bodily excretions (e.g., nasal exudates, urine, feces, or blood). Transmission can occur through mechanical transfer by footwear, hands, or shared equipment (e.g., stall-cleaning equipment) or via biologic vectors such as rodents, insects, or clinic cats or dogs. Care should be taken to

deter patient access to waste containers during stall cleaning. Appropriate disposal methods, such as autoclaving and incineration, will depend on the suspected infectious agent, as well as local regulations. Proper disinfection of equine bedding often becomes problematic because of large volumes. Effective methods may include autoclaving, composting, landfill disposal, or steaming.

The bottom line is that, prior to disposal, veterinary medical waste should be treated in accordance with state and local rules and regulations to eliminate the threat of pathogen transmission to other animals and to protect public health and the environment.

Wildlife Reservoirs

Control of insects, ticks, rodents, and other wildlife is an important part of a biosecurity program at equine hospitals. Both

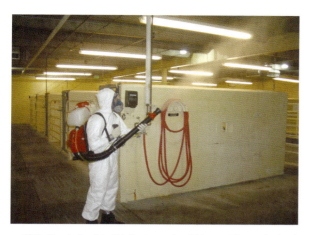

Figure 62-2 Directed mist disinfection using Virkon with a solo backpack mister during annual "bug out" at CSU large animal hospital.

insects (e.g., flies and mosquitoes) and rodents (e.g., mice, rats) can serve as biologic or mechanical vectors for dissemination of pathogens.[36,39] Similarly, pets, such as clinic cats or dogs, can serve as biologic or mechanical vectors for infectious agents, as well as a source of antimicrobial-resistant bacteria.[79,80] Previous epidemiologic investigations have linked cats to *Salmonella enterica* outbreaks,[81] and other reports suggest a clinic cat to reduce the risk of *Salmonella* transmission based on their impact on rodent and wild birds in the hospital.[82] Wildlife can also serve as a source of pathogens for domestic animals, for example, feces of the opossum may contain the infective form of *Sarcocystis neurona*, which is the causative agent for equine protozoal myeloencephalitis (EPM).[83] West Nile virus is spread via mosquito bites,[84,85] EIA is spread by tabanid flies,[86] flies have been shown to carry *Salmonella*,[87-89] and certain insects are proposed vectors for the spread of vesicular stomatitis virus.[90,91] For this reason, pest management should be incorporated into a comprehensive infection control program.

Monitoring Biosecurity Protocol Effectiveness

A comprehensive infection control program includes monitoring the effectiveness of implemented protocols through patient and environmental assessment. There are multiple reasons to monitor an infection control program, including assessing its effectiveness and efficiency, as well as to provide feedback to stakeholders as a means of enhancing protocol compliance. With the emergence and reemergence of infectious diseases, it is imperative to ensure existing protocols are adequate. Monitoring may lead to a permanent policy change or to a temporary change in order to mitigate a transient risk. For example, emergence of VS in the southwestern United States every few years poses a risk to equine hospitals in the area as admission of a case to the general patient population could result in quarantine of the facility. In this situation, a temporary alteration in biosecurity protocols, such as requiring certificates of veterinary inspection or visual inspection prior to entry into the facility, can aid in risk mitigation. Cleaning effectiveness can be monitored in many ways, including visual inspection (although a poor indicator of microbiologic cleanliness because a visually clean surface can still harbor pathogens[92,93]) and environmental cultures once stalls have been cleaned. Increased environmental contamination may indicate a lack of protocol compliance or failure of existing protocols to mitigate the pathogen of interest. Early detection will allow corrective measures to be implemented prior to the occurrence of increased nosocomial infections. Monitoring and reporting of environmental contamination

or the occurrence of nosocomial infections as part of a surveillance program can promote hospital personnel awareness of the potential hazards of reduced biosecurity efforts and encourage continued compliance with biosecurity protocols. The principle of surveillance and monitoring for control of nosocomial infections in veterinary hospitals has been previously described in detail.[6,94,95]

Patient Monitoring

The ultimate goal of a comprehensive surveillance system is to detect all occurrences of nosocomial infection and disease. However, achieving such a goal may not be possible because of limited resources or diagnostic modalities. A number of methods can be employed to monitor for nosocomial infections among hospitalized patients, including weekly clinician rounds, regular analysis of computerized clinical data for predefined clinical signs (i.e., syndromic surveillance), or full microbiologic monitoring for specific agents. The principles behind syndromic surveillance include monitoring of clinical signs suggestive of infection in hospitalized patients without specific microbiologic diagnosis. Syndromic surveillance can be incorporated into a computerized medical record system so that any trends (e.g., increased frequency of catheter-associated infections, fever in hospitalized patients) can be quickly recognized. This will allow the person overseeing the biosecurity program to further investigate and potentially implement corrective actions before the situation escalates. Monitoring patients and providing feedback to stakeholders can result in increased awareness among hospital personnel and improved compliance with infection control protocols, thus enhancing program effectiveness beyond the disease being surveyed.

Experience with infection control in human health care settings also suggests that it is possible to be more efficient and as effective if specific high-risk or high-cost problems are targeted.[54] As such, targeted surveillance is more often used in human health care facilities and is becoming more commonly used in veterinary hospitals. It allows a facility to focus its efforts on a particular type of patient (e.g., all patients versus inpatients versus critical care patients), a specific pathogen (e.g., *Salmonella* or MRSA), or a specific syndrome (e.g., colic, diarrheic, or febrile patients). Patient monitoring may be an active process (e.g., performing fecal cultures on all inpatients on admission for *Salmonella*) or a passive process (e.g., summarizing laboratory tests to identify MRSA isolates). The specific focus and methods for surveillance need to be matched to the needs and resources of each facility while accommodating their level of risk aversion. The major benefit of targeted surveillance is the decreased cost of and effort needed for data collection. The downside is an inability to detect potential problems in patients that are not being monitored and an inability to make an etiologic diagnosis.

A combination of different monitoring methods can be used in patient surveillance. For example, at the CSU-VTH, all large animal inpatients are monitored for *Salmonella* shedding based on fecal cultures performed twice weekly throughout the period of hospitalization. Other potential nosocomial infections are passively monitored based on syndromic surveillance, which may or may not be followed-up with bacteriologic cultures. The type of patient monitoring to incorporate into a biosecurity program will be facility specific and likely reflect the availability of resources, the level of risk aversion of the stakeholders, previous disease outbreak experiences, and disease prevalence in the area.

Environmental Monitoring

Environmental monitoring is used to assess veterinary biosecurity program effectiveness and contributes to the comprehensiveness of a biosecurity program.[94,96] Contamination of the environment near where patients are managed or samples are processed is not an uncommon finding.[96] Environmental surveillance can be more efficient than monitoring every patient and can identify important reservoirs for exposure. For example, if individual patient *Salmonella* fecal cultures are not feasible, periodic monitoring of the environment can provide a less expensive alternative. The detection methods used for environmental testing must be appropriately validated and optimized. Focusing efforts on high-traffic areas, such as examination areas and alleyways, or on identification of an environmentally persistent pathogen (e.g., *Salmonella*) can be used to monitor the overall efficacy of the biosecurity program and identify possible sources of infectious agents.

Incorporating environmental surveillance into a biosecurity program requires consideration of sample type, method of sample collection, detection method, laboratory selection, and available resources (both financial and personnel). Environmental samples can be collected using multiple methods, including electrostatic wipes or sterile sponges that are cultured for specific microorganism[96,97] or contact plates (e.g., Rodac plates) to enumerate nonspecific bacterial growth.[98-100] Identification of specific microorganisms relies on the services of a qualified laboratory, whereas nonspecific bacterial counts can be performed with limited training of personnel and with a minimal cost.

The type of sample collection device used for testing the environment should be considered as the various options likely will have different sensitivities. For example, in a recent study, electrostatic wipes were a more sensitive collection method compared to sterile sponges for detection of *Salmonella enterica* in a large animal veterinary hospital environment.[97] These differences can be attributed to both the collection method (the device used and the size of the surface area sampled), as well as the culture method. In general, sampling a larger surface area will not only provide a more representative sample but will likely be a more sensitive method for organism detection. To gain meaningful information, environmental testing should be performed regularly to establish a baseline level of environmental bacterial contamination to which future findings can be compared. In this way, potential environmental reservoirs of microorganisms can be detected and cleaning effectiveness can be continually monitored.

Use of Outdoor Exercise Areas at Equine Hospitals

Although pasture or open paddocks in many ways may be optimal housing environments for equine patients, they are impossible to thoroughly decontaminate. Therefore the use of pasture or paddock should be reserved for horses without suspect or confirmed infectious disease. If it is preferred that a patient with a suspected or confirmed infectious disease have exercise, then they may be exercised by being led in hand on cleanable surfaces. If these surfaces become soiled they must be immediately cleaned and disinfected. If the use of a pasture or paddock is unavoidable, methods for "cleaning" include removing all feces and resting the pasture, allowing sufficient time for infectious agents to die-off before the introduction of other horses to the pasture or paddock.[70] The amount of time needed will vary, depending on several factors, including the pathogen, type of pasture or paddock, and climate. The survival time of *Streptococcus equi* subsp. *equi* on wood under laboratory conditions was reported to be 63 days at 2° C (35.6° F) and 48 days at 20° C (68° F) with a measurable decline in bacterial count occurring after 7 days.[101] Alternatively, the dirt in the paddock can be removed and replaced after use by an infectious disease case. If the goal is to allow horses to graze, there are other options for grazing infectious disease cases such as cultivating raised grass beds.

Specific Aspects of Biosecurity

Application of the concepts of biosecurity and biocontainment is important not only in veterinary hospitals but also for ambulatory practices, equine breeding facilities, training and boarding facilities, and other facilities that house horse populations such as racetracks or those hosting equine events.

Summary of Biosecurity in Equine Veterinary Hospitals

In a veterinary clinic, large numbers of animals, with potentially enhanced susceptibility to infection, are concentrated in a small area, thus increasing the risk of transmission of pathogens from one animal to another, particularly if animals with infectious disease are housed in proximity to animals with increased susceptibility to infection such as immune-compromised patients or neonatal foals. In addition, intensive management or care of patients increases the possibility of exposure to pathogens because of frequent contact between medical personnel and a number of sick equine patients. Design of the facility can impact the ability to control spread of pathogens. Specifically, factors, such as ability to segregate patients by risk level, type of surfaces, airflow, and air-exchange rate, can influence the success of implemented biosecurity procedures.[95] These factors should therefore be taken into consideration when designing equine hospital facilities.

It is important to recognize that nosocomial infections are an inherent risk of hospitalization. This fact should be communicated clearly to clients. At the CSU-VTH, information about nosocomial infection is part of the admission form that is signed by clients when their horse is admitted to the clinic. The amount of effort aimed at preventing nosocomial disease in an equine clinic depends on specific circumstances such as size of the operation, type of cases managed, type of clientele, financial resources available for this purpose, prevalence of various infectious diseases in the region and risk aversion as perceived by clients and practice management. For example, a two-veterinarian clinic may not need and probably will not be able to justify as extensive a biosecurity program as would be appropriate for a large referral hospital. In general, clients who are highly educated about their horses and willing to pay for advanced medical care are likely to expect high-quality care in all aspects of patient management and would choose a provider who fulfills these criteria. This includes more comprehensive infection control efforts. As mentioned earlier, because nosocomial infections are an inherent risk of hospitalization, high quality care cannot be achieved without efforts to prevent these infections. Facilities with a large patient load likely have a larger number of personnel and a larger facility to manage, therefore a written protocol is indicated to allow for uniformity in procedures and to ensure all personnel are informed about the protocols. There are two comprehensive biosecurity programs for VTHs at Colorado State University and the University of California-Davis, which have recently been published.[6,95]

Biosecurity in Equine Ambulatory Practice

The equine ambulatory practitioner moves between horses that are managed as separate groups such as those owned or trained by different individuals at a single property (i.e., boarding facility) or at equine events (i.e., racetrack). They also move between different facilities, such as the veterinary hospital and a farm; between farms; and between farms and equine events such as shows or other competitions. These movements could result in the transfer of pathogens between groups of horses at the same facility or between different facilities if precautions to avoid transmission are not implemented. By way of example, consider equine influenza virus. The predominant methods of spread of equine influenza virus, in decreasing order of importance, are movement of live infectious horses, fomites, and aerosols (local spread). Veterinarians likely accept that horse-to-horse contact plays a role in transmission of contagious equine disease agents, however, they also need to accept and thus take actions to reduce the risk that they themselves could result in pathogen transmission. There have been reports that suggest the most likely way that equine influenza virus moved from a quarantine station to the general horse population in Australia was on the clothing or equipment of a groom, veterinarian, farrier, or other person who had contact with an infected horse and subsequently left the quarantine station without taking biosecurity measures.[102]

Horses in the community setting (e.g., outside of the veterinary hospital) are likely more resistant to developing disease if exposed to pathogens (i.e., we generally believe that a larger pathogen challenge is required to cause disease in normal animals than in patients in a veterinary hospital, although few studies confirm this assumption). In addition, the time between acquiring a pathogen on clothing, footwear, or equipment and contacting other horses likely reduces the transferred pathogen load, especially for those pathogens that are less environmentally persistent such as some viruses.[103]

Although much of the emphasis on biosecurity for equine practices has been related to the control of transmission of pathogens in veterinary hospitals, the ambulatory practitioner is also obligated to take reasonable precautions to reduce the risk they pose when moving between groups of horses, whether at the same facility or different facilities. Based on recent equine disease outbreaks the equine industry is much more aware of biosecurity practices and thus will expect the veterinarian visiting their facility to have taken reasonable precautions to avoid spread of contagious equine pathogens. In addition, because of the heightened awareness among the equine industry, there is an opportunity for the veterinary practitioner to serve as a source of information related to biosecurity at equine facilities, including private farms and competition venues. Thus the ambulatory veterinarian has several incentives to understand and implement biosecurity practices for themselves and their client's horses, including serving as an example to others when it comes to taking precautions to protect the health of their patients.

The ambulatory equine practitioner should develop a list of every day protocols that become routine infection control practices. These protocols should be followed by the practitioner, thus setting an example for those with whom they work; in addition, they should be practiced by their assistants and clients. These procedures should be employed when working with horses that appear healthy at facilities where no active contagious disease is occurring. For example, practicing good hand hygiene between groups of horses that are maintained separately from each other (i.e., managed by different owners or trainers or residing on different facilities) should be a routine practice. If hands are soiled (e.g., blood, nasal secretions, feces, placental fluid, etc), they should be washed with soap and water as described in the previous section of this chapter. If hands are not grossly soiled and soap and water are unavailable, then use of an alcohol-based hand sanitizer is indicated. Hand hygiene should be performed before touching door handles or the steering wheel of the practice vehicle, as well as before touching objects such as a cell phone or pager. Clean outerwear dedicated to the practice of veterinary care should be worn each day. If the veterinarian's or their assistant's outerwear becomes soiled while providing veterinary care, a change of attire is indicated. Footwear should be cleaned with soap and water if there is fecal or soiled bedding present on the soles prior to entering the

practice vehicle. No sharing of equipment between groups of horses should occur unless sanitized, and there should be no reuse of needles and syringes. Some clients may ask practitioners to implement even more stringent procedures for everyday practice such as using outer clothing and footwear dedicated to their facility. The practitioner should comply with these requests. Optimally the practitioner should park their practice vehicle away from the horse housing area to avoid moving material from one premises to another on the tires or undercarriage of the vehicle. The practice vehicle, including the interior footmats, should be washed whenever visibly dirty, prior to going on the next call.

The ambulatory practitioner should be prepared to manage the risk the examination of a horse with contagious disease poses to a subsequent patient's care. For example, while on a call to do a purchase examination, a call comes in to examine a horse at a neighboring premises that has a fever and swelling of the head and neck area (i.e., a strangles suspect). Having a "biosecurity kit" that the practitioner can carry in the practice vehicle for themselves and an assistant can facilitate safe examination of a suspected or confirmed case of contagious disease and minimize the chances of carrying contamination to other horses.[104] A "biosecurity kit" should contain items used for implementing barrier nursing precautions. For example, examination gloves (at least one pair per horse examined), coveralls dedicated to a given animal's examination or that of a group of animals of equal status, a covering for the upper body that is impervious to secretions (e.g., nasal discharge), durable water resistant footwear covers, and some type of head covering. Once the barrier precautions are removed, a spray container of disinfectant for the soles of footwear and hand sanitizer or hand soap with a water source is a must.

If a contagious disease is highly likely or confirmed (i.e., a suspected outbreak of infectious disease), then additional materials, such as disinfectants, gloves, footbaths/footmats, cautionary signs, etc., should be obtained that would allow ongoing efforts at containing the disease to a given horse or farm. Detailed information has been previously published and is available from the American Association of Equine Practitioners (AAEP), including sources and indications for use of biosecurity supplies.[103,104]

Protection of Resident Horses and Control of Infectious Diseases at Equine Events

Biosecurity programs for equine facilities can have multiple goals, including reducing the risk of pathogen introduction and, if introduced, reducing the spread of pathogens among horses in the facility. The control measures, such as reducing risk of exposure, that were discussed earlier in the section on hospital infection control also relate to the protection of horses on equine operations. In general, horses that comprise the general equine population, analogous to the "community" for human health discussions, are less susceptible to infectious diseases than those in a hospital population because normal horses are not experiencing the stresses and other risk factors that hospitalized horses encounter. Therefore use of fewer precautions will likely be effective at minimizing infectious disease risk in a population of healthy horses. However, lack of basic biosecurity precautions can result in pathogen introduction and subsequent spread among the general horse population. Outbreaks of equine infectious diseases can have an impact through the cost incurred in the diagnosis and treatment of sick horses, the implications of stopped horse movement to contain an outbreak and the lost use and potentially lost lives of affected horses.[105]

Infection control for horses in the general equine population can be implemented at many different levels. The owner of the horse could institute control measures based on the risk their horse is likely to incur, taking into account its use, signalment, and other aspects of its management. For example, a horse ridden alone on trail rides has a different level of risk than a horse attending a group event where the health status of horses with which it can come into contact is unknown. An equine facility manager, such as the manager of a boarding facility, could implement infection control practices that are applied to all horses residing at that facility. Finally, event organizers responsible for shows or other venues where horses come together on a temporary basis to compete or perform could have biosecurity requirements and response plans for disease outbreaks to mitigate the risk of infectious diseases occurring among horses at the event. Each of these decision makers needs to consider the risks the horses they oversee face and how best to manage that risk based on their risk-aversion level.

In general, considerations should be given to the development of a vaccination and parasite control program, requirements for horses entering a facility or property (both returning resident horses and nonresident horses), isolation of new arrivals and returning resident horses (e.g., from a show or event), monitoring of horses for infectious disease (e.g., taking daily rectal temperatures of resident horses), infection control strategies to be used by those who work with horses (e.g., dedicated attire, working from low risk to high risk), and the development of a response plan should a suspected or confirmed contagious disease be identified. For diseases that are reportable to state or federal animal health officials, the response to disease detection will be regulated by animal health officials.

Various recommendations have been made related to the use of one or more infection control practices on equine operations. In general, these practices include reducing the risk of exposure or optimizing resistance if an animal is exposed. For example, the implementation of vaccination on a population basis, having entry requirements for visitors and nonresident horses, monitoring for signs of infectious disease, and pursuing a diagnosis if disease is detected. If disease is detected, the initial response may be to consider it a contagious disease risk. This response can be further refined based on diagnostic testing and detection of subsequent cases, thereby tailoring the response to the detected problem.[106]

A study based on the National Animal Health Monitoring Survey (NAHMS) Equine 2005 data found that 78.5% of participating U.S. equine operations with greater than or equal to five resident horses had some risk of exposure to nonresident horses in the previous year.[107] As the size of the operation increased so too did the risk for exposure to nonresident horses, as well as the likelihood for implementing biosecurity measures. This study suggested that the most at-risk equine facilities defined as operations with resident horses having contact with nonresident horses were more likely to implement biosecurity practices aimed at multiple aspects of infection control (e.g., vaccination, entry requirements, and response to detected disease).[107] A recent survey of select Colorado equine boarding facilities found that many facilities had the opportunity to implement additional infectious disease control measures with 22.6% of respondents deemed to have less than adequate biosecurity at their facility.[108] Among respondents, 6.6% regularly employed isolation of resident equids returning from travel and among facilities that regularly receive new equids, only 50% reported requiring isolation of these equids from resident horses.[108]

There have been recent additions to the available resources on equine biosecurity for equine owners and facility managers. An *Equine Biosecurity Risk Calculator* has been developed as an educational resource by Equine Guelph (University of Guelph) in partnership with CSU, sponsored by the AAEP Foundation and Vétoquinol Canada, Inc.[109] This risk calculator survey takes

approximately 10 minutes to complete, offers equine owners and farm managers the opportunity to assess their risk, and provides educational information related to control of equine infectious diseases. The *Equine Biosecurity Principles and Best Practices Guide* was developed by the Alberta Veterinary Medical Association and the Alberta Equestrian Federation as a way to interactively educate horse owners while encouraging discussions with veterinarians regarding biosecurity on their farms.[110] A *Horse Venue Biosecurity Workbook* has been developed, based on the equine influenza outbreak that occurred in Australia in 2007, by Animal Health Australia in conjunction with equine industry groups, including the Australian Horse Industry Council.[111] This workbook is a self-assessment guide for all horse venues, including race courses, show grounds, pony clubs, and boarding facilities, and it provides a way for managers to assess risk and offers options for managing identified risks. A *Biosecurity Toolkit for Equine Events* has also been developed by the California Department of Food and Agriculture.[112] This toolkit consists of sections focusing on options for preventing the introduction of pathogens to an event, an infection control plan, and options for heightened control efforts should an outbreak of a contagious equine disease occur related to an equine event. The recent (2011) multistate EHV-1 outbreak that was traced to horses that attended a large western performance event in Ogden, UT, highlights the potential for equine disease to be transmitted among horses attending competitions or other sites where horses commingle and provides the impetus for facility and event managers to incorporate infection control strategies into facility management and event planning. Table 62-2 provides a list of equine biosecurity resources and Web sites.

The adoption of biosecurity practices on an equine operation is a balance of perceived benefit versus the cost/impact of implementation. The benefits of a biosecurity program can be hard to realize because it is difficult to measure the cost of an outbreak averted. Specific biosecurity plans need to be tailored to the facility or venue based on potential risks for infectious disease entry and spread, risk aversion of the decision makers, control options available, and the available support both financial and for adherence to the biosecurity program.

Equine Owners

Protection of Resident Horses

In general, horses residing at their home facilities (e.g., horse farms, stables, stud farms, and similar facilities) are typically healthy. As such, a biosecurity program for these facilities tends to focus primarily on preventing the entry of an infectious agent onto the premises and secondarily on controlling the spread of an infectious agent should it enter the establishment. To some degree, all of the control measures previously discussed can be implemented on any equine facility. However, because the general equine population is less likely to be susceptible to common infectious agents, fewer biosecurity precautions will likely be needed to effectively keep this population healthy. Nonetheless, lack of minimum biosecurity practices can lead to the introduction of a new disease agent to a susceptible population, sometimes with serious emotional and financial consequences.[42]

In general, all resident horses should be vaccinated on a regular basis. The type of vaccines and frequency of administration should be determined by an attending veterinarian based on published evidence of efficacy, knowledge of local disease risks, and consideration of factors such as geographic region, size of the facility, extent of movement of people and horses onto and off the operation, and the age of the resident equine population. Vaccination principles with specific recommendations related to the core and risk based vaccine recommendations

Table 62-2 Biosecurity Resources

Resource	Web site
AAEP Vaccination Guidelines[114]	www.aaep.org/vaccination_guidelines.htm
Biosecurity Tool Kit for Equine Events[112]	www.cdfa.ca.gov/ahfss/Animal_Health/Equine_Biosecurity.html
Equine Biosecurity Principles and Best Practices[110]	www.albertaequestrian.com/Biosecurity
Equine Biosecurity Risk Calculator (Equine Guelph)[109]	www.equineguelph.ca/Tools/biosecurity_2011.php
Equine infectious disease outbreak: AAEP Control Guidelines[103]	www.aaep.org/control_guidelines_nonmember.htm
Hand hygiene in health care settings: Hand hygiene basics[57]	www.cdc.gov/handhygiene/Basics.html
Hand hygiene in health care settings: Guidelines[58]	www.cdc.gov/handhygiene/Guidelines.html
Horse Venue Biosecurity Workbook (Animal Health Australia)[111]	www.horsecouncil.org.au/_Upload/Files/Horse%20Venue%20Biosecurity%20Workbook.pdf
Biosecurity supplies*	www.gemplers.com (Disinfection Mat, Footbath Mat, Virkon S†)
	www.eNasco.com (Entrance Disinfection Mat, face shields, protective eyewear)
	www.qcsupply.com (Knot-a-Boot‡)

*Not an endorsement; provided to allow readers to quickly find resources in an emergency. The authors' encourage readers to develop their own product preferences and suppliers.

†Virkon S, Antec International, Sudbury, Suffolk, United Kingdom.

‡Knot-a-Boot, Continental Plastic Corp, Delavan, WI.

have been previously published by the AVMA and AAEP.[113,114] All new arrivals, including resident horses returning from competitions, breeding facilities, or sales, should be quarantined for a period that exceeds the maximum incubation period for the disease of concern. According to a survey conducted by the U.S. Department of Agriculture Veterinary Services in 2005, among a representative sample of equine operations in 28 states, approximately one-third of equine operations that added resident equids routinely isolated new arrivals. The majority of those that isolated newly arrived horses used a separation period of more than 2 weeks, with an average length of quarantine of 28.5 days.[115] Any traffic to and from equine facilities should be minimized or controlled. For example, any commercial vehicles that are likely to have visited other farms can be restricted from entering horse stabling areas. Visitors can be asked to wear clean clothing, wash their hands before contact with the horses on the premises, or step on a disinfectant footmat before entering the stabling area. It may be advisable to ask the medical history for all horses coming onto the operation and specifically inquire about recent episodes of respiratory infection or diarrhea. Similarly, all visiting horses on arrival should be inspected for clinical signs of infectious disease, such as diarrhea or nasal discharge, denying facility access to animals showing such signs. It may also be helpful to require all visiting horses to be from premises with active parasite control programs and be vaccinated against specified pathogens. Premises owners could require documentation of an active parasite control and vaccination program, as well as require testing of new arrivals for diseases of concern.

Protection of Traveling Horses

An equine owner should be concerned with the possible exposure of horses to pathogens at sales, competitions, training stables, breeding facilities, or anywhere horses congregate from multiple different sources. In addition to difficulties in controlling exposure to possible pathogens in these situations, traveling horses may have a compromised immune system and therefore may be more likely to develop clinical disease when exposed to common pathogens.[116] Principles of biosecurity for these horses are similar to those discussed for resident horses, with day-to-day hygiene and use of efficacious vaccines playing major roles in maintaining health.

Although it is often difficult to restrict traffic around traveling horses (e.g., at sale barns or competitions), it is possible to limit direct contact to only essential personnel. It is also possible to provide stall-side hand sanitizers and options for footwear sanitation to further minimize trafficking of pathogens. Stalls at equine events can be thoroughly cleaned and disinfected between uses either by the event coordinators or by the participants, although the efficacy of these actions may be hindered by porous construction materials (e.g., wood) and dirt stall floors. In addition, good ventilation and temperature control can help reduce stress on the respiratory tract of horses and reduce circulation of pathogens. Owners or trainers of travelling horses should involve their veterinarian in developing a plan for infection control that includes vaccination, as well as ways to reduce exposure risk and monitor for disease occurrence.

Conclusions

Biosecurity and infection control are important aspects of the day-to-day operation of any equine facility and are especially important for equine hospitals. A successful infection control program requires the commitment and participation of all personnel. It is essential that the people in decision-making roles, such as clinicians (in the hospital) and owners, trainers, or managers (in an equine facility), educate personnel about biosecurity and observe compliance with infection control measures. Leadership by example is the best way to ensure compliance of all personnel. Additionally, educational efforts should be undertaken to make sure all personnel understand the importance of biosecurity and their role in maintaining the facility as a safe place for horses and their human caregivers.

The complete reference list is available online at www.expert-consult.com.

Infectious Diseases and International Movement of Horses

63

Peter J. Timoney

We are living in an era in which the world has become a "global village," with "shrinking" national borders and liberalization of trade between countries. The populace of discrete countries can no longer consider themselves remote from the risk of incursion of a wide variety of infectious diseases of public health and veterinary significance.[1,2] It is widely acknowledged that increasing globalization, whether with respect to movement of people or trade in animals or animal products, provides greater opportunities for the rapid and widespread dissemination of a variety of diseases from country to country and within countries, a situation that is historically unprecedented. The ever-increasing volume of international movement has given rise to a major paradigm shift in the geographic distribution of many diseases. Fewer and fewer diseases can now be regarded as "geographically restricted" or "compartmentalized" to certain areas of the world.

The list of human and animal pathogens that have been accidentally introduced or reintroduced into regions or countries where they were never previously known to occur or from which they were eradicated in the past is expanding.[3] Examples of the more important human diseases and disease agents spread through international travel include tuberculosis, severe acute respiratory syndrome (SARS virus), influenza, malaria, cholera, Lassa fever, and Ebola virus. The roster of animal diseases with convincing evidence of spread through international movement or trade in animal products is also extensive and includes foot-and-mouth disease, hog cholera, exotic Newcastle disease, equine influenza, glanders, canine parvovirus, West Nile virus (WNV), and more recently, highly pathogenic avian influenza (H5N1 virus). Some animal disease pathogens (e.g., WNV, Venezuelan equine encephalomyelitis [VEE] virus, and *Burkholderia mallei*) are important zoonoses and can give rise to significant morbidity and mortality in humans, as well as in various animal species.

Many transboundary animal disease incursions are relatively transient in duration; the diseases are effectively controlled and eradicated within a limited time after their introduction. However, this is not always the case. Some disease pathogens are highly adaptable and very successful in establishing themselves in a new geographic environment. This is well illustrated by the behavior of WNV over the past 10 to 15 years both in Europe and in the Western Hemisphere. The virus has been confirmed in an increasing number of European countries, including but not necessarily limited to Hungary, Greece, Italy, Spain, and Portugal; in some of these countries there is evidence of overwintering of the virus. An analogous situation exists in various countries in the Western Hemisphere in which WNV has adapted itself remarkably well and become endemic since its first known introduction into North America (United States)

in 1999 and now has resurged again in 2012 in humans in the United States.[4] It took only 5 years for WNV to become established in 48 of the 50 states in the United States.

Growth of Horse Industries Worldwide

The horse is unique not only because of the longevity of the species and significant financial value of individual animals, but also, more importantly, because of the frequency with which horses are shipped between countries and between continents for various commercial purposes. Frequently taken for granted, the advent of commercial jet aircraft transportation has been the single most important factor in facilitating the unparalleled growth in international trade in equids, semen, and embryos that has taken place over the past 50 years or so.[5] Air travel has revolutionized the speed and ease with which horses can be shipped between or within countries and has largely replaced other means of transporting horses over considerable distances by land or by sea. In today's world, the horse can truly be considered no less an "international jetsetter" than its human counterpart.

Changing trends in the equine industry worldwide have contributed significantly to the evolving nature of the international trade in equids, semen, and embryos. In the process, however, such changes have inevitably increased the risk of spread of various equine diseases. Before elaborating on specific factors involved in the international dissemination of equine diseases in detail, it is important to appreciate the transformation that the equine industry in many countries has undergone over the past 50 to 60 years. Since the 1960s, there has been an unprecedented upsurge in the growth of the horse industry in many countries, both for commercial and recreational purposes. Consideration of the increased prominence of the equine industry worldwide must acknowledge the resurgence of interest in the horse through leisure activities. The 2005 Economic Impact Study carried out in the United States identified recreation as the single largest equine-related activity, involving 3.9 million horses of an estimated national equid population of 9.2 million animals.[6] The most significant factor in this development was the favorable economic climate enjoyed by these countries over this period. National economics flourished from changes in the global market structure under various multinational trade agreements.[7] Among the industries to benefit has been the equine industry, with a resultant increase in the volume of international trade in equids and semen. The trend toward globalization of the equine industry received further impetus after establishment of the World Trade Organization

(WTO) in January 1995.[8] The primary goal of the WTO is to promote freer economic exchange between member countries through reduction or elimination of protectionist barriers to trade.[9] Regrettably, continued growth in the horse industry worldwide has slowed in the last several years as a consequence of the recession that has significantly impacted the national economies of many countries. Notwithstanding the current economic downturn, emergent equine industries are being developed in the Republic of Korea and the People's Republic of China.

Basis for International Movements and Trade in Equine Germplasm

An appreciation of the nature of international movement of equids is fundamental to understanding how trade in horses, semen, and embryos can contribute to the spread of equine diseases.[5] Horses are shipped internationally for various reasons. Some are intended for permanent entry and others for temporary entry into the importing country. Most frequently, horse travel between countries is for the purpose of competing in a particular performance event. Among the more prominent and better known performance activities are racing, show jumping, dressage, eventing, driving, polo vaulting, reining, and endurance riding.

Shipment of stallions and mares for breeding purposes is another important facet of the international movement of equids. This is especially significant in the case of the Thoroughbred industry worldwide, which does not allow the use of artificial insemination (AI) or embryo transfer in the breed. Over the years, significant growth has occurred in the practice of "shuttling" stallions, Thoroughbreds and Standardbreds between countries in the Northern and Southern Hemispheres.[10] Horses are also shipped internationally to be sold at a commercial sale or in the case of a change in ownership.

A final category of horse movement that applies primarily to countries other than the United States is the shipment of horses for processing, primarily for human consumption. Several hundred thousand horses are shipped annually from Eastern Europe, Northern Africa, and certain countries in South America to various countries in Western Europe, including but not exclusive of Italy, Germany, France, and Belgium, for this purpose.[3]

As with live animal movements, the international trade in equine semen and embryos has expanded significantly in recent years.[5] This is largely the result of the acceptance of AI in all the major horse breeds except Thoroughbreds.[11]

Economic Impact

A major factor contributing to the importance of international trade in equids, semen, and embryos has been the increased socioeconomic significance of the equine industry in a growing number of countries worldwide. The horse has joined the list of animal and plant commodities that are traded globally.[3]

To date, relatively few countries have attempted to assess the impact of their respective industries on their national economies. Limited studies have been done in the United Kingdom, Ireland, and Mexico, all of which underscore the important cultural and economic value of the horse in these countries.[12] Australia and the United States have carried out comprehensive studies of their respective equine industries.[6,13-15] The American Horse Council Foundation commissioned an economic impact study of the horse industry in the United States in the mid-1990s[6] and again 10 years later.[14] Comparison of the findings of the two studies revealed that the U.S. equid population had increased considerably over the intervening period, from an estimated 6.9 million in the mid-1990s to 9.2 million in 2005. Both impact studies dramatically demonstrated the major contribution of the horse industry to the national economy. In the 2005 study, the combined contributions of the direct, indirect, and induced effects of the industry (in terms of Gross Domestic Product) were assessed at more than $102 billion.[6] The industry provides considerable employment, estimated at 1.4 million full-time equivalent jobs annually. Until the widespread financial recession in the last few years, revenue from the sale of equids had risen steadily, grossing in excess of $2 billion at its peak.

Changing Trends

Not surprisingly, changing trends in the horse industry over the past 40 to 50 years, most of them commercially driven, have been a major influence on the evolving nature of international trade in equids, semen, and embryos.[7] As already mentioned, horses are most frequently transported between countries to compete in various performance events, racing, show jumping, and other types of equestrian sports. The number of highly prestigious and lucrative equine competitive events has proliferated around the world in the past 15 to 20 years.[3] This is well illustrated by the increase in number of major equestrian events held under the aegis of the International Equestrian Federation (FEI); these events have nearly doubled over the past 8 years alone. Attracted by the considerable prize monies involved, owners are shipping their horses many thousands of miles, sometimes from the Northern to the Southern Hemisphere, or vice versa, to compete in international equestrian or racing events. Transporting horses over significant distances for competition purposes has inherent risks (e.g., traumatic injuries, shipping fever). Nonetheless, the number of prestigious international events will likely continue to increase, with escalation in the volume of movement of horses, despite the inherent health risks involved.

Another important economic trend that has grown in volume, especially over the past 20 years, is the practice of dual-hemisphere breeding of stallions, in which a stallion fulfills a breeding season in both hemispheres in the same calendar year.[10] This is more popular and economically more advantageous, for both stallion and mare owner alike, than transporting mares between hemispheres for breeding purposes (e.g., shipping a mare from the Southern to the Northern Hemisphere to be bred in Southern Hemisphere time). The vast majority of "shuttle stallions" are shipped from the Northern to the Southern Hemisphere. While many of them are Thoroughbreds, Standardbred stallions are also shuttled. They originate principally in Ireland, the United Kingdom, France, the United States, Canada, and Japan and travel primarily to Australia and to a lesser extent, New Zealand, Argentina, Chile, Brazil, Columbia, Peru, Venezuela, and South Africa.

As noted, acceptance of AI by an increasing number of breed registries has been another major development in the horse industry in recent years.[11] Technical advances in preserving the fertilizing capability of equine sperm and the viability of equine embryos have provided the basis for the expanding trade in fresh-cooled and especially frozen semen being shipped internationally. There is greater demand among breeders for access to particular preeminent bloodlines among those breeds in which AI is permitted.

In summary, continued proliferation in the number of prestigious equestrian and racing events, dual-hemisphere breeding of stallions, and the legalized use of AI in all the major horse breeds, except the Thoroughbred, are the principal, economically driven trends in the equine industry, and these trends are responsible for the sustained growth in international trade in equids, semen, and embryos worldwide.

Factors Influencing Global Distribution of Equine Diseases

A diversity of related and unrelated factors have been identified with the potential to influence the global distribution of equine infectious diseases.[3,5,10] These include the international trade in equids, semen, and embryos; multinational trade agreements; emergent diseases; variants of established equine pathogens; climatic disturbances; availability of new vectors; migration of amplifying/reservoir hosts or vectors of specific pathogens; disease spread from feral equids; reliability of preexport laboratory testing; and acts of agroterrorism.

International Trade in Equids, Semen, and Embryos

Movement of equids and trade in semen represent the most important factors responsible for the spread of equine diseases.[3,16-19] With the progressive growth in international trade in equids, semen, and embryos, the risk of dissemination of a variety of equine diseases, both within and between countries, has increased commensurately. This has been amply borne out by the significant number of times that specific diseases have been introduced or reintroduced into countries or geographic regions of the world through the importation of equids or semen. Most vulnerable to the risk of disease incursions are countries with a significant import trade in equids, semen, and embryos such as the United States.

The risk of incursion of transboundary equine diseases can be influenced in part by whether the equids being imported are approved for temporary or permanent entry into a country.[3] An exception would be those diseases transmitted primarily by the respiratory route, such as equine influenza, equine herpesvirus-1 (EHV-1) and -4 (EHV-4)–related diseases, strangles, and glanders. Spread of respiratory infections can occur irrespective of whether importation is temporary or permanent. On the other hand, in the case of equine diseases characterized by the carrier state, the risk of transfer of these diseases is much greater in horses taking up permanent residence in a country. This applies to vector-borne diseases, such as equine infectious anemia (EIA) and equine piroplasmosis (EP), as well as infections transmitted by the venereal route such as contagious equine metritis (CEM), equine viral arteritis (EVA), and dourine *(Trypanosoma equiperdum)*.

Clearly, the mode(s) of transmission of individual equine diseases has an important influence on how successfully they can be transmitted to and spread within a naïve or unprotected equine population in an importing country. Any shipment of equids may include one or more animals incubating or subclinically infected with a particular agent or that are asymptomatic carriers of a specific pathogen. Examples include equine herpesviruses (EHV-1, EHV-3, and EHV-4), equine arteritis virus, EIA virus, *Streptococcus equi* subsp. *equi*, *Taylorella equigenitalis*, *Burkholderia mallei*, *Salmonella* spp., *T. equiperdum*, *Theileria equi*, and *Babesia caballi*.[3,7]

Respiratory transmission by an acutely infected equid is widely considered one of the most efficient means of disease transfer. Respiratory-borne diseases, such as equine influenza virus (EIV), equine rhinopneumonitis caused by EHV-1 or EHV-4, and strangles, have been spread repeatedly between countries through international movement of horses (Table 63-1). Venereal transmission is also of major significance with respect to imported breeding animals, both stallions and mares, which may be carriers of specific pathogens (e.g., EAV, EHV-3, *T. equigenitalis*, *T. equiperdum*, and certain serotypes of *Klebsiella pneumoniae* and *Pseudomonas aeruginosa*).

A further category of carriers are equids persistently infected with disease agents such as EIA virus, *T. equi*, and *B. caballi*,

Table 63-1 Epidemics of Equine Influenza Resulting from International Movement of Equids, 1963-2012

Virus Strain	Importing Country	Year	Source
Equine-2 influenza A virus	United States	1963	South America
Equine-2 influenza A virus	Western Europe	1965	North America
Equine-1 influenza A virus	England, Ireland	1977	Continental Europe
Equine-1 influenza A virus	Singapore, Malaysia	1977	Europe
Equine-2 influenza A virus	England, Ireland	1979	Continental Europe
Equine-2 influenza A virus	South Africa	1986	United States
Equine-2 influenza A virus	India	1987	France
Equine-2 influenza A virus	Jamaica	1989	United States
Equine-2 influenza A virus	Hong Kong	1992	England and Ireland
Equine-2 influenza A virus	United Arab Emirates (Dubai)	1995/96	United States
Equine-2 influenza A virus	Puerto Rico	1997	United States
Equine-2 influenza A virus	Philippines	1997	United States
Equine-2 influenza A virus	South Africa	2003	United States
Equine-2 influenza A virus	Japan	2007	United States/Europe
Equine-2 influenza A virus	Australia	2007	Japan

Modified from Timoney PJ: Equids and equine semen: international trade vs. disease control. In Proceedings of Eighth International Conference on Equine Infectious Diseases, Newmarket, England, 1999, R&W Publications.

which are primarily vector-borne infections but can also be transmitted iatrogenically. Besides the potential for many equine diseases to be introduced and effectively spread by respiratory, venereal, or vector-borne routes, agents can be transferred between countries by other means, which, although less frequently encountered, should not be overlooked. A limited number of pathogens (e.g., EHV-1 and EHV-4, *T. equigenitalis*) can be introduced into a country through the importation of a pregnant mare that is harboring these organisms in utero. In such cases, the potential for spread of these pathogens is at the time of foaling.[3]

A final means of introduction of a disease agent is through importation of an equid infested with the intermediate state of a parasite such as the larvae of the botfly, *Cochliomyia hominivorax*, the cause of screwworm myiasis.[3] In sporadic but repeated cases, horses imported into the United States from certain South American countries (e.g., Argentina, Venezuela) have been found infested with these larvae on postentry inspection.

Even though most of the international spread of equine diseases results from the movement of equids, usually horses, trade in semen is also of proven importance in the global dissemination of certain equine pathogens, including EAV, *T. equigenitalis*, *K. pneumoniae*, and *P. aeruginosa*.[3,16,17] Imported virus-infective semen, primarily from Warmblood stallions in Europe, was responsible for extensive and economically significant outbreaks of EVA in the United States and in Argentina in 2010, in some cases associated with abortion and the death of young foals.[16,18]

Over the past 40 years, numerous outbreaks or epidemics of particular equine diseases have resulted from the importation of an infected animal(s) or infective semen[3] (Table 63-2). African horse sickness (AHS) and VEE are the two most dreaded equine diseases, and both have been responsible for devastating epidemics. The most recent epidemics of AHS outside the endemic areas in sub-Saharan Africa occurred during 1987-1991 in Spain, Portugal, and Morocco, causing

Table 63-2 Disease Outbreaks and Epidemics Related to International Movement of Equids and Semen, 1959-2012

Disease	Importing Country	Year	Source
African horse sickness	Middle East, Southwest Asia, India	1959	Extension from epidemic in Africa
	Spain, Cyprus	1987	Imported zebra from Namibia
	Morocco, Portugal	1989	Extension from epidemic in Spain
Contagious equine metritis	England, Ireland	1977	Imported carrier animal
	Australia	1977	Imported carrier stallions from Europe
	Brazil	1977	Imported carrier animal from Europe
	United States	1978	Imported carrier animal from Europe
	Japan	1980	Imported carrier animal from Europe
	England	1996	Imported carrier stallion from Europe
	United States	2000	Imported carrier stallion from Denmark
	South Africa	2011	Imported carrier stallion from Europe
Equine herpesvirus myeloencephalopathy	United States	2006	Imported horses from Germany
Equine infectious anemia	England	1974	Imported carrier mare from Italy
	Ireland	2006	Imported plasma from Italy
Equine viral arteritis	United States	1986/87	Imported carrier stallion or semen from Europe
	England	1993	Imported carrier stallion from Europe
	South Africa	1994-1998	Imported semen from Europe
	United States	1996-2005	Imported carrier stallions or semen from Europe
	Argentina	2010	Imported semen from the Netherlands
Glanders	United Arab Emirates (Dubai)	2004	Middle East
	Germany	2006	Imported horse from Brazil
	Kuwait	2009/10	Imported horses from Syria
	Bahrain	2010	Imported horses from Syria and Kuwait
	Lebanon	2011	Imported horses from Syria
Piroplasmosis	United States	1959	Imported Cuban horses with *Babesia caballi*
	United States	2009/2010	Imported horses from Mexico
Venezuelan equine encephalomyelitis	United States	1971	Extension from epidemic in South America, Central America, and Mexico

Modified from Timoney PJ: Equids and equine semen: international trade vs. disease control. In Proceedings of Eighth International Conference on Equine Infectious Diseases, Newmarket, England, 1999, R&W Publications.

significant economic losses and having a major impact on international trade in equids from affected countries.[19] The source of the original outbreak in Spain in 1987 was traced to the importation of 10 zebras from Namibia, which transited through Portugal en route to a safari park near Madrid.

Equine influenza has frequently been spread through international movement and has occasionally been responsible for widespread epidemics of disease in immunologically naïve or inadequately protected horses. Such occurrences have had a major economic impact on the racing industries in affected countries. The first recorded introduction of EIV into the racing population in Hong Kong in 1986 resulted in the cancellation of seven race meetings and financial losses totaling almost $1 billion.[20] Similarly, the disease had a major impact on the racing industry in South Africa after it was first introduced in 1992[21] and reintroduced in 2003.[22] The latter epidemic affected an estimated 3700 horses in training (40% of the country's racehorse population) at Cape Town, Johannesburg, and Port Elizabeth and approximately 3000 other equids. Loss in revenue to the equine industry from this epidemic was estimated at more than 60 million rand. The most recent major epidemic of EIV occurred in Australia in 2007.[23] This was traced to the importation of a number of subclinically infected shuttle stallions from Japan. Breaches in biosecurity at a postentry quarantine station led to escape of the virus and very extensive spread of the disease among the horse populations in southern Queensland and New South Wales. Estimated economic impact of this epidemic exceeded 1 billion dollars.

The widespread occurrence of CEM in Kentucky in 1978 exemplifies the major economic impact that introduction of a transboundary equine disease can have on a previously unexposed naïve breeding population.[3] The disease was traced to the importation of two carrier stallions from Europe in the fall of 1977 and resulted in major disruption to the 1978 breeding season and an estimated financial loss to the state's Thoroughbred breeding industry of at least $4 million. More recently, there was a second major CEM event in the United States that was first discovered in late 2008.[24] The source of *T. equigenitalis* was believed to have been a carrier stallion imported from Denmark in 2000. Approximately 1100 stallions and mares were exposed during the occurrence, with the cost to the industry and the government of several million dollars.

Experience over the years has repeatedly reaffirmed the ease with which various equine diseases have been disseminated globally through the international trade in equids and semen.[5] Such incursions have had major financial repercussions for the horse industry in affected countries. Aside from significant disruption to racing or other equine performance events and perhaps to a country's breeding industry, occurrences of transboundary diseases can have a long-term effect on international trade. This can best be illustrated by the restrictions on importation of equids that many countries impose on any country or region thereof affected with AHS. In addition to equine health and economic consequences, the introduction of certain transboundary equine diseases (e.g., VEE, glanders) can have a major impact on public health.

Multinational Trade Agreements

In an era of increasing globalization, facilitation of trade between countries through the reduction or elimination of restrictive trade practices has been the goal of various bilateral and multinational trade agreements. The European Union Free Trade Area, the North American Free Trade Agreement (NAFTA), and the World Trade Organization (WTO) are among the major world trading groups, markets, and agreements.[3] Formation of the WTO at the Uruguay Round of Multilateral Trade Negotiations in 1994 marked a significant change in how its member countries could regulate for the control of infectious diseases of plants and animals under the organization's Sanitary and Phytosanitary Agreement.[8] The key provisions of that agreement are aimed at facilitating international trade in animals, including animal germplasm, by reducing preimport and post-import health requirements among participating countries.[7]

It could be rightly argued that easing trade restrictions and related testing requirements enhances the risk of introducing transboundary diseases while limiting a country's ability to protect its equine industry from the incursion of various equine pathogens. Currently, there is no compelling justification for reducing existing preentry and postentry health requirements for equids imported into the United States on the pretext of furthering international trade. To do so would undoubtedly heighten the risk of introducing a range of equine diseases, some transboundary and others presently endemic in the United States equid population. An example in point is the number of stallions and mares imported from Europe over the past 15 years that turned out to be carriers of CEM on postentry quarantine and testing. All had been tested in their respective countries of origin and were certified negative for the carrier state prior to export. The potential economic consequences for the domestic horse industry from any such incursions could far outweigh the financial benefits to be gained from facilitating international trade.

Emergent Diseases

Over the past 40 to 50 years, several previously unrecognized diseases have been described that can affect horses and other members of the family *Equidae*.[2,5,7] The list of "new" or emergent equine pathogens continues to grow, as it does for humans and other animal species. It currently includes several bacterial diseases, such as CEM, Potomac horse fever, equine granulocytic ehrlichiosis, equine proliferative enteropathy, and nocardioform placentitis and abortion, and a number of viral diseases, including equine encephalosis, Getah virus infection, Hendra virus infection, Nipah virus infection, and Salem virus infection. The geographic distribution of most of these diseases has remained essentially the same as when they were originally identified. A notable exception is CEM, which has been spread to various countries worldwide through the international movement of carrier stallions and mares.[3]

Additional equine diseases will undoubtedly be discovered. Containing these diseases and preventing their dissemination globally will require the cooperation and combined efforts of horse industries and animal health officials in the country or countries in which they are initially recognized.

New Variants of Established Pathogens

Natural mutation of certain equine pathogens has given rise to variants and strains of enhanced virulence for the horse, as illustrated by several examples in the past 20 years. In 1989 a novel strain of EIV (H3N8), the Jilin'89 strain of equine-2 influenza A virus, emerged in China.[25] Thought to be of avian origin, this particular virus strain was responsible for tens of thousands of cases and numerous deaths in the indigenous equid population. If it had spread outside China, this strain of H3N8 could have had devastating consequences for other unprotected equine populations.

Significant outbreaks of equine encephalomyelitis in southwestern Mexico in 1993 and again in 1996 provided the first confirmed evidence of the emergence of a strain of VEE virus subtype IE with the capability to cause illness and associated mortality not only in humans but also in equids.[26] Before these outbreaks, the endemic IE virus subtype was not considered to have the potential to cause widespread disease in

equids. Clearly, similar variants of this subtype of VEE virus may reemerge in the future and spread to other geographic areas, which could include Central America and the United States.

The most recently recognized example of emergence of a variant of an established equine pathogen is the identification of strains of EHV-1 with enhanced neuropathogenicity for the horse. These neuropathogenic strains of the virus appear to have evolved as a result of a single-point mutation in the viral DNA polymerase gene.[27] Such strains have been shown to cause higher clinical attack rates and greater case-fatality rates than virus strains lacking this mutation. Available evidence from outbreaks of equine herpesvirus myeloencephalopathy in the United Kingdom, France, and the United States indicates that the frequency of this disease is increasing in these countries. Because of the high percentage of horses that can become latent carriers of this infection, these neuropathogenic strains of EHV-1 will inevitably become more widely disseminated through the international movement of equids and there is evidence to indicate this is already occurring.

Climate Disturbance Effects

There is mounting evidence that climate-related phenomena, such as El Niño–southern oscillation and global warming, can have an influence on the occurrence and distribution of certain diseases, especially vector-borne diseases such as AHS, equine encephalosis, and the equine viral encephalomyelitides.[28,29] The increased temperatures and altered rainfall directly linked to such phenomena are likely to affect the range and biologic behavior of arthropod vectors and intermediate, amplifying/reservoir hosts, as well as the viability and maturation rates of infective agents in those vectors.[30]

African horse sickness, equine encephalosis, and vesicular stomatitis are diseases affecting the horse that can be spread through windborne carriage of infected insect vectors such as *Culicoides* spp. Study of the climatic patterns for the western region of South Africa, where most epidemics of AHS have occurred, has shown that all but 1 of the 14 epidemics of the disease recorded since 1803 have been in El Niño years.[31] Such years were characterized by an earlier period of drought followed by heavier rainfall than usual. The higher-than-normal temperatures customary of the drought period lead to significant increases in the vector population and favor the transmission of AHS.

Although not yet conclusively proved, climate phenomena can and will have an influence on the global distribution and incidence of various vector-borne diseases of equids and other species.

Availability of New Vectors

The inadvertent introduction of a particular arthropod vector (e.g., species of mosquito, midge, or tick) into a country or geographic region for the first time can have significant consequences if the arthropod becomes successfully established in its new environment and is shown to be competent to transmit specific vector-borne diseases present in the country or region. In the past 20 to 30 years, the United States has been the recipient of two mosquito species, *Aedes albopictus (Stegomyia albopicta)* or Asian tiger mosquito and *Ochlerotatus japonicus*, neither of which was previously known to occur in the country.[32,33] Both mosquito species have been found to be competent vectors of certain equine viral encephalomyelitides, especially Eastern equine encephalomyelitis (EEE) and West Nile encephalitis.[7] Since their known introduction, the two mosquito species have established themselves and are currently becoming widely distributed in an increasing number of states.

The United States is not unique in respect to the availability of new vectors. Other countries in both the Northern and the Southern Hemisphere have had similar experiences.[3] Such incursions, mostly of species of mosquito, have been short-lived in some cases, whereas in other cases the new vector has become permanently established in its new habitat as exemplified by *Aedes albopictus* in northeastern Italy.

Migration of Amplifying/Reservoir Hosts or Vectors of Specific Pathogens

Migration of amplifying/reservoir hosts or vectors of specific pathogens can influence the geographic distribution and occurrence of particular diseases of humans, equids, and other livestock species and wildlife. Evidence indicates that migrating birds can be responsible for infrequent cases or reintroduction of certain diseases into countries in which they did not previously occur.[34-36] This has been starkly illustrated by the recent rapid global spread of the highly pathogenic avian influenza virus (H5N1). Birds are also thought to be responsible for the occasional reintroduction of WNV into various countries in southern Europe and the Middle East from the African continent.[37] There is little doubt that migratory birds have been primarily responsible for the spread of this virus from the United States into Mexico, Central America, and certain Caribbean countries over the past several years. Birds have also been implicated in the transfer of EEE and Western equine encephalomyelitis (WEE) viruses between southern and northern hemispheres of the Americas, and vice versa.

The distribution and occurrence of other equine arthropod-borne diseases can be influenced by the migration of the relevant vectors.[3] African horse sickness, equine encephalosis, and vesicular stomatitis are diseases that can be spread over considerable distances through wind-borne carriage of infected *Culicoides* spp. Wind-borne carriage of infected mosquitoes may similarly account for the periodic incursions of Japanese encephalitis virus into the Cape York Peninsula of northeastern Queensland, Australia, from Papua, New Guinea (P.M. Ellis, personal communication, 2000).

Reliability of Preexport Testing

Without detracting from the value of preexport testing that involves laboratory tests required by the importing country, as well as live animal inspection, it must be acknowledged that the certifications of health and freedom from contact with various infectious diseases accompanying horses being shipped are not always reliable. Of continuing concern is the need for a greater harmonization between the laboratory testing conducted prior to export and that carried out in the importing country. There have been repeated instances where CEM carrier stallions and mares and equine arteritis virus carrier stallions and infective semen were only detected on postentry laboratory examination. The importance of a thorough clinical examination performed on all horses prior to shipment cannot be overemphasized. Horses should not arrive after a transatlantic flight with overt signs of strangles or other respiratory diseases. The consequences of such disease introductions can be significant as was amply demonstrated by the series of outbreaks of equine herpesvirus myeloencephalopathy that occurred in 2006 and which were traced back to a shipment of infected horses from Germany.

Disease Spread from Feral Equids

In countries with feral equid populations, there is the potential risk of spread of certain diseases to domestic horses. This was well exemplified by the reintroduction of AHS into the Iberian peninsula in 1987, where the source of virus was a group of zebra imported into Portugal from Namibia en route to Spain.

Agroterrorism

Before the terrorist attacks on the United States in September 2001 and the subsequent anthrax letter incidents, little consideration was given to the need to prevent and respond to a bioterrorist attack against the U.S. agricultural industry and equine population in particular.[38] Regrettably, past events serve to underscore the reality of the threat posed to agricultural industries. Whereas the transfer of diseases between countries occurs most often accidentally or inadvertently, such incursions could also be deliberate, the consequence of an act of bioterrorism.

In view of the major economic importance of the U.S. equine industry, certain transboundary diseases could have a huge financial impact if deliberately introduced into the unprotected equine population. Of the entire array of equine infectious diseases, AHS and VEE have the potential to cause the most serious and devastating epidemics of disease among all categories of horses. Neither causal agent would require to be "weaponized" to achieve such an outcome. Were they to occur, such disease events would also cripple the ability of the United States to export equids or semen throughout the world.

Clearly, the potential threat of agroterrorism should neither be underappreciated nor oversensationalized. Widespread acceptance of the reality of the threat is the important issue, as well as the awareness that a national emerging response plan has been developed to deal with any bioterrorist-related health emergency involving the horse or other livestock industries.

Reducing the Risk of International Spread of Equine Diseases

Historically, veterinary regulatory authorities worldwide have responded to the threat of infectious disease spread inherent in international trade by formulating import policies that maximize disease prevention safeguards but minimize facilitation of trade. It has become increasingly difficult, however, for countries to uphold policies based on overly restrictive import controls in today's global economic climate. They are perceived in conflict with the overall goal of the WTO, which is to eliminate or reduce unjustified protectionist barriers to trade among member countries.[9]

It is freely accepted that the economic viability and success of the horse industry worldwide is critically dependent on the ability to ship horses within a state, a country, or internationally, without excessive restrictions on movement. With the aim of reducing the level of risk of disease spread from such movements, regulatory authorities have developed specific control measures to prevent the introduction and potential dissemination of a range of equine diseases into the importing country. To assist in formulation of their animal health import policies, the Office International des Epizooties (OIE), now the World Organization for Animal Health as recognized by the WTO, has developed a Terrestrial Animal Health Code that provides countries worldwide with principal control standards for preventing the spread of specific diseases listed by the OIE, including those of equids.[39] Regardless of country of origin or destination, horses are shipped internationally under license/permit issued by the appropriate regulatory agent in the exporting country. This documentation serves as a means of individual animal identification, certification of health and freedom from contact with various equine diseases, and a declaration that the exporting country or its region/zone has been confirmed free of evidence of certain diseases within a particular time frame.

Preexport Requirements

In addition to certification of freedom of the exporting country or region/zone from specified equine diseases (e.g., AHS, VEE, glanders), current regulations governing the import of equids into the United States and most other countries require similar certification with respect to the premises of origin of the horse(s) being exported, other premises within a stated radius of that location, and most importantly, the individual animal(s) being exported. Horses must be held in preexport quarantine for a specified period, during which they are subjected to the necessary clinical examination and laboratory tests prescribed by the importing country. Of critical importance to ensuring the integrity of sampling and testing of horses for export is the need for some form of permanent individual identification such as a unique animal identification number (microchip) or alternative system of permanent identification (iris scanning, retinal scanning). Poor or inferior systems of animal identification increase the potential for willful substitution of horses before shipment and enhance the disease risks involved.

Postimport Requirements

Assuming all the preexport certification and testing meet the requirements of the importing country, the horse(s) being shipped are approved for temporary or permanent entry into that country. Where the United States is the country of destination, the U.S. Department of Agriculture (USDA) requires that all horses imported from non–AHS-affected countries are, transported immediately after arrival in a federally sealed conveyance to a USDA-approved quarantine station closest to the port of entry. The animals are held in isolation for up to 42 hours, during which they are clinically monitored and serologically tested for evidence of dourine, glanders, EIA, and EP. Subject to a satisfactory health report and negative serologic findings for these diseases, horses are released from quarantine and shipped to their state(s) of destination.

Intact male or female horses over 731 days of age originating in a CEM-affected country and approved for permanent entry into the United States are required to undergo additional testing to confirm their freedom from *T. equigenitalis*, the causal agent of CEM. To accomplish this, such individuals are shipped in a sealed conveyance to a state that is federally approved to accept and quarantine stallions and mares from CEM-affected countries. They are quarantined on a premises approved for that purpose in accordance with federal and state guidelines and subjected to the necessary testing for CEM. They are released from quarantine once they have been confirmed not to be carriers of *T. equigenitalis*.

Some in the international community advocate that the importing country accept the reliability of laboratory testing conducted in the exporting country, thereby obviating the need for a period of postentry quarantine and repeat laboratory testing in the country of destination. However, experience has shown that failure to provide adequate post-entry screening of equids for specific infections can pose an unacceptable disease risk for the horse industry in the importing country such as the United States. For example, over the past 15 years alone, a total of 36 stallions and mares imported into the United States from Europe were confirmed carriers of *T. equigenitalis* on postentry quarantine and testing. All the animals involved were tested in the countries of origin and certified free of evidence of this bacterium. If this transboundary disease had been reintroduced into the United States breeding population through any of these importations, it could have had major economic repercussions for the horse breeding industry. Another example of the existing federal postimport inspection and testing program successfully preventing the introduction of a transboundary disease is screwworm myiasis. In repeated but infrequent cases, horses imported from certain South American countries and certified free from this parasite were confirmed infested with the larvae of *Cochliomyia hominivorax* in postentry quarantine.

In addition, horses shipped from various European countries have occasionally been found to be clinically affected with diseases, such as strangles or EHV-1 and EHV-4–related diseases, on arrival in the United States. Collectively, these incidents bring into question the reliability of preimport laboratory testing and clinical veterinary inspection conducted by the exporting country. Also, they reaffirm the importance of maintaining the current system of postentry safeguards that has served the horse industry well over the years and has helped to minimize the risk of introduction of various transboundary diseases.

Clearly, a balance must be struck between allowing movement of equids and providing the necessary safeguards to prevent the spread of various equine diseases. In light of the risks associated with international trade in horses and semen, countries need to have in place adequate postentry risk management strategies. Countries can no longer be passive to the health risks involved.

Monitoring Surveillance and Reporting of Diseases

Surveillance of equine diseases at a national level and prompt reporting to the relevant authorities and industry organizations are critical to the effectiveness of national and international equine health control programs. Essential to any disease or early-warning monitoring program is the availability of adequate diagnostic capability for the disease(s) under surveillance. Accuracy and timeliness of a laboratory diagnosis of the suspected disease are of paramount importance.

In any national reporting system, primary consideration should be given to the equine diseases listed by the OIE, together with a number of those listed as multispecies diseases. In addition to OIE notification of occurrences of listed diseases and any newly emergent disease problem, an informal disease-reporting system is supported by a growing number of countries worldwide. It requires that each participating country provide interim and quarterly reports of any confirmed occurrences of a range of equine diseases, many but not all listed by the OIE, to the International Collating Center at the Animal Health Trust in the United Kingdom.

The value of timely exchange of accurate, up-to-date information on occurrences of specific equine diseases at an international level cannot be overemphasized. Such sharing of information facilitates the process of risk assessment analysis between countries and enhances opportunities for reduction or elimination of unjustified restrictions on international trade in equids, semen, and embryos. At a national level, monitoring, surveillance, and reporting serves as a means of early detection of a disease that has already gained entry, whether a transboundary or endemic disease. It cannot be overemphasized how important a role the practicing veterinarian and the horse owner play in ensuring the success of any surveillance and reporting system and in helping to monitor the health integrity of their equine industry.

Industry Initiatives

No program for the national or international control of equine infectious diseases can expect to be successful if it lacks the participation and support of the horse industry. With this in mind, several international groups have been formed over the years that represent the racing, equestrian sports, and breeding sectors of the industry. They include the Federation of Horseracing Authorities Permanent Liaison Committee on the International Movement of Horses, the FEI, and an International Thoroughbred Breeders' Federation. These respective organizations or groups are broadly representative of the international community of countries with significant horse-breeding/performance industries. Their overall goal is to enlist industry involvement in identifying specific equine health or related issues that adversely affect international movement of horses and to seek ways to resolve them.

Within the realm of industry initiatives, the FEI has recently sought the support of the OIE in seeking to obtain a more equitable balance between facilitation of international movement of high-value performance horses and meeting the testing requirements of importing countries. It has been recognized for many years that the risk of disease transfer is not necessarily equivalent among different categories of horses. For several reasons, high-value performance horses can be considered a lower risk category. Because of the frequency with which they travel internationally, they are tested more often and monitored more closely for a range of the most important diseases. Additionally, their vaccination status for diseases of significance is likely to be current. The goal of this initiative is to establish a strategic framework for countries and regions to harmonize their approach to sanitary conditions for the international movement of performance horses. Objectives are to (1) maintain the high health status of performance horses and minimize the risk of transboundary disease transmission while removing unjustified health requirements; (2) ensure the welfare of the horses during transportation; and (3) educate government regulatory authorities, industry, and stakeholders on OIE standards and biosecurity requirements relating to the international movement of performance horses.

Yet, another example of an industry initiative is the concept of establishing an "equine disease-free zone" in countries wishing to host an internationally recognized performance event but are unable to do so because of the disease status of their resident equine population. The aims of developing such a facility are twofold: (1) to enable equine athletes from other countries to compete in an international event without the risk of being exposed to a disease or diseases endemic in the host country and (2) to protect the host country's equine population from a disease introduced by a competing country's horses. Proof of concept that this was achievable was the "Equine Disease-Free Facility" that was developed in Guangdong Province in PR China. It enabled the country to host the equine program of the 2010 Asian Games. The detailed advance planning, discussions, and negotiations that took place between the relevant international agencies and ruling bodies and the national and provincial animal health authorities in China were crucial to ensuring the success of this unique initiative. Under similar circumstances in the future, other countries may adopt the same approach if intent on hosting international performance events.

Greater control over the international spread of equine diseases is an achievable goal. However, attaining it is only possible if horse industries and animal health regulatory authorities worldwide work cooperatively together toward that end.

The complete reference list is available online at www.expertconsult.com.

CHAPTER

64 Immunoprophylaxis

W. David Wilson, Nicola Pusterla, and Debra C. Long

Immunoprophylaxis is the prevention of infectious disease through induction or enhancement of antigen-specific protective immune responses. Immunity can be passively acquired by natural or exogenous transfer of humoral or cellular factors from animals previously immunized through natural exposure or vaccination. Active induction of responses is through administration of vaccines containing (1) inactivated or live pathogens modified to attenuate their pathogenicity, (2) microbial components, (3) inactivated microbial products such as toxoids, (4) genetic material encoding for expression of protective antigens, and (5) genetically engineered noninfectious particles. Recent advances have focused on the packaging of viruses with adjuvants, cytokines, and various molecules to direct the immune response. Furthermore, needleless administration and orally and mucosally delivered vaccines are the intense focus of the next generation of vaccines. In addition to route of administration, new polymers and drug delivery systems consisting of micelles, nanoparticles/microparticles, and nanospheres/microspheres are being developed to offer safer, yet enhanced immune targeting.[1] Because of the major changes in the animal pharmaceutical and biological industry since the first edition of this text was published, most vaccine trade names have been removed from this chapter. The reader is encouraged to read vaccine labels and refer to original studies to verify the formulation of a product.

Active Immunization

Basic Principles

Active immunization typically involves administration of a primary series of injections of one or more doses of vaccine to "prime" the immune system and generate effector proteins (antibodies) and cells. Typically, "booster" doses of vaccine are administered periodically to enhance the level of specific antibody and effector T cells. During priming, development of the T helper (Th) response occurs that can (1) bias the immune response toward (or away from) a humoral (Th2) or cellular (Th1) response; (2) bias the immune response toward (or away from) effector cytokines, such as interferon-gamma (IFN-γ; Th1) or interleukin 4 (IL-4; Th2); and most importantly, (3) provide the induction of Th cells that enhance the proliferative capacity and intensity of the secondary response. Without T-cell helper responses, the effector immune response will not provide adequate protection. In addition, an antibody isotype switch occurs to enhance the specificity and activity of effector antibodies.

On subsequent exposure to the specific pathogen, memory cells can be recruited to quickly generate specific antibodies and effector cells, such as cytotoxic T lymphocytes (CTLs), to neutralize the pathogen before it causes disease. Some vaccines are capable of inducing sterile immunity, in which case infection and replication of the pathogen are completely blocked as in the action of neutralizing antibody for preventing encephalitis virus infection of the CNS. Other vaccines induce clinical protection without completely blocking infection or replication of the organism, although the latter is typically at a much reduced level.

Types of Vaccines

Inactivated Vaccines

Most of the vaccines currently licensed for use in horses in North America and Europe are traditional vaccine formulations such as bacterins, toxoids, or inactivated viral vaccines.[2] Inactivated pathogen vaccines are the most common form of equine vaccine in current use and are comprised of microorganisms that have been treated with heat or chemicals to inactivate them while preserving their immunogenicity (Table 64-1). Phenol, formaldehyde, and β-propiolactone are among the inactivating agents used most frequently in the preparation of inactivated bacterial and viral vaccines.[3] Inactivated vaccines are inherently biologically safe because they have, in theory, no residual virulence and have a high stability in storage. They are typically suitable and safe for use in pregnant mares, debilitated or immunocompromised animals, geriatric horses, and colostrum-deprived foals. However, such vaccines typically require multiple doses and regular boosters, and efficacy frequently depends on use of potent adjuvants and high antigenic

mass. Compared with vaccines of other types, disadvantages often associated with inactivated vaccines include slow onset of immunity, increased risk of local and allergic complications (high antigenic mass and inclusion of adjuvants are two factors that increase the likelihood of reactions), need for multiple doses in the primary series, need for parenteral (typically intramuscular [IM]) administration, need for regular boosters at frequent intervals to maintain reasonable immunity, and shorter duration of immunity than achieved with MLVs. Further, because inactivated vaccines are known to be weak inducers of cell-mediated immunity, they are not very efficient in eliminating virus-infected cells.[4]

Protein or Subunit Vaccines

Extracted and purified proteins naturally produced by pathogens can be used to formulate inactivated vaccines. Such vaccines can be developed only if the immunogens responsible for inducing the protective immune response are known. These vaccines often need high antigenic mass and strong adjuvants to stimulate the immune system. The major advantage of subunit vaccines is their inherent biologic safety because there is no risk of residual virulence. These vaccines have been associated with fewer injection site reactions than vaccines containing whole bacterial products. Equine influenza virus and tetanus vaccines containing influenza hemagglutinin (HA) and neuraminidase (NA) and tetanus subunit proteins with an immune-stimulating complex (ISCOM) adjuvant are marketed in Europe and South Africa. These vaccines have demonstrated both experimental and field efficacy.[5-8] Some recombinant tetanus toxoids and vaccines against strangles based on the M protein of *Streptococcus equi* subsp. *equi* (SeM) are also described. The cell surface protein (CSP) of *Streptococcus equi* subsp. *zooepidemicus* has been isolated, produced as a recombinant protein, and shown to induce protection in a mouse model of infection.[9]

DNA Vaccines

The basis for deoxyribonucleic acid (DNA) immunization is that host cells take up plasmid DNA, which is expressed *in vivo* in transfected cells, theoretically in a manner identical to that occurring in natural infection.[10,11] Consequently, if administered correctly, DNA vaccines could stimulate both humoral and cellular immunity. Plasmid DNA vaccines offer many of the

Table 64-1 Types of Equine Vaccines Licensed in North America

Disease/Virus	Dead Vaccines		Live Vaccines		DNA Vaccine
	Inactivated	Subunit	Modified Live	Recombinant	
Tetanus	X*				
Equine western encephalitis	X				
Equine eastern encephalitis	X			X	
Equine Venezuelan encephalitis	X		X		
West Nile	X			X, X (chimera)†	X†
Equine influenza	X		X	X	
Equine herpesvirus 1	X		X		
Equine herpesvirus 4	X				
Strangles	X†	X	X		
Equine viral arteritis			X		
Rabies	X				
Equine neorickettsiosis (Potomac horse fever)	X				
Botulism	X*				
Rotavirus‡	X				
Equine Rhinitis A‡	X				

*Inactivated toxoid.

†Licensed but not currently marketed.

‡Conditionally licensed.

potential benefits of live vaccines without the same inherent risks such as reversion to virulence. Because the vaccine consists of a single gene, it will not induce infection or disease. Plasmid DNA vaccines typically induce expression of only one or a few of the many protein antigens present in the parent microorganism, thereby raising the possibility of developing companion diagnostic tests to differentiate vaccinated animals from animals that are carriers of the disease. Further, DNA vaccines may be able to overcome maternally derived immunity in neonates or in very young animals.[10] To date, no adverse effects have been associated with the use of DNA vaccines; however, safety concerns, including the potential integration of plasmid DNA into the host genome or the generation of anti-DNA antibodies, are of some concern.

A DNA vaccine expressing the HA protein of equine H3N8 influenza virus generates both homologous and heterologous immune responses and protects against clinical disease and viral replication by homologous H3N8 virus in horses. This vaccine uses a needle-free delivery system.[12]

Modified Live Vaccines

Modified live vaccines (MLVs) consist of attenuated microorganisms that replicate *in vivo*, thereby eliciting an immune response similar to that induced by natural infection, but without the associated clinical signs typically seen with natural exposure to the specific pathogen. Modified live vaccines typically induce rapid onset of immunity that includes both humoral and cell-mediated responses, produce a long-lasting duration of immunity, and require fewer doses to immunize the host. Depending on the route of administration, some MLVs are capable of inducing local mucosal responses. Compared with killed vaccines, MLVs generally contain a lower antigenic mass and usually do not require inclusion of an adjuvant; therefore they are less likely to induce adverse local reactions. Because the mutations responsible for attenuation of virulence in MLVs often are poorly defined, one of the major concerns is the possibility that the vaccine organism regains its virulence or combines with a wild strain to generate a more pathogenic reassortant that could induce clinical disease, death, and possibly outbreaks. Therefore modified pathogens with multiple mutations on different genes are more suitable candidates for MLVs because they are less likely to revert to virulence than pathogens with single mutations. Lack of safety data in immunocompromised or pregnant horses compromises the appropriateness and, in some instances, precludes the use of such vaccines in these animals.

Attenuation usually is achieved by in vitro passage through one or more cell types, selection of spontaneous or induced temperature sensitive mutants, use of reassortants obtained by co-infection of the same cell with two different viruses with segmented genomes, or use of chemicals that induce mutations.[10,13,14] Several MLVs are currently marketed for use in horses, including vaccines for prevention of equine influenza, strangles, equine herpesvirus 1 (EHV-1), and equine viral arteritis (EVA).

Recombinant Vaccines

Viruses and bacteria can be genetically engineered to serve as carriers or vectors for the expression of foreign proteins through the use of recombinant technology. A prerequisite to using this technology is thorough definition of the protective antigens of the specific pathogen of interest. Such vectors allow the introduction of the transgene into host cells, leading to production of protein antigens and stimulation of both B-cell and T-cell responses.[15] Adenoviruses and herpesviruses are being considered and evaluated as potential vaccine vectors, and a recombinant modified vaccinia Ankara virus (rMVA) vaccine for equine influenza has already shown efficacy in challenge studies in

horses.[16,17] In contrast to many poxviruses, which have a very broad vertebrate host range, the canarypox and fowlpox viruses are host restricted to certain avian species and produce an abortive infection in mammals. Canarypox and fowlpox are therefore ideal candidate vectors for mammalian vaccines because they express the inserted foreign genes in the absence of productive replication. Avian poxvirus–vectored vaccines have the potential to induce a broad array of immune responses in the absence of an adjuvant, although the canarypox-vectored West Nile virus (WNV) and influenza vaccines currently marketed for use in horses do contain a polymer adjuvant.[18-20] It appears that canarypox virus recombinants do not trigger a neutralizing response against the vector, which would preclude an immune response against the transgene when subsequent booster doses of vaccine are administered.

Chimera vaccines are similar to live vectored vaccines in that they use components of one viral agent to transport genes encoding for expression of important protective antigens of the pathogen of interest. In the case of chimera vaccines, the vector and the pathogen of interest are typically in the same family. To date, this technology has been applied most extensively to immunize against dengue, Japanese encephalitis (JE), and WNV, all of which are flaviviruses, using the highly attenuated 17D vaccine strain of the related flavivirus, yellow fever virus (YF), as the vector. The premembrane (prM) and envelope (E) structural proteins of the pathogen of dengue, JE, or WNV are exchanged for the homolog proteins of YF 17D using complementary DNA (cDNA) templates encoding for these proteins.[21] A single dose of the nonadjuvanted YF-WNV chimeric vaccine generated using this technology induces solid protection in horses subjected to intrathecal challenge with virulent WNV. This formulation is also part of an inactivated vaccine against WNV.[22]

Vaccine Augmentation

Marker Vaccines

Vaccines that differentiate infected animals from vaccinated animals (DIVA) are needed in situations in which the differentiation between a naturally infected and a vaccinated animal is important. Such vaccines can be subunit, gene-deleted, vectored, or DNA vaccines and are always used in conjunction with a diagnostic test. Presently one such combination exists in Australia where the vaccine used was canarypox recombinant influenza vaccine that only has the HA gene. A corollary enzyme-linked immunosorbent assay (ELISA) was developed to differentiate vaccinated from infected horses.

Vaccine Adjuvants

Vaccine adjuvants are chemicals, microbial components, or mammalian proteins that enhance the immune response to a vaccine. When developing a vaccine, it is essential to know what type of immune response will provide optimal protection and then select an adjuvant that will help induce that type of immune response without unacceptable adverse effects. Adjuvants in development or already incorporated in animal vaccines include aluminum salts, oil emulsions, liposomes, microparticles, saponins, ISCOMs, nonionic block co-polymers, cytokines, and a wide variety of bacterial derivatives. Adjuvants can be broadly divided into two classes based on their principal mechanisms of action: vaccine delivery systems and immunostimulatory adjuvants. Some vaccines contain proprietary adjuvants, the composition of which has not been made public.

The mechanism of action of most adjuvants remains poorly understood because immunization often activates a complex

Table 64-2 Adjuvants Used in Veterinary Medicine With Induced Immune Responses

Adjuvant	Immune Response		
	Cell Mediated (Th1)	Antibody Mediated (Th2)	CTL
Aluminum salts (alum)	X	X	
Oil emulsions		X	
Liposomes		X	X
Nanoparticles	X	X	X
Saponins	X	X	X
ISCOMs	X	X	X
Nonionic block co-polymers		X	X
Cytokines	X	X	
Bacterial products		X	X

Th1, T-helper cell type 1; *Th2*, T-helper cell type 2; *CTLs*, cytotoxic T lymphocyte; *ISCOMs*, immune-stimulated complexes.

cascade of responses, and the primary effect of the adjuvant is difficult to discern clearly. In general, adjuvants appear to exert their effect by enhancing antigen presentation, improving antigen stability, or acting as immunomodulators.[23,24] A single adjuvant may have more than one mechanism of action. Adjuvants that influence antigen presentation can affect this complex process by improving antigen uptake by antigen-presenting cells (APCs), the cells that process antigens and present epitopes to T cells in association with major histocompatibility complex (MHC) molecules. Some adjuvants appear to trap the antigen at the injection site and provide a continuing supply to local APCs, whereas others may work by saturating Kupffer cells in the liver and subsequently may increase the amount of antigen reaching the APCs. Most adjuvants can effectively stimulate Th cells and humoral immunity (Table 64-2). Some, such as liposomes, also appear to deliver antigens to pathways that lead to the presentation of MHC class I molecules and the induction of a CTL response. Immunomodulation is another mechanism of action of adjuvants and is achieved by altering the cytokine network. Adjuvants can influence the type of immunity by enhancing some cytokines and reducing the concentration of others, which may shift the immune response toward a Th1 (cell-mediated) or Th2 (humoral) response. By shifting the balance of cytokines, adjuvants, such as saponins, may stimulate cell-mediated immunity to an antigen that would normally induce only antibodies.

One particular type of adjuvant deserving special mention is the mucosal adjuvant. Mucosal immunity has a critical role in resistance to a wide variety of pathogens such as equine influenza and *Streptococcus equi* subsp. *equi*. Generating mucosal immunoglobulin A (IgA) responses with killed vaccines is challenging, and the only effective mucosal adjuvants defined to date are the bacterial exotoxins of enteric bacterial pathogens such as cholera toxin or the labile toxin of *Escherichia coli*.

In addition to enhancing the immune response, adjuvants can also increase the adverse effects of the vaccine. Adverse effects are influenced by the interactions of the specific adjuvant and antigen.[25] Systemic, nonspecific adverse effects can include lethargy, anorexia, fever, arthritis, uveitis, and soreness. More often, however, adjuvants cause local reactions, including inflammation and more rarely, granulomatous or sterile abscesses. Although most of these reactions are minor and transient, severe inflammation can trap antigens at the injection site and prevent them from being recognized by the immune system. Further, local inflammation and granulomas after vaccination have been linked to the development of vaccine-associated tumors in small animals and a myoblastic fibrosarcoma with multifocal osseous metaplasia has been reported in a horse at the site of influenza vaccination.[25a]

Regulatory Aspects of Vaccination

Licensing and Safety of Vaccines

Most countries of the world that have ministries of animal health have vaccine adverse event reporting. In the United States, the United States Department of Agriculture (USDA) Animal and Plant Health Inspection Service (APHIS) is the federal agency charged with licensing and overseeing the production and use of veterinary vaccines and other biologic products marketed in the United States. The Canadian Department of Agriculture has similar authority in Canada. The Veterinary Medicine Directorate of the National Office of Animal Health has a system for adverse event reporting in the United Kingdom. These agencies license the facilities in which vaccines are produced and regularly inspect them to ensure that facilities and production methods meet established standards. All vaccines are checked for potency, stability, and safety before licensing and at regular intervals thereafter. Safety is established by testing for sterility, toxicity, freedom from extraneous organisms and other material (i.e., purity), and confirmation of the identity of the antigens or organism(s) included in the vaccine. Both "in-house" and field safety studies involving several hundred animals (typically >500 in the case of horses) are also completed before final licensing to confirm that the risk of inducing local or systemic adverse reactions is at an acceptably low level.

The starting point in potency tests is to determine the immunogenicity of a vaccine or the minimum dose of antigen that induces a defined immune response, either determined serologically or in challenge studies. Because organisms included in live attenuated or vectored vaccines inevitably die over time, a substantial excess of the organism above the minimum immunizing dose is included in the marketed product to ensure that at least this minimal amount of antigen is present in the vaccine up to the expiration date, assuming appropriate storage and handling of the product. Potency of each batch (serial) of vaccine is therefore tested before and after accelerated aging. Similarly, excess antigen is also in inactivated vaccines, even though they are considerably more stable than live vaccines. Vaccines must not be used after the stated expiration date, even though most will retain potency beyond that date if stored properly. Because live vectored vaccines are governed by the same regulations as MLVs, they typically contain substantially higher amounts of the live vector than the minimum dose needed to immunize horses. These higher amounts not only add to the expense of vaccine production, but they also may be responsible for some of the systemic reactions observed occasionally in horses after administration of recently released serials of the canarypox-vectored WNV vaccine that presumably contain higher titers of the vector as a result of minimal "die-off" after release. These systemic adverse effects may include fever, lethargy, inappetence, tachycardia, abdominal discomfort, hyperemic mucous membranes, and mildly delayed capillary refill time.

The USDA has traditionally placed more emphasis on documentation of the purity, stability, and safety of veterinary vaccines than on their efficacy.[26,27] Consequently, vaccines for use in horses are typically safe when stored, handled, and administered according to label directions. Many vaccines, however, particularly those directed at pathogens of the respiratory and gastrointestinal tracts, have been found to be of questionable efficacy in the field. Furthermore, published data documenting the efficacy of equine vaccines in well-controlled blinded challenge or field studies have been sparse until recently. For those vaccines for which challenge data were available, duration of immunity (DOI) was rarely established because challenge was typically performed a few weeks after completion of the primary series, when immunity would be expected to be maximal. Without data to define DOI, label directions for revaccination were often arbitrary or ambiguous. Similarly, efficacy studies were not typically performed on foals; therefore the potential inhibitory effects of maternally derived antibodies and the age at which to commence primary immunization were typically not established. Fortunately, "the bar has been raised" considerably during recent years, to the extent that solid challenge data, including information on DOI, are available for virtually all new equine vaccines granted full licenses during the last decade. It is hoped that this type of information will be generated in the future for vaccines that were first licensed many years ago.

In addition to full licenses, the USDA has the prerogative to grant conditional licenses to vaccines or antibody products that have met requirements for purity, safety, and stability but have not had efficacy documented in either experimental challenge or field studies. Other criteria used in the granting of a conditional license include a determination that the disease is an imminent and significant threat, that currently available measures for prevention and treatment are inadequate, and that the vaccine or plasma product has a reasonable expectation of efficacy. For vaccines, this expectation of efficacy is typically based on documentation of a detectable serologic response in vaccinated animals and a reasonable likelihood that this serologic response will be protective. Conditional licenses are issued for a limited period and are renewable while the manufacturer works toward documentation of efficacy to support granting of a full license. Each respective state department of agriculture decides whether to allow marketing of a particular conditionally licensed product in that state. In contrast, an inactivated rotavirus vaccine has been marketed under conditional licenses for many years without apparent progress in documenting efficacy to support granting of a full license. A vaccine for equine viral arteritis is fully licensed for use in the United Kingdom (UK) and Europe, whereas in the United States this vaccine is regulated under a conditional license and its use determined by each respective state veterinarian. Additionally, an equine rhinitis A virus vaccine was granted a conditional license in late 2012.

Adverse Events

Although uncommon, the possibility always exists for adverse reactions (including anaphylaxis) associated with administration of a vaccine; therefore vaccines should be administered by, or under the direct supervision of, a veterinarian. Adverse reactions should be reported to the vaccine's manufacturer and to the agency in charge of adverse event reporting. Anaphylaxis constitutes a life-threatening emergency requiring prompt treatment with epinephrine 5 mL of a 1:10,000 dilution intravenously (IV) or in less acute situations, 2 to 5 mL of a 1:1000 dilution IM or subcutaneously (SC). A recent study reported development of immunoglobulin E (IgE) antibodies against nontarget antigen components of equine viral vaccines.[28] This work documented IgE antibodies by ELISA before and after vaccination. In addition, horses were tested via intradermal inoculation for sensitivity to bovine serum albumin, a common component of most equine vaccines. Over the 5-year period, high IgE–responder horses showed gradually increasing bovine serum albumin-specific serum IgE levels and positive skin test reactivity, yet none had an adverse event. Nonantigen protein components of vaccines may sensitize horses for future adverse responses to vaccination. Local irritant tissue reactions occur more frequently, particularly when polyvalent combination vaccines are used. These reactions are usually self-limiting, but resolution can be promoted by parenteral or oral administration of nonsteroidal antiinflammatory drugs (NSAIDs), topical application of warm compresses or the cutaneously absorbed NSAID, diclofenac (Boehringer Ingelheim Vetmedica Inc, St.

Joseph, MO), and gentle exercise. Significant reactions in the neck muscles may make the horse reluctant to lower or raise its head; therefore feed and water buckets should be positioned accordingly. The incidence of local reactions can be reduced by administration of the vaccine deep in the semimembranosus and semitendinosus muscles of the hindleg rather than in the neck, and by allowing the horse to exercise after vaccination. In addition, horses that repeatedly react to polyvalent vaccines may benefit from administration of NSAIDs before administration of the vaccine, administration of the individual antigenic components separately in different sites, or use of a different brand of vaccine containing a different adjuvant or administered by a different route such as intranasal rather than IM.

If unacceptable reactions occur repeatedly, the need for continued annual or more frequent revaccination against individual antigens should be carefully reevaluated, taking into account risk of disease, balanced against the risk of an adverse reaction. Many of the horses that experience adverse reactions have received many doses of many vaccine antigens, repeated over many years. In these horses the vaccination protocol should be "pared down" so that only the most essential antigens are administered and the maximum possible interval between boosters is employed. For diseases, such as rabies and tetanus, for which resistance can reasonably be correlated with circulating antibody titer, one possible approach to define the maximum or optimal interval between booster doses would be to measure the antibody titer to define the need for revaccination. The introduction in recent years of commercially available ELISA testing for antibodies to the SeM protein (Equine Diagnostic Solutions, Lexington, KY) and neutralizing antibody testing for almost all viral diseases, including equine influenza, EHV-1 and 4, Eastern equine encephalitis (EEE), Western equine encephalitis (WEE), and WNV provided by state and federal laboratories has made it possible to refine vaccination protocols for these diseases in horses that experience adverse reactions to vaccination.

Safety of Vaccines in Broodmares

Consideration of vaccine safety in broodmares must take into account risks to the pregnancy and safety to the fetus. Potential adverse effects of vaccines on pregnancy are difficult to document, even when large numbers of mares are used, unless obvious problems occur. Because fetal organogenesis occurs early in gestation and this period is also characterized by substantial embryonic loss, even in normal mares, it is sound practice to avoid administering vaccines to mares during the first 60 days of gestation unless conditions of imminent risk prevail.

Few vaccines carry specific label recommendations for use in pregnant mares, and little published data exist to document the safety of equine vaccines during pregnancy. Of the available fully licensed vaccines, the two EHV-1 vaccines (Pneumabort-K + 1b, Zoetis, Madison, NJ; and Prodigy, Merck, Millsboro, DE) are marketed and labeled for use in pregnant mares as an aid to prevention of EHV-1 abortion. Several other vaccines include directions for use in pregnant mares. Although not specifically labeled for administration during pregnancy, widespread use in practice over many years has failed to document that any of the inactivated vaccines currently marketed for use in horses poses an unacceptable risk to pregnant mares. Therefore pregnant mares are routinely vaccinated with inactivated vaccines directed against tetanus, EEE, WEE, WNV, influenza, EHV-4, strangles and to a lesser extent Equine neorickettsiosis (EN), rabies, and Venezuelan equine encephalomyelitis (VEE), botulism, and rotavirus. Similarly, adverse impacts on pregnancy have not been documented for intranasally vaccines marketed for strangles and influenza, MLVs marketed for EHV-1, and recombinant WNV vaccines. A canarypox-vectored influenza vaccine marketed in the UK is labeled for use during pregnancy. In contrast, the modified live-virus EVA and VEE vaccines and live–anthrax spore vaccines should not be used in pregnant mares. Protection of mares against the potential abortigenic effects of EVA infection is therefore best accomplished by completing the primary immunization series before the mare enters the broodmare band and by administering subsequent boosters during the open period before rebreeding.[29]

The practice of booster-vaccinating mares against multiple diseases to maximize colostral transfer of antibodies to the foal results in the typical broodmare receiving multiple doses of many vaccine antigens and adjuvants during her lifetime. In addition to stimulating high levels of antibody against a range of antigens for the benefit of the foal, this practice may also predispose these mares to a higher rate of local and systemic adverse reactions, an issue that not only warrants further investigation but also may force horse owners and veterinarians to consider strategies for revaccination carefully.

Passive Immunization

Use of Exogenous Antibodies

Passive immunization through administration of exogenous plasma or serum products from immune donors is commonly practiced as a means of providing temporary protection from infection during a defined period of risk. Plasma and serum products from hyperimmunized donors are also used as an adjunct to the treatment of specific disease conditions such as tetanus, botulism, WNV infection, endotoxemia, neonatal septicemia, and hypoalbuminemia secondary to other diseases (see appropriate chapters covering these diseases for further information). The degree and duration of protection depend on the amount of total and specific immunoglobulin administered; however, the rapid decay of exogenous antibodies inevitably provides only temporary protection.

By far the major indication for passive immunization through the use of plasma products is the treatment of partial or complete failure of passive transfer (FPT) of maternal antibodies in neonatal foals. Although the definitions of "complete" and "partial" FPT remain the subject of debate, most veterinarians agree that a plasma transfusion using 1 to 2 liters (20-40 mL/kg) of high–immunoglobulin G (IgG) plasma is indicated for foals with postnursing total serum IgG concentrations of less than 400 mg/dL. Some veterinarians also recommend transfusing foals with serum IgG concentrations between 400 and 800 mg/dL, particularly if other risk factors or signs suggestive of sepsis are present. All plasma products that make specific label claims must be licensed by the USDA to ensure purity, potency, sterility, stability, safety, and efficacy in treating the label indication. The sole indication for products marketed as immunoglobulin supplements is the treatment of FPT. USDA licensing requires documentation that at the recommended dose, these products increase the total IgG concentration by 400 mg/dL. USDA-licensed plasma products for IV administration contain at least 2500 mg/dL of IgG. In addition, concentrated serum-derived IgG products are labeled to contain at least 30 g of IgG per 250-mL bottle. Oral preparations should contain at least 30 g of IgG per 300-mL bottle and may be administered to foals less than 24 hours of age to prevent FPT.

Several USDA-licensed tetanus antitoxin products have been available in North America for many years as adjuncts to the prevention of tetanus (see later section on tetanus). Some plasma products are licensed for protection against specific diseases such as *Rhodococcus equi*, the J5 core antigen of *E. coli*, *Clostridium botulinum* type B toxin,[30,31] or *Streptococcus equi*. One conditionally licensed plasma product is marketed as an aid in the treatment and control of WNV infection. Companies that sell plasma products often infer efficacy for prevention or treatment of specific diseases by stating that the plasma donors were hyperimmunized against specific infectious agents. In order to be a USDA licensed and labeled biological product for prevention or treatment of a specific disease, evidence of efficacy, in vitro or in vivo, must be provided. A labels that claims efficacy based solely on the vaccination status of the plasma donor does not indicate that efficacy in preventing or treating the specific disease has been proved in controlled studies; therefore, practitioners should view these implied efficacy claims with caution.

Passive Transfer of Maternal Immunity

Passive transfer of maternal antibodies from the mare to the foal through colostrum constitutes by far the most important form of passive immunization in horses. The epitheliochorial placentation present in the mare prevents transfer of maternal immunoglobulins to the fetus during gestation, rendering the foal essentially agammaglobulinemic at birth. Therefore protection of the foal against specific infectious diseases that it is likely to encounter during the first few months of life, as its own immune system matures, relies heavily on postnatal absorption of specific antibodies and perhaps other factors that the dam has concentrated in colostrum during late gestation. The duration of protection afforded by maternally derived antibodies (MDAs) depends on many factors, the most important of which are the characteristics of the specific infectious agent, the challenge dose, and the magnitude of the postnursing titer of specific antibody. The latter is influenced by the dam's history of disease exposure and vaccination, age, parity, normalcy of gestation, and prepartum leakage of colostrum (i.e., factors that influence concentration of specific antibody in colostrum). Above all, interval between foaling and nursing, the volume of colostrum ingested, and ingestion of macromolecules other than colostrum before ingesting colostrum play major roles in determining passive transfer of specific MDAs. Although several immunoglobulin isotypes are present in colostrum, the subisotypes of IgG are absorbed into the systemic circulation of the foal in much higher concentration than either immunoglobulin M (IgM) or IgA.[32] Specific IgA, however, is secreted continuously in milk and may provide passive protection against pathogens, such as *S. equi* and enteric organisms, by helping coat the pharyngeal and intestinal mucosa, thereby neutralizing pathogens.[32,33] When foals ingest adequate amounts of high-quality colostrum during the first 12 hours after birth, titers of specific antibody in the serum of the foal are typically very similar to the serum titer in the dam at the time of foaling. Whereas the rate of decay of specific subisotypes of IgG varies to some extent, the overall half-life of decline of maternal IgG antibodies is typically between 25 and 40 days.[34-40] Thus the magnitude of the postnursing antibody titer and the sensitivity of the assay used to detect passively transferred antibodies will determine persistence of these antibodies at measurable levels in the serum of foals. Use of ELISA and other sensitive assays has made it possible to detect persistence of MDAs for 6 months or longer in some cases.[35,40]

Whereas passively acquired MDAs are important for protecting the foal against infection with many pathogens, they play a particularly critical role in prevention of infection with enteric pathogens, such as rotavirus, *E. coli*, and other Enterobacteriaceae, to which neonates are particularly susceptible. Passive transfer of immunity to these and other agents (e.g., botulism) that affect foals can be enhanced by stimulating either a primary or an anamnestic response in the mare during late gestation. This is typically an important focus of immunization programs for mares and can be accomplished through planned exposure if the infectious agent does not pose a threat to the mare, as is the case with rotavirus, or more appropriately through administration of booster doses of vaccines to mares, 30 to 60 days before foaling. Maintaining consistent vaccination protocols for mares will maximize the likelihood that a uniformly high level of colostral antibody transfer and passive protection will be achieved within the foal crop. Whereas intranasally administered vaccines may afford good protection to the mare, they are typically less effective than parenterally administered inactivated vaccines in stimulating high levels of circulating IgG, the isotype that is passively transferred to the foal in highest concentration. Parenteral vaccines are therefore preferred over intranasal vaccines for vaccination of mares during late gestation.

It is widely assumed that pregnant mares are fully capable of mounting appropriate cellular and humoral immune responses to vaccines; however, this issue has received little research attention. Whereas mares that have been primed before breeding appear to mount appropriate anamnestic responses to vaccines administered during late gestation, it appears that the humoral response to primary vaccination with at least the inactivated WNV vaccine is downregulated during gestation. In one study, more than 75% of naïve mares, vaccinated for the first time against WNV while pregnant, failed to mount a detectable serologic response to two doses of an inactivated WNV vaccine administered 4 weeks apart.[41] Consequently, their foals failed to acquire any WNV antibodies through colostrum and were rendered potentially susceptible to infection. Preliminary evidence suggests this apparent pregnancy-associated suppression of serologic responses to primary immunization also applies to inactivated rabies vaccines; however, it is not known whether responses to other inactivated vaccine antigens are similarly affected. Nevertheless, it is wise to complete primary immunization before breeding and administer booster doses of selected antigens late in gestation rather than attempting to complete the primary series during gestation, regardless of the vaccine. The common practice of administering booster doses of multiple antigens to mares during late gestation raises the possibility that "competition" between multiple antigens will compromise the response to some or all of them and increase the risk of an adverse local or systemic reaction. Although these issues have not been addressed in controlled research studies, it is nevertheless good practice to administer no more than four antigens at one time and to allow an interval of 3 to 4 weeks between administration of vaccines containing additional antigens.

Vaccination of Foals and Influence of Maternal Antibodies on Vaccine Responses

Whereas foals are considered to be immune competent at birth and are capable of mounting both humoral and cellular immune responses to a range of antigens, continued maturation of the immune system after birth is believed to be necessary to achieve optimal immune function. However, few studies have been done to determine the age at which various elements of the innate and adaptive immune system become fully competent and optimal responses to vaccines can be achieved. Maternal antibodies and perhaps other important immune effectors (e.g., lymphocytes) that are concentrated in colostrum and are passively transferred to the foal play a crucial role in defense against pathogens encountered during the first few months of life while endogenous immune function continues to mature.

In addition to passively protecting the foal, maternal antibodies have been shown to exert a profound inhibitory effect on the immune response of foals to antigens, including those contained in vaccines. Several studies reported by groups in Holland, Ireland, and the United States during the 1990s brought this issue into focus by demonstrating that foals less than 6 months of age consistently failed to mount serologic responses to inactivated influenza vaccines.[36,38,40,42-45] Of potentially greater concern was the finding that not only a high proportion of foals vaccinated under the cover of MDAs failed to seroconvert in response to the recommended primary series of two or three doses of influenza vaccine, but also many failed to respond to multiple additional doses administered during the next year, suggesting induction of a potentially detrimental "immunotolerance-like" phenomenon.[42,43,46] Our studies confirmed an apparent lack of response of foals to multiple doses of inactivated influenza vaccines when the HA inhibition (HI) test was used to detect serologic responses. When the same samples were retested using sensitive isotype-specific ELISA tests, it was found that 6-month-old foals did mount a response that included all IgG subisotypes but that was less vigorous for the more important virus neutralizing IgGa and IgGb subisotypes than for the less effective IgG(T) subisotype.[40] Whereas there appeared to be some differences in responses to different vaccines containing different adjuvants, this "misdirection" of isotype responses in favor of IgG(T), likely influenced by MDAs, was consistently observed.[40] Subsequent studies, in which titers of total, rather than antigen-specific, IgG subisotypes were determined, documented that the age-related increase in concentrations of IgGb lagged significantly behind increases in concentrations of other isotypes and remained below adult levels beyond 6 months of age.[47]

Maternal antibody interference has now been documented as a significant issue for many other antigens, including tetanus, EEE, WEE, EHV-1, EHV-4, and WNV contained in vaccines administered to foals.[39,40,48-51] Even low levels of antibody, below those detectable by many routine serologic tests and below those thought to be protective, can completely block the serologic response to some vaccines, resulting in a potentially prolonged period of susceptibility before the foal is capable of responding appropriately to vaccines.[50] These findings also indicate that it is not typically feasible to test samples from foals serologically to predict whether they will respond to particular vaccines. We now recommend that primary immunization with most vaccines containing inactivated antigens should be delayed until foals are 6 months of age or older and with the exception of rabies vaccine, three doses of vaccine should be included in the primary series rather than the two doses routinely recommended by vaccine manufacturers. Typically, the third dose stimulates a serologic response of greater magnitude and durability than two doses and may also contribute to a higher "set point" for the response to subsequent booster doses.[40,41,50,52] Studies that partition mares based on parity are needed because there may be less inhibition of responses in foals of disease-naïve mares than in those from mares that have had many foals and have been vaccinated repeatedly. Work with equine arteritis virus indicates that in areas with high seroprevalence, vaccination of foals should start at 8 months.[53]

If maternal antibody interference was not an issue, the approach to vaccination of foals would be greatly simplified because primary vaccination against all important diseases could be completed before MDAs had declined to nonprotective levels. In effect, the "window of susceptibility" would be eliminated. A more realistic goal is to maximize the beneficial effects of MDAs while minimizing their negative impact on primary immunization. To best meet this goal, it is necessary to decide which one (or both) of the following is the primary focus:

1. To protect the foal and weanling against specific high-risk infectious diseases that affect this age group and have the

potential to cause significant disease, either directly or by predisposing to other secondary infections.
2. To initiate primary immunization to protect against disease later in life.

Assessing risk takes into account both the incidence of disease (i.e., the likelihood that the foal will become infected) and the risk of serious sequelae or death if the horse does become infected. If the disease affects the foal early in life, as with rotavirus infection, there is usually insufficient time to induce a protective immune response by actively immunizing the foal. Under these circumstances, the approach should be to maximize the degree of protection passively transferred from the dam through colostrum. Other diseases, such as rabies, affect horses of all ages, but the risk of acquiring infection is generally low.

Diseases of moderate to high risk to young foals but low risk to adults include rotavirus infection (on certain breeding farms in certain years) and in geographic areas, such as Kentucky and some other eastern states, type B botulism. For these diseases, the following approach is appropriate:

- Booster vaccinate the dam before foaling to maximize uniformity of passive transfer.
- Ensure good passive transfer of maternal antibodies.
- Introduce management practices to reduce exposure to the infectious agent.
- Vaccinate the foal if risk continues beyond the first few months of life.

Diseases of moderate to high risk for weanlings and older horses but lower risk to young foals born to vaccinated mares include EHV-4, EHV-1, strangles, influenza, tetanus, EEE, WEE, and WNV. For these diseases, the following approach is appropriate:

- Vaccinate the dam before foaling to maximize uniformity of passive transfer.
- Ensure good passive transfer of maternal antibodies.
- Start foal vaccination after the risk of MDA interference is no longer present in most foals. When several vaccine types are available for a particular disease, the vaccine that is least subject to MDA interference should be used. Introduce management practices to reduce exposure to the infectious agent while primary vaccination is being completed.
- If a two-dose primary series is recommended for adult horses, use three or more doses of vaccine in the primary series to improve the chances that foals that do not respond to earlier doses will respond to additional doses administered later.
- In the primary series, it is recommended that the first two injections be administered 30 days apart and the second and third dose be administered a minimum of 60 days apart.

Diseases of low risk to foals in most circumstances include influenza, rabies, EN, and EVA. For these diseases, the following approach is appropriate:

- Vaccinate the dam before foaling if the disease is a significant risk to adult horses and a vaccine shown to be safe for use in pregnant mares is available. If the available vaccines are not considered safe for use in pregnant mares, administer boosters before breeding.
- Ensure good passive transfer of maternal antibodies.
- Start foal vaccination after the risk of MDA interference is no longer present in any foal (typically 9 months to 1 year of age).

Concept of Core and Noncore Vaccines

Fully licensed vaccines are now available in North America as aids to the prevention of tetanus, viral encephalomyelitis (EEE, WEE, VEE), WNV infection, influenza, EHV-1 and EHV-4 infection, strangles, rabies, EVA, EN, and type B botulism. In addition, conditionally licensed vaccines are available to immunize horses against rotavirus and equine rhinitis A virus infection. Tetanus, rabies, and viral encephalomyelitis caused by EEE, WEE, and WNV pose a threat to horses in all geographic areas and are therefore considered to be "core" diseases against which all horses in North America should be vaccinated. The abortogenic potential of EHV-1 warrants inclusion of this disease in the core for all pregnant broodmares. Although influenza is not routinely included as a core disease, vaccination against this highly contagious respiratory tract infection is strongly recommended for all horses that are likely to be co-located with horses from other facilities during transportation or at sales, shows, trail rides, races, or other events. The remaining diseases for which vaccines are available are considered "noncore." Noncore does not mean that these vaccines can be overlooked; rather, the concept is that the individual farm or horse risk should be assessed when deciding whether to incorporate a vaccine into the annual program. Indications for use of vaccines against these diseases are discussed in the relevant sections that follow.

Vaccination Recommendations for Specific Diseases

Tetanus

All horses are at risk for developing tetanus, an often-fatal disease caused by a potent neurotoxin elaborated by the anaerobic, spore-forming bacterium *Clostridium tetani*. These organisms are present in the intestinal tract and feces of horses, other animals, and humans and are ubiquitous in soil. Tetanus is expensive to treat and has a high mortality rate; therefore all horses should be actively immunized using tetanus toxoid as part of the core vaccination program. Active immunization reduces the need to administer tetanus antitoxin, the use of which is associated with risk of inducing potentially fatal serum hepatitis. Protection against tetanus appears to be mediated by circulating antibodies, and these antibodies are transferred efficiently through colostrum. The many available vaccines are typically formalin-inactivated, adjuvanted toxoids that are inexpensive and safe and that induce an excellent serologic response and solid, long-lasting immunity. Manufacturers recommend administration of a primary series of two doses of toxoid at 3- to 6-week intervals, followed by annual boosters. Titers of specific antibody increase within 14 days after administration of the second dose in the primary series and in adult horses, persist at detectable levels for 12 months or longer, depending on the adjuvant system used in the vaccine.[54,55]

No published challenge studies are available to document the speed of onset or duration of protection induced by tetanus toxoid preparations currently licensed in North America; conclusions regarding their efficacy are therefore based on the serologic response obtained in laboratory animals. However, a challenge study conducted in Europe almost 60 years ago found that horses were resistant to challenge 8 days after receiving a single injection of tetanus toxoid, before antibody could be detected in their serum.[56] A second study demonstrated that a series of three doses of tetanus toxoid induced protection lasting for at least 8 years and perhaps for life, even when antibodies could no longer be detected.[57] A recent study in Europe documented that protective levels of antibody (>0.2 IU/mL as measured by tetanus toxin-binding ELISA) persist for at least

18 months after revaccination of horses previously primed with a 2-dose series of a tetanus toxoid/influenza ISCOM vaccine.[5] In contrast, tetanus has been documented in vaccinated horses in North America,[58] although survival was strongly associated with previous vaccination. Thus it would not be prudent to recommend extension of the annual interval for revaccination with tetanus toxoid products available in North America, pending publication of data documenting duration of immunity. Vaccinated horses that sustain a wound or have surgery more than 6 months after receiving their previous tetanus booster should be revaccinated with tetanus toxoid.

The annual booster for pregnant mares should be administered 4 to 8 weeks before foaling to protect the mare if she sustains foaling-induced trauma and to enhance concentrations of specific immunoglobulins in colostrum. Colostrum-derived antibodies significantly interfere with the immune response of foals vaccinated with tetanus toxoid until they are about 6 months of age.[40,55] If a foal received appropriate transfer of colostral antibodies from a vaccinated mare, that foal should receive its primary series of three doses of tetanus toxoid beginning at age 6 months or older. Foals born to nonvaccinated mares should receive this initial three-dose series starting at 1 to 4 months of age. The three-dose primary series is recommended for foals because a high proportion of foals fail to seroconvert in response to two doses of tetanus toxoid, regardless of whether maternal antibodies are detectable at administration of the first dose.[40,55] Optimally, the interval between the first two doses of vaccine should be approximately 4 weeks and the interval between the second and third doses should be 2 to 5 months. Yearlings should be revaccinated in the early spring rather than waiting 1 year since the third booster.

Tetanus antitoxin is produced by hyperimmunization of donor horses with tetanus toxoid. Administration of one vial of antitoxin (1500 IU) to nonvaccinated horses induces immediate passive protection that lasts no longer than 3 weeks.[55] More prolonged protection may be accomplished with higher doses. In addition to the use of high doses of tetanus antitoxin to treat tetanus, indications frequently cited include administration to newborn foals born to nonvaccinated mares and to nonvaccinated horses that sustain an injury. In these cases the concurrent administration of tetanus antitoxin and tetanus toxoid at different sites using separate syringes has been advocated, followed by administration of additional doses of toxoid at 4- to 6-week intervals to complete the primary series.[59] Because a small but significant number of horses experience serum sickness and fatal hepatic failure (serum hepatitis) several weeks after receiving tetanus antitoxin,[60,61] a preferred approach to the nonvaccinated horse that sustains a puncture or deep laceration is to thoroughly clean and debride the wound, initiate active immunization by administering tetanus toxoid, and institute a course of antimicrobial treatment with penicillin or an alternate antimicrobial that is active against C. tetani.

Equine Encephalomyelitis

The encephalomyelitis viruses (EEE, WEE, VEE) are transmitted by mosquitoes and infrequently by other bloodsucking insects to horses from wild birds or rodents, which serve as natural reservoirs for these viruses. Risk of exposure and geographic distribution of the encephalomyelitis viruses vary by season and from year to year with changes in distribution of insect vectors and wildlife reservoirs. The distribution of EEE has historically been restricted to the eastern, southeastern, and some southern states, whereas outbreaks of WEE have been recorded in the western and midwestern states, with sporadic cases in the Northeast and Southeast United States. Because EEE or WEE (or both) is endemic in most areas of North America, vaccination against these diseases should be part of the core vaccination program for all horses. Venezuelan equine encephalomyelitis occurs in South and Central America but has not been diagnosed in the United States or Mexico for many years; therefore routine vaccination of horses in these regions against VEE is not recommended at this time, unless transportation to endemic areas is planned.

Although correlates for protection against EEE, WEE, and VEE are not well established, circulating antibodies are assumed to be important because infection is acquired by vascular injection (mosquito bites), and current inactivated vaccines are protective.[62,63] Available vaccines are inactivated, adjuvanted, bivalent whole-virus products containing EEE and WEE, or trivalent products that also contain VEE. Veterinarians and horse owners often use combination products containing other antigens, such as tetanus, influenza, WNV, or equine herpesviruses, for primary or booster immunization of horses against encephalomyelitis viruses.

Primary immunization of nonvaccinated adult horses is accomplished by administration of 2 doses of inactivated vaccine 3 to 6 weeks apart. In endemic areas, it is recommended to vaccinate foals and all new arrivals with three injections. In these areas, all young horses should receive encephalitis vaccines biannually until the age of 4 years. In areas where EEE is not a threat and mosquito vectors are active for less than 6 months of the year, annual revaccination in the spring, before the peak insect vector season, is recommended. Inactivated encephalomyelitis vaccines are considered to be safe for use in pregnant mares; therefore booster vaccination 4 to 8 weeks before foaling is routinely recommended to enhance colostral concentrations of specific immunoglobulins. Neutralizing antibodies to WEE and EEE are transferred passively to foals through colostrum and decline with an estimated half-life of 33 and 20 days, respectively. Maternally derived antibodies (MDAs) appear to confer protection and are detectable in the serum of many foals from vaccinated mares for at least 3 months and up to 7 months, depending on the postnursing titer.[34,39,64,65]

Several studies have shown that MDAs exert a profound inhibitory effect on the ability of foals to mount serologic responses to inactivated bivalent WEE/EEE vaccines, which likely accounts for some of the reported cases of vaccine failure and resultant clinical EEE in vaccinated horses, particularly those less than 2 years of age.[34,39,46,50,64] Studies have shown that 3-month-old foals born to immune mares consistently failed to mount a serologic response to two doses of inactivated bivalent WEE/EEE vaccine, and the majority had not responded even after administration of a third dose.[41,50] Whereas many 6-month-old foals failed to seroconvert after administration of two doses of vaccine, most responded following administration of a third dose.[50] Based on these data, inclusion of a third dose in the primary series, 2 to 5 months after administration of the second dose, is strongly recommended for foals and yearlings.

WEE has a lower mortality rate than EEE, and prevalence of WEE in many western states is sufficiently low that the risk of foals acquiring infection during their first year of life is also low. Therefore primary vaccination of foals in areas where mosquitoes die off in the winter and the risk of infection is low is best completed when foals are 6 month of age or older, to minimize the potential for maternal antibody interference.

West Nile Virus

As of April 2013, four WNV vaccines are licensed and marketed for use in horses in North America. All vaccines have met USDA requirements for safety with tests each involving more than 640 horses. Vaccine efficacy was assessed with either parenteral or intrathecal (direct injection into the central nervous system [CNS]) challenge models. The parenteral challenge models have shown that vaccination significantly reduced the magnitude of viremia in experimentally infected, vaccinated horses compared to nonvaccinated control horses for as long as 12 months after primary vaccination with two doses of vaccine.[31,51,52] Although viremia was reliably induced in nonvaccinated control horses in these challenge models, clinical disease was not. Therefore these vaccines are labeled as aids to the prevention of viremia due to WNV infection. In contrast, an intrathecal challenge model that reliably induced severe clinical disease was used to test the efficacy of more recently licensed vaccines. These findings support the results of field studies that provide clear evidence that, when used according to manufacturer recommendations, available licensed WNV vaccines reduce the risk of disease and death after natural challenge, although clinical disease may not be fully prevented with all vaccines.[60-62]

Directions for primary immunization using all products currently licensed include administration of two doses of vaccine 3 to 6 weeks apart (consult the specific label). Optimal protection cannot be expected until 2 weeks after administration of the second dose, although significant protection was obtained as early as 26 days after administration of the first dose of the canarypox vectored WNV vaccine.[66] Vaccine manufacturers recommend revaccination of previously vaccinated horses on an annual basis or more frequently when local conditions are conducive to a prolonged period of potential exposure to infected mosquito vectors. Annual revaccination is best completed in the spring (late February through early April), before the onset of the insect vector season. In areas where the mosquito season is prolonged, revaccination twice annually, once in the spring and again in the late summer or early fall (late July through early September), may be necessary to maximize protection.

None of the licensed vaccines currently marketed in the United States carry label recommendations for administration to pregnant mares; therefore it is recommended that mares be vaccinated before breeding whenever possible. It is well recognized, however, that pregnant mares are at risk of acquiring infection from infected mosquitoes. Consequently, it has become accepted practice by many veterinarians to administer vaccines to pregnant mares on the reasonable assumption that the risk of adverse consequences of WNV infection greatly exceeds the reported adverse effects of use of vaccines in pregnant mares. Thousands of doses of WNVs have been administered safely to pregnant mares, and a recent study failed to document vaccine-associated adverse effects in a large population of pregnant mares.[67]

Booster vaccination of previously primed pregnant mares should be accomplished 4 to 6 weeks before foaling.[41] A significant proportion of naïve pregnant mares failed to seroconvert when the primary series of an inactivated vaccine was administered during the second half of gestation. If subsequently proven, this preliminary observation adds further justification to the recommendation that the primary series is best completed before breeding.

Although one study concluded that MDAs do not significantly interfere with the response of foals to an inactivated WNV vaccine,[41] most WNV vaccine products are now combined with other vaccines for other encephalitides; therefore, foal vaccination schedules should follow the same recommendation as those for EEE, WEE, and tetanus. As with other vaccines, delaying of the third dose until 2 or more months after the second dose increases the likelihood that foals with high MDA levels, which may have attenuated the response to the first dose of vaccine, will become primed and protected. A booster should be administered during the spring of the yearling year, after which the recommendations for vaccination of adult horses should be followed. It is prudent to follow the same guidelines as those for the other encephalitides for the first few years of life to induce full protection quickly in endemic areas.

Equine Influenza

Infection of the respiratory tract of horses with the orthomyxovirus, influenza A/equine/2 (H3N8), remains one of the most common causes of rapidly spreading outbreaks of respiratory disease. The influenza A/equine/1 subtype (H7N7) has not been recognized as a cause of clinical disease for many years and is likely extinct in nature. Influenza is endemic in the equine populations of the United States and much of the world, with only a few exceptions. Rigorous investigations in countries, such as New Zealand and Iceland, have never found evidence of infection in resident horses, and there are some countries, such as Singapore, Japan, South Africa, and Australia, that have previously had infected horses, but which have apparently eliminated the virus through rigorous control efforts. Rapid national and international transportation of horses facilitates spread of the virus. Concentrating young horses at racetracks, training facilities, boarding stables, breeding farms, shows, or similar athletic events increases the risk of infection, as does a low serum concentration of specific antibody.[68] Older horses are generally less susceptible to infection but may become ill when partial protection is overwhelmed by exposure to horses excreting large amounts of virus. Although the disease is endemic in many countries and infection cycles continuously, explosive outbreaks occur at intervals of several years when the immunity of the equine population wanes and sufficient antigenic drift has occurred to generate a new viral strain. In contrast to herpesviruses, equine influenza virus is not maintained in asymptomatic carrier horses and does not circulate constantly, even in large groups of horses. Rather, the disease is introduced sporadically by a symptomatic or asymptomatic infected horse. This epidemiologic finding and the rapid elimination of the virus by the equine immune response suggest that infection can be avoided by preventing entry of the virus into an equine population (e.g., by quarantine of newly arriving horses for at least 14 days) and by appropriate vaccination.[69]

Equine influenza virus is highly contagious and spreads rapidly through groups of horses in aerosolized droplets dispersed by coughing. Contaminated buckets, grooming or feeding equipment, tack, and transport vehicles may serve as fomites because the virus can survive for hours on such objects. Severity of clinical signs of influenza, which include nasal discharge, fever, lethargy, anorexia, cough, and myalgia, depends on the degree of existing immunity and other factors. Infected horses shed virus for up to 10 days in their nasal secretions. Inactivated vaccines do not induce sterile immunity; therefore, recently vaccinated horses can become infected, shed virus, and contribute to interepidemic persistence of infection within the equine population and propagation of infection during outbreaks.[70]

Immunity to the same (homologous) strain of virus following natural infection persists for more than a year and involves both local and systemic humoral and cellular mechanisms. These include induction of large amounts of virus-specific neutralizing IgG and secretory IgA antibody in nasal secretions, high levels of circulating IgG antibodies, and genetically restricted antigen-specific CTLs that kill infected cells.[71-75] Memory CTLs can be detected in peripheral blood for at least 6 months after infection, and solid immunity persists even when circulating antibody titers have declined to low or nondetectable levels.[72,73,76,77] Similarly, protection induced by the licensed modified live intranasal influenza vaccine is presumably mediated through induction of local immune responses in the respiratory tract because this vaccine does not typically induce high levels of circulating antibody.[78,79] Except possibly for ISCOM vaccines, inactivated vaccines administered by IM injection have limited potential to induce CTL or nasal secretory IgA responses and induce only low levels of neutralizing antibody in nasal secretions.[71,77,80] The degree of protection induced by inactivated influenza vaccines is highly correlated with postvaccination titers of circulating antibody, predominantly of the IgGa and IgGb subisotypes, as measured by HI or single radial hemolysis (SRH) tests.[68,81-84] SRH levels of 100 mm^2 or greater are considered to be at least partially protective; however, levels greater than 140 mm^2 are required for successful prevention of disease.[83] The partial protection induced by inactivated vaccines is of limited duration (a few weeks up to about 7 months, depending on the vaccine) and is manifested as a reduction in clinical signs and attenuation of viral shedding in horses exposed to infection.[69,71]

The magnitude of the serologic response to inactivated influenza vaccines depends on many factors, including the preparation of antigen contained in the vaccine, antigenic mass, the nature of the adjuvant, history of previous vaccination or infection, interval since the last dose of vaccine, antibody titer at the time of vaccination, age, and maternal antibody status. Relatedness of the vaccine strain to circulating field strains of influenza virus is another important determinant of efficacy, at least for inactivated influenza vaccines.[81,85,86] There are three types of influenza virus (types A, B, and C) that are differentiated by their highly conserved internal proteins (matrix protein and nucleoprotein); horses are only infected by some Type A influenza viruses. The more variable surface glycoproteins, HA and NA, contain the major antigenic determinants and are used to characterize subtypes of influenza virus (e.g., H3N8). Three distinct subtypes of influenza virus have been isolated from horses since 1956. These are represented by the following prototype strains: influenza A/equine/Prague/56 (H7N7), which is sometimes referred to as A1 equine influenza; influenza A/equine/Miami/63 (H3N8), which is sometimes referred to as A2 equine influenza; and influenza A/equine/Jilin/89 (H3N8). Only strains that evolved from the Miami/63 isolate are currently circulating in horse populations, but this virus has evolved into genetically and antigenically distinguishable clusters: a so-called "Eurasian" lineage and an "American" lineage. The American lineage further evolved during the 1990s into Kentucky, Florida, and South America sublineages.[87] For the Florida sublineage, there are two clades indentified: clade I represented by Ohio 03 and South Africa 03 and clade II as represented by Richmond 07. According to the World Organization for Animal Health (OIE) surveillance panel, clade I representatives of the Florida sublineage are present in North America, Europe, South Africa, and Japan, whereas clade II representatives are present in Europe, India, and China.

By generating antigenically heterologous viruses, antigenic drift reduces the degree and duration of protection conferred by previous infection or vaccination because of the specificity of immunoglobulins and allows horses with high titers to become infected and develop clinical signs of disease if the vaccine strain is not closely related to the drifted infectious field strain.[88] Although antigenic drift of equine influenza virus is slower than that of human influenza viruses, it is recommended that inactivated equine influenza vaccines include viral antigens from isolates obtained within the most recent 5 years. An expert surveillance panel meets annually to recommend strains that should be included in influenza vaccines in subsequent years (www.equiflunet.org.uk). In the past, federal regulations in the USA made updating of equine influenza vaccines through inclusion of recently isolated strains so costly and time-consuming that vaccines typically lagged more than the recommended 5 years behind the antigenic drift of field viruses, resulting in suboptimal protection. Recent changes in vaccine licensing regulations should make more frequent updating of equine influenza vaccines feasible. Even though the modified live intranasal vaccine marketed in the United States contains only a 1991 H3N8 strain of North American lineage, it has been

shown to protect against challenge with Eurasian strains and recently isolated North American strains.

The short-lived immunity after vaccination with inactivated equine influenza vaccines was the impetus for past recommendations for frequent revaccination, at intervals as short as 2 months. However, too short an interval between revaccination may compromise efficacy because influenza vaccination in the horse with a high titer inhibits development of an optimal anamnestic response.[89] An additional consideration that potentially limits the efficacy of influenza vaccines is the phenomenon termed "original antigenic sin," whereby horses exposed to a drifted field A/equine/2 virus will mount an anamnestic immune response directed more strongly against the strain with which they were vaccinated initially than against the drifted field virus.[90]

A considerable amount of published efficacy data, based both on challenge studies and on field epidemiology studies, has been available for many years in Europe to support the use of influenza vaccines. In contrast, information regarding the efficacy of influenza vaccines marketed in North America has remained sparse until recently. Large cross-sectional and prospective longitudinal epidemiologic studies conducted during 3 consecutive years in the early 1990s at a Thoroughbred racetrack in Saskatchewan failed to document any reduction in risk of influenza in recently vaccinated horses.[68] Furthermore, a double-masked, randomized field trial conducted by the same researchers showed that vaccination of horses with the then-leading influenza vaccine marketed for use before an anticipated influenza epidemic did not significantly reduce the risk of developing respiratory tract disease or reduce the severity of disease, although the duration of clinical disease was shortened in vaccinates.[70] Serologic testing performed during these studies indicated that vaccine failure was caused by failure of the influenza vaccines in use at the time to induce protective antibody titers. Indeed, many horses failed to mount a detectable serologic response, a finding that was subsequently confirmed in a field study involving 173 horses on six premises in northern Colorado during 1997 and 1998 using aluminum hydroxide–adjuvanted vaccines containing an inactivated Miami/63 H3N8 strain.[91] In contrast, Newton[92] found that 73% of previously vaccinated 2-year-old Thoroughbreds in England achieved a protective SRH antibody titer of 140 mm^2 2 weeks after administration of a booster dose of a European-licensed inactivated aluminum hydroxide–adjuvanted influenza vaccine containing a more recent H3N8 isolate and likely also a higher antigenic mass.

Fortunately, vaccine manufacturers in North America have responded to the challenge of producing more efficacious equine influenza vaccines during the last 15 years by incorporating more relevant recent viral strains, by increasing antigenic mass of relevant strains, by eliminating the seemingly irrelevant H7N7 strain, by modifying adjuvant systems, and by introducing novel technologies. An important advance occurred in 1999 when Heska Corporation marketed an attenuated live, cold-adapted influenza vaccine for intranasal administration. This vaccine, which contains a Kentucky/1991 strain of North American lineage, was found to be highly efficacious in blinded, controlled challenge studies conducted 5 weeks, 6 months, and 1 year after administration of a single dose to naïve horses.[79] Subsequently, the intranasal vaccine was shown to cross-protect against European H3N8 strains, as well as against North American strains isolated during the late 1990s and early 2000s, and to induce a rapid onset of protection within 7 days of administration of a single dose to naïve horses.[78,93] Although horses challenged 1 year after administration of a single dose showed a significant but only partial reduction in severity of clinical signs and virus shedding, a more marked reduction in clinical signs and viral shedding was found when the challenge was performed 6 months after vaccination.[79] Based on these results, revaccination at 6-month intervals is recommended. Field experience indicates that this regimen induces solid clinical protection after natural challenge. Currently, the intranasal vaccine is licensed for use in nonpregnant horses 11 months of age or older, primarily because this was the youngest age of the horses used in the challenge studies for licensing. Horses may shed small amounts of vaccinal virus for several days after vaccination with the intranasal vaccine, but the amount of virus shed is so low that in-contact horses generally will not become infected or immunized with vaccinal virus shed by recently vaccinated horses, and the likelihood of reversion to virulence is extremely low.[94]

In the years since the intranasal vaccine was licensed in North America as the first equine influenza vaccine with documented efficacy based on independent published challenge studies, several manufacturers have updated their inactivated vaccines and demonstrated efficacy in challenge studies. Inactivated influenza vaccines containing one or more relevant H3N8 strains are currently marketed by several manufacturers. Each of these vaccines contains at least one American-type and one Eurasian-type strain of equine influenza virus. These companies also market a large number of multicomponent combination vaccines that contain the same inactivated influenza antigens as in their single-component products but also contain tetanus, WEE and EEE virus, EHV, or WNV antigens.

A study in which naïve 9-month-old horses were challenged by aerosol with a recent influenza H3N8 strain (KY/99), 16 weeks after the last dose of a three-dose vaccination series (0, 4, and 16 weeks), documented that the three vaccines tested reduced clinical signs and viral shedding in vaccinated horses compared with nonvaccinated control horses.[95] There were differences in antibody titer induced by the vaccines; horses vaccinated with the vaccine that induced the highest serum antibody titers experienced less fever, nasal discharge, and viral shedding than horses vaccinated with other products. Based on these findings, the authors concluded that the vaccine containing both American and Eurasian strains developed, formulated, and efficacy-tested according to European Union guidelines was the most effective inactivated influenza vaccine available in North America at that time. The initial two doses of this vaccine are administered IM; subsequent doses may be administered IM or intranasally. It is proposed, but not proved, that administration of booster doses by the intranasal route may provide a stronger local mucosal immune response. This vaccine is licensed for use in horses older than 6 months of age, including pregnant mares. Vaccines in these studies have been updated; one now contains KY/97 strain and the others contain the KY/93 and KY/2002 North American strains and the Newmarket/93 Eurasian H3N8 strains. The recent updates to these vaccines should further improve their efficacy.

The injectable canarypox-vectored recombinant equine influenza vaccine has been used with success in Europe for several years. This vaccine induces strong protection in challenge studies and shows great potential to have a positive impact on influenza prevention in North America.[19] The vaccine incorporates the HA gene from the Ohio 03 and Newmarket 93 H3N8 strains into the same vector delivery platform as the efficacious recombinant WNV vaccine and contains a carbomer polymer adjuvant in the diluent. Consequently, this vaccine invokes a broad array of humoral and cellular immune responses. It is likely that the vectored influenza vaccine will be able to circumvent the inhibitory effect of maternal antibodies, an issue that significantly impacts primary immunization of foals using inactivated influenza vaccines.

Vaccination Protocols for Influenza

Influenza should be considered a core vaccine on all facilities that are not totally closed to preclude contact with "outside" horses from other locations. Pending availability of published efficacy data for other equine influenza vaccines, we advocate use of the intranasal MLV (Flu-Avert) as a central component of control programs for equine influenza in North America. Incorporation of the MLV into a program that has relied on inactivated vaccines can occur when routine administration of inactivated vaccines would otherwise be scheduled.

As with other diseases, the full benefit of vaccination against influenza can be realized only if the primary vaccination series is completed, or booster doses of vaccine administered, several weeks before anticipated exposure. The following five issues should be considered when planning an influenza vaccination program: (1) primary vaccination of adult horses, (2) routine revaccination, (3) vaccination of pregnant mares, (4) primary vaccination of foals, and (5) vaccination in an outbreak.

Primary Vaccination of Adult Horses

The following schedules are for primary immunization of for adult horses that have not previously been vaccinated:

1. Intranasal MLV vaccine: administer a single dose intranasally. A second dose administered 3 months later may be beneficial, particularly for horses vaccinated at less than 11 months of age.
2. Inactivated IM-administered vaccines: administer two doses, 3 to 6 weeks apart according to label directions. Although not specifically recommended by some manufacturers, administration of a third dose of vaccine, 3 to 5 months after the second dose, is indicated because it significantly enhances the magnitude of the primary response and duration of persistence of antibodies at protective levels.
3. Canarypox-vectored vaccine: administer two doses, 4 to 6 weeks apart, and revaccinate again 5 months later.

Routine Revaccination

Improvements in injectable vaccines and introduction of new vaccine types during the past 15 years has extended the duration of clinical protection achievable through vaccination; therefore a routine revaccination interval of 6 months appears to be appropriate for most of the influenza vaccines currently marketed in North America. This "routine" protocol should be customized, by adjusting timing of boosters or inclusion of an additional booster, to achieve maximum protection during periods when the risk of exposure is high. For example, strategic revaccination 1 month before being placed at high risk of exposure, such as at a show or sale or being transferred to a training or boarding facility, is justified to maximize protection.

Vaccination of Pregnant Mares

For a mare to produce colostrum that contains a high level of antibodies against equine influenza, she should be revaccinated 4 to 8 weeks before foaling with a vaccine that stimulates a robust serologic response. Although the intranasally administered vaccine induces good protection, it does not routinely stimulate high levels of circulating antibody, at least when used for primary immunization. An inactivated injectable vaccine is therefore recommended for prefoaling booster vaccination of pregnant mares at this time.[41] The canarypox-vectored recombinant vaccine will likely also prove suitable for booster vaccination of pregnant mares.

Vaccination of Foals

The antibody status of a mare at the time of foaling is the main determinant of the postnursing circulating antibody titer in her foal and therefore has a profound impact on the ability of the foal or weanling to respond to influenza vaccines administered during the first year of life. Foals born to seronegative, nonvaccinated mares respond appropriately to influenza vaccines;

therefore primary vaccination can commence at 3 months of age or younger if significant risk of exposure to influenza exists. In contrast, maternal antibodies completely block the serologic response of foals to a primary immunization series comprised of two or more doses of inactivated influenza vaccines when the first dose is administered at 6 months of age or younger.[36,38,40,42-45,50] Interference from MDAs may persist until 9 months of age or beyond for foals with high antibody titers after nursing.[41]

In a study to investigate the finding that many yearling horses had low or undetectable levels of HI antibody despite having received multiple doses of inactivated subunit influenza vaccine during the first year of life, Cullinane et al[43] found that a substantial number of foals vaccinated at 3 months of age not only failed to respond serologically but also failed to respond to four or more additional doses of either an inactivated subunit or a whole-virus vaccine administered over the next year. This result suggested that early vaccination in the presence of maternal antibody had induced immunotolerance to influenza vaccines, at least as defined by lack of serologic responses. Similar results were obtained in our laboratory when the responses of 3-month-old antibody-positive foals to inactivated whole-virus influenza vaccines were assessed using the HI test. However, when the same samples were retested using a sensitive ELISA assay that detects subisotypes of IgG, evidence of induction of tolerance was not found. Instead, misdirection of the immune response in favor of IgG(T), rather than the IgGa and IgGb subisotypes believed to be important for protection, was documented.[40] In the same study the response of 6-month-old foals from seropositive mares was superior to that of 3-month-old foals, both in terms of the percentage of foals seroconverting and the magnitude of the resulting antibody titers, and the response of yearlings was clearly superior to that of 6-month-old foals.[50] Whereas 60% of the yearlings seroconverted to influenza A/equine/2 after two doses of vaccine, all seroconverted after three doses, and more than 50% developed HI titers of more than 1:1000. Based on these data, it was concluded that titers will likely persist at a protective level for a much longer duration after a three-dose primary series than after a two-dose series. This conclusion is also supported by results of studies in Europe, to the extent that administration of a third dose, 3 to 5 months after the second dose, is now strongly recommended. Because the inhibitory effects of MDAs on responses to inactivated influenza vaccines may persist up to 9 months of age in foals born to mares with high titers, primary vaccination of foals from immune mares should be delayed as long as possible, and preventive measures should focus on preventing introduction of infected horses.* Studies in Newmarket, UK, have shown that influenza virus infection is rare in Thoroughbred yearlings before they enter training, suggesting that the risk of influenza is low in horses less than 1 year of age born to mares in herds that are well vaccinated.[86,97,98] Therefore little justification appears to exist for vaccinating young foals from vaccinated mares against influenza, as recommended in the past.[65,99,100]

The intranasal MLV (Flu-Avert I.N.) is licensed for vaccination of horses 11 months of age or older. Whereas this vaccine has been shown to be safe in foals as young as 2 months of age,[101] published data regarding the potential for MDAs to interfere with the response are lacking. Unpublished observations suggest that MDAs interfere with the response of foals age 3 to 6 months, whereas foals with MDA vaccinated at 7 months of age were protected against virulent challenge (Holland and Chambers, personal communication). Pending publication of well-controlled studies, it is recommended that if the first dose of Flu-Avert I.N. vaccine is administered before 11 months of age, a second dose should be administered at 11

months of age or older.[102] The live canarypox-vectored recombinant influenza vaccine is licensed in Europe and North America for use in pregnant mares and foals as young as 4 months of age.[77] The recombinant vaccine has been shown to efficiently prime foals in the presence of maternally derived immunity against influenza as was evidenced by a clear anamnestic antibody response when a secondary vaccination with the same vaccine was performed. The canarypox-vectored recombinant influenza vaccine therefore offers a unique opportunity to overcome the limitations of early life vaccination in the face of maternally derived immunity in foals.[103] If the foal experiences failure of passive transfer of maternal antibodies, or if the mare is seronegative for influenza, the manufacturer recommends commencing vaccination at 4 months of age and including an additional dose in the primary series.

Vaccination in an Outbreak

Definitive diagnosis of equine influenza infection should be pursued during outbreaks of suspected viral respiratory disease because specific measures can then be initiated to contain spread of the disease. Rapid (same-day) diagnosis of influenza can be accomplished using the highly sensitive and specific polymerase chain reaction (PCR) or antigen-capture ELISA tests. In addition, virus isolation should be pursued during outbreaks to characterize new isolates and assess efficacy of current vaccines.

The decision whether to vaccinate in an outbreak depends on many factors, most importantly the age, vaccination status, and size of the population of horses at risk; the elapsed time since onset of the outbreak; the rapidity with which a diagnosis can be confirmed; the layout of the physical facilities; and availability of personnel. Outbreaks of influenza at racetracks and similar facilities typically take 1 month or more to spread through the entire population; therefore sufficient time exists to enhance immune protection of many at-risk horses while implementing other management strategies to minimize disease spread.[93] It is prudent to booster-vaccinate those horses that have been on a regular influenza vaccination program but have not been revaccinated within the previous 3 months. It is also important to induce protection as quickly as possible in horses that have not previously been vaccinated. Of the vaccines currently available, Flu-Avert I.N. induces protection most rapidly, within 7 days of administration of a single intranasal dose; therefore this is currently the product of choice for vaccination of naive horses and those of unknown vaccination status during an outbreak. No evidence suggests that adverse effects will occur when the intranasal vaccine is administered to horses that are incubating infection, although vaccination of horses that are already clinically ill is not recommended. Alternatively, an accelerated vaccination schedule using the canarypox-vectored vaccine with a primary intervaccination interval of 14 days and booster at 105 days has shown to confer long-lasting protective antibody levels.[104] All 14 vaccinates demonstrated high SRH antibodies 14 days following V2, thereby achieving 100% herd immunity to homologous viral challenge. High levels of rapidly acquired herd immunity are critical in containing an outbreak of such a highly contagious pathogen as equine influenza virus. In a strategic vaccination program, it is important that horses remain protected for a sufficient period of time to allow control programs to succeed. An accelerated 14-day primary course intervaccination interval and booster at 105 days achieves both of these objectives.

Future Influenza Vaccines

In addition to the modified canarypox virus vector described earlier,[19] a rMVA vector that delivers genetic material encoding for relevant HA antigens of an H3N8 influenza virus has been developed.[16,17] The rMVA system is designed to focus the CTL response on the recombinant antigen and was initially tested in a prime-boost strategy in which the priming dose consisted of a DNA plasmid encoding for expression of the HA antigen. The intent of this DNA prime-rMVA boost regimen was to invoke both cellular and humoral immune responses involved in protection.[16] A subsequent study showed that the rMVA system was capable of inducing virus-specific lymphoproliferative and IFN-γ messenger ribonucleic acid (mRNA) responses; antigen-specific IgGa, IgGb, and IgA antibodies; and protection from challenge, both with and without a priming dose of the DNA vaccine. These data indicate that vaccination of horses with rMVA alone, or as part of a prime-boost regimen, is an effective means of inducing protective immunity to influenza virus infection.[17] Considerable research has been performed to document the efficacy of the DNA vaccine used in these studies against equine influenza. However, the delivery system used (multiple sublingual, conjunctival, and subcutaneous injections delivered with a gene gun under general anesthesia) is impractical for use in the field.[17,105] Licensing of a naked plasmid DNA vaccine that can be conveniently administered to horses by IM injection to prevent WNV infection clearly documents the potential for development of a DNA vaccine to prevent influenza in horses in the future. Additionally, a DNA vaccine expressing the hemagglutinin protein of H3N8 influenza virus was recently shown to protect ponies against challenge when administered subdermally using a needle-free delivery system.[3,12]

Equine Herpesvirus (Rhinopneumonitis)

The respiratory tract is the primary route of infection for both equine herpesvirus type 1 (EHV-1) and equine herpesvirus type 4 (EHV-4), which are agents often cited as important causes of primary and secondary respiratory tract disease. Seroepidemiologic studies indicate that the vast majority of foals become infected with EHV-1 and EHV-4 during the first few months of life, but the clinical disease syndrome resulting from these infections is not well defined. Similarly, surveillance studies involving racehorses document that seroconversion to both EHV-1 and EHV-4 occurs sporadically during the course of a racing season but is not clearly associated with outbreaks of respiratory disease that follow an epidemiologic pattern consistent with an infectious agent. EHV-1 and EHV-4 are spread by aerosolized secretions from infected horses, by direct and indirect (fomite) contact with nasal secretions, and in the case of EHV-1, by aborted fetuses, fetal fluids, and placentas associated with abortions. Management practices are therefore of primary importance for control of clinical disease caused by equine herpesviruses.

Viremia occurs frequently after infection with EHV-1, potentially leading to paralytic neurologic disease (equine herpes myeloencephalopathy or EHM) secondary to vasculitis of the spinal cord and brain, abortion of virus-infected fetuses, or birth of infected nonviable foals. In contrast, manifestations of infection with EHV-4 (rhinopneumonitis) are generally confined to the respiratory tract because EHV-4 does not typically infect endothelial cells or produce a cell-associated viremia.[106] As with herpesvirus infections in other species, horses typically fail to clear primary infections with either EHV-1 or EHV-4, the result being that most horses in the population remain latently infected with both viruses.[107,108] Latently infected horses do not show clinical signs but may experience recrudescence of infection, with or without clinical signs, an increase in antibody titer, and shedding of the virus when stressed. Consequently, many horses have detectable levels of SN antibody to both EHV-1 and EHV-4 in their serum.[108,109] These features of the epidemiology of herpesvirus infections seriously compromise efforts to control these diseases and explain why outbreaks of EHV-1 or EHV-4 can occur in closed populations of horses.

Whereas most mature horses have antibodies to EHV-1 and EHV-4 and do not show respiratory signs when they become infected, horses do not appear to become resistant to the abortogenic or neurologic forms of infection with EHV-1, even after repeated exposure.[110]

Correlates for protection against EHV-1 and EHV-4 infection have been investigated extensively but are not yet clearly defined. Infection with EHV-1 induces a strong humoral response, but protection from reinfection is short lived and is not achieved until the horse has experienced multiple infections with homotypic virus. No clear relationship exists between protection from EHV-1 infection and concentrations of circulating antibody induced by vaccination or infection, but the duration and amount of virus shedding from the nasopharynx are reduced in animals with high levels of circulating neutralizing antibody.[106] Mucosal immunity and cell-mediated responses likely play a role at least as important as circulating neutralizing antibodies in protection against EHV-1 infection[111] because the presence of MHC class I–restricted CTL precursors in peripheral blood is correlated with protection. Because EHV-4 replication is largely confined to epithelial cells of the upper respiratory tract, it is likely that mucosal immunity is important in protection. Whereas circulating antibodies alone do not prevent EHV-4 infection, high levels of vaccine-induced circulating virus-neutralizing antibody greatly reduce virus shedding and clinical signs after challenge infection.[106]

The principal indication for use of equine herpesvirus vaccines is prevention of EHV-1–induced abortion in pregnant mares. Consistent vaccination appears to reduce the frequency and severity of herpesvirus-induced disease. Although convincing evidence is lacking, field experience suggests that, whereas the incidence of sporadic EHV-1–induced abortions in individual mares has not changed, the incidence of abortion storms caused by EHV-1 has declined significantly since the introduction and widespread use of EHV-1 vaccines in the United States.[107,110] Outbreaks of abortion and associated perinatal foal death, however, do continue to occur on occasion in herds of vaccinated mares. Of the vaccines currently licensed for use in pregnant mares in North America, only inactivated monovalent EHV-1 vaccines containing abortogenic strains of EHV-1 carry a label claim for preventing abortion, whereas at least one bivalent EHV-1/EHV-4 vaccine is licensed for prevention of abortion in Europe. One of the vaccines available in North America (Pneumabort-K + 1b) incorporates both the 1p and 1b subtypes of EHV-1 to reflect the documented increase in the proportion of EHV-1 abortions caused by the 1b subtype that occurred during the 1980s as compared to earlier years.[112] Pregnant mares should be vaccinated during the fifth, seventh, and ninth months of gestation. Many veterinarians also recommend a dose during the third month of gestation. Similarly, vaccination of mares with an inactivated EHV-1/EHV-4 vaccine at the time of breeding and again 4 to 6 weeks before foaling is commonly practiced to enhance concentrations of colostral immunoglobulin for transfer to the foal. However, no published reports document the effectiveness of this approach in raising titers of specific antibody in mares that have already been vaccinated against EHV-1 three times during the previous 5 months. Vaccination of barren mares and stallions with either a bivalent EHV-1/EHV-4 vaccine or a monovalent EHV-1 vaccine before the start of the breeding season and thereafter at 6-month intervals is recommended, with the goal of increasing herd immunity in an attempt to reduce viral shedding and challenge to pregnant mares on breeding farms.[107]

A modified live-virus EHV-1 vaccine has been used as an aid to prevention of EHV-1 abortion by some practitioners for many years, even though this vaccine is not currently labeled for this use. However, several recent developments have created a renewed interest in the potential for use of MLVs for protecting horses against manifestations of EHV-1 and EHV-4 infection. Sequencing of the EHV-1 genome has made it possible to document the nature of the mutation encoding for attenuation, mediated through truncation of the glycoprotein, gp2, of the KyA strain.[113] Similar studies may soon yield information regarding the mutation underlying attenuation of the RAC-H strain from which Rhinomune was derived. In addition, studies in Europe have documented the efficacy of an intranasally administered, temperature-sensitive, live EHV-1 vaccine in preventing abortion, neurologic disease, and respiratory disease after experimental challenge with virulent EHV-1.[111,114] This renewed interest in MLVs, as well as ongoing investigation of recombinant vaccines expressing the major EHV glycoprotein antigens, will likely lead to improved approaches to immunoprophylaxis in the near future.

Because currently available inactivated vaccines do not block infection with equine herpesviruses, the most we can hope for when using inactivated vaccines is reduction of severity of clinical signs and attenuation of virus shedding to help protect herd mates. Challenge studies in weanlings age 5 to 8 months have clearly demonstrated the efficacy of an inactivated whole-virus EHV-1/EHV-4 vaccine in reducing clinical manifestations and virus shedding induced by virulent EHV-1 challenge administered 2 weeks after completion of the two-dose primary series.[115] Efficacy was clearly correlated with vaccine-induced antibody levels at the time of challenge in this study. Studies investigating the serologic response of 3- and 5-month-old foals to this same vaccine documented failure of a high proportion of foals to seroconvert, suggesting that this vaccine is likely to be less effective in protecting younger foals than in protecting the foals age 5 to 8 months cited in the previous challenge study.[51]

Specific antibodies against both EHV-1 and EHV-4 are passed in colostrum.[37,48,49,51,116] Field studies with EHV-1 MLVs indicate that colostral antibodies exert a profound inhibitory effect on serologic responses to vaccination up to at least 5 months of age.[48,117,118] However, a cytotoxic cellular immune response to both EHV-1 and EHV-4 was induced in a substantial percentage of foals vaccinated with an EHV-1 MLV in the presence of maternal antibody, even though humoral responses were often absent.[119] It is uncertain whether these responses would provide protection against natural challenge. Recent studies with two commercially available, inactivated bivalent EHV-1/EHV-4 vaccines and one inactivated EHV-4/influenza vaccine have shown that the majority of foals from EHV-vaccinated mares do not mount a detectable neutralizing antibody response to vaccines administered at 3 and 4 months of age, even when three doses are administered in the primary series.[49-51] An increased proportion of foals responded when vaccinated with a three-dose series starting at 5 or 6 months of age, but a substantial number still failed to seroconvert.[50,51] Some foals with low or undetectable levels of serum-neutralizing antibody at the time of vaccination failed to mount a serologic response, suggesting that low levels of antibody, below the lower limit of detection of the serum-neutralizing test based on EHV-1 antigen, are capable of inhibiting the serologic response to inactivated EHV-1/EHV-4 vaccines.[51] The failure of a large proportion of foals less than 6 months of age to mount serologic responses to inactivated EHV-1/EHV-4 vaccines and the influence of antibody titer at the time of vaccination on failure to respond has been confirmed using sensitive glycoprotein D (gD) and G (gG) ELISAs in studies on commercial stud farms in Australia.[120] In parallel studies, these researchers concluded that mares were the source of infection for foals, and that intensive use of inactivated EHV-1/EHV-4 vaccines on breeding farms in Australia had minimally impacted the infection rate of young foals and weanlings with EHV-1 and EHV-4.[108,109,121]

Considering the uncertainty regarding the role of EHV-1 and EHV-4 as causes of clinically important respiratory disease, the lack of published data regarding the efficacy of available vaccines in preventing infection and establishment of latency, and results of a recent study documenting the poor serologic responses of naïve horses to a number of killed-EHV respiratory vaccines currently marketed in North America,[122] there appears to be little rationale to support the common practice of frequent revaccination of foals, weanlings, yearlings, and young performance horses against EHV-1 and EHV-4.[123] Furthermore, an obvious dilemma in designing a vaccination strategy to prevent EHV-1 and EHV-4 infection in foals and weanlings is that if primary immunization is delayed until 6 months of age or older to reduce the likelihood of maternal antibody interference, foals are likely to encounter field infection before completion of the three-dose primary series. Thus it is unreasonable to expect a high degree of efficacy for vaccination programs designed to protect foals and weanlings against EHV infection using available vaccines. Despite these uncertainties, many practitioners elect to vaccinate against both EHV-1 and EHV-4. Under these circumstances, a reasonable compromise would be to start foal vaccination at 4 to 6 months of age using two doses of an inactivated bivalent vaccine or an EHV-1 MLV administered 3 to 4 weeks apart, followed by administration of a third dose 8 to 12 weeks later. Revaccination at 4 to 6 month intervals thereafter using either an inactivated bivalent vaccine or an EHV-1 MLV appears appropriate for yearlings and young performance or show horses that experience contact with other horses. Frequent vaccination of nonpregnant mature horses, except those on breeding farms, with EHV vaccines is generally not indicated.

There is no evidence that current vaccines can prevent equine herpesvirus-1 myeloencephalopathy (EHM) in the field. Although a preliminary study indicated some benefit associated with vaccination with a MLV,[124] no specific recommendation can be made in terms of vaccination for the prevention of EHM at this time. However, based on the presumed similar pathogenic mechanism between EHV-1 abortion and neurologic disease,[125,126] some parallels likely exist in terms of the requirement for immunologic protection. The control of cell-associated viremia is thought to be critical for the prevention of EHV-1 abortion and presumably, neurologic disease. Therefore the goal of any vaccination program aimed at the prevention of EHV-1 abortion or neurologic disease is to stimulate those immune responses that can reduce or eliminate cell-associated viremia. Several recent studies have investigated the protective effect of commercially available killed and MLV vaccines by experimentally infecting horses with neurotropic EHV-1 strains.[127,128] Collectively, these studies demonstrated that commercial vaccines significantly suppressed EHV-1 disease and nasal viral shedding, and one vaccine suppressed days of viremia, which appears to be a key element in controlling EHM.

Future Vaccination Strategies to Prevent Herpesvirus Infection

To be completely effective in blocking primary infection and establishing a lifelong carrier state with EHV-1 and EHV-4, future vaccination strategies should be directed at inducing a strong mucosal immune response in the upper respiratory tract during the first few weeks of life, at a time when high levels of maternal antibodies are present. Promising progress toward this goal was reported by Patel et al,[129] who documented that intranasal administration of a single dose of temperature-sensitive EHV-1 MLV to MDA-positive foals aged 1.4 to 3.5 months afforded partial but significant protection against febrile respiratory disease, viremia, and virus shedding after intranasal challenge with virulent EHV-1 performed 8 weeks after vaccination. The recent third International Havemeyer Workshop on EHV-1 highlighted the need to improve vaccines, with MLV considered more likely to succeed in inducing a protective immune response.[130]

The goals of future vaccine candidates will be to stimulate both humoral and cell mediated immunity, to differentiate infected from vaccinated horses, to provide minimal gaps in immunity, to induce a rapid onset and long-lasting immunity, to be effective in the presence of maternally derived antibody to prevent early life infection, to provide a wide clinical and virologic cross-protection, to be proved safe and effective against the development of EHM, to suppress reactivation of latent EHV-1 infection, and to be used safely in the face of an outbreak.

Streptococcus equi subsp. *equi* Infection (Strangles)

Strangles is a highly contagious disease caused by the bacterium *Streptococcus equi* subsp. *equi* (*S. equi*). Strangles primarily affects young horses (weanlings and yearlings), although horses of any age can become infected if not protected by previous exposure to the organism or by vaccination. The organism is transmitted by direct contact with infected horses or subclinical carriers, or indirectly by contact with water troughs, feed bunks, pastures, stalls, trailers, tack, or grooming equipment contaminated with nasal discharge or pus draining from lymph nodes of infected horses. The organism survives for only a few weeks in the environment. Because *S. equi* is a clonal organism, there is minimal antigenic variation between different isolates, even though isolates vary in their pathogenicity. Most horses develop a solid immunity during recovery from strangles, which persists in more than 75% of animals for 5 years or longer.[129] The acquired immune response is directed predominantly at the cell wall SeM and involves a combination of circulating opsonophagocytic antibodies and local antibodies produced in the nasopharynx.[131-133] The predominant opsonophagocytic antibodies are of the IgGb subisotype but also include IgGa and IgA, whereas IgGb and subsequently mucosal IgA predominate in nasopharyngeal secretions.[32,131]

Licensed strangles vaccines include one inactivated, adjuvanted cell wall SeM extract and one attenuated live vaccine derived from a nonencapsulated mutant of *S. equi* for intranasal administration.[134] Infection of horses with *S. equi* continues to cause troublesome outbreaks of strangles throughout North America, despite the availability and widespread use of these vaccines, indicating that their efficacy is suboptimal.[135] M-protein vaccines induce a good opsonophagocytic antibody response in serum but a minimal mucosal IgA response, which likely accounts for the incomplete protection observed when they are used in the field.[131,136] However, vaccination using injectable SeM vaccines significantly reduces the attack rate and severity of strangles in herds with endemic infection.[136-138] The live intranasal vaccine induces a relevant mucosal immune response and partial or complete protection but may do so without inducing a strong serologic response.[135,139,140]

Vaccination against *S. equi* is not routinely recommended for pleasure or performance horses kept in low-risk situations, but it is a consideration for horses that are resident on, or being transported to, premises such as breeding farms where strangles is a persistent endemic problem or where a high risk of exposure is anticipated. The bacterial MLV is generally preferred over inactivated injectable vaccines for primary vaccination of foals and weanlings and for routine use in older horses that are at high risk for infection. On breeding farms, efforts should be concentrated on preventing infection of foals and weanlings by booster vaccinating broodmares 4 to 6 weeks before foaling to maximize colostral content of antibodies. Whereas the intranasal vaccine is safe for use in mares at all stages of pregnancy and can be used in mares during an outbreak, it does not reliably stimulate high levels of circulating antibody. For this reason, IM-administered inactivated SeM products are preferred for prefoaling booster immunization of mares. Antibodies of the IgG and IgA class recognizing the SeM are passively transferred to the foal through colostrum and are also present in the milk of immune mares.[33] Antibodies of predominantly the IgGb isotype are absorbed from colostrum and redistribute to the nasopharyngeal mucosa.[32] These IgGb antibodies, along with the SeM-specific IgA antibodies that are present in milk and passively coat the pharyngeal mucosa of nursing foals, provide protection to most nursing foals up to the time of weaning.[32,33,133] Resistance of nursing foals to strangles during the first few months of life appears to be mediated by IgGb antibodies in nasal secretions and milk and not by IgA.[33] Serologic (ELISA) responses to M-protein vaccines are poor in foals, most likely because of the inhibitory effect of maternal antibodies.

The intranasal MLV may be less susceptible than the inactivated extract vaccines to MDA interference, but this issue has not been investigated, and the manufacturer does not recommend administration of this vaccine to horses less than 9 months of age. Considering that on farms where strangles is endemic, foals often become infected around the time of weaning, at 4 to 8 months of age, it is difficult to protect them if vaccination is delayed until 9 months of age. Therefore a reasonable compromise on breeding farms where the risk of strangles infection is high and mares are on a regular vaccination program would be to begin foal vaccination using the intranasal live vaccine as early as 4 months of age. The recommended two-dose primary series administered 2 to 3 weeks apart should be followed by a third dose 3 months later and boosters at 6- to 12-month intervals thereafter, depending on risk of infection. The intranasal vaccine has been administered to foals as young as 5 or 6 weeks of age during outbreaks. If used in this manner, a third dose of the vaccine should be administered 2 to 4 weeks before the foal is weaned to optimize protection during this high-risk period. Although there are few reports of adverse effects attributable to use of the intranasal strangles vaccine in young foals, the inability of foals to mount an adequate mucosal IgA response during the first month of life and the potential for interference by maternal antibodies suggest that foals are unlikely to benefit fully from intranasal strangles vaccine administered before 4 months of age. When an inactivated M-protein vaccine is used for primary vaccination of foals, it is recommended that the initial series begin at 4 to 6 months of age, using three doses administered at 3- to 6-week intervals, followed by semiannual boosters for as long as high-risk conditions prevail.

Outbreaks of strangles generally persist for several months to more than 1 year, particularly on breeding farms, where each foal crop adds new susceptible animals to the population. Thus strangles vaccines are frequently administered during an outbreak in an attempt to bring outbreaks under control, as an adjunct to management practices designed to reduce spread of infection. Whereas all horses, except those that are clinically ill or incubating infection, can be vaccinated under these circumstances, the likelihood of preventing strangles is greatest for horses that have not yet been exposed and can be kept isolated from infected horses until the vaccination protocol can be completed. Horses that have been vaccinated previously will generate a response more rapidly than naive horses. Similarly, the attenuated live intranasal vaccine is preferred over inactivated vaccines for immunization of naïve horses in an outbreak because it is likely to generate a protective immune response more rapidly.

Injectable strangles vaccines tend to cause local reactions at the site of injection more often than other equine vaccines, particularly when administered in the muscles of the neck. In addition, purpura hemorrhagica, a serious and sometimes life-threatening systemic immune complex (Arthus-type) vasculitis manifested as edema with or without petechial hemorrhages on mucosal surfaces, has been observed with low frequency in the weeks after administration of strangles vaccines. Inactivated extract vaccines are implicated more often than the intranasal live vaccine, but all strangles vaccines have the potential to induce purpura hemorrhagica. The antigen present in immune complexes is SeM, along with antibodies of the IgA class. Because a high serum IgG titer against *S. equi* appears to be associated with an increased risk of developing purpura hemorrhagica, routine testing for specific IgG antibodies using a commercially available ELISA test has been recommended as a means of preventing vaccine-associated purpura hemorrhagica. Horses with titers of 1600 or greater in the SeM ELISA should not be vaccinated.[135] A recent study investigated the factors associated with likelihood of horses having a high serum *S. equi* SeM-specific antibody titer.[141] This study indicated that older horses, horses other than Thoroughbreds and Warmbloods, and horses that had been vaccinated with an attenuated-live intranasal *S. equi* vaccine between 1 and 3 years previously had an increased likelihood of having a serum SeM-specific antibody titer ≥1600. Recommendations of when to vaccinate horses after an *S. equi* outbreak largely depend on how long horses maintain a serum SeM-specific antibody titer ≥1600, which can range from 9 to 27 months. Therefore the recommendation is to wait 2 years after an outbreak before vaccinating horses against *S. equi* and to test for *S. equi* SeM-specific antibody titer 12 to 24 months following the outbreak.[141]

The bacterial MLV for intranasal administration will cause injection site abscesses if inadvertently injected IM. To avoid inadvertent contamination of other vaccines, syringes, and needles, it is advisable and considered good practice to administer all parenteral vaccines before handling and administering the intranasal strangles MLV. Other reported adverse responses after administration of the intranasal MLV include nasal discharge, submandibular or retropharyngeal lymphadenopathy with or without abscessation, limb edema, internal abscesses (bastard strangles), and purpura hemorrhagica. The overall frequency of adverse events is low but appears to be higher than reported to the manufacturer (4.8 per 10,000 doses). On the other hand, the majority of reported adverse events occur in horses on farms with endemic or epidemic strangles. Thus it is often uncertain whether the adverse event was caused by the vaccine or by a wild strain of *S. equi*.

Rabies

Rabies is an infrequently encountered neurologic disease of horses that results when horses are inoculated with the rabies virus through the bite of infected (rabid) wildlife. Even though the incidence of rabies in horses is low, the disease is invariably fatal and has considerable public health significance. Wildlife species that serve as the natural reservoirs for infection with this rhabdovirus differ among regions of North America. All horses kept in areas where rabies is endemic in the wildlife population are at risk and should be vaccinated. Therefore vaccination of horses against rabies is recommended using one of the three inactivated, tissue culture–derived products currently licensed for use in horses. These vaccines induce strong serologic responses after a single dose. Although correlates for protection against infection with rabies virus in horses are not well defined, it is logical to assume that protection correlates with titers of circulating antibody because infection is usually acquired by systemic injection through bites by rabid animals. In humans, postvaccination antibody titers are used to predict protection and to assess the need for postexposure vaccination or administration of immune serum. In dogs, however, postvaccination serologic test results were not found to be completely predictive

of resistance to challenge exposure during tests performed with certain inactivated vaccines.[142] Published results of challenge studies to assess efficacy of rabies vaccines licensed for use in horses in North America are not available.

Label directions on inactivated rabies vaccines licensed for use in horses suggest administration to foals age 3 months or older using one dose of vaccine in the primary series, followed by a second dose at 1 year of age. Thereafter, annual revaccination is recommended. None of the licensed vaccines carries a specific label approval for use in pregnant mares; therefore it is recommended that mares be revaccinated before breeding whenever possible. However, it should be recognized that some veterinarians administer the killed-virus vaccine to pregnant mares and do not encounter adverse consequences. Because rabies antibodies persist in serum for a prolonged period, foals born to mares that are revaccinated while open acquire substantial titers of rabies antibody after ingesting colostrum.

Documentation of rabies in reportedly vaccinated horses, most of which were less than 2 years old, has brought into question the efficacy of label recommendations for primary vaccination of foals against rabies.[143] Recent studies show that the serologic response of most 3-month-old foals from antibody-positive mares is completely blocked, even when a two-dose primary vaccination series is used. Although the response to the first dose of vaccine is typically blocked in 6-month-old foals from antibody-positive mares, these foals appear to seroconvert after administration of a second dose administered 4 weeks later. Primary vaccination of foals from vaccinated mares should therefore be delayed until they are 6 months of age or older and should include two doses of inactivated vaccine administered approximately 4 weeks apart, followed by a third dose at 1 year of age. For foals from nonvaccinated mares, the primary vaccination series can be started as early as 3 months of age and may comprise only one dose, although a two-dose series will likely induce more durable protection.

Equine neorickettsiosis (Potomac Horse Fever)

Equine neorickettsiosis, also known as Potomac horse fever, is caused by *Neorickettsia risticii* (formerly *Ehrlichia risticii*) and was originally described in 1979 as a sporadic disease affecting horses residing in the northeastern United States near the Potomac River. Equine neorickettsiosis is known to occur in 43 states, three provinces in Canada (Nova Scotia, Ontario, Alberta), South America (Uruguay, Brazil), Europe (The Netherlands, France), and India. The disease does not appear to be directly contagious, and it now appears that accidental ingestion of aquatic insects harboring metacercariae infected with *N. risticii* is at least one mode of transmission.[144] Incidence of EN is seasonal, occurring between late spring and early fall in temperate areas, with most cases in July, August, and September at the onset of hot weather. The disease may affect individual horses sporadically or cause outbreaks involving multiple horses. Foals appear to be at low risk for the disease. If EN has been confirmed on a farm or in a particular geographic area, it is likely that cases will occur in future years. Documentation of the involvement of operculate freshwater snails and aquatic insects such as caddis flies and mayflies in the life cycle of *N. risticii* has permitted formulation of focused control measures directed at minimizing exposure of horses to the habitats occupied by these species during the summer and fall months, when disease risk is highest in endemic areas.[144] Risk reduction is best accomplished by turning off barn lights at night, by covering hay or storing it indoors, by preventing horses from drinking at natural water sources like ponds or streams, and by staying informed about local hatches of aquatic insects.[145]

Recovery after natural infection with *N. risticii* induces a strong antibody response and durable protection from reinfection lasting 20 months or longer. However, the presence of antibodies does not necessarily correlate with protection, and cell-mediated responses likely play a crucial role.[146] A β-propiolactone inactivated host cell-free *N. risticii* vaccine protects mice against homologous challenge.[147] Only one inactivated EN vaccine for IM administration is currently licensed and available for use in horses as an aid to prevention of equine monocytic ehrlichiosis. The high rate of serious complications and mortality associated with this disease has been considered adequate justification for vaccinating horses residing in or traveling to endemic areas. In a series of studies in which ponies were challenged IV with *N. risticii* approximately 4 weeks after completion of the two-dose primary vaccination series using a formalin-inactivated, aluminum hydroxide–adjuvanted vaccine that is no longer marketed, Ristic et al[148] reported that 78% of experimentally infected ponies were protected against all clinical manifestations of disease except fever and 33% were protected against all signs, including fever. A published non-controlled field study involving the same vaccine documented induction of serologic responses in most vaccinated horses and a substantial reduction in disease prevalence, morbidity, and mortality compared with data collected in a previous year when horses were not vaccinated.[146,149]

In contrast to the results of the previous studies, an epidemiologic investigation involving a large number of horses in New York State failed to demonstrate any clinical or economic benefit from annual vaccination with vaccines available at that time.[150,151] Failure of a substantial number of individual horses to mount an immune response to inactivated EN vaccines, heterogeneity of *N. risticii* isolates, the presence of only one *N. risticii* strain in vaccines, and much more rapid waning of immunity after vaccination than after natural infection likely account for the observed failure of vaccines to provide protection against field infection.[146,152] Despite the lack of documented efficacy of approved vaccines to prevent infection in the field setting, many practitioners who work in endemic areas believe that severity of disease is attenuated and mortality is reduced in vaccinated horses when vaccines are administered at 4- to 6-month intervals, with administration of one booster timed to precede the anticipated period of peak challenge.

If vaccination is elected, a primary series of two doses should be administered 3 to 4 weeks apart. The manufacturer recommends revaccination at 6- to 12-month intervals, although a 4-month revaccination interval appears to be necessary to achieve a reasonable likelihood of protection of horses in endemic areas because protection after vaccination is incomplete and short lived. Because the disease has a distinct seasonal pattern, revaccination in the late spring, about 1 month before the first cases are expected, followed by a second dose about 4 months later, appears to be a reasonable approach for strategic immunization to maximize the chances of protection during the period of peak challenge. The only available vaccine is licensed for use in stallions and pregnant mares and can be administered to gestating mares 4 to 6 weeks before foaling to maximize passive transfer of specific antibodies to foals through colostrum. Whereas approximately 67% of foals from antibody-positive mares were antibody negative by 12 weeks of age, antibody was detectable in 33% of foals up to 5 months of age. On the basis of these findings, the low risk of clinical disease in young foals, and the apparent susceptibility to infection of two foals vaccinated earlier than 12 weeks of age, Sessions and Dawson[149] recommended that vaccination of foals from antibody-positive dams should begin with a two-dose primary series starting at 3 to 5 months of age, followed by administration of one subsequent booster dose 8 to 12 weeks later. However, the efficacy of this recommendation requires further study. Vaccination of foals in endemic areas is further complicated by the distinct seasonal incidence of disease in July, August, and September, when the majority of foals are 2 to 6 months of age and may be subject to maternal antibody interference with vaccination.

Botulism

Three forms of botulism—toxicoinfectious botulism (shaker foal syndrome), forage poisoning, and wound botulism—have been observed in horses as a result of the action of the potent toxins produced by the soil-borne, spore-forming bacteria of *Clostridium botulinum*. "Wound botulism" results from vegetation of spores of *C. botulinum* and subsequent production of toxin in contaminated wounds. "Shaker foal syndrome" results from toxin produced by vegetation of ingested spores in the intestinal tract. "Forage poisoning" results from ingestion of preformed toxin produced by decaying plant material or animal carcasses present in feed. Currently, toxicoinfection with *C. botulinum* type C is being investigated as a cause of "equine grass sickness," a largely fatal, pasture-associated dysautonomia affecting horses mainly in Great Britain, continental Europe, and Australia.

Botulinum toxin is the most potent biologic toxin known and acts by blocking transmission of impulses at motor end plates, resulting in weakness progressing to paralysis, inability to swallow, and frequently death. Of the eight distinct toxins produced by subtypes of *C. botulinum*, types A, B, and C are associated with most outbreaks of botulism in horses. Almost all cases of shaker foal syndrome are caused by type B. Shaker foal syndrome is a significant problem in foals age 2 weeks to 8 months in Kentucky and in the mid-Atlantic seaboard states and occurs sporadically in other areas.[153-155] A toxoid vaccine directed against *C. botulinum* type B is licensed for use in horses in the United States, with its primary indication being the prevention of shaker foal syndrome. A similar toxoid is available to protect foals in endemic areas in Australia.[156] For primary vaccination, mares should be vaccinated during gestation with a series of three doses administered 4 weeks apart, scheduled so that the last dose will be administered 4 to 6 weeks before foaling to enhance concentrations of specific immunoglobulin in colostrum. Subsequently, mares should be revaccinated annually with a single dose 4 to 6 weeks before foaling.

Passively derived colostral antibodies appear to protect the foal for 8 to 12 weeks.[154,156] Maternal antibodies do not appear to interfere with the response of foals to primary immunization against botulism[157]; therefore a primary series of three doses of vaccine, administered 4 weeks apart, can be started when foals in endemic areas are 2 to 3 months of age or older. MDAs directed against *C. botulinum* type B do not confer 100% protection; therefore the clinician must be aware of the status of transfer of passive immunity of each foal. Failure of transfer of specific immunity to botulinum toxin, insufficient specific antibody production by the dam in response to the vaccination, overwhelming toxin production, and loss of passive immunity by the time of exposure to the toxin may be reasons for vaccine failure. Other horses can be immunized using a primary series of three doses of vaccine administered at 4-week intervals, followed by annual revaccination. Currently, no licensed vaccines are available for preventing botulism caused by *C. botulinum* type C or other subtypes of toxins, and cross-protection between the B and C subtypes does not occur; thus routine vaccination against *C. botulinum* type C is not currently practiced. A type C toxoid approved for use in mink was used successfully in horses under special license to protect them during an outbreak of forage poisoning caused by contaminated alfalfa cubes in southern California.

Horses and foals with clinical botulism may be treated with botulinum antitoxin administered IV. Antitoxin is not effective against toxin that has been translocated to motor end plates.

Therefore clinical signs may progress for 12 to 24 hours after administration of the antitoxin or until all internalized toxin has attached to motor end plates.

Equine Viral Arteritis

Equine viral arteritis (EVA) is a contagious disease of equids caused by equine arteritis virus (EAV) and is found throughout the world. All breeds appear to be susceptible to the virus, but the prevalence of infection, as determined by seroconversion, is much higher in some breeds, notably Standardbreds, than in others. Despite the high seroprevalence of infection in Standardbreds, clinical disease is rarely observed in this breed, indicating that subclinical infection is common.[29,158] Conversely, Thoroughbreds and most other breeds have a low seroprevalence of infection but are likely to show fulminant clinical signs when they become infected. EVA is of special concern because the virus can cause abortion in pregnant mares, result in death of young foals, and establish a long-term carrier state in stallions.[29,159] Outbreaks of EVA are infrequent and sometimes difficult to diagnose because of clinical similarity to several other diseases (e.g., equine rhinopneumonitis, influenza, equine infectious anemia, purpura hemorrhagica). Clinical signs vary in severity and may include fever; anorexia; depression; edematous swelling of the eyelids, face, limbs, trunk, mammary glands, and genitalia; lacrimation and conjunctivitis; rhinitis and nasal discharge; skin rash; and infrequently, pneumonia and death of young foals. Aerosolized droplets of respiratory secretions containing virus can transmit the virus from horses with acute clinical disease. Of perhaps greater concern is transmission of the virus from subclinically infected carrier stallions to mares through semen during natural breeding or artificial insemination with fresh, chilled, or frozen semen. Carrier stallions are primarily responsible for maintenance of EAV in populations of horses. Identification of these individuals through serologic testing, followed by PCR testing or virus isolation from semen, forms the cornerstone of eradication measures.

An MLV based on an attenuated strain of EAV was developed by researchers in Kentucky in 1969.[160] This vaccine was first used extensively in the field during the 1984 outbreak of EVA in Kentucky and proved to be safe and very helpful in bringing the outbreak under control.[29] Subsequently, this vaccine was developed further and licensed for commercial use, with the primary indications being (1) to prevent infection and establishment of the carrier state in previously unexposed stallions and (2) to protect nonpregnant mares being bred to carrier stallions. The vaccine has also been shown to be effective in controlling outbreaks of the disease in concentrated populations of performance horses at racetracks. Primary immunization involves administration of a single dose of vaccine, with boosters administered annually thereafter.

Vaccination of stallions, nonpregnant mares, and prepubertal colts is a safe and effective means of controlling EVA. Strategic use of the MLV has formed the cornerstone of a highly successful program to control EVA in the Kentucky Thoroughbred breeding population during the past 20 years. Annual revaccination of breeding stallions, 28 days before the start of breeding season, is highly recommended as a means of preventing establishment of the carrier state. Mares being bred to carrier stallions should be revaccinated annually at least 21 days before breeding. Vaccinated mares may shed virus transiently after being bred to carrier stallions; therefore isolation of these individuals for 21 days after breeding is recommended.[29] The vaccine is not recommended for use in pregnant mares, especially during the last 2 months of gestation, or in foals less than 6 weeks of age, except in emergency situations when there is a high risk of exposure. Apparent infection of the fetus with the modified live vaccine strain after vaccination of pregnant

mares has been documented in rare instances.[161,162] A recently published study in which 73 pregnant mares were vaccinated during mid- to late-gestation concluded that it is safe to vaccinate healthy pregnant mares up to 3 months before foaling and during the immediate postpartum period. Vaccinating mares during the last 2 months of gestation was associated with a risk of abortion.[163] The authors concluded that, when faced with substantial risk of natural exposure to EAV, the risk associated with vaccination must be weighed against the much greater risk of widespread abortions in unprotected populations of pregnant mares.

Foals born to seropositive mares become seropositive after ingesting colostrum. The MDAs decay with a mean half-life of approximately 32 days, with the result that foals are generally seronegative by 7 months of age. Maternal antibodies are unlikely to interfere with the response to vaccine administered at 8 months of age or older.[35] Establishment of the carrier state appears to depend on the high levels of androgens circulating in intact stallions and can be prevented by vaccinating colts, preferably prior to puberty, before they are used for breeding.[29] In breeds or in areas where EAV is prevalent, vaccination of intact males between 8 and 12 months of age should therefore be strongly encouraged to prevent them from becoming carriers when exposed to EAV later in life through breeding or aerosol contact. Routine vaccination of Standardbred colts would be a logical approach to reducing the number of stallions that later become chronic carriers and would likely result in a substantial reduction in the incidence of infection in this breed.

Horses vaccinated with the MLV can be expected to become seropositive for life. Titers resulting from vaccination with the MLV currently licensed in North America or the inactivated vaccines licensed in Europe and in Japan cannot be distinguished from titers resulting from natural infection. Therefore vaccination may complicate testing of horses for export. Although only a few countries currently restrict the importation of horses that test positive for neutralizing antibodies against EAV, several countries restrict entry of seropositive stallions because of the likelihood that they are chronically infected and may shed the virus in semen. It is advisable to collect a blood sample for serologic testing before administering the first dose of vaccine. Coordination of vaccination with state and federal regulatory officials, along with results of serologic tests that provide evidence the horse was seronegative before vaccination, may be helpful in resolving disputes but do not guarantee that entry will be granted into foreign countries or onto breeding farms. Development and marketing of a DIVA vaccine that allows vaccinated horses to be distinguished from inapparent infected carriers would greatly facilitate control, and even eradication, of EAV from horse populations.

Rotaviral Diarrhea

Equine rotavirus is one of the most important causes of infectious diarrhea in foals during the first few weeks of life and often causes outbreaks involving the majority of the foal crop on individual farms.[164-166] Older foals and adult horses are more resistant to infection. Equine rotavirus is transmitted via fecaloral contamination and causes diarrhea by damaging the tips of villi in the small intestine, resulting in cellular destruction, maldigestion, and malabsorption. Equine group A rotavirus strains are icosahedral, nonenveloped viruses possessing a genome of 11 segments of double-stranded RNA (dsRNA). The two outer capsid proteins, VP7 and VP4, elicit neutralizing antibodies independently and are used to differentiate equine group A rotavirus strains into G-types (glycoprotein) and P-types (protease-sensitive).[167] Molecular genome analysis suggests strongly that the vast majority of the currently circulating equine group A rotavirus strains are highly conserved, with only limited genetic diversity.[168] A conditionally licensed inactivated rotavirus A vaccine containing the G3 (H2) serotype in a metabolizable oil-in-water emulsion is available and is indicated for administration to pregnant mares in endemic areas as an aid to prevention of diarrhea in their foals caused by infection with rotaviruses of serogroup A. Foal vaccination is not indicated. Label recommendations call for a three-dose series of the vaccine to be administered during each pregnancy at 8, 9, and 10 months of gestation. This protocol induces significant increases in serum concentrations of neutralizing antibody in vaccinated mares and in concentrations of antibodies of the IgG, but not IgA, subclass in the colostrum and milk of vaccinated mares.[169,170] After nursing, the concentration of passively derived rotavirus-specific antibody of the IgG subclass in the serum of foals up to 90 days of age from vaccinated mares is significantly higher than that measured in serum of foals born to nonvaccinated mares. A field study showed this vaccine to be safe and provided circumstantial evidence of at least partial efficacy. An approximately twofold higher incidence of rotaviral diarrhea was found in foals from nonvaccinated mares compared with those from vaccinated mares, although this difference did not prove to be statistically significant.[169] Similarly, a controlled field study in Argentina, in which an inactivated aluminum hydroxide–adjuvanted vaccine containing the SA11 (G3P2), H2 (G3P12), and Lincoln (G6P1) strains was administered to 100 mares at 60 days and again at 30 days before foaling, demonstrated a substantial reduction in the incidence and severity of rotaviral disease in foals from vaccinated mares compared with foals from nonvaccinated mares.[171]

Challenge studies involving two inactivated rotavirus vaccines administered in a similar manner to pregnant mares in Japan showed that their foals were not completely protected against infection but had a substantial reduction in severity of clinical signs after challenge.[172] The major correlate for protection against rotaviral infection appears to be mucosal immunity, predominantly mucosal IgA, in the gastrointestinal tract. Studies of the immunoglobulin isotype responses of mares and of antibodies passively transferred to their foals after parenteral vaccination of their dams with inactivated rotavirus vaccines indicate that this approach is unlikely to provide foals with intestinal mucosal protection in the form of IgA.[170] Consequently, it is not surprising that current protocols do not provide complete protection. In addition, because the vaccine available in the United States contains only the G3 serotype of the A serogroup, it cannot be expected to protect against infection with all field strains.

Anthrax

Anthrax is a serious and rapidly fatal septicemic disease caused by proliferation and spread of the vegetative form of *Bacillus anthracis* in the body. *B. anthracis* is acquired through ingestion or contamination of wounds by soil-borne spores of the organism and is encountered only in limited geographic areas where alkaline soil conditions favor survival of the organism. A Sterne's strain, nonencapsulated, live-spore vaccine has been used to vaccinate horses. A primary series consisting of two doses of that vaccine should be administered subcutaneously 2 to 3 weeks apart, followed by annual revaccination. Adverse systemic or local effects may occasionally occur. Little objective information is available regarding use of this vaccine in horses, but clinical evidence suggests that it provides protection; however, vaccination of pregnant mares is not recommended.[173] Because it is a live bacterial product, appropriate caution should be used during storage, handling, and administration of the vaccine. Concurrent administration of antimicrobial drugs that are effective against *B. anthracis* is contraindicated if the vaccine is to function as intended.

Equine Rhinitis A Virus

Two rhinitis viruses, equine rhinitis A virus (formerly known as equine rhinovirus 1, genus *Aphthovirus*, family *Picornaviridae*), and equine rhinitis B virus (formerly known as equine rhinovirus 2, genus *Erbovirus* family *Picornaviridae*), have been identified in horses.[174-179] Seroprevalence studies confirm that both viruses are active in horse populations worldwide, with prevalence ranging from 20% to 90%, depending on the age group and use of the horses sampled.[175,176,180] The rhinitis viruses have been largely overlooked as potential causes of clinically apparent respiratory disease for many years; however, recently investigated outbreaks of contagious respiratory disease, as well as challenge studies, suggest that ERAV and ERBV may indeed be important pathogens of horses, causing disease of both lower and upper respiratory tract.[177,179,180] Clinical manifestations include pyrexia, nasal discharge, cough, lethargy, anorexia pharyngitis and submandibular lymphadenopathy.[177,179] It has also been suggested that ERAV may play a causative role in inflammatory airway disease.[180] A unique feature of ERAV is persistent shedding in urine, but only transient shedding in nasal secretions, after infection of the respiratory tract.[174]

An inactivated ERAV vaccine (Equine Rhinitis A Vaccine, Boehringer Ingelheim) was granted a conditional license in late 2012 while efficacy and potency tests are in progress. The vaccine is labeled for vaccination of healthy horses 4 months of age or older. The manufacturer recommends a primary vaccination series of three 1 mL doses administered intramuscularly at 3 to 4 week intervals, followed by revaccination annually or prior to anticipated exposure. Pending publication of more data regarding vaccine efficacy, as well as the role of ERAV as a cause of respiratory disease, these authors are unable to provide recommendations regarding use of this vaccine.

Miscellaneous Infections

Many vaccine candidates are under development for pathogens that can have profound effects on the health of equids. Most of these are in development for human diseases. The most common quests for vaccines involve *Candida*, *Cryptococcus*, and *Aspergillus* infections.[181] Most of these are subunit vaccines designed to induce development of opsonizing antibodies, neutralizing antibodies, and/or CD4 Th1 cell stimulation against major antigens of these organisms.

The complete reference list is available online at www.expertconsult.com.

65 Antimicrobial Therapy

Jennifer L. Davis and Mark G. Papich*

Principles of Therapy

Antibiotic therapy for horses has always been challenging because of their poor oral absorption, the large volumes required for administration, and the high cost of some drugs. The risk of some adverse drug reactions that affect the gastrointestinal (GI) tract is a greater concern in horses than in other animals. Despite these drawbacks, it is essential that horses with serious infections receive appropriate therapy to prevent a chronic or life-threatening condition. Drug-resistant bacterial infections are an emerging problem, and the use of highly active drugs has become more important than ever before. Foals, in particular, need highly active drugs because they may be immunocompromised at the time of treatment. Drug treatment for foals has additional challenges because of differences in drug disposition in foals versus adults. Differences in oral absorption, volumes of distribution, metabolism, and clearance between foals and adults must be considered when selecting antibacterial dosage regimens.

To assist veterinarians in prescribing effective antibiotics for their equine patients, pharmacokinetic-pharmacodynamic relationships have been used to provide guidelines for effective use. The selection of the most appropriate drug has been facilitated by new approaches to bacterial identification and susceptibility testing. This chapter reviews some of these concepts that guide antibiotic therapy for equine patients and provide important strategies for effective dosing.

Microbial Susceptibility

Many microbes have predictable susceptibility patterns. Therefore, if the infectious agent can be accurately identified, rational antimicrobial therapy can be selected. For those bacteria and fungi that are usually highly susceptible, empiric-therapy antimicrobial agents may be chosen initially before susceptibility results are available.

Streptococcus and Pasteurella

Streptococcus and Pasteurella bacteria are consistently susceptible to β-lactam antibiotics such as the penicillins and cephalosporins. Resistance among Streptococcus spp. to trimethoprim-sulfonamide (TMS) combinations and chloramphenicol appears to be increasing. Trimethoprim-sulfonamide combinations for the horse may include either trimethoprim-sulfadiazine or trimethoprim-sulfamethoxazole; these drugs are also referred to as potentiated sulfonamides. (See Appendix D for dosing information.) Many of the fluoroquinolones (e.g., enrofloxacin, orbifloxacin, marbofloxacin) used in veterinary medicine have low activity, which is reflected in high minimum inhibitory (MIC)

values against Streptococcus spp., whereas Pasteurella organisms are frequently susceptible to fluoroquinolones, as well as other drugs. Aminoglycosides have good activity against Pasteurella spp. but not against streptococci, therefore they should be combined with a penicillin.

Actinobacillus

Actinobacillus spp. have historically been susceptible to many of the β-lactam antibiotics and the potentiated sulfonamides, although resistance has been documented in the last several years. One report of postoperative wound infection showed that 100% and 60% of the isolates were resistant to penicillin and TMS, respectively.[1] This resistance to penicillin may be caused by the production of β-lactamases by some strains.[2] Susceptibility to the cephalosporins and aminoglycoside antibiotics is usually anticipated.

Staphylococcus

Staphylococcus spp. that do not produce β-lactamase have a predictable susceptibility pattern to many of the penicillins and cephalosporins. Staphylococcus spp. are usually susceptible to oxacillin and dicloxacillin, but these are not typically administered to horses. Most staphylococci are sensitive to the fluoroquinolones and aminoglycosides. The majority of strains are also sensitive to chloramphenicol, TMS, or erythromycin, but resistance is possible. Susceptibility of β-lactamase–positive staphylococci is less predictable. The β-lactamase will inactivate penicillins, aminopenicillins (e.g., ampicillin, amoxicillin), and some of the extended-spectrum penicillins (e.g., ticarcillin). The addition of a β-lactamase inhibitor (clavulanate or sulbactam) or the use of β-lactamase–resistant β-lactam antibiotics, such as cephalosporins (e.g., cefadroxil, cefpodoxime, cefazolin), will increase activity to include β-lactamase–producing strains of staphylococci.

Recent reports have raised concerns of staphylococcal resistance in horses.[3-5] The isolated methicillin-resistant Staphylococcus aureus (MRSA) strains colonized both horses and people who were in contact with the horses (see Chapter 29). Evidence for human-to-animal transmission was reported. These strains were resistant to other antibiotics, in addition to β-lactams. Methicillin-resistant Staphylococcus aureus has been reported more often in some referral centers. These MRSA strains present an important problem for veterinarians because they are resistant to all β-lactam antibiotics, regardless of whether they are combined with a β-lactamase inhibitor. Some of these strains remain sensitive to chloramphenicol, tetracyclines, and TMS, but there may be cases for which the only active drugs are the glycopeptide vancomycin or the oxazolidinone linezolid (Zyvox). Vancomycin has been used sporadically in the treatment of equine MRSA as an intravenous (IV) infusion at doses of 4.3 to 7.5 mg/kg body weight every 8 hours (q8h).[6,7] There are no reports of clinical use of linezolid in horses, and at the time of this writing, its use is considered to be cost prohibitive.

*The authors acknowledge and appreciate the original contributions of these authors, whose work has been incorporated into this chapter.

Instituting appropriate hygiene measures and the use of topical antibiotics (i.e., mupirocin) are also recommended, particularly in hospital situations.[8]

Anaerobic Bacteria

If bacteria are anaerobic, predictable susceptibility patterns also are available. In horses, anaerobic bacteria causing infection include *Clostridium*, *Fusobacterium*, *Peptostreptococcus*, and *Bacteroides* spp.[9] These bacteria are usually sensitive to penicillin, chloramphenicol, metronidazole, or one of the second-generation cephalosporins such as cefotetan or cefoxitin. If the anaerobe is from the *Bacteroides fragilis* group, resistance may be more of a problem as the result of the production of a β-lactamase that inactivates first-generation cephalosporins, penicillins, and ampicillin/amoxicillin. The incidence of resistant strains of *Bacteroides* has increased in recent years.[10] Because many anaerobic infections in horses may be caused by *B. fragilis*,[11] metronidazole is a logical choice for treatment. This drug is consistently active against anaerobes, including *B. fragilis*, and doses have been established from pharmacokinetic studies. Chloramphenicol also has consistent activity against many anaerobic bacteria. Clindamycin frequently has good activity against anaerobic bacteria, although resistance has increased over the last several years. In small animals, up to 17% of *Bacteroides* spp. and 20% of *Clostridium* spp. are reported to be resistant.[10] However, clindamycin should never be used in the horse because of the likely development of a severe, often fatal, diarrhea. The activity of first-generation cephalosporins, TMS, or fluoroquinolones against anaerobic bacteria is unpredictable. None of the aminoglycosides is active against anaerobic bacteria.

Pseudomonas, Enterobacter, Klebsiella, and Escherichia coli

If the organism is *Pseudomonas aeruginosa*, *Enterobacter*, *Klebsiella*, *Escherichia coli*, or *Proteus*, resistance to many common antibiotics is possible, and a susceptibility test is advised. Many *E. coli* isolates are resistant to common antibiotics such as penicillins, aminopenicillins, first-generation cephalosporins, and tetracyclines. Based on susceptibility data, gram-negative enteric bacteria are usually expected to be susceptible to fluoroquinolones and aminoglycosides. However, some reports suggest that resistance to fluoroquinolones may be increasing in small animals,[12,13] and a similar trend has been reported in foals.[14] Resistance to gentamicin among equine pathogens is increasing and has been documented in veterinary teaching hospitals for more than 15 years.[15] Amikacin is the most active of the aminoglycosides against gram-negative bacteria in horses, including *P. aeruginosa*, and may be more suitable for the treatment of resistant gram-negative infections. *Pseudomonas aeruginosa* is inherently resistant to many drugs, but it may be susceptible to fluoroquinolones, aminoglycosides, or extended-spectrum penicillins (e.g., ticarcillin, piperacillin). If a fluoroquinolone is used to treat *P. aeruginosa*, a large dose is necessary because the MICs of *Pseudomonas* spp. are higher than for other gram-negative organisms. Although pharmacokinetic studies have documented effective plasma concentrations for most gram-negative bacteria from typical doses of fluoroquinolones, no studies have used high enough doses to produce plasma concentrations considered to be effective against *Pseudomonas* spp. Moreover, the high doses recommended for treating *Pseudomonas* in dogs have not been tested for safety in clinical studies in horses. Of the currently available fluoroquinolones (human or veterinary drugs), ciprofloxacin is the most active against *P. aeruginosa*, but it is not absorbed well orally in horses[16] and has been associated with the development of

severe colitis and other adverse effects after both oral and IV administration.[17]

The extended-spectrum cephalosporins (second-, third-, and fourth-generation cephalosporins) have been used in horses for some of the refractory gram-negative infections. They have greater activity against gram-negative bacteria than first-generation cephalosporins such as cefazolin. Only ceftazidime has consistent activity against *P. aeruginosa*. Because the extended-spectrum cephalosporins are expensive, use of drugs, such as cefotaxime and ceftazidime, has been limited in horses. However, one of the veterinary drugs, ceftiofur, has been frequently used in horses, and some dosing regimens may be effective (see section on Cephalosporins).

Fungi

Systemic fungal infections in horses can be difficult to treat because of the lack of availability of affordable treatments and the difficulty involved in culturing and identifying the organisms. However, some generalizations about susceptibilities can be made. Many of the yeast and yeastlike infections in horses have good susceptibility to the triazole antifungals—fluconazole, itraconazole, and voriconazole—including the organisms that cause candidiasis, histoplasmosis, blastomycosis, and coccidioidomycosis. Fluconazole is a rational treatment for these pathogens because it has excellent oral bioavailability and produces sustained plasma and tissue concentrations.[18] This drug is now available in a generic human formulation, which has decreased its cost for effective therapy. Some *Candida* spp. have developed resistance to fluconazole however, and alternative therapies may be necessary. *Aspergillus* spp. are typically sensitive to itraconazole and voriconazole but not to fluconazole. *Fusarium* spp. present a very difficult treatment dilemma in that they are resistant to many of the available drugs. Only voriconazole and amphotericin B demonstrate significant in vitro antifungal activity against *Fusarium* spp. If systemic treatment for dermatophytosis is required, griseofulvin can be used and is labeled for use in the horse.

Bacterial Susceptibility Testing

Agar Disk Diffusion Test

When bacterial resistance is likely, a susceptibility test is recommended. Bacterial susceptibility to drugs has traditionally been tested with the agar disk diffusion (ADD) test, also known as the Kirby-Bauer test. With this test, paper disks impregnated with the drug are placed on an agar plate and the drug diffuses into the agar. The zone of inhibition around the disk is correlated to the bactericidal or bacteriostatic activity of the drug against the bacteria. The ADD must be performed according to strict procedural standards for inoculation size, depth of agar, and incubation time set by the Clinical and Laboratory Standards Institute (CLSI).[19,20] The ADD test results are qualitative and determine only resistance or sensitivity for the bacteria tested. If this test is performed using standardized procedures, it is valuable; at times, however, it may overestimate the degree of susceptibility.

Minimum Inhibitory Concentration Determination

Laboratories typically measure the MIC of an organism directly with an antimicrobial dilution test. The test is most often performed by inoculating the wells of a plate with the bacterial culture and adding multiple dilutions of antibiotics across the rows of the plate. The MIC is recorded by observing the lowest concentration required to inhibit bacterial growth. In some laboratories, other methods to measure the MIC are being used such as the E-test (epsilometer test) by AB Biodisk (Solna, Sweden). The E-test is a quantitative technique that identifies the MIC by direct measurement of bacterial growth along a concentration gradient of the antibiotic contained in a test strip.

When the MIC is measured, resistance and susceptibility are determined by comparing the organism's MIC to the drug's breakpoint, as standardized by CLSI.[19-21] If bacteria have an MIC equal to or below the "susceptible" breakpoint, treatment with this drug should produce a cure unless there are other factors independent of the drug's activity. An MIC equal to or above the "resistant" breakpoint indicates that the organism is resistant regardless of the dose administered or location of the infection. An MIC in the "intermediate" range means that the organism is resistant to the drug unless dosing modifications are used, or unless the drug concentrates at the site of infection, as with topical treatment, or in the lower urinary tract for drugs excreted via the kidney.

Even though we believe that an MIC determination is valuable to guide therapy, some limitations exist. One important limitation for interpreting susceptibility information for pathogens infecting horses is that interpretive criteria to establish susceptibility breakpoints are available for only a small number of drugs used in horses (ceftiofur, gentamicin; see Tables 1 and 2 in the CLSI M-31 document under Group A[21]). For other drugs, human interpretive criteria are used.

Pharmacokinetic-Pharmacodynamic Optimization of Doses

To achieve a cure, the drug concentration at the site of the infection should be maintained above the MIC, or some multiple of the MIC, for at least a portion of the dose interval. Antibacterial dosage regimens are based on this assumption (see Appendix D.) However, drugs vary with respect to the magnitude of the peak concentration and the time above the MIC that is needed for a clinical cure. Pharmacokinetic-pharmacodynamic (PK-PD) relationships of antibiotics attempt to describe how these factors can correlate with clinical outcome.[22,23] Parameters that describe the plasma concentration versus time profile may be used as pharmacokinetic factors to predict antibiotic cures (Fig. 65-1). The "C_{max}" is the maximum

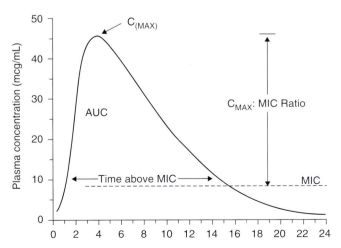

Figure 65-1 Plasma concentration versus time profile and minimum inhibitory concentration *(MIC)*. Relationship between MIC and pharmacokinetic terms are shown; see text. C_{max}/MIC ratio, Maximum (peak) plasma concentration; *AUC*, area under the curve.

plasma concentration attained during a dosing interval. The C_{max} is related to the MIC by the C_{max}/MIC ratio. The "AUC" is the total area under the curve. The AUC for a 24-hour period is related to the MIC value by the AUC_{24}/MIC ratio. The duration of effective plasma concentrations is determined by the time (T) above MIC measured in hours (T > MIC), or reported as the percentage of the T above the MIC during a 24-hour dosing interval.[24]

Antibiotics can be bactericidal, bacteriostatic, or both, depending on the drug and the organism. For a drug that is bactericidal, its action may be either concentration dependent or time dependent. If concentration dependent, the clinician should administer a high enough dose to maximize the C_{max}/MIC ratio or the AUC_{24}/MIC ratio. If time dependent, the drug should be administered frequently enough to maximize the T > MIC. For bacteriostatic drugs, the drug concentration should be kept above the MIC at the site of action for as long as possible during the dosing interval. Examples of how these relationships affect drug regimens for some drugs used in horses are described next.

Aminoglycosides

Aminoglycosides are concentration-dependent bactericidal drugs, therefore the higher the drug concentration, the greater the bactericidal effect. An optimal bactericidal effect occurs if a high enough dose is administered to produce a peak of 8 to 10 times the MIC. This can be accomplished by administering a single IV dose once daily because a significant postantibiotic effect has been demonstrated. This regimen is at least as effective, and perhaps less nephrotoxic, than lower doses administered more frequently.[25,26] Current dosing regimens in horses employ this strategy. The single daily dose is related to the drug's volume of distribution (Vd) using the equation Dose = C_{max} × Vd. A once-daily dose for gentamicin in adult horses using these guidelines is 4 to 6.8 mg/kg.[27] For amikacin, the recommended dose is 8 to 10 mg/kg. The efficacy of these regimens has not been tested for conditions encountered in veterinary medicine, but the relationships are supported by studies in experimental animals. These regimens assume some competency of the immune system. If the animal is severely immunocompromised, the clinician may consider a more frequent interval for administration and/or synergistic combinations with β-lactam antibiotics.

Fluoroquinolones

Fluoroquinolone antibiotics are rapidly bactericidal and exhibit a significant postantibiotic effect. As reviewed in several papers,[22,28-30] either the C_{max}/MIC ratio or the AUC_{24}/MIC ratio may predict clinical cure in studies of laboratory animals and in a limited number of human clinical studies. There are no published studies involving horses (or dogs and cats) to indicate which of these parameters will better predict clinical cure or what the respective target ratios might be. However, studies in experimental animals have demonstrated that a C_{max}/MIC ratio of 8 to 10 or an AUC_{24}/MIC ratio greater than 100 to 125 has been associated with a cure. The cited AUC/MIC ratio above 125 refers to administration to critically ill, neutropenic human patients. In other patients, the ratio to achieve a cure may not be that high. Wright et al[29] presented evidence that AUC_{24}/MIC ratios as low as 30 to 55 are associated with a clinical cure. This difference may reflect the severity of illness in the subjects of these investigations, but it also may be organism specific. With clinical doses used for many infections in veterinary medicine, the AUC/MIC ratios are often lower than 125, and clinical cures are still observed. An examination of the current use of the fluoroquinolones in veterinary medicine suggests that, in immunocompetent animals, AUC/MIC ratios of 50 to 60 are likely to be effective.[30]

Current guidelines recommend doses of fluoroquinolones to achieve C_{max}/MIC ratios above these threshold levels, which have been associated with a lower incidence of the development of resistance.[31] Sensitive bacteria from horses might be expected to have an MIC for enrofloxacin of 0.125 µg/mL or less based on available information.[32] Pharmacokinetic studies available from horses showed that to achieve desirable PK-PD indices administering enrofloxacin, IV doses of 5 mg/kg once daily or 7.5 to 10 mg/kg orally may be adequate.[33-36] Monitoring of plasma concentrations in hospitalized equine patients after oral and injectable administration of enrofloxacin confirmed that these doses are adequate to achieve targeted plasma concentrations for bacteria with MICs less than or equal to 0.5 µg/mL.[37]

β-Lactam Antibiotics

β-Lactam antibiotics, such as penicillins, potentiated aminopenicillins, and cephalosporins, are slowly bactericidal. Their concentration should be kept above the MIC throughout most of the dosing interval (long T > MIC) for the optimal bactericidal effect.[24] In general, the goal is to maintain plasma concentrations above the MIC for at least 50% of the dosing interval. For gram-negative organisms, however, no postantibiotic effect (PAE) exists for β-lactam antibiotics, and reduced efficacy of cephalosporin antimicrobial therapy has been reported when T greater than MIC is less than 80% of the dosing interval.[24,38] In neutropenic patients, maintaining concentrations greater than the MIC for 90% to 100% of the dosing interval is required for maximal bactericidal action against gram-negative organisms and streptococci.[24] For the treatment of some gram-negative bacteria, some regimens for penicillins and cephalosporins require administration three to four times per day to meet this target. Some of the third-generation cephalosporins have longer half-lives, and less frequent dosing intervals have been used for these drugs (e.g., cefotaxime, ceftiofur). Because the MICs are lower for gram-positive bacteria and antibacterial effects occur at concentrations below the MIC (PAE), longer dose intervals may be possible for infections caused by gram-positive compared with gram-negative bacteria.

Bacteriostatic Drugs

Drugs, such as the tetracyclines, macrolides (erythromycin and derivatives), sulfonamides, and chloramphenicol derivatives, act in a bacteriostatic manner against most bacteria. However, against susceptible gram-positive bacteria, the macrolides appear to be bactericidal and can demonstrate a PAE. Chloramphenicol also can produce a bactericidal effect if the organism is very susceptible.

Bacteriostatic drugs are most effective when concentrations of the drug at the site of the infection are maintained above the MIC for the entire dosing interval. In this way, they act in a time-dependent manner. However, the most predictive PK-PD index for antibacterial success is the AUC/MIC ratio. Many of the bacteriostatic drugs must be administered frequently or demonstrate a long half-life to achieve this goal. A property of some of these drugs is that they persist in tissues for a prolonged time, allowing infrequent dosing intervals. The macrolide derivative azithromycin (Zithromax, Pfizer) has shown tissue half-lives as long as 70 to 90 hours in cats and dogs, permitting infrequent dosing. Accumulation and persistence of azithromycin in polymorphonuclear leukocytes (PMNs) and macrophages of foals has also been demonstrated.[39] Concentrations of clarithromycin can be maintained with twice-daily dosing in foals.[40] Tissue concentrations of TMS persist long enough to allow once-daily dosing for many infections, although a study in equine joint infections showed that twice daily was more effective.[41]

Tissue Penetration of Drugs

For most tissues, antibiotic drug concentrations in the serum or plasma can predict the drug concentration in the extracellular space (interstitial fluid) because no physical barrier impedes drug diffusion from the vascular compartment to extracellular tissue fluid.[42] Pores (fenestrations) or microchannels in the endothelium of capillaries are large enough to allow drug molecules to penetrate. One important limitation involves drugs that are highly protein bound in the blood[43]; examples of drugs for which this may be important in equine medicine include doxycycline and itraconazole.

For most antimicrobial drugs, the plasma drug concentrations produce tissue fluid concentrations in lung, pleural space, skin, abdominal fluid, joint fluid, soft tissues, and bone that are similar to steady-state plasma drug concentrations. For example, gentamicin reached concentrations in lymph fluid of horses that closely paralleled plasma concentrations.[44] Rapid equilibration between the extracellular fluid and plasma is possible because of high surface area/volume (SA/V) ratio (i.e., the surface area of the capillaries is high relative to the volume into which the drug diffuses).

Some caution is advised when interpreting tissue concentrations reported in pharmacokinetic papers. Tissue concentrations in homogenized tissues reflect the total tissue content (intracellular and extracellular drug concentration) rather than the drug concentration in interstitial fluid. Drug concentrations from homogenized tissues will also reflect both protein-bound and protein-unbound drug, as well as drug bound to the tissues. It is only the unbound form of the drug that is microbiologically active. Therefore homogenized tissue drug concentrations often overestimate the actual drug at the site, or they may underestimate the drug concentrations in extracellular fluid if the drug has low lipophilicity.

Drug diffusion into an abscess or cavitated lesion may be delayed because the volume into which the drug must diffuse is higher, resulting in a lower SA/V, lower drug concentrations, and slower equilibrium between plasma and tissue. Therefore observed slow equilibrium or a low peak drug concentration in this case is more a factor of the geometry of the tissue (low SA/V), than a physical barrier to diffusion. For an abscess or granuloma, penetration by antibiotics also is impaired because drug penetration relies on simple diffusion from the plasma compartment, and the site of infection may lack an adequate blood supply.

Tissues once assumed to present a barrier to drug diffusion actually attain adequate drug penetration. For example, it is a common misconception that drug penetration into synovial fluid of joints is impaired in horses. Penetration of ampicillin and gentamicin is adequate from the vascular compartment to synovial fluid in horses,[45] but equilibrium is often delayed because of the synovial volume (low SA/V). After equilibrium is achieved, synovial fluid concentrations either parallel plasma drug concentrations or decline more slowly. β-Lactam antibiotics and aminoglycosides penetrated inflamed joints more rapidly and achieved higher concentrations than in healthy joints,[46] most likely from increased blood flow to the joint. However, penetration during chronic inflammation could be impeded by the presence of pus and fibrosis.

When the SA/V ratio is small and the drug's elimination from the plasma is rapid, some drugs may not have sufficient time to diffuse adequately into infected sites.

Impaired Diffusion into Tissues

Tissues that lack pores or channels may inhibit penetration of some drugs. In some tissues a lipid membrane (e.g., tight junctions in capillaries) presents a barrier to drug diffusion. In these cases, a drug must be sufficiently lipid soluble or must be actively carried across the membrane to reach effective concentrations in tissues. These tissues include the central nervous system (CNS), eye, and prostate. Lipophilic drugs (e.g., macrolides, fluoroquinolones, tetracyclines, trimethoprim, chloramphenicol) may be more likely to diffuse through lipid membranes for treating infections in these tissues. Many clinicians believe that drug penetration across these barriers is not important when treating inflammatory diseases because these barriers will be breached and drugs will be able to diffuse freely into the affected area. However, this is not always the case. In a study analyzing amikacin concentrations in the CSF of the horse, drug was not detected in any of the horses with a normal blood-brain barrier (BBB).[47] In one horse that developed septic meningitis during the study, drug was not detectable until 4 hours after the second injection and reached a peak of only 0.97 μg/mL, which did not occur until 8 hours after the fifth injection.

Box 65-1 summarizes drugs known to penetrate into the cerebrospinal fluid (CSF) and aqueous humor of horses. A barrier also exists between plasma and bronchial epithelium (blood-bronchus barrier).[48] This restricts penetration of some drugs in the bronchial secretions and epithelial fluid of the airways. However, disposition of drug into lung tissue not separated by the blood-bronchus barrier is not impaired (e.g., when treating pneumonia).

Intracellular Drug Penetration

Most bacterial infections are located extracellularly, and a cure can be achieved with adequate drug concentrations in the extracellular (interstitial) space rather than intracellular space. Intracellular infections, however, present a different problem. For drugs to reach intracellular sites, they must either diffuse passively or utilize a transport process. One of the most important equine intracellular organisms is *Rhodococcus equi*. Drugs traditionally used for treatment of *R. equi* pneumonia in foals include erythromycin and rifampin because these drugs are known for their ability to achieve high concentrations intracellularly.[49] Treatment of rickettsial infections in horses also requires intracellular penetration. Infections caused by *Neorickettsia risticii* and *Anaplasma phagocytophilum* have been treated most often with tetracyclines because they are known to attain sufficient intracellular concentrations. Other intracellular organisms include *Chlamydia* and *Mycobacterium*. *Staphylococci* and *Salmonella* spp. may become resistant to treatment in some cases because of intracellular survival.

Examples of drugs that accumulate in leukocytes, fibroblasts, macrophages, and other cells are fluoroquinolones, tetracyclines, macrolides (erythromycin, clarithromycin), and the azalides (azithromycin).[50] β-Lactam antibiotics and aminoglycosides do not reach effective concentrations within cells. Doxycycline, despite high protein binding in horses, achieves leukocyte concentrations 17 times greater than maximum plasma concentrations.[51] This may explain why doxycycline is efficacious in the treatment of many bacterial infections, despite the low plasma concentrations. The erythromycin derivative azithromycin (Zithromax) achieves particularly high concentrations of active drug intracellularly. In equine studies the oral absorption of azithromycin in foals was 33%, and the concentrations achieved in phagocytes were 200 times the corresponding plasma concentrations.[39]

Local Factors That Affect Antibiotic Effectiveness

Local tissue factors may decrease antimicrobial effectiveness. For example, pus and necrotic debris may bind and inactivate vancomycin or aminoglycoside antibiotics, causing them to be ineffective. Cellular material also can decrease the activity of topical agents such as polymyxin B. Foreign material in a wound, such as material surgically implanted, can protect bacteria from antibiotics and phagocytosis by forming a biofilm (glycocalyx) at the site of infection.[52,53] Cations can adversely affect the activity of antimicrobials at the site of infection. Two important drug groups diminished in activity by cations (e.g., Mg^{+2}, Al^{+3}, Ca^{+2}) at the site of infection are fluoroquinolones and tetracyclines. Cations, such as magnesium, iron, and aluminum, also can inhibit oral absorption of these drugs.

The acidic environment of infected tissue may decrease the effectiveness of erythromycin, other macrolides, fluoroquinolones, and aminoglycosides. Penicillin and tetracycline activity is not affected as much by tissue pH, but hemoglobin at the site of infection will decrease the activity of these drugs. An anaerobic environment decreases the effectiveness of aminoglycosides because oxygen is necessary for drug penetration into bacteria. Trimethoprim-sulfonamide combinations are sometimes not effective in vivo despite in vitro results that suggest susceptibility.[54] Tissues may contain thymidine and para-aminobenzoic acid (PABA), which are inhibitors of the action of trimethoprim and sulfonamides, respectively.

Effective antibacterial drug concentrations may not be attained in tissues that are poorly vascularized (e.g., extremities during shock, sequestered bone fragments, endocardial valves). An abscess rarely responds to antibiotic therapy alone because several factors hamper successful therapy: poor blood supply, material in tissue fluid and pus that may inactivate drugs, and a small SA/V ratio of the infected site.

Box 65-1 Summary of Drugs Studied in Cerebrospinal Fluid (CSF) and Aqueous Humor in the Horse*

Drugs That Penetrate Intact Blood-Brain Barrier
Chloramphenicol (39%)
Ciprofloxacin (23%)
Enrofloxacin (25%)
Fluconazole (39%)
Metronidazole (31%)
Orbifloxacin (25%)
Streptomycin (4%)
Sulfamethoxazole (30%)
Trimethoprim (27%)

Drugs That Do Not Penetrate Intact Blood-Brain Barrier
Amikacin
Ceftiofur

Drugs That Penetrate Intact Blood-Aqueous Barrier
Chloramphenicol (16%)
Ciprofloxacin (4%)
Doxycycline (10.5%)
Enrofloxacin (12%)
Fluconazole (37%)
Streptomycin (10%)
Voriconazole (41%)

Drugs That Do Not Penetrate Intact Blood-Aqueous Barrier
Cephalexin
Itraconazole

*The value in parentheses represents the percentage of drug found in the CSF or aqueous humor compared with that found in plasma or serum.

Absorption of Antimicrobials in Horses

One of the challenges presented for antibiotic therapy in horses is actually delivering the drug into the animal. Injectable drugs can cause pain and irritation. Many oral drugs are poorly absorbed, which presents risks because unabsorbed drug in the intestine may disrupt the normal bacterial population and cause diarrhea and enteritis.

Injectable Drugs

Many injectable solutions can be administered IV, which delivers high concentrations to tissues rapidly. Intramuscular (IM) administration also is suitable for some drugs, although pain and muscle injury from injection can be important drawbacks. The absorption rate from an IM injection usually is sufficient to achieve high concentrations rapidly, and absorption usually is complete. For some drugs, slow release of the drug from the IM injection may effectively prolong the dosing interval either due to disruption of blood flow at the injection site after IM administration and slower uptake into the circulation, or with specialized formulations designed to produce slow release of the drug from the injection such as ceftiofur crystalline free acid. Because the rate of absorption determines the terminal half-life in these cases, half-life is prolonged. Pharmacokineticists refer to this as the "flip-flop effect." Systemic availability (% F) may be falsely overestimated in studies in which the flip-flop effect is observed.

As in cattle,[55] the site of IM injection also affects drug absorption. In studies comparing different IM sites, injections in the neck muscle of horses showed faster and more complete drug absorption compared with injections in the gluteal or hamstring muscles (semitendinosus).[56]

Oral Absorption

As reviewed by Baggot,[57] oral absorption is low for many drugs in horses. Drugs, such as aminopenicillins (ampicillin, amoxicillin), cephalosporins, and macrolide antibiotics, are not absorbed as rapidly or to as great an extent compared with administration of these drugs in small animals or humans. This limits the use of the oral route for many drugs in horses. For example, oral amoxicillin is absorbed well enough in humans, dogs, and cats to be a useful and practical route of administration. However, systemic availability of oral amoxicillin in adult horses is only 2% to 10%.[58,59] Ampicillin also is not a good option for oral administration in horses because of poor availability.[60] Even though oral absorption is poor for these drugs in adult horses, there may be an advantage for oral administration in foals because they appear to exhibit higher oral absorption. For example, compared with the poor absorption cited for adult horses, oral absorption of amoxicillin in foals is 36% to 42%.[61]

For cephalosporins, the same pattern is observed. Cefadroxil is absorbed better in the foal than in adult horses.[62,63] Oral absorption of cephalexin is low in horses (5%), but at 30 mg/kg orally q8h, concentrations can be maintained above the MIC of susceptible bacteria.[64]

Modification of some drugs has improved oral absorption in horses. Esters and salts of erythromycin have improved oral absorption in horses. Erythromycin base administered to horses is rapidly degraded into inactive metabolites in the equine stomach and intestine, and systemic availability of erythromycin is poor.[65] However, if erythromycin is administered as an ester prodrug such as erythromycin estolate, it is absorbed as the intact ester and converted to the active drug after absorption. Oral absorption is also improved if erythromycin is administered as a phosphate salt, whereby it resists degradation in the stomach and intestine and is absorbed as active erythromycin.[66] Similarly, the ester prodrug cefpodoxime proxetil (Simplicef, Pfizer) has been shown to have greater bioavailability than other cephalosporins in horses and foals.[67]

The effect of food on the oral absorption of drugs in veterinary medicine is often overlooked. Most pharmacokinetic studies administer drugs to horses that have been fasted before and after drug administration. However, this may not be possible or practical in field conditions. Significantly decreased drug absorption has been demonstrated for several oral antibiotics in the horse when they are administered with feed. When healthy foals were given microencapsulated erythromycin base, they had decreased plasma concentrations and systemic bioavailability when they were allowed to eat hay up until the time of drug administration compared with those that were fasted.[65] Trimethoprim-sulfachlorpyridazine combinations were shown to bind to feed constituents and cecal contents in vitro.[68] In addition, systemic bioavailability was significantly decreased when the drug was administered as a topical dressing compared with nasogastric intubation.[69] Oral bioavailability of rifampin decreased from 68% when it was administered 1 hour before feeding to 26% when administered 1 hour after feeding.[57] The extent of oral absorption of doxycycline increased by approximately 50% when it was administered by nasogastric tube to a fasted horse versus a fed horse.[51] Whenever possible, feeding schedules should be taken into account when dosing with oral antibiotics.

Local Drug Administration

Direct drug administration has been used to provide high concentrations of drugs in bones and joints of horses and decrease reliance on high systemic doses. Intraarticular administration of aminoglycosides, such as gentamicin and amikacin, as well as ceftiofur, to horses produces high synovial drug concentrations.[65,70-72,74] Because of the low SA/V ratio in joints and delayed equilibrium, drug clearance from joint fluid after this administration is slower than from the plasma and may provide effective concentrations for at least 24 hours. High concentrations in the limbs can also be achieved by regional limb perfusion.[73] In this technique, an infected limb is perfused with an antibiotic, and the drug concentration is kept high by applying a temporary tourniquet to the limb proximal to the site of drug administration.[77] Regional limb perfusion of equine limbs allows high concentrations to be achieved in bone and joints of limbs without high doses and systemic exposure to the drug.

Considerations for Antimicrobials in Foals

In some cases, drug dosages for foals are similar to adults because of similarity in drug distribution and clearance. In other cases, doses should be modified because of differences in oral absorption, clearance, and distribution. When treating foals, equine practitioners should consult specific references to administer the safest and most effective dose.

Drug absorption and disposition in the foal are different than in the adult horse. In general, neonatal foals have a higher volume of distribution, a lower clearance, and a longer half-life than adult horses. Systemic bioavailability for some oral antibiotics is also often increased in neonatal foals, especially for the β-lactam antibiotics. A well-designed study on the absorption of cefadroxil in foals over 0.5 to 5 months showed that the oral absorption rate becomes faster with age, but bioavailability decreased from 99.6% at 0.5 months to 14.5% at 5 months.[62] Amoxicillin also is absorbed better in foals than adult horses.[42,61] The differences in bioavailability between foals and adults may be caused by an increased intestinal permeability in young foals, a change in gastric pH as the foal ages and the diet changes,[75] or a difference in intestinal transport carriers.

The horse's age also affects drug distribution due to a larger extracellular fluid compartment observed in young animals that leads to a larger volume of distribution of water-soluble drugs. A larger volume of distribution for neonatal foals may necessitate higher doses to achieve adequate plasma concentrations. The best example of this property is amikacin. In adult horses an appropriate dose for amikacin is 8 to 10 mg/kg once daily.[76] However, because foals have a higher volume of distribution, a larger proportion of the administered dose is distributed to extracellular fluid. For example, the volume of distribution in foals has been measured at 0.5 to 0.7 L/kg[77,78] versus 0.17 and 0.26 L/kg in adults.[47,79] Therefore the dose of amikacin for foals should be increased to 20 to 25 mg/kg once daily. Gentamicin doses are also proportionately higher in foals than adults.

When treating foals, some antibiotics may also be more likely to distribute across diffusion barriers, such as the BBB, that they might not cross normally. In foals younger than 2 weeks of age, CSF protein concentrations are elevated compared with adults, which may be caused by a more permeable BBB.[80] Because the BBB may not be fully mature at birth, it may cause increased drug penetration into the CSF.[75]

Drug metabolism and elimination may be impaired in young foals because of a deficiency in hepatic drug metabolism capacity. This has been demonstrated in foals receiving chloramphenicol, which is extensively metabolized by the liver and is mostly excreted through the biliary system into the feces. When IV chloramphenicol was administered to foals at 1, 3, 7, 14, and 42 days of age, its clearance increased and elimination half-life decreased with increasing age.[81] Neonatal foals have minimal capacity to metabolize enrofloxacin to ciprofloxacin, whereas in adult horses, ciprofloxacin concentrations are about 17% of the enrofloxacin concentrations.[82]

In some cases, drug dosages for foals are similar to adults because of similarity in drug distribution and clearance. In other cases, doses should be modified because of differences in oral absorption, clearance, and distribution. Equine practitioners should consult specific references when treating foals to administer the safest and most effective dose.

Adverse Drug Reactions in Horses

Various adverse drug reactions caused by antimicrobials have been reported in the horse (Box 65-2). This section discusses the more severe reactions. Antimicrobial-associated diarrhea is the most frequently reported adverse effect of antibacterial drug administration to the horse. The mechanism is most likely related to a change in the GI and colonic microbial flora. Alterations in GI motility may also occur with the administration of some antibiotics, like erythromycin. The organisms most often associated with the disease are *Salmonella* and *Clostridium* spp. The lincosamides (clindamycin and lincomycin) should never be used in horses because they have been associated with a severe, often-fatal diarrhea. These antibiotics have even been used as an experimental model for colitis in the horse.[83] Other antibiotics associated with colitis are listed in Box 65-2.

The kidney is a frequent site for drug toxicity because many drugs are renally excreted and often become concentrated within the renal tubules. The aminoglycoside antibiotics are frequently associated with nephrotoxicity in many species, although the incidence has decreased with the implementation of once-daily dosing regimens. Aminoglycoside-induced nephrotoxicosis can be reversible with aggressive fluid therapy. Administration of IV calcium may also be beneficial.[84]

Box 65-2 Adverse Drug Reactions Associated With Antimicrobial Use in the Horse

Antibiotic-Associated Colitis
Severe or Frequent
Ciprofloxacin
Clindamycin
Lincomycin
Neomycin
Oxytetracycline
Erythromycin (in adults)
Moxifloxacin
Florfenicol
Tylosin

Mild or Infrequent
Trimethoprim-sulfonamide combinations
Penicillin
Doxycycline

Nephrotoxicity
Aminoglycosides
Polymyxin B
Tetracyclines
Amphotericin B
Imipenem
Cephalosporins (rare)

Hepatotoxicity
Isoniazid

Cardiotoxicity
Doxycycline (intravenous)
Tetracycline (intravenous)
Tilmicosin (intravenous)
Monensin
Lasalocid sodium

Bone or Cartilage Effects in Growing Animals
Tetracyclines (not doxycycline)
Fluoroquinolones

Teratogenic Effects
Griseofulvin
Chloramphenicol
Sulfonamides
Pyrimethamine

Immune-Mediated Hemolytic Anemia
Penicillins
Cephalosporins
Trimethoprim-sulfamethoxazole

Neuromuscular Blockade
Aminoglycosides
Tetracyclines

Bone Marrow Suppression
Chloramphenicol
Trimethoprim-sulfa combinations
Pyrimethamine

Cardiotoxicity is another often-fatal complication that has been associated with antimicrobial use in the horse. Intravenous doxycycline causes collapse and sudden death in horses when administered as a bolus or constant-rate infusion. Even at very low doses, doxycycline causes supraventricular tachycardia, systemic arterial hypertension, and clinical signs of discomfort.[85] Rapid IV administration of oxytetracycline may also cause collapse and death. This has historically been attributed to chelation of calcium and subsequent hypocalcemia or neuromuscular blockade, but it is more likely caused by a reaction to the drug vehicle.[86] Changes in serum calcium levels have not been observed with IV doxycycline, and no reaction occurs when the vehicle has been administered alone, so the mechanism of cardiotoxicity remains unclear.[85] The ionophore antibiotics are also cardiotoxic to horses, and extreme care should be taken whenever cattle or sheep being fed grain with these feed additives are on the premises. Tilmicosin, a macrolide antibiotic used in cattle and swine for the treatment of respiratory disease, is cardiotoxic to horses, as well as humans.

Drugs may induce injury to the articular cartilage and bone of foals. The most well-documented example is caused by the fluoroquinolone class of antimicrobials. Enrofloxacin and ciprofloxacin decrease cartilage and tendon cell proliferation and adherence in vitro at concentrations that are achieved in vivo.[87,88] Administration of enrofloxacin at 10 mg/kg/day for 7 days causes severe cartilage damage and lameness in foals.[82] Some musculoskeletal effects have also been observed in adult horses, including inflammation of the tarsal plantar ligament, superficial digital flexor tendonitis, and tarsal sheath effusion.[89] These effects were observed, however, only with chronic administration of three to five times the recommended dose.

Alternative Uses of Antimicrobials in the Horse

Several antimicrobial agents have biologic activity unrelated to their effects on microbes. Tetracycline has been used frequently in foals for the treatment of flexural and angular limb deformities.[90,91] The proposed mechanism of action is chelation of intramuscular calcium, leading to relaxation of muscle tissue and tendons. However, differences were not detected in plasma calcium or ionized calcium concentrations after 50 to 67 mg/kg of oxytetracycline was administered to 4- or 5-day-old foals.[92] This is in the range of doses used for treatment of limb deformities in foals, typically 2 or 3 g per foal. The same study did not detect any deleterious effects on renal or hepatic parameters in healthy foals after two consecutive doses at this level, and drug clearance was not prolonged from such a large dose in the young foal.

Tetracyclines also have the ability to prevent neutrophil chemotaxis and apoptosis in vitro,[93,94] although the clinical relevance is questionable at drug concentrations achieved in vivo after oral administration.[95,96] Doxycycline decreases the production of proinflammatory cytokines, such as matrix metalloproteinases (MMP-8, MMP-9), interleukin-1 (IL-1), IL-6, and tumor necrosis factor alpha (TNF-α), from inflammatory cells.[97-99] Doxycycline inhibits MMPs from the horse[100] and has been successfully used for the treatment of melting corneal ulcers. It also inhibits staphylococcal exotoxin-induced cytokines and chemokines and improves the prognosis in a mouse model of endotoxemia.[101] This action by doxycycline is accomplished by attaining sufficiently high intracellular concentrations in leukocytes to interfere with intracellular processes. Doxycycline and minocycline inhibit MMP production in equine synoviocytes, with minocycline being more effective at lower concentrations.[102]

Metronidazole reduces the clinical severity and GI inflammation in people with Crohn's disease.[103] It has been recommended for the treatment of colitis and other nonspecific causes of diarrhea in people, although no reports are available to demonstrate a similar effect in horses. Both metronidazole and ciprofloxacin decrease leukocyte migration through the intestinal cell wall and inhibit intestinal T-helper type 1 (Th1) cytokine production, thereby decreasing inflammation.[103]

Low doses of erythromycin are often used as a prokinetic drug in the horse. It acts by stimulating motilin receptors in the GI tract and promoting GI motility.[104] This may also contribute to the diarrhea seen with administration of erythromycin in adult horses and foals. This prokinetic property has not been attributed to other macrolides.

Polymyxin B is a cationic polypeptide antibiotic effective against gram-negative bacteria. Its use as an antibiotic has been limited because of its nephrotoxic effect at therapeutic doses. Polymyxin B is often used in equine medicine, however, as a treatment for endotoxemia. At doses below those needed for antibacterial effects, it binds to the lipid A moiety of the lipopolysaccharide and alters its structure so that it cannot interact with the horse's white blood cells and initiate the inflammatory cascade.[105,106] At doses of 1000 to 6000 IU/kg, IV polymyxin B significantly reduces fever, tachycardia, and serum TNF-α when administered before or 1 hour after challenge with endotoxin.[107] A more recent study[108] demonstrated that polymyxin B should be administered to horses at a dose of 6000 IU/kg (1 mg/kg) and repeated at 8-hour intervals for up to 5 treatments to treat endotoxemia. At this dosage regimen, it did not accumulate and was safe. Nevertheless, it is essential that the horse be well hydrated during therapy and that serum creatinine levels are monitored to prevent the development of acute renal failure.

Update on Antibiotics Used in Horses

Fluoroquinolone Antimicrobials

The fluoroquinolone (FQ) class of antibiotics work via inhibition of deoxyribonucleic acid (DNA) gyrase (topoisomerase II), which is required for bacterial DNA replication, transcription, repair, and recombination. Resistance is mediated through chromosomal mutations in DNA gyrase (gyrA), which confers cross-resistance to other FQs. Fluoroquinolones distribute well to the tissues and penetrate well intracellularly. Enrofloxacin reaches the highest concentration in the cells as the result of high lipid solubility. Enrofloxacin is metabolized in vivo to ciprofloxacin, which has higher antibacterial activity than other FQs. Elimination is via the kidney, and these drugs are often highly effective for treating resistant urinary tract infections (UTIs). Four FQs are labeled for use in small animals (enrofloxacin, marbofloxacin, orbifloxacin, and difloxacin). There are currently no FQ antibiotics labeled for use in the horse; however, research into the safety and efficacy of these compounds continues because of their favorable spectrum of activity against gram-negative enteric bacteria. Enrofloxacin, and to a lesser extent marbofloxacin and orbifloxacin, continue to be used in horses. Ciprofloxacin pharmacokinetics were investigated following IV and oral administration to adult horses.[17] This study confirmed the previously reported low oral bioavailability of the drug (average 10.5%), and it also elucidated numerous adverse effects associated with both oral and IV administration, including mild transient diarrhea to severe colitis, endotoxemia, and laminitis, necessitating euthanasia of three out of the eight study horses. Other adverse effects associated with IV administration were agitation and excitement followed by lethargy; sweating; muscle fasciculation; increased flehmen response; lip smacking; periorbital edema; patchy edema involving the face, neck, and/or cranial thorax; and transient loss of appetite. The conclusions of this study were that the high incidences of adverse events preclude oral and rapid IV administration of ciprofloxacin.

Levofloxacin pharmacokinetics have also been studied in stallions.[109] Levofloxacin is the active enantiomer of ofloxacin and has increased activity against topoisomerase IV. Bioavailability after IM administration approached 100%, and IV or IM administration produced plasma concentrations expected to be therapeutic for bacteria with MICs less than or equal to 0.1 μg/mL following a dose of 4 mg/kg.

New information is also available on the use of fluoroquinolones via nonsystemic routes. Topical administration of moxifloxacin resulted in better penetration through healthy equine corneas and reached higher measurable aqueous humor-concentrations than ciprofloxacin, suggesting moxifloxacin might be of greater value in the treatment of deep corneal or intraocular bacterial infections caused by susceptible organisms.[110] Systemic administration of enrofloxacin (7.5 mg/kg IV q24h) has also been shown to produce aqueous humor concentrations above the reported MIC for *Leptospira pomona*, making it a possible treatment for equine recurrent uveitis caused by this organism.[111] Inhaled marbofloxacin has also been studied.[112] Aerosolization of 300 mg of marbofloxacin (25 mg/mL) produced concentrations in the bronchoalveolar lavage (BAL) fluid 5.5 times higher than systemic administration, with minimal systemic absorption and no effect on pulmonary function.

The pharmacokinetics of certain FQs have also been investigated in donkeys. Marbofloxacin (2.2 mg/kg IV) has a slower systemic clearance, longer elimination half-life, and a larger AUC in donkeys compared to horses.[113] In contrast, danofloxacin (1.25 mg/kg) was more rapidly cleared, had a larger volume of distribution, and following IM administration, reached a lower C_{max} in donkeys compared with horses.[114]

Macrolides and Derivatives

The macrolide antibiotics are considered bacteriostatic and work through inhibition of protein synthesis at the level of the 50s ribosomal subunit. Because of their high intracellular concentrations, these drugs are most frequently used in equine medicine for the treatment of intracellular pathogens such as *R. equi* and *Lawsonia intracellularis*. Erythromycin is the prototypical macrolide; however, it has many disadvantages, including adverse GI effects, poor bioavailability, and a short half-life. Because of poor absorption and adverse effects associated with erythromycin, new drugs have been developed that have better pharmacokinetic properties and improved spectrum of activity and are better tolerated. Clarithromycin exhibits a broader spectrum of activity, better tolerability, and higher intracellular accumulation than erythromycin. Azithromycin has a similar gram-positive spectrum as erythromycin, but it has some activity against anaerobes and other intracellular bacteria, better oral absorption, and persistence in the tissues and cells. Tilmicosin, a cattle and swine antibiotic, is not advisable to use in the horse due to negligible oral absorption, severe injection site reactions following subcutaneous administration, and cardiotoxicity after intravenous administration.[115] Tulathromycin, another cattle and swine antibiotic, has also been studied in foals.[116] Although the pharmacokinetics are favorable, with a long half-life, large volume of distribution, and accumulation in BAL cells,[116] this drug has been determined not to be effective in the case of *R. equi* pneumonia as a result of the inherent resistance of *R. equi* to the drug (MIC$_{90}$ > 64 μg/mL).[117]

The pharmacokinetics of clarithromycin have been investigated in foals, and a dose of 7.5 mg/kg orally q12h is suggested for the treatment of *R. equi* pneumonia.[40] Based on pharmacokinetic data[39,118] and anecdotal clinical experience, veterinarians have used azithromycin in foals at a dose of 10 mg/kg once daily initially, followed by 10 mg/kg orally every other day after clinical improvement is observed.

Clinical experience with azithromycin and clarithromycin in the field indicates that they are safe for use in foals for the treatment of *R. equi* or *L. intracellularis* infections. However, given the chronic nature of these diseases and the need for extended treatment, another drug, gamithromycin, has recently been evaluated.[119] A single dose of gamithromycin (6.6 mg/kg IM) maintained pulmonary epithelial lining fluid (PELF) concentrations above the MIC$_{90}$ for *S. zooepidemicus* and phagocytic cell concentrations above the MIC$_{90}$ for *R. equi* for approximately 7 days. Clinical efficacy and safety of this drug have not

been reported; however, it has recently been approved for use in cattle in the United States. Because of the increase in resistance of *R. equi* to macrolide antibiotics over the last 10 years, another drug, telithromycin, has been studied.[120] Telithromycin is a synthetic ketolide antibiotic that is used for the treatment of macrolide resistant *R. equi* in humans. However, based on the reported pharmacokinetics, a dose of 15 mg/kg PO q12h would still be inadequate to treat 50% of macrolide resistant *R. equi* isolates from foals and its use does not appear to have any advantage over the other more commonly used drugs.

Typically, macrolide antibiotics are not used in adult horses because of the risk of antibiotic-associated colitis. However, azithromycin has been used clinically by the author in a limited number of cases with no severe adverse effects, and the pharmacokinetics and safety have been studied in the adult horse.[121] Bioavailability was similar to foals; however, a dose of 10 mg/kg orally (PO) q24h produced mild decreases in appetite and alterations in fecal consistency in some horses. Therefore the safety of this compound in this age of horse needs further investigation.

β-Lactam Antibiotics

The β-lactam antibiotics include the penicillins, cephalosporins, and carbapenems. They have excellent activity against most gram-positive bacteria and very few associated side effects. They are considered bactericidal and time dependent. Postantibiotic effects have been associated with some drugs in this class. The mechanism of action involves penetration of the outer cell wall and binding to penicillin-binding proteins (PBP). This interferes with cell wall synthesis and opens channels through the cell wall to create pores that allow fluid into the cell, causing cell swelling and death. In general, the β-lactam antibiotics have low plasma protein binding, distribute well to the extracellular fluid in most tissues, and are excreted renally. With a few exceptions, they have a very short half-life and require frequent dosing. β-Lactams do not distribute well to protected sites such as the CNS, the eye, or the prostate.

Procaine penicillin and potassium penicillin are still frequently used in horses, and there are little new data available on this group of drugs. Dosages are listed in Appendix D. Ampicillin trihydrate suspension (Polyflex) is administered IM, usually at a dose of 6.6 to 22 mg/kg q12h or q24h (most common). Ampicillin sodium is administered to horses IV at 10 to 20 mg/kg q6h to q8h and IM at 10 to 22 mg/kg q12h. Our laboratory performed computer simulations and Monte Carlo predictions (unpublished studies) to indicate that ampicillin sodium at a dose of either 22 mg/kg IM q12h or 22 mg/kg IV q8h achieves sufficient plasma concentrations to meet PK-PD criteria for MIC values of less than or equal to 2.0 μg/mL, which may be high enough for many *Enterobacteriaceae*. *Streptococcus* spp. have a much lower MIC range (usually ≤0.25 μg/mL) and can be treated with much lower doses.

The cephalosporin antibiotics have many advantages in animals, including a broad spectrum of activity and a good safety profile. Cephalosporins studied in horses for clinical use include the first-generation cephalosporins: cephalexin, cefazolin, cephapirin, and cefadroxil; the second-generation cephalosporin: cefoxitin; and the third-generation cephalosporins: ceftiofur, cefpodoxime, and ceftriaxone.

Oral absorption of first-generation cephalosporins is somewhat limited, but this route can be used in some cases, as with cephalexin. First-generation cephalosporins have a spectrum that is limited to highly susceptible gram-negative bacilli (*Enterobacteriaceae*), streptococci, and *Staphylococcus* spp.

Perhaps the most frequently used cephalosporin in horses is ceftiofur. Ceftiofur is metabolized quickly to an active metabolite, desfuroylceftiofur (and other metabolites). Ceftiofur was approved for use in horses for treatment of respiratory tract infections caused by *Streptococcus equi* subsp. *zooepidemicus* at a dose of 2.2 to 4.4 mg/kg q24h IM. Higher doses or more frequent intervals have been recommended for treating gram-negative organisms (e.g., *Klebsiella, Enterobacter, Salmonella*). Because these organisms are inherently more resistant, higher plasma concentrations are needed for efficacy. The susceptibility breakpoint for ceftiofur use in horses is very low (≤0.25 μg/mL), and organisms other than streptococci may be classified in vitro as resistant. In septic neonatal foals, doses as high as 10 mg/kg IV q6h have been used. However, more recent studies in foals[122,123] have shown lower doses (5 mg/kg IV, subcutaneous [SC] q12h) are sufficient for the treatment of most bacteria cultured from septic neonates (MIC$_{90}$ < 0.5 μg/mL). Constant rate infusion of ceftiofur has also been shown to be safe in foals at doses up to 20 mg/kg/day. This dose rate is adequate for the treatment of bacteria with MICs up to 4 μg/mL. Toxicity studies have shown that horses tolerate ceftiofur doses up to 11 mg/kg/day IM, with pain at the injection site and decreased feed consumption as the most common adverse effect at the highest dose.

A new formulation of ceftiofur has been approved for use in horses (ceftiofur crystalline free acid [CCFA], Excede). This formulation is designed to be a sustained-release formulation that will provide 10 days worth of therapeutic concentrations against streptococci (MIC < 0.2 μg/mL) following a 2-dose regimen (6.6 mg/kg IM, repeated 96 hours later).[124] The main adverse effect associated with this formulation has been injection site reactions, which can be minimized by splitting the dose into two different injection sites.[125] Extralabel dosing of the drug has been used in clinical practice, mainly through the use of prolonged dosing regimens. For treatment of streptococci, the recommended dosing regimen for CCFA is 6.6 mg/kg IM on day 1 and 4, then every 7 days after. For more resistant bacteria (MIC ≤ 1 μg/mL), the recommended dosing regimen is 6.6 mg/kg IM every 4 days. All of these regimens are for adult horses, as the pharmacokinetics differs in foals. Investigations in healthy neonatal foals showed that subcutaneous administration of CCFA had a lower AUC, shorter observed time to maximum concentration, and a higher observed C$_{max}$ compared to adult horses.[123] Based on that study, administration at a dose of 6.6 mg/kg body weight SC q72h would provide protection against bacteria isolated from neonatal foals, based on an MIC of 0.5 μg/mL and SC administration resulted in minimal injection site inflammation. Weanling age foals (4-6 months old) also exhibit different pharmacokinetics, including higher peak plasma concentrations and AUC compared to adults; however, these differences were not significant enough to necessitate a difference in dosing regimen.[126] Therefore administration of 6.6 mg/kg IM in weanling foals provided plasma and PELF concentrations above the therapeutic target of 0.2 μg/mL for at least 4 days and would be expected to be an effective treatment for pneumonia caused by *Streptococcus equi* subsp. *zooepidemicus* at doses similar to the adult label.

An ester formulation of cefpodoxime, cefpodoxime proxetil, has been examined for use in horses.[67] This third-generation cephalosporin was recently registered for use in dogs (Simplicef, Pfizer). Cefpodoxime has higher activity against gram-negative bacteria than first-generation cephalosporins and is more active than many other third-generation cephalosporins against *Staphylococcus*. However, it is not active against *Pseudomonas aeruginosa*, enterococci, or MRSA. In a study in horses and foals, oral absorption was good enough that a dose of 10 mg/kg q6h to q12h produced plasma concentrations that would potentially treat infections in horses.[67] When testing susceptibility for cefpodoxime, the breakpoint for susceptibility is lower than for other third-generation cephalosporins.[21] Therefore a bacterial isolate may be reported as sensitive to cefotaxime or

ceftazidime, which has a breakpoint of ≤8 μg/mL, but resistant to cefpodoxime, which has a breakpoint of ≤2 μg/mL.[21] Specific disks are suggested for testing bacterial isolates, rather than relying on the results from other cephalosporins.

The carbapenems are the newest class of β-lactam antimicrobials. They have an extended spectrum of activity, including gram-negatives, and are associated with more of a postantibiotic effect. Clinical use in horses is limited because of cost; however, imipenem has been used in foals at a dose of 5 mg/kg IV infused over 20 minutes q6h to q8h. A pharmacokinetic study in adult horses suggests a dose of 10 to 20 mg/kg by slow IV infusion q6h would be necessary to maintain adequate plasma concentrations.[127] The author has used meropenem in adult horses. Because of its short half-life, a constant rate infusion of 10 μg/kg/min (15 mg/kg/day) is recommended.

Aminoglycosides

The aminoglycosides include gentamicin, tobramycin, amikacin, and kanamycin. Among these, gentamicin and amikacin are used most often in horses, with amikacin often preferred in neonates. Aminoglycosides are considered the drug of choice for severe gram-negative infections. They also have activity against staphylococci. Their primary mechanism of action includes binding to the 30S ribosomal subunit, causing the formation of nonfunctional proteins. Aminoglycosides have high water solubility, low protein binding, and poor oral absorption. They distribute well to the extracellular fluid but do not penetrate intracellularly or into the CNS, eye, or prostate. Aminoglycosides have a long postantibiotic effect, allowing for once daily dosing, which is important in preventing toxicity. These drugs are excreted via glomerular filtration; they are also reabsorbed/sequestered in the proximal tubular epithelium. Gentamicin or amikacin are often used in combination with a β-lactam antibiotic (e.g., penicillin, ampicillin) to produce a synergistic broad-spectrum bactericidal effect. The β-lactam–associated inhibition of bacterial cell wall synthesis enhances the uptake of aminoglycosides into bacteria, accounting for the synergy of this combination. Note, however, that these drugs should not be mixed in the same vial or syringe before dosing because admixing these drugs produces in vitro inactivation of the aminoglycoside.

Although the pharmacokinetics of amikacin have been extensively studied in neonatal foals, the pharmacokinetics in adult horses using currently recommended once daily dosing intervals have only been recently investigated. A study investigating the disposition of amikacin in adult horses showed that a daily dose of 10 mg/kg IV distributed well into extracellular fluids, including peritoneal fluid, synovial fluid, and interstitial fluid, and would be expected to be therapeutic against bacteria with an MIC of ≤4 μg/mL.[76] This dose is much lower than that recommended for foals (20-25 mg/kg), mainly the result of differences in total body water content, resulting in a larger volume of distribution in foals. Similarly, doses of gentamicin vary between adult horses (4-6.6 mg/kg/day) and foals (8-12 mg/kg/day).

Recent shortages in drug availability of amikacin have led to an increased use of tobramycin in horses. A daily dosing regimen of 4 mg/kg IV has been found to be effective.[128] The author has also administered the drug IM and intraarticularly with no adverse effects. Tobramycin is expected to be more efficacious than gentamicin but less efficacious than amikacin against most gram-negative bacteria and staphylococci.

Trimethoprim-Sulfonamides

Trimethoprim is most frequently combined with sulfadiazine or sulfamethoxazole for administration to horses. The effectiveness of these combinations is attributed to their synergistic effect in inhibiting folic acid metabolism in bacteria. Sulfonamides are competitive inhibitors of dihydrofolate synthesis. Trimethoprim inhibits the enzyme dihydrofolate reductase. Complete reviews are available on these combinations, with some specifically for use in horses.[54]

Tissue concentrations of TMS persist long enough to allow once-daily or twice-daily dosing for many infections. Studies performed in cattle and horses appear to support a T > MIC parameter as being the most important for clinical success.[129-132] In these studies, drug concentrations (of the combination) associated with clinical success persisted in plasma or tissue fluids for the duration of the dose interval. Most published dosage regimens for TMS are designed to take these pharmacokinetic properties into account (see Appendix D).

A susceptibility test should always measure inhibition of the combination, not the individual drugs. The spectrum of activity is broad. Trimethoprim-sulfonamide combinations are active against many pathogens that infect horses, including *Pasteurella* spp., *Proteus*, and *Salmonella* spp. Occasionally, staphylococci, *Corynebacterium*, *Klebsiella*, *E. coli*, and streptococci are susceptible. *Pseudomonas*, *Enterococcus* spp., and *Bacteroides* are usually resistant. The activity of TMS against anaerobic bacteria can be variable. Trimethoprim-sulfonamide has good activity against anaerobic bacteria in vitro, but clinical results are not as good because thymidine and para-aminobenzoic acid (PABA) (inhibitors of trimethoprim-sulfonamide activity) may be present in anaerobic infections.

Tetracyclines

Tetracyclines are considered broad spectrum and have activity against gram-positive and gram-negative bacteria, *Chlamydia*, rickettsia, spirochetes, mycoplasma, L-form (cell wall deficient) bacteria, and some protozoa. Of this group, doxycycline is the most active. The mechanism of action involves binding to the 30S ribosomal subunit and blocking protein synthesis. This binding is reversible, making tetracyclines bacteriostatic. Resistance is widespread among staphylococci, streptococci, *Pseudomonas* spp., and *Enterobacteriaceae*. Enterococci are not susceptible to tetracyclines. Resistance is plasmid-mediated and relates to a failure of the active transport system necessary to penetrate the bacterial cell.

Oral absorption of the tetracyclines can be erratic because these drugs are excellent chelators, and cations in the stomach can bind the drugs and prevent oral absorption. These drugs should be given on an empty stomach. The one exception is doxycycline, which is less affected by feeding status. Tetracyclines distribute well to most tissues, with the exception of the CNS and the eye, and are mainly eliminated by the kidneys. Doxycycline is again an exception, in that a significant amount of excretion is through the intestine. Tetracyclines accumulate within cells, making them ideal for intracellular infections. They are considered the first choice antibiotic for infections caused by *Neorickettsia risticii*, *Anaplasma phagocytophilum*, and *Lawsonia intracellularis*.

Recent work on tetracyclines has focused on the pharmacokinetics of oral doxycycline in foals. Oral absorption is presumed to be higher in foals based on a higher C_{max} and AUC compared to adult horses.[133] Oral administration at a dosage of 10 mg/kg q12h would maintain serum, PELF, and BAL cell activity above the MICs of *Rhodococcus equi*, β-hemolytic streptococci, and other susceptible bacterial pathogens (MIC < 3 μg/mL) for the entire dosing interval. Other areas of research have focused on the use of these drugs as antiinflammatory agents, as previously discussed. Doxycycline has been shown to accumulate in synovial fluid, suggesting a possible role in the treatment of osteoarthritis.[134] Doxycycline concentrations have

also been detected in the preocular tear film, further supporting its use in cases of ulcerative keratomalacia.[135]

Chloramphenicol

Chloramphenicol and its derivatives, thiamphenicol and florfenicol, reversibly bind to the 50S ribosome subunit, resulting in protein synthesis inhibition. They are bacteriostatic. Competitive antagonism may occur when co-administered with macrolide antibiotics, since they share the same site of action. These antimicrobials are broad spectrum, with activity against gram-positive and gram-negative bacteria, as well as anaerobes, *Rickettsia*, *Chlamydia*, and *Mycoplasma* spp. Activity against *Enterobacteriaceae* is unpredictable, and activity against *Pseudomonas* is poor. Resistance, particularly among gram-negative bacteria, occurs via acetylation and inactivation of chloramphenicol by bacterial enzymes. Chloramphenicol undergoes extensive metabolism by the liver. This metabolism is deficient in very young animals, resulting in a prolonged half-life. It distributes well to most tissues of the body, and drug concentrations may persist longer in the tissues than in the plasma or serum. Currently, there is not enough information to recommend the use of florfenicol in the horse, as administration of a single dose (IV, IM, PO) resulted in loose feces in all horses studied.[136]

Metronidazole

Metronidazole is a nitroimidazole antimicrobial with activity against protozoa and anaerobic bacteria but no activity against other bacteria. The mechanism of action involves the reduction of the nitro group on the antibiotic by nitroreductases produced by susceptible bacteria. This results in the formation of highly reactive intermediates that disrupt bacterial DNA. These antibiotics are only active in anaerobic conditions because oxygen will compete with the antibiotic for electrons necessary in the nitroreductase reaction. Metronidazole is well absorbed following oral administration, and different feeding regimens do not affect bioavailability.[137] Metronidazole also has excellent distribution into tissues, including the CNS and abscesses. It has quick onset of action and is rapidly bactericidal. One of the main uses in equine medicine is against *Bacteroides fragilis*, a β-lactamase–producing anaerobic bacteria that is often resistant to penicillin.

Miscellaneous Antibiotics

Rifampin

Rifampin inhibits DNA-dependent ribonucleic acid (RNA) polymerase in susceptible organisms, suppressing RNA synthesis. It has no effect on the mammalian enzyme. Its action is bacteriostatic or bactericidal, depending on the susceptibility of the bacteria and the concentration of the drug. Bacterial resistance to rifampin develops rapidly, therefore it is usually administered with another antimicrobial. However, recent evidence suggests that co-administration of rifampin with other macrolide antibiotics may result in decreased bioavailability of the macrolide. Both tulathromycin and clarithromycin have been shown to have a significantly reduced bioavailability when coadministered with rifampin,[138,139] which is thought to be the result of inhibition of an unknown intestinal uptake transporter.[140]

Aztreonam

Aztreonam is a monobactam antibiotic that is active against many gram-negative bacterial pathogens, although activity is very limited against gram-positive or anaerobic bacteria. It has a very low incidence of nephrotoxicity, therefore it is used in human neonatal septicemia in those patients that cannot tolerate aminoglycosides. A single-dose pharmacokinetic study has been published examining a dose of 30 mg/kg IV of aztreonam in foals.[141] The short half-life and development of diarrhea in several foals in the study will likely preclude its clinical use in the horse.

Fosfomycin

Fosfomycin inhibits bacterial cellular wall synthesis and has shown an additive or synergistic action with β-lactam drugs, aminoglycosides, macrolides, and fluoroquinolones. It has in vitro activity against gram-positive and gram-negative bacteria. The pharmacokinetics in horses suggest that a 20 mg/kg dose administered SC would produce clinically relevant plasma concentrations for up to 10 hours after dosing.[142] More information is necessary before clinical use is recommended.

Antifungal Drugs

Azoles

The azole antifungals can be divided into two main groups, the imidazoles and the triazoles, according to the number of nitrogen molecules on the azole ring. They are fungistatic, and their mechanism of action involves inhibition of fungal cytochrome P-450, which results in an inhibition of ergosterol in the fungal cell wall. The specificity of these drugs for fungal versus animal cytochrome P-450 is highly variable. The imidazoles tend to be less specific, whereas the newer triazoles are more specific, for fungal enzymes.

Imidazoles

The imidazoles are a group of broad-spectrum antifungal drugs that include miconazole and ketoconazole. Miconazole is only available as a topical cream and is frequently compounded for ophthalmic use. Ketoconazole is not absorbed after oral administration in the horse unless it is first dissolved in 1 N hydrochloric acid and dosed intragastrically.[143]

Triazoles

The triazole group includes fluconazole, itraconazole, and the newest drug, voriconazole. All three drugs have been studied in horses, and their pharmacokinetic properties vary widely. Fluconazole is a highly water-soluble drug that has almost 100% bioavailability in the horse.[18] It has excellent tissue penetration and reaches therapeutic concentrations in the plasma, CSF, synovial fluid, aqueous humor, and urine for the treatment of susceptible yeasts and fungi. The half-life after oral administration is approximately 38 hours, and a loading dose of 14 mg/kg orally followed by 5 mg/kg orally once a day is recommended. Fluconazole has recently become available in generic formulations and is now less expensive than other antifungal drugs. Unfortunately, the spectrum of activity of fluconazole is narrower than for the other azole antifungals. It is active against the organisms that cause histoplasmosis, blastomycosis, coccidioidomycosis, and conidiobolomycosis.[18,144] It is active against yeasts, including some *Candida* spp., although resistance may be increasing. Fluconazole has virtually no in vitro activity against filamentous fungi such as *Aspergillus* and *Fusarium* spp.

Itraconazole has a similar spectrum of activity to fluconazole, but it is active against some *Aspergillus* spp. Most *Fusarium* strains, however, are still resistant.[145] Itraconazole is effective in horses for the treatment of mycotic rhinitis, osteomyelitis, and guttural pouch mycosis.[146-148] It has been used safely for up to 6 months in the horse. The pharmacokinetics of itraconazole in horses are much less favorable than for fluconazole.[145] There are three formulations of itraconazole currently marketed: an oral capsule, an oral solution, and an IV solution. Bioavailability of the oral capsules is approximately 12%, and its absorption is highly variable because its dissolution relies on the acid environment of the stomach. The oral solution has better bioavailability, approximately 60%, but at the recommended dose of 5 mg/kg, 250 mL of solution is needed per dose for an adult horse because of the low concentration of the drug in the formulation. The IV formulation is prohibitively expensive. Itraconazole is practically insoluble in water and is only soluble and stable at a low pH. Compounded forms of itraconazole are available, but they are often unstable and have even poorer absorption than the marketed formulations. The compounded formulations should not be used in horses.

Voriconazole is the newest triazole antifungal. It has improved activity against *Aspergillus* and *Fusarium* spp. compared with other triazoles and an excellent safety profile in humans. Preliminary pharmacokinetic data on voriconazole in the horse shows excellent bioavailability and a long elimination half-life.[149] The drug penetrates well into the aqueous humor after systemic administration, as well as after topical administration of the IV formulation. A preliminary single-dose study showed that an oral or IV dose of 4 mg/kg q24h produces therapeutic plasma concentrations.[149] A subsequent study showed voriconazole concentrations in urine, aqueous humor, synovial and peritoneal fluids, and CSF higher than the therapeutic target of 0.5 µg/mL can be achieved by the use of 4 mg/kg administered orally once daily.[150]

Polyenes

The polyene antifungals include nystatin and amphotericin B. They have the advantage of being fungicidal by binding to ergosterol in the fungal cell wall, creating pores in the membrane. Nystatin is too toxic to administer parenterally and is not absorbed orally. Its main use in veterinary medicine is a topical ophthalmic preparation for the treatment of fungal keratitis.

Amphotericin B is used only sporadically in equine medicine. It has the broadest spectrum of activity of all the antifungal drugs, including against many *Candida* spp., *Aspergillus* spp., *Histoplasma* spp., *Blastomyces* spp., and *Coccidioides immitis*. It is also frequently used to treat *Fusarium* spp. in humans. No pharmacokinetic data are available on amphotericin B in the horse, but it has been given as an IV infusion at doses of 0.38 to 1.4 mg/kg.[151,152] Its use is often limited by its toxicity. Infusion reactions and nephrotoxicity are common.

Griseofulvin

Griseofulvin is a fungistatic drug with a limited spectrum of activity. It is used almost solely for the treatment of dermatophytosis. Its action depends on incorporation into skin and keratin, so it requires a long duration of therapy. It should not be used in pregnant mares; teratogenic effects have been reported in a mare treated in the second month of gestation.[153]

Terbinafine

Terbinafine is a selective inhibitor of fungal squalene epoxidase, thereby increasing the extracellular concentration of squalene to levels toxic to fungal cells and inhibiting cell wall function because of decreased synthesis of ergosterol. It has activity against many dermatophytes, as well as some *Aspergillus* spp. The pharmacokinetics of this drug have been studied in horses.[154] Although absorption is low, therapeutic concentrations against some fungi that affect horses were reached in the plasma following a dose of 30 mg/kg PO. The author has used this drug in clinical cases for up to 14 days with no reported adverse effects.

Antiviral Drugs

Cyclic Amines

Amantadine and rimantadine are cyclic amines used in the treatment of influenza virus infection. The mechanism of action of these drugs involves inhibiting the uncoating of viral RNA in infected cells and thus effectively preventing viral replication. In vitro testing suggests that amantadine suppresses viral replication at concentrations of 300 ng/mL, whereas rimantadine is more potent and has activity at concentrations as low as 30 ng/mL.[155,156]

Intravenous amantadine at a dose of 15 mg/kg may produce fatal seizures with few premonitory signs. Doses of 10 mg/kg were better tolerated but may still cause serious adverse effects in horses with lowered seizure thresholds. The bioavailability of oral amantadine was too variable to determine a dosing regimen that would be adequate for treatment in the majority of horses because of large interindividual variation.[155] The safety and efficacy of amantadine should be further investigated before its clinical use is recommended.

Rimantadine shows greater promise as an antiviral drug in horses. Rimantadine is available in a generic form as a 100-mg tablet. A multidose study examining the effects of oral rimantadine at a dose of 30 mg/kg q12h showed adequate absorption of the drug, with plasma concentrations maintained above the estimated effective concentration (30 ng/mL) throughout the dosing interval. No adverse effects were reported. In addition, in challenge studies using influenza virus A2, prophylactic rimantadine administration was associated with a significant decrease in rectal temperature and lung sounds.[156]

Nucleoside Analogs

Acyclovir is an acyclic guanosine derivative that has been used clinically in the horse for the treatment of equine herpesvirus type 1 (EHV-1).[157,158] Intravenous acyclovir is the treatment of choice for herpes simplex encephalitis in humans, possibly because it crosses the BBB, with CSF concentrations approximately 50% of serum concentrations. Even though the oral form is now generic and inexpensive, oral absorption in horses is low and variable.[159,160] In vitro efficacy of acyclovir against EHV-1 strains has also been documented, but susceptibility varies with the strain of virus tested. Based on the results of simulated multiple IV doses, twice-daily (q12h) IV infusions of acyclovir (10 mg/kg) would result in plasma concentrations greater than 0.3 µg/mL for the entire treatment interval.[156] This study demonstrated that IV infusion of acyclovir results in plasma concentrations exceeding the concentration that inhibits plaque formation in vitro, suggesting clinical applicability for this drug in cases of EHV-1 infection in horses. However, a single dose of 20 mg/kg of acyclovir administered orally did not result in concentrations greater than the lower limit of detection.

To increase the absorption of the nucleoside analogs, they are often administered as a prodrug. For example, valacyclovir is a prodrug of acyclovir and famciclovir for penciclovir. The pharmacokinetics of these drugs have been evaluated as a potential therapy for EHV-1–induced neurologic disease. Valacyclovir is well absorbed in horses. Several treatment regimens have been reported, including 27 mg/kg PO q8h for 2 days followed by 18 mg/kg PO q12h[161] or 40 mg/kg PO q8h.[162] Administration of 40 mg/kg PO q8h for 4 days resulted in therapeutic plasma concentrations of acyclovir in the plasma; however, concentrations in the nasal mucus and CSF were below the reported half maximal effective concentration (EC50) for EHV-1.[163] Clinical experience with valacyclovir has shown that it can reduce fever and neurologic signs if started within 2 days of infection. If treatment is delayed beyond this,

the drug ganciclovir (2.5 mg/kg IV q8h for 1 day, then q12h for 1 week) can be used. Oral dosing of famciclovir resulted in plasma concentrations of penciclovir expected to be therapeutic against EHV-1, using a dose of 20 mg/kg famciclovir.[164] Clinical experience with this drug is currently limited, and multiple-dose pharmacokinetics have not been published.

Neuraminidase Inhibitors

Oseltamivir is a drug active against many influenza strains, including the common equine influenza strains. An investigation into the efficacy of oseltamivir against experimental infections with equine influenza in adult horses showed that 2 mg/kg administered PO q12h for 5 days, used as treatment or prophylaxis, shortens the period of virus excretion and pyrexia, and decreases the number of *Streptococcus equi* subsp. *zooepidemicus* organisms recovered from BALs collected 7 days after inoculation.[165] However, virus excretion and pyrexia were not prevented and pharmacokinetic studies suggest shorter dosing intervals (<10 hours) may be necessary to maintain therapeutic concentrations.[166]

Antiprotozoal Drugs

Treatment of Equine Protozoal Myeloencephalitis

The number of antiprotozoal drugs available for use in the horse has increased over the past decade, mainly because of the increasing prevalence of equine protozoal myeloencephalitis (EPM). Folate synthesis inhibitors such as pyrimethamine, trimethoprim and sulfonamides; and the triazine derivatives: diclazuril, toltrazuril, and ponazuril can be used. Nitazoxanide, a drug previously approved for use in horses for the treatment of EPM, is no longer commercially available in the United States.

Folate Synthesis Inhibitors

Trimethoprim, sulfonamides, and pyrimethamine were the first drugs used to treat EPM. Each drug prevents protozoal synthesis of folic acid; however, they act at different levels and on different enzyme substrates. Sulfonamides inhibit dihydrofolate synthesis through competitive inhibition of PABA, whereas trimethoprim and pyrimethamine inhibit dihydrofolate reductase. Because pyrimethamine and trimethoprim inhibit the same enzyme in the pathway, the use of both drugs is not necessary, and pyrimethamine is often chosen over trimethoprim because of its more potent effects on protozoa than bacteria. Pyrimethamine is coccidiocidal at concentrations of 1 µg/mL, whereas trimethoprim requires concentrations of 5 µg/mL for coccidiocidal activity. Sulfonamides have very little antiprotozoal action when used alone, but synergism occurs when they are used in combination with either trimethoprim or pyrimethamine.[167]

These drugs are inexpensive and generally safe but require longer treatment periods than the triazine derivatives, and clinical signs may return if therapy is discontinued too early. Few adverse effects have been associated with long-term treatment with these drugs, although anemia and pancytopenia may result from folate deficiency.[168] Congenital defects, including weakness, recumbency, and skin lesions, have been reported in foals born to mares being treated for EPM with sulfonamides, pyrimethamine, and folic acid.[169]

Triazine Derivatives

The triazine-derivative antiprotozoals include diclazuril, toltrazuril, and ponazuril. Ponazuril was the first drug approved for use in horses for the treatment of EPM in the United States and is commercially available in the United States. It is an active metabolite of toltrazuril (toltrazuril sulfone). Ponazuril comes in a convenient paste formulation and is recommended for treatment at a dose of 5 mg/kg once daily for 28 days; however, dosing may be extended for another 28 days or until maximal improvement has been noted (see Chapter 55). Some clinicians recommend increasing the dose (up to 35 mg/kg PO q24h) for the initial 4 days of treatment and then following up with the regular treatment dose for the additional 28 days to prevent recrucescence of disease later. Ponazuril is 90% effective at blocking merozoite production in vitro at concentrations of 1 µg/mL and is more than 95% effective at concentrations of 5 µg/mL.[167] Diclazuril has demonstrated similar effectiveness in vitro and reaches therapeutic concentrations in the CSF after oral administration.[170] A Food and Drug Administration (FDA)-approved formulation of diclazuril has recently come on the market in the United States as an alfalfa-based antiprotozoal pellet used as a top-dress on feed and indicated for the treatment of EPM caused by *S. neurona* in horses. This formulation is labeled for a dosage rate of 1 mg/kg for 28 consecutive days.

Treatment of Other Protozoal Diseases

Other protozoal diseases occur infrequently in the horse. Equine piroplasmosis is rare but has been reported in the southeastern United States. Treatment involves administration of imidocarb dipropionate (2.2 mg/kg IM q24h for two doses). This regimen is reasonably effective for treatment of *Babesia caballi*, but higher doses for longer periods may be necessary to treat *Theileria equi* (see Chapter 56).[171] Adverse effects of imidocarb at higher doses include colic, hypersalivation, diarrhea, and death. Imidocarb should not be administered to donkeys because they tend to have severe reactions to the drug. Addition of parvaquone or buparvaquone may help with therapy but, when given alone, may cause treated horses to become carriers. *Giardia* is an infrequent cause of diarrhea in foals and should respond to treatment with metronidazole.

The complete reference list is available online at www.expertconsult.com.

CHAPTER

Immunotherapy

66

Maria Julia Bevilaqua Felippe

As our understanding of immune responses and the pathogenesis of infectious disease has increased over the last two decades, there has been a concomitant increased interest in immunotherapeutics. Immunomodulators are substances that enhance or suppress immune responses (Table 66-1). This diverse group of therapeutic agents includes both nonspecific immunomodulators and drugs with highly selective targets within the immune system. For treatment of horses, recommendations are difficult because of the limited number of studies evaluating their efficacy in that species.

Immunostimulants

Induction of Nonspecific Immune Responses

Many immunostimulants activate innate immunity and promote release of endogenous immune mediators (e.g., cytokines) as an aid in the treatment of immunodeficiency conditions, chronic infections, or cancer. In the 1890s, Dr. William Coley, a surgeon at New York Memorial Hospital, used killed *Streptococcus pyogenes* and *Serratia marcescens* (Coley's vaccine) to treat sarcomas, carcinomas, lymphomas, melanomas, and myelomas in his patients.[1] This treatment originated from the observation that tumors regressed when spontaneous acute infections occurred, especially with high fever. Coley and others initially used live bacteria to induce infection and fever; however, fatal infections eventually led to the use of an inactivated organism.

Immunostimulants induce a nonspecific activation of the immune system, unless they are associated with antigens (e.g., adjuvants in vaccines), and may amplify different effectors of the immune response, including phagocytosis and intracellular

killing of organisms, antigen presentation, cytotoxic and antiviral activity, cytokine release, and antibody production.[2] Immunomodulators predominantly activate macrophages and dendritic cells in the liver, spleen, skin, and lungs.[3] The route of administration is designed to bring the drug into contact with antigen-presenting cells (APCs). In the horse, pulmonary intravascular macrophages are likely important for recognition of foreign antigens in circulation.[4,5] These large, mature, permanent resident macrophages of the pulmonary capillary lumen phagocytose particulate material in the circulation, including bacteria, endotoxins, fibrin, and leukocytes. These cells likely secrete inflammatory mediators that result in alterations in systemic vascular resistance and permeability, are chemoattractants for neutrophil margination into the pulmonary vascular system, and produce additional proinflammatory mediators.

The innate immune response is a nonspecific recognition of and subsequent response to pathogens. Signal transduction pathways activate oxidative burst activity and the production of cytokines and chemokines. These responses initiate microbial defenses and inflammation. Toll-like receptors (TLRs) are type I transmembrane proteins expressed in cells responsible for this first encounter with a pathogen and the presentation of processed peptide to lymphocytes: macrophages, dendritic cells, and in some species, mucosal epithelial cells and dermal epithelial cells. In addition, certain types of TLRs are present in the cytosol for the recognition of processed viral or bacterial components (e.g., ribonucleic acid [RNA], deoxyribonucleic acid [DNA]). Therefore activation of TLRs may be induced in conditions in which an immune response is desired (e.g., vaccination). Blocking of TLR pathways may be beneficial to prevent life-threatening inflammation (e.g., sepsis).[6] In addition to TLRs, other important innate receptors, including

Table 66-1 Immunomodulators

Component	Origin	Mechanism of Action	Immunologic Effect
Immunostimulants			
Bacterial Derivatives			
Propionibacterium acnes	Inactivated *P. acnes* extract	TLR2 receptor–mediated activation of NF-κB on monocytes and macrophages Th1-type response of lymphocytes	Cytotoxic, antitumoral, and antiviral effects Promotes neutrophil and macrophage attraction and activity
Mycobacterium spp.	Deproteinated *Mycobacterium* spp. cell wall extract	TLR2 and TLR4 receptor–mediated activation of NF-κB on macrophages and dendritic cells increase expression of co-stimulatory molecules on APCs.	NK-cell cytotoxic and antitumoral activities Promotes neutrophil and macrophage attraction and activity
Exogenous Cytokines			
Interferon alpha (IFN-α)	Human recombinant molecule Human natural purified molecule	Increase expression of antiviral components (PKR, Mx) Increase in MHC class I expression on infected cells Inhibits gene transcription	Potent antiviral effect Inhibits cell proliferation Proapoptosis effect Promote IFN-α secretion
Granulocyte colony-stimulating factor (G-CSF)	Canine recombinant molecule Human recombinant molecule	Myeloid stimulation factor	Promotes myeloid cell production and maturation of macrophages and dendritic cells
Viral Derivatives			
Parapoxvirus ovis	Chemically inactivated *Parapoxvirus ovis* strain D 1701	CD14-mediated inflammatory response of APCs	Promotes cytokine secretion NK-cell cytotoxicity Antiviral and phagocytic activity
Other Immunostimulants			
Levamisole	Synthetic anthelmintic	Unknown	Phagocytic activity Antibody production
Caprine serum fraction	Purified serum protein fraction	Unknown	Unknown
Immunosuppressants			
Inhibitors of Gene Expression			
Glucocorticoids	Synthetic molecules	Binding to cytosolic glucocorticoid receptor promotes its translocation into nucleus to bind to glucocorticoid responsive elements Binding to and neutralization of proinflammatory transcription factors (NF-κB, AP-1, CREB)	Potent antiinflammatory effect Antiphagocytic activity Inhibit APC maturation and activation Inhibit T-cell activation Inhibit antibody production
Kinase and Phosphatase Inhibitors			
Cyclosporine A	Fungal polypeptide	Binding to cyclophilin inhibits phosphorylation of NFAT and its translocation to the nucleus	Inhibits T-cell activation and proliferation
Inhibitors of Nucleotide Synthesis			
Azathioprine	Purine analog precursor	Inhibits de novo pathway of purine synthesis; inhibits synthesis of DNA and RNA	Inhibits cell proliferation Inhibits T-cell activation
Alkylating Agents			
Cyclophosphamide	Metabolite of nitrogen mustard	Alkylate DNA bases	Mutagenic, cytotoxic, antiproliferative, and chemotherapeutic effects
Chlorambucil	Metabolite of nitrogen mustard	Alkylate DNA bases	
Vinca Alkaloids			
Vincristine	Vinca alkaloid	Binding to tubulin in the mitotic spindle prevents purine synthesis	Inhibit cell proliferation Thrombopoietic effect
Passive Immunotherapy			
Regular plasma	Pooled alloimmune plasma from horse donors	Passive transfer of immunoglobulins Binding of donor immunoglobulin to the Fc receptors of phagocytes in liver and spleen Saturation of endosome receptors involved in immunoglobulin degradation	Increases opsonization capacity Inhibits removal of antibody-bound red cells or platelets by phagocytes Accelerates catabolism of autoantibodies
Hyperimmune plasma	Pooled alloimmune plasma from antigen-specific vaccinated horses	Binding of immunoglobulins to organism's antigenic targets	Neutralizes the effects of and toxins
Antiserum-antitoxin	Serum concentrate of antigen-specific immunoglobulins	Binding of immunoglobulins to antigenic targets	Neutralizes the effects of toxins

TLR, Toll-like receptor; *NF-κB*, nuclear factor kappa B; *APCs*, antigen-presenting cells; *Th1*, T-helper cell type 1; *PKR*, protein kinase R; *MHC*, major histocompatibility complex; *NK*, natural killer; *AP*, activator protein; *CREB*, cAMP response element–binding protein; *NFAT*, nuclear factor of activated T lymphocyte.

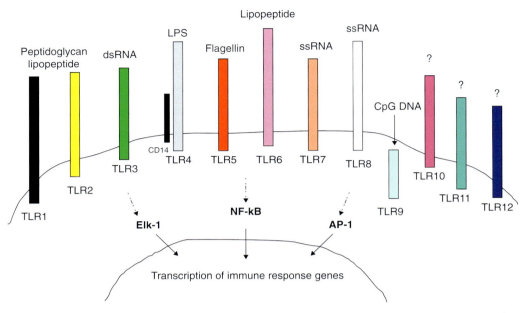

Toll-like receptors (TLRs) recognize pathogen-associated molecular patterns (PAMPs)

Figure 66-1 Toll-like receptors. Each toll-like receptor *(TLR)* recognizes a different pathogen-associated molecular pattern *(PAMP)*; together, they can identify a wide range of organisms, including gram-positive and gram-negative bacteria, viruses, fungi, and parasites. The binding to a TLR results in activation of signaling pathway cascades and the translocation of transcriptional factors (NF-κB, Elk-1, AP-1) into the nucleus, with subsequent cell activation and inflammatory cytokine expression. Immunomodulators may mimic the natural activation of antigen-presenting cells (APCs) through TLR receptor and consequently promote the availability of proinflammatory signals. *LPS,* Lipopolysaccharide; *dsRNA,* double-strand ribonucleic acid; *ss,* single-strand; *CpG,* cytosine-phosphate-guanosine; *NF,* nuclear factor; *AP,* activator protein.

nucleotide-binding oligomerization domain-containing protein (NOD), retinoic acid-inducible gene RIG-like receptors (RLR), mannose, and complement receptors, are expressed in the cytosol or surface of APCs.

The contribution of TLRs to the immune response was first observed with *Aspergillus fumigatus* infection of *Drosophila.*[7,8] Since then, as many as 13 TLRs have been identified, but their expression varies among species.[9] Each TLR recognizes a different pathogen-associated molecular pattern (PAMP); therefore together they can mediate response to a wide range of organisms (Fig. 66-1). In addition, TLRs may recognize low-molecular-weight synthetic molecules.

After antigen processing of an immunostimulant, intracellular signaling pathways for expression of proinflammatory genes and endogenous cytokines (interleukin-1 [IL-1], IL-6, tumor necrosis factor alpha [TNF-α], and interferon alpha [IFN-α]) are activated (Fig. 66-2). These mediators, while promoting the desirable immune responses, exert adverse systemic effects, including transient fever, lethargy, and decreased appetite.[10] Toxic effects of these crude or live bacterial products include increased vascular permeability, hypotension, pulmonary edema, diarrhea, hypersensitivity reactions with infiltrative/granulomatous cell reaction, autoantibody production, and collapse.

The use of immunostimulants in equine medicine is promoted for the preventive or adjunctive therapy of respiratory diseases and other infectious diseases, acquired immunosuppression secondary to stress (transportation, training, weaning), immunosuppressive treatment, infiltrative diseases, metabolic/endocrine diseases, malnutrition, or any condition that has reduced the ability of the immune system to fight against opportunistic and pathogenic organisms. Immunostimulants are also recommended for antitumor treatment (e.g., sarcoids) in the horse.

Bacterial Particles

Propionibacterium acnes

Propionibacterium acnes is a gram-positive bacterium studied since the 1950s (when it was known as *Corynebacterium parvum*) for its antitumoral and antiviral properties. Immunostimulatory activity has been demonstrated in vitro and in vivo in humans and mice. These actions include (1) stimulation of monocytes and macrophages with production of inflammatory cytokines (IL-1, IL-6, and TNF-α), chemokine production (IL-8), phagocytosis and reactive oxygen species activity; (2) activation of CD8⁺ T cells (cytotoxic T lymphocytes [CTLs]), natural killer (NK) cells, and lymphokine-activated killer (LAK) cells with IL-2 and IFN-α–dependent cytotoxicity; (3) increase in resistance to intracellular bacteria and viruses in mice; (4) in vivo antitumoral effect; and (5) potential adjuvant with antigens.[11-14] The recognition of *P. acnes* PAMP is mediated by the TLR2 and TLR9 on monocytes and macrophages. Activation results in nuclear factor kappa B (NF-κB) activation and expression of IL-6, IL-8, and IL-1 and the generation of a T-helper cell type 1 (Th1) immune response.[15-17] When added to murine bone marrow cell cultures, *P. acnes* promoted the differentiation of monocytes into mature dendritic cells that expressed IL-12 and high levels of co-stimulatory (CD80 and CD86) and antigen-presentation (major histocompatibility class II [MHC II]) molecules.[18]

Propionibacterium acnes (Eqstim, Neogen, Lexington, KY) is licensed for adjunctive therapy in the treatment of viral and bacterial infections of the respiratory tract of the horse in association with other conventional therapy. In healthy young horses, a series of three intravenous (IV) injections of *P. acnes* extract resulted in immunomodulatory responses.[19] It is suspected that the bacterial extract is rapidly taken up by the intravascular pulmonary macrophages, which in turn produce

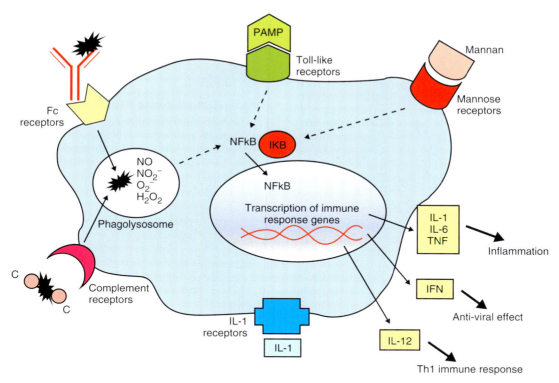

Figure 66-2 Innate immunity. Antigen-presenting cells (APCs) display different mechanisms to detect antigens and pathogens at first encounter: Fcγ and complement receptors facilitate the phagocytosis of antibody-bound and complement (C)–bound organisms, respectively; on phagocytosis, reactive nitrogen and oxygen species (NO, NO_2^-, O_2^-, H_2O_2) are produced for the killing of the pathogen; toll-like receptors (TLRs) recognize specific pathogen-associated molecular patterns *(PAMPs)*; mannose receptors bind to mannan on fungal and bacterial organisms; and the interleukin-1 *(IL-1)* receptor recognizes the IL-1 cytokine, which is released by activated inflammatory and epithelial cells to signal for "danger." Activation of APCs by these mechanisms results in translocation of nuclear factor kappa B *(NFκB)* into the nucleus, with subsequent signaling for the transcription of proinflammatory cytokines, including IL-1, IL-6, tumor necrosis factor alpha *(TNFα)*, interferon-alpha *(IFNα)*, and IL-12. *Th1,* T-helper cell type 1.

inflammatory cytokines and clinical effects (indicated by mild fever). In peripheral blood, nonopsonized phagocytosis is increased. In bronchoalveolar lavage (BAL) fluid, there is a decrease in total leukocyte counts, especially lymphocytes, with a proportional increase in macrophages. The CD4/CD8 T-lymphocyte ratio and LAK cell activity are increased in peripheral blood and BAL fluid after 3 days of administration of this immunostimulant. Peripheral blood mononuclear cells exhibit an increase in IFN-γ and the NK-lysin antimicrobial peptide for up to 7 days after treatment.[20]

An open, randomized clinical trial demonstrated that administration of two doses of *P. acnes* before shipping reduced the incidence of transport-stress–induced respiratory disease by more than 60% compared with horses in a placebo-treated group.[21] In two blinded, randomized clinical studies of horses with naturally occurring respiratory disease treated with conventional therapy, 79% and 96% of the horses that received *P. acnes* recovered within 14 days of treatment, compared with 47% and 35%, respectively, of the horses from the placebo group.[22]

The effect of *P. acnes* was tested in equine neonates and foals, resulting in an improvement in IFN-γ production by peripheral blood lymphocytes when administered in the first month of life but not in the first week of life; no effect was observed in the production of IFN-γ by BAL cells at the same age periods.[23] Treatment of foals with *P. acnes* resulted in significantly less intracellular proliferation of *R. equi* within ex vivo-infected monocyte-derived macrophages compared to control foals.[24]

Bacille Calmette-Guérin Vaccine and Mycobacterium Cell Wall Extracts

Microbiologists Calmette and Guérin from the Pasteur Institute took 13 years to attenuate a strain of *Mycobacterium bovis* by 230 serial passages in culture. This resulted in a loss of virulence without loss of immunogenic properties in the attenuated strain. Since then, genetic drift has resulted in different strains of bacille Calmette-Guérin (BCG), which induce the distinct immunogenic and therapeutic effects observed at present.[25] BCG was originally created for use as a vaccine against *Mycobacterium tuberculosis* in humans. Use as a nonspecific immunomodulator began in the 1970s for treatment of superficial bladder cancer.[26,27] Currently, BCG cell wall fractions and recombinant BCG (rBCG) combined with foreign antigens (viral, bacterial, or parasitic particles) or cytokines (e.g., human IFN-α gene) are available for clinical use and research.[28] The recombinant forms are studied for their application as adjuvants in specific immune responses.

Low-dose BCG vaccine and inactivated *Mycobacterium* preparations have a potent immunomodulatory effect on macrophages and dendritic cells primarily via TLR2 and TLR4.[29,30] In addition to enhanced production of the cytokines IL-12, IL-1, and TNF-α, BCG-stimulated dendritic cells promote the upregulation of CD80, CD86, and CD40, which are important co-stimulatory molecules for T-cell activation. BCG vaccine–stimulated monocytes and macrophages induce Th1-type CD4+ T-cell proliferation in vitro.[31] BCG vaccine stimulates NK-cell cytotoxicity and IFN-γ production via monocyte and macrophage IL-12 secretion. A comparable direct effect of BCG vaccine on NK cells in the absence of APCs has also been demonstrated in vitro.[32,33] In addition, BCG vaccine stimulates the expression of integrins, IL-1α and IL1β, IL-8, macrophage inflammatory protein 1α (MIP-1α) and MIP-1β and resistance to apoptosis in neutrophils.[34] Together, the immunostimulatory effects promote neutrophil and macrophage attraction and activation, which subsequently induces Th1-type CD4+ T-cell activation and NK-cell cytotoxic response.

Although the mechanisms of action of BCG vaccine have been widely studied in other species, to date there are limited in vitro or in vivo data describing the effects of this immunomodulator in the horse. Different components of the mycobacterial cell wall act as potent macrophage stimulants, including muramyl dipeptide and lipoarabinomannan. Equimune I.V. (Bioniche Animal Health Research) is an emulsion of deproteinized *Mycobacterium* cell wall fraction that claims to have reduced toxic effects without loss of immunostimulatory activity. It is indicated as a single-dose immunostimulant for the treatment of equine respiratory disease complex resulting from viral or bacterial infection.

Adverse reactions to BCG vaccine (live-attenuated form of *Mycobacterium*) are more common in children. These reactions may include persistent local abscess at the site of injection and regional suppurative lymphadenopathy.[35] Adverse reactions to intravesical instillation of BCG live-attenuated vaccine for the treatment of superficial bladder carcinoma in human patients include disseminated BCG infection in distant organs: granulomatous hepatitis, miliary pulmonary disease, pulmonary granulomas, renal abscess, and retroperitoneal lymphadenopathy.[36] In addition, sepsis and hypersensitivity reactions (fever, pancytopenia, anaphylaxis, hepatitis, renal insufficiency) have been reported.[37] Pulmonary toxicity could be septic and secondary to mycobacteremia, which induces sensitization before a second BCG exposure. Hypersensitivity reactions a few weeks after immunotherapy may be observed in patients with disseminated pulmonary and hepatic granulomas, characterized by noncaseating epithelioid granuloma with Langhans-type giant cells and lymphocytes. In these cases, cultures for mycobacteria from blood and affected tissues are negative.[38]

A randomized, double-blind clinical study in horses with naturally occurring respiratory disease and treated with conventional therapy suggested that 83% of horses receiving one IV dose of purified *Mycobacterium* spp. cell wall extract recovered from respiratory clinical signs in a shorter time (7 days) than the placebo group (36%).[39] Live BCG vaccine or preparations of BCG cell wall fraction (Regressin-V, Bioniche Animal Health) have been used with quantifiable success (about 60%-70%) for intratumoral treatment of sarcoids in horses.[40] This therapy is more efficacious for treatment of facial lesions and in horses with a positive delayed hypersensitivity reaction to purified protein derivative before treatment and leukocytosis after the first injection.[41] Nonresponsive cases are associated with lesions elsewhere on the body (limbs, body wall), large size, or the presence of multiple sarcoid lesions.

In horses, adverse effects after immunotherapy with mycobacterial preparations include reaction at the injection site, fever, lethargy, and decreased appetite, likely related to the induced endogenous cytokine release. An acute reaction with pancytopenia, fever, hypotension, tachycardia, and tachypnea has been observed in a horse treated intralesionally for a sarcoid lesion (Felippe, unpublished data). This horse had been previously treated with a BCG formula several months before this reaction. Four horses with a history of cough developed severe inflammatory reaction in the respiratory tract after immunomodulator administration. These horses had interstitial pneumonia, multifocal pulmonary granulomas, and bronchiolitis, with subsequent development of lung fibrosis despite glucocorticoid therapy.[42] Another report describes an adult horse that developed severe interstitial pneumonia, pleuritis, granulomatous lymphadenopathy, and hepatopathy after the administration of a live BCG vaccine for the treatment of equine sarcoids.[43] Because of these types of adverse reactions, veterinary *Mycobacterium* compounds have been removed from the market in some countries.

Unmethylated Cytosine-Phosphate-Guanosine Motifs

Cytosine-phosphate-guanosine (CpG) motifs are unmethylated dinucleotides present in high frequency in bacterial but not in vertebrate genomes. Cytosine-phosphate-guanosine motifs are recognized by TLR-9 expressed primarily in APCs.[44] Synthetic oligodeoxynucleotide (ODN) motifs can mimic natural CpGs and stimulate macrophages, dendritic cells, and B cells. In general, CpG-ODN motifs induce a Th1-type immune response, with both cellular and humoral components.[45] Therefore CpG-ODNs can be potentially used as immunomodulators for treatment of immune-mediated disorders or as adjuvants in vaccines.[46-48]

In murine B cells, CpG motifs induce robust T-cell–independent B-cell proliferation; enhance production of IL-6, IL-10, and antibodies; promote isotype switching; and prevent B-cell apoptosis.[49] In monocytes, macrophages, and dendritic cells, CpG motifs induce the production of large quantities of IL-12 and smaller quantities of IFN-α, TNF-α, and IL-6.[50] There is maturation of dendritic cells with upregulation of cell surface MHC II molecule and co-stimulatory molecules, including CD86.[51] Therefore these APCs become more capable of presenting processed antigen to T cells and promoting their activation. The increased production of IL-12 by APCs results in potent stimulation of NK cells and T cells, with subsequent IFN-γ release.

There is species specificity in the recognition of CpG motifs, and certain CpG motifs may have dissimilar effects on immune cells according to their sequence.[52] CpG-ODN–induced proliferation in vitro correlates well with in vivo responses, and this method is used to screen different motifs for clinical application.[53] Other synthetic products that contain a bicyclic heterobase in which the C in CpG is replaced by R (rybofuranosyl, RpG) are also studied.[54]

The effect of CpG seems conditional to the types of CpG tested and responding cells. In foals, CpG-ODNs have been tested as an enhancer of immune response in early age. Isolated peripheral blood mononuclear cells of neonatal foals stimulated in vitro with CpG-ODN responded with increased expression of IFN-γ, IL-6, and IL-12(p35/p40); the magnitude of response was less for newborn foals than for older foals.[55] In other studies, purified foal neutrophils have been shown to respond to B-class CpG 2142 stimulus with enhanced reactive oxygen species and greater mRNA expression of IFN-γ, IL-8, IL-12p35, and IL-17 than controls, but with decreased TNF-α expression.[56,57] When co-cultured with other leukocytes, foal neutrophils were significantly activated at birth by CpG and produced IL-6, IL-8, IL-12p40, and IL-23p19 at similar magnitudes to those at 2 months of age. Sequential in vivo administration of CpG in equine neonates failed to modulate the cytokine expression of peripheral blood mononuclear cells isolated from foals at different ages, and subsequently infected in vitro with *Rhodococcus equi*.[58] CpG-ODN 2135 significant increased IL-12p40 and IFN-α messenger RNA (mRNA) expression in adult horse dendritic cells but not macrophages, in comparison to nonstimulated cells in vitro.[59] In contrast, foal APCs did not respond to CpG-ODN stimulation with increased cytokine mRNA expression up to 3 months of age, despite the fact that TLR-9 mRNA expression and NF-κB activation (NF-κB p65) in foal dendritic cells and macrophages were comparable to adult horse cells.

Other reported applications of CpG-ODNs in the horse tested their immunomodulatory properties in vaccination and hypersensitivity conditions. The addition of a CpG-ODN 2007 formulated with 30% Emulsigen (MVP Technologies, Omaha, NE) to a commercial killed influenza virus vaccine induced significantly greater influenza-specific antibody response in comparison to vaccine alone or saline.[60] The effect of CpG-ODN was not as apparent in disease protection because vaccination with or without CpG-ODN equivalently improved protection against virus challenge. Some types of allergic conditions may benefit from a shift away from the Th2-type immune response, and CpG-ODNs have been extensively studied in immune-mediated diseases for this reason. A-class CpG-ODN 2216 bound to gelatin nanoparticles has been shown to induce upregulation of IL-10 and IFN-γ and downregulation of IL-4 in horses affected with recurrent airway obstruction.[61]

As with many other immunomodulating agents, CpG motifs may be toxic and promote an undesirable, exacerbated immune response. Toxic responses to CpG motif have been demonstrated in mice after repeated administration of high doses of CpG motifs. A lethal synergism is observed when CpG motif administration is followed by endotoxin (lipopolysaccharide [LPS]) challenge.[62] Despite promoting B-cell activity, CpG does not induce an anti-DNA antibody response or accelerate autoimmune disease. Further studies of the use of this immunomodulatory agent are necessary to identify CpG sequences with biologic effect, the type of response generated, potential clinical applications, and safety in the horse.

Exogenous Cytokines

Cytokines are proteins or glycoproteins secreted by immune cells and other cells in direct contact with microorganisms. Their effect is primarily autocrine or paracrine, and they function as messengers or mediators of the immune system. Interleukins and other cytokines may be administered as immunomodulating agents to stimulate enhanced immune activity in the treatment of infectious, neoplastic, and autoimmune diseases.

Interferon-α

Endogenous IFNs are multifunctional proteins that play important roles in antiviral defense and cell proliferation/viability by binding to cell surface receptors on virus-infected cells and inducing transcription of specific genes. High IFN levels can control the rate of virus replication in early infection.[63] Type I IFNs are produced primarily by the innate immune system leukocytes (e.g., IFN-α) or fibroblasts (e.g., IFN-α and IFN-β) after viral infection.[64] Viral binding to extracellular receptors or the presence of viral products (double-strand RNA [dsRNA]) bound to cytoplasmic receptors can induce expression of type I IFNs. Type II IFNs (IFN-γ) are produced by NK cells and T cells (in response to cytokines IL-12 and IL-18). Both types of IFN promote an "antiviral state" by interfering with the mechanisms of cell proliferation, translation, and subsequently, viral replication. In addition, IFNs make infected cells more susceptible to apoptosis (procaspase activity) and to recognition by CD8+ cytotoxic T cells by enhancing the expression of MHC I on infected cells.

One of the most important antiviral activities of IFNs is induction of proteins that prevent proliferation or promote destruction of RNA molecules in the cell. These include the dsRNA-dependent protein kinase R (PKR), which controls transcription and translation of other genes with antiviral effect (e.g., NF-κB). The gene 2′-5′-oligoadenylate synthetase inhibits protein synthesis by promoting ribonuclease (RNase) activity. The Mx proteins interfere with virus polymerase and upregulate adenosine deaminase (ADAR), which is important for RNA editing, effectively inhibiting viral multiplication. Caspase proteins promote apoptosis.[65] Interferons are so important in the

control of viral infection and replication that many viruses have developed mechanisms to inhibit the IFNs.[66]

Besides the potent direct antiviral effects of IFN-α, this cytokine promotes cell-mediated immunity. It enhances the cytotoxic effects of NK cells and LAK cells by increasing levels of perforins and granzymes (apoptotic effect), production of IFN-γ, and cell proliferation. Once IFN-γ secretion is enhanced, this stimulation is self-sustained with cell-to-cell contact for a time, even in the absence of additional IFN-α.[67] Interferon gamma induces activation and maturation of APCs, potentiated even further by IL-12 and IL-15. Interleukin-12 drives CD4+ T cells into a Th1-type response, resulting in additional IFN-γ production. Interleukin-15 supports the survival and proliferation of activated and memory T cells.[68] In addition, IFN-γ induces the production of reactive oxygen (O_2-, superoxide; $OH-$, hydroxyl; H_2O_2, hydrogen peroxide; $HClO-$, hypochlorite) and reactive nitrogen (NO, nitric oxide; NO_2, nitrogen dioxide; HN_2, nitrous acid) products in phagocytes for effective microbial killing.[69]

Commercially available IFN-α is found in natural (in vitro purified human IFN-α with multiple subtypes) and recombinant forms (*Escherichia coli* clone expressing human IFN-α-2a subtype DNA). The natural form of IFN-α may provide broader biologic function compared with the single recombinant subtype. Low-dose IFN-α therapy is more efficient in antiviral activity than high doses, which may induce an excessive inflammatory response, downregulation of IFN receptors, and production of neutralizing antibodies. Studies using IFN-α as an adjuvant for influenza peptide vaccines in mice revealed a potential benefit in the induction of CTL activity.[70]

Interferon-α has been used therapeutically via oral or parenteral (subcutaneous [SC], intramuscular [IM]) routes in people and horses for its antiviral and antiproliferative (antitumoral) activities. Parenteral high-dose human IFN-α-2a has been used to treat human patients with chronic hepatitis C, West Nile virus (WNV) infection, hairy cell leukemia, chronic myelogenous leukemia, and acquired immunodeficiency syndrome (AIDS)–related Kaposi's sarcoma.[71-75] Adverse effects associated with parenteral high-dose IFN-α-2a treatment include fever, fatigue, and myalgia. Contrasting results of in vitro experiments question the susceptibility of WNV to IFN-α. There is evidence of both resistance and susceptibility of the virus to the cytokine.[76] Nevertheless, human patients infected with WNV treated with high parenteral doses of IFN-α had rapid recovery and fewer sequelae.[77] Polyethylene glycol-conjugated IFN-α (PEG IFN-α) for treatment of mice resulted in increased survival, reduced viremia, clearance of the virus by day 2 postinfection, and prevented exacerbated inflammatory response by macrophage and splenic CD4, CD8, and B cells in comparison to nontreated infected mice.[78]

Oral IFN-α acts directly on oropharyngeal-associated lymphoid tissues by activating the antiviral state in those cells.[79] In horses, low-dose oral administration of natural human IFN-α has been used for the treatment of inflammatory airway disease and viral respiratory diseases.[80] In a double-blind, randomized, block-design study of horses with inflammatory airway disease (characterized by poor performance and exudate in the upper and lower airway), natural human IFN-α given orally reduced airway inflammation, pharyngeal lymphoid hyperplasia, nasal discharge, and cough compared with horses receiving placebo. The cytokine profile of BAL fluid cells returned to normal in horses that received oral IFN-α. A commercially available recombinant IFN-α-2a, which contains only one subtype of IFN-α, failed to reduce virus shedding and respiratory disease in experimental herpesvirus type 1 infection in horses.[81] A double-blind, randomized clinical trial testing the effect of oral treatment with natural or recombinant human IFN-α on inflammatory airway disease revealed that both IFN-α forms decreased the time to recovery and number of relapses compared with placebo.[82] In horses, IFN-α has been used parenterally for the treatment of WNV; however, to date, randomized, placebo-controlled trials have not been completed. Another study examined how IFN-α could act as an adjuvant for an adenovirus-based vaccine expressing Venezuelan equine encephalitis virus structural protein.[83] The expression of IFN-α with the vaccine reduced the antibody response to the vaccine; however, adenovirus-delivered IFN-α alone protected mice from disease when administered 24 hours prior to challenge but not when administered 6 hours after challenge, suggesting a role for IFN-mediated antiviral response in Venezuelan equine encephalitis.

Other Cytokines: Present and Future

The two most common cytokines studied in cancer immunotherapy in human patients (e.g., renal cell carcinoma) are IL-2 and IFN-α, which can be used independently (high doses) or in combination (lower doses).[84,85] Because only a small percentage of patients respond to cytokine therapy alone, this mode of treatment is often combined with traditional chemotherapy.[86] Effective response and toxicity are both dose dependent with this cytokine; therefore, to minimize systemic effect, peripheral blood or tumoral infiltrating lymphocytes (TILs) can be activated and expanded with cytokines (IL-2) in vitro and returned to the patient for a potentiated effect against tumor cells.[87] Hyporesponsive lymphocytes from the malignant effusion of lung cancer patients can be reactivated into CTLs when treated in vitro with IL-2 (or IL-15) and anti-CD3 antibodies.[88]

The use of cytokines in combination with conventional antibiotic therapy or as vaccine adjuvants has been beneficial in the treatment and prevention of infection with intracellular bacteria. The use of IL-12 alone has limited clinical application, but it has promising adjunctive properties to induce Th1-type immune response when paired with peptides in vaccines. In murine models, intranasal administration of IL-12 in combination with an antibiotic or antifungal medication improves survival and clearance of *Mycobacterium avium*, *Francisella tularensis*, influenza virus, or cryptococcal infection.[89-92] In human patients with asthma, treatment with IL-12 with the objective to inhibit Th2-type and promote Th1-type responses failed to improve airway hyperreactivity.[93] Work with a cytokine fusion protein consisting of allergen (or allergen complementary DNA [cDNA]) fused to IL-12 or IL-18, or allergen cDNA fused with IL-18 cDNA, reveals redirection of immune responses into a Th1 type and reduction of airway hyperreactivity in a mouse model.[94]

The antitumor effect of the plasmid DNA-encoding IL-12 has been observed in murine tumor models; however, many of these therapies failed when applied to human patients with cancer. In horses with metastatic melanoma, a randomized double-blind, placebo-controlled study described the use of intratumorally-injected cytokine-encoding plasmid DNA (IL-18–encoding plasmid DNA, IL-12–encoding plasmid DNA, or empty plasmid DNA as control). Significant tumor regression could be shown in both the treatment groups receiving IL-18 and IL-12–encoding plasmid DNA, whereas placebo-treated control patients showed tumor growth over the course of the treatment.[95,96]

The use of other cytokines to induce Th1-type immune response in clinical patients has had limited effect. Administration of IFN-γ to prevent *Pseudomonas aeruginosa* infection in a stress mouse model revealed recovery of IL-12 secretion but did not improve bacterial clearance or reduce mortality.[97]

Neonatal mice treated with fms-like tyrosine kinase 3 (Flt-3) ligand, a hematopoietic growth factor for dendritic cells, B cells, and NK cells, demonstrated a 100-fold increase in the innate resistance to herpes simplex virus type 1 and *Listeria*

monocytogenes.[98] The dendritic cell induction was independent of mature T and B cells and their cytokines. This finding has important implications in neonatal immune defense because the adaptive immune system is not well developed.

Granulocyte-macrophage colony-stimulating factor (GM-CSF) is a cytokine used to reconstitute myeloid cells in the bone marrow and promote macrophage and dendritic cell development. This cytokine has also been evaluated as an adjuvant in vaccines or in combination with other cytokines (IFN-γ) to promote dendritic cell maturation for use in cancer immunotherapy. In the horse, subcutaneous administration of recombinant human granulocyte colony-stimulating factor (G-CSF) stimulates in vitro bone marrow cells from Standardbred horses with familial neutropenia and accelerates bone marrow production of neutrophils in foals with alloimmune neonatal neutropenia.[99,100] Response to G-CSF is immediate, and in the presence of normal myeloid precursors in the bone marrow, neutrophil counts may be within normal reference ranges within 48 hours of administration.

Other Immunomodulators

Parapoxvirus ovis

The use of poxvirus as an immunostimulant originated from observations related to the smallpox eradication program, in which vaccinated human patients had improvement in viral diseases and tumors. In vitro studies using murine, human, bovine, ovine, and swine cells suggest that the Parapoxvirus envelope contains proteins that promote the activation of NK cells, enhance phagocytic activity, and increase the release of IFN-α, IL-2, TNF-α, and GM-CSF.[101] The mechanism of stimulation of APCs involves the CD14 molecule, with production of antiinflammatory IL-10 and Th2-type IL-4 cytokines.[102] Pretreatment with *Parapoxvirus ovis* protected mice in a dose-dependent manner from lethal vesicular stomatitis virus and herpes simplex virus type 1 infections.[103]

Administration of inactivated *Parapoxvirus ovis* (ecthyma virus or Orf virus) strain D 1701 is indicated for the prophylaxis of stress-induced respiratory diseases caused by transportation, hospitalization, and weaning; for the metaphylaxis and therapy of infectious diseases; and to enhance immunization response. In the horse, a blinded field study suggested that prophylactic administration of *Parapoxvirus ovis* to foals 6 and 4 days before weaning, and at 5 days thereafter, assisted in preventing and reducing the incidence of respiratory disease from 24% to 7.9%.[104] In a controlled field trial, Thoroughbred foals from the same farm received three doses of the immunotherapeutic drug or placebo immediately after birth and 24 or 48 hours later. These foals were monitored for 4 weeks, and 20% to 30% of the foals from the placebo group developed respiratory infections, whereas the foals in the groups receiving the immunomodulator did not. *Parapoxvirus ovis* was suggested to minimize but not to prevent respiratory clinical signs (based on nasal exudate scores) in horses naturally challenged by contact with virulent equine herpesvirus type 1 (EHV-1) or type 4 (EHV-4).[105] Young horses under stress induced by weaning, transportation, and commingling that were treated with this immunomodulating agent were more resistant to EHV-1 and EHV-4 infection, as well as development of respiratory clinical signs, when receiving *Parapoxvirus ovis*, compared with horses receiving placebo.[104]

Another placebo-controlled, randomized study tested the effect of inactivated *Parapoxvirus ovis* in the incidence of pneumonia in foals.[106] Foals received a dose of *Parapoxvirus ovis* or placebo at birth, 24 hours after, and 8 days later. A three-dose treatment of *Parapoxvirus ovis* starting at birth did not change the incidence of clinical or ultrasonographic evidence of pneumonia. Nevertheless, there was a significant effect on the number of IFN-γ–secreting cells in foals 7 to 14 days old but not in younger foals.

Inactivated *Parapoxvirus ovis* stimulation significantly increased IFN-α and IFN-β gene expression in peripheral blood mononuclear cells in vitro and enhanced the effect of the concanavalin A mitogen in their cytokine production.[107] Treatment of horses with a three-dose regimen of the immunostimulant resulted in elevation of IFN-γ gene expression in blood cells collected at 24 hours after the first dose. Also, intradermal inoculation led to an increased gene expression of IFN-γ, IFN-β, IL-15, and IL-18 in biopsied tissues.

A placebo-controlled, randomized study tested the effect of inactivated Parapoxvirus *ovis* treatment on neutrophil, macrophage, and lymphocyte function during ex vivo exposure to *Rhodococcus equi*.[24] Overall, *Parapoxvirus ovis* significantly increased neutrophil phagocytosis and oxidative burst activity and induced greater TNF-α production in monocyte-derived macrophages and IL-12p40 production in BAL macrophages in comparison to controls.

Levamisole Phosphate

Levamisole phosphate is a synthetic anthelmintic with reported immunomodulatory properties that have been rarely observed and poorly characterized in vitro and in vivo. In horses, the effect of levamisole was tested in pregnant mares with weekly injections starting 4 to 6 weeks before parturition. Colostrum of mares receiving the immunostimulant had greater immunoglobulin G (IgG) and IgG(T) concentrations than did colostrum from control mares.[108] In sick foals, levamisole has been administered in the attempt to improve cell-mediated responses and phagocytic activity.

Oral administration of the anthelmintic levamisole leads to the formation of amphetamine-like metabolites known as *aminorex* and *rexamino;* therefore, in the horseracing industry, administration of levamisole has an impact in drug testing; yet, analysis of urine chiral isomer distribution may differ from aminorex originated from a synthetic, racemic form and the one formed from levamisole administration.[109]

Caprine Serum Fraction

Caprine serum fraction is a sterile, filtered, purified, and standardized fraction of goat serum preserved in phenol and thimerosal (Pulmo-Clear, Colorado Serum Co, Denver). It is recommended as an immunomodulator for adjunctive therapy of lower respiratory tract disease in horses. A clinical efficacy trial in horses with unspecified lower respiratory tract disease suggested improvement in airway inflammation, as evaluated by endoscopic examination score after two doses of the immunomodulator.[110] Phenotypic analysis of leukocyte subpopulations, phagocytosis, and oxidative burst activity; LAK cell activity; and IL-2 receptor (IL-2R) expression were evaluated in peripheral blood and BAL fluid leukocytes after administration of two IM injections of placebo or caprine serum fraction to six healthy yearling fillies. The results suggested immunomodulatory activity with an increase in CD4+/CD8+ T-lymphocyte ratio in peripheral blood. The cellularity of BAL fluid, especially B lymphocytes and macrophages, was reduced after administration of the immunomodulator. Other immune function tests, including LAK cell activity, phagocytosis, and oxidative burst activity and IL-2R expression, were unchanged.

Acemannan

Acemannan immunostimulant consists of long-chain mannan polymers interspersed with acetyl groups and is derived from the pulp of the Aloe vera plant. In vitro studies have demonstrated immunostimulatory effects on macrophages (increased secretion of IL-1α, IL-6, TNF-α, nitric oxide, phagocytosis) and

the stimulation of CTLs.[111,112] Commercially available products for topical use in veterinary medicine are indicated for wound healing.

Imiquimod

One study investigated the efficacy of imiquimod 5% cream for the treatment of equine aural plaques; although a long-term treatment was required, the treatment was favorable for the majority of horses; some adverse effects included marked local inflammation and exudation.[113]

Echinacea angustifolia

Standardized *Echinacea angustifolia* has been evaluated as an immunomodulator in horses. Findings suggest increased phagocytic capacity of neutrophils and increased numbers of lymphocytes, red cells, and hemoglobin in the peripheral blood compared with placebo groups.[104-114]

Ginseng

One study reported that powdered ginseng fed to horses for 28 days increased the antibody titer response to equine herpersvirus-1 inactivated vaccine, in comparison to control-vaccinated horses that did not receive ginseng in their diet.[115]

Vaccination

The objective of a vaccine is to stimulate a protective immune response to an infectious organism (Fig. 66-3). Often, protection requires both mucosal and circulatory humoral and cellular immune responses. Long-term protection with immunologic memory is fundamental.

Types of Vaccines

Vaccines come in a variety of types, including inactivated whole pathogen, protein vaccines, recombinant subunit vaccines, DNA vaccines, modified live vaccines, and recombinant vector vaccines.[116] Different vaccine types elicit different levels of humoral and cellular immune response (Fig. 66-4). The choice of vaccine depends on the type of desired immune response, accessible technology, and costs of production. Limited information on marketed vaccines is available regarding the type of immune response induced by a specific vaccine, the actual efficacy and duration of immunity induced when using products from different companies, the efficacy of multivalent vaccines, and proper vaccination schedules for different age and risk groups. Seroconversion, measured as a clinical response, only indicates vaccine antigen recognition and humoral response and does not necessarily equate with protective immunity. In the last decade, veterinary professionals became more demanding for scientific evidence of efficacy in disease prevention of commercially available vaccine products.

Vaccine Adjuvants

An adjuvant is a substance used to increase the immunogenicity of purified peptides or carbohydrates, improve antigen presentation in lymphoid tissues by inducing the expression of major histocompatibility molecules and co-stimulatory molecules, modulate antigen-specific immune response toward a Th1-type or Th2-type response, and decrease the dose of antigen and frequency of administration necessary to achieve vaccine efficacy.[117] Importantly, in the absence of an adjuvant, purified antigens may induce tolerance.

In veterinary medicine, many adjuvants have been used in commercially available vaccines.[118] Aluminum salts (alum) are

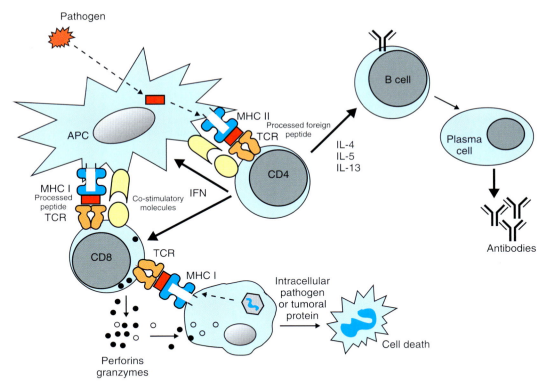

Figure 66-3 Adaptive immunity. Immature dendritic cells phagocytose pathogens in the periphery and become activated with upregulation of major histocompatibility complex class II *(MHC II)* and co-stimulatory molecules (CD86, CD40). They migrate to the regional lymph node and present the processed pathogen to the CD4[+] T cell receptor via MHC II (signal 1); the binding of co-stimulatory molecules with its ligands (CD86 with CD28, and CD40 with CD40 ligand) confirms T-cell activation (signal 2). According to the antigen-presenting cell *(APC)* activation status, CD4[+] T cells differentiate into Th1-type or Th2-type immune cells. Th1-type CD4[+] T cells secrete interferon-gamma *(IFNγ)* and promote the activation of CD8[+] T cells into cytotoxic T cells (CTLs). The CD8[+] T cells can also be activated by APCs via MHC class I antigen presentation of processed antigen (cross-presentation); this process is required for immunity against intracellular pathogens and tumoral cells and for response to vaccines. Th2 CD4[+] T cells secrete cytokines (IL-4, IL-5, IL-13) that promote B-cell differentiation into plasma cells, with subsequent antibody secretion. Therefore, activation of APCs is essential for the development of acquired immunity, and immunomodulators may be used to augment (e.g., adjuvants) or diminish (e.g., glucocorticoids) this process. *TCR,* T-cell receptor.

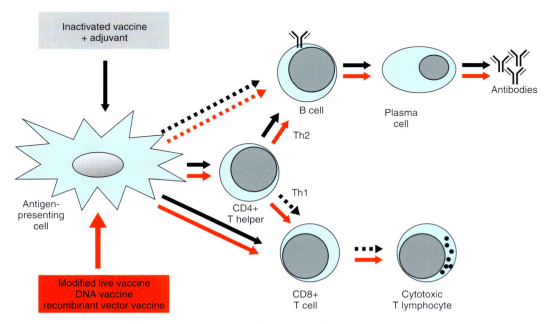

Figure 66-4 Immune response to vaccines. Different vaccine types elicit different levels of humoral and cellular immune response. Inactivated vaccines *(black arrows)* are known to induce high levels of antibodies and depend on the activation of the immune cells by adjuvants. Modified live vaccines, DNA vaccines, and recombinant vector vaccines *(red arrows)* have been shown to induce both antibody production and, importantly, cellular immunity with activation of antigen-specific cytotoxic T lymphocytes (CTLs) that recognize infected cells. The development of CTLs with the use of inactivated vaccines is questionable *(interrupted black arrows)* and may depend on the type of adjuvant.

safe, widely used adjuvants that induce primarily short-lived Th2-type humoral responses.[119] Bacterial structures provide important source of adjuvants, and they are recognized by TLRs in APCs.[120] Freund's complete adjuvant (killed mycobacterium mixed with water-in-oil emulsion) induces strong Th1-type cellular immune responses with potential adverse effects. In contrast, Freund's incomplete adjuvant (water-in-oil emulsion without the killed mycobacterium) has a weaker effect on the immune response with a faint cytokine response. However, it induces stronger Th2-type responses than alum and releases antigen slower that oil-in-water emulsions. Water-in-oil emulsion adjuvants often cause reactions at the injection site. Cholera toxin and *E. coli* exotoxin are promising adjuvants for transcutaneous or mucosal immunizations, with potential to induce humoral and cell-mediated responses. Attenuated *Salmonella enterica* serovar *Typhimurium* expressing key proteins of pathogens has also been tested in vaccine constructs.[121] Synthetic unmethylated CpG-ODNs that mimic bacterial CpG are being widely studied as adjuvants in vaccines to induce a Th1-type immune response.

Liposomes and archaeosomes are lipid vesicles that can be combined with antigens and incorporated in endosomes of APCs to induce both Th1-type and Th-2 type immune responses.[122] Microparticle adjuvants are made of nontoxic polymers, and they may be used for long-term release of antigens in an adverse environment (gastrointestinal tract, nasal passages).[123] When associated with immunomodulators, they can induce both humoral and cell-mediated immune responses. Protein carriers (toxoids, keyhole limpet hemocyanin KLH) can be linked to antigens that are poorly immunogenic or cannot be recognized by the immune system.[124] Saponins are adjuvants originating from plants (Quil A, QS21, and other purified fractions) that can induce both Th1-type and Th2-type responses. Saponins can be associated with cholesterol and phospholipids and form immune-stimulating complexes (ISCOMs), which induce robust Th1-type immune responses.[125] Vaccination against influenza using a product containing ISCOM as adjuvant resulted in greater resistance to disease and reduction of viral shedding than unvaccinated horses when infectious challenge was performed at the time of revaccination 12 months after the initial two doses.[126] For tetanus toxoid vaccine using the same adjuvant, immunity was measured for 24 months after an initial series of three doses of vaccine.

Neonatal Vaccination

The equine fetus is capable of responding to foreign antigens in utero. However, the naïve immune system of the equine neonate takes approximately 2 to 3 months to expand its lymphocyte population in lymphoid tissues, peripheral blood, and organs.[127] During this period, maternal antibodies absorbed from colostrum passively immunize against a large number of pathogens that can be neutralized by humoral mechanisms. Control of intracellular pathogens may be a challenge to the neonate and young foal. Neutralizing antibodies alone may not be sufficient to eliminate or control infection.

Herd management on breeding farms include vaccination of mares 4 to 6 weeks before foaling with killed vaccines to increase the concentration of specific antibodies in colostrum. Paradoxically, there is evidence that maternal antibodies absorbed from colostrum, despite their crucial role in neonatal protection, interfere with the foal's humoral response to vaccine antigens (maternal antibody interference).[128] Questions about the effect of circulating maternal antibodies in the foal's immune response include (1) the potential effect of maternal antibodies on the equine neonatal cellular immune response and response to pathogens during natural exposure, (2) intrinsic limitations of the equine neonate in recognition of certain

vaccine compounds versus others, (3) response to inactivated versus recombinant vector vaccination in foals, and (4) differences in half-lives of maternal antibodies that may affect vaccination schedules. Ideally, a vaccine should induce a rapid immune response that mimics the protective, long-term response that results from natural infection; should bypass maternal antibody interference; and should be immunogenic in the neonate. Successful examples of immunization of equine neonates include the protective humoral response by foals as young as 1-day-old to a recombinant canarypox-vectored equine influenza vaccine and the primary and anamnestic response measured in foals vaccinated with KLH, a highly antigenic protein, in the presence of maternal antibodies.[23,129]

Molecular Vaccines

A vaccine containing DNA is usually composed of naked or plasmid DNA that is directly injected into the target cell. Recombinant vaccines often include a viral vector that promotes endogenous production of a putative protective antigen. These vaccines have developed into several subtypes, one of which involves splicing together genetic material from more than one organism (chimera). Advances in the use of DNA vaccines or recombinant vector vaccines will likely contribute to safe and successful immunization strategies for diseases that require cellular immunity and protection at the point of pathogen encounter (i.e., mucosal vaccines).[130-132] Deoxyribonucleic acid vaccines against equine influenza and *Rhodococcus equi* have been developed and studied, and results have shown limited but promising immune response and protection, including in equine neonates.[133,134]

Cancer Vaccines

Many challenges must be overcome before vaccines can be designed to successfully induce a specific immune response that reverses the progression of tumors.[135] Some cancer vaccines include a cancer-associated antigen and an adjuvant to enhance immune response.[136] For horses, vaccines made from the crude purification of tumor cells have been used as immunotherapy for melanomas, sarcoids, and papillomas, with variable results. Other examples of cancer vaccines studied in human and veterinary medicine include idiotype vaccines (monoclonal antibodies against immunoglobulin expressed on B-cell lymphoma), DNA vaccines (DNA from cancer cells inserted in plasmids that are injected in the patient), heat shock protein-peptide vaccines (cancer antigens associated with heat shock proteins), vector vaccines (virus vectors that encode antigens similar to cancer antigens), genetically altered tumor cells (tumor cells transfected with genes encoding cytokines that activate CTLs or the expression of co-stimulatory molecules), and dendritic cell vaccines (fusion of tumor cells from the patient with APCs).[137-141]

Immunotherapy for Hyposensitization

Immunotherapy may be used in treatment of immunoglobulin E (IgE)–mediated allergies to induce long-term tolerance by the administration of small but increasing concentrations of the known allergen at regular intervals over months to years.[142] The mechanisms involved in successful immunotherapy are not completely understood but may include redirection from a Th2-type response to a Th1-type immune response. Th2-type cytokines (IL-4, IL-13) favor the production of IgE, whereas IFN-γ inhibits the production of those cytokines and promotes the secretion of allergen-specific IgG.[143] Alternatively, immunotherapy increases the secretion of IL-10 by regulatory CD4+CD25+ cells. In horses, immunotherapy has been used to treat atopy or skin hypersensitivity, with variable results (50%-80% response).[144] Although immunotherapy may be an efficient method to minimize clinical signs of hypersensitivity, its future in equine medicine will depend on the development of improved testing for the identification of relevant allergens. DNA vaccines containing vectors encoding specific antigens may substitute protein allergen vaccines. Novel adjuvants that induce Th1-type responses may also be used.[145]

Passive Immunity

Passive immunity is the transfer of preformed antibodies from the immunized individual (donor) to a recipient (patient). Plasma-containing polyvalent immunoglobulins may be used therapeutically to replace deficits of endogenous immunoglobulin production (failure of transfer of immunoglobulins through colostrum in neonates, humoral immunodeficiencies) or to transfer large amounts of specific immunoglobulins from donors immunized with relevant antigens (hyperimmune plasma). Immunoglobulin replacement may prevent and help fight infections or the effects of toxins.

Transfer of Nonspecific Antibodies

Intravenous plasma transfusion with normal plasma is routine practice in neonatal foals with failure of transfer of passive immunity from colostrum and in foals with sepsis. Plasma transfusion increases total serum IgG levels and opsonization capacity in foals.[146,147] In general, serum IgG protective levels are greater than 400 to 500 mg/dL; however, in foals, the goal is to reach concentrations greater than 800 mg/dL because of the high exposure to pathogens in the environment (antibody consumption), short half-life of donor immunoglobulin, and time necessary for endogenous production of immunoglobulins by the foal (4-5 weeks).[148,149]

Circulating antibodies participate in immune defense by neutralizing antigens, facilitating phagocytosis (opsonization), and promoting antibody-dependent cell cytotoxicity (ADCC) by NK cells (Fig. 66-5). Phagocytosis is an essential component of the innate immune system and is facilitated by the presence of opsonins, which may function through C3 receptors (for complement) or Fcγ receptors (for immunoglobulins) on phagocytes. Complement activity in presuckle foals is approximately 13% of adult activity, increasing to 64% by 1 month of age and 85% by 5 months.[150] In foals with sepsis, plasma transfusion is essential to improve opsonization capacity.[151] Recent studies have demonstrated significant individual variation in the opsonic capacity of plasma from different adult horses.[152] This variability is independent of IgG concentrations. The use of pooled plasma from different donors may decrease this variability in the total opsonization capacity.

Transfer of Antigen-Specific Antibodies

Rhodococcus equi

Intravenous administration of commercially available *Rhodococcus equi* hyperimmune plasma obtained from donors vaccinated with *R. equi* antigens increases specific antibody levels against *R. equi* in the serum of foals for 60 days after transfusion.[153] Hyperimmune plasma transfusion provides some benefits in the control of disease on enzootic farms.[154] Using a cell culture model of infection, the use of plasma enriched with specific antibodies for the opsonization of *R. equi* increased oxidative burst activity of phagocytes and the secretion of TNF-α by

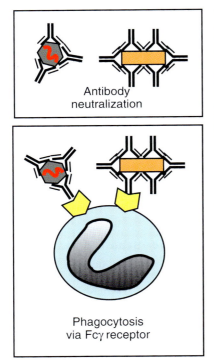

Antibody neutralization

Phagocytosis via Fcγ receptor

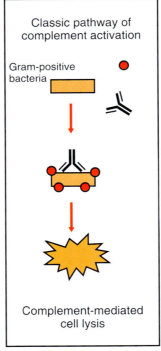

Classic pathway of complement activation

Gram-positive bacteria

Complement-mediated cell lysis

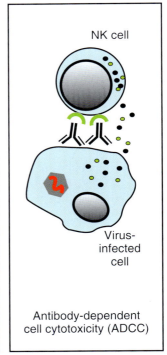

NK cell

Virus-infected cell

Antibody-dependent cell cytotoxicity (ADCC)

Figure 66-5 Mechanisms of antibody-mediated protection. Antibodies can neutralize pathogens by direct binding. They also facilitate phagocytosis (opsonization), and antibody-bound pathogen is phagocytosed via the Fcγ receptor on the cell membrane of neutrophils and macrophages. Antibodies can also activate complement via the classic pathway, which results in cell destruction. In addition, antibody-bound infected cells can be recognized by FcγRIII receptors on natural killer (NK) cells and activate antibody-dependent cell cytotoxicity (ADCC) using perforins and granzymes for target cell destruction.

macrophages in comparison to nonopsonized bacteria and plasma depleted of *R. equi*–specific antibodies. The addition of hyperimmune plasma to broth also decreased the extracellular bacterial viability when compared with broth alone[155] (see Chapter 31).

West Nile Virus

Antibodies against WNV are commercially available for horses in the form of hyperimmune plasma. A trial in hamsters has been performed to test for efficacy of passive transfer against viral challenge in a dose-dependent manner. Plasma transfusion before and 1 day after challenge neutralized the inoculated virus efficiently. A plaque reduction neutralization test (PRNT) using serum from horses that received IV plasma transfusion indicated that 2 mL of plasma/kg body weight provides a titer of 30, which is higher than protective levels obtained after vaccination (PRNT titer of 5). Additional studies are necessary to validate the efficacy of hyperimmune plasma transfusion for treatment of horses with WNV encephalitis (see Chapter 21).

Endotoxemia

In the adult horse with colitis and endotoxemia, the benefit of hyperimmune plasma to the LPS core antigen of *E. coli*, obtained from horses vaccinated with the J5 *E. coli* vaccine, in survival and clinical outcome is controversial. Using an established equine endotoxin challenge model, pretreatment with hyperimmune equine plasma produced from horses immunized against *E. coli* had no significant effect on peak total plasma TNF-α concentration and corresponding clinical signs of endotoxemia but significantly reduced the bioavailable (unbound) TNF-α measured by the bioassay compared to saline-treated controls.[156] It is possible that a reduction in TNF bioactivity was achieved by the binding of factors present in the plasma. In a double-blinded, coded fashion prospective study, critically ill and septic foals receiving commercially available hyperimmune equine plasma or equine plasma specifically rich in antiendotoxin antibodies revealed an increase in survival rate to discharge in the group treated with the latter product.[157] Although plasma transfusion may be beneficial in treatment of endotoxemia, other plasma factors may play a role in this positive effect (see Chapter 11).

Clostridium botulinum

Plasma with high concentrations (>5000 IU and >20,000 IU) of *Clostridium botulinum* type B antitoxin is commercially available for treatment of horses with botulism. In addition, polyvalent hyperimmune plasma is available at the University of Pennsylvania, New Bolton Center.[158] Intravenous administration of botulinum antitoxin is most efficient in the initial phase of disease to neutralize neurotoxins before they bind to the presynaptic membranes at the neuromuscular junctions (see Chapter 43).

Clostridium tetani

Tetanus antitoxin is commercially available for the treatment of tetanus or prevention of disease in nonvaccinated foals and horses with an unknown history of vaccination (see Chapter 44). Combined active-passive method (tetanus toxoid vaccine and tetanus toxoid antiserum) for simultaneous protection and immunization is efficient for prevention of tetanus in the horse.[159] Administration of tetanus antitoxin at high doses intravenously or into the subarachnoid space may be efficacious to block neurotoxins before they bind to gangliosides at the presynaptic inhibitory motor nerve endings.[160] In adult horses, there is a risk of hepatitis secondary to antitoxin administration (serum hepatitis); such a response has not been observed in foals.[161]

Snake Venoms

Snake antivenin for IV use is more often accessible in areas where encounters with poisonous snakes are likely; in general, polyvalent antivenin contains antibodies against toxins of local snakes. The neutralizing ability of the antiserum results primarily from IgG(T).[162] The relatively small amount of venom injected during the bite rarely causes death of a large horse, and local swelling and secondary bacterial infection can be treated with conventional therapy. However, an incident involving a foal or pony may be life-threatening, and early administration of antivenin is recommended.

Transfusion-Induced Immunomodulation

In addition to providing immunoglobulins for protection, antibodies may modulate immune responses by neutralizing circulating foreign antigens in the recipient. At high doses, plasma IgG may compete for Fc-receptor binding on phagocytic cells, resulting in decreased phagocytic function.[163] This effect is desired in the control of inflammatory responses and in the prevention of removal of erythrocytes or platelets with autoantibodies on their surface. Plasma transfusion has been used in horses for this effect in the treatment of immune-mediated anemia or thrombocytopenia.

Plasma transfusion with high concentrations of immunoglobulins accelerates the catabolism and elimination of autoantibodies and is therapeutic in humoral-mediated autoimmune diseases.[164] The clearance of IgG depends on plasma concentrations, and low concentrations may increase plasma half-life up to 10 times. During IgG degradation by endocytosis, immunoglobulins that do not bind endosome receptors are degraded; immunoglobulins that are bound to receptors are protected from degradation and return to circulation (recycled). If there is excess IgG, receptors become saturated, and a large number of IgG molecules are not protected from degradation. Therefore a single dose of plasma with high concentration of IgG induces the accelerated degradation of antibodies.

Transfusion-induced immunomodulation has been studied in human patients who receive whole-blood transfusion. The donor-blood immune cells and antigens (foreign) may be able to modulate the immune system of the recipient in a very complex form.[165] In general, blood transfusion promotes immunotolerance, which can be clinically observed by prolonged graft survival, increased tumor recurrence, and increased susceptibility to infections. Studies in mice and people indicate decreased macrophage function, IL-2 secretion, NK-cell activity, and peripheral blood CD4/CD8 T-cell ratio. Nevertheless, antigens expressed on cells and proteins (antibodies) of the blood donor stimulated antibody production by the recipient's immune system.[166] Antiidiotype antibodies may be produced after whole-blood or plasma transfusion. The recipient may build a humoral and cellular response against the donor antigens. The variable region (idiotype) of the new antibodies becomes antigenic, which then induces antiidiotype antibody production.

Whole-blood transfusion–associated graft-versus-host disease is also a concern. Lymphocytes from the donor may not be recognized and may be destroyed by the recipient's immune system (patients with immunosuppression, neonates) and become engrafted.[167] When activated, donor cells may recognize the recipient cells as foreign and build a T-cell–mediated and NK-cell–mediated immune response against the recipient's cells. Tissue destruction at many levels occurs in the recipient: liver, bone marrow, gastrointestinal tract, and skin. In response to the inflammatory process, the recipient's own cytokines amplify the engrafted-cell effect.[168] Clinical signs associated with this type of response are observed 1 to 3 weeks after blood transfusion and may include fever, pancytopenia, hepatitis, diarrhea, skin rash, hemorrhage, and death.

Immunosuppressants

Immunosuppressive therapy is important in treatment of autoimmune disorders mediated by autoreactive B lymphocytes or T lymphocytes (CD4+ or CD8+ cells). Production of autoantibodies or reactive T lymphocytes can result from molecular mimicry of microbes and self-epitopes, failure of the antiidiotype control mechanism, or development of new epitopes on self-proteins from tissue injury caused by viruses, bacterial exotoxins, or antibiotics.

The ideal immunosuppressant drug would induce longterm, specific inflammatory or immune nonresponsiveness with short-term administration; maintain competent immune response to infectious organisms; and induce minimal adverse systemic effects. Therapeutic use of monoclonal antibodies directed against specific targets of the immune response may eventually allow design of these ideal drugs. The mechanism of action of immunosuppressant drugs has become more specific, largely because of advances in management of organ transplantation patients, with the development of drugs that target defined molecules or response pathways. The combination of drugs to target different sites of cellular metabolism has increased the success of immunosuppressive therapy.

Based on their primary mechanism of action, immunosuppressants may be classified as (1) inhibitors of gene expression or transcription (glucocorticoids), (2) phosphatase (cyclosporine, tacrolimus, rapamycin) and kinase (leflunomide) inhibitors, (3) inhibitors of nucleotide synthesis (azathioprine), (4) alkylating agents (cyclophosphamide, chlorambucil), and (5) monoclonal antibodies (against T-cell receptor, IL-2R).[169,170]

Inhibitors of Gene Expression or Transcription

Glucocorticoids

Glucocorticoids are potent antiinflammatory and immunosuppressant medications that are frequently used to treat inflammatory, allergic, autoimmune, and neoplastic (lymphoma, lymphosarcoma) diseases and to prevent allograft rejection in transplantation. Their effect, duration, and intensity depend on individual pharmacokinetic and pharmacodynamic parameters.[171] Frequently used glucocorticoids in horses include hydrocortisone, dexamethasone, prednisolone, methylprednisolone, isoflupredone, triamcinolone, beclomethasone, and fluticasone.[172-174] In addition to applications in antiinflammatory therapy, glucocorticoids in horses have been used for the treatment of a broad range of diseases that directly involve the immune system: atopy or skin hypersensitivity reactions, contact dermatitis, inflammatory airway disease, recurrent airway obstruction, immune-mediated hemolytic anemia, immune-mediated thrombocytopenia, immune-mediated myositis, uveitis, purpura hemorrhagica, vasculopathy, pemphigus foliaceus, and lymphomas or lymphosarcomas.[175-178]

Glucocorticoids should be used judiciously in the treatment of primary infectious processes (e.g., bacterial, viral, or protozoal meningitis) and in neonates because of their immunosuppressive effect. Chronic treatment with glucocorticoids may lead to susceptibility to infection, hypokalemia, adrenal suppression, hyperglycemia, gastrointestinal ulceration, delayed wound healing, growth suppression, osteoporosis, myopathy, and hypertension. Therefore many studies focus on identifying strategies to inhibit the proinflammatory mediators selectively and treat inflammation or autoimmune diseases without adverse effects.

Box 66-1 Effects of Glucocorticoid Suppressor Mechanisms

- *Migration of inflammatory cells to the site of inflammation:* Reduce the expression of chemotactic proteins and adhesion molecules: macrophage chemotactic protein (MCP-1), intercellular adhesion molecule (ICAM-1), vascular cellular adhesion molecule (VCAM-1), E-selectin, and migration inhibition factor (MIF).
- *Neutrophils, monocytes, and macrophages:* Inhibit phagocytosis, expression of complement and immunoglobulin receptors, bactericidal and fungicidal activity, chemotactic response, and secretion of cytokines (IL-1, IL-6, IL-8, IL-12, IFN-β, TNF-α) and other products (prostaglandins, nitric oxide).
- *T cells:* Suppress proliferative response, IL-2 secretion, and the upregulated expression of the co-stimulatory molecule CD40L ligand on activated CD4+ T cells. Although glucocorticoids decrease cytokine secretion in general, the reduced production of IL-12 and resistant production of IL-10 by monocytes and macrophages result in decreased secretion of IFN-γ and increased production of IL-4, favoring a Th2-type response. In addition, glucocorticoids inhibit early T-cell receptor (TCR) signaling and the transcription of protease granzymes in cytotoxic T cells.
- *Antibodies:* Suppress production of new antibodies.
- *Dendritic cells:* Impair T-cell–mediated terminal maturation of dendritic cells and consequently decrease dendritic cell secretion of IL-1β, IL-6, and TNF-α and expression of co-stimulatory molecule CD86.
- *Eosinophils:* Promote apoptosis.

Glucocorticoids are lipophilic and pass freely through cell membranes. They bind to a cytosolic glucocorticoid receptor (GR), which is a transcription factor that subsequently translocates to the nucleus and regulates gene transcription by binding to glucocorticoid-responsive elements.[179] Importantly, glucocorticoids bind to and inhibit proinflammatory transcription factors NF-κB, activator protein-1 (AP-1), and cyclic adenosine monophosphate (cAMP) response element–binding protein (CREB). In certain cell types, glucocorticoids can increase the synthesis and function of the NF-κB inhibitory protein (iκB-alpha), which prevents NF-κB translocation into the nucleus. This results in repression of transcription and protein synthesis of cytokines, chemokines, inflammatory enzymes, and adhesion molecules[180] (Box 66-1).

Phosphatase and Kinase Inhibitors

Cyclosporine

Cyclosporine is a cyclic polypeptide with immunosuppressive effects. It binds to the cytoplasmic receptor cyclophilin and subsequently to the catalytic domain of the cytoplasmic phosphatase calcineurin.[181] This binding results in the inhibition of dephosphorylation of transcription factors, importantly the nuclear factor of activated T lymphocyte (NFAT), which prevents its translocation to the nucleus. Therefore the production of key elements of T-cell activation and proliferation (IL-2, IL-4, CD40L, TNF-α, IFN-γ, c-myc) is suppressed. Cyclosporine has been used in the horse for intravitreal treatment of recurrent uveitis. Potential adverse effects of cyclosporine include vasoconstriction, hypertension, nephrotoxicity, and hepatotoxicity. Significant bone marrow suppression is not usually observed.

Tacrolimus

Tacrolimus is a macrolide antibiotic that binds to the cytoplasmic FK-binding protein (FKBP), and the resultant protein complex inhibits calcineurin. The NFAT transcription factor is inhibited, and transcription of IL-2, IL-2R, IL-3, IL-4, IL-5, IFN-γ, TNF-α, and GM-CSF is impaired. Tacrolimus is considered to be a more powerful immunosuppressive drug than cyclosporine.

Rapamycin (or Sirolimus)

Rapamycin is a macrolide antibiotic that binds to FKBP and blocks translation of mRNA into proteins required for progression through the G1 phase of the cell cycle. Therefore rapamycin inhibits the proliferative signal generated by IL-2R (late T-cell function inhibitor) and induces cell cycle arrest or apoptosis.

Mycophenolate Mofetil

Mycophenolate mofetil (MMF) is a prodrug of mycophenolic acid that inhibits an important enzyme (inosine monophosphate dehydrogenase [IMPDH]) involved in the de novo biosynthesis of guanosine. This drug is a very specific T- and B-lymphocyte proliferation inhibitor.[182] The most significant adverse effects are diarrhea and gastric ulceration.

Leflunomide

Leflunomide is a synthetic isoxazole prodrug of malononitriloamide, which inhibits a critical tyrosine kinase (DHODH) involved in de novo biosynthesis of pyrimidine. Therefore it inhibits cell proliferation, importantly of T and B cells.

Inhibitors of Nucleotide Synthesis

Azathioprine

Azathioprine is a prodrug of 6-mercaptopurine, a purine analog that is incorporated into the DNA of lymphocytes and inhibits the de novo pathway of purine synthesis. Therefore it inhibits the synthesis of DNA and RNA and consequently, lymphocyte activation and proliferation. Azathioprine has been used in horse for the treatment of immune-mediated anemia, immune-mediated thrombocytopenia, vasculopathy, and pemphigus foliaceus.[183,184] The use of azathioprine allows reduction in glucocorticoid dose when the two are combined in therapy. Because proliferation of many cell types can also be inhibited, adverse effects associated with azathioprine treatment include leukopenia, alopecia, and hepatotoxicity. Pharmacokinetic studies of azathioprine in horses suggest that the drug has low bioavailability and a short terminal half-life, which may limit its usefulness in horses.[185]

Alkylating Agents

Cyclophosphamide and Chlorambucil

The metabolites of the nitrogen mustard derivatives, cyclophosphamide (phosphoramide and acrolein) and chlorambucil (phenylacetic acid mustard), alkylate DNA bases. The results are mutagenic, cytotoxic, antiproliferative, and chemotherapeutic effects. The mutagenic effect increases the risk of development of secondary malignancies. Cyclophosphamide has a greater effect on B cells and therefore is used in the treatment of autoantibody-mediated diseases. In horses, these drugs have been used for the treatment of lymphosarcoma.[186] Adverse effects associated with cyclophosphamide and chlorambucil therapy include anemia, leukopenia, and alopecia.

Vinca Alkaloids

Vincristine

Vincristine is a vinca alkaloid with antitumor, immunosuppressive, and thrombocytopoietic effects. It binds to tubulin in the mitotic spindle and prevents purine synthesis by inhibiting glutamic acid utilization, thus it inhibits cell proliferation. In horses, vincristine has been used for the treatment of immune-mediated thrombocytopenia and fibrosarcoma.[187] Mild neurologic adverse effects (proprioceptive deficits, ileus) may occur.

Monoclonal Antibodies

The development of species-specific monoclonal antibodies (mAbs) and the identification of appropriate antigenic targets have contributed to the advance in the use of mAbs in medicine.[188] The great advantage of mAbs is the specificity of response, which may minimize adverse effects. Examples of mAbs used in the treatment of human cancer are rituximab (targets CD20 on non-Hodgkin's lymphoma), trastuzumab (targets HER2/neu on breast cancer), and daclizumab (targets IL-2Rα on cutaneous T-cell lymphoma and hairy B-cell leukemia). The use of mAbs linked to cytotoxic drugs or radioisotopes is currently being investigated. These antibodies would deliver toxins to specific cancer cell targets and minimize systemic exposure (e.g., gemtuzumab for treatment of myelogenous leukemia).[189]

In autoimmune disorders (e.g., T-cell–mediated psoriases), IV single-dose injection of anti–IL-12 mAbs is well tolerated and induces concentration-dependent improvement of psoriatic lesions.[190] The anti–IFN-γ (infliximab), which blocks this crucial inflammatory mediator in its early signaling, has been approved for the treatment of human rheumatoid arthritis, Crohn's disease, ankylosing spondylitis, and vasculitis.[191]

The complete reference list is available online at www.expertconsult.com.

Infectious Disease Rule-Outs for Medical Problems*

Maureen T. Long and Debra C. Sellon

Respiratory Problems

Cough

Pleuropneumonia (1, 28, 45)
Pharyngeal or laryngeal abscess (1, 28, 25)
Pulmonary abscess (1)
Guttural pouch empyema or mycosis (1, 28, 52)
Bacterial pneumonia (1, 28, 45)
Equine influenza (12, 13)
Equine herpesvirus (12, 14)
Equine viral arteritis (12, 15)
African horse sickness (12, 16)
Equine rhinovirus (1, 12, 17)
Equine adenovirus (1, 12, 17)
Hendra virus (12, 17)
Strangles (27, 28)
Nocardiosis (27, 45)
Rhodococcus equi (27, 31)
Tuberculosis (27, 33)
Glanders (27, 36)
Pneumocystosis (27, 46, 53)
Pneumocystis carinii infection (46, 53)
Coccidioidomycosis (46, 47)
Pythiosis, zygomycosis (46, 55)
Pulmonary aspergillosis (46, 56)
Cryptococcosis (54, 57)
Parascaris equorum larval migration (54, 62)
Lungworms (54, 62)

Nasal Discharge

Lymphoid pharyngeal hyperplasia (1)
Bacterial pneumonia (1)
Pleuropneumonia (1)
Guttural pouch mycosis (1)
Lung abscess (1)
Guttural pouch empyema, chondroids (1, 28)
Equine influenza (13)
Equine herpesvirus (14)
Equine viral arteritis (15)
African horse sickness (16)
Equine adenovirus (17)
Equine rhinovirus (16)
Hendra virus (16)
Strangles (28)
Nocardiosis (30)
Rhodococcus equi (31)
Tuberculosis (45)

Glanders (36)
Coccidioidomycosis (47)
Ascarid migration (62)
Nasal fungal infection (54, 60)
Pulmonary aspergillosis (52)
Cryptococcosis (53)
Surra *(Trypanosoma evansi)* (60)
Dourine *(Trypanosoma equinum)* (60)
Besnoitiosis (60)
Ascarid migration (57)
Lungworm infection (57)

Respiratory Noise

Arytenoid chondritis (1)
Guttural pouch empyema (1, 28)
Strangles (1, 28)
Conidiobolomycosis (1, 51)

Rhinitis, Sinusitis

Glanders (36)
Conidiobolomycosis (46, 51)
Aspergillosis (1, 52)
Cryptococcus (1, 53)

Pleural Effusion

Pleuropneumonia (1)
African horse sickness (16)

Dyspnea

Pneumonia (1, 28, 45)
Pleuropneumonia (1, 28, 45)
Aspiration pneumonia (1)
Interstitial pneumonia (1)
Endocarditis (2)
Myocarditis (2)
Neonatal septicemia (6)
Influenza (13)
Equine herpesviruses (14)
Adenovirus (17)
Hendra virus (17)
Rhinovirus (1, 17)
Streptococcal diseases (28)
Corynebacterium pseudotuberculosis (45)
Rhodococcus equi (31)
Mycobacteria (27, 45)
Glanders (36)
Anaerobic infection (45)
Pneumocystosis (46, 53)

---

*Numbers in parentheses refer to chapters in which diseases are discussed.

Pulmonary aspergillosis (52)
Pulmonary habronemiasis (57)
Lungworms (57)
Ascarid migration (57)

Gastrointestinal Problems

Diarrhea in Adult Horses

Aeromonas spp. (3)
Mycobacterial infections (27)
Endotoxemia (11)
Salmonellosis (35)
Neorickettsia risticii infection (40)
Enteric clostridia (41)
Histoplasmosis (53)
Cryptosporidiosis (60)
Giardiasis (60)
Parasitism (54, 57, 58, 60)
Cyathostomiasis (57)
Cestodes (58)

Diarrhea in Foals

Aeromonas spp. (3)
Neonatal septicemia (6)
Rotavirus (18)
Coronavirus (18)
Rhodococcus equi (31)
Lawsonia intracellularis (34)
Endotoxemia (11)
Salmonellosis (35)
Clostridium perfringens type A, B, or C (41)
Clostridium difficile (41)
Tyzzer's disease (42)
Cryptosporidiosis (60)
Giardiasis (60)
Gastrointestinal parasites (57, 58, 60)
Strongyloidosis (58)

Abdominal Pain

Peritonitis (3)
Abdominal abscess (3)
Neonatal septicemia (6)
Oophoritis (8)
Equine viral arteritis (15)
African horse sickness (16)
Rabies (19)
West Nile virus (21)
Purpura hemorrhagica (*Streptococcus zooepidemicus* subsp. *equi*)
   (28)
Corynebacterium pseudotuberculosis (45)
Anthrax (45)
Rhodococcus equi (31)
Lawsonia intracellularis (3, 34)
Endotoxemia (11)
Salmonellosis (35)
Neorickettsia risticii infection (40)
Enteric clostridia (41)
Botulism (43)
Tetanus (44)
Pythiosis (51)
Piroplasmosis (56)
Ascarid impaction (57)
Strongylosis (57)
Cestodes (58)

Dysphagia

Guttural pouch mycosis (1)
Guttural pouch empyema (1, 28)
Pharyngeal or laryngeal infection or abscess (1, 28)
Oral infection (3)
Bacterial meningitis or encephalitis (4, 20, 21)
Rabies (19)
Alphaviruses (20)
West Nile virus infection (21)
Strangles (28)
Botulism (43)
Tetanus (44)
Equine protozoal myeloencephalitis (55)
Sarcocystosis (60)
Tick paralysis (59)

Icterus

Cholangiohepatitis, cholangitis (3)
Hepatic abscess (3, 28, 30)
Equine viral arteritis (15)
Equine infectious anemia (23)
Leptospirosis (32)
Anaplasma phagocytophilum infection (39)
Neorickettsia risticii infection (40)
Tyzzer's disease (42, 45)
Piroplasmosis (56)
Surra (60)
Dourine (60)
Ascarids (57)

Oral Ulcerations or Vesicles

Equine herpesvirus (14)
Equine viral arteritis (15)
Vesicular stomatitis (24)
Jamestown Canyon virus (26)
Mycobacterial infections (27)

Hepatomegaly, Hepatic Inflammation

Equine infectious anemia (23)
Rhodococcus equi (31)
Mycobacterial infections (27)
Leptospirosis (32)
Endotoxemia (11)
Tyzzer's disease (45)
Echinococcosis (61)

Abdominal Mass

Abdominal abscess (3, 27, 28, 45)
Strangles (28)
Corynebacterium pseudotuberculosis (45)
Rhodococcus equi (31)
Mycobacterium spp. (27, 45)
Echinococcus infection (60)

Abdominal Effusion

Abdominal abscess (3)
Peritonitis (3)
Streptococcal infections (28)
Rhodococcus equi (31)
Coccidioidomycosis (47)
Verminous arteritis (57)
Corynebacterium pseudotuberculosis (60)

Central Nervous System Problems

Cortical Signs

Parasite migration (4, 57, 60)
Brain abscess, meningitis (4, 28, 45)
Neonatal septicemia (6)
Equine herpesvirus type 1 (14)
Rabies (19)
Eastern equine encephalitis (20)
Western equine encephalitis (20)
Venezuelan equine encephalitis (20)
Japanese encephalitis virus (21)
West Nile virus (21)
Borna disease (22)
Main Drain virus (26)
Snowshoe hare virus (26)
Jamestown Canyon virus (26)
Equine encephalosis (26)
Glanders (36)
Candidiasis (49)
Cryptococcus neoformans (60)
Equine protozoal myeloencephalitis (55)
Piroplasmosis (56)

Brainstem Signs

Temporohyoid osteoarthropathy (1)
Guttural pouch mycosis or empyema
  (1, 28)
Parasite migration (4, 61)
Brainstem abscess (4, 28)
Equine herpesvirus type 1 (12, 14)
Rabies (12, 19)
West Nile virus (12, 21)
Borna disease (12, 22)
Equine protozoal myeloencephalitis (55)

Spinal Cord or Peripheral Nerve Signs

Vertebral body abscess (4-6, 27-29, 35)
Diskospondylitis (4)
Equine herpesvirus type 1 (14)
Rabies (19)
West Nile virus (21)
Borna disease (22)
Equine infectious anemia (23)
Rhodococcus equi (31)
Lyme disease (33)
Anaplasma phagocytophilum (39)
Botulism (43)
Tetanus (44)
Protozoal myeloencephalitis (55)
Dourine (60)
Surra (60)
Tick paralysis (59)

Urinary Tract Problems

Dysuria, Stranguria, Pollakiuria

Cystitis (9)
Urethritis (9)
Pyelonephritis (9)
Urinary calculi (9)
Habronemiasis (60)

Incontinence

Parasite migration (4, 62)
Equine herpesvirus type 1 (14)
Rabies (19)
Protozoal myeloencephalitis (55)

Hematuria

Seminal vesiculitis (8)
Cystitis (9)
Urinary tract infection (9)
Urolithiasis (9)
Corynebacterium pseudotuberculosis (45)
Leptospirosis (32, 34)
Endotoxemia (11)
Salmonellosis (35)
Enteric clostridia (41)
Habronemiasis (60)

Renal Failure

Pyelonephritis (9)
Urolithiasis (9)
Leptospirosis (32)
Endotoxemia, sepsis (11)
Protozoal myeloencephalitis (55)

Musculoskeletal Problems

Myositis, Increased Muscle Enzyme Activity

Sarcocystosis (5, 60)
Equine influenza (13)
Equine herpesviruses (14)
African horse sickness (16)
Strangles (28)
Streptococcal infections (28)
Clostridial myonecrosis (42)
Anaerobic bacterial infections (45)
Surra (60)

Lameness, Stiffness, Arthritis

Aortoiliac thrombosis (2)
Septic arthritis (5)
Osteomyelitis (5)
Bacterial tenosynovitis (5)
Neonatal septicemia (6)
Rabies (19)
West Nile virus (21)
Borna disease (22)
Purpura hemorrhagica (strangles) (28)
Streptococcal infections (28)
Staphylococcal infections (29)
Corynebacterium pseudotuberculosis (45)
Rhodococcus equi (31)
Lyme disease (33)
Endotoxemia (11)
Brucellosis (37)
Neorickettsia risticii infection (40)
Clostridial myonecrosis (42)
Tetanus (44)
Coccidioidomycosis (47)
Candidiasis (49)
Equine protozoal myeloencephalitis (55)

Muscle Fasciculations

Rabies (19)
West Nile virus (21)
Borna disease (22)
Anthrax (45)
Endotoxemia (11)
Botulism (43)
Tetanus (44)

Cardiovascular Problems

Cardiomyopathy, Myocarditis, Endocarditis

Bacterial endocarditis (2)
Inflammatory valvulitis (2)
Equine influenza (13)
Equine herpesvirus (14)
African horse sickness (16)
Streptococcal infections (1, 28)
Rhodococcus equi (31)
Anaplasma phagocytophilum (39)

Reproductive Problems

Abortion, Infertility, Early Embryonic Loss, Birth of Weak Foals

Endometritis (8)
Pyometra (8)
Oophoritis (8)
Salpingitis (8)
Neospora spp. (8)
Nocardioform placentitis (8)
Aeromonas hydrophila (8)
Chlamydiosis (8)
Mycoplasma infection (8)
Bacterial placentitis (8)
Fungal placentitis (8)
Equine herpesvirus type 1 (14)
Equine viral arteritis (15)
Equine infectious anemia (23)
Streptococcal infections (28)
Rhodococcus equi (31)
Mycobacterial infections (45)
Leptospirosis (32)
Salmonellosis (35)
Brucellosis (37)
Contagious equine metritis (38)
Neorickettsia risticii infection (40)
Coccidioidomycosis (47)
Candidiasis (49)
Aspergillosis (52)
Piroplasmosis (56)
African animal trypanosomiasis (60)
Surra (60)
Dourine (60)

Scrotal/Preputial Enlargement

Epididymitis (8)
Equine herpesvirus type 3 (8)
Orchitis (8)
Streptococcal infections (8, 28)
Corynebacterium pseudotuberculosis (45)

Glanders (36)
Dourine (60)
Habronemiasis (57)
Onchocerciasis (57)

Hemolymphatic Problems

Enlarged Lymph Nodes

Upper respiratory tract infection (1)
Equine influenza (13)
Equine herpesviruses (14)
Equine rhinovirus (16)
Equine adenovirus (17)
Strangles (28)
Corynebacterium pseudotuberculosis (45)
Rhodococcus equi (31)
Mycobacterial infections (45)
Glanders (36)
Pythiosis (51)
Histoplasmosis (60)
Cryptococcosis (53)
Blastomycosis (53)

Lymphangitis

Epizootic lymphangitis (53)
Corynebacterium pseudotuberculosis (45)
Rhodococcus equi (31)
Glanders (36)
Sporotrichosis (48)

Anemia

Equine infectious anemia (23)
Streptococcal infection (28)
Corynebacterium pseudotuberculosis (45)
Anaplasma phagocytophilum (39)
Clostridial myonecrosis (42)
Piroplasmosis (babesiosis) (56)
Dourine (60)
Surra (60)
African animal trypanosomiasis (60)
Gastrointestinal parasitism (57, 58, 60)

Petechial Hemorrhages

Neonatal septicemia (6)
Equine viral arteritis (15)
Equine infectious anemia (23)
Purpura hemorrhagica (strangles) (28)
Endotoxemia, septicemia, bacteremia (11)
Salmonellosis (35)
Anaplasma phagocytophilum (39)
Neorickettsia risticii infection (40)
Equine protozoal myeloencephalitis (55)
African animal trypanosomiasis (60)
Surra (60)

Ventral Abdominal or Limb Edema

Pleuritis, pleuropneumonia (1)
Pericarditis (2)
Thrombophlebitis (2)
Bacterial endocarditis (2)

Equine herpesvirus (14)
Equine viral arteritis (15)
Equine infectious anemia (23)
Purpura hemorrhagica (strangles) (28)
Corynebacterium pseudotuberculosis
   (45)
Anthrax (45)
Mycobacterial infections (45)
Endotoxemia (11)
Anaplasma phagocytophilum (39)
Monocytic ehrlichiosis (43)
Protozoal myeloencephalitis (55)
Dourine (60)
Surra (60)
African animal trypanosomiasis (60)
Gastrointestinal parasitism (57, 58, 60)

Hypoalbuminemia

Mycobacterial infections (45)
Lawsonia intracellularis (36)
Salmonellosis (35)
Enteric clostridia (41)
Gastrointestinal parasitism (57, 58, 60)
Cyathostomiasis (57)
Equine herpesvirus type 2 (14)
African animal trypanosomiasis (60)

Thrombocytopenia

Equine viral ateritis (15)
African horse sickness (16)
Equine infectious anemia (23)
Endotoxemia (11)
Salmonellosis (35)
Anaplasma phagocytophilum (39)
Neorickettsia risticii infection (40)
Enteric clostridia (41)
Babesiosis (57)
Trypanosomiasis (60)

Ocular Problems

Uveitis

Neonatal septicemia (6)
Viral infection (10)
Setaria infection (10)
Verminous migration (10, 57)
Uveitis (10, 34)
Streptococcal infections (28)
Rhodococcus equi (31)
Leptospirosis (32)
Lyme disease (33)
Anaplasma phagocytophilum (39)
Onchocerciasis (57)

Keratitis

Temporohyoid osteoarthropathy
   (1)
Neonatal septicemia (6)
Bacterial keratitis (10)
Fungal keratitis (10, 52)
Equine herpesviruses (13)
Dourine (60)
Onchocerciasis (57)

Conjunctivitis

Chlamydiosis (10)
Thelazia (10)
Equine influenza (13)
Equine herpesviruses (14)
Equine viral arteritis (15)
African horse sickness (16)
Equine adenovirus (17)
Streptococcal infections (28)
Lyme disease (33)
Blastomycosis (53)
Epizootic lymphangitis (53)
Protozoal myeloencephalitis (55)
Surra (60)
Dourine (60)
Besnoitiosis (57)
Onchocerciasis (57)
Habronemiasis (57)

Corneal Edema

Equine herpesvirus type 2 (14)
Leptospirosis (32)
Aspergillosis (52)
Onchocerciasis (57)

Blindness

Guttural pouch empyema (1)
Brain abscess (4)
Meningitis (4)
Toxoplasmosis (10)
Echinococcosis (10, 60)
Equine leukoencephalomalacia (10)
Rabies (19)
Alphavirus encephalitides (20)
Japanese encephalitis (21)
West Nile virus (21)
Aspergillosis (52)
Equine protozoal myeloencephalitis (55)

Skin Problems

Hair Loss

Dermatophilosis (30)
Dermatophytosis (50)
Besnoitiosis (60)
Pinworms (57)
Onchocerciasis (57)
Lice (59)
Mite infestation (59)
Culicoides hypersensitivity (59)

Pruritus

Malassezia infection (7)
Folliculitis (7)
Besnoitiosis (7, 60)
Rabies (19)
Dermatophilosis (30)
Dermatophytosis (50)
Onchocerciasis (57)
Pinworms (57)
Culicoides hypersensitivity (59)
Pediculosis (59)

Lice (59)
Mites (59)

Crusting, Scaling

Bacterial folliculitis (7)
Malassezia infection (7)
Poxvirus (7, 26)
Besnoitiosis (7, 61)
Dermatophilosis (7, 30)
Dermatophytosis (7, 50)
Onchocerciasis (7, 62)
Culicoides hypersensitivity (7, 59)
Mite infestation (7, 64)

Ulcers, Fistulas, Granulomatous Lesions

Leishmaniasis (7)
Equine sarcoid (25)
Staphylococcal infections (29)
Corynebacterium pseudotuberculosis (45)
Nocardiosis (27, 45)
Mycobacterial infections (45)
Glanders (36)
Brucellosis (37)
Sporotrichosis (48)
Pythiosis (46, 51)
Basidiobolomycosis (46, 51)
Mucormycosis (46, 51)
Habronemiasis (60)
Myiasis (59)

Papulonodular Lesions

Bacterial furunculosis (7)
Molluscum contagiosum (7)
Leishmaniasis (7)
Papillomatosis (25)

Dermatophytosis (50)
Fly or tick bites (59)
Warbles (59)
Straw itch mites (59)

Large Nodular Dermatoses or Abscesses

Equine sarcoid (7, 25)
Streptococcal infections (28)
Staphylococcal infections (29)
Corynebacterium pseudotuberculosis (45)
Nocardiosis (27, 45)
Rhodococcus equi (31)
Mycobacterial infections (45)
Glanders (36)
Coccidioidomycosis (47)
Sporotrichosis (48)
Zygomycosis (51)
Pythiosis (51)

Sudden Death

Collapse and Sudden Death

Guttural pouch mycosis (acute hemorrhage) (1)
Septic thromboembolism (2)
Ruptured pulmonary or abdominal abscess (3)
Neonatal septicemia (6)
Hendra virus (26)
Anthrax (45)
Salmonellosis (35)
Neorickettsia risticii infection (40)
Enteric clostridia (41)
Clostridial myonecrosis (42)
Tyzzer's disease (foals) (45)
Botulism (43)

Laboratories Molecular Testing for Infectious Diseases

B

Maureen T. Long

Since the 1990s, a rapid explosion in molecular-based diagnostics has occurred in veterinary medicine. Contemporaneous with this expansion, training in diagnostic medicine is declining because of loss of state and federal support of veterinary training and lack of interest in veterinary students, who primarily track into clinical programs.[1,2] Most molecular diagnostic tests presently emphasize the polymerase chain reaction (PCR) format. The most current application is a real-time format; most companies have now developed formats that can perform a 40-cycle PCR test in 35 to 45 minutes in a high-throughput format once nucleic acids are extracted.[3] With robotics, samples can be processed and results obtained within a very short window of time. Regardless of technologic advances that apply, the same basic concepts apply when submitting samples for diagnostic testing that are based on either high-throughput or new technologies.[4,5]

Understanding Older and Newer Formats for Detection of Infection

Table 1 lists the basic definitions of PCR methods. A basic understanding of the different PCR test formats is needed for continuing education of practitioners and diplomates.[1] Although it is not necessary for the practitioner to be a molecular biologist, Table 1 provides a short review of the definitions of molecular testing.

Proper Procedures: Collection, Transport, Storage

The main advantage of genomic strategies for testing is that a live organism is not needed for diagnosis. Although diagnosis based on molecular techniques does not require a live organism, DNA and RNA are subject to the same microbiologic, biochemical, and physical factors as live organisms for degradation.[6] In some situations, genomic DNA may be robust in its survival for forensic purposes; however, overgrowth and chemical contamination of a small microbiologic sample could result in false-negative reactions for any of the aforementioned molecular techniques. A sample collected using the correct media that is solely dedicated for PCR testing should be taken. For blood, ethylenediamine tetraacetic acid (EDTA) or purple top tubes are best. Use of EDTA as an anticoagulant for testing of virus in plasma or buffy coat is applicable for most genomic techniques and viral culture techniques. However, if one wishes to culture plasma (e.g., that of a foal) for bacteria, EDTA is bacteriostatic, and a blood culture bottle must also be collected. Anticoagulants such as heparin can inhibit PCR reactions especially when a kit extraction method is used, which is likely to be the typical formats in most diagnostic laboratories.

For detection of nasal or respiratory pathogens, wooden swabs contain formalin, which can inhibit PCR (fixed tissue methods are performed on paraffin, and formalin has been removed in the paraffin process). Plastic, polypropylene sticks with Dacron or rayon swabs, *not* those with calcium alginate, are essential for nasal swabbing.[7] Cotton allows bacteria and virus to become embedded in fibers, and frequently the extraction method calls for direct extraction off the swab. This step inactivates most viruses and bacteria because of the detergent used in the first lysis step. Finally, use of a transport medium is best for viruses because this inhibits overgrowth of bacteria that may inactivate and break down nucleic acids needed for the successful detection of viruses. The proteins in the viral medium also assist in keeping the virus in a biologically active state, so this is preferable for viral culture also.

Most testing has been validated on specimens that have been collected under the best conditions without inhibitors and contamination stored appropriately. Specimens requiring storage before shipping to a laboratory should not be stored, and the *most* optimal time for testing by PCR is less than 3 days in a sample stored consistently at 4°C. If one cannot ship a horse sample within the allotted time, the sample should be allowed to sit in a refrigerator for 20 minutes and then the plasma drawn off and placed in a new tube without any anticoagulants. For horses, the sample should *not* be centrifuged. The white blood cells of horses settle in this time and do not form a buffy coat that is adhered to red blood cells (RBCs). This allows collection of as few RBCs as possible.[8] This is essential because as RBCs lyse in older samples, heavy protein contamination occurs, and these particular proteins (iron) are toxic to many PCR reactions. Many laboratories historically have indicated shipment at either 4°C or not to exceed 75°C. The latter is not appropriate for blood or nasal specimens because of the potential for hemolysis or bacterial overgrowth, respectively. All samples should be shipped on ice packs *(no wet ice)* overnight for arrival within 24 hours. One should not ship expecting successful Saturday delivery, and it is our experience that samples become lost more frequently with weekend deliveries.

Standardization

There is no federal body or international body that consistently provides methodologic standardization for infectious diseases. Several organizations exist to which laboratories may belong or adhere to and can be accredited for quality assurance and control standards; however, these organizations, owing to their mission and funding constraints, usually focus on either

Table 1 Basic Description of Polymerase Chain Reaction Methods

Technique	Description	What Is a Positive Test	Advantage	Disadvantage
Conventional PCR	Basic amplification of target that is part of the genome originating from DNA	Gel-based test that in most laboratories is based on analysis of correct target by size only. May be inherently inaccurate depending on system. For closely related bacteria, parasites, and fungi, restriction enzyme digest of targets needs to be frequently performed. Ultimately confirmation with a probe (Southern blot) confirms specificity, but many laboratories do not perform routinely	Faster than culture of organism. Does not require live organism in most cases	Slow and less sensitive than real-time. Less automation available. May be less specific if analysis of end product not performed
Conventional reverse transcriptase PCR	Basic amplification of target that is part of the genome originating from RNA. An extra step is utilized before PCR, where a viral reverse transcription enzyme transcribes the RNA into cDNA for amplification	Gel-based test that in most laboratories is based on analysis of correct target by size only. May be inherently inaccurate depending on system. For closely related bacteria, parasites, and fungi, restriction enzyme digest of targets needs to be frequently performed. Ultimately confirmation with a probe (Southern blot) confirms specificity, but many laboratories do not perform routinely	Faster than culture of organism. Does not require live organism in most cases	Slow and less sensitive than real-time. Less automation available. May be less specific if analysis of end product not performed
Real-time PCR	Still basic PCR amplification, but coupled to a fluorochrome and light detection system. The target is DNA	The use of a probe in addition to primers provides specificity within the assay	Very fast analysis. Same cycle number is more sensitive than conventional PCR but still may be less sensitive than nested PCR. More specific because of probe that binds to generated target	Still can have contamination issues. May have false-positive issues owing to high sensitivity
Real-time reverse transcriptase PCR	Still basic PCR amplification, but coupled to a fluorochrome and light detection system. The target is RNA where a viral reverse transcription enzyme transcribes the RNA into cDNA for PCR amplification	Use of a probe in addition to primers provides specificity within the assay	Very fast analysis. Same cycle number is more sensitive than conventional PCR. More specific because of probe that binds to generated target	Still can have contamination issues. May have false-positive issues owing to high sensitivity

laboratory maintenance as a form of quality assurance or a subset of diseases for a given set of syndromes. There is a relative lack of standardization in both human and veterinary molecular diagnostic testing, and it is estimated that in herpes simplex virus testing alone, there is a 7.9% false-positive rate and a 14% false-negative rate when proficiency testing is examined.[9]

International Standards

The World Organization for Animal Health (OIE), based in France, is an intergovernmental agency whose main mission is to track contagious animal diseases.[8] The Web site of this organization, http://www.oie.int/eng/en_index.htm, contains some of the most up-to-date information regarding world disease outbreaks in animals. Within the last several years, the focus has included veterinary pathogens with public health significance, animal welfare, food safety, and ethical use of antimicrobials. In terms of infectious diseases, this body has generated an important document, "Terrestrial Animal Health Code." This is a reference document and historically has been used by governmental veterinary officers, epidemiologists, and import/export services. However, *any* practitioner that is involved with the international shipment of animals should be familiar with these principles for disease control. Since the 1960s, this body has strived to develop standards, guidelines, and recommendations that contribute to preventing the transfer of infectious agents

between countries. The guidelines for testing focus on what many countries consider foreign animal diseases (FADs) should exposure or outbreak occur in their country. The tests included in international trade are for horses, cattle, swine, goats, and bees, and the diseases affecting horse and horse movement include:

Vesicular stomatitis virus (VSV), vesicular swine disease (VSD), Rift Valley fever, African horse sickness (AHS), echinococcosis, leptospirosis, rabies, leishmaniasis, contagious equine metritis, dourine, equine encephalomyelitis viruses (eastern, western, and Venezuelan), equine infectious anemia, equine influenza, equine piroplasmosis, equine rhinopneumonitis, glanders, equine viral arteritis, horse mange, epizootic lymphangitis, Japanese encephalitis virus, trypanosomiasis, Bunyavirus diseases, salmonellosis, mange, West Nile virus (WNV), *Campylobacter jejuni*, cryptosporidiosis, Hendra and Nipah viruses, and listeriosis.

Generally, the regulated equine diseases do not have PCR as a trade test; however, PCR methodologies and their recommended reagents are listed in the OIE for several equine tests. As of this writing, the OIE is in the process of adopting PCR for screening of horses for AHS. With adoption of this format as a gold standard, this could revolutionize the South African horse industry because of worldwide embargos of horses from AHS endemic areas in Africa. In addition, the OIE has developed several criteria that are based on the very tough international standards developed for trading countries called ISO/IEE compliance in 1999.[9]

North American Standards

The American Association of Veterinary Laboratory Diagnosticians (AAVLD) is a nonprofit organization that works to communicate through the diagnostic laboratory system information regarding the diagnosis of animal diseases (http://www.aavld.org/mc/page.do). A main tenet of their mission is to assist laboratories in establishing uniform diagnostic techniques and improvement of existing techniques. Only public supported laboratories can be part of this system, and the laboratories must be integrated. Table 2 lists all of the North American accredited laboratories and the tests available by PCR. The AAVLD laboratories must provide in their inspections evidence for quality assurance and quality control of their tests but do not standardize individual techniques. Because these are public institutions, in-state testing is usually subsidized and therefore much less expensive than a private laboratory. By the same token, overnight service may not be available through these laboratories.

The United States Department of Agriculture Animal Health inspection service provides proficiency testing and several laboratories below to the National Animal Health Laboratory Network. This is a state and federal partnership to protect mainly against FADs. Currently, there is no certification for any equine disease except for VSV. Public and private laboratories can be approved to run regulated tests by APHIS (http://www.aphis.usda.gov/animal_health/lab_info_services/approved_labs.shtml), which for horses includes contagious equine metritis, equine infectious anemia, equine viral arteritis, and VSV.

Private Laboratories

There is no accreditation that an outside laboratory can seek that provides protocol-based guidelines for laboratories to follow except for proficiency in regulated tests. One private laboratory has dry card testing available, whereby blood and other fluid samples are spotted on the card and tested. This type of testing is appropriate only for infections that are highly represented in fluid samples and for which there is a high amount of agent in the sample.[10] This would include blood, cerebrospinal fluid (CSF), and joint fluid, which usually is not where equine infectious agents are in abundance during clinical stages of disease. Many of these laboratories trademark their testing protocols, and understandably the primers and targets are kept as trade secrets; thus, further standardization and independent validation are not likely except through proficiency laboratory testing. Table 3 lists private molecular testing laboratories.

Interpretation of Polymerase Chain Reaction Results

Given the problems with inappropriate sampling and handling and lack of standards for these new techniques, what can be said regarding interpretation of test results? There is no question that molecular medicine has dramatically revolutionized infectious disease diagnosis, treatment, and especially biosecurity. In the long run, molecular-based assays are more efficient and allow for minimal exposure of laboratory personnel and

veterinarians to many infectious agents.[11] Ultimately, nothing will take the place of isolation of an infectious agent as confirmation of active infection from a properly collected and handled sample, but the efficiency and accuracy with good sampling and laboratory standardization make testing strategy of PCR diagnostics the most common in the future.

Given that sampling, handling, and all quality assurance for a particular laboratory are reliable, one must understand what a positive or a negative genomic-based test means. For instance, a positive PCR test result means that nucleic acids that belong to the genome of that particular pathogen were detected in the sample. This agent may or may not be live, infectious, or capable of replication in that sample. At least three different scenarios may be occurring in regard to the sample tested: (1) the pathogen is present and directly is causing the clinical signs observed, (2) the pathogen is present but is not responsible for the clinical signs observed, or (3) the pathogen is not present but the reaction mixture is binding to some other target in the assay. By the same token, a negative sample has failed to detect the nucleic acids of the infectious agent. A negative result can reflect at least three different scenarios in regard to the sample tested: (1) the pathogen was absent at the time of testing, (2) the pathogen is present but not detectable within the limits of sensitivity, and (3) there was some type of inhibition of the positive reaction. The mere results cannot be interpreted without understanding the context in which testing was performed in the first place unless this is used for regulatory purposes. In the absence of case criteria, the results by themselves are not confirmatory for disease causation. This is especially true for negative tests—hence repeated sampling is recommended should the case criteria create a high degree of suspicion for that disease. In the end, a comprehensive investigation using multiple samples employing different detection formats may be the only way to confirm disease causation in an outbreak or new emergence of disease in a group of animals. There is no "magic bullet" when it comes to testing.

Status of Molecular Testing for Particular Diseases

Vesicular Diseases

Vesicular diseases are highly infectious agents that usually have very high morbidity with low mortality. However, their intensive infectiousness and painful nature when involved in outbreaks in hoofed livestock result in economic catastrophe. Investigatory laboratories around the world have developed several PCR assays that detect simultaneously (called a multiplex reaction) several vesicular viruses.[12] These assays will likely revolutionize early detection of outbreak spread but so far have several issues. Both conventional and real-time formats are available, and the OIE investigatory laboratories are working on some of these assays. The initial assays focused on detection of foot and mouth disease virus (FMDV) and SVD. No incorporation was made for VSV, a disease affecting cattle and horses of economic importance with disease activity in the United States. The VSV PCR is still run as a separate assay format. In addition, many subtypes of FMDV exist, and not all of the techniques available incorporate primers and probes that detect all subtypes. The most comprehensive assay in the literature is a "conventional" PCR format, and this was validated by testing "spiked" samples and experimentally inoculated swine.[13] Limited multiplex real-time PCR formats have been developed, but these were validated on a limited number of samples. Development of these tests is crucial for rapid disease surveillance. In experimental inoculation, virus detection (SVD, VSV, and FMDV) was possible even with multiplex conventional reverse transcriptase PCR in either blood or serum by the first and second

Table 2 Comprehensive Listing All AAVLD Laboratories within the United States That Perform Testing via Molecular Diagnostics

Location and Web site	EEE	WEE	WNV	EHV-1	EHV-2	EHV-3	EHV-4	INFA	EVA	S. EQUI	R. EQUI	SALM	CDIFF	CPERF	PHF	LAWSO	LEPTO	ROTA	SNEUR	NOCAD	ANA	LYME	LIST
Arizona Veterinary Diagnostic Laboratory http://microvet.arizona.edu/AzVDL/index.shtml	✓	✓	✓	✓			✓																
Arkansas Veterinary Diagnostic Laboratory http://www.arlpc.org/lab.asp			✓	✓				✓															
California Animal Health & Food Safety Laboratory System http://cahfs.ucdavis.edu/			✓	✓				✓															
College of Veterinary Medicine & Biomedical Sciences Veterinary Diagnostic Laboratories http://www.dlab.colostate.edu/			✓	✓		✓	✓		✓					✓	✓						✓		
Connecticut Veterinary Medical Diagnostic Laboratory http://www.patho.uconn.edu/																						✓	
Kissimmee State Veterinary Diagnostic Laboratory http://www.doacs.state.fl.us/ai/labs/			✓																				
University of Georgia Veterinary Diagnostic Laboratories http://www.vet.uga.edu	✓		✓																				
Purdue University www.addl.purdue.edu			✓									✓	✓	✓	✓	✓	✓						✓
Iowa State University Veterinary Diagnostic and Production Animal Medicine http://www.vetmed.iastate.edu/departments/VDPAM/vdl.aspx			✓							✓													
Kansas State Veterinary Diagnostic Laboratory http://www.vet.ksu.edu/depts/dmp/service/index.htm			✓											✓	✓		✓				✓		

Continued

Table 2 Comprehensive Listing All AAVLD Laboratories within the United States That Perform Testing via Molecular Diagnostics—cont'd

Location and Web site	EEE	WEE	WNV	EHV-1	EHV-2	EHV-3	EHV-4	INFA	EVA	S. EQUI	R. EQUI	SALM	CDIFF	CPERF	PHF	LAWSO	LEPTO	ROTA	SNEUR	NOCAD	ANA	LYME	LIST
Kentucky State University Livestock Disease Diagnostic Laboratory http://ces.ca.uky.edu/lddc/	✓	✓	✓	✓	✓	✓	✓		✓			✓			✓	✓	✓						✓
Louisiana State University Louisiana Animal Disease Diagnostic Laboratory http://laddl.lsu.edu/	✓		✓	✓		✓	✓	✓	✓	✓	✓												
Michigan State University http://www.animalhealth.msu.edu	✓		✓	✓			✓	✓	✓						✓			✓	✓		✓		
Veterinary Diagnostic Laboratory of Minnesota http://www.vdl.umn.edu								✓								✓		✓					
Mississippi Veterinary Research and Diagnostic Laboratory System, Mississippi State University http://www.cvm.msstate.edu	✓																		✓				
Veterinary Medical Diagnostic Laboratory, University of Missouri http://www.cvm.missouri.edu/vmdl	✓		✓	✓			✓	✓	✓			✓				✓	✓				✓	✓	
Nebraska State Veterinary Diagnostic Center http://nvdls.uni.edu			✓										✓			✓	✓						✓
Animal Health Diagnostic Center, College of Veterinary Medicine Cornell University http://diaglab.vet.cornell.edu/				✓						✓				✓	✓						✓		✓
North Carolina Department of Agriculture & Consumer Services Rollins Laboratory http://www.ncvdl.com/	✓		✓																				
Department of Veterinary Diagnostic Services, North Dakota State University http://www.vdl.ndsu.edu/			✓											✓									

Ohio Animal Disease Diagnostic Laboratory http://www.ohioagriculture.gov/addl	✓		✓				✓	✓	✓
Veterinary Diagnostic Laboratory, Oregon State University http://www.vet.orst.edu/		✓	✓	✓			✓		✓
Department of Agriculture, Pennsylvania Veterinary Laboratory http://www.padls.org	✓	✓	✓			✓	✓		✓
Clemson Veterinary Diagnostic Center http://www.clemson.edu/lph	✓	✓							
Oklahoma Animal Disease Diagnostic Laboratory, Oklahoma State University http://www.cvm.okstate.edu	✓	✓	✓	✓	✓		✓		
Texas Veterinary Medical Diagnostic Laboratory (TVMDL), TVMDL–College Station http://tvmdlweb.tamu.edu		✓					✓	✓	
Washington Animal Disease Diagnostic Laboratory, Washington State University http://wwwvetmed.wsu.edu/depts_waddl	✓	✓	✓				✓		
Wisconsin Veterinary Diagnostic Laboratory http://www.wvdl.wisc.edu	✓	✓						✓	✓
Wyoming State Veterinary Laboratory http://wyovet.uwyo.edu/		✓	✓	✓				✓	✓

Table 3 Private Molecular Testing Laboratories by Alphabetical Order (Non–AAVLD-Certified)

a. Equine Diagnostic Solutions
1501 Bull Lea Rd. Suite 104
Lexington, KY 40511

Pathogen	Sample Requested
Sarcocystis neurona	CSF
Streptococcus equi	Nasal swabs, nasal cultures, nasal washes, guttural pouch washes, abscess material
EHV1 (neuropathogenic strain ID)	Blood, nasal swab
EHV4	Blood, nasal swab
Equine influenza	
Rhodococcus equi	
Salmonella	

b. IDEXX Laboratories
2825 KOVR Drive
West Sacramento, CA 95605

Pathogen	Comprehensive Panel	Standard Panel	Culture*
Equine rotavirus	•	•	
Equine coronavirus	•		
Cryptosporidium spp.	•		
Salmonella spp.	•	•	•
Clostridium perfringens enterotoxin A	•	•	
Rhodococcus equi	•		
Clostridium difficile toxin A	•	•	
Clostridium difficile toxin B	•	•	
Neorickettsia risticii	•		
Lawsonia intracellularis	•	•	
Salmonella spp.	•	•	•
EHV-1	•	•	
EHV-4	•	•	
EHV-1 neuropathic strains	•	•	
Streptococcus equi	•	•	•

c. Lucy Whittier Real-time PCR Research and Diagnostics Core Facility
3110 Tupper Hall
One Shields Avenue
UC Davis, SVM
Davis, CA 95616-8737

Bacteria	Sample Type
Anaplasma phagocytophilum (tick fever, formerly E. equi)	Tick, whole blood (LTT), CSF, spleen, liver
Borrelia burgdorferi (Lyme disease)	Tick, CSF, synovial fluid, skin biopsy, urine
Clostridium difficile toxins A and B (quantitative load)	Feces, bacterial isolate, colon tissue
Clostridium perfringens	Feces
Corynebacterium pseudotuberculosis (pigeon fever)	Whole blood (LTT), abscess swab, skin biopsy, soil
Lawsonia intracellularis	Feces, fecal swabs, ilium, tonsillar tissue
Lawsonia intracellularis IPMA serology	Serum
Leptospira spp.	Urine, CSF, aqueous humor
Listeria monocytogenes	CSF, whole blood (LTT), feces, placenta
Methicillin resistance gene MecA	Culture, urine, nasopharyngeal swab
Neorickettsia helminthoeca (salmon poisoning)	Lymph node aspirates, feces, spleen, liver
Neorickettsia risticii (Potomac horse fever)	Please submit both feces and whole blood (LTT). Both samples must be from same animal. Additional options include tissue (intestine or colon), or bone marrow.
Rhodococcus equi (vapA gene)	Tracheal swab, tracheal wash, feces
Rickettsia spp. (including RMSF)	Tick, whole blood (LTT)
Salmonella spp.	Feces, fecal swabs, GI tissue, bile, environmental samples
Streptococcus equi subsp. equi (strangles, quantitative load)	Guttural pouch lavage, nasal swab/wash, tracheal swab/wash

Fungi	Sample Type
Aspergillus fumigatus	Fluids or tissues at site of infection
Candida albicans	Fluids or tissues at site of infection
Coccidioides immitis (valley fever)	Fluids or tissues at site of infection
Coccidioides posadasaii (valley fever)	Fluids or tissues at site of infection
Cryptococcus neoformans	Fluids or tissues at site of infection
Macrorhabdus ornithogaster	Feces, fecal swabs
Microsporum canis	Fluids or tissues at site of infection
Sporothrix schenckii	Soil, culture, skin biopsy, sputum, synovial fluid, CSF, or swab of lesion
Trichophyton mentagrophytes	Fluids or tissues at site of infection

Table 3 Private Molecular Testing Laboratories by Alphabetical Order (Non–AAVLD-Certified)—cont'd

Parasites	Sample Type
Babesia caballi (equine piroplasmosis)	Whole blood (LTT)
Babesia conradae	Whole blood (LTT) or spleen tissue
Cryptosporidium spp.	Feces
Giardia spp. (*lamblia* and *intestinalis*)	Feces, GI tract tissue
Leishmania	Whole blood (LTT)
Neospora hughesi and *N. caninum*	Aborted material, brain, heart
Sarcocystis neurona	CSF, brain tissue
Theileria equi (equine piroplasmosis, formerly *Babesia equi*)	Whole blood (LTT)

Virus	Sample Type
Equine arteritis virus (EVA)	Nasal swab or wash, nasopharyngeal swab, (trans) tracheal wash, lung tissue, semen, placenta, conjunctival swab
Equine coronavirus	Feces
Equine herpesvirus 1 (quantitative load) and genotype (neuropathogenic and non-neuropathogenic). Both samples must be from same animal	By order of preference: (1) nasal swab or wash, (trans) tracheal wash or nasopharyngeal swab, (2) whole blood (LTT), (3) CSF, (4) marrow, placenta, lung, or liver
Equine herpesvirus 1 transcript; presence or absence of active replication	Available only when EHV1 DNA is positive
Equine herpesvirus 2	Nasal swab or wash, nasopharyngeal swab, (trans) tracheal wash, or lung tissue
Equine herpesvirus 4	Nasal swab or wash, nasopharyngeal swab, (trans) tracheal wash, or lung tissue
Equine herpesvirus 5	Nasal swab or wash, nasopharyngeal swab, (trans) tracheal wash, or lung tissue
Equine influenza A (H3N8)	Nasal swab or wash, nasopharyngeal swab, (trans) tracheal wash, or lung tissue
Equine rhinitis A virus	Nasal swab or wash, nasopharyngeal swab, (trans) tracheal wash, or lung tissue
Equine rhinitis B virus	Nasal swab or wash, nasopharyngeal swab, (trans) tracheal wash, or lung tissue
Equine rotavirus	Feces or fecal/rectal swabs
West Nile virus	CSF, brain, spinal cord, choanal swab, liver, kidney, spleen

Equine Panels	Sample Type
Respiratory panel: EHV-1 (quantitative load) and genotype (neurotropic, and non-neurotropic), EAV, influenza A, EHV-4, *S. equi*	Nasal swab or wash, tracheal swab, guttural pouch lavage, lung
Vector-borne panel: *A. phagocytophilum*, *Bartonella* spp., *Rickettsia* spp., *B. burgdorferi*	Tick, whole blood*
GI/diarrhea panel: *C. difficile* toxins A and B (quantitative load), *L. intracellularis*, *N. risticii*, *Salmonella* spp.	Feces

Fungus Panel	Sample Type
Fungus breakout panel: *Aspergillus fumigatus*, *Candida albicans*, *Cryptococcus neoformans*, *Microsporum canis*, *Trichophyton mentagrophytes*, *Coccidioides immitis*	Fluids, tissue
Biosecurity and infectious disease control (≥10 samples must be submitted together to qualify for discounted pricing)	Sample type
Salmonella spp.: Any fresh samples will undergo a 20-hour selenite enrichment step before testing	Fresh or pre–selenite-enriched feces, fecal swabs, gastric reflux, bedding, surface swabs/washes/gauze
Equine herpesvirus 1: quantitative load and genotype (neurotropic and non-neurotropic)	Nasal swab, nasal wash, tracheal wash
IDC enteric panel: *Salmonella* spp., *Clostridium difficile* toxin A, *Clostridium difficile* toxin B. Fresh samples will be tested for *C. difficile* before undergoing a 20-hour selenite enrichment step and testing for *Salmonella* spp.	Feces, fecal swabs
IDC respiratory panel: EHV-1 (quantitative load) and genotype (neurotropic and non-neurotropic), EAV, influenza A, EHV-4, *S. equi*	Nasal swab or wash, tracheal wash, guttural pouch lavage

*Whole blood not recommended for *B. burgdorferi*.

day after inoculation and before vesicular lesions. Testing of nasal swabs was ultimately more sensitive for VSV. Consistent with the OIE handbook, testing of vesicular lesions in clinically affected animals is the sample of choice for viral culture and conventional and real-time reverse transcriptase PCR.

Diarrheal Diseases

PCR protocols are described in the literature for many diarrheal pathogens. Specifically, diagnostics for horses include *Salmonella enterica*, *Clostridium perfringens* A toxins, *Lawsonia intracellularis*, rotavirus, and several miscellaneous pathogens (see Table 2). Regarding *Salmonella* PCR in the horse, its excellent sensitivity is most useful for identification of subclinical shedders and environmental contamination during an outbreak.[14] Standard microbial culture methods are still required to obtain the isolates and confirm actual presence of the organism. A clinically ill horse that tests positive by PCR but negative by repeated culture should be interpreted with caution. Given the ultrasensitivity of this technique and the ability for bacterial elements to mobilize between fecal bacteria, only validated PCR techniques for *Salmonella* should be used. For horses, there is little standardization between the few laboratories that use PCR for detection of *Salmonella*.

Detection and typing of C. perfringens in the human field have advanced beyond PCR to microarray to elucidate the complexities involved in differentiation of possible clostridial food-borne and water-borne poisoning. In horses, much attention has been given to the beta-2 C. perfringens toxin as an important cause of diarrhea in adult horses and foals; however, only in the pig has active transcription of beta-2 toxins in the positive strains been documented, and only in the pig has correlation been strong to disease.[15-20] One study has provided a wider epidemiologic correlation in horses. At the molecular level, although the toxin is present in C. perfringens type A isolates garnered from equine clinical cases, the expression of this toxin is extremely low compared with the pig.[15] Well-designed case-control and molecular epidemiology studies are paramount for further analysis of this toxin in horses. The most commonly used technique is a conventional PCR protocol that detects the presence of the toxin genes (not activity or expression).[16] Many AAVLD laboratories now offer this technique, and it has largely supplanted biologic assays, which use rodents. This is usually performed on C. perfringens isolates rather than directly on fecal samples, although this is likely the more practical approach. Interpretation is very important because C. perfringens is a common component of fecal flora.

Respiratory Diseases

Molecular techniques have greatly altered the efficiency of diagnosis of equine respiratory pathogens. Nowhere is this more apparent than for the diagnosis of Streptococcus equi subsp. equi. Because S. equi subsp. equi is in many cases the notifiable pathogen and one that control is directly correlated to biocontainment practices, differentiation and early identification of S. equi subsp. equi in an outbreak of respiratory disease is crucial. Historically, S. equi subsp. equi is differentiated from S. equi subsp. zooepidemicus on the basis of sugar fermentation. Conventional PCR was first performed with the 16S ribosomal gene and sequencing or in terms of the more easily differentiated superoxide dismutase A gene.[21] In addition, other genes, such as the SePE-I gene (pyrogenic mitogen), have been characterized and found present in S. subsp. equi but not S. subsp. zooepidemicus.[21] Both of these genes have also been characterized using a real-time format.[22] In this format, real-time PCR was able to detect and identify correctly all cultivatable S. equi subsp. equi isolates. In addition, six additional samples meeting the case criteria were positive for S. equi subsp. equi, two of which were identified as S. equi subsp. equi and four of which were identified as S. equi subsp. zooepidemicus. This technique did not identify two S. equi subsp. zooepidemicus isolates. Sequencing demonstrated that the target gene had molecular differences not previously described for S. equi subsp. zooepidemicus. These results compare with previously reported results for conventional PCR. Isolation and identification of S. equi subsp. equi–positive horses can be greatly enhanced by multiple sampling. Three consecutively obtained nasal swabs increase sensitivity of detection to 85%, which is equal to a single guttural pouch flushing.

Influenza testing has remarkable efficiency for detection of influenza A in human patients. With vaccination in horses, the window of positive testing is restricted mainly to the period of clinical signs, although even vaccinated horses shed virus during an outbreak.[23] Because most outbreaks in horses are currently caused by equine-2 H3N8 influenza strains, the specificity of most viral testing is unquestioned. Virus isolation is considered the gold standard, but real-time reverse transcriptase PCR and antigen test kits are supplanting this very specialized culturing because it must be done in egg cultures (a real art).[24,25] Real-time PCR was more sensitive than five antigen detection kits and viral isolation.[26,27] In addition, viral detection using real-time was correlated with quantization by tissue culture techniques.

There are many different PCR techniques for detection of equine herpesviruses (EHV). EHV 1 through 4 as a group all are detectable by conventional PCR.[28-33] Real-time methods have been described for EHV-1 and EHV-4, and several simultaneous detection assays (multiplex) are in the literature.[28,30,34-38] Assays that target DNA of the polymerase gene of EHV appear to be most sensitive.[34] Use of RNA targets to examine latency has been described, which may allow study of pathogenesis.[39,40] Location of virus and amount for latent infections in biopsy specimens of pharyngeal tissues with conventional nested PCR (double round of PCR essentially) currently defines latency.[41-43] In vaccinated horses, viral shedding of EHV-1 (non-neurotropic) and EHV-4 is extremely short and must be performed when horses are febrile if early identification of emergence is to be obtained.

Central Nervous System Pathogens

One of the most frustrating areas of diagnostic medicine is diagnosis of infectious encephalitis. The primary indigenous U.S. etiologies for encephalitis include WNV, western equine encephalomyelitis, eastern equine encephalomyelitis, various Bunyaviruses, EHV-1, rabies virus, various parasitic infections, and various fungal infections. FADs include Venezuelan equine encephalomyelitis virus, Murray Valley virus, Semliki forest virus, Japanese encephalitis virus, Hendra virus, Nipah virus, Powassan virus, Kunjin virus, and Borna virus. Although various private laboratories and even AAVLD laboratories have published sequences on the detection of the U.S. arboviruses, the U.S. Centers for Disease Control and Prevention (CDC) has recommended primers/probes for real-time PCR detection. For the purposes of standardization, these targets are used by the respective state Departments of Health for surveillance and communication of public health threat.[44-47] Although a conventional nested PCR test has been described and shown to be more sensitive for detection of WNV in horse tissues, this technique is fraught with greater probability of false-positive results. Also, use of the real-time format is more amenable to automation (hence, more rapid results). Although one article compared nested PCR with the real-time format, many of the samples in the literature are not controlled for sampling site of tissue. In our laboratory with experimental inoculation and in studies where field specimens were evaluated, the highest viral load for WNV was seen in thalamus and pons/medulla. Should these sections of brain be consistently evaluated, real-time PCR is likely reliable in horse brain. There is no question that the use of the CDC primers for detection of eastern equine encephalitis virus is sensitive and reliable. Horses have high viral load in thalamus, pons, and medulla. The same samples used for diagnostic testing for WNV also can be used for eastern equine encephalitis and western equine encephalitis testing. In arbovirus testing, plasma and serum are not appropriate for testing in horses with neurologic disease.

With neurotropic EHV-1, in our experience, there are high amounts of nasal shedding of virus and a high viral load in the hindbrain of neurologically affected horses. Several real-time PCR techniques have been developed and validated by OIE laboratories and investigators.[34,42] Currently, the recommended protocol is to screen for EHV-1 using a generalized target for EHV-1 glycoprotein B gene. This gene is highly conserved and can be used to differentiate EHV-1 from EHV-4. In cases in which EHV-1 presence is questionable, the OIE nested protocol is considered the PCR gold standard. When EHV-1 is identified, a special PCR protocol (a single nucleotide polymorphism assay) is run for the differentiation of the strain associated with neurologic disease from the other EHV-1 not usually associated with central nervous system disease. The specific viral mutation (ORF 30) accounts for only approximately 80% to 85% of equine herpes myeloencephalitis cases. Regardless, field investigation, outbreak details, and recent molecular studies have indicated that horses affected with equine herpes myeloencephalitis shed high amounts of virus early in the course of disease, and early quarantine and detection of nasal shedding within the exposed population is paramount to control. Automated, rapid molecular assays are essential for containment of outbreaks.

Miscellaneous Polymerase Chain Reaction–Based Assays of Diagnostic Utility

Cyathostomin Infection

One of the most exciting areas of diagnostic investigation with PCR techniques is for detection and differentiation of cyathostome infection in horses.[48] There are approximately 43 cyathostomin species. Not only will PCR allow differentiation of these species, but it is also being developed to detect egg and L3 and L4 stages of infection in horse feces.[49,50] PCR protocols also have been used to detect helminth resistance. A PCR technique for detection of *Anoplocephala* has been described.[20,51] This technique is sensitive and will likely aid in detection of another equine parasite that is notoriously difficult to identify. Furthermore, this technique will likely contribute to our understanding of the relationship between acute abdominal disease in horses and infection. *Habronema* infection can be extremely difficult to confirm in premortem biopsy sections, especially in the Southeast United States where diagnosis is complicated by fungal infection.[51-53] An extremely sensitive technique has been developed for detection in feces. This technique needs to be validated for peripheral tissue sections.

Molecular tests that detect pathogen fungi are also a much needed area for diagnosis of infection in the equine. Several PCR techniques have been developed for detection of *Pneumocystis jiroveci* in human immunodeficiency virus infection. Because *Pneumocystis* organisms are considered host-species specific, these techniques must be validated for equine infections. Likewise, invasive *Aspergillus* infections are another area of interest for molecular detection formats. These techniques would likely be most useful for tissue invasion rather than detection of primary respiratory infection because *Aspergillus* can be a transtracheal wash contaminant. *Candida* infection occurs in the blood of equine neonates. These infections can be extremely hard to diagnose. Other pathogenic yeasts for which PCR techniques are highly applicable include *Cryptococcus neoformans*, *Coccidioides immitis*, *Histoplasma*, and *Blastomyces dermititidis*. The differentiation of *Pythium insidiosum* infection from mucormycotic fungi in horses is extremely useful because the former is highly resistant to treatment, whereas the latter can be removed by surgical excision/debulking and respond to antifungal therapies.

Conclusion

Faster, more discriminating identification of equine pathogens is possible through development of molecular assays. However, standardization of molecular techniques between laboratories, validation with appropriate sampling, and use of appropriate controls for quality assurance is necessary for expert and quality results in this rapidly expanding service for stakeholders. Ultimately, it is up to the equine practitioner to have a basic understanding of the methods and interpret the disease in the face of appropriate case criteria.

The complete reference list is available online at www.expertconsult.com

Diagnostic Test Kits

Maureen T. Long

The following table lists assays developed for common equine infectious diseases. The reader is referred to the Web site of each manufacturer, the product insert literature, and the scientific literature for validation of each test. Many of these tests are regulated and may require a permit from the United States Department of Agriculture or a respective country for use and reporting of results.

Becton Dickenson Worldwide Headquarters]
1 Becton Drive
Franklin Lakes, New Jersey, 07417
United States
Phone: 201-847-6800
http://www.bd.com/

Centaur Inc.
P.O. Box 25667
Overland Park, KS 66225-5667
http://www.centaurunavet.com
Sales@centaurunavet.com

DENKA SEIKEN USA INC
1999 South Bascom Av
Suite 905
Campbell, CA 95008

Fuller Laboratories
1135 E. Truslow Avenue
Fullerton, California 92831
Chris_Shapiro@FullerLabs.com
Lee@Fullerlabs.com

Disease	Type of Assay	Manufacturer
African horse sickness	ELISA	Prionics
Anaplasma antibody	IFA slides	Fuller Laboratories
Babesia caballi	cELISA	VMRD, Inc
Babesia equi	cELISA	VMRD, Inc
Babesia	IFA slides	Fuller Laboratories
Borrelia	IFA slides	Fuller Laboratories
Babesia	IFA slides	Centaur Inc.
Borrelia	IFA slides	Centaur Inc.
EHV1/EHV4	ELISA	SVANOVIR
EHV1/EHV4	ELISA	Prionics
EIAV	AGID	VMRD, Inc
EIAV	AGID	Synbiotics
EIAV	cELISA	VMRD, Inc
EIAV	ELISA	Synbiotics
EIAV	ELISA	IDEXX
EIAV	ELISA	Centaur Inc.
EIAV	ELISA	IDvet
EVA	ELISA	IDvet
EVA	ELISA	Prionics
GI parasites	ELISA	Synbiotics
Influenza	ELISA	IDEXX
Influenza	ELISA	Synbiotics
Influenza	ELISA	IDvet
Leptospira	IFA slides	Fuller Laboratories
Leptospira	ELISA	Prionics
Neospora caninum	ELISA	VMRD, Inc
Neospora spp.	IFA slides	Centaur Inc.
Neorickettsia risticii	IFA slides	Centaur Inc.
Neorickettsia risticii	IFA slides	Fuller Laboratories
Neorickettsia risticii	IFA slides	Centaur Inc.
Rotavirus	Human immunochromatographic assay	Becton-Dickinson
Rotavirus	Human immunochromatographic assay	Eiken Chemical Co, Ltd
Rotavirus	Human immunochromatographic assay	TFB, Inc
Rotavirus	Human immunochromatographic assay	DS Pharma Biomedical Co, Ltd
Rotavirus	Human immunochromatographic assay	Sekisui Medical Co, Ltd
Rotavirus	Latex agglutination assay	Sekisui Medical Co, Ltd
Rotavirus	Latex agglutination assay	Denka Seiken Co, Ltd
WNV	IgM ELISA	IDEXX
WNV	IgM ELISA	IDvet
WNV	cELISA	IDvet

[a]*EHV*, Equine herpesvirus; *EIAV*, equine infectious anemia virus; *EVA*, equine viral arteritis; *WNV*, West Nile virus.

[b]*ELISA*, Enzyme Linked Immunoabsorbent Assay; *IFA*, immunofluorescent antibody; *cELISA*, competitive ELISA; *AGID*, agarose gel immune diffusion.

D Antimicrobial Drug Formulary

Jennifer L. Davis and Mark G. Papich*

Drug	Brand Name	Dosing Information
Antibiotics		
Amikacin	Amiglyde-V	*Adult:* 8-10 mg/kg IM or IV q24h *Foals:* 20-25 mg/kg IM or IV q24h
Ampicillin	Amp-Equine, generic	10-20 mg/kg IM or IV q6-8h. Higher doses should be used for anaerobic infections. Doses up to 25 to 40 mg/kg q6-8h have been used for refractory infections.
Amoxicillin	Amoxil, Amoxi-ject, Amoxitabs	10-20 mg/kg IV or IM q6h; 20-30 mg/kg PO q4-6h. Not absorbed well orally, except in foals.
Azithromycin	Zithromax	For *Rhodococcus equi:* 10 mg/kg PO q24h for 7 days, then q48h for 21 days. May cause diarrhea in adult horses.
Cefadroxil	Cefa-Tabs	30 mg/kg PO q12h. Oral absorption is adequate only in young foals, not adults.
Cefazolin	Ancef, Kefzol	10-22 mg/kg IV or IM q6-8h
Cefepime	Maxipime	*Adult:* 2.2 mg/kg IV or IM q8h *Foals:* 11 mg/kg IV q8h
Cefoxitin	Mefoxin	20 mg/kg q4-6h IV or IM
Cefotaxime	Claforan	*Foals:* 25-40 mg/kg IV q6h
Cefpodoxime proxetil	Simplicef	*Foals:* 10 mg/kg PO q8-12h. More frequent dosing should be used for *Salmonella* or *Escherichia coli* infections.
Ceftiofur	Naxcel	Gram-positive infections: 2.2 mg/kg IV or IM q12-24h *E. coli* infections: 4.4-5 mg/kg IV or IM q12h Doses up to 11 mg/kg/day have been used for refractory infections.
Ceftiofur crystalline free acid	Excede	6.6 mg/kg IM at 0 and 96 hours for treatment of *Streptococcus zooepidemicus.* For longer treatment periods, repeat dosing every 7 days after initial 10-day regimen. For other bacteria with MIC up to 1 µg/mL, repeat dosing every 4 days after initial 2 doses. *Foals:* 6.6 mg/kg SC q72h for bacteria with MIC ≤0.5µg/mL
Cephalexin	Keflex, generic	30 mg/kg PO q8h or 10 mg/kg IV q8h
Cephapirin	Cefadyl, generic*	20-30 mg/kg IM or IV q4-8h
Chloramphenicol	Chloromycetin, generic	35-50 mg/kg PO q6-8h or 25 mg/kg IV q6-8h
Clarithromycin	Biaxin	For *Rhodococcus equi:* 7.5 mg/kg PO q12h. May cause diarrhea in adult horses.
Doxycycline	Vibramycin, generic	10 mg/kg PO q12h or 20 mg/kg PO q24h. Do not administer IV.
Enrofloxacin	Baytril, Baytril-100	5-7.5 mg/kg IV q24h. 7.5-10 mg/kg PO q24h.
Erythromycin	Generic	Erythromycin base alone by itself is poorly absorbed. For *Rhodococcus equi:* Erythromycin estolate: 25 mg/kg PO q6-8h Erythromycin phosphate: 37.5 mg/kg PO q12h Erythromycin gluceptate injection: 5 mg/kg IV q4-6h

*Discontinued in the United States.

Continued

*The authors acknowledge and appreciate the original contributions of these authors, whose work has been incorporated into this chapter.

Drug	Brand Name	Dosing Information
Florfenicol	Nuflor	Do not administer to horses until more safety data become available.
Gamithromycin	Zactran	6 mg/kg IM every 7 days for *Streptococcus zooepidemicus* and *Rhodococcus equi*. Clinical efficacy not proved.
Gentamicin	Gentocin	*Adult:* 4.4-6.6 mg/kg IV or IM q24h *Foals:* (<2 weeks) 12-14 mg/kg IV or IM q24h
Imipenem	Primaxin	*Adult:* 10-20 mg/kg IV q6h, constant rate infusion 16 μg/kg/min *Foals:* 5 mg/kg IV infused over 20 minutes q6-8h.
Marbofloxacin	Zeniquin	2 mg/kg IV, IM, SC, or PO q24h
Meropenem	Merrem	10 μg/kg/min as a constant rate infusion
Metronidazole	Flagyl, generic	10-20 mg/kg PO q6-8h
Orbifloxacin	Orbax	5-7.5 mg/kg PO q24h
Oxytetracycline	LA-200, other forms	*Ehrlichiosis:* 3.5 mg/kg IV q12h or up to 10 mg/kg IV or IM q24h (give IV slowly) *Foals* (flexural limb deformities): As much as 44 and up to 70 mg/kg IV (2-3 g per foal) with 2 doses given 24 hours apart have been used.
Penicillin G	Generic	Sodium or potassium penicillin G: 22,000 U/kg IV q6-8h Procaine penicillin G: 22,000 U/kg IM q12h Doses up to 44,000 U/kg q6h or 22,000 IU/kg q3h have been used for refractory cases.
Rifampin	Rifadin	10 mg/kg PO q24h *Rhodococcus equi:* 5-10 mg/kg PO q12h. Always use in combination with a macrolide or azalide.
Sulfonamides	Generic	See Trimethoprim-sulfonamides.
Ticarcillin	Timentin	44 mg/kg IV or IM q6-8h Ticarcillin also is used intrauterine in mares.
Tilmicosin	Micotil	Do not use in horses until more safety data become available.
Tobramycin	Nebcin, generic	4 mg/kg IV q24h
Trimethoprim-sulfadiazine or trimethoprim-sulfamethoxazole	Tribrissen, Uniprim, Bactrim	15 mg/kg IV q12h or 20-30 mg/kg PO q12-24h. Formulations contain a ratio of sulfonamide to trimethoprim of 5:1.
Vancomycin	Vancocin	4.3-7.5 mg/kg as IV infusion q8h

Antifungals

Drug	Brand Name	Dosing Information
Amphotericin B	Fungizone	0.1-0.6 mg/kg as IV infusion q24h. Start at low doses and increase gradually.
Fluconazole	Diflucan, generic	Loading dose: 14 mg/kg PO followed by 5 mg/kg PO q24h.
Griseofulvin	Fulvicin U/F	Microsize particle: 5 mg/kg PO q24h
Itraconazole	Sporanox	Ultramicrosize particle: 2.5 mg/kg Oral solution: 5 mg/kg PO q24h Oral capsules: 7.5-10 mg/kg PO q24h. Absorption is low and variable. IV solution*: 1.5 mg/kg IV q24h
Terbinafine	Lamisil, Terbinex	20-30 mg/kg PO q24h
Voriconazole	Vfend	2-4 mg/kg PO q24h or 1 mg/kg IV q24h. Use higher doses for *Fusarium* spp.

Antiprotozoals

Drug	Brand Name	Dosing Information
Pyrimethamine	Daraprim	1 mg/kg PO q24h. Used in combination with a sulfonamide for the treatment of EPM.
Trimethoprim-sulfonamide combinations	Tribrissen, Uniprim, Bactrim	See above.
Ponazuril	Marquis	5 mg/kg PO q24h. Treatment recommended for a minimum of 28 days for EPM.
Diclazuril	Protazil	1 mg/kg PO q24h as a top dress on feed. Treatment recommended for a minimum of 28 days for EPM.

Drug	Brand Name	Dosing Information
Antivirals		
Acyclovir	Zovirax	10 mg/kg IV q12h diluted in 1 L 0.9% sodium chloride and infused over 1 hour.
Famciclovir	Famvir	20 mg/kg PO. Dosing interval not yet determined.
Ganciclovir	Cytovene	2.5 mg/kg IV q8h for 1 day, then 2.5 mg/kg IV q12h for 1 week
Oseltamivir	Tamiflu	2 mg/kg PO twice daily for 5 days
Rimantadine	Flumadine	30 mg/kg PO q12h
Valacyclovir	Valtrex	27 mg/kg PO q8h for 2 days followed by 18 mg/kg PO q12h for 1-2 weeks OR 40 mg/kg PO q8h

IM, Intramuscular; *q24h,* every 24 hours; *IV,* intravenous; *PO,* oral; *MIC,* minimum inhibitory concentration; *SC,* subcutaneous; *EPM,* equine protozoal myeloencephalitis.

Index

A

AAEP (American Association of Equine Practitioners), 151-152
  biosecurity information, 541
AAT (African animal trypanosomiasis), 505, 507
AAVLD (American Association of Veterinary Laboratory Diagnosticians), 606
abdominal effusion, 599
abdominal masses, 599
abdominal pain, 599
aberrant hosts, 220f
aberrant parasites, 509-510
abortions, 93. *See also* placentitis
  ascendant placentitis, 94
  bacterial causes, 94-98
    Chlamydophila, 99
    Escherichia coli, 95f
    leptospirosis, 305-306, 309
    Mycoplasma equigenitalium or *subdolum*, 99
    samples and tissue selection, 259b
  brucellosis (*See* brucellosis)
  diagnostic approach, 98
  etiology
    Chlamydophila, 99
    coccidiomycosis, 405
  infectious, 93-99
  infectious causes, 93-99, 277
  mare reproductive loss syndrome (MRLS), 515
  parasitic causes, 99
  pathogens associated with, 99
  rule-outs, 601
  viral causes, 98-99
    equine arteritis virus, 175-176
    equine herpesvirus, 98, 155, 157, 160-161
    equine viral arteritis, 98-99, 174
abscesses
  central nervous system (CNS) infections, right brain hemisphere, 56f
  corneal, 424
    fungal, 113f
    mycotic keratitis (keratomycosis), 424f
  Corynebacterium pseudotuberculosis, 378-379
    external, 375, 378-379
    kidneys, 376f
    pectoral, 373f, 375f
    spleen, 377f
    triceps, 378f
  intracranial, 56-57
    clinical findings, 56
    diagnosis, 56-57
    etiology, 56
    therapy, 57
  lung, 382f
  ovarian, 93f
  pulmonary, 7
    Rhodococcus equi, 296f
    Streptococcus equi, 7
  skin, 603

abscesses *(Continued)*
  spine, 57-58, 58f (*See also* vertebral infections)
    clinical findings, 58
    diagnosis, 58
    etiology and epidemiology, 57-58
    therapy, 58
  spleen, 335f
  Streptococcus equi equi (strangles), 6-7, 269-270, 270f
    abscess rupture sites, 269f
    lymph node abscesses, 273
  subcutaneous, 82
  testicular, 102f
Absidia corymbifera, 420
acaricidal treatments, 496
accessory sex glands, 102-104
acemannan, 591
acid-base abnormalities, 72
acid-fast stains, 257
acid-stable picornavirus (ASP), 195
acoustic nerve. *See* vestibulocochlear/acoustic nerve (CN VIII)
ACTH (adrenocorticotropic hormone), 72
Actinobacillus species, 26, 32, 42-43, 72
Actinobacillus equuli, 46-47, 57-58, 64
Actinobacillus lignieresii, 57-58
Actinomyces species, 1
Actinomyces bovis, 337-338
actinomycetomas, 381
active immunization, 551-553
  DNA vaccines, 552-553
  inactivated vaccines, 552
  modified live vaccines, 553
  principles of, 551-552
  protein or subunit vaccines, 552
  recombinant vaccines, 553
ACVIM (American College of Veterinary Internal Medicine), 151-152
adaptive immunity, 592f
adenosine, 166
adenoviruses, 43, 189-192
  clinical findings, 190-191
  diagnosis, 191
    laboratory testing, 191
    pathologic findings, 192
    public health considerations, 192
    serology, 191
    therapy and prevention, 192
    virus isolation, 191
  epidemiology, 189
  equine adenovirus type 1 (EAdV1), 189
  etiology, 189
  immunity, 190
  ocular manifestations of, 116t
  pathogenesis, 189-190
  severe combined immune deficiency (SCID), 189, 190f-191f
adrenal insufficiency, 75
adrenocorticotropic hormone (ACTH), 72
A/equine/Fontainebleau/79, 5-6
A/equine/Kentucky/81, 5-6
A/equine/Newmarket/2/93, 5-6
A/equine/Prague/56, 5-6

A/equine/Saskatoon/90, 5-6
Aeromonas species, 44
aflatoxicosis
  clinical findings, 425
  diagnosis, 427-428
  epidemiology, 423
  pathogenesis, 424
  therapy, 433
African animal trypanosomiasis (AAT), 505, 507
African horse sickness (AHS)
  clinical findings, 183-185
    dikkop (cardiac) form, 184, 184f-185f, 187f
    dunkop (pulmonary) form, 184, 184f, 186f-187f
    horsesickness fever form, 185
    of large intestines, 187f
    mixed form, 184-185
    of stomach, 187f
  diagnosis, 185-186
  distribution and transmission, 182
  epidemiology, 182-183
  etiology, 182
  ocular manifestations of, 116t
  outbreaks due to international movement of horses, 547t
  overview, 181-182
  pathogenesis, 183
  pathologic findings, 186-188
    dikkop (cardiac) form, 186
    dunkop (pulmonary) form, 186
    macroscopic, 186-188
    microscopic, 186-188
    mixed form, 186
  prevention, 188
  public health considerations, 188
  therapy, 188
agalactia, 272
agar gel immunodiffusion (AGID), 139
agroterrorism, 549
AHS. *See* African horse sickness (AHS)
Alberta Equestrian Federation, 542
Alberta Medical Association, 542
alkylating agents, 585t, 597
allergies, 80, 485
alopecia, 80
  base of tail, 484-485
  Culicoides hypersensitivity, 502f
  dermatophilosis, 284f-285f
  Onchocerca cervicalis, 486f
  rule-outs, 602
Alphaherpesvirinae, 152
alphaviruses, 116t
  Eastern equine encephalitis (EEE), 210-214
  life cycle, 211
  location/hosts/disease manifestation, 210t
  reported North American, 210t
  Venezuelan equine encephalitis (VEE), 215-217
  western equine encephalomyelitis (WEE), 214-215
alveoli, 2, 446, 447f

Note: Page numbers followed by "f" refer to illustrations; page numbers followed by "t" refer to tables; page numbers followed by "b" refer to boxes.

Amblyomma maculatum, 495
American Association of Equine
    Practitioners (AAEP), 151-152
    biosecurity information, 541
American Association of Veterinary
    Laboratory Diagnosticians (AAVLD),
    606
American College of Veterinary Internal
    Medicine (ACVIM), 151-152
American Veterinary Medical Association
    (AVMA), 208-209
aminoglycosides, 573, 580
amphoteracin B, 410
ampicillin, susceptibility testing, 264f
AMR (antimicrobial resistance), 532
Amycolatopsis species, 95
anaerobic infections, 387-390
    clinically significant obligately anaerobic
        bacteria, 374f
    culturing of, 259
    diagnosis, 389-390
    epidemiology, 388
    etiology, 387-388
    of oral cavity/pharynx, 42
    pathogenesis and clinical signs, 388-389
    public health considerations, 390
    of respiratory tract, 388
    therapy, 390
anaphylactic reactions, 504
Anaplasma marginale, 344
Anaplasma phagocytophilum. See equine
    granulocytic anaplasmosis/ehrlichiosis
anatomy. *See under specific infection/disease
    or body area*
anemia, 601. *See also* equine infectious
    anemia (EIA)
    with equine piroplasmosis (EP), 473
    hemolytic, 427f
    nagana, 504
    tick-related, 495
aneurysm formation, 17
Animal and Plant Health Inspection Service
    (APHIS), 179
Anocentor nitens, 495
Anoplocephala, 613
Anoplocephala magna, 449, 490, 490f,
    507-508
Anoplocephala perfoliata, 14, 449, 451f,
    490-491, 490f-491f, 507-508
    age/gender differences in incidence, 492
    epidemiology, 491-492
    ileocecal intussusception with, 492b, 493f
    life cycle, 491
    prevalence, 492, 492b
Anoplocephaloides mamillana, 490
ant bites, 504
anterior enteritis, 43
anterior mesenteric artery, strongyle
    infection of, 476
anthelmintic therapy, 14. *See also* parasitic
    infections
    acaricides, 475
    Anoplocephala perfoliata, 494
    efficacy
        nonstrongylid nematodes, 483t
        Paracaris infection, 482
        strongylids, 478t
    equine piroplasmosis (EP), 474
    nematodes
        efficacy, 478t
        nonstrongylid nematodes, 483t
    respiratory infections, 13-14
    species resistance to
        ascarids, 483
        cyathostomin, 479

anthrax, 383-385
    clinical findings, 384
    diagnosis, 384
    epidemiology, 383
    etiology, 383
    pathogenesis, 383-384
    pathologic findings, 385
    prevention, 385
    public health considerations, 385
    treatment, 384-385
    vaccine recommendations, 570
antibiotic therapy. *See also* therapy *or*
        treatment *under specific infection/disease*
    broad spectrum, for THO, 20
    cyclosporine, 596
    factors affecting effectiveness, 575
    immunomodulators, 585t
    b-Lactam, 8
    neonatal sepsis, 74t
    oral, 75
    rapamycin (sirolimus), 597
    resistance to, 7
    skin diseases, 78-79
    systemic, 69t
        uterine infections, 91t
    tacrolimus, 596
    update on, 578-582
        aminoglycosides, 580
        azteronam, 581-582
        β-Lactam antibiotics, 579-580
        chloramphenicol, 581
        fluoroquinolones (FQs), 578-579
        fosfomycin, 582
        macrolides and derivatives, 579
        metronidazole, 581
        rifampin, 581
        tetracyclines, 581
        trimethoprim-sulfonamides, 580-581
antibodies/immunoglobulins
    antibody detection, 147-148
        blastomycosis, 436
        Cryptococcus species, 437
        equine protozoal myeloencephalitis
            (EPM), 464
        Sarcocystis neurona, 462
    antibody-mediated immune responses,
        554t
    anti-equine IgG/IgM detection, 139f
    antiviral, 138f
    enzyme-linked immunosorbent assay
        (ELISA) method for detecting, 139f
    exogenous antibodies, 556
    IgG, 471-472
    immunoglobulin A (IgA), 1, 2f, 71
    immunoglobulin G (IgG), 1, 14, 71
    immunoglobulin M (IgM), 71
    immunotherapy, antibody-mediated
        protection, 594f
    indirect fluorescent antibody test, 346,
        526b-527b
    maternal antibodies, 557-558
    monoclonal antibodies, 597
        equine infectious anemia (EIA), 137f
    passive immunity
        endotoxemia antibodies, 595
        transfer of antigen-specific antibodies,
            594-595
        transfer of nonspecific antibodies, 594
        West Nile virus antibodies, 595
    release of antigens, dermatophilosis, 284
    role of, 290-291
    suppressor mechanisms, 596b
    testing before vaccination, 179-181
    upper respiratory tract, 1
    in uterine secretions, 85

antibody detection, 147-148
    blastomycosis, 436
    Cryptococcus species, 437
    equine protozoal myeloencephalitis
        (EPM), 464
    Sarcocystis neurona, 462
    viral sensitivity and specificity, 140
antibody-mediated immune responses, 554t
antibody-mediated protection, 594f
antiendotoxin therapy, 75
antifungal therapy, 582. *See also* fungal
        infections
    azoles, 582
    Candida albicans
        azoles, 410-411
        polyenes, 410
    candidiasis, 410-411
    choice of, 431-432
    griseofulvin, 582
    guttural pouch mycosis, 18
    imidazoles, 582
    minimal inhibitory concentration (MIC)
        values, 408
    neonatal sepsis, 75
    polyenes, 582
    susceptibility testing, 425-426
    systemic, uterine infections, 91t
    terbinafine, 582
    triazoles, 582
antigen detection, 145-147. *See also*
        pathologic findings *under specific
        infection/disease or pathogen*
    antibody detection, 147-148
    blastomycosis, 436
    common antigen tests, 355
    Cryptococcus species, 437
    ELISA-based assays, 148
    hemagglutination inhibition, 147, 147f
    Histoplasma species, 442-443
    immunoassays, 146
    immunofluorescence, 146
    reverse transcriptase-polymerase change
        reaction, 146-147
    single radial hemolysis, 147-148
    virus isolation, 145-146
antigenic drift, 5-6
antigen-specific responses, 1
antimicrobial resistance (AMR), 532
antimicrobial therapy. *See also* therapy *or*
        treatment *under specific infection/disease
        or pathogen*
    absorption of, 576
        injectable drugs, 576
        local drug administration, 576
        oral absorption, 576
    adverse reactions associated with,
        577-578, 577b
    alternative uses for, 578
    antibiotics (*See* antibiotic therapy)
    antifungal (*See* antifungal therapy)
    antiprotozoal (*See* antiprotozoal therapy)
    antiviral (*See* antiviral therapy)
    bacterial susceptibility testing, 572-573
    central nervous system infections, 54
    clostridial enteritis, 356-357
    Corynebacterium pseudotuberculosis,
        378-379, 379t
    delivery of
        antimicrobial-impregnated
            polymethylmethacrylate (PMMA)
            beads, 67, 68b
        constant-rate infusion system, 65f
        IV regional limb perfusion, 65f, 67, 68b
        plaster of Paris beads, 67-68
        techniques for synovial infections, 65

antimicrobial therapy *(Continued)*
  drug formulary, 615t-617t
  drugs that penetrate/do not penetrate
      blood-brain and blood-aqueous
      barriers, 575b
  for foals, 576-577
  fungal *(See* antifungal therapy)
  judicious use of antimicrobials, 532
  Lawsonia intracellularis, 320
  multidrug-resistant bacteria, 531-532
  osteomyelitis, 67
  parasitic *(See* anthelmintic therapy)
  peritonitis, 46
  pharmacokinetic-pharmacodynamic
      optimization of doses, 573-574
    aminoglycosides, 573
    bacteriostatic drugs, 574
    β-Lactam antibiotics, 574
    fluoroquinolones, 573-574
  plasma concentration versus time profile
      and minimum inhibitory
      concentration, 573f
  principles of, 571
  resistance to *(See* drug resistant/sensitive
      organisms)
  as risk factor for *Clostridium difficile*
      infection, 352
  septic foals, 74-75
  susceptibility testing, 263-264, 571-572
    Actinobacillus species, 571
    anaerobic bacteria, 572
    fungi, 572
    indications, 263
    interpretation, 264
    methods, 263-264
    patterns of microorganisms, 74t
    Pseudomonas, Enterobacter, Klebsiella,
        Escherichia coli, 572
    Staphylococcus species, 571-572
    Streptococcus and *Pasteurella,* 571
  synovial infections, 64
  tissue penetration of drugs, 574-575
    impaired diffusion into tissue, 575
    intracellular, 575
  urinary tract infections, 109
  viral *(See* antiviral therapy)
antiprotozoal therapy. *See also* protozoal
    infections
  for equine piroplasmosis, 584
  equine protozoal myeloencephalitis,
      465-466, 583-584
    Diclazuril, 466
    folate inhibitors, 466
    folate synthesis inhibitors, 583
    Ponazuril, 465-466
    triazine derivatives, 583-584
antiseptics, 530, 538t
antiviral antibodies, 138f
antiviral therapy, 585t. *See also* viral infections
  cyclic amines, 583
  equine influenza, 149-150
  neuraminidase inhibitors, 583
  nucleoside analogs, 583
aortic infective endocarditis, 27f. *See also*
    infective endocarditis (IE)
aortitis, 39
aortoiliac thrombosis, 40f
APHIS, 471
APHIS (Animal and Plant Health
    Inspection Service), 179
Aphthovirus, 6
apoptosis, 596b
aquatic insects, ingestion of. *See* Potomac
    horse fever (PHF)/equine
    neorickettsiosis (EN)

arboviruses, 240
  Murray Valley encephalitis, 255
aroa, 218t-219t
arterial thrombosis, 39, 114f
arteritis
  arterial, 39
  verminous, 476f
  viral *(See* equine viral arteritis (EVA))
arthritis
  rule-outs, 600
  septic
    candidiasis, 410
    in foals, 64
arthroscopy, debridement of septic/
    contaminated joints, 64
arthrospores, 413
artificial insemination, 545
arytenoid chondritis, 5, 6f
ascarids (roundworms), 481, 482f, 483
ascending placentitis, 94-95, 94f
Ascomycota, 446
aseptic peritonitis, 46
aspartate transaminase (AST), 60
aspergillosis
  clinical findings, 424-425
    aflaxotoxicosis, 425
    central nervous system aspergillosis,
        425
    corneal scrapings, 426f
    disseminated aspergillosis and
        hemolytic anemia, 426f
    endometritis and placentitis, 425
    mycotic keratitis (keratomycosis),
        424-425, 424f
    nasal or sinus aspergillosis, 425
    pulmonary aspergillosis, 425
  diagnosis, 425-428
    aflatoxicosis, 427-428
    biopsies, 426
    central nervous system aspergillosis,
        427
    culturing, 425
    endometritis and placentitis, 427
    immunohistochemical techniques, 426
    mycotic keratitis (keratomycosis),
        426-427
    nasal and sinus aspergillosis, 427
    pulmonary aspergillosis, 427
    real-time (RT) polymerase chain
        reaction (PCR) test, 425
    serology, 425
    susceptibility testing, 425-426
  epidemiology, 422-423
    aflatoxicosis, 423
    endometritis and placentitis, 423
    mycotic keratitis (keratomycosis),
        422-423
  etiology, 421-422
  ocular manifestations of, 117
  pathogenesis, 423-424
    aflaxotoxicosis, 424
    endometritis and placentitis, 424
    keratomycosis, 423-424
  pathologic findings
    brain, 427f
    branching hyphae, 427f
    conidospores, 422f
  therapy, 428-433
    aflatoxicosis, 433
    azole antifungal drugs, 428-430
    chitin synthesis inhibitors, 430
    endometritis and placentitis, 433
    mycotic keratitis (keratomycosis),
        430-432
    nasal and sinus aspergillosis, 432

aspergillosis *(Continued)*
    polyene antifungal drugs, 428
    pulmonary aspergillosis, 432
    systemic, 429t
    topical (keratomycosis), 430t
  virulence, 422
Aspergillus species, 57-58, 61, 94, 398f, 410,
    421-422
  identification of, 395-396
    Gomori's methenamine silver stain,
        396f
    Gram stain, 395f
Aspergillus flavus, 423
Aspergillus fumigatus, 17-18, 422
Aspergillus parasiticus, 423
Aspergillus species, 422-423
AST (aspartate transaminase), 60
ataxia, 106-107, 162f. *See also* lameness/gait
    disturbances
atlanto-occipital collection of cerebrospinal
    fluid, 51f
attack risk table, 525t
attributable fraction (AF), 524b
attributable risk (AR), 523, 524b
aural plaques, 246, 246f
autonomic function disturbances, 370
avermectins, 496
avian influenzas, 521f
AVMA (American Veterinary Medical
    Association), 208-209
azathioprine, 597
azole antifungal drugs, 428-431
azoles, 582
azteronam, 581-582

B

Babesia species, 468, 470
Babesia bovis, 471-472
Babesia caballi, 471-472, 495, 584
Babesia equi. See Theileria equi
babiosis. *See* equine piroplasmosis (EP)
Bacille-Calmette-Guérin vaccine, 587-588
Bacillus species, 46
Bacillus abortus, 338f. *See also* brucellosis
Bacillus anthracis, 383. *See also* anthrax
Bacillus piliformis. See Tyzzer's disease
bacteremia, 259
  definition, 70
  ocular involvement, 76
  sampling protocols, 260
bacterial infections. *See also* antibiotic
    therapy; antimicrobial therapy; specific
    infection/disease or pathogen
  abortion caused by, 94-98
    Chlamydophila, 99
    Escherichia coli, 95f
    Mycoplasma equigenitalium or
        subdolum, 99
  aerobic, 42
  anaerobic bacteria, 572 (*See also*
      anaerobic infections)
  central nervous system, 48t
  Clostridium species, treatment of, 43
  conjunctivitis, causative agents, 111b
  crusting/scaling dermatoses, 79-80
  cultures, 1-2
  keratitis, 112
  laboratory diagnosis
    antimicrobial susceptibility testing,
        263-264
    broth microdilution antimicrobial
        susceptibility testing, 264f
    direct microscopic examination,
        257-258

bacterial infections (Continued)
  fastidious organisms (specialized media/ culture requirements), 261b
  gram-stain reactions and morphology, 257t, 258f
  interpretation of isolation and identification results, 261-262
  Kinyoun acid-fast stain, 258f
  Kirby-Bauer disc dilution antimicrobial susceptibility testing, 264f
  molecular methods, 262-263
  normal flora, 259b
  sampling for bacterial cultures, 258-261, 259b
  serologic diagnosis, 264-265
  submission of samples, 261
  transportation of samples, 261
  meningitis and meningoencephalitis, 55-56
  MRSA (methicillin-resistant *Staphylococcus aureus*), 79-80, 531-532
  ocular manifestations/complications of systemic, 116
  opportunistic bacteria, 107
  oral cavity, 42
  pathogen detection methods
    polymerase chain reaction, 262-263, 262f
    toxin gene detection, 263
  pathogen morphology, 257t
  pneumonia, 7
  respiratory tract, 7
  rhinitis, 4
  skin
    dermatophilosis (See dermatophilosis)
    infectious, 82b
    subcutaneous, 83
    streptococcal (See streptococcal infections)
    tick-borne, 495
  urinary tract, 107f
    cystitis, 106f
    pathogens reported in, 106
bacterial myositis, 60-61
  primary, 60-61
    clinical findings, 60
    diagnosis, 60-61
    etiology, 60
    therapy, 61
bacterial particles, 586-589
  Propionibacterium acnes, 586-587
  unmethylated cytosine-phosphate-guanosine motifs, 588-589
Bacterioides species, 387
Bacterioides fragilis, 389
bacteriostatic drugs, 574
bacteriotherapy, 357-358
Bacteroides species, 10-11, 46
Bacteroides fragilis, 1
Baerman procedure, 454
BAL (bronchoalveolar lavage), 1-2, 446-447, 448f
balanitis, 101f
balloon occlusion/catheter technique, 19
BALT (bronchial-associated lymphoid tissue), 1
barrier gowns, 535
barrier nursing precautions, 534-535, 535f
Basidiobiosis species, 415-416, 419. See also *Pythium* species
basidiobolomycosis, 419, 420f
Basidiobolus species. See zygomycosis
Basidiobolus ranarum, 415, 419, 419f
Basidiomycota, 446

bastard strangles, 270
BBB (blood-brain barrier), 49-50
  drugs that penetrate/do not penetrate, 575b
BD. See Borna disease (BD)
bee stings, 504
Berne virus (torovirus), 203
Besnoitia bennetti, 80, 512f
besnoitiosis, 80, 511
Betacoronavirus, 201-202
β-Lactam antibiotics, 574, 579-580
biofilm, 89
biopsies
  aspergillosis, 426
  blastomycosis, 434-435
  corneal, 427
  dermatophilosis lesions, 286
  endometrial, 86
  muscle, 61
  osteomyelitis, 67
  skin, 78, 80
    Onchocerca cervicalis, 451f
    Onchocerca cervicalis infection, 486f
  parasitic infections, 455
  tissue for fungal cultures, 395
biosecurity. See also environmental management
  aborted fetal and placental material, 155
  African horse sickness (AHS), 188
  alphavirus vector control, 214
  application of concepts, 540-543
    equine ambulatory practices, 540-541
    protection of resident horses, 542-543
    summary of, 540
    traveling horses/protection at events, 541-543
  in breeding operations, 105-106
  cleaning methods, 539
  at competitions, 543
  control measures for reducing airborne pathogens, 543
  education of personnel, 543
  environmental infection control, 537
    cleaning of surfaces, 537
    disinfection, 537
  equine herpesvirus (EHV), 167-168, 168b
  equine viral arteritis (EVA), 178-181
    husbandry and control programs, 179-181
    immunity, 178-179
  ethics of infection control, 136-137, 530
  exposure to pathogens, 541
  guidelines for breeding stallions shedding EAV/EVA, 180f
  hand hygiene, 534, 541
  Hendra virus (HeV), 192-195
  importance of, 531-532
    hospital/practice protection, 532
    judicious antimicrobial use, 532
    patient protection, 531
    personnel protection, 531-532
  level of, 531
  monitoring protocol effectiveness, 539-540
    environmental monitoring, 539-540
    patient monitoring/surveillance, 539
  MRSA control/prevention, 282
  outdoor exercise areas at hospitals, 540
  preventive measures, 533-540
    antiseptics and disinfectants, 538t
    barrier gowns, 535
    barrier nursing precautions, 534-535, 535f
    biosecurity kits, 541

biosecurity (Continued)
  daily attire, 534
  disinfection methods, 539f
  face/eye protection, 535
  footbaths/footmats, 536-537
  footwear hygiene, 535
  gloves, 535
  hand hygiene, 534
  movement/traffic flow management (personnel), 535
  separation/isolation, 535-536
  transmission routes, 534
  program development, 532-533
    corrective action plan, 533
    critical control point identification (CCP), 533
    critical control point monitoring, 533
    critical limits for preventive measures, 533
    hazard analysis/identification, 532-533
  program evaluation, 533
  protocol compliance, 537
  resources/Web sites, 543t
  rotavirus, 201
  safety measures for necropsies, coccidiomycosis, 406
  veterinarian's role in, 531
  waste management and disposal, 537-538
  wildlife reservoirs/control, 538-539
biting flies, 499-501
  stable fly (*Stomoxys calcitrans*), 500
  tabanids, 500
biting midges, 501-503
black fly (*Simulium* species), 500-501
bladder
  paralysis of, 106, 106f
  stones in, 107f
  urolithiasis in, 106-107
Blastomyces dermatitidis, 433, 435f
blastomycosis, 433-436
  clinical findings, 434
  diagnosis, 434-436
    antibody detection, 436
    antigen detection, 436
    biopsy, 434-435
    culturing, 435
    cytology, 434
    molecular identification of yeasts, 435
  endemic areas, 434f
  epidemiology, 433-434
  etiology, 433
  pathogenesis, 434
  prevention, 436
  therapy, 436
blepharitis, 110-111
blindness, 56f, 425, 602
  cortical, 48-49
blockades, inflammatory cell activation, 128
blocking ELISA, 148
blood-aqueous barrier, drugs that penetrate/ do not penetrate, 575b
blood-brain barrier (BBB), 49-50
  drugs that penetrate/do not penetrate, 575b
blood cultures, 259-260
  specimen collection and transport, 394
blood loss, treatment of, 18
blood smears, 455
boarding facilities, infection control methods, 542
body fluids, 192-193
  culturing, 397
  specimen collection and transport, 395

bone infections. *See also* osteo—*entries*
debridement of, 64f
effects of antimicrobial therapy on
growing, 577b
etiology, 57-58
Rhodoccus equi, 293
septic arthritis, 76
septic osteomyelitis and osteitis,
66-70
antimicrobial-impregnated
polymethylmethacrylate (PMMA)
beads, 68b
clinical findings, 66
diagnosis, 66-67
etiology and pathogenesis, 66
supportive care for severe lameness,
69-70
systemic antibiotics for, 69t
therapy, 67-69
bone marrow suppression, 577b
Boophilus species, 495
Borellia burgdorferi, 311, 312f. *See also* Lyme
disease
Borna disease (BD)
about, 226-227
clinical findings, 229-230, 230f
diagnosis, 230-231
antemortem, 230-231
postmortem, 231
epidemiology, 227-228
etiology, 227
pathogenesis, 228-229
pathologic findings, 230f-231f, 231-232
prevention, 232
public health considerations, 232
therapy, 232
worldwide distribution, 228f
Borrelia burgdorferi, 312f, 495. *See also* Lyme
disease
botfly *(Gasterophilus species)*, 504, 510-511,
510f
botulism, 261, 367f
botulinum toxin, 364
clinical findings, 365
diagnosis, 365
epidemiology, 364
etiology, 364
mammalian species affected by, 364t
ocular manifestations of, 117t
pathogenesis, 364-365
pathologic findings, 365-366
pressure sores, 366f
prevention, 367, 367b, 568-569
public health considerations, 367
therapy, 366-367
lateral recumbency, 367f
slinging a horse, 367f
types A, B, C, D, 364
Bovicola equi, 499f
bovine papillomavirus (BPV), 244
BPV (bovine papillomavirus), 244
brain infections, 48-49
aspergillosis, 427f
equine protozoal myeloencephalitis
(EPM), 462
brainstem signs
rabies, 205-206
rule-outs, 600
breathing. *See also* respiratory diseases
depth of, 3
physiologic considerations, 2
breeding industry, 545
broodmares
botulism vaccination for, 366-367
safety of vaccines in, 555-556

breeding industry *(Continued)*
international trade in equids, semen,
embryos, 546-547
breed predilection to disease
clostridial myonecrosis, Quarter Horses,
361
equine adenovirus, 189
equine encephalosis virus (EEV),
251-252
equine viral arteritis (EVA), 171
bronchial-associated lymphoid tissue
(BALT), 1
bronchoalveolar lavage (BAL), 1-2, 446-447,
448f
bronchopneumonia, 7, 190
pathogenesis of, 7
Rhodoccus equi, 293f
broodmares. *See under* mares
broth microdilution antimicrobial
susceptibility testing, 264f
Brucella species, 26, 57-58
Brucella abortus, 337
Brucella suis, 337
brucellosis
diagnosis, 338
etiology and epidemiology, 337
pathogenesis and clinical findings,
337-338
fistulous withers, 338f
prevention and public health
considerations, 339
therapy, 338-339
buffy coat smear, 3
Bulinus species, 512
Bunyviridae, 255
Burkholderia mallei, 333. *See also* glanders
bursatti *(Habronema* species), 486
bursitis, septic, 337

C

Cache Valley virus, 255
caddisfly larvae, 348f
calcfluor white stains, 396
California group *(Bunyviridae)*, 255
cancer vaccines, 593
Candida species, 94
description, 408
Gram stain, 396f
identification of, 396
urinary tract infections, 106
Candida albicans, 75, 409f
virulence, 409
Candida parapsilosis, 88f
candidiasis, 410
candidiasis (thrush)
arthritis, hock (foal), 410f
clinical findings, 409-410
systemic infection, 409-410
thrush, 409
diagnosis, 410
epidemiology, 408-409
etiology, 408
oral, 72-74
pathogenesis, 409
risk factors, 408-409
therapy
antifungal, 410-411
supportive, 411
topical, 411
virulence factors, 409
canine heartworm, 510
caprine serum fraction, 591
cardiac catheterization, pericarditis, 34-35
cardiac dysrhythmias, 39-41

cardiac (dikkop) form of African horse
sickness, 184, 184f-185f, 186, 187f
cardiomyopathy, 601
cardiotoxicity, 577b
cardiovascular system
cardiac complications in inflammatory
response syndrome and sepsis, 39
caudal vena cava thrombosis syndrome, 39
facial arteries and veins, 14
infective endocarditis (IE), 21-30
jugular thrombophlebitis, 36-39
myocarditis, 30-31
pericarditis, 31-36
rule-outs, 601
cardiomyopathy, myocarditis,
endocarditis, 601
toxic ingestions, pyrrolizidine alkaloid
toxicity, 41f
carriers/carrier state. *See also* hosts/host
factors
contagious equine metritis (CEM),
341-342
equine viral arteritis (EVA), 171-173
inapparent, 472
salmonellosis, 326
Streptococcus equi, 275-276
detection of, 275
treatment of, 275-276, 275b
CARS (compensatory antiinflammatory
response syndrome), 70
cartilage damage
due to synovial infections, 63
effects of antimicrobial therapy on
growing, 577b
caseous exudates, 296f
categorical data
cumulative incidence, 523-525, 524b
relative risk, 523, 524b
epidemiologic measures of disease
frequency, 519-520
cause-fatality rate, 520b
cumulative incidence, 519-520, 519b
incidence rate, 520, 520b
mortality rate, 519b
prevalence, 519, 519b
relationship between prevalence and
incidence, 520, 521b
outbreak investigations, 523-525
prevalence comparisons
odds ratio, 523, 524b
reality of difference, 525
proportions, 518
rates, 518-519
ratios, 518
using, 523-525
cat fleas, 504
catheterization
staphylococcus infections with, 280
for urinary tract infection diagnosis, 108
caudal vena cava thrombosis syndrome, 39
causal factors of disease, 517
categorical data, 518-519
data types, 518
identifying, 517-525
interval data, 518
measuring, 517-520
population-at-risk, 518
causative agents. *See specific pathogen/agent,
or under specific infection/disease*
cause-fatality rate, 520b
causes of, 7
CCA (common carotid artery), 18-19
CCP (critical control point), 533
CDCP (Centers for Disease Control and
Prevention), 612

CDI (*Clostridium difficile* infection). *See* clostridial enteritis; *Clostridium difficile*
cecal microflora, 44
cefoxitin, 281
cELISA (competitive enzyme-linked immunosorbent assay), 473
cell/egg cultures, 133-134
cell-mediated immune responses, 554t
cellophane (Scotch) tape test, 454
cellular immunity, 291
cellulitis, 61-63
  ascending, 83
  clinical findings, 62
  diagnosis, 62
  etiology, 61-62
  therapy, 62-63
CEM. *See* contagious equine metritis (CEM)
central nervous system (CNS) infections. *See also* brain infections; spinal cord infections; spinal infections
  abscesses
    intracranial, 56-57
    right brain hemisphere, 56f
    spinal, 57-58
  aspergillosis
    clinical findings, 425
    diagnosis, 427
  bacterial meningitis and meningoencephalitis, 55-56
  cerebrospinal fluid collection and analysis, 49-53
  cryptococcosis, 440
  economic impact of, 47
  equine protozoal myeloencephalitis (EPM), 459, 464-465
  helminth and dipterin parasites infecting, 509-510
  neuroanatomy, 48-50
    blood-brain barrier and cerebrospinal fluid, 49-50
    brain and meninges, 48-49
    cranial nerves, 49
    meninges, 48f
  neuro-ophthalmic infectious diseases, 114-116
    Horner's syndrome, 115-116
    vestibular disease, 114-115
  parasitic, 58
  pathogenesis, 50-51
    entry of pathogens, 50
    immune response to, 50-51
  pathogens, 48t, 612-613
  rabies (*See* rabies (RABV))
  rule-outs, 600
    brainstem signs, 600
    cortical signs, 600
    spinal cord or peripheral nervous system signs, 600
  signs of meningitis, 76
  spinal cord, 49 (*See also* spinal cord infections)
  therapeutic considerations (in general), 54-55
    antimicrobial agents, 54
    glucocorticoids, osmotic agents, diuretics, 54-55
    supportive therapy, 55
  vascularization, 49
cephalic tetanus, 369
cerebellitis, 47
cerebrospinal fluid (CSF)
  analysis, 53
  appearance, 53
  biochemical parameters, 53

cerebrospinal fluid (CSF) (*Continued*)
  cellular evaluation, 53
  characteristics, 49-53
  collection techniques, 49-53
    atlanto-occipital (AO), 51f
    lumbosacral (LS), 52f
  immunologic testing/molecular diagnostics, 53
  laboratory diagnosis, 49-53
  protein concentration, 53
  xanthochromic cerebrospinal fluid, 164f
cestodes
  Anoplocephala perfoliata, 490f-491f
    ileocecal intussusception with, 493f
    prevalence in U.S. states and other countries, 492b
  clinical findings, 492-493
  diagnosis, 493
  epidemiology, 491-492
  etiology, 490-491
    life cycle, 491
    morphology, 490-491
  pathogenesis, 492
  pathologic findings, 494
  prevalence by species of, 490
  prevention, 494
  tapeworm species, 494
  therapy, 494
CFT (complement fixation test), 473
Chandipura virus, 204
chi-square test, 525t
chitin synthesis inhibitors, 430
Chlamydophila species, 99
chlorambucil, 597
chloramphenicol, 581
chondroids, 16f, 17
Chorioptes species, 83, 497
Chorioptes bovis mite, 497f
chorioptic mange, 497-498
  diagnosis, 497
  epidemiology, 497
  etiology, 497
  pathogenesis and clinical findings, 497
  prevention, 497-498
  therapy, 497
chronic granulomatous pneumonia, 11
circle of Willis, 18-19
circling (symptom), 56f
Citrobacter diversus, 94
CK (creatinine kinase), 60
Cleopatra species, 512
climate disturbance effects on disease, 548
Clinical and Laboratory Standards Institute (CLSI), 263
  minimal inhibitory concentration (MIC) values for antifungal agents, 408
  standardized testing of antifungal drugs, 399
clinical findings. *See under specific infection/disease or pathogen*
clitoral fossa culture, 341, 341f
clitoral sinus, yeast colonization of, 437
clostridial enteritis, 260-261
  classification of isolates based on toxin production, 354t
  clinical findings, 354-355
  diagnosis, 355-356
    Clostridium difficile, 355-356
    Clostridium perfringens, 356
    Gram staining, 352f
  epidemiology and pathogenesis, 352-354
    Clostridium difficile, 352-354
    Clostridium perfringens, 354
  etiology, 352
  pathologic findings, 354t

clostridial enteritis (*Continued*)
  prevalence in healthy horses, 354t
  prevention, 358
    outbreak control, 358
    sporadic clostridial colitis, 358
    transmission to other horses, 358
  public health considerations, 358-359
  shedding by nondiarrheic horses, 353t
  species found in intestinal tract, 353b
  treatment, 356-358
    antimicrobial therapy, 356-357
    fecal transplantation, 357-358
    probiotics, 357-358
    toxin adsorption, 357
clostridial myonecrosis (gas gangrene), 61, 359-361
  clinical findings, 360
    skin and muscle sloughing, 361f
  diagnosis, 360
    Gram stain, 360f
  epidemiology, 359
  etiology, 359
  at injection sites, 361f-362f
  pathogenesis, 359-360
  prevention, 361
  Quarter Horses, 361
  therapy, 360-361
Clostridium species, 1, 10-11, 46, 60-61, 258-259
  pathogenic, 352, 353b, 359
Clostridium botulinum. *See* botulism
Clostridium botulinum hyperimmune plasma, 595
Clostridium difficile, 43-44, 260-261, 352-354, 516, 532-533
  diagnosis, 355-356
  epidemiology and pathogenesis, 352-354
Clostridium perfringens, 43-44, 260-261, 354, 356, 612-613
  diagnosis, 356
  epidemiology and pathogenesis, 354
  types A, B, and C, 354
Clostridium perfringens enterotoxin (CPE), 354
Clostridium piliformis (or *piliforme*). *See* Tyzzer's disease
Clostridium septicum, 354
Clostridium sordelli, 354
Clostridium tetani, 368, 595. *See also* tetanus
CLSI (Clinical and Laboratory Standards Institute), 263
  MIC (minimal inhibitory concentration) values for antifungal agents, 408
  standardized testing of antifungal drugs, 399
CNS. *See* central nervous system (CNS) infections
CN VII (facial nerve), 14
  damage to, 19, 20f
  paralysis of, 114f
CN VIII (vestibulocochlear/acoustic nerve), 14, 19
  damage to, 20f
coagulase-negative staphylococci (CoNS), 278-280
coagulase-positive staphylococci (CPS), 278, 280-281
coagulopathies
  management of, 124
  neonatal sepsis, 76-77
Coccidioides species, 94, 399
Coccidioides immitis, 4, 393-394, 399, 405
  identification of, 396
  life cycle of, 400f
Coccidioides posadasii, 405

coccidiomycosis
  anatomic locations of, 402f
  clinical findings, 402-404
    noncomestic horses, 404
  diagnosis and pathologic findings,
    404-405
    immunodiffusion serologic test, 404f
    lung radiograph, 403f
    parietal pleura with granulomata, 403f
    serologic tests, 404t
  epidemiology and epizootiology, 401-402
  equids with naturally acquired, 400b
  etiology, 400-401
  geographic distribution, 401f
  histopathologic appearance in spleen, 401f
  histopathologic appearance of, 401f
  pathogenesis, 402
  prevention and public health
    considerations, 405-406
  safety measures for necropsies, 406
  therapy, 405
coccidiosis, enteric, 507-508
coital exanthema, 104-105
Coley's vaccine, 584
colic
  ascarids in small intestine, 482f
  in foals with rotavirus, 200-201
  tapeworm-related, 492-493
colitis
  bacterial, samples and tissue selection,
    259b
  etiology
    Clostridium difficile infection, 353
    pinworm infection, 485
    related to antimicrobial therapy, 577b
    sporadic clostridial colitis, 358
collapse and sudden death, 603
colliculus seminalis, 103f
Colorado State University Veterinary
    Teaching Hospital (CSU-VTH), 533
  monitoring methods, 539
  outbreak precautions, 531
colostrum, 77
comet tail artifacts, 9
common antigen tests, 355
common carotid artery (CCA), 18-19
compensatory antiinflammatory response
    syndrome (CARS), 70
competitive enzyme-linked immunosorbent
    assay (cELISA), 473
complement fixation test (CFT), 473
computed tomography (CT). *See* diagnosis
    under specific infection/disease
conidiobolomycosis, 419
Conidiobolus species, 416-417, 419. *See also*
    zygomycosis
Conidiobolus coronatus, 419
conidospores, 422f
conjunctiva
  conjunctivitis, 602
    bacterial/fungal, 111b
    primary, 111
  depigmentation of, 118
  hyperemia, 110f, 113f, 185f
  normal flora, 259b
CoNS (coagulase-negative staphylococci),
    278-280
constrictive pericarditis, 34f
contagious equine metritis (CEM), 554t,
    556. *See also Taylorella equigenitalis*
  clinical findings, 340
    purulent vaginal discharge, 340f
  diagnosis, 340-341
    clitoral fossa culture, 341, 341f
    penis/prepuce cultures, 341, 342f

contagious equine metritis (CEM)
  (Continued)
    terminal urethra culture, 343f
    urethral sinus culture, 342f
  epidemiology, 339-340
  etiology, 339
  import requirements, 341-343
  outbreaks due to international movement
    of horses, 547t
  pathogenesis, 340
  prevention and control, 343
  public health considerations, 343
  purulent discharge and endometritis, 340f
  therapy, 104, 343
contagiousness (infectivity), 515-516
contamination
  of equipment, 412, 412f
  mechanisms of, 1
  prevention measures, 535 (*See also*
    biosecurity)
control of infection. *See* biosecurity
core vaccines, 558
cornea
  abscesses, 424
    fungal, 113f
    mycotic keratitis (keratomycosis), 424f
  edema, 113f-114f, 602
  fungal hyphae, 111f
  fungal infections, 394
    aspergillosis, 426f
    mycotic keratitis (*See* mycotic keratitis
      (keratomycosis))
  keratitis, 602
    bacterial, 112
    fungal, 112-114
    primary, 111
    viral, 112
  pedicle grafts, 113f
  ulcers, 20, 76, 110f, 113f
    culturing methods, 261
    with edema and vascularization, 114f
    melting, 113f
  vascularization of, 113f
coronaviruses, 43, 201-203
  in adult horses, 202
  diagnosis, 203
  epidemiology and clinical findings, 202
  etiology, 201-202
  husbandry/infection control, 203
  subfamilies, 201-202
  torovirus, 203
coronitis, 241f
corpus hemorrhagicum, 87f
cortical blindness, 48-49
cortical signs, rule-outs, 600
corticosteroid therapy
  contraindications for, 113-114, 129, 432
  neonatal sepsis, 78
Corynebacterium species
  antimicrobial agents for, 109
  urinary tract infections, 106
Corynebacterium equi. See Rhodococcus equi
Corynebacterium pseudotuberculosis, 60-61,
    94, 373
  clinical findings, 375-376
    external abscesses, 375
    flies on exudate, 374f
    internal infections, 375-376
    pectoral abscess, 375f
    pectoral abscesses, 373f
    secondary pneumonia, 378f
    triceps abscess, 378f
    ulcerative lymphangitis, 376
    ventral midline dermatitis, 374f
  clinicopathologic data, 376t

Corynebacterium pseudotuberculosis
  (Continued)
  diagnosis, 377-378
    culture, 377
    serology, 377
    ultrasonography, 375f-378f, 377-378
  epidemiology, 373-374
  etiology, 373
  orchitis, 102f
  pathogenesis, 374
  therapy, 378-379
    antimicrobial drugs, 379t
    external abscesses, 378-379
    internal infections, 379
    prevention, 379
    ulcerative lymphangitis, 379
coughing, 598
  pneumonia-related, 7-8
  on tracheal palpation, 3
CPE *(Clostridium perfringens* enterotoxin),
    354
CPS (coagulase-positive staphylococci), 278,
    280-281
cracked heels. *See* pastern dermatitis
cranial nerve function
  abnormalities, 462f
  CN VII (facial nerve), 14
    damage to, 19, 20f
    paralysis of, 114f
  CN VIII (vestibulocochlear/acoustic
    nerve), 14, 19
    damage to, 20f
  deficits with Borna disease, 229
  equine protozoal myeloencephalitis
    (EPM), 461
creatinine kinase (CK), 60
critical control point (CCP), 533
Crotalaria, 11
crusting/scaling dermatoses, 79-81, 603
  bacterial, 79-80
  clinical findings, 79
  Culicoides hypersensitivity, 502f
  dermatophilosis (*See* dermatophilosis
    (rain rot))
  dermatophytosis (*See* dermatophytosis
    (ringworm))
  diagnosis, 79
  fungal, 80
  infectious
    nonpuritic, 79b
    puritic, 79b
  muzzle lesions, 241f
  nonpuritic, 79b
  parasitic, 80
  prevention, 80
  puritic, 79b
  therapy, 79-80
  viral, 80-81
    molluscum contagiosum, 81
    poxvirus, 80-81
cryosurgery, warts, 246
cryotherapy
  cellulitis, 62
  prevention of laminitis, 70
  sarcoids, 249
cryptococcosis, 116-117, 437
  clinical findings, 437-438
  diagnosis, 436
    biopsy, 437
    culturing, 437
    cytology, 437
    endoscopy, 436
    radiography and computed tomography,
      436
    serology, 437

cryptococcosis *(Continued)*
  epidemiology, 437
  etiology, 436-440
  pathogenesis, 437
  pathologic findings, 439-440
    central nervous system, 440
    gastrointestinal tract, 440
    reproductive tract, 440
    respiratory tract, 440
    subcutaneous tissue, 440
  subcutaneous tissue, 440
  therapy, 440
  virulence factors, 436
    capsules, 436
    melanin, 436
    thermotolerance, 436
Cryptococcus species, 4, 410, 438f-439f
  antibody detection, 437
  antigen assays, 437
  diagnosis, 438f
  identification of, 396
Cryptococcus gatti, 4, 395
Cryptococcus neoformans, 4, 94, 439f, 446
  Gram stain, 396f
  identification of, 395
  ocular manifestations of, 4, 116-117
cryptosporidiosis, 508-509
Cryptosporidium species, 43, 449, 507-508
Cryptosporidium parvum, 452f
CSF. *See* cerebrospinal fluid (CSF)
CSU-VTH (Colorado State University
    Veterinary Teaching Hospital), 533
  monitoring methods, 539
  outbreak precautions, 531
CTLs (cytotoxic T lymphocytes), 235
Culex species, 211
Culex pipiens, 220
Culex tarsalis, 214, 220
Culicoides species, 118, 182, 251-252
Culicoides bolitinos, 183
Culicoides variipennis, 182
Culiseta melanura, 211
culture media, 259-260
culturing, 44
cumulative incidence, 519-520, 519b
cumulative incidence comparisons
    comparing attributable risk (AR) and
      attributable fraction (AF), 523, 524b
    relative risk, 523, 524b
cutaneous leishmaniasis, 82
cutaneous onchocerciasis, 486
Cyathostominae (cyathostomes,
    cyathostomins, small stronglyes,
    trichonemes), 478-481
  clinical findings, 479
  diagnosis, 479
  epidemiology, 479
  etiology, 478-479
  pathogenesis, 479
  pathologic findings, 479
  prevention, 480-481
  public health considerations, 481
  therapy, 479-480
Cyathostominae species, 477f, 478, 479f
cyathostomin infection, 613
cyclic amines, 583
cyclophosphamide, 597
cyclosporine, 596
cystitis, 106-107
  sabulous, 106-107
cysts
  Besnoitia, 512f
  parasitic, 80
  warbles, 504
cytidine, 166

cytokines, 590
cytomegalovirus (equine herpesvirus-2), 6
cytotoxic T lymphocytes (CTLs), 235

D

daily attire, 534
dead-end hosts, 459, 531-532
death, sudden, 384, 603
  neonatal, 305-306, 309
demodectic mange, 498
  diagnosis, 498
  epidemiology, 498
  etiology, 498
  pathogenesis and clinical findings, 498
  therapy, 498
Demodex species, 111
Demodex caballi, 498
Demodex equi, 498
dendritic cell suppressor mechanisms, 596b
denervation of laryngeal nerve, 17-18
dengue, 218t-219t
depigmentation, 245
Dermacentor niten, 470-471
Dermatobia hominis, 504
dermatology. *See* skin infections
dermatophilosis (rain rot), 283-284, 285f
  antimicrobial therapy
    systemic, 286
    topical, 287
  clinical findings, 284-285
    after rainfall, 285f
    alopecia, 284f-285f
    clinical findings, paintbrush appearance
      of crusts, 284f
    dry skin and scaling, 285f
    paintbrush appearance of crusts, 284f
    sensitivity to touch, 285f
    on unpigmented areas, 286f
  diagnosis, 285-286
    cultures, 286
    cytology, 286, 286f
  etiology and epidemiology, 283
  host factors, 284
  pathogenesis, 283-284
    climatic conditions and host factors,
      284
    immune response to *Dermatophilus*,
      284
    skin trauma and insect bites, 284
    virulence of strains, 283-284
  pathology, 286
  prevention, 287
  public health considerations, 287
  rainfall factors, 283-284
  resistance to, 284
  therapy, 286
Dermatophilus congolensis, 283
  aggravation of lesions by *Staphylococcus*,
    284-285
  cytology, 286f
  virulence, 283-284
  virulence of strains, 283-284
dermatophyte cultures, 396-397, 397f
  dermatophyte test medium (DTM), 412f,
    413
dermatophytes, about, 393-394
dermatophytosis (ringworm). *See also*
    Trichophyton equinum
  clinical findings, 412-413
    alopecia patches/pruritis, 412f
  diagnosis, 413-414
    culturing, 413-414
      dermatophyte test medium (DTM),
        412f, 413

dermatophytosis (ringworm) *(Continued)*
    direct examination of hair, 413
    pathology, 414
    Wood's lamp, 413
  epidemiology, 411-412
  etiology, 411
  fungal pathogens, 80
  pathogenesis, 412
    environmental factors, 412
    host factors and immune response,
      412
    virulence factors, 412
  prevention, 414
  public health considerations, 414
  therapy, 414
    environmental control, 414
    systemic, 414
    topical, 414
dermatoses
  large nodular/mass, 82-83, 82b
    diagnosis, 83
    etiology, 82-83
    therapy, 83
  nodular/masses, 82-83
  papulonodular, 81-82
descemetroceles, ruptured, 113f
deworming programs, horses/donkeys/mules,
  14
diagnosis. *See under specific infection/disease
    or pathogen*
diagnostic test kits, 614, 614t
diagnostic test properties, 525-527
  estimation of sensitivity and specificity,
    526-527, 526b
  evaluation of characteristics of, 528
  measurement types, 525
  test accuracy, 526-527
diarrhea
  adult horses, 599
    acute diarrhea, 44-45
    chronic, 45-46
    Gastrodiscus, 513
    laboratory diagnosis, 44-45
    parasitic, 44
    rule-outs, 599
  clostridial, 353t, 354-355, 357
  Clostridium perfringens, 357
  Clostridium perfringens enterotoxin (CPE),
    354
  coronaviruses, 201-203
  equine proliferative enteropathy (EPE),
    318f
  foals, 42-43, 599
    bacterial, 42-43
    Escherichia coli, 42-43
    protozoal, 43
    rule-outs, 599
    Strongyloides infection, 484
    viral disorders, 43
  giardia, 584
  molecular testing, 611-612
  Neorickettsia risticii, 349-350
  probiotics for prevention, 358
  rotavirus, 198-201
  salmonellosis, 331
  torovirus, 203
  vaccine recommendations, 569-570
DIC (disseminated intravascular
    coagulation), 354t
Diclazuril, 466
Dictyocaulus arnfeildi, 13-14
Dictyocaulus arnfeildi eggs, 451f
diet/nutrition
  food allergies, 80
  grain component, 44

diet/nutrition *(Continued)*
 toxic ingestion (*See* toxic ingestions)
 for urinary tract infection treatment/
  prevention, 109
differential diagnosis. *See* diagnosis *under
 specific infection/disease;* rule-outs
diffuse peritonitis, 46
dikkop (cardiac) form of African horse
 sickness, 184, 184f-185f, 186, 187f
direct microscopic examination, 257-258
Dirofilaria immitis, 118, 510
dirofilariasis, 118
dirty mucus, 1
disease agent characteristics, 515-516
disease control. *See* biosecurity
disease distribution factors, 546-549
 agroterrorism, 549
 effects of climate disturbance, 548
 emergent diseases, 548
 growth of horse industries, 544-545
 international trade in equids, semen,
  embryos, 546-547
 migration of amplifying/reservoir hosts,
  vectors, pathogens, 549
 multinational trade agreements, 547-548
 new variants of pathogens, 548
 preexport testing reliability, 549
 spread from feral equids, 549
disease ecology, 515-517
disinfectants, 538t, 539f
 for footbaths, 536
 surface cleaning, 537
diskospondylitis, 58f
disseminated aspergillosis and hemolytic
 anemia, 426f
disseminated intravascular coagulation
 (DIC), 46, 354t
distal limb edema, 345f
distribution of disease. *See* epidemiology
 *under specific infection/disease or
 pathogen*
distributive shock, 123
diuretics, 54-55
DNA
 amplified, 134f
 papovaviruses, 81-82
 testing for EHV-1, 3
DNA probes, 263
DNA vaccines, 552-553
dogs, African horse sickness (AHS) in,
 183-184
Dohle bodies, 71
donkeys, 13
 besnoitiosis, 511
 deworming, 14
 dourine, 505
 enteric coccidiosis, 507-508
 as reservoir hosts for equine lungworm,
  489
 Taylorella asinigenitalis, 337
dourine, 105, 505-506
DPJ (duodentitis/proximal jejunitis), 43
drainage (therapy)
 abdominal, 46-47
 pleural cavity, 11
Draschia megastoma, 487f
drug resistant/sensitive organisms
 Dermatophilus congolensis, 286
 equine arteritis virus (EAV), to physical
  and chemical agents, 169-170
 Florida study, 74
 fungi, 399
 MRSA (*See* methicillin-resistant
  Staphylococcus aureus (MRSA))
 multidrug-resistant bacteria, 531-532

drug resistant/sensitive organisms
 (Continued)
 resistance to (*See* drug resistant/sensitive
  organisms)
 staphylococcal, 280
 Staphylococcus aureus (*See* methicillin-
  resistant *Staphylococcus aureus*
  (MRSA))
 streptococcal organisms, 85
 ticks, 496
DTM (dermatophyte test medium), 412f,
 413
dumb form of rabies, 205
dunkop (pulmonary) form of African horse
 sickness, 184, 184f, 186, 186f-187f
duodentitis/proximal jejunitis (DPJ), 43
dysphagia, 599
 Borna disease, 230
 causes of, 7
 guttural pouch mycosis, 17f
 with guttural pouch mycosis, 17-18
 medical therapy, 18
dyspnea, 598-599
dysrhythmias, 39-41
dysuria, 108, 600

E

EAdV1 (equine adenovirus type 1), 189
ears
 dropped, 114f
 middle ear infections, 48
 sarcoids, 248f
 tick infestations, 495
 otitis externa, 495
 vestibulocochlear/acoustic nerve (CN
  VIII), 14, 19, 20f
 warts (papillomavirus), 245f
eastern equine encephalitis (EEE), 210t,
 516
 clinical findings, 212, 212f
 diagnosis, 212-213
 epidemiology, 211
 etiology, 210-214
 ocular manifestations of, 116t
 pathogenesis, 211-212
 pathologic findings, 213, 213f
 prevention, 213-214
 public health considerations, 214
 therapy, 213
 vaccine recommendations, 559
EAV. *See* equine arteritis virus (EAV)
Echidnophaga gallinacea, 504
Echinacea angustifolia, 591
echinococcosis, 118, 510
ectoparasites
 biting flies (*See* flies/larvae)
 hypodermiasis (warbles) (*See under* flies/
  larvae)
 mites (*See* mites/mange)
 mosquitoes (*See* mosquitoes/mosquito
  bites)
 nonbiting flies (*See under* flies/larvae)
 pediculosis (*See* lice (pediculosis))
 poultry lice (*See under* lice (pediculosis))
 stinging insects (*See* insect bites/stings)
 ticks (*See* ticks/tick-borne diseases)
 in wounds (*See* wound infections)
edema
 African horse sickness (AHS)
  cardiac form, 185f
  conjunctival, 185f
  lungs, 186, 186f
  corneal, 113f-114f
  distal limb, 345f

edema *(Continued)*
 distal limbs, purpura hemorrhagica, 271f
 ventral abdominal or limb, 601-602
EEE. *See* eastern equine encephalitis (EEE)
Efficacy of Nosocomial Infection Control
 (SENIC), 530
EGA. *See* equine granulocytic anaplasmosis/
 ehrlichiosis
egg/cell cultures, 133-134
EHM (equine myeloencephalopathy), 547t
EHM (myeloencephalopathy), 3
Ehrlichia equi. See equine granulocytic
 anaplasmosis/ehrlichiosis
Ehrlichia risticii. See Neorickettsia risticii
ehrlichiosis. *See* equine granulocytic
 anaplasmosis/ehrlichiosis
EHV. *See* equine herpesvirus (EHV)
EI. *See* equine influenza (EI)
EIA. *See* equine infectious anemia (EIA)
EIA (enzyme immunosorbent assay), 516
Eikenella corrodens, 57-58
Eimeria species, 449
Eimeria leuckarti, 452f, 507-508
Eimeria solipedum, 507-508
Eimeria uniungulsti, 507-508
electron microscopy, 138
ELEM (equine leukoencephalomalacia), 117
ELISA. *See* enzyme-linked immunosorbent
 assay (ELISA)
EMAs (equi merozoite antigens), 471-472
emergencies. *See also* trauma
 synovial infections, 64
 tachydysrhythmia, 33t
emergent diseases, 548
employees/personnel, 531. *See also*
 biosecurity
 biosecurity measures
  barrier gowns, 535
  daily attire, 534
  face/eye protection, 535
  footbaths/footmats, 536-537
  footwear hygiene, 535
  gloves, 535
  hand hygiene, 534
  movement/traffic flow management,
   535
 education on biosecurity management for,
  543
 infection control, 536 (*See also*
  biosecurity)
 MRSA colonization in, 283t
 zoonotic infection protection, 531-532
empyema
 guttural pouches, 15f, 16-17
  clinical findings, 16
  diagnosis, 16
  etiology, 16
  medical therapy, 16-17
  surgical therapy, 17
 subdural, 47
EN (equine neorickettiosis). *See
 Neorickettsia risticii*
encephalitis. *See also* central nervous system
 (CNS) infections; flavivirus
 encephalitides; myeloencephalitis
 eastern equine encephalitis (*See* eastern
  equine encephalitis (EEE))
 fulminant, 59
 Japanese encephalitis (JE), 218t-219t,
  220
  human encephalitis cases, 221
  life cycles, 220f
 kokobera encephalitis, 218t-219t
 meningitis and meningoencephalitis,
  55-56

encephalitis *(Continued)*
  modoc encephalitis, 218t-219t
  Murray Valley encephalitis, 254f, 255
  Nigerian equine encephalitis, 256
  Ntaya encephalitis, 218t-219t
  paramyxovirus, 255-256
  rhombencephalitis, 47
  Rio Bravo encephalitis, 218t-219t
  seabird encephalitides, 218t-219t
  Sondweni encephalitis, 218t-219t
  tick-borne, 218t-219t
  verminous, 58
encephalomyelitis. *See* West Nile virus
    (WNV)
encephalosis, 251-252
endemic diseases, 521
  African horse sickness (AHS), 182
  blastomycosis, 434f
  coccidiomycosis, 401-402, 401f
  rabies, 203-204
endocarditis. *See* infective endocarditis (IE)
endocrine adaptations to illness, 72
endometritis, 92f
  with contagious equine metritis, 340f
  diagnosis, 427
  epidemiology, 423
  fungal, 88f
    aspergillosis, 423-425
    candidiasis in, 410
  pathogenesis, 424
  therapy, 433
  in utero treatment, 90t
endophthalmitis, 9-10
endothelial dysfunction, 123
endotoxemia, 125f-126f, 331
endotoxemia antibodies, 595
endotoxins
  lipopolysaccharide (LPS), 120f
  mediators of inflammatory response to,
      122t-123t
  role in gram-negative sepsis of, 70
enophthalmos, 17-18
enteric clostridial infections. *See* clostridial
    enteritis
enteric coccidiosis, 507-508
enteric infections, 260-261
enteritis, 43, 259b, 484
Enterobacter species, 64
  microbial susceptibility, 572
  placentitis, 94
  urinary tract infections, 106
Enterobacteriaceae species, 63, 66
Enterobus vermicularis, 485
enterococcal infections, 385-386
Enterococcus species
  antimicrobial agents for, 109
  urinary tract infections, 106
enterocolitis
  in foals, 43
  quinidine, 114f
environmental management. *See also*
    biosecurity
  ascarid contamination, 483
  dermatophilosis, 284
  epidemiology and, 516-517
  fly control, 499-500
  infection control, 537
    cleaning of surfaces, 537
    disinfection, 537
  insect control, 502-503
  maintenance of clean, 77
  mosquito control, 501
  pinworm control, 485
  skin infections and, 78, 80
  tick control, 496

environmental management *(Continued)*
  transmission of strongylosis, 476
  unsanitary, 71
Environmental Protection Agency (EPA),
    Medical Waste Tracking Act (MWTA),
    537-538
environment characteristics, 516-517
  individual, 516
  population aggregate, 516-517
enzyme immunosorbent assay (EIA), 516
enzyme-linked immunosorbent assay
    (ELISA), 3, 18, 44, 138-139, 138f-139f,
    528b. *See also* laboratory diagnosis
  Anoplocephala perfoliata diagnosis, 493
  blocking ELISA, 148
  competitive enzyme-linked
      immunosorbent assay (cELISA), 473
  ELISA-based assays, 148
  indirect, 138
  polymerase chain reaction- (PCR-ELISA),
      477
eosinophilic granulomas, 417-418
eosinophil suppressor mechanisms, 596b
EP. *See* equine piroplasmosis (EP)
EPA (Environmental Protection Agency),
    MWTA (Medical Waste Tracking Act),
    537-538
EPDs (extrapulmonary disorders), 292
EPE. *See* equine proliferative enteropathy
    (EPE)
epidemic curve associations, 521f-522f
  equine influenza (EI), 546t
epidemic diseases, 521
epidemiology. *See also under specific
    infection/disease or pathogen*
  attack risk table, 525t
  categorical data, 523-525
  cumulative incidence, 523-525
  causation of disease, 517
  chi-square test, 525t
  comparing groups, 522-525
  definition, 515
  diagnostic test properties, 525-527
    estimation of sensitivity and specificity,
        526-527, 526b
    evaluation of characteristics of, 528
    measurement types, 525
    test accuracy, 526-527
  disease agent characteristics, 515-516
  disease ecology, 515-517
  environment characteristics, 516-517
    individual, 516
    population aggregate, 516-517
  epidemic curve associations, 521f-522f
  epidemiologic approach, 515
  five Ws of, 515
  host characteristics, 516
  identifying causal factors, 517-525
    categorical data, 518-519
    data types, 518
    interval data, 518
    measuring disease, 517-520
    population-at-risk, 518
  interpretation of test results, predictive
      values, 527-528, 527b-528b
  measurement data, 522-523
    reality of difference, 522-523
  measures of disease frequency, 519-520
    cause-fatality rate, 520b
    cumulative incidence, 519-520, 519b
    incidence rate, 520, 520b
    mortality rate, 519b
    prevalence, 519, 519b
    relationship between prevalence and
        incidence, 520, 521b

epidemiology *(Continued)*
  outbreak management, 529
  predictive values, 528b, 528f
  prevention strategies, 528-529
  principles of, 515
  probability of new cases of disease, 516f
  temporal patterns of disease, 520-522
  using tests in combination, 528
epididymis, infections of, 102, 102f
  epidiymitis, 102
epidural abscesses, 47
epiphysitis, septic, 69f
epistaxis
  endoscopic examination, 18
  with guttural pouch mycosis, 17
epizootic lymphangitis, 117
EPM. *See* equine protozoal
    myeloencephalitis (EPM)
EPM (equine protozoal myeloencephalitis),
    117
equi merozoite antigens (EMAs), 471-472
equine adenovirus type 1 (EAdV1), 189
equine ambulatory practices, 540-541
equine arteritis virus (EAV). *See also* equine
    viral arteritis (EVA)
  Bucyrus strain, 169, 174f
  clinical findings of equine viral arteritis
      (EVA) after inoculation of, 175f-176f
  equine arteritis virus antigen in fetus,
      178f
  genetic strains, 172-173
  guidelines for breeding to stallions
      shedding, 180f
  mortality, 175
  virulence determinants, 170
*Equine Biosecurity Principles and Best
    Practices Guide* (Alberta Medical
    Association and Alberta Equestrian
    Federation), 542
Equine Biosecurity Risk Calculator, 542
equine dysautonomia (grass sickness), 366
equine encephalosis virus (EEV), 251-252
equine granulocytic anaplasmosis/
    ehrlichiosis
  clinical findings, 345-346
    distal limb edema, 345f
    icteric sclera, 345f
    petechiation of nasal septum mucosa,
        345f
  diagnosis, 346
    microscopic and molecular, 346f
  epidemiology, 344
  etiology, 344
  ocular manifestations of, 117t
  pathogenesis, 344-345
  pathologic findings, 346
    inclusions in neutrophilic and
        eosinophilic granulocytes, 346f
  prevention, 347
  therapy, 346-347
equine herpesvirus (EHV)
  alpha types, 151, 516
  classifications of
    alpha (EHV-1, EHV-3, EHV-4), 6
    gamma (EHV-2, EHV-5), 6
  clinical findings, 159-161
    abortion, 160
    foals/young horses, 160f
    myeloencephalopathy, 162f, 164f
    neonatal foals, 160
    neurologic, 161
    respiratory, 159-160
    stallions, 160
  control, 167-168
  demonstration of infection, 161-163

equine herpesvirus (EHV) *(Continued)*
  description/overview, 151-152
  diagnosis 161-165
    case selection for sampling, 161
    cerebrospinal fluid (CSF) analysis, 164, 164f
    direct immunofluorescence (IF) tests, 161
    hematology, 163
    histopathology, 163
    history and clinical signs, 161
    of latent and lytic cycles, 164t
    of latent infection, 164-165
    polymerase chain reaction, 162-163
    serology, 163-164
    tests used for, 163t
    virus isolation, 163
  epidemiology, 155-156
    latency, 156
    reactivation from latency, 156
  equine herpesvirus-2 (cytomegalovirus), 6
  equine herpesvirus myeloencephalopathy (EHM), 3
  etiology, 152-155
    glycoproteins, 155
    lytic and latent infection cycles, 153-154
    viral genomes, 152
    viral proteins, 155
    viral replication, 152-153
    virology overview, 152
  management guidelines, 168b
  myeloencephalopathy (EHM), 3
  pathogenesis and pathologic findings, 155, 157-159
    central nervous system (CNS), 157
    immune evasion, 159
    immunology, 158-159
    respiratory tract, 157
    uterus, 157
    viremia, 157
    virulence, 157-158
  prognosis, 160
  treatment, 165-166
    abortion, 165
    myeloencephalopathy, 165-166
    ocular, 165
    respiratory, 165
  type 1 (EHV-1), 3
    latency and reactivation, 154f
    life cycle, 158
    regulation of, 153f
    transmission of, 156f
  type 2 (EHV-2)
    diagnostic methods, 3-4
    ocular manifestations of, 116t
  type 3 (EHV-3), 104, 104f
    abortion caused by, 98
  type 4 (EHV-4), 3
    life cycle, 158
  type 5 (EHV-5), 11-12
  vaccination, 166-167
  vaccine recommendations, 564-566
  viral genomes, 153f
equine herpesvirus-2 (cytomegalovirus), 6
equine herpesvirus myeloencephalopathy (EHM), 3, 47, 162f, 164f, 165-166
equine industry trends/changes, 544-545.
  See also international movement of horses
  growth of, 544-545
equine infectious anemia (EIA)
  about, 232-233
  branding of reactors, 238, 238f
  clinical findings, 236-237, 236f

equine infectious anemia (EIA) *(Continued)*
  diagnosis, 237
  epidemiology, 233-235
    prevalence, 233-234
    transmission, 234-235, 234f
  etiology, 233
  fly vectors, 499-500
  monoclonal antibodies, 137f
  ocular manifestations of, 116t
  outbreaks due to international movement of horses, 547t
  pathogenesis, 235-236
    anemia, 235
    immune control, 235-236
    thrombocytopenia, 235
  pathologic findings, 233f, 237, 237f
  prevention, 238
  public health considerations, 238
  therapy, 238
equine influenza (EI), 5-6
  Australian epidemic (2007), 531
  clinical findings, 144
    nasal discharge, 144f
  diagnosis, 145-148
    antigen detection, 145-147, 147f
    nasal mucosal swab, 146f
    single radial hemolysis (SRH) assay, 148f
  diagnostic procedures, 3
  epidemics, 546t
  epidemiology, 142-143
  etiology, 141-142
  genetic reassortment of parental viruses, 141f
  immunity to, 144-145
  influenza A components, 141f
  international movement of horses and spread of, 546t
  ocular manifestations of, 116t
  pathogenesis, 143-144
  pathologic findings, 148-149
  prevention, 150-151
    husbandry, 150-151
    vaccination, 150
  public health considerations, 151
  therapy, 149-150
    antiviral, 149-150
    medical, 149
  vaccination protocols, 562-563
    in an outbreak, 563
    foals, 562-563
    future vaccines, 563-564
    pregnant mares, 562
    primary series for adult horses, 562
    routine revaccination, 562
  vaccine recommendations, 560-564
equine leukoencephalomalacia (ELEM), 117
equine monocytic ehrlichiosis, 44
equine *Morbillivirus. See* Hendra virus (HeV)
equine myeloencephalopathy (EHM), 547t
equine neorickettiosis (EN). *See*
  Neorickettsia risticii; Potomac horse
  fever (PHF)/equine neorickettsiosis
  (EN)
equine pastern dermatitis (EPD), 83
  clinical findings, 83
  diagnosis, 83
  therapy, 83
equine piroplasmosis (EP), 117, 495
  with African horse sickness (AHS), 188
  antiprotozoal therapy, 584
  clinical findings/pathology, 472-473
    acute infection, 472
    Babiesa caballi merozoites in
      erythrocytes, 468f

equine piroplasmosis (EP) *(Continued)*
  chronic infection, 472
  inapparent carriers, 472
  pathophysiology, 473
    Theileria equi merozoites in
      erythrocytes, 468f
  complement fixation test (CFT), 473
  diagnosis, 473-474
    microscopy, 473
    polymerase chain reaction (PCR), 474
    serology, 473-474
  epidemiology, 470-471
  etiology, 468-469
  immunity to, 471
  life cycles
    Babesia caballi, 469, 469f
    Theileria equi, 469, 470f
  outbreaks, 468, 470-471
  outbreaks due to international movement
    of horses, 547t
  pathogenesis and immunity, 469,
    471-472, 475
    placental, 471
  prevention, 475
  public health considerations, 475
  therapy, 474
    effects of no treatment, 467-468
  transmission of, 475
equine proliferative enteropathy (EPE)
  clinical findings, 317-318
    diarrhea, 318f
    small intestinal wall thickness, 319f
    ventral and distal limb edema, 317f
    ventral and sheath edema, 318f
    weight loss, 318f
  diagnosis, 318-319
  epidemiology, 316-317
  etiology, 316
  pathogenesis, 317
  pathologic findings, 319-320
    cytoplasm, 320f
    hyperplasia of crypt glands, 320f
    ileal-cecal junction lesions, 319f
    ileum wall thickening, 319f
  prevention, 320-321
  therapy, 320
equine protozoal myeloencephalitis (EPM),
    47, 117, 461, 464f-465f, 509, 515-516.
    See also Sarcocystis neurona
  clinical findings, 461-462
    acute recumbency, 462f
    cranial nerve abnormalities, 462f
    muscle atrophy, 461f
  diagnosis, 462-464
    immunoblot test, 463f
    laboratory diagnosis, 463
  differential diagnosis, 456
  epidemiology, 457-459
  etiology, 456-457
  pathogenesis, 459-461
  pathologic findings, 456, 464-465
    myelitis in spinal cord, 464f
    necrosis of spinal cord, 464f-465f
    spinal cord infiltration, 465f
  prevention, 467
  public health considerations, 467
  therapy, 465-467
    antiprotozoal, 583-584
      folate synthesis inhibitors, 583
      triazine derivatives, 583-584
    antiprotozoal drugs, 465-466
    supportive, 466-467
equine recurrent uveitis (ERU), 114f
  leptospirosis, 305-307, 307f, 309-310
  treatment, 310

equine reorickettsiosis. *See* Potomac horse fever (PHF)/equine neorickettsiosis (EN)
equine rhinitis A virus, vaccine recommendations, 570
equine rhinoviruses. *See* rhinoviruses
equine viral arteritis (EVA), 4, 160. *See also* equine arteritis virus (EAV)
  abortion caused by, 98-99
  clinical findings, 174-176, 175f-176f
  diagnosis of, 4, 176-177
    equine arteritis virus antigen in fetus, 178f
    histopathology, 177
    serology, 177
    viral nucleic acid detection, 177
    virus isolation, 176-177
  epidemiology, 170-173
    carrier state/molecular epidemiology, 171-173
    outbreaks, 170-171
    seroprevalence and breed predilection, 171
    transmission, 171
  etiology, 169-170
    molecular properties, 169-170
    resistance to physical and chemical agents, 170
  genome organization and expression, 170f
  guidelines for breeding to stallion shedding virus, 180f
  ocular manifestations of, 116t
  outbreaks due to international movement of horses, 547t
  pathogenesis, 172f-173f, 173-174
  pathology, 177-178
  prevention, 178-181
    husbandry and control programs, 179-181
    immunity, 178-179
    vaccination, 179
  public health considerations, 181
  T cell-resistant groups, 174f
  therapy, 178
  vaccine recommendations, 569
equinum*Microsporum equinum autotrophicum*, 411
Equus burchelli, 182
Equus caballus, 244
Erbovirus, 6
ERU. *See* equine recurrent uveitis (ERU)
ERU (equine recurrent uveitis), 114f
Escherichia coli, 1, 57-58, 64, 72, 94
  abortion caused by, 95f
  diarrhea in foals due to, 42-43
  microbial susceptibility, 572
  urinary tract infections, 106
  virulence, 107
esophagus, 42
  infectious disorders, 42
  normal flora, 42
ethics of infection control, 530
etiology. *See under specific infection/disease or pathogen*
ETs (exfoliative toxins), 279-280
Eubacterium species, 1
eumycetomas, 381
EVA. *See* equine viral arteritis (EVA)
events, biosecurity measures at, 168, 541-543
examinations. *See under specific infection/disease or pathogen*
exfoliative toxins (ETs), 279-280
exogenous antibodies, 556

exogenous cytokines, 585t, 589-590
  interferon-α, 589-590
  present and future of other cytokines, 590
external parasites. *See* specific infection/disease or parasite
extrapulmonary disorders (EPDs), 292
exudates
  arytenoid chondritis in, 6f
  caseous, *Rhodoccus equi*, 296f
  chronic sinusitis with, 5f
  Escherichia coli, 95f
  guttural pouch, inspissation of, 3f
eyelids
  blepharitis, 110-111
  blepharospasm, 9-10
  Histoplasma capsulatum farciminosum (HCF), 444-445
  mite infestations, 498
  retraction of, 369
  sarcoids, 248f
eye protection (personnel), 535
eyes. *See ocular* entries
eyeworm, 502-503

F

face/eye protection, 535
face fly, 502-503
facial nerve (CN VII), 14
  damage to, 19, 20f
  paralysis of, 114f
FADs (foreign animal diseases), 605-606, 612
failure of passive immunity (FPT), 71
  ensuring adequate, 77
Fasciola, morphology, compared to *Gastrodiscus*, 513t
Fasciola hepatica, 449, 452f
fastidious organisms (specialized media/culture requirements), 261b
fecal tests, 44-45, 449
  aerobic cultures, 44
  anaerobic cultures, 44-45
  cultures, 44-45, 453
  fecal egg count reduction (FECR) test, 480b
  fecal flotation, 449-453
    Anoplocephala perfoliata, 493
    ascarid diagnosis, 482
    Cryptosporidium oocysts, 508
    Dictyocaulus arnfieldi, 13
    Gastrodiscus, 513
  fecal microbiota transplantation, 357-358
  fecal sedimentation, 453-454
  fecal smears, 454
feral equids, disease spread by, 549
fetal necropsies, 381
fetuses, equine arteritis virus antigen in, 178f
fibrin, 33f
  in anterior chamber, 110f, 113f-114f
  removal of, 411
fibrinoeffusive idiopathic pericarditis, 35f
fibroblastic sarcoid, 248-249, 248f
filamentous fungi, 394
Filobasidiella neoformans, 4-5
fire ants (*Solenopsis* species), 504
fistulas
  guttural pouch, 18
  rule-outs, 603
fistulous withers, brucellosis, 337-338, 338f
flashing of nictitans, 369f
flatworms, 449

flavivirus encephalitides, 254f, 255
  clinical findings, 223-224
  diagnosis, 224-225
    Japanese encephalitis, 225
    West Nile virus, 224-225
  epidemiology, 220-222
    geographic and seasonal distribution, 221
    hosts and reservoirs, 221
    intrinsic risk factors, 221-222
    life cycle and transmission, 220
    vectors, 220-221
  etiology, 218-220
  genomic organization of *Flavivirus*, 219f
  immune responses, 223
  impact of, 217
  neuronal injury, 223
  pathogenesis, 222-223
  pathologic findings, 225
  Powassan virus, 255
  prevention, 226
  public health considerations, 226
  taxonomic structure, vectors, hosts, distribution, significance, 218t-219t
  therapy, 225-226
  virus translation, 220f
  West Nile virus and Japanese encephalitis life cycles, 220f
fleas, cat and poultry, 504
flies/larvae, 503-504
  biting, 499-501
    stable fly (*Stomoxys calcitrans*), 500
    tabanids, 500
  black fly (*Simulium* species), 500-501
  botfly (*Gasterophilus* species), 504
  horn fly (*Haematobia irritans*), 500
  horseflies, 234f
  hypodermiasis (warbles), 504
    clinical findings and diagnosis, 504
    epidemiology, 504
    etiology, 504
    prevention, 504
    therapy, 504
  louse fly (*Hippobosca*), 504
  myiasis (maggots), 503-504
  nonbiting, 503
  sandfly (*Phlebotomus* and *Lutzomyia*), 504
  species affecting equines, 499-500
  transmission of equine infectious anemia virus, 234
  tsetse fly (*Glossina*), 504
  wound myiasis, 503-504
flora
  bacterial, 108
  colonic flora modulation with salmonellosis, 331
  genital, 381
  ocular, 110
  reproductive tract, 388
flora/microflora
  bacterial, 108, 259b
  gastrointestinal tract
    cecal microflora, 44
    colonic flora modulation with salmonellosis, 331
    esophagus, 42
    gastrointestinal tract, 259b
    large intestine, 44
    small intestine, 42
    stomach, 42
  genitourinary tract, 259b
  ocular, 110, 259b
  oral cavity, 1, 42
  pharynx, 42

flora/microflora *(Continued)*
  respiratory system, 1
    nasal cavities, 259b
  skin infections, 259b
fluconazole, 410
flukes, 449, 453-454, 512-514, 513f
fluoroquinolones (FQs), 573-574, 578-579
flushing. *See* lavage/flushing
flying foxes (pteropid bats), 192-193
fly larvae deposition, 503
fly worry, 499-500
foals
  abscesses, 56f
  African horse sickness (AHS), 188
  antimicrobial therapy, 74-75, 576-577
  ascarid impactions, 482-483
    colic due to, 482f
    S. equi zooepidemicus with, 482
  birth of weak, 601
  botulism prevention, 367, 367b
  Candida albicans, 409f-410f
  candidiasis (thrush), 410f
  clostridial enteritis, 354-355
  diarrhea
    bacterial, 42-43
    Escherichia coli, 42-43
    infectious, 42-43
    protozoal, 43
    rule-outs, 599
    Strongyloides infection, 484
    viral, 43
  diarrhea in, 42-43
    bacterial disorders, 42-43
    protozoal, 43
    viral, 43
  ensuring rapid gastrointestinal (GI) intake, 77
  enteric coccidiosis, 508
  enterocolitis, 43
  equine herpesvirus (EHV), 160f
  frenzy syndrome, 484
  giardia, 584
  leptospirosis, 307
  monitoring of, 77
  musculoskeletal infections in, 60
    pain management, 70
  neonatal (*See also* neonatal sepsis)
    equine herpesvirus (EHV), 160
    piroplasmosis, 472
    septic arthritis, 64
    vaccination for, 593
  osteomyelitis
    causes, 66
    clinical findings, 66
    treatment of septic, 68
  pneumocystis infections, 447
  respiratory infections
    parasitic, 13
    pneumonia, 14
    viral, 6
  Rhodococcus equi immunity, 291
  rotaviruses, 198, 198f, 200-201
  septic
    gastric ulcers in, 75
    jugular venous thrombosis in, 76-77
    survival rates, 77
    survival rate studies, 77
  suckle reflex, 77
  tetanus, 369
  tick-related syndromes, 495
  Tyzzer's disease, 362-363
  vaccination protocols
    equine influenza (EI), 562-563
    influences on vaccine response, 557-558
    rabies, 209b

focal infections, neonatal sepsis, 75-76
folate inhibitors, 466
folliculitis, 79f
  bacterial, 79
  dermatophytosis (ringworm), 411
  Staphylococcus species, 79f
food allergies, 80
footbaths (employees/personnel), 536
footbaths/footmats, 536-537
footwear hygiene protocols, 535-537, 541
forage mites, 498-499
forage poisoning, 364
foreign animal diseases (FADs), 605-606, 612
fosfomycin, 582
fossa glandis, 342f
FPT (failure of passive immunity), 71
  ensuring adequate, 77
FQs (fluoroquinolones), 573-574, 578-579
Francisella tularensis, 495
frenzy syndrome, 484
fulminant (peracute) infections, 472
fungal antigen detection, 398
fungal hyphae identification, 426
fungal infections. *See also specific infection/ disease or pathogen*
  about fungi, 393-394
  antifungal susceptibility testing, 398-399
  Ascomycota and Basidiomycota, 446
  of central nervous system, 48t
  crusting/scaling dermatoses, 80
  culturing, 1-2
  diagnosis
    calcofluor white staining, 396
    direct examination, 395-396
    fungal antigen detection, 398
    Gomori's methenamine silver (GMS), 396, 448f
    Gram stain, 395-396, 395f-396f
    India ink identification, 395, 395f
    methylene blue, 396
    periodic acid-Schiff stains, 396
    potassium hydroxide (KOH) treatment, 395
  drug-resistant species, 399
  host susceptibility, 394
  infectious, 82b
  laboratory diagnosis, 393-394
    culture and identification, 396-397
    dermatophyte test media, 397f
    interpretation of culture results, 398
    laboratory safety, 394
    Microsporum gypseum, 397f
    serology, 399
    specimen collection and transport, 394-395
  molecular testing, 398, 613
  mycotic, 7
  ocular manifestations/complications of systemic, 116-117
  pathogen sources, 394
  predisposing conditions, 80
  terms used in mycology, 393b
  therapy, antifungal susceptibility testing, 398-399
  yeasts, 411, 613
  zygomycotic, 82-83
fungal isolates, from diseased eyes, 110
fungal myositis, 61
  primary, 61
    clinical findings, 61
    diagnosis and therapy, 61
    etiology, 61
fungi
  filamentous, 394
  nematode-trapping, 480

fungi *(Continued)*
  saprophytes/transients, 394
  species identification, 397
furious form of rabies, 205
Fusobacterium species, 1, 10-11

G

gait disturbances. *See* lameness/gait disturbances
Galumna species, 491
Game Ready Equine system, 62-63
Gammaherpesvirinae, 152
gamonts, 469
Garm's technique, 17
gas gangrene. *See* clostridial myonecrosis (gas gangrene)
gastric ulcers
  role of *Candida albicans* in, 410
  in septic foals, 75
Gastrodiscus species, 512, 513f
Gastrodiscus aegyptiacus, 512-514, 513f
  morphology, compared to *Fasciola*, 513t
gastrointestinal diseases/infections, 599. *See also* small intestine; stomach; specific infection/disease or pathogen
  ascarids, 482f
  cryptococcosis, 440
  cyathostominae (cyathostomes, cyathostomins, small stronglyes, trichonemes), 478-481
    clinical findings, 479
    diagnosis, 479
    epidemiology, 479
    etiology, 478-479
    pathogenesis, 479
    pathologic findings, 479
    prevention, 480-481
    public health considerations, 481
    therapy, 479-480
  cyathostomin larvae, 477f, 479f
  Draschia megastoma, 487f
  equine adenovirus type 1, 190
  nematodes, 475-485
  normal flora, 259b
  oxyuris equi, 485f
  oxyurosis, 484-485
  parascorosis, 481-483
  parasitic infections, *Gastrodiscus aegyptiacus* (fluke), 512-514
  Pascaris equorum, 481f
  rule-outs, 599
    abdominal effusion, 599
    abdominal masses, 599
    abdominal pain, 599
    diarrhea (adult horses), 599
    diarrhea (foals), 599
    dysphagia, 599
    hepatomegaly or hepatic inflammation, 599
    icterus, 599
    oral ulcers or vesicles, 599
  strongylinae, 475-478
  Strongyloides westeri, 483f
  strongyloidosis, 483-484
  strongylosis, 475-481
gastrointestinal (GI) intake, foals, ensuring rapid, 77
gastrointestinal (GI) rupture
  organisms associated with, 46
  prognosis, 47
gastrointestinal (GI) tract
  acid suppression, 75
  effects of neonatal sepsis, 76

gastrointestinal (GI) tract *(Continued)*
 intestine (*See* large intestine; small
  intestine)
 oral cavity, 42
 parasitic infections
  Anoplocephala perfoliata, 490f, 492b,
   493
  cestode species, 490
  nematodes (*See* nematodes)
geldings. *See also* penis
 urinary tract infections, 106
 urine scalding due to, 108
gene expression or transcription inhibitors,
  585t, 596
 gluocorticoids, 596
genetic factors, in drug resistance, 278-279
genetic reassortment, equine influenza, 141f
genital papillomas, 245
genitourinary diseases/infections. *See also*
  kidneys; mares; stallions
 bacterial infections, samples and tissue
  selection, 259b
 normal flora, 259b
genome organization and expression, equine
  viral arteritis (EVA), 170f
genomes, viral, 153f
genomic testing strategies, 604. *See also*
  molecular testing
germplasm
 changing trends, 545
 economic impact, 545
germplasm trade, 545
getah virus, 252-253
GI. *See* gastrointestinal (GI) tract
giardia, 584
*Giardia duodenalis (G. lamblia, G.
  intestinalis)*, 509
Giardia intestinalis, 452f
giardiasis, 509
Giemsa stains, 361-362
ginseng, 591
glanders
 clinical findings, 334-335
  nasal exudate, 335f
  ulcers and swollen cutaneous
   lymphatics, 334f
 diagnosis, 335-336
  intradermal mallein test, 336f
 epidemiology and pathogenesis, 334
 etiology, 333-334
 outbreaks, 547t
 pathologic findings
  granulomas and ulcers in nasal septum,
   335f
  pulmonary granulomas, 335f
  spleen abscesses, 335f
  swollen sheath, 335f
 prevention, 336
 public health considerations, 336
 therapy, 336
glomerulonephritis, 272
glossitis, 509f
gloves, 535
glucocorticoids, central nervous system
  (CNS) infections, 54-55
glucocorticoid suppressor mechanisms, 596b
glycoproteins, 155
GMS (Gomori's methenamine silver), 396
Gomori's methenamine silver (GMS), 396,
  448f
gram-negative bacteria, 113f
 cell wall components, 120f
Gram stain, 72, 74, 257, 395-396
 Aspergillus species, 395f
 Candida species, 396f

Gram stain *(Continued)*
 Clostridial species screening, 43-45
 clostridial enteritis, 352f
 clostridial myonecrosis (gas gangrene),
  360f
 clostridial species, 352f
 Clostridium difficile, 352f
 Cryptococcus neoformans, 396f
 fungal infections, 395-396, 395f-396f
 peritoneal infections, 46
 reactions and morphology, 257t, 258f
granulocytic anaplasmosis. *See* equine
  granulocytic anaplasmosis/ehrlichiosis
granuloma formation, sinuses, 4
granulomatous lesions, rule-outs, 603
grass sickness (equine dysautonomia), 366
grease heel. *See* pastern dermatitis
Grévy's zebra, 404
griseofulvin, 582
group comparisons (epidemiology),
  522-525
Guillain-Barré syndrome, 231
guttural pouch, 14-20
 anatomy, 14, 14f-15f
 chondroids, 268f
 chondroids of, 16f
 clinical examination, 15-16
 empyema of, 15f, 16-17
  clinical findings, 16
  diagnosis, 16
  etiology, 16
  medical therapy, 16-17
  surgical therapy, 17
 endoscopy, 15-16
 endoscopy techniques, 18f
 functions of, 15
 inspissation of exudate, 3f
 mycosis, 17-19
  clinical findings, 17-18
  diagnosis, 18
  medical therapy, 18
  prognosis, 18-19
  surgical therapy, 18-19
 mycosis of, 17f
 pathogenesis of diseases, 14-15
 retropharyngeal lymph node and purulent
  material, 16f
 streptococcal infections, 275-276
 temporohyoid osteoarthropathy (THO),
  19-20
  for ostectomy, 20f
 vestibulocochlear and facial nerve
  damage, 20f

H

H3N8 equine influenza viruses, 6
H7N7 influenza virus, 5-6
Habronema species, 486, 613
Habronema microstoma, 500
habronemiasis, 118, 487-489, 488f-489f
 clinical findings, 487
 diagnosis and pathologic findings,
  487-488
 etiology and epidemiology, 487
 lesions of penis, 101f
 pathogenesis, 487
 prevention, 489
 pulmonary, 487
 therapy, 488
HACCP (Hazard Analysis and Critical
  Control Point) system, 532
Haematobia irritans, 373, 374f
Haemophilus species, 26
Halicephalobus deletrix, 449

Halicephalobus gingivalis encephalomyelitis,
  58-59
 clinical findings, 59
 diagnosis, 59
 etiology and epidemiology, 59
 pathogenesis, 59
 prevention and control, 59
 zoonotic potential, 59
 therapy, 59
hand hygiene, 534, 541
Hazard Analysis and Critical Control Point
  (HACCP) system, 532
HBOs (hyperbaric oxygen chambers),
  62-63
HCF. *See Histoplasma capsulatum
  farciminosum* (HCF)
HCV (hepatitis C virus), 217
heart disease. *See also* cardio — *entries*
 African horse sickness (AHS), dikkop
  (cardiac) form, 184, 184f-185f, 186,
  187f
 aortic infective endocarditis, 27f (*See also*
  infective endocarditis (IE))
 cardiac complications of, pyrrolizidine
  alkaloid toxicity, 41f
 cardiac dysrhythmias, 39-41
 cardiomyopathy, 601
  rule-outs, 601
 cardiotoxicity, related to antimicrobial
  therapy, 577b
 constrictive pericarditis, 34f
 endocarditis (*See* infective endocarditis
  (IE))
 fibrinoeffusive idiopathic pericarditis, 35f
 myocarditis (*See* myocarditis)
 nocardiosis (*See* nocardiosis)
 pericarditis (*See* pericarditis)
 sepsis
  cardiac complications in, 39-41
  myocardial, 41f
 septic fibrinoeffusive pericarditis, 33f-35f
 tachycardia, in pleuropneumonia, 9
Helicobacter pylori, 42
helminth infections, 449. *See also* parasitic
  infections; protozoal infections
 laboratory diagnosis, 449
 species visible to naked eye, 507-508
Helsoma duryi, 512
hemagglutination inhibition assay (HI),
  139-140, 147, 147f
hematogenous multifocal or diffuse
  placentitis, 95
hematuria, 600
hemodynamic changes, in systemic
  inflammatory response syndrome,
  123
hemolymphatic disorders, 601-602
 rule-outs, 601-602
  anemia, 601
  enlarged lymph nodes, 601
  hypoalbuminemia, 602
  lymphangitis, 601
  petechial hemorrhages, 601
  thrombocytopenia, 602
  ventral abdominal or limb edema,
   601-602
hemolytic anemia, 427f
hemorrhage
 African horse sickness (AHS), ocular,
  185f
 of caudal auricular artery, 17
 fatal, guttural pouch mycosis, 18-19
hemorrhages
 ecchymotic, *Clostridium difficile*, 355f
 petechial, 601

hemorrhagic pulmonary infarction, 9-10
Hendra virus (HeV), 192-195, 192f, 530-532
  Australian outbreak, 193t
  clinical findings, 194
  diagnosis, 194
    antigen detection, 194
    quantitative real-time polymerase chain reaction, 194
    serology, 194
    virus isolation, 194
  epidemiology, 192-193
  etiology, 192
  lung lesions, 194f
  pathogenesis and pathology, 193-194
  prevention, 194-195
    vaccination, 194-195
  public health considerations, 195
  therapy, 194
hepatic inflammation, 599
hepatitis C virus (HCV), 217
hepatomegaly, 599
hepatoxicity, related to antimicrobial therapy, 577b
herd immunity, 516-517
herd testing, for *S. equi*, 4
herpesviruses. *See also* equine herpesvirus (EHV)
  abortion caused by, 95
  outbreaks, 547t
Heterobilharzia americana, 449, 452f
HI (hemagglutination inhibition assay), 139-140
Hippobosca (louse fly), 504
histopathology. *See under specific infection/disease or pathogen*
Histoplasma species, 8, 94, 443f
Histoplasma capsulatum farciminosum (HCF), 444-446, 444f-445f
  clinical findings, 444-445
  diagnosis, 445
    animal incubation, 445
    culturing, 445
    cytology, 445
    intradermal testing, 445
    pathology and histology, 445
    serology, 445
  epidemiology, 444
  etiology, 444
  pathogenesis, 444
  prevention, 446
  therapy, 445-446
Histoplasma species, 442
histoplasmosis, 440-444
  clinical findings, 442
    mycotic keratitis, 442
  diagnosis, 442-443
    culturing, 442
    cytology, 442
    histopathology, 442
    intradermal testing, 443
    laboratory tests, 442, 443t
    serology, 442-443
    thoracic radiography, 442
  epidemiology, 441
  etiology, 440-441
  geographic prevalence, 441f
  pathogenesis, 441
  pathology, 443-444
    mycotic keratitis, 443-444
  therapy, 444
    mycotic keratitis, 444
  virulence factors, 440-441
Histoplasmosis capsulatum, 8
history taking, skin infections, 78

hoofs, sloughed hoof capsule (arterial thrombosis), 127f
Horner's syndrome, 17-18, 115-116
horn fly *(Haematobia irritans)*, 374f, 500
horseflies, 234f
Horserace Betting Levy Board (UK), Code of Practice, 151-152
horsesickness fever form of African horse sickness, 185
hospital infection control. *See* biosecurity
hospital protection, 532
host characteristics, 516
hosts/host factors. *See also* carriers/carrier state; reservoir hosts; vectors; *specific infection/disease or pathogen*
  alphaviruses, 210t
  dead-end hosts, 459, 531-532
  dermatophilosis (rain rot), 284
  dermatophytosis (ringworm), 412
  flavivirus encephalitides, 218t-219t, 221
  host characteristics, 516
  host defenses
    mucosal, 107
    peptides, 2
    suppression of, 345
  host health, 2f
  host susceptibility, 394
    fungal infections, 394
  intermediate hosts, *Sarcocystis neurona*, 458-459
  Leptospira species, 304t
  migration of amplifying/reservoir hosts, vectors, pathogens, 549
houseflies, 374f
husbandry. *See* biosecurity; prevention *under specific infection/disease*
hydatidosis, 61
hydrocyanic acid, 106-107
hygiene procedures, 533-534. *See also* biosecurity
  footwear hygiene, 535
  hand hygiene, 534, 541
  prevention of *Streptococcus equi equi* (strangles), 276
  udder hygiene, 77
hyoid apparatus, 20f
hyperbaric oxygen chambers (HBOs), 62-63
hyperemia, 114f
  conjunctival, 110f
  corneal, 113f-114f
hyperglycemia, in neonatal sepsis, 71
hyperplasia, crypt glands, equine proliferative enteropathy (EPE), 320f
hyperplasia of crypt glands, equine proliferative enteropathy (EPE), 320f
hyperplasias, lymphoid pharyngeal hyperplasia, 5
  grading of, 5b
hyperthermia, sarcoids, 249
hypertonic baths, 62-63
hyphae, fungal, 111f
hypoalbuminemia, 602
Hypoderma lineatum, 504
hypodermiasis (warbles), 504
  clinical findings and diagnosis, 504
  epidemiology, 504
  etiology, 504
  prevention, 504
  therapy, 504
hypoglycemia, 71
hypomelanosis, 245
hypoproteinemia, 427f
hypopyon, 110f, 113f
  Rhodococcus equi, 293f

hyposensitization, 593-594
hypotension, sepsis-related, 70
hypoxemia, 13
hytadid cyst formation, 510

I

ICA (internal carotid artery), 18-19
icteric sclera, 345f
icterus, 599
IE. *See* infective endocarditis (IE)
IFAT (indirect fluorescence assay test), 473
Ig—. *See* antibodies/immunoglobulins
ileal-cecal junction lesions, 319f
ileocecal intussusception, *Anoplocephala perfoliata*, 492b, 493f
ileum wall thickening, equine proliferative enteropathy (EPE), 319f
ileus, 427f
imaging studies. *See specific technique, e.g.* radiography, *or* diagnosis *under specific infection/disease or pathogen*
imidazoles, 582
imiquimod, 591
immune control, 235-236
immune exclusion, 1
immune-mediated hemolytic anemia, related to antimicrobial therapy, 577b
immune-mediated polysynovitis, 292f
immune-mediated spread of infection, 271-272
  streptococcal infections
    agalactia, 271-272
    glomerulonephritis and myocarditis, 272
    myositis, 271-272
    purpura hemorrhagica, 271, 271f
immune protection, 1-2
immune response
  Babesia bovis and *Babesia caballi*, 471-472
  Dermatophilus congolensis, 284
  dermatophytosis (ringworm), 412
  equine herpesvirus, 158-159
  to equine piroplasmosis infection, 471
  pathogens of central nervous system, 50-51
  to vaccines, 592f
immunity, 290-291
  ascarids, 483
  dermatophytosis (ringworm), 412
  EAV/EVA, 178-179
  to equine influenza, 144-145
  equine piroplasmosis (EP), 471-472
  innate, 587f
  lack of development of, dermatophilosis, 286
  passive (*See* passive immunity)
  Strongylides species, 484
immunization. *See also* vaccines/vaccination
  active, 551-553
    DNA vaccines, 552-553
    inactivated vaccines, 552
    modified live vaccines, 553
    principles of, 551-552
    protein or subunit vaccines, 552
    recombinant vaccines, 553
  goals of, 1
  passive, 556-557
    exogenous antibodies, 556
    passive transfer of maternal immunity, 556-557
immunoassays, 146, 417
immunoblot test, 463f
  Sarcocystis neurona, 462f

immunoblot (Western blot) test, 473-474, 527b
  EPM (equine protozoal myeloencephalitis), 463
immunodiffusion serologic test, 404f
immunofluorescence, 136-137, 137f, 146
immunoglobulins. *See* antibodies/ immunoglobulins
immunohistochemical techniques, aspergillosis, 426
immunohistochemistry, 136-137, 417
immunohistological stain, 417f
immunohistological stains, 417f
immunology
  equine granulocytic anaplasmosis/ ehrlichiosis, 345
  factors in maintaining host health, 2f
immunomodulators, 585t, 590-591
  acemannan, 591
  caprine serum fraction, 591
  Echinacea angustifolia, 591
  ginseng, 591
  imiquimod, 591
  levamisole phosphate, 591
  Parapoxvirus ovis, 590-591
immunoprophylaxis, 551-553
  active immunization, 551-553
    DNA vaccines, 552-553
    inactivated vaccines, 552
    modified live vaccines, 553
    principles of, 551-552
    protein or subunit vaccines, 552
    recombinant vaccines, 553
  core and noncore vaccines, 558
  influences on vaccine response on foals, maternal antibodies, 557-558
  licensing and safety of vaccines, 554-555
    adverse events, 555
    safety of vaccines in broodmares, 555-556
  passive immunization, 556-557
    exogenous antibodies, 556
    passive transfer of maternal immunity, 556-557
  vaccine augmentation, 553-554
    adjuvants, 553-554, 554t
    marker vaccines, 553
  vaccine recommendations for specific diseases, 558-570
    anthrax, 570
    botulism, 568-569
    equine encephalomyelitis viruses (EEE, WEE, VEE), 559
    equine herpesviruses, 564-566
    equine influenza, 560-564
    equine rhinitis A virus, 570
    equine viral arteritis (EVA), 569
    Potomac horse fever (PHF), 567-568
    rabies, 567
    rotaviral diarrhea, 569-570
    Streptococcus equi equi (strangles), 566-567
    tetanus, 558-559
    West Nile virus, 559-560
immunostaining methods, 137f
immunostimulants, 584-591, 585t
  induction of nonspecific immune responses, 584-586
immunosuppressants, 596-597
  glucocorticoid suppressor mechanisms, 596b
  inhibitors of gene expression or transcription, 596
  phosphatase and kinase inhibitors, 596-597

immunosuppression
  oral candidiasis with, 410-411
  pneumocystis infections with, 446-447
immunotherapy. *See also* vaccines/ vaccination
  adaptive immunity, 592f
  antibody-mediated protection, 594f
  Bacille-Calmette-Guérin vaccine and *Mycobacterium* cell wall extracts, 587-588
  bacterial particles, 586-589
    Propionibacterium acnes, 586-587
    unmethylated cytosine-phosphate-guanosine motifs, 588-589
  exogenous cytokines
    interferon-α, 589-590
    present and future of other cytokines, 590
  for hyposensitization, 593-594
  immune response to vaccines, 592f
  immunomodulators, 585t, 590-591
    acemannan, 591
    caprine serum fraction, 591
    Echinacea angustifolia, 591
    ginseng, 591
    imiquimod, 591
    levamisole phosphate, 591
    Parapoxvirus ovis, 590-591
  immunostimulants, 584-591
    induction of nonspecific immune responses, 584-586
  immunosuppressants, 596-597
    glucocorticoid suppressor mechanisms, 596b
    inhibitors of gene expression or transcription, 596
    phosphatase and kinase inhibitors, 596-597
  innate immunity, 587f
  passive immunity, 594-596
    Clostridium botulinum hyperimmune plasma, 595
    Clostridium tetani (tetanus antitoxin), 595
    endotoxemia antibodies, 595
    snake antivenin (IV), 595-596
    transfer of antigen-specific antibodies, 594-595
    transfer of nonspecific antibodies, 594
    West Nile virus antibodies, 595
  sarcoids, 250
  toll-like receptors, 586f
  vaccination, 591-594
    cancer vaccines, 593
    molecular vaccines, 593
    neonatal, 593
    types of vaccines, 591
    vaccine adjuvants, 591-593
importation requirements, 339. *See also* international movement of horses
impression smears, 455
inactivated vaccines, 552
inapparent carriers
  equine piroplasmosis (EP), 472
  Streptococcus equi, 272
  treatment of dourine and, 506
incidence rate, 520, 520b-521b
incontinence, urinary, 106-107, 600
  urine scald secondary to, 108f
India ink test, 395, 395f, 438f
indirect enzyme-linked immunosorbent assay (ELISA), 138
indirect fluorescence assay test (IFAT), 473
indirect fluorescent antibody test, 346, 526b-527b

individual risk factors for disease, 516-517
infection control. *See* biosecurity; prevention *under specific infection/disease or pathogen*
infections. *See also specific infection/disease or pathogen*
  in adult horses, causes of, 60
  definition, 70
  fulminant (peracute), 472
  geographic location and pathogens, 72, 74
  opportunistic, 448
  systemic, 61
infectious diseases. *See specific infection/ disease or pathogen*
infectious waste management, 537-538
infective endocarditis (IE), 21-30
  clinical findings, 25-26, 25t
  diagnosis, 26-28
  echocardiograms, 28f-29f
  electrocardiogram exercise, 25f
  etiology and pathogenesis, 21-25
  location of lesions in, 22t
  with myocarditis, 27f
  prognosis, 28-30
  therapy, 30
  vegetations in, 22f-24f
infectivity (contagiousness), 515-516
infertility, rule-outs, 601
inflammation/inflammatory response
  chronic, arytenoid chondritis, 6f
  effects on airway of, 2
  with fungal infections, 395
  mediators of systemic, 122t-123t
  to pulmonary intravascular macrophages, 2
  with salmonellosis, 331
  systemic inflammatory response syndrome (*See* systemic inflammatory response syndrome (SIRS))
inflammatory cell activation, 121
inflammatory cell migration, 596b
inflammatory mediators, 121-123
influences on vaccine response on foals, maternal antibodies, 557-558
influenza. *See* equine influenza
influenza A, 141f. *See also* equine influenza
inhaled irritants/toxins, pulmonary effects, 11
inhibitors of gene expression or transcription, 596
injections, intramuscular (IM), prevention of clostridial myonecrosis, 361
injection sites, clostridial myonecrosis (gas gangrene) at, 361f-362f
innate immunity, 587f
innate immunity response, 290
inoculated rapid sporulation media, 397f
insect bites/stings
  allergies, 80
  control/repellents, 538-539
    dermatophilosis prevention, 287
  Dermatophilus transmission, 284
  venomous insects, 504
insecticides. *See* therapy *under specific insect, e.g.* lice/pediculosis
in situ hybridization, 138
interferon-α, 589-590
interleukin-8 (IL-8), 70
intermediate hosts, *Sarcocystis neurona*, 458-459
internal carotid artery (ICA), 18-19
International Animal Health Code, guidelines for countries with African horse sickness, 188

International des Epizooties (OIE),
470-471, 605
  Web site, 473
international movement of horses
  availability of new vectors, 548-549
  basis for movement and trade in
    germplasm, 545
    changing trends, 545
    economic impact, 545
  disease distribution factors, 546-549
    agroterrorism, 549
    effects of climate disturbance, 548
    emergent diseases, 548
    growth of horse industries, 544-545
    international trade in equids, semen,
      embryos, 546-547
    migration of amplifying/reservoir hosts,
      vectors, pathogens, 549
    multinational trade agreements,
      547-548
    new variants of pathogens, 548
    preexport testing reliability, 549
    spread from feral equids, 549
  diseases spread by, 544
  equine influenza epidemics due to, 546t
  import requirements, contagious equine
    metritis (CEM), 339
  outbreaks related to, 547t
  risk reduction, 549-551
    industry initiatives, 550-551
    postimport requirements, 550
    preexport requirements, 550
    surveillance and reporting of diseases,
      550
  test for glanders, 335
interstitial pneumonia, 11-13
  clinical findings, 12
  diagnosis, 12
  epidemiology, 11
  etiology, 11-12
  histopathology, 12f
  prognosis, 11, 13
  radiography, 12f
  therapy, 12-13
intestinal larvae, 14
intestines. *See* large intestine; small intestine
intracranial abscesses, 56-57
  clinical findings, 56
  diagnosis, 56-57
  etiology, 56
  therapy, 57
intradermal mallein test, 336f
intramuscular (IM) injections, prevention of
  clostridial myonecrosis, 361
in utero infections, dourine, 505
iris prolapses, 113f
irradiation therapy, sarcoids, 250
irrigation, guttural pouch empyema, 16-17
isolated worm recovery, 455-456
isolation methods, 535-536. *See also*
  biosecurity
isolation of live viruses (cell/egg cultures,
  animal inoculation), 133-134
itraconazole, 411
ivermectin, 14
Ixodes species, 312f. *See also* ticks/tick-borne
  diseases
Ixodes scapularis, 311

J

Japanese encephalitis (JE), 218t-219t, 220,
  220f
  human encephalitis cases, 221
  life cycles, 220f

JE. *See* Japanese encephalitis (JE)
Johne's disease, 390
Johnson grass, 106-107
joint infections
  bacterial cultures, 258, 260
  effusion with *Rhodoccus equi*, 292f
  laceration of metatarsophalangeal joint,
    64f
  Rhodoccus equi, 293, 296f
  sepsis, 65-66
    tarsocrural joint with septic epiphysitis,
      69f
  synovial infections, 63-66
Juga yrekaensis snail, 348, 348f
jugular thrombophlebitis, 36-39
  clinical findings, 36
  diagnosis, 37
    laboratory diagnosis, 37
    ultrasonography, 37
  etiology and pathogenesis, 36
  prevention, 37-39
  prognosis, 37
  therapy, 37
jugular thrombosis, 37f-38f
jugular venous thrombosis, in septic foals,
  76-77

K

keratinases, 412
keratitis, 602
  bacterial, 112
  fungal (*See* mycotic keratitis
    (keratomycosis))
  primary, 111
  viral, 112
keratomycosis. *See* mycotic keratitis
  (keratomycosis)
key to microfilariae, 453b
kidneys. *See also* urinary tract infections
  (UTIs)
  Corynebacterium pseudotuberculosis
    abscesses, 376f
  nephrotoxins, 109, 577b
  pyelonephritis, 107, 107f
  renal failure, 600
  renal insufficiency, 473
  treatment of urinary tract infections, 109
  ultrasonography of, 108
kinase inhibitors, 585t, 596-597
kinases, 166
Kinyoun acid-fast stain, 258f
Kinyoun staining, 257
Kirby-Bauer disc dilution antimicrobial
  susceptibility testing, 264f
Kirby-Bauer test, 263
Klebsiella species, 57-58, 64
  microbial susceptibility, 572
  placentitis, 94
  urinary tract infections, 106
Klebsiella pneumoniae, transmission of, 104
KOH (potassium hydroxide) treatment, 395
kokobera encephalitis, 218t-219t
Kunjin virus, 254f, 255
kunkers, 415, 416f, 419-420

L

laboratory diagnosis. *See also* diagnosis *under
  infection/disease, or specific pathogen;
  molecular testing; sample collection*
  agar gel immunodiffusion (AGID), 139
  animal inoculation, 133-134
  Anoplocephala perfoliata, 451f
  Anoplocephala perfoliata diagnosis, 493

laboratory diagnosis *(Continued)*
  antibody detection, 147-148
  antimicrobial susceptibility testing,
    263-264
  aspartate transaminase (AST), 60
  bacterial cultures, 60-61
  bacterial susceptibility testing
    agar disk diffusion test, 572
    minimum inhibitory concentration
      determination, 572-573
  Baerman procedure, 454
  bioassays, 44-45
  blood smears, 455
  broth microdilution antimicrobial
    susceptibility testing, 264f
  buffy coat smear, 3
  Candida albicans, 410
  cellophane (Scotch) tape test, 454
  cerebrospinal fluid collection, 49-53
  Clostridium difficile, 355
  Clostridium perfringens, 356
  competitive enzyme-linked
    immunosorbent assay (cELISA), 473
  creatinine kinase (CK), 60
  Cryptosporidium parvum, 452f
  culture and identification, 396-397
  culture and sensitivity (C&S), 61
    staphylococcal infections, 281
  cultures, 1-2
  cytology, 1-2, 9, 13
  dermatologic, 79-80
  dermatophyte cultures, 397f
  diagnostic test kits, 614t
  diagnostic test properties, 525-527
    estimation of sensitivity and specificity,
      526-527, 526b
    evaluation of characteristics of, 528
    measurement types, 525
    test accuracy, 526-527, 526b
  Dictyocaulus arnfieldi eggs, 451f
  Diff-Quick, 286
  direct fecal smear, 454
  direct microscopic examination, 257-258
  Eimeria leuckarti, 452f
  electron microscopy, 138
  ELISA (*See* enzyme-linked
    immunosorbent assay (ELISA))
  equine herpesvirus (EHV), 163t
  equine piroplasmosis (EP), 472-474
  equine viral arteritis (EVA)
    histopathology, 177
    serology, 177
    viral nucleic acid detection, 177
    virus isolation, 176-177
  Fasciola hepatica egg, 452f
  fastidious organisms (specialized media/
    culture requirements), 261b
  fecal cultures, 44, 453
  fecal egg count reduction (FECR) test,
    480b
  fecal flotation, 449-453
  fecal sedimentation, 453-454
  fungal infections, 393-394
  Giardia intestinalis, 452f
  Gram stain (positive and negative), 72,
    74
    Clostridial species screening, 43-45
    peritoneal infections, 46
  gram-stain reactions and morphology,
    257t, 258f
  gross fecal examination, 449
  helminths, 449
  hemagglutination inhibition, 147
  hemagglutination inhibition assay (HI),
    139-140

laboratory diagnosis *(Continued)*
  hematology, 8, 13
  Heterobilharzia americana, 452f
  histopathology, 136
  immunoassays, 146
  immunodiffusion serologic test, 404f
  immunofluorescence/
    immunohistochemistry, 136-137, 146
  immunostaining methods, viral antigen
    detection in tissue, 137f
  impression smears, 455
  indirect enzyme-linked immunosorbent
    assay (ELISA), 138
  indirect fluorescence assay test (IFAT),
    473
  indirect fluorescent antibody test, 346,
    526b-527b
  inoculated rapid sporulation media, 397f
  in situ hybridization, 138
  interpretation of culture results, 398
  interpretation of isolation and
    identification results, 261-262
  interpretation of test results, 527-528
    predictive values, 527-528, 527b-528b
  intradermal mallein test, 336f
  isolated worm recovery, 455-456
  isolation of live viruses, 133-134
  key to microfilariae, 453b
  Kinyoun acid-fast stain, 258f
  Kirby-Bauer disc dilution antimicrobial
    susceptibility testing, 264f
  laboratory safety, 394
  lactophenol aniline blue, 397f-398f
  Leishmania species, 452f
  McMaster's procedure, 454-455
  microarray detection of viruses, 137-138
  Microsporum gypseum, 397f
  modified Wright's stain, 133f
  molecular methods, 262-263
  National Veterinary Services Laboratory,
    44
  nematode larvae identification, 453b
  neutralization of virus infectivity, 139
  normal flora, 259b
  Onchocerca cervicalis, 451f
  overview, 132
  Oxyuris equi eggs, 451f, 455f
  parasitic infections, 449-456
  Pascaris equorum eggs, 450f
  peritonitis, 46
  polymerase chain reaction *(See*
    polymerase chain reaction (PCR)
    testing)
  preexport testing reliability, 549
  protozoal organisms, 449
  reverse transcriptase-polymerase change
    reaction, 146-147
  safe handling of *Coccidioides immitis,* 394
  sample collection, transport, storage, 604
  sample transportation, 261
  sampling for bacterial cultures, 258-261,
    259b
  serology, 4, 138-140, 264-265, 399
    serologic interpretation, 140
    serologic response detection, 138-140
  silver stained (Warthin-Starry stain), 363
  single radial hemolysis, 147-148
  in situ detection of virus in tissue sections,
    136-137
  skin biopsy, 455
  specimen collection and transport,
    394-395
  staphylococcal infection, 280-281
  strongyles, 450f, 454f
  Strongyloides westeri eggs, 451f

laboratory diagnosis *(Continued)*
  submission of samples, 261
  surra, 506-507
  swabbing procedures, 3
  synovial fluid analysis, 63
  Theileria equi, 455f
  total nucleated cell count (TNCC), 43-44
  transtracheal wash analysis, 10f
  urine, 108
  using tests in combination, 528
  viral characterization, 135-136
  viral nucleic acids detection (polymerase
    chain reactions), 134-136
  virus isolation, 145-146
  Western blot (immunoblot) test, 473-474,
    527b
lacerations
  metatarsophalangeal joint, 64f
  near joints, 64
Lactobacillus species, 42
lactophenol aniline blue, 397f-398f
Lagenidium hyphae, 417
lagophthalmos, 114f
lameness/gait disturbances
  ataxia, 106-107, 222
    equine herpesvirus (EHV), 162f
  cellulitis, 62
  equine protozoal myeloencephalitis
    (EPM), 461-462
  rule-outs, 600
  synovial infections, 63
  with tetanus, 369
  West Nile virus, 222-224
laminitis of support limb, 70
large intestine, 44-46
  acute diarrhea in adult horses, 44-45
    diagnosis, 44-45
    etiology, 44
    therapy, 45
  chronic diarrhea in adult horses, 45-46
    diagnosis, 45
    etiology, 45
    prognosis, 45-46
    therapy, 45
  normal flora, 44
large nodular dermatoses, 603
large nodular/mass dermatoses, 82-83, 82b
  diagnosis, 83
  etiology, 82-83
  therapy, 83
larvae, fly. *See* flies/larvae
laryngeal nerve
  denervation of laryngeal nerve, 17-18
  signs of, 17-18
laser therapy
  pythiosis, 418
  sarcoids, 249
latency cycle, equine herpesvirus, 156
latency phase of infections, 516
  equine herpesvirus, reactivation from, 156
lavage/flushing
  abdominal, 46-47
  bladder, 109
  bronchoalveolar, 1-2
  guttural pouch, 16, 18
  guttural pouch mycosis, 18
  joint, 411
  peritoneal, 47
  seminal vesicles, 103f
  uterine, 87-89
    endometritis and pyometra, 92f
    guidelines for, 89t
Lawsonia intracellularis, 43, 316f, 613. *See
  also* equine proliferative enteropathy
  (EPE)

leflunomide, 597
Leishmania species, 449, 452f, 504, 507
Leishmania braziliensis, 82
Leishmania siamensis, 82
leishmaniasis, 82, 82f
  diagnosis, 82
  etiology, 82
  therapy, 82
Leptospira species, 94, 258
  genomospecies identified with serovars of,
    303t
  placentitis related to, 95
  serovars and hosts identified in horses,
    304t
leptospirosis
  abortions/stillbirths/neonatal deaths
    clinical findings, 306
    diagnosis, 309
    epidemiology, 305
  clinical findings, 306-307
    systemic disease in adults and foals, 307
  diagnosis, 307-309
    animal inoculation/serologic response,
      308
    culturing, 308
    direct detection methods, 307-308
    DNA methodology, 308
    immunohistochemical staining, 308f
    of leptospires, 308f
    serology, 308-309
  epidemiology, 304-305
    risk factors, 305
    seroprevalence, 304-305
  equine recurrent uveitis
    clinical findings, 306-307
    diagnosis, 307f, 309
    epidemiology, 305
    therapy for, 310
  etiology, 303-304
  pathogenesis, 305-306
  pathologic findings, 309-310
  prevention, 310-311
  public health considerations, 311
  spirochete classification, 303f
  ultrastructure of leptospires, 303f
leukocyte re-programming, 121-123
leukoencephalomalacia, 117
leukopenia, 71
  in equine herpesvirus, 158-159
levamisole phosphate, 591
lice (pediculosis), 499
  Bovicola equi, 499f
  clinical findings, 499
  diagnosis, 499
  epidemiology, 499
  etiology, 499
  prevention, 499
  species of equine, 499
  therapy, 499
licensing and safety of vaccines, 554-555
  adverse events, 555
  safety of vaccines in broodmares, 555-556
lichenification, *Culicoides* hypersensitivity,
  502f
life cycles
  cestodes, 491
  equine piroplasmosis (EP)
    Babesia caballi, 469, 469f
    Theileria equi, 469, 470f
  tick species, 495
ligands, toll-like receptor (TLR) ligands,
  119t
limb edema, 601-602
  equine proliferative enteropathy (EPE),
    317f

lintiviruses, 233
lipopolysaccharide (LPS), 120f
lipopolysaccharide scavengers, 128
lips
   dropped, 114f
   orthopoxvirus, 256
Listeria monocytogenes, 386
listeriosis, 386-387
liver
   ascarid migration to, 482
   Corynebacterium pseudotuberculosis,
      375f-376f
liver disease
   Dirofilaria immitis, 510
   hytadid cyst formation, 510
liver fluke, 449, 512-513
live virus isolation, 133-134
   cell/egg cultures and animal inoculation,
      133-134
local tetanus, 369-370
louse fly (*Hippobosca*), 504
lower respiratory tract. *See also* respiratory
      diseases
   bronchopneumonia, 7
   clinical findings, 7-8
   diagnosis, 8
   etiology and epidemiology, 7
   guttural pouch (*See* guttural pouch)
   pneumonias (*See* pneumonia)
   pulmonary abscesses, 7
   relationship to upper, 2f
   therapy, 8
LPS (lipopolysaccharide), 120f
lumbosacral collection of cerebrospinal
      fluid, 52f
lungs
   African horse sickness (AHS), septal
      edema of lungs, 186f
   ascarid migration to, 482
   aspergillosis, 427f
   lungworm, 489
      clinical findings, 489
      diagnosis and pathologic findings, 489
      etiology, epidemiology, pathogenesis,
         489
      therapy and prevention, 489
   pneumocystis infections, 448
   purpura hemorrhagica, 271f
   severe combined immuno-deficiency
      (SCID), 448
Lutzomyia, 504
Lyme disease. *See also Borrelia burgdorferi*;
      ticks/tick-borne diseases
   clinical findings, 313
      lymphohistiocytic cutaneous nodules,
         314f
      muscle wasting and pain, 313f
   diagnosis, 314
   epidemiology, 311-313
   etiology, 311
   ocular manifestations of, 117t
   pathologic findings, 314
   prevention, 315
   public health considerations, 315
   risk in United States of, 312f
   therapy, 314-315
lymphangitis, 601
   ulcerative, 407
lymph nodes
   enlarged, 269, 601
   glanders, 334f
   pythiosis, 416
lymphoid follicles in perilimbal region, 111f
lymphoid pharyngeal hyperplasia, 5
   grading of, 5b

lysis-centrifugation blood culture methods,
      260
Lyssavirus, 204, 239, 256
lytic infection cycles, 152-153
   equine herpesvirus, 153-154

M

macrolides and derivatives, 579
macrophages, 596b
maggots. *See* myiasis (maggots)
magnetic resonance imaging (MRI). *See*
      diagnosis *under specific infection/disease*
Main Drain virus, 255
Malassezia equina, 80
Malassezia pachydermatis, 80
malevolent sarcoids, 248
Maltese cross formation (merozoites), 469
mammary glands, agalactia, *Streptococcus*
      equi equi (strangles), 272
mandible deviation, 462f
mange. *See* mites/mange
mare reproductive loss syndrome (MRLS),
      32, 515
mares. *See also* contagious equine metritis
      (CEM); endometritis; vagina
   abortion (*See* abortion)
   broodmares
      botulism vaccination for, 366-367
      safety of vaccines in, 555-556
   contagious equine metritis (CEM),
      337
   endometritis/pyometra, 92f
   imported, 343
   mastitis
      bacterial, 101f
      in lactating/nonlactating mares, 100f
   pregnant (*See also* placenta)
      early embryonic loss, 601
      equine arteritis virus antigen in fetuses,
         178f
      equine herpesvirus, 167-168
      equine influenza (EI), 562
      passive transfer of maternal immunity,
         556-557
      transplacental transmission of disease,
         234, 350
      in utero infections, 505
   reproductive tract infections
      infectious vaginitis, 93
      mastitis, 99-100
      in nonpregnant mares, 84-93
      oophoritis, 93
      ovarian abscess and adhesions, 93f
      persistent mating-induced endometritis
         (PMIE), 87f
      postpartum metritis, 93
      pyometra, 92-93, 93f
      systemic antimicrobial therapy, 91t
      uteroplacental thickness measurement,
         96f
   transport/shipment of, 545
   udder hygiene, 77
   urinary tract infections, 106
   uterus (*See* uterine infections)
   vulva, normal and abnormal
      conformation, 85f
marker vaccines, 553
MARS (mixed antiinflammatory response
      syndrome), 70
Mastadenovirus, 189
mastitis, 99-100
   bacterial, 101f
   in lactating/nonlactating mares, 100f
McMaster's procedure, 454-455

measurement data, 522-523
   reality of difference, 522-523
measures of disease occurrence, 517-520
medical therapy. *See under specific infection/*
      disease or pathogen
Medical Waste Tracking Act (MWTA),
      537-538
Megasphaera species, 1
melanin, 436
Melanoides tuberculata, 512
melis, 333
meninges, 48-49
meningitis and meningoencephalitis, 47
   bacterial, 55-56
      clinical findings, 55
      diagnosis, 55-56
      etiology, 55
      prevention, 56
      therapy, 56
   neonatal sepsis, 76
      ocular complications, 76
mentation, 125f
merozoites, 469
   equi merozoite antigens (EMAs),
      471-472
methicillin-resistant *Staphylococcus aureus*
      (MRSA), 79-80, 278, 279t, 531-532
   colonization in personnel and horse
      owners, 283t
   first identification in horses, 278-279
   indicators of, 281
   prevention, 282
   prognosis, 282
   risk factors, 279
   screening for, 281
   skin and tissue infections, 280f
   strains of, 279
   wound and postoperative infections, 280
methylene blue stain, 396
metritis. *See also* contagious equine metritis
      (CEM); endometritis
   postpartum, 93
metronidazole, 10-11, 581
microarray detection of viruses, 137-138
microbial susceptibility testing, 571-572
   Actinobacillus species, 571
   anaerobic bacteria, 572
   fungi, 572
   Pseudomonas, Enterobacter, Klebsiella,
      Escherichia coli, 572
   Staphylococcus species, 571-572
   Streptococcus and *Pasteurella*, 571
Microsporum canis, 411
Microsporum gypseum, 397f, 411, 499-500
middle ear infections, 48
midges, 501-503
   clinical findings and diagnosis, 501-502
   epidemiology and clinical findings, 501
   therapy and prevention, 502-503
migration of amplifying/reservoir hosts,
      vectors, pathogens, 549
minimal inhibitory concentration (MIC)
      values for antifungal agents, 408
miosis, 17-18
mites/mange, 496-499
   catching mite samples, 497
   Chorioptes bovis mite, 497f
   chorioptic mange, 497-498
      diagnosis, 497
      epidemiology, 497
      etiology, 497
      pathogenesis and clinical findings,
         497
      prevention, 497-498
      therapy, 497

mites/mange *(Continued)*
    demodectic mange, 498
        diagnosis, 498
        epidemiology, 498
        etiology, 498
        pathogenesis and clinical findings, 498
        therapy, 498
    poultry mites, 504
    psoroptic mange, 496-497
        diagnosis, 496
        epidemiology, 496
        etiology, 496
        pathogenesis and clinical findings, 496
        prevention, 497
        therapy, 496-497
    sarcoptic mange, 496
        diagnosis, 496
        epidemiology, 496
        etiology, 496
        pathogenesis and clinical findings, 496
        public health considerations, 496
        therapy, 496
    trombiculids and forage mites, 498-499
        diagnosis, 498
        epidemiology, 498
        etiology, 498
        pathogenesis and clinical findings, 498
        public health considerations, 499
        therapy, 498
mitral regurgitation, 22-24, 32f
mixed antiinflammatory response syndrome
    (MARS), 70
mixed form of African horse sickness,
    184-186
MLST (multilocus sequence typing), 263
MMF (mycophenolate mofetil), 597
MNPF (multinodular pulmonary fibrosis), 7,
    11-13
MOD (multiple organ dysfunction), 41
modified live vaccines, 553
modified Wright's stain, 133f
modoc encephalitis, 218t-219t
mold identification, 397
molecular epidemiology, bacterial
    pathogens, 263
molecular testing. *See also* polymerase chain
    reaction (PCR) testing
    bacterial pathogen detection methods,
        262-263
        polymerase chain reaction, 262-263,
            262f
        toxin gene detection, 263
    Blastomyces dermatitidis, 435
    blastomycosis, 435
    Borna disease, 227
    central nervous system pathogens,
        612-613
    collection, transport, storage procedures,
        604
    cyathostomin infection, 613
    description of polymerase chain reaction
        methods, 605t
    diarrheal diseases, 611-612
    equine granulocytic anaplasmosis/
        ehrlichiosis, 346f
    fungal infections, 398
    Histoplasma species, 443
    interpretation of PCR results, 606
    laboratories in United States doing,
        607t-611t
    Neorickettsia risticii, 351f
    newer and older formats for, 604
    polymerase chain reaction format, 604
    private laboratories, 606
    pythiosis, 417

molecular testing *(Continued)*
    respiratory diseases, 612
    standardization, 604-606
        international standards, 605-606
        North American standards, 606
    vesicular diseases, 606-611
molecular vaccines, 593
molluscum contagiosum, 79
Moniezia expansa, 491
monitoring/surveillance systems
    biosecurity protocol effectiveness,
        539-540
    environmental monitoring, 539-540
    patient monitoring/surveillance, 539
monoclonal antibodies, 597
monocytes, 596b
Mononegavirales, 227
Moraxella species, 110-111
mortality, 519b. *See also specific infection/
    disease*
mosquitoes/mosquito bites, 501
    epidemiology and public health
        considerations, 501
    mosquito-borne viruses, 218t-219t
    therapy and prevention, 501
movement/traffic flow management
    (personnel), 535
moxidectin, 14
MRLS (mare reproductive loss syndrome),
    32, 515
MRSA. *See* methicillin-resistant
    Staphylococcus aureus (MRSA)
Mucor species, 94
mucormycosis, 420
mucormycotic fungi, 613
mucus
    production of, 2
    respiratory, 1
mucus membranes, color of, 9
mud fever. *See* pastern dermatitis
mules, 13
    deworming, 14
    as reservoir hosts for equine lungworm,
        489
multilocus sequence typing (MLST), 263
multinational trade agreements, 547-548
multinodular pulmonary fibrosis (MNPF), 7,
    11-13
multiorgan dysfunction syndrome (MODS),
    70
multiple organ dysfunction (MOD), 41
Murray Valley encephalitis (MVE) virus,
    254f, 255
Musca domestica, 373, 374f
muscle fasciculations, 601
muscle infarction, 271-272
muscle infections, 60-61
    clostridial myonecrosis, 61
    primary bacterial myositis, 60-61
        clinical findings, 60
        diagnosis, 60-61
        etiology, 60
        therapy, 61
    primary fungal myositis, 61
        clinical findings, 61
        diagnosis and therapy, 61
        etiology, 61
    primary parasitic myositis, 61
        clinical findings, 61
        diagnosis and therapy, 61
        etiology, 61
    secondary parasitic myositis, 61
        clinical findings, 61
        diagnosis and therapy, 61
        etiology, 61

muscles
    atrophy/wasting, 61
        equine protozoal myeloencephalitis
            (EPM), 461f
        Lyme disease, 313f
    infarction/necrosis, 61
musculoskeletal system, 600-601. *See also*
    bone infections
    bacterial infections, samples and tissue
        selection, 259b
    rule-outs, 600-601
        lameness, stiffness, arthritis, 600
        muscle fasciculations, 601
        myositis, increased muscle enzyme
            activity, 600
muzzle
    orthopoxvirus, 256
    warts (papillomavirus), 245f
MVE (Murray Valley encephalitis) virus,
    254f, 255
MWTA (Medical Waste Tracking Act),
    537-538
mycelia, 17
mycetomas, nocardia-induced, 381
mycobacterial infections, 390-392
Mycobacterium species, 391, 587-588
    cell wall extracts, 587-588
Mycobacterium avium, 57-58
Mycobacterium bovis, 390, 407
Mycobacterium equie. See *Rhodoccus equi*
Mycobacterium tuberculosis, 390
mycolata, 287
mycology terminology, 393b. *See also* fungal
    infections
Mycoplasma equigenitalium, 99
Mycoplasma felis, 32
Mycoplasma subdolum, 99
mycosis fungoides, 61
mycotic infections. *See* fungal infections;
    specific infection/disease or pathogen
mycotic keratitis (keratomycosis), 111f,
    112-114
    aspergillosis, 117, 422-423
    clinical findings, 424-425, 424f
        fungal hyphae in corneal scraping,
            426f
        stromal abscesses, 424f
    diagnosis, 426-427
        corneal biopsy and staining, 427
        culturing, 426-427
        cytology, 426
    epidemiology, 422-423
    etiology
        Aspergillus species, 422-423
        Histoplasma species, 442
    fibrosis and scar formation, 432
    histoplasmosis, 442-444
    pain management, 432
    pathogenesis, 423-424
    prognosis, 432
    therapy, 430-432
        azole antifungal drugs, 431
        choice of antifungal medications,
            431-432
        contraindications for corticosteroid
            treatment, 432
        control of uveitis/ocular pain, 432
        duration of, 432
        histoplasmosis, 444
        polyene antifungal drugs, 430
        povidone-iodine solution, 431
        silver sulfadiazine, 431
        surgical, 432
        thiabendazole, 431
        topical antifungals, 430t

mycotoxins, contaminated ryegrass, 522f
myelitis, 47, 464f
myeloencephalitis, 47, 54. *See also* equine
protozoal myeloencephalitis (EPM)
myeloencephalopathy, 3, 47, 54
myeloencephalopathy (EHM), 3
myiasis (maggots), 503-504
  clinical findings, 503
  diagnosis, 503
  etiology and epidemiology, 503
  public health considerations, 503-504
  therapy and prevention, 503
myocarditis, 30-31, 272, 601
  clinical findings, 31, 31f
  diagnosis, 31
  echocardiogram, 32f
  etiology and pathogenesis, 30
  M-mode echocardiogram, 33f
  prognosis, 31
  therapy, 31
myonecrosis. *See* clostridial myonecrosis (gas
gangrene)
myopathies, 271-272
myositis, 509f
  increased muscle enzyme activity, 600
  infectious, 61
  primary bacterial, 60-61
    clinical findings, 60
    diagnosis, 60-61
    etiology, 60
    therapy, 61
  primary fungal, 61
    clinical findings, 61
    diagnosis and therapy, 61
    etiology, 61
  primary parasitic, 61
    clinical findings, 61
    diagnosis and therapy, 61
    etiology, 61
  secondary parasitic, 61
    clinical findings, 61
    diagnosis and therapy, 61
    etiology, 61
  with *Streptococcus equi equi* (strangles),
    271-272

N

nagana, 504
NAHMS (National Animal Health
  Monitoring Survey), 542
nares
  Besnoitia lesions, 511, 512f
  orthopoxvirus, 256
nasal aspergillosis, 425
  clinical findings, 425
  diagnosis, 427
  therapy, 432
nasal cavities. *See also* rhinitis
  normal flora, 259b
  polyps, 420f
  swelling of mucosa, 17-18
  zygomycosis, 419
nasal discharge, 4, 9, 598
  acute myocarditis, 31f
  equine influenza, 144f
  glanders exudate, 335f
  purulent, 16
  rule-outs, 598
nasal glanders, 334-335
nasal septum, petechiation of, 345f
nasopharynx, pharyngeal hyperplasia, 5b
National Animal Health Monitoring Survey
  (NAHMS), 542
National Veterinary Services Laboratory, 44

necrosis/necrotic changes. *See also* clostridial
  myonecrosis (gas gangrene); tumor
  necrosis factor (TNF)
  in allantochorion, 97f
  focal, 427f
  spider bites, 504
  of spinal cord, 464f-465f
nematodes, 59, 61, 475-485
  anthelmintic therapy
    efficacy, 478t
    nonstrongylid nematodes, 483t
  ascarids, 482f
  cyathostominae (cyathostomes,
    cyathostomins, small strongyles,
    trichonemes), 478-481
    clinical findings, 479
    diagnosis, 479
    epidemiology, 479
    etiology, 478-479
    larvae, 477f, 479f
    pathogenesis, 479
    pathologic findings, 479
    prevention, 480-481
    public health considerations, 481
    therapy, 479-480
  Draschia megastoma, 487f
  fecal egg count reduction (FECR) test,
    480b
  identification of, 453b
  Nippostrongylus brasiliensis, 492
  nonenteric, 485-489
    habronemiasis, 487-489, 488f
    habronemiasis (lacrimal gland), 489f
    lungworm, 489
    Onchocerca cervicalis, 486f
    onchocerciasis, 485-487
  Oxyuris equi, 485f
  oxyurosis, 484-485
  Parascaris equorum, 481f
  parascorosis, 481-483
  species identification, 477
  species infecting equines, 449
  strongylinae, 475-478
  Strongyloides westeri, 483f
  strongyloidosis, 483-484
  strongylosis, 475-481
neonatal foals. *See also* foals
  Candida albicans, 408
  death of (leptospirosis), 305-306, 309
  equine herpesvirus (EHV), 160
  immunity in, 291
  piroplasmosis, 472
  septic arthritis, 64
  vaccination protocols, 593
neonatal sepsis, 70. *See also* foals; sepsis
  blood cultures, 72
  clinicopathologic findings, 71-72
  coagulopahy, 76-77
  definitions, 70
  etiology/causative organisms, 72-74
  focal infection and sequelae, 75-76
  frequency of bacterial isolates, 73t
  gastrointestinal involvement, 76
  meningitis, 76
  ocular involvement, 76
  pathophysiology, 70
  physical examination findings, 71
  predisposing factors, 70-71
  preventive strategies, 77
  prognosis/outcomes, 77
  respiratory involvement, 76
  risk factors, 71, 78
  routes of infection, 71
  secondary infections with, 75-76
  septic arthritis and osteomyelitis, 76

neonatal sepsis *(Continued)*
  therapy, 74-77
    antacid, 75
    antiendotoxin, 75
    antifungal, 75
    antimicrobial, 74-75
    cardiovascular support, 75
    corticosteroid, 78
    recommended antimicrobial dosages, 74t
    reported antimicrobial susceptibility
      patterns of microorganisms, 74t
    umbilical involvement (omphalitis), 76
Neorickettsia risticii, 44, 347, 349f, 516-517.
  See also Potomac horse fever (PHF)/
  equine neorickettsiosis (EN)
Neospora species, 457
nephrotoxins, 109, 577b
nervous system. *See also* central nervous
  system (CNS) infections
  bacterial infections, 259b
  symptoms of Borna disease, 226-227
nested polymerase chain reaction, 134-136
neuraminidase inhibitors, 583
neuritis, 47
neuroanatomy, 48-50
  blood-brain barrier and cerebrospinal
    fluid, 49-50
  brain and meninges, 48-49
  central nervous system vascularization, 49
  cranial nerves, 49
  meninges, 48f
neurologic disorders
  pressure sores of recumbent horses with,
    366f
  protozoal myeloencephalitis (*See* equine
    protozoal myeloencephalitis (EPM))
neurologic signs, 106-107
  Borna disease (BD), 230
  equine herpesvirus (EHV), 161
  facial nerve paralysis with ocular
    complications, 114f
  rabies (*See* rabies (RABV))
neuromuscular blockade, 577b
neuro-ophthalmic infectious diseases,
  114-116
  Horner's syndrome, 115-116
  vestibular disease, 114-115
neurotoxins. *See* botulism; tetanus
neutralization of virus infectivity, 139
neutrophil activation, 123-124, 596b
neutrophil chemotaxis, 85-86
nictitans
  flashing of, 369f
  prolapse of, 369
Nigerian equine encephalitis, 256
Nipah virus, 255
Nippostrongylus brasiliensis, 492
Nocardia species, 258f, 379-383
Nocardia asteroides, 381
nocardioform placentitis, 95-96
nocardiosis, 379-383
  clinical findings, 380-381
    abortion, 381
    disseminated nocardiosis, 380-381
    localized cutaneous and subcutaneous
      nocardiosis, 381
    mycetomas, 381
    pulmonary nocardiosis, 380
    ulcerative skin lesions, 381f
  diagnosis, 381-382
    direct examination, 381
    isolation and identification, 382
    molecular identification, 382
    radiography, 380f
    serology, 382

nocardiosis *(Continued)*
  epidemiology, 380
  etiology, 379-380
  pathogenesis, 380
  pathologic findings, 381
    lung abscessation, 382f
    lung photomicroscopy, 382f
  public health considerations, 383
  therapy, 382-383
nodular/masses dermatoses, 82-83
  Histoplasma capsulatum farciminosum
    (HCF), 444
  sarcoids, 248
nonbiting, 503
nonbiting flies, 503
noncore vaccines, 558
noncytopathic viral growth, 133
nonenteric nematodes, 485-489
  habronemiasis, 487-489, 488f-489f
  lungworm, 489
  Onchocerca cervicalis, 486f
  onchocerciasis, 485-487
nonseptic polysynovitis, 292-293
nonsteroidal antiinflammatory drugs
  (NSAIDs)
  neuritis, 18
  SIRS, 129
nonulcerative infectious keratitis, 113-114
normal flora, 259b
nosocomial infections
  coagulase-negative staphylococci, 280
  informing clients of risk of, 540
  pathogens, 532
  risk management, 531
Ntaya encephalitis, 218t-219t
nucleic acid amplification and polymerase
  chain reaction, 294-295
nucleoside analogs, 583
nucleotide synthesis inhibitors, 585t, 597

O

occult sarcoids, 248
Occupational Safety and Health
  Administration (OSHA), General Duty
  Clause, 531
ocular diseases/infections, 602
  bacterial, 261
  bacterial isolates
    from diseased eyes, 110
    from normal eyes, 110
  blepharitis, 110-111
  blindness, 56f
    cortical, 48-49
  conjunctival (*See* conjunctiva)
  corneal (*See* cornea)
  denervation of laryngeal nerve in, 17-18
  endophthalmitis, 9-10
  equine recurrent uveitis, leptospirosis and,
    305-307, 309
  eyeworm, 502-503
  fungal infections, specimen collection and
    transport, 394
  habronemiasis
    conjunctival, 488
    lacrimal gland, 487, 489f
  hypopyon, 110f
  impact of, 109-110
  keratitis (*See under* cornea)
  lymphoid follicles in perilimbal region,
    111f
  miotic pupils, 113f
  mycotic keratitis (keratomycosis)
    fibrosis and scar formation, 432
    pain management, 432

ocular diseases/infections *(Continued)*
  neuro-ophthalmic infectious diseases,
    114-116
    Horner's syndrome, 115-116
    vestibular disease, 114-115
  rule-outs, 602
    blindness, 602
    conjunctivitis, 602
    corneal edema, 602
    keratitis, 602
    uveitis, 602
  ruptured descemetrocele, 113f
  uveitis, 76
    with corneal ulcer, 113f
    equine recurrent uveitis (ERU), 114f
    with mycotic keratitis (keratomycosis),
      432
    primary, 114
    Rhodococcus equi infection, 114f
ocular flora, 110
  bacterial isolates
    from diseased eyes, 110
    from normal eyes, 110
  fungal isolates, from diseased eyes, 110
ocular manifestations of diseases/infections
  African horse sickness (AHS), 185f
  aspergillosis (*See* mycotic keratitis
    (keratomycosis))
  equine viral arteritis (EVA), 116t
  icteric sclera, 345f
  rabies, 208f
  Rhodoccus equi, 293f
  systemic diseases, 116-118
    bacterial, 116
    candidiasis, 410
    fungal, 116-117
    meningitis, 76
    neonatal sepsis, 76
    parasitic, 117-118
    systemic inflammatory response
      syndrome (SIRS), 113f
    viral, 116
Office International des Epizooties (OIE),
  184
OIE (International des Epizooties),
  470-471, 605
  Web site, 473
OIE (Office International des Epizooties),
  184
Onchocerca species, 485, 507
Onchocerca cervicali, 118
Onchocerca cervicalis, 449, 451f, 485, 486f
Onchocerca reticulata, 449, 485
onchocerciasis, 118, 485-487
  clinical findings, 486
  diagnosis and pathologic findings, 486
  etiology and epidemiology, 485
  pathogenesis, 485-486
  therapy, 486-487
oomycetes, pythiosis, 82b
oophoritis, 93
ophthalmic disorders. *See* ocular diseases/
  infections
oral cavity, 42
  bacterial flora, 1
  candidiasis (thrush), 72-74, 409, 409f, 411
  infectious disorders, 42
  normal flora, 42, 259b
  purpura hemorrhagica, 271f
  rule-outs, vesicular stomatitis virus, 242
  ulcers or vesicles
    rule-outs, 599
    vesicular stomatitis viruses (VSVs),
      241f
Orbivirus, 182

orbiviruses, 251-252
orthomyxoviruses, 5-6
orthopedic implants, infected, 68
orthopedic infections. *See* bone infections
orthopoxvirus, 256
osmotic agents, 54-55
ostectomy, 20, 20f
osteitis, septic, 66-70
osteomyelitis, 58f. *See also* bone infections;
  vertebral infections
  culture and sensitivity (C&S), 67
  debridement, 67
  prognosis, 68-69
  of scapulohumeral joint, 69f
  septic, 66-70
    antimicrobial-impregnated
      polymethylmethacrylate (PMMA)
      beads, 68b
    clinical findings, 66
    diagnosis, 66-67
    etiology and pathogenesis, 66
    supportive care for severe lameness,
      69-70
    systemic antibiotics for, 69t
    therapy, 67-69
  vertebral (*See* spinal infections)
Otobius megnini, 495
outbreaks
  abortion storms, 160
  African horse sickness (AHS), 183
  anthrax, 383-384
  botulism type C, 364
  Clostridium perfringens infection, 358
  due to transportation of infected animals,
    555-556
  equine herpesvirus, 168
  equine infectious anemia, 233-234
  equine influenza, 143, 563
  equine piroplasmosis, 468, 470-471
  equine viral arteritis, 170-171
  glomerulonephritis, 277
  Hendra virus (HeV), 192
    Australian outbreak, 193t
  investigations, attack risk table, 523-525
  management of, 529
  mare reproductive loss syndrome
    (MRLS), 515
  nosocomial infections, 531
  point-source outbreaks of neurologic
    signs, 522f
  related to international movement of
    horses, 547t
  rotavirus (on-farm), 199
  rules/regulations for management of, 531
  streptococcal infections, 274-276
    guttural pouch infections, 275-276
    outbreak investigations, 274-275
  Venezuelan equine encephalitis (VEE),
    217
  vesicular stomatitis viruses (VSVs), 239,
    242, 244
outdoor exercise areas, 540
outerwear, 541
ovarian abscesses and adhesions, 93f
owners of horses
  biosecurity measures for, 542-543
  MRSA colonization in, 283t
  protection of resident horses, 541-543
oxacillin, 281
oxytocin therapy, 87f
Oxyuris equi, 485f, 507-508
Oxyuris equi eggs, 451f, 455f
oxyurosis, 484-485
  clinical findings, 484-485
  diagnosis, 485

oxyurosis *(Continued)*
etiology and epidemiology, 484
pathogenesis, 484
pathologic findings, 485
prevention, 485
public health considerations, 485
therapy, 485

P

pain/pain management
abdominal pain, 599
cellulitis, 62
guttural pouch mycosis, 18
Lyme disease, 313f
musculoskeletal infections, 69-70
mycotic keratitis (keratomycosis), 432
salmonellosis, 331-332
synovial infections, 63
uveitis/ocular pain, 432
pandemic diseases, 521f
Panton-Valentine leukocidin (PVL), 279-280
papillomavirus, 81b
papillomaviruses, 81-82
about, 244
aural plaques, 246
bovine papillomavirus (BPV), 244
equine warts, 244-246
infections/noninfectious, 81b
papilloma virus type 2, 82
sarcoids, 246-251
papular dermatitis, 80
orthopoxvirus, 256
papulonodular dermatoses, 81-82, 603
bacterial etiology, diagnosis, treatment, 81
leishmaniasis, 82, 82f
papillomavirus, 81-82
infections/noninfectious, 81b
Parafilaria multipapillosa, 449
paramyxoviruses, 255-256
Paranoplocephola mamillana, 449
Parapoxvirus ovis, 590-591
Parascaris equorum, 13-14, 481f, 507-508
parascorosis, 481-483
clinical findings, 482
diagnosis, 482
etiology and epidemiology, 481
pathogenesis, 481
pathologic findings, 482
prevention, 483
public health considerations, 483
therapy, 482-483
parasitemia, 468-469
parasitic infections. *See also* anthelmintic
therapy; antimicrobial therapy;
helminth infections; protozoal
infections
aberrant parasites, 509-510
abortion caused by, 99
babesiosis (piroplasmosis), 117
besnoitiosis, 80
blepharitis, 111
of central nervous system, 48t, 58-59
Halicephalobus gingivalis
encephalomyelitis, 58-59
cestodes (*See* cestodes)
conjunctivitis, causative agents, 111b
crusting/scaling dermatoses, 80
deworming programs, horses/donkeys/
mules, 14
diarrhea in adult horses and, 44
dirofilariasis, 118
echinococcosis, 118

parasitic infections *(Continued)*
equine protozoal myeloencephalitis
(EPM), 117
habronemiasis, 118
laboratory diagnosis, 449-456
Anoplocephala perfoliata, 451f
Baerman procedure, 454
blood smears, 455
cellophane (Scotch) tape test, 454
Cryptosporidium parvum, 452f
Dictyocaulus arnfieldi eggs, 451f
direct fecal smear, 454
Eimeria leuckarti, 452f
Fasciola hepatica egg, 452f
fecal cultures, 453
fecal flotation, 449-453
fecal sedimentation, 453-454
Giardia intestinalis, 452f
gross fecal examination, 449
helminths, 449
Heterobilharzia americana, 452f
impression smears, 455
isolated worm recovery, 455-456
key to microfilariae, 453b
Leishmania species, 452f
McMaster's procedure, 454-455
nematode larvae identification, 453b
Onchocerca cervicalis, 451f
Oxyuris equi eggs, 451f, 455f
Pascaris equorum eggs, 450f
protozoans, 449
skin biopsy, 455
strongyles, 450f, 454f
Strongyloides westeri eggs, 451f
Theileria equi, 455f
nematodes (*See* nematodes)
ocular manifestations/complications of
systemic, 117-118
onchocerciasis, 118
piroplasmosis (*See* equine piroplasmosis
(EP))
pneumonia, 13-14 (*See also* anthelmintic
therapy; parasitic pneumonia)
prevalence by species of, 490
prevention, *Anoplocephala perfoliata*, 494
selective treatment, 481
setariasis, 118
tapeworm (*See* cestodes)
thelaziasis, 118
toxoplasmosis, 117-118
parasitic myositis
primary, 61
clinical findings, 61
diagnosis and therapy, 61
etiology, 61
secondary, 61
clinical findings, 61
diagnosis and therapy, 61
etiology, 61
parasitic pneumonia, 13-14
clinical findings, 13
body condition, 13
diagnosis, 13
etiology, 13
prognosis, 14
therapy, 13-14
paratuberculosis, 390
parenteral injection site infections. *See*
clostridial myonecrosis (gas gangrene)
parietal pleura with granulomata, 403f
Pascaris equorum eggs, 450f
passive immunity, 594-596
Clostridium botulinum hyperimmune
plasma, 595

passive immunity *(Continued)*
Clostridium tetani (tetanus antitoxin), 595
endotoxemia antibodies, 595
snake antivenin (IV), 595-596
transfer of antigen-specific antibodies, 594-595
transfer of nonspecific antibodies, 594
West Nile virus antibodies, 595
passive immunization, 556-557, 585t
exogenous antibodies, 556
passive transfer of maternal immunity, 556-557
passive transfer of maternal immunity, 556-557
pastern dermatitis, 83
Pasteurella species, 1, 571
Pasteurella multocida, 32
pastures/paddocks
management for parasitic infection
control, 494, 540
mite infestations, 498
pathogenesis. *See under specific infection/
disease or pathogen*
pathogens. *See* etiology *under specific
infection/disease;* specific infection/
disease or pathogen
pathogens variants, 548
pathophysiology. *See under specific infection/
disease or pathogen*
patient protection, 531
patterns of disease, 520-522
PcP. *See* pneumocystis infections
PCR. *See* polymerase chain reaction (PCR)
testing
pedicle grafts, corneal, 113f
pediculosis. *See* lice (pediculosis)
Pelodera strongylides, 83
penicillin resistance. *See* drug resistant/
sensitive organisms
penis
culturing of penis/prepuce, 341, 342f
contagious equine metritis (CEM), 342f-343f
habronemiasis infection, 101f, 488f
infectious diseases, 100-102
prepuce, 100-102
priapism, 212f
peptide-conjugated phosphorodiamidate
morpholino oligomer (PPMO), 178
Peptostreptococcus species, 10-11
percutaneous centesis, 16
performance, poor performance syndrome, 160
performance horses, lower airway infections, 7
pericardiocentesis, 35b
pericarditis, 31-36
clinical findings, 34
constrictive, 34f
diagnosis, 34-36
echocardiography, 34
electrocardiography/radiography/cardiac
catheterization, 34-35
laboratory diagnosis, 35-36
etiology and pathogenesis, 31-33
fibrinoeffusive idiopathic, 35f
prognosis, 36
septic fibrinoeffusive, 33f-35f
periorchitis, 102f
peritoneal infections, 46-47
diagnosis, 46
etiology and clinical findings, 46
prognosis, 47
therapy, 46-47
peritoneal lavage, 47

peritonitis, 46
persistent mating-induced endometritis (PMIE), 87f
personnel. *See* employees/personnel
Peruvian horse sickness virus (PHSV), 252
petechial hemorrhages, 113f, 601
   Clostridium difficile, 355f
Pfeifenrauchen (chewing movements), 229, 230f
PFGE (pulse-field gel electrophoresis), 263
phaeohyphomycotic fungi, pyogranuloma with, 83f
phagocytes, alveolar macrophages, 1-2
pharmacokinetic-pharmacodynamic optimization of drug doses, 573-574
pharyngeal lymphadenopathy, diagnosis of, 3
pharyngitis, 6
pharynx
   aerobes/anaerobes of, 42
   flora/microflora, 42
   lymphoid pharyngeal hyperplasia, 5, 5b, 5f
   pharyngeal hyperplasia, 5
   pharyngeal lymphadenopathy, 3
   pharyngitis, 6
   retropharyngeal lymph nodes, 16f
PHF. *See* Potomac horse fever (PHF)/equine neorickettsiosis (EN)
Phlebotomus, 504
phosphatase inhibitors, 585t, 596-597
phosphorylation, 166
PHSV (Peruvian horse sickness virus), 252
phycomycoses, 61
phycomycosis, 415. *See also* pythiosis; zygomycosis
Physa acuta, 512
physical therapy, cellulitis, 62
physiology. *See under specific infection/disease or pathogen*
PIMs (pulmonary intravascular macrophages), 2
pinworms *(Oxyuris equi)*, 484-485
pipesmoking movement, 229, 230f
piroplasmosis. *See* equine piroplasmosis (EP)
PIRO system, 120
Piry virus, 204
placenta
   handling aborted placental material, 155
   normal/abnormal, 97f
   transplacental transmission of disease, 234, 350, 471
   uteroplacental thickness measurement, 96f
placentitis. *See also* abortion; mares
   abortion caused by, 94-98
   ascendant, 94-95, 94f
   aspergillosis
      clinical findings, 425
      diagnosis, 427
      epidemiology, 423
      etiology, 423-424
      pathogenesis, 424
      therapy, 433
   clinical findings, 425
   coccidiomycosis, 405
   etiology, aspergillosis, 423-424
   hematogenous multifocal or diffuse, 95
   Leptospira species, 95
   necrotic changes in allantochorion, 97f
   nocardiform, 95-96, 381
   pathogenesis and diagnosis, 96-97
   treatment, 97

plaque reduction neutralization test, 225f
plaques, aural, 246
plasma concentration versus time profile and minimum inhibitory concentration, 573f
pleural effusion, 598
pleurodynia, clinical findings, 8
pleuropneumonia, 8-11, 9f
   etiology and epidemiology, 8
   indwelling thoracic tube placement, 11f
   pleural effusion and pulmonary consolidation with, 9f
plymyarian-meromyarian musculature, 59
PMIE (persistent mating-induced endometritis), 87f
Pneumocystis species, 446
Pneumocystis carinii (P. jirovecii), 397, 446
pneumocystis infections, 446-448
   clinical findings, 447
   diagnosis, 447-448
   epidemiology, 446
   etiology, 446
   pathogenesis, 446-447
   pathologic findings, 448
   prevention, 448
   public health considerations, 448
   therapy, 448
pneumonia, 8-14
   aspiration, 7
   bacterial
      etiology and epidemiology, 7
      samples and tissue selection, 259b
      Streptococcus pneumoniae, 277
      Streptococcus zooepidemicus, 277
   bronchopneumonia, 7, 190
      pathogenesis of, 7
      Rhodococcus equi, 293f
   chronic granulomatous, 11
   clinical findings, 8-9
   coughing related to, 7-8
   diagnosis, 9-10
   etiology and epidemiology, 7
   foals/young horses, 14
   interstitial, 11-13
      clinical findings, 12
      diagnosis, 12
      epidemiology, 11
      etiology, 11-12
      histopathology, 12f
      prognosis, 11, 13
      radiography, 12f
      therapy, 12-13
   Klebsiella pneumoniae, 104
   mechanisms of contamination, 1
   parasitic, 13-14
      clinical findings, 13
      diagnosis, 13
      etiology, 13
      prognosis, 14
      therapy, 13-14
   pleuropneumonia, 8-11, 9f
      etiology and epidemiology, 8
      indwelling thoracic tube placement, 11f
      pleural effusion and pulmonary consolidation with, 9f
   rhinopneumonitis, vaccine recommendations for, 564-566
   Rhodococcus equi, 516
      survival rates, 77
   secondary, *Corynebacterium pseudotuberculosis*, 378f
   septic myocardial dysfunction, antimicrobial therapy, 41f

pneumonia *(Continued)*
   Streptococcus pneumoniae
      clinical findings and therapy, 277
      etiology, 277
      pathogenesis, 277
      public health considerations, 277
      therapy, 10-11
pneumonthorax, 9
pododermatitis in Draft horses, 83
point-source epidemics, 521
polioencephalomyelitis, 223-225
pollakiuria, 600
poll evil, 338
polyene antifungal drugs, 428, 430, 582
polymerase chain reaction (PCR) testing, 3, 44, 134-136, 134f, 281. *See also* molecular testing
   Anoplocephala perfoliata diagnosis, 493
   aspergillosis, 425
   bacterial pathogen detection methods, 262f
   bacterial pathogens tested for, 263
   Borna disease (BD), 231
   clostridial myonecrosis, 360
   contagious equine metritis (CEM), 337-338
   description of testing methods, 605t
   equine adenovirus type 1, 189
   equine protozoal myeloencephalitis (EPM), 464
   fungal infections, 398
   gel analysis of, 134f
   molecular testing format, 604
   pneumocystis infections, 447-448
   real-time, 134-136, 425
   reverse transcriptase-polymerase change reaction, 146-147
   rotavirus, 199-200
   staphylococcal infections, 281
polyps, nasal, 420f
polysynovitis, 292-293, 292f
Ponazuril, 465-466
poor performance syndrome, post-equine herpesvirus, 160
population-at-risk, 516-518
postoperative infections, 280
postpartum metritis, 93
postpartum uterine lavage, 89t
potassium hydroxide (KOH) treatment, 395
Potomac horse fever (PHF)/equine neorickettsiosis (EN), 44, 516, 567-568. *See also Neorickettsia risticii*
   clinical findings, 350
   diagnosis, 350-351
      molecular detection, 351f
   epidemic curve, 521f
   epidemiology, 347-349
      caddisfly larvae, 348f
      snails, 348f
      trematodes, 348f
   etiology, 347
   pathogenesis, 349-350
   pathologic findings, 351
   prevention, 351
   therapy, 351
   vaccination recommendations, 44, 567-568
   whole blood or serum tests for, 44
poultry fleas, 504
poultry mites, 504
povidone-iodine solution, 431
Powassan virus, 255
poxvirus, 80-81

PPMO (peptide-conjugated phosphorodiamidate morpholino oligomer), 178
practice protection, 541-542
Prascaris equorum (ascarids/roundworms), 481
predictive values, 528b, 528f
preexport testing reliability, 549
prepuce
  culturing of, contagious equine metritis (CEM), 342f
  infectious diseases of, 100-102
pressure sores of recumbent horses, 366f
prevalence of a disease, 519, 519b
  comparisons
    odds ratio, 523, 524b
    reality of difference, 525
  relationship to incidence, 520, 521b
prevention, 533-540. *See also* biosecurity; specific infection/disease or pathogen
  antiseptics and disinfectants, 538t
  barrier gowns, 535
  barrier nursing precautions, 534-535, 535f
  biosecurity kits, 541
  cryptosporidiosis, 508-509
  daily attire, 534
  disinfection methods, 539f
  face/eye protection, 535
  footbaths/footmats, 536-537
  footwear hygiene, 535
  gloves, 535
  hand hygiene, 534
  immunoprophylaxis (*See* immunoprophylaxis)
  movement/traffic flow management (personnel), 535
  separation/isolation, 535-536
  strategies for, 528-529
  transmission routes, 534
priapism, 212f
probiotics, diarrhea prevention, 358
prognosis. *See specific infection/disease or pathogen*
program development
  critical control point (CCP)
    identification, 533
    monitoring, 533
  critical limits for preventive measures, 533
  hazard analysis/identification, 532-533
propagated epidemics, 521
prophylaxis. *See* biosecurity; immunoprophylaxis; prevention; specific infection/disease or pathogen
Propionibacterium acnes, 586-587
proprioceptive deficits
  Borna disease (BD), 230f
  equine herpesvirus (EHV), 162f
proprioceptive deficits Borna disease (BD), 229
protein (subunit) vaccines, 552
proteolytic bacteria, 42
Proteus mirabili, 94
protozoal infections. *See also* antiprotozoal therapy; helminth infections; parasitic infections; specific infection/disease or pathogen
  causes of diarrhea in foals, 43
  of central nervous system, 48t
  laboratory diagnosis, 449
  myeloencephalitis (*See* equine protozoal myeloencephalitis (EPM))
proximal enteritis, 43
pruritis, 602-603
  midge-related, 501
  mite infestation-related, 497

pruritis (*Continued*)
  Onchocerca cervicalis, 486f
  as symptom of parasitic infection, 80
Przewalski's horses, 404
Pseudallescheria boydii, 82-83
Pseudomonas species, 8, 32, 64
  microbial susceptibility, 572
  placentitis, 94
Pseudomonas aeruginosa, 94
  transmission of, 104
  urinary tract infections, 106
Psoroptes cuniculi, 496
Psoroptes equi, 496
Psoroptes natalensis, 496
Psoroptes ovis, 496
psoroptic mange, 496-497
  diagnosis, 496
  epidemiology, 496
  etiology, 496
  pathogenesis and clinical findings, 496
  prevention, 497
  therapy, 496-497
PTE (pulmonary thromboembolism), 10
pteropid bats (flying foxes), 192-193
ptosis, 17-18
public health considerations. *See also* biosecurity; zoonotic diseases; specific infection/disease or pathogen
  flavivirus encephalitides, 217
  fly vectors, 503
  mosquitoes, 501
pulmonary —. *See respiratory entries*
pulmonary clearance mechanisms, 1
pulmonary definition mechanisms, 1-2
pulmonary findings, 7-8
pulmonary infections. *See* respiratory diseases
pulmonary intravascular macrophages (PIMs), 2
pulmonary thromboembolism (PTE), 10
pulse-field gel electrophoresis (PFGE), 263
punch biopsies, 78
puncture wounds, 368
pupils, miotic, 113f-114f
purpura hemorrhagica, 271, 271f
purulent vaginal discharge, 340f
PVL (Panton-Valentine leukocidin), 279-280
pyelonephritis, 107-108
pyogranuloma, 83f
pyogranuloma with phaeohyphomycotic fungi, 83f
pyometra, 92-93, 92f-93f
pyrantel pamoate, 14
pyrrolizidine alkaloid toxicity, 41f
pythiosis, 82b, 415-419
  clinical findings, 415-416
    lesions, 416f
  diagnosis, 416-417
    culturing, 417
    cytology, 416-417
    immunohistochemistry, 417
    molecular assays, 417
    serology, 417
  etiology and epidemiology, 415
  pathologic findings, 417-418
    immunohistological stain, 417f
    subcutaneous lesions, 416f
  therapy, 418-419
    immunotherapy, 418
    medical, 418-419
    surgical, 418
Pythium species, 61, 415. *See also Basidiobiosis* species
Pythium insidiosum, 415, 416f-417f

Q
quarantines. *See also* biosecurity
  contagious equine metritis (CEM), 338
  Streptococcus equi equi, 274-275
quinidine toxicity, 114f

R
rabies (RABV), 531-533
  clinical findings, 205, 206f
  diagnosis, 205-206
  differential diagnosis, 205
  distribution of reservoirs, 204f
  epidemiology, 204-205
  equine cases in United States and Puerto Rico, 203-204, 205f
  etiology, 204
  ocular manifestations of, 116t
  overview, 203-204, 204f
  pathogenesis, 205
  pathologic findings, 206-208, 206f-208f
  prevention, 208-209
    approved vaccines, 208t
    vaccination protocol, 209b
  public health considerations, 209
  therapy, 208
  in vaccinated animals, 209
  vaccine recommendations, 567
radio-frequency current-induced hyperthermia, 249
radiography. *See* diagnosis *under specific infection/disease*
rain rot. *See* dermatophilosis (rain rot)
rapamycin (sirolimus), 597
rates of disease incidence, 518-519
real-time (RT) polymerase chain reaction (PCR) test, 134-136, 425
recombinant vaccines, 553
recumbent horses
  acute recumbency, 462f
  botulism, 365
  pressure sores of, 366f
renal —. *See* kidneys
reproductive tract infections, 601
  abortion (*See* abortion)
  anaerobic flora, 388
  anatomy, normal and abnormal vulva conformation, 85f
  biosecurity in breeding operations, 105-106
  cryptococcosis, 440
  equine herpesvirus (EHV), 160
  equine venereal diseases, 104-105
  laboratory diagnosis, endometrial cytology, 87f-88f
  mares (*See under* mares)
  rule-outs, 601
    abortion, infertility, early embryonic loss, birth of weak foals, 601
    scrotal/preputial enlargement, 601
  stallions (*See under* stallions)
reservoir hosts, 516-517. *See also* epidemiology *under specific* disease/ infection; hosts/host factors
  aberrant, 220f
  African horse sickness (AHS), 182
  Brucella abortus, 337
  equine granulocytic anaplasmosis/ ehrlichiosis, 344
  equine lungworm
    donkeys as, 489
    mules as, 489
  Gastrodiscus, 512
  Hendra virus, pteropid bats, 192

reservoir hosts (Continued)
  humans, 510
  Sarcocystis neurona, 456, 458, 467 (*See also* equine protozoal myeloencephalitis (EPM))
  sarcocystosis, 509
  vertebrate, 240
  wildlife reservoirs/control, 538-539
resistance to drugs. *See* drug resistant/sensitive organisms
respiration
  depth of, 3
  physiologic considerations, 2
respiratory diseases, 1-2, 598-599. *See also pulmonary entries;* specific infection/disease or pathogen
  anatomy and physiology, 2, 2f
  aspergillosis
    clinical findings, 425
    diagnosis, 427
    therapy, 432
  chronic infections, 335
  clearance of debris, 1
  cryptococcosis, 440
  endoscopy, 3
  epithelial protection of, 2
  equine adenovirus type 1, 190
  equine herpesvirus (EHV), 159-160
  Histoplasma capsulatum farciminosum (HCF), 444-445
  infectious, 3
    clinical findings, 3
    diagnostic approach, 3-4
    upper respiratory tract, 4-7
  laboratory diagnosis
    buffy coat smear, 3
    cytology, 1-2, 9, 13
    enzyme-linked immunosorbent assay (ELISA) test, 3
    hematology, 8, 13
    polymerase chain reaction (PCR), 3
    serology, 4
    swabbing procedures, 3
    transtracheal wash analysis, 10f
  lower (*See* lower respiratory tract)
  mechanisms of removal of pathogens, 1
  molecular testing, 612
  neonatal sepsis effects on, 76
  normal flora, 1
  odors (diagnostic), 9
  propagated outbreaks of, 522f
  pulmonary abscesses, 7
  pulmonary blastomycosis, 433-434
  pulmonary definition mechanisms, 1-2
  pulmonary (dunkop) form of African horse sickness, 184, 184f, 186, 186f-187f
  pulmonary granulomas (glanders), 335f
  rhinoviruses (*See* rhinoviruses)
  Rhodococcus species, 292
  rule-outs/differential diagnosis, 598-599
    cough, 598
    dyspnea, 598-599
    nasal discharge, 598
    pleural effusion, 598
    respiratory noise, 598
    rhinitis/sinusitis, 598
  severe combined immune deficiency (SCID), 190f-191f, 471
  transtracheal wash procedure, 3
  upper (*See* upper respiratory tract)
respiratory distress, 448f
respiratory failure, 366-367
respiratory noise, 598
retropharyngeal lymph nodes, 16f

Retroviridae, 233
rhabdomyolysis, 271-272
Rhabdoviridae, 204, 239
rhinitis, 4-5, 598
  diagnosis of, 3-5
  differential diagnosis, 598
  equine rhinitis A and B, 195-197
    clinical findings, 196-197
    diagnosis, 197
    epidemiology, 196
    equine rhinitis A virus (ERAV), 195-197
    equine rhinitis B virus (ERBV), 4
    equine rhinitis B virus 2 (ERBV2), 4, 6, 195-197
    etiology, 195-196
    laboratory findings and virus isolation, 197
    organism detection, 197
    pathogenesis, 196
    pathologic findings, 197
    prevention, 197
    public health considerations, 197
    serology, 197
    therapy, 197
  radiography, 4-5
  therapy, 5
rhinopneumonitis, vaccine recommendations for, 564-566
rhinoviruses
  diagnostic methods, 4
  serogroups A and B (ERAV/ERBV), 4, 6
  serotypes 1, 2, and 3, 195
Rhodococcus equi, 3, 6, 46, 57-58, 63-64, 66, 293f, 484, 516, 531-532
  clinical findings, 291-293
    abdominal, 292
    in adult horses, 293
    body systems, 293
    bone and joint diseases, 293
    caseous exudates, 296f
    extrapulmonary disorders (EPDs), 292
    immune-mediated polysynovitis, 292f
    nonseptic polysynovitis, 292-293
    pulmonary diseases, 292
  diagnosis, 293-296
    complete blood count (CBC), 295
    culturing, 294, 294f
    cytology, 294, 294f
    imaging studies, 293f, 295-296, 296f
    nucleic acid amplification and polymerase chain reaction, 294-295
    serology, 295
  epidemiology, 288-289
  etiology, 287-288
  hyperimmune plasma sources, 290b
  immunity, 290-291
    cellular immunity, 291
    innate immunity response, 290
    in neonatal foals, 291
    role of antibody, 290-291
  intravenous administration of hyperimmune plasma, 594-595
  mechanisms of disease, 289-290
  pathogenesis, 289-291
  pathologic findings, 296-297
    pulmonary abscesses, 296f
  pneumonia survival rates, 77
  prevention, 299-302
    active immunization, 301-302
    chemoprophylaxis and immunostimulants, 301
    decreasing exposure, 299-300

Rhodococcus equi (Continued)
    early detection, 300
    passive immunization, 301
  prognosis, 299
  public health considerations, 302
  therapy, 297-299
    antibiotics, 297t
    antimicrobial, 297-299
  virulence, 287f
Rhodococcus rubropertinctus, 95
Rhodococcus equi, 114f
rhombencephalitis, 47
rickettsial infections, 48t. *See also* bacterial infections; specific infection or pathogen
rifampin, 581
ringworm. *See* dermatophytosis (ringworm)
Rio Bravo encephalitis, 218t-219t
risk factors/risk management, 549-551. *See also* biosecurity
  antimicrobial therapy as, 352
  candidiasis (thrush), 408-409
  comparing attributable risk (AR) and attributable fraction (AF), 523, 524b
  cumulative incidence comparisons relative risk, 523, 524b
  defining by risk, 168b
  Equine Biosecurity Risk Calculator, 542
  flavivirus encephalitides, 221-222
  individual risk factors for disease, 516-517
  international movement of horses, 549-551
    industry initiatives, 550-551
    postimport requirements, 550
    preexport requirements, 550
    surveillance and reporting of diseases, 550
  leptospirosis, 305
  Lyme disease, 312f
  methicillin-resistant *Staphylococcus aureus* (MRSA), 279
  MRSA, 279
  neonatal sepsis, 70-71, 78
  nosocomial infections
    informing clients of risk of, 540
    risk management, 531
  outbreaks
    attack risk table, 523-525, 525t
    population-at-risk, 516-518
  salmonellosis, 323-326
  staphylococcal infections, 280
  steroid use with fungal infections, 80
  vesicular stomatitis viruses (VSVs), 240-241
risus sardonicus, 369
RNA (ribonucleic acid), 5-6
rodent control, 538-539
Ross River virus, 253-255, 254f
rotaviruses, 43, 198-201, 199f-200f
  clinical findings, 199
  diagnostic options, 200
  epidemiology, 198-199
  etiology, 198
  field testing procedures, 199
  in foals, 198f
  multidrug-resistance, 532-533
  pathogenesis, 199
  pathologic findings, 200
  prevention, 201
    husbandry/infection control, 201
    public health considerations, 201
  therapy, 200-201
  vaccine recommendations, 569-570
roundworms (ascarids), 481, 482f, 483
rubivirus, 210t

rule-outs. *See also* diagnosis *under specific infection/disease or pathogen*
  cardiovascular system, 601
    cardiomyopathy, myocarditis, endocarditis, 601
  central nervous system (CNS), 600
    brainstem signs, 600
    cortical signs, 600
    spinal cord or peripheral nervous system signs, 600
  collapse and sudden death, 603
  dermatophytosis (ringworm), 411-412, 414
  gastrointestinal diseases/infections, 599
    abdominal effusion, 599
    abdominal masses, 599
    abdominal pain, 599
    diarrhea (adult horses), 599
    diarrhea (foals), 599
    dysphagia, 599
    hepatomegaly or hepatic inflammation, 599
    icterus, 599
    oral ulcers or vesicles, 599
  hemolymphatic disorders, 601-602
    anemia, 601
    enlarged lymph nodes, 601
    hypoalbuminemia, 602
    lymphangitis, 601
    petechial hemorrhages, 601
    thrombocytopenia, 602
    ventral abdominal or limb edema, 601-602
  musculoskeletal system, 600-601
    lameness, stiffness, arthritis, 600
    muscle fasciculations, 601
    myositis, increased muscle enzyme activity, 600
  ocular diseases/infections, 602
    blindness, 602
    conjunctivitis, 602
    corneal edema, 602
    keratitis, 602
    uveitis, 602
  pythiosis, 416
  reproductive tract infections, 601
    abortion, infertility, early embryonic loss, birth of weak foals, 601
    scrotal/preputial enlargement, 601
  respiratory diseases, 598-599
    cough, 598
    dyspnea, 598-599
    nasal discharge, 598
    pleural effusion, 598
    respiratory noise, 598
    rhinitis/sinusitis, 598
  rotavirus, 200
  skin disorders, 602-603
    crusting/scaling, 603
    hair loss, 602
    large nodular dermatoses or abscesses, 603
    papulonodular lesions, 603
    pruritis, 602-603
    ulcers, fistulas, granulomatous lesions, 603
  sporotrichosis, 407
  urinary tract disorders, 600
    dysuria, stranguria, pollakiuria, 600
    hematuria, 600
    incontinence, 600
    renal failure, 600
  vesicular stomatitis viruses, 242
Ruminococcus flavefaciens, 44
ruptured descemetrocele, 113f

S
sabulous cystitis, 106-107
Salem virus, 255-256
sales, biosecurity measures at, 543
Salmonella species, 44, 57-58, 64, 260, 516
  geographic location, 72
  isolation for infection, 536
Salmonella enterica, 60, 266, 531-533, 538-540, 613
Salmonella enterica enteritidis, 44
salmonellosis
  clinical findings, 327-328
  with *Clostridia perfringens* infection, 359
  diagnosis, 328-329
    clinical pathology, 328
    detection of organism, 328-329
    serologic testing, 329
  epidemiology, 322-326
    carrier horses, 326
    prevalence, 323, 325
    risk factors, 323-326
    source of infection, 322-325
  etiology, 321-322
  pathogenesis, 326-327
  pathologic findings, 329-330
  prevention, 332-333
    optimizing resistance, 332-333
    reducing exposure, 332
  public health considerations, 333
  therapy, 330-332
    antimicrobial therapy, 330
    colonic flora modulation, 331
    environmental management, 331
    fluid and colloidal therapy, 330
    pain management, 331-332
    treatment for endotoxemia and inflammation, 331
sample collection. *See also* laboratory diagnosis
  bacterial cultures, 258-261, 259b
    appropriate samples for, 258
    blood cultures, 259-260
    botulism and tetanus, 261
    clostridial enteritis, 260-261
    enteric infections, 260-261
    indications, 258
    joint cultures, 260
    methods, 258-259
    ocular infections, 261
    submission of, 261
    suspected anaerobic infections, 259
    wound cultures, 260
  catching mite samples, 497
  equine herpesvirus (EHV), 161
  molecular testing, 604
  parasites, 507
  submission of samples, 258-259
  transport media, 259
sandfly (*Phlebotomus* and *Lutzomyia*), 504
saprophytes, 394
Sarcocystis species, 61
Sarcocystis falcatula, 456
Sarcocystis neurona, 538-539
  in brain of horse, 458f
  epidemiology, 457-458
  immunoblot test, 462f
  life cycle, 457f
  monocyte infection, 458f
  reservoir hosts, 458, 467 (*See also* equine protozoal myeloencephalitis (EPM))
  life cycle, 456
  schizogonic stages, 458f

sarcocystosis, 509, 509f
sarcoids, 246-251
  clinical findings, 247-248, 248f
  diagnosis, 248-249
  epidemiology, 247
  etiology, 246-247
  pathogenesis, 247
  pathologic findings, 249, 249f
  therapy, 249-251
    carbon dioxide laser, 249
    chemotherapy, 250-251
    cryotherapy, 249
    hyperthermia, 249
    immunotherapy, 250
    irradiation, 250
    photodynamic, 250
    prevention, 251
    public health considerations, 251
    surgical resection, 249
Sarcoptes scabei equi, 496
sarcoptic mange, 496
  diagnosis, 496
  epidemiology, 496
  etiology, 496
  pathogenesis and clinical findings, 496
  public health considerations, 496
  therapy, 496
schizophrenia, 231
SCID (severe combined immune deficiency), 189-190, 190f-191f, 471
SCID (severe combined immuno-deficiency), 448, 448f
scinitgraphy, osteomyelitis, 67
scleral injection, with SIRS, 113f
scleral pearls, 511, 512f
scolex, 492
Scotch (cellophane) tape test, 454
scratches. *See* pastern dermatitis
screwworms, 503
scrotal/preputial enlargement, 601
seabird encephalitides, 218t-219t
secretory cells, 2
seizures, 48-49
semen, international transport of, 545
seminal vesiculitis, 103f
Senecia, 11
SENIC (Efficacy of Nosocomial Infection Control), 530
separation methods, 536. *See also* isolation methods; quarantines
sepsis
  Actinobacillus species, 42-43
  bacterial, ocular manifestations of, 117t
  cardiac complications in, 39-41
  definitions associated with, 70
  early identification of, 77
  in foals (*See* neonatal sepsis)
  gram-negative, 113f
  modified sepsis score, 72
  myocardial, 41f
  neonatal (*See* neonatal sepsis)
  scoring systems for, 72
  SIRS-related, 127
  synovial, 64
  of tarsocrural joint with septic epiphysitis, 69f
septic arthritis
  Candida albicans, 411
  candidiasis, 410
  in foals, 64
  middle carpal joint, 64f
septicemia, 259-260, 259b

septic fibrinoeffusive pericarditis, 33f-35f
septic foals
  jugular venous thrombosis in, 76-77
  survival rates, 77
  studies, 77
septic myocardial dysfunction, 41f
septic osteitis/osteomyelitis, 63-64
septic peritonitis, 46
septic shock
  definition, 70
  systemic inflammatory response syndrome
    with, 123
serology, 264-265. *See also* diagnosis *under
    specific infection/disease or pathogen;*
    laboratory diagnosis
  indications, 264-265
  interpretation of, 140, 265
  response detection, 138-140
serous nasal discharge, 144f
setariasis, 118
severe combined immune deficiency
    (SCID), 189-190, 190f-191f, 471
  Arabian horses, 190
severe combined immuno-deficiency
    (SCID), 448, 448f
  sexually transmitted diseases (STDs). *See*
    venereal diseasescontagious equine
    metritis (*See* contagious equine
    metritis (CEM))
sheath, glanders, 335f
sheath edema, equine proliferative
    enteropathy (EPE), 318f
shedding (of pathogens)
  Borna disease (BD), 232
  cryptosporidiosis, 508-509
  equine arteritis virus (EAV)
    guidelines for breeding to stallions
      shedding, 180f
    isolation of shedding stallions, 181
  equine herpesvirus, 154-155, 157,
      159-161, 166
  equine viral arteritis, guidelines for
    breeding to shedding stallions with,
    180f
shedding, clostridial pathogens, by
    nondiarrheic horses, 353t
shock
  distributive, 123
  septic
    definition, 70
    systemic inflammatory response
      syndrome with, 123
  toxic shock syndrome toxin-1 (TSST-1),
    279-280
signs/symptoms. *See under specific infection/
    disease or pathogen*
silver stain (Warthin-Starry stain),
    361-363
silver sulfadiazine, 431
single radial hemolysis, 147-148
sinus infections
  aspergillosis, 425
    clinical findings, 425
    diagnosis, 427
    therapy, 432
  Cryptococcus species, 438f
  sinusitis, 4-5, 598
    chronic, 5f
    differential diagnosis, 598
    radiography, 4-5
    therapy, 5
sirolimus (rapamycin), 597
SIRS. *See* systemic inflammatory response
    syndrome (SIRS)
skin biopsies, 455

skin infections, 602-603. *See also specific
    infection/disease or pathogen*
  allergies/sensitivity, *Onchocerca* species,
    485
  contagious infections, 78
  crusting/scaling dermatoses, 79-81
  Culicoides hypersensitivity, 502f
  dermatophilosis (*See* dermatophilosis)
  diagnostic methods, 78
  dry skin and scaling, 285f
  environmental factors, 78
  equine pastern dermatitis (EPD), 83
  folliculitis, 79f
  history taking, 78
    questions for, 78b
  infectious, 82b
  large nodular/mass dermatoses, 82-83
    clinical findings, 83
    diagnosis, 81
    etiology, 82-83
    infectious/noninfectious, 82b
    pyogranuloma with
      phaeohyphomycotic fungi, 83f
    therapy, 83
  mange (*See* mites/mange)
  normal flora, 259b
  papulonodular dermatoses, 81-82
    bacterial etiology, diagnosis, and
      treatment, 81
    leishmaniasis, 82
    papillomavirus, 81-82
  parasitic
    Habronema species, 486 (*See also
      parasitic infections*)
    Onchocerca cervicalis, 486f
  ringworm (*See* dermatophytosis
    (ringworm))
  rule-outs, 602-603
    crusting/scaling, 603
    hair loss, 602
    large nodular dermatoses or abscesses,
      603
    papulonodular lesions, 603
    pruritis, 602-603
    ulcers, fistulas, granulomatous lesions,
      603
  samples and tissue selection, bacterial
    infections, 259b
  sarcoids (*See* sarcoids)
  sensitivity to touch, 285f
  sloughing on distal limbs, purpura
    hemorrhagica, 271f
  specimen collection and transport, fungal
    infections, 394
  therapies, 78-79
  tick infestation syndromes, 495
  trauma to, 284
  unpigmented areas, 286f
  warts (*See* warts (papillomavirus))
sling use, 367f
  complications of, 165-166
  tetanus, 371
small intestine, 42-44
  diseases in adult horses, 43-44
    clinical and laboratory findings, 43-44
    etiology and pathophysiology, 43
    therapy, 44
  equine proliferative enteropathy findings,
    319f
  infectious disorders causing diarrhea in
    foals, 42-43
    bacterial, 42-43
    protozoal, 43
    viral, 43
  normal flora, 42

snails, 348f
snake antivenin (IV), 595-596
soap bubble lesions, 439-440
soil contamination, *Clostridium piliformis (or
    piliforme)*, 362-363
Sondweni encephalitis, 218t-219t
SP (acid-stable picornavirus), 195
spider bites, 504
spinal cord infections, 49
  equine protozoal myeloencephalitis
    (EPM), 461, 464f-465f
  rule-outs, 600
spinal infections
  abscesses, 57-58, 58f (*See also* vertebral
    infections)
    clinical findings, 58
    diagnosis, 58
    etiology and epidemiology, 57-58
    therapy, 58
  vertebrae, 57-58
  vertebral osteomyelitis, 57-58, 58f
    clinical findings, 58
    diagnosis, 58
    etiology and epidemiology, 57-58
    therapy, 58
spirochete classification, 303f
spleen abscesses
  Corynebacterium pseudotuberculosis, 377f
  glanders, 335f
spontaneous abortion. *See* abortion;
    brucellosis
sporadic clostridial colitis, 358
sporadic diseases, 521, 521f
sporogony, 469
Sporothrix schenckii, 406
  identification of, 396
sporotrichosis
  clinical findings, 407
    nodules/ulcerations of lymphatics, 407f
  diagnosis, 407-408
  epidemiology and pathogenesis, 406-407
  etiology, 406
  public health considerations, 408
  therapy, prognosis, prevention, 408
stable fly *(Stomoxys calcitrans)*, 500
staff. *See* employees/personnel
staining methods
  acid-fast stains, 257
  calcofluor white stain, 396
  corneal biopsy and staining, mycotic
    keratitis (keratomycosis), 427
  Giemsa stain, 361-362
  Gomori's methenamine silver stain
    Aspergillus species, 396f, 448f
  Gram stain, 72, 74, 257, 395-396
    Aspergillus species, 395f
    Candida species, 396f
    Clostridial species screening, 43-45
    clostridial enteritis, 352f
    clostridial myonecrosis (gas gangrene),
      360f
    clostridial species, 352f
    Clostridium difficile, 352f
    Cryptococcus neoformans, 396f
    fungal infections, 395-396, 395f-396f
    peritoneal infections, 46
    reactions and morphology, 257t, 258f
  immunohistochemical staining,
    leptospirosis, 308f
  immunohistological stain, pythiosis, 417f
  immunohistological stains, pythiosis, 417f
  immunostaining methods, viral antigen
    detection in tissue, 137f
  Kinyoun acid-fast stain, 257, 258f
  methylene blue, 396

staining methods (Continued)
modified Wright's stain, 133f
periodic acid-Schiff stains, 396
silver stain (Warthin-Starry stain), 361-363
Wright's stain, 257
Ziehl-Neelsen staining, 257
stallions. See also penis
contagious equine metritis (CEM), 337
effects of equine herpesvirus on, 160
equine arteritis virus (EAV)
infertility with, 176
isolation of shedding, 181
testing for antibodies before vaccination, 179-181
vaccinated stallions, 179
equine arteritis virus-infected, castration of, 172
equine viral arteritis (EVA)
guidelines for breeding to shedding stallions with, 180f
role of carrier stallion in, 172f
imported, 343
reproductive tract infections
accessory sex glands, 102-104
balanitis, 101f
habromiasis lesions of penis, 101f
inflammation of colliculus seminalis, 103f
prepuce and penis, 100-102
seminal vesiculitis, 103f
testes and epididymis, 102, 102f
transport/shipment of, 545
urinary tract infections, 106
standardization, molecular testing, 604-606
international standards, 605-606
North American standards, 606
standards of practice, outbreak management, 531
Standard Starts Index, 77
staphylococcal infections
clinical findings, 280
with methicillin-resistant species, 280
diagnosis, 280-281
etiology, 278
pathogenesis, 279-280
prevention, 282
prognosis, 282
public health considerations, 282-283
risk factors for infection development, 280
treatment, 281-282
Staphylococcus species, 4, 46, 63
aggravation of Dermatophilus lesions by, 284-285
antimicrobial agents for, 109
resistance to, 278-279
coagulase-negative staphylococci (CoNS), 278-280
coagulase-positive staphylococci (CPS), 278, 280-281
drug-resistant (See drug resistant/sensitive organisms)
ecology of, 281
folliculitis, 79f
groups of, 278
MRSA (See methicillin-resistant Staphylococcus aureus (MRSA))
urinary tract infections, 106
virulence, 279
Staphylococcus aureus, 32, 60-61, 82-83, 337-338, 531-532
Staphylococcus epidermidis, 279
Staphylococcus equi equi, 60, 110-111

Staphylococcus pseudintermedius, 279
methicillin-resistant (MSRP), 278
steroid use, as risk factor in fungal infections, 80
stiffness, rule-outs, 600
stillbirths, 305-306, 309
stomach, 42
Draschia megastoma granuloma, 487f
infectious diseases, 42
infectious disorders, 42
normal flora, 42
ulcers
role of Candida albicans in, 410
in septic foals, 75
stomatitis, vesicular. See vesicular stomatitis viruses (VSVs)
Stomoxys calcitrans, 373, 500
strangles. See Streptococcus equi equi (strangles)
stranguria, 600
streptococcal infections (in general)
antimicrobial agents for, 109
diagnosis, blood agar cultures, 266f
overview, 265
Streptococcus species, 1, 32, 46-47, 57-58, 63-64
antimicrobial susceptibility, 571
Lancefield's study and classification, 265
placentitis, 94
transmission routes, 266
Streptococcus equi
clinical findings
limb edema, 271f
muscle infarcts, 272f
petechial hemorrhages, 271f
skin sloughing on distal limbs, 271f
complications of, 7
diagnosis
interpretation of SeM-specific ELISA, 273t
nasal wash procedure, 272b
environmental persistence, 272
pathologic findings, cerebral abscesses, 270f
prevention, control of transmission, 275t
pulmonary abscess formation, 7
therapy, guttural pouch infections, 275b
Streptococcus equi equi (strangles), 3-4, 3f, 6-7, 56-57, 60-61, 265-276, 516, 532-533
clinical findings, 267f, 269-272
abscess rupture sites, 269f
submandibular lymph node enlargement, 269f
complications of spread of infection, 269-272
immune-mediated, 271-272
internal infection, 269-270
diagnosis, 272
cultures, 272
endoscopy, 268f
polymerase chain reaction (PCR) assay, 272
serology, 272
epidemiology, 267-268
transmission, 267-268
etiology, 265-267
lymph node manifestations, 269
pathogenesis, 268
prevention, 273-276
control of outbreaks, 274-276
hygiene measures, 276
quarantine and bacteriologic screening, 274
vaccination, 273-274

Streptococcus equi equi (strangles) (Continued)
public health considerations, 276
therapy, 272-273
with complications, 273
drugs of choice, 273
with early clinical signs, 272-273
with lymph node abscessation, 273
tracheostomy, 270f
transmission, 272
vaccine recommendations, 566-567
Streptococcus faecalis, 385
Streptococcus pneumoniae, 277
clinical findings and therapy, 277
etiology, 277
pathogenesis, 277
public health considerations, 277
Streptococcus zooepidemicus, 4, 7, 42, 258, 265, 276-277, 531-532
acute mastitis, 101f
clinical findings, 277
etiology, epidemiology, pathogenesis, 276-277
placentitis, 94
prevention, 277
public health considerations, 277
secondary to ascarid infection, 482
therapy, 277
urinary tract infections, 106
Streptomyces nodosus, 410
stress factors, dermatophytosis (ringworm), 412
stress response, in neonatal sepsis, 72
strongyles, 450f, 454f
Strongylinae, 475-478
Strongyloides species, 475-476
larval stage infections, 476
Strongyloides westeri, 483-484, 483f
Strongyloides westeri eggs, 451f
strongyloidosis, 483-484
clinical findings, 484
diagnosis, 484
etiology and epidemiology, 483-484
pathogenesis, 484
pathologic findings, 484
prevention, 484
public health considerations, 484
therapy, 484
strongylosis, 475-481
strongylinae (large strongyles, strongylins), 475-478
clinical findings, 477
diagnosis, 477
epidemiology, 476
etiology, 475-476
pathogenesis, 476-477
pathologic findings, 478
prevention, 478
public health considerations, 478
therapy, 478
Strongylus species, 477f, 507-508
Strongylus vulgaris, 476f-477f
stylohyoid bone
ostectomy of, 20
thickened, 20f
subcutaneous lesions, 416f
bacterial abscesses, 82
subdural empyema, 47
subunit (protein) vaccines, 552
suckle reflex, 77
Sudan grass, 106-107
sudden death, rule-outs, 603
collapse and, 603
summer sores (Habronema species), 486
sunburn, differential diagnosis, 242

support limb laminitis, 70
surgical therapy. *See* therapy *under specific infection/disease or pathogen*
surra, 499-500, 505-507
surveillance and reporting of diseases, 550
susceptibility testing, aspergillosis, 425-426
swallowing problems. *See* dysphagia
swamp cancer *(Habronema species)*, 486
swamp fever. *See* equine infectious anemia (EIA)
sweat glands, increased activity of, 17-18
sweating, patchy, 17-18
symptoms/signs. *See under specific infection/ disease or pathogen*
synovial infections, 63-66
  clinical findings, 63
  diagnosis, 63-64
    imaging techniques, 63-64
    synovial fluid analysis, 63
  etiology and pathogenesis, 63
  septic synovitis
    distal interphalangeal joint with osteomyelitis, 66f
    scapulohumeral joint, 69f
  therapy, 64-66
    constant-rate infusion system, 65f
    intravenous regional limb perfusion, 65f, 68b
systemic diseases/infections
  Candida albicans, 72-74
  candidiasis, 409-410
  clostridial myonecrosis (gas gangrene), 359-361
  with ocular manifestations/complications, 116-118
    bacterial, 116
    fungal, 116-117
    parasitic, 117-118
    viral, 116, 116t
  tickborne, 495
  Tyzzer's disease, 361-363
systemic inflammatory response syndrome (SIRS), 70
  clinical findings and diagnosis, 125-126, 125f-127f
    scleral injection, 126f
  endotoxemia, 125f
  epidemiology, 120-121
  etiology, 119-120
  lipopolysaccharide, 120f
  mediators of, 122t-123t
  pathogenesis, 121-125
    acute-phase response, 125
    coagulopathy, 124
    complement activation, 124-125
    endothelial dysfunction, hemodynamic changes, and shock, 123
    inflammatory cell activation, 121
    inflammatory mediators, 121-123
    neutrophil activation, 123-124
  septic jugular thrombosis, 126f
  therapy, 126-131
    blockade of inflammatory cell activation, 128
    corticosteroids, 129
    future directions for, 131
    lipopolysaccharide scavengers, 128
    management of coagulopathies, 130
    mediator-directed, 129
    nonsteroidal antiinflammatory drugs (NSAIDs), 129
    source control, 127-128
    supportive care, 129-130
  toll-like receptor (TLR) ligands, 119t

T
Tabanus species, 234, 499-500
Tabanus fuscicostatus, 234f
tachycardia, in pleuropneumonia, 9
tachydysrhythmia, agents used for emergency treatment of, 33t
tachypnea, in pleuropneumonia, 9
tack, transmission of disease by, 247
tacrolimus, 596
tail blocks, bacterial cystitis after, 106f
tapeworm, 449, 494. *See also* cestodes
Taylorella asinigenitalis, 337
Taylorella equigenitalis, 337, 516. *See also* contagious equine metritis (CEM)
T cell-resistant groups, equine viral arteritis (EVA), 174f
T cell responses, equine protozoal myeloencephalitis (EPM), 461
T cell suppressor mechanisms, 596b
teat lesions, vesicular stomatitis virus, 241-242
teeth, pleuropneumnonia with toxic line around incisors, 9f
temporal patterns of disease, 520-522
temporohyoid osteoarthropathy (THO), 19-20, 20f
  etiology, 19
  for ostectomy, 20f
  therapy, 20
temporohyoid osteoarthropathy for ostectomy, 20f
teratogenic effects of antimicrobials, 577b
terbinafine, 582
terminal urethra culture, 343f
testicular infections, orchitis, 102, 102f
tetanus. *See also Clostridium tetani*
  antitoxin, 595
  clinical signs, 369-370
    classification of severity, 369b
    contraction lines, 370f
    flashing of nictitans, 369f
    tetanic spasms, 370f
  diagnosis, 370
  epidemiology, 368
  etiology, 368
  laboratory diagnosis, 261
  ocular manifestations of, 117t
  pathogenesis, 368-369
  prevention, 372
  prognosis, 372
  therapy, 371-372
    drugs for sedation/muscle relaxation, 371t
  vaccine development, 368
  vaccine recommendations, 558-559
tetracyclines, 581
Theileria species, 468. *See also* equine piroplasmosis (EP)
  epidemiology, 470
Theileria annulata, 495
Theileria equi, 455f, 469, 495, 584
Thelazia lacrimalis, 118
thelaziasis, 118
therapy, 7-8
therapy/treatment. *See under specific infection/disease or pathogen*
thermotolerance, 436
thiabendazole, 431
THO (temporohyoid osteoarthropathy), 19-20, 20f
  etiology, 19
  for ostectomy, 20f
  therapy, 20
thoracic radiography, 3

thoracic tube placement, 11, 11f
thoracocentesis, 9
Thoroughbred horses, equine encephalosis virus (EEV), 251-252
thrombocytopenia, 235, 602
thrombophlebitis. *See* jugular thrombophlebitis
thrombosis
  aortoiliac, 40f
  arterial, 39, 114f
  caudal vena cava thrombosis syndrome, 39
  jugular venous, 37f-38f, 76-77, 113f
thrush. *See* candidiasis (thrush)
thymidine, 166
tick paralysis, 495
ticks/tick-borne diseases, 495-496. *See also specific infection/disease or pathogen*
  clinical findings, 495
  dermatophilosis, 284
  diagnosis, 495
  epidemiology, 495
  equine granulocytic anaplasmosis/ ehrlichiosis, 344
  etiology, 495
  flavivirus encephalitides, 218t-219t
  identified species, 495
  pathogenesis, 495
  pathologic findings, 495
  piroplasmosis (*See* equine piroplasmosis (EP))
  piroplasms, 468-469
  public health considerations, 496
  therapy and prevention, 496
tissue collection
  bacterial laboratory diagnosis, 258-259
  culturing, 397
  fungal infections, specimen collection and transport, 395
tissue penetration of drugs, 574-575
  impaired diffusion into tissue, 575
  intracellular, 575
TLR (toll-like receptor) ligands, 119t
T lymphocytes, function of, 1-2
TNCC (total nucleated cell count), 43-44
TNF (tumor necrosis factor), α and b, 70
togaviruses, 210-211
  Getah virus, 252
  Semliki Forest complex of, 253
toll-like receptor (TLR) ligands, 119t
toll-like receptors, 586f
tongue
  atrophy and self-mutilation of, equine protozoal myeloencephalitis (EPM), 462f
  swelling of, 509f
  ulcers/vesiculation, vesicular stomatitis virus, 242f
topical antifungals, 430t
torovirus (Berne virus), 203
torticollis, 230
total nucleated cell count (TNCC), 43-44
toxic granulation, 71
toxic ingestions
  cardiac complications of, pyrrolizidine alkaloid toxicity, 41f
  pulmonary diseases associated with, 11
  pyrrolizidine alkaloid toxicity, 41f
  quinidine, 114f
  Sudan and Johnson grasses, 106-107
toxic shock syndrome toxin-1 (TSST-1), 279-280
toxin gene detection, 263
toxins
  antimicrobials as, 577b
  bioassays for detecting, 44-45

toxins *(Continued)*
  clostridial, 364-365
    botulinum neurotoxin, 364-365
Toxoplasma gondii, 111
toxoplasmosis, 117-118
transcription inhibitors, 596
transfaunation, 357-358
transient fungi, 394
transmission of pathogens (in general), 534,
    540-541, 548. *See also* biosecurity;
    pathogenesis *or* epidemiology *under*
    specific disease; prevention *under specific*
    infection/disease or pathogen
transportation
  of horses
    for human consumption, 545
    international movement (*See*
        international movement of horses)
    pleuropneumonia related to, 7
  of laboratory samples, 261, 507, 604
transtracheal aspirate (TTA), 3
transtracheal wash procedure, 10f
trauma. *See also* emergencies
  bone, 66
  infections related to, 60-62
  skin, dermatophilosis, 284
  synovial structures, 63-64
traveling horses, 541-543
treatment/therapy. *See under specific*
    infection/disease or pathogen
trematodes, 348f
triazoles, 582
Trichinella species, 61
  larvae in horse meat, 61
trichinellosis, 61
Trichodesma, 11
Trichophyton species, 110-111
Trichophyton bullosum, 411
Trichophyton equinum, 80, 412f, 531-532.
    See also dermatophytosis (ringworm)
Trichophyton equinum autotrophicum, 411
Trichophyton equinum equinum, 411
Trichophyton equinum verucosum, 411
Trichophyton mentagrophytes, 80, 411
Trichosporon species, 88f
trigeminal nerve (CN V), 6
  abnormality with equine protozoal
    myeloencephalitis, 462f
trimethoprim-sulfonamides, 580-581
Triodontophorus tenuicolli, 476-477
trismus, 369
trombiculid mites, 498-499
  diagnosis, 498
  epidemiology, 498
  etiology, 498
  pathogenesis and clinical findings, 498
  public health considerations, 499
  therapy, 498
Trypanosoma species, 504
Trypanosoma brucei brucei, 505, 507
Trypanosoma congolense, 507
Trypanosoma congolense Nannomonas, 505
Trypanosoma equiperdum, 506f
Trypanosoma evansi, 507
Trypanosoma vivax Duttonella, 505
trypanosomiasis, 505-507
  African animal trypanosomiasis (AAT),
    507
  dourine, 505-506
  surra, 506-507
tsetse fly *(Glossina)*, 504, 507
TSST-1 (toxic shock syndrome toxin-1),
    279-280
TTA (transtracheal aspirate), 3
tumor necrosis factor (TNF), α and b, 70

Tyzzer's disease, 361-363
  clinical findings, 363
  diagnosis, 363
  epidemiology and pathogenesis, 362-363
  etiology, 361-362
  pathologic findings, 363
    liver, 362f
  prevention, 363
  therapy, 363

U

Uasin Gishu disease, 80
udder seeking, reduction of bacterial load
    for, 77
ulcers/ulcerations
  corneal, 20, 76, 110f, 113f-114f
    culturing methods, 261
    with edema and vascularization, 114f
    melting ulcer, 113f
  gastric
    role of *Candida albicans* in, 410
    in septic foals, 75
  glanders, 334f-335f
  oral cavity
    rule-outs, 599
    vesicular stomatitis viruses (VSVs),
      241f-242f
  rule-outs, 603
  skin, 381f, 502f
  sporotrichosis, nodules/ulcerations of
    lymphatics, 407f
  ulcerative cutaneous lesions, zygomycosis,
    419f
  ulcerative lymphangitis, 376, 379, 407
  zygomycosis, ulcerative cutaneous lesions,
    419f
ultrasonography. *See* diagnosis *under specific*
    infection/disease
umbilical care, 77
  for sepsis prevention, 77
University of Florida studies, 411-412
  drug resistance, 74
  Neonatal Intensive Care Unit, 77
  neonatal sepsis, 72
University of Guelph, 542
unmethylated cytosine-phosphate-guanosine
    motifs, 588-589
upper respiratory tract. *See also* respiratory
    diseases
  arytenoid chondritis, 5, 6f
  lymphoid pharyngeal hyperplasia, 5
  relationship to lower, 2f
  rhinitis and sinusitis, 4-5
  strangles, 6-7
  therapy, 7
  viral diseases, 5-6
uracil, 166
ureters, ectopic, 107
urethra
  contagious equine metritis (CEM)
    terminal urethra culture, 343f
    urethral sinus culture, 342f
  urethritis, 106
  urolith in, 107f
urethral mucosa, 108
urethral sinus culture, 342f
urethritis, 106
urinary incontinence, 106-107, 108f, 600
urinary obstructions, 106-107
urinary tract infections (UTIs), 600. *See also*
    kidneys
  anatomic division of, 106
  bladder paralysis/recurrent bacterial
    cystitis, 106f

urinary tract infections (UTIs) *(Continued)*
  clinical findings, 108
  diagnosis, 108
    urinalysis (UA), 258, 262
  etiology, 106-107
  pathogenesis, 107
  predisposing factors, 106
  pyelonephritis, 107f
  rule-outs, 600
    dysuria, stranguria, pollakiuria, 600
    hematuria, 600
    incontinence, 600
    renal failure, 600
  therapy, 109
  upper, 107
  urine scald with incontinence, 108f
  urolithiasis, 107f
urine acidification, 109
urine retention, 106-107
urine scald, 108, 108f
urolithiasis, 106-107
  bladder lavage for treating, 109
  surgical treatment, 107
U.S. Centers for Disease Control and
    Prevention (CDCP), 383, 534, 612
U.S. Department of Agriculture (USDA)
  Animal Health inspection services, 606
  contagious equine metritis (CEM),
    342-343
  equine protozoal myeloencephalitis
    incidence, 459
  Equine Viral Arteritis: Uniform Methods
    and Rules, 179
  Veterinary Services, 542-543
uterine infections, 84-92
  diagnosis, 86-87
  etiology, 84
  lavage and flushing
    endometritis and pyometra, 92f
    guidelines for, 89t
  in nonpregnant mares, 84-92
  pathogenesis, 85-86
    immunity/uterine defense, 85-86
    physical barriers, 85
    physical clearance of infection, 86
  prevention, 91-92
  therapy, 87-91
    antimicrobial therapy, 89-90
    colostrum infusion, 91
    lavage and flushing, 87-89
    plasma infusion, 90-91
  viremia (equine herpesvirus), 157
uteroplacental thickness measurement, 96f
uterus
  neutrophil chemotaxis, 85-86
  ultrasonography after insemination, 87f
UTIs. *See* urinary tract infections (UTIs)
uveitis, 76, 602
  with corneal ulcer, 113f
  equine recurrent uveitis (ERU), 114f
    treatment, 310
  with mycotic keratitis (keratomycosis),
    432
  pain management, 432
  primary, 114
  Rhodococcus equi infection, 114f

V

vaccine adjuvants, 591-593
vaccines/vaccination, 591-594. *See also*
    immunization; immunoprophylaxis;
    immunotherapy
  African horse sickness (AHS), 182, 188
  anthrax, 383, 385

vaccines/vaccination *(Continued)*
augmentation of vaccines, adjuvants, 553-554, 591-593
Bacille-Calmette-Guérin vaccine, 587-588
Borna disease (BD), 232
botulism, 367b
Brucella, 338-339
cancer vaccines, 593
Clostridium perfringens infection, 358
Coley's vaccine, 584
core and noncore, 558
dermatophytosis (ringworm), 413
development of new, 570
equine herpesvirus (EHV), 166-167
equine influenza protocols, 150-151, 562-563
in an outbreak, 563
foals, 562-563
future vaccines, 563-564
pregnant mares, 562
primary series for adult horses, 562
routine revaccination, 562
equine piroplasmosis (EP), 475
equine protozoal myeloencephalitis (EPM), 467
equine rhinoviruses, 197
equine viral arteritis (EVA), 179
equine warts, 246
flaviviruses, 226
glanders, 336
Histoplasma capsulatum farciminosum, 446
immune response to, 592f
influences on vaccine response in foals, maternal antibodies, 557-558
Lawsonia intracellularis, 320
Lawsonia intracillularis, 320-321
leptospirosis, 310-311
licensing and safety of, 552t, 554-555
adverse events, 555
safety of vaccines in broodmares, 555-556
Lyme disease, 315
molecular vaccines, 593
neonatal, 593
passive immunization, 556-557
exogenous antibodies, 556
passive transfer of maternal immunity, 556-557
Potomac horse fever (equine neorickettsiosis), 44, 351
principles and recommendations, 542-543
pythiosis, 418
rabies (RABV)
approved vaccines, 208t
occurrence in vaccinated animals, 209
vaccination protocol, 209b
recommendations for specific diseases, 558-570
anthrax, 570
botulism, 568-569
equine encephalomyelitis viruses (EEE, WEE, VEE), 559
equine herpesviruses, 564-566
equine influenza, 560-564
equine rhinitis A virus, 570
equine viral arteritis (EVA), 569
Potomac horse fever (PHF), 567-568
rabies, 567
rotaviral diarrhea, 569-570
Streptococcus equi equi (strangles), 566-567
tetanus, 558-559
West Nile virus, 559-560
Rhodococcus equi, 301

vaccines/vaccination *(Continued)*
rotaviruses, 201
salmonella, 332
tetanus, 372
development of vaccine, 368
types of vaccines, 591
vaccine adjuvants, 591-593
vaccine augmentation, 553-554
adjuvants, 553-554, 554t
marker vaccines, 553
West Nile virus, 221, 226
vacuolization, 71
vagina, 85
contagious equine metritis (CEM), vaginal discharge, 340f
vaginitis
candidiasis, 410
infectious, 93
Varicellovirus, 152
vectors, 517. *See also* hosts/host factors
alphaviruses, 211
arthropod, 240
Corynebacterium pseudotuberculosis, 374f
equine granulocytic anaplasmosis/ ehrlichiosis, 344
introduction of new, 548-549
migration of, 549
Neorickettsia risticii, 348
rabies vectors, 204-205, 204f
vesicular stomatitis viruses (VSVs), 240t
West Nile virus, 221
Veillonella species, 1
venereal diseases/venereal transmission of disease
coital exanthema, 104-105
contagious equine metritis, 104
dourine, 105
equine herpesvirus (EHV) type 3, 104, 104f (*See also* equine herpesvirus (EHV))
Pseudomonas aeruginosa and *Klebsiella pneumoniae* transmission, 104
Venezuelan equine encephalitis (VEE), 210t, 215-217, 531-532, 612
clinical findings, diagnosis, pathologic findings, 217
endemic cycle, 216f
epidemiology, 216-217
etiology, 215-216
ocular manifestations of, 116t
outbreaks due to international movement of horses, 547t
pathogenesis, 217
prevention, 217
vaccine recommendations, 559
venomous insects, 504
ventral abdominal edema, 601-602
verminous arteritis, 476f
verrucous sarcoids, 245, 248, 248f. *See also* warts (papillomavirus)
vertebral infections
etiology, 57-58
osteomyelitis, 57-58, 58f
clinical findings, 58
diagnosis, 58
etiology and epidemiology, 57-58
therapy, 58
vesicular diseases, 606-611
oral, 599
orthopoxvirus, 256
seminal vesiculitis, 103f
vesicular stomatitis viruses (VSVs), 241f
clinical findings, 241-242, 241f-242f
diagnosis, 242-243

vesicular stomatitis viruses (VSVs) *(Continued)*
epidemiology, 239-241
risk factors, 240-241
transmission, 240, 240t
in United States, 239-240
etiology, 239
pathogenesis, 241
prevention, 243
public health considerations, 243-244
therapy, 243
Vesiculovirus, 239
vestibular disease, 114-115
vestibulocochlear/acoustic nerve (CN VIII), 14, 19, 20f
veterinarians, role in biosecurity of, 531
Viborg's triangle, 16-17
vinca alkaloids, 585t, 597
vincristine, 597
viral antigens, 139f, 177
viral arteritis. *See* equine viral arteritis (EVA)
viral characterization, 135-136
viral genomes, 152, 153f
viral infections, 5-6. *See also* antimicrobial therapy; antiviral therapy; specific infection/disease or pathogen
abortion caused by, 98-99
equine herpesvirus (EHV), 98
equine viral arteritis (EVA), 98-99
of central nervous system, 48t
conjunctivitis, causative agents, 111b
crusting/scaling dermatoses, 80-81
molluscum contagiosum, 81
poxvirus, 80-81
diarrheal diseases
coronaviruses, 201-203
rotavirus, 198-201
torovirus, 203
equine influenza (*See* equine influenza (EI))
fluid analysis for, 1-2
foreign animal diseases (FADs), 612
keratitis, 112
laboratory diagnosis
agar gel immunodiffusion (AGID), 139
electron microscopy, 138
enzyme-linked immunosorbent assay (ELISA), 138f-139f, 139
hemagglutination inhibition assay (HI), 139-140
histopathology, 136
immunofluorescence and immunohistochemistry, 136-137
immunostaining methods, 137f
indirect enzyme-linked immunosorbent assay (ELISA), 138
isolation of live viruses (cell/egg cultures, animal inoculation), 133-134
microarray detection of viruses, 137-138
modified Wright's stain, 133f
neutralization of virus infectivity, 139
overview, 132
polymerase chain reaction (PCR), 134f
serologic interpretation, 140
serologic response detection, 138-140
in situ hybridization, 138
in situ virus detection, 136-137
viral characterization, 135-136
viral nucleic acids detection (polymerase chain reactions), 134-136
molluscum contagiosum, 79

viral infections *(Continued)*
  ocular manifestations/complications of
    systemic, 116, 116t
  respiratory tract, 3, 7
  rotavirus, 43
  shedding, equine herpesvirus, 154-155,
    157, 159-161, 166
  tick- and mosquito-borne, 218t-219t
  transmission of, 251
  upper respiratory tract, 7
  zoonotic, 531-532
viral nucleic acids detection (polymerase
    chain reactions), 134-136
viral proteins, 155
viral replication, 152-153
viremia
  eastern equine encephalitis, 214
  equine herpesvirus, 157-158
virology
  equine herpesvirus, 152
  virus in tissue sections *(in situ)* detection,
    136-137
  virus isolation, 145-146
vision. *See ocular entries*
voriconazole, 411
vulva, normal and abnormal conformation,
  85f
vulvovaginitis, *Candida albicans*, 410

W

warbles. *See* hypodermiasis (warbles)
Warthin-Starry stain (silver stain), 361-363
warts (papillomavirus), 244-246
  clinical findings, 245, 245f
  diagnosis, 245
  epidemiology, 244
  etiology, 244
  pathogenesis, 244-245
  pathologic findings, 245
  prevention, 246
  public health considerations, 246
  therapy, 245-246
  verrucous sarcoid, 248f
waste management and disposal, 537-538
weanlings, parasitic infections of, 13. *See
    also* foals
weight loss, 318f, 425
Western blot (immunoblot) test, 473-474,
  527b
  equine protozoal myeloencephalitis
    (EPM), 463
western equine encephalitis (WEE), 210t,
  214-215
  clinical signs, 215
  diagnosis, 215
  epidemiology, 214-215
  etiology, 214
  ocular manifestations of, 116t

western equine encephalitis (WEE)
    (Continued)
  pathogenesis, 215
  pathology, 215
  prevention, 215
  treatment, 215
  vaccine recommendations, 559
  variants, 214
West Nile virus (WNV), 47, 255, 515-516,
  612
  antibodies, 595
  diagnosis, 225f
  differential diagnosis, 213
  epidemic curve, 521f
  human susceptibility, 221-222
  life cycle, 220f
  ocular manifestations of, 116t
  United States distribution, 222f
  vaccine recommendations, 559-560
white blood cell count, 258
Whitehouse approach, 16f
wildlife reservoirs, biosecurity control
    measures, 538-539
withers, fistulous, 338f
withers, fistulous, brucellosis, 337-338,
  338f
WNV. *See* West Nile virus (WNV)
Wood's lamp, 413
World Assembly of Delegates of OIE,
  185-186
World Organization for Animal Health. *See*
    International des Epizooties (OIE)
wound infections/wound care
  bacterial cultures, 260
  clostridial myonecrosis, 360
  MRSA, 280
  myiasis, 503-504
    clinical findings, 503
    diagnosis, 503
    etiology and epidemiology, 503
    public health considerations, 503-504
    therapy and prevention, 503
  prevention of fly larvae deposition, 503
  puncture wounds, 368
wound myiasis, 503-504
Wright's stain, 257

X

xanthochromic cerebrospinal fluid, 164f

Y

Yaoundé encephalitis, 218t-219t
yeasts/yeast infections, 393-394. *See also*
    fungal infections
  differentiation of, 396
  fungal infections, 411, 613
yellow fever, 217, 218t-219t

Z

zebras
  African horse sickness (AHS), 182
  coccidiomycosis, 404
  Gastrodiscus aegyptiacus, 512
Ziehl-Neelsen staining, 257
zoonotic diseases/pathogens, 531-532.
    See also public health considerations
  African horse sickness (AHS), 188
  anthrax, 385
  brucellosis, 337, 339
  clostridial infections, 359
  control of, 531 (*See also* biosecurity)
  cryptosporidiosis, 508-509
  dermatophytosis (ringworm), 414
  echinococcosis, 510
  emergence of, 530
  equine piroplasmosis (EP), 475
  equine rhinoviruses, 197
  flavivirus encephalitides, 218
  giardiasis, 509
  histoplasmosis, 443t
  human fatalities, 532
  identification of, 532-533
  leptospirosis, 311
  MRSA, 282-283
  protection of personnel from, 531-532
  rabies, 209
  removal of designation (pneumocystis),
    448
  Rhodococcus equi, 301
  Ross River virus, 254-255
  salmonellosis, 333
  surra, 507
  Tyzzer's disease, 362f
  vesicular stomatitis viruses (VSVs), 244
  West Nile virus, 221-222
zygomycosis, 82-83, 419-421. *See also*
    Conidiobolus species
  clinical findings, 419-420
    basidiobolomycosis, 419
    conidiobolomycosis, 419
    mucormycosis, 420
    nasal polyps, 420f
    ulcerative cutaneous lesions, 419f
  diagnosis, 420
  etiology and epidemiology, 419
  pathologic findings, 420
    basidiobolomycosis lesions, 420f
  prognosis, 421
  therapy, 420-421
    topical, 421